Veterinary Medic le to Dog and Cat Breeds

Jerold S. Bell, DVM
Clinical Associate Professor of Genetics
Department of Clinical Sciences
Tufts Cummings School of Veterinary Medicine
North Grafton, MA

Kathleen E. Cavanagh, DVM
B.Sc. Specialized, Genetics
Masters of Educational Technology
President, Matrix Multimedia, Ridgeville, Ontario

Larry P. Tilley, DVM
Diplomate, ACVIM (Internal Medicine)
President, VetMed Consultants, Lexington, MA
Consultant, New Mexico Veterinary Referral Center
Santa Fe, New Mexico

Francis W. K. Smith, DVM
Diplomate, AVCIM (Cardiology & Internal Medicine)
Vice-President, VetMed Consultants, Lexington MA
Clinical Assistant Professor
Department of Clinical Sciences
Tufts Cummings School of Veterinary Medicine
North Grafton, MA

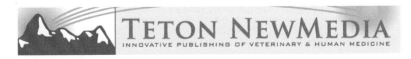

TETON NEWMEDIA
INNOVATIVE PUBLISHING OF VETERINARY & HUMAN MEDICINE

Executive Editor: Carroll C. Cann
Development Editor: Susan L. Hunsberger
Design and Production: www.fiftysixforty.com
Photographers, Dog Images: Neale Photography, DigitalDean Photography, Ellen Pankey, Ironwood Coonhounds, Agi Hejja/Alida Greendyk, Nancy Bartol, Hollow Creek Kennel, Bluetick1Kennels, Mary Kvarnstrom, Blackstar Icelandics, Michael Work
Photographers, Cat Images: Lark Studios and Chanan Studios

Teton NewMedia
P.O. Box 4833
Jackson, WY 83001
1-888-770-3165
tetonnm.com

Copyright© 2012 Teton NewMedia

ISBN# 1-59161-002-8

Printed in the United States

Print Number 5 4 3 2 1

Library of Congress Cataloging-in-Publication Data on file

Preface

This book is designed to provide the veterinary practitioner, student, breeder, and pet owner with a complete and quick reference to the diagnosis and management of breed related medical conditions of dogs and cats. Our goal in creating this textbook is also to provide up-to-date information in an easy-to-use format. Prior to the publication of this book, this information could be found scattered throughout a variety of clinical resources.

One objective of this book is to make information quickly available. To this end, we have organized the breeds alphabetically. At the end of the book, there are appendices that contain quick reference to conditions by breed, available genetic tests, and registries.

This book is not an indictment on the health of purebred dogs and pedigreed cats. The majority of genetic disease that is seen in dogs and cats appears equally in purebred, designer cross-bred, and random-bred individuals. However, the improved genetic health of all dogs and cats is dependent on breeder selection of genetically healthy parents. Indeed, it is the ethical responsibility of breeders to do so. This book provides the information necessary to make those breeding decisions.

This first edition constitutes an important, up-to-date medical reference source for the reader. We strived to make it complete yet practical and easy to use. Our dreams are realized if this text helps you to quickly locate and use the information that is essential to high-quality veterinary medical care. We would appreciate your input so that we can make future editions even more useful. If you would like to see any changes in content or format, additions, or deletions, please let us know. Send comments to the following:

Teton New Media
P.O. Box 4833
Jackson, WY 83001

Jerold S. Bell

Kathleen Cavanagh

Larry P. Tilley

Francis W.K. Smith Jr.

Dedication

There are many people who influence your professional development and the direction you take in your life. I have as a role model my father A. Milton Bell, who was a dental practitioner and later an educator who passed on the practical knowledge he gained from his years of practice. I would like to recognize the influence of Professor Joseph Rosen, the late Dr. Herman M. Slatis, Dr. E. James Potchen, and Dr. Alexander de Lahunta. To my sons and daughters James and Leslie, Elizabeth and Bill, and my grandchildren Erin, Derek, Kevin, Leah, and Jacob; you inherit the world we made for you. I dedicate this effort to my beloved wife and life partner, Candice.

Jerold S. Bell

I would like to thank my family (Dave, Kevin, and Patrick, and my now deceased father Ray) for their patience, while considerable family time was dedicated to the research, writing and reviews for this project. My Burmese cat was 24 years old in 2010 as I wrote this, and was a constant companion to me at the computer while working on the book over the years. Her loving and gentle, warm presence epitomized the deep human-animal bond that inspires us to help our 4-legged friends live a long, healthy, and fulfilling lifespan, hopefully free of genetic and other disorders.

Kathleen Cavanagh

To my wife, Jeri, my son, Kyle, my grandson, Tucker, in honor of that secret correspondence within our hearts; to family and animals who represent the purity of life.

Larry Patrick Tilley

To my wife, May, my son, Ben, and my daughter, Jade, I cherish our time together and your constant love and support. To my father, Frank, thanks for being my perfect role model.

Francis W.K. Smith Jr.

Acknowledgements

We would like to acknowledge and thank our families for their support of this project and the sacrifices they made to allow us the time to complete the book.

In addition to thanking veterinarians who have referred patients to us, we would like to express our gratitude to each of the veterinary students, interns, and residents whom we have had the privilege of teaching. Their curiosity and intellectual stimulation have enabled us to grow and have prompted us to undertake the task of writing this book.

We would like to thank the cat and dog fancy, breeders and breed clubs, committed veterinarians, genetics researchers, educators, genetic testing facilities, animal health associations, foundations, and many others worldwide who work together to provide optimal health and welfare, through research and application of new knowledge towards canine and feline health. Without their dedication, the field would not be advancing. Our sincere thanks go out to all for their continuing support of this exciting field of endeavor.

Finally, a special thank you goes to Carroll Cann and to all the rest of the staff at Teton New Media and everyone in the production and editing departments. They are all meticulous workers and kind people who have made the final stages of preparing this book both inspiring and fun. An important life goal of ours has been fulfilled: to provide expertise in small animal internal medicine and to teach the principles contained in this textbook to veterinarians, students, breeders, and pet owners everywhere.

Jerold S Bell DVM

Kathleen E Cavanagh DVM

Larry P Tilley DVM

Francis W K Smith Jr. DVM

Table of Contents

Section 3: Cat Breeds

Section 1

How to use this Book

Each species section of the book has a foreword that provides orientation to the content of the section. All chapters are consistent in layout and presentation. Appendices have been provided where there is a need for summary information applicable to all breeds. The sections on genetic concepts and genetic counselling are designed as a concise review only. Standard genetics texts should be consulted for in-depth material. The glossary (terms definitions list) is limited primarily to genetic terms and conformation/color terms. A standard medical dictionary should be consulted for terms not defined. Where conditions have been covered in detail in internal medicine texts, coverage herein is cursory. Internal medicine texts should be referred to during case management.

This book is not meant to be a breed promotion book, but rather a presentation of scientific facts. This is especially difficult in one section of the chapters, the Recognized Behavior Issues and Traits. Reported breed characteristics are collated from many sources, including cat fancy organizations, kennel clubs and lay breed books whose mission is to promote breeds. For this reason, and because temperament and personality traits of an individual cannot be generalized to a population, this section should be interpreted in a general way only.

As with all published works, because of advances in knowledge, this is a work that represents the state of our understanding as of the year of publication only. As we continue to update the resource in the next few years, we hope to hear from readers to help us identify gaps in content, and hear from those carrying out research who are aware of new findings in order to help us maintain a state-of-the-art fact finder book. As a first edition, this is a first pass through the literature and first proof of concept. If any reader would like to provide input on format, content or concept, please contact us to help us make our next edition even better. Our goal is to provide regular updates to maintain contemporary content. Our next edition will include some additional rare breeds, and updates on active areas of research.

We hope that this new textbook provides an effective, concise source of information to help your practice achieve a best practices quality approach to the care of dog and cat breeds.

The authors

Genetic Concepts

Any trait or disorder that has a hereditary component is genetic. *Congenital* disorders are those present at birth. Some congenital disorders are hereditary, and others are not. Those occurring spontaneously may be caused by environmental exposures to infections, or compounds such as drugs or toxins. Genetic disorders will sometimes only be evident much later in life, even though the genetic coding for the disorder is present at birth. The age of onset of a trait or disorder does not differentiate whether it is genetic or environmental. Some disorders can be caused by either a genetic or acquired *(phenocopy)* origin, and need to be differentiated in order to determine if genetic counseling is warranted. For example, the neurological incoordination disorder cerebellar hypoplasia in cats can be a hereditary disease, but can also be caused by in-utero infection with feline panleukopenia virus.

As our understanding of genetic mechanisms evolves, we are finding out that a lot more disorders have genetic influences than previously thought. The inheritance of genes that cause liability or susceptibility to disease can present as *breed predispositions*. Identifying specific, testable genes for these disorders will be helpful in their control.

Genes are pieces of deoxyribonucleic acid (DNA). *Coding genes* produce proteins and enzymes. *Regulatory genes* act to turn coding genes on or off. Genes are contained on paired *chromosomes* that are either *autosomes*, or *sex chromosomes*. Females have two X sex chromosomes, and males have an X and a Y. Dogs have 38 pairs of autosomal chromosomes, and cats have 18 pairs. One gene in each gene pair comes from the father and the other from the mother. If the two genes in a pair are identical, they are referred to as *homozygous*, and if they are different, they are called *heterozygous*. The location of a gene on the chromosome is called its *locus*, and each gene in a gene pair is called an *allele*.

The interaction of the two alleles determines the expression of the gene. The type of gene combinations for a particular locus (i.e. AA, Aa or aa) is the *genotype*. The appearance or expression of the genes at particular loci (i.e. black or brown) is the *phenotype*. The phenotypic expression of the gene pair is determined by how the two genes in the pair interact. A *dominant* gene (only requiring one copy in the pair) is always expressed, while a *recessive* gene requires a homozygous pair for expression. When two heterozygous carriers of a recessive gene are bred together, on average you can expect 25% affected, 50% carrier, and 25% normal offspring. The actual observed percentages within litters will vary. Many dominant traits are *homozygous lethal* during fetal development; such as Chinese Crested dogs homozygous for the hairless gene (HH), the gene for polycystic kidney disease in Persian and related cat breeds, and the Manx gene (MM) in cats.

Co-dominance or *incomplete dominance* is when heterozygous alleles show an intermediate phenotype. An example is a bi-colored cat (Ss) as an intermediate between that seen with homozygous solid color (SS) and the recessive van pattern (a white cat with color only on its tail and the top of the head) seen with the homozygous ss genotype. The merle color pattern in dogs is also an example. Most merle dogs have the Mm genotype, with mm producing normal coloration. Double dominant MM merle dogs are mostly white, and can be born blind, deaf, or with other severe abnormalities.

Sex-linked (also referred to as *X-linked*) disorders are controlled by genes on the X-chromosome. As males have only one X chromosome, a single defective gene on it will cause a genetic defect. For females to be affected with an X-linked recessive disorder, they have to be homozygous for the defective gene. Hemophilia A & B are examples of X-linked recessive disorders.

Genetic traits and disorders can be caused by the action of a single gene pair *(monogenetic disorders)*, or several pairs of genes *(complex or polygenic inheritance)*. Complexly inherited traits can involve *qualitative* genes (that can show dominance and recessiveness), or *quantitative* genes (that can act in an *additive* fashion). Many complexly inherited disorders are *threshold traits*, where a *genetic load* of genes and possibly additional environmental effects combine to cross a threshold level to produce the phenotype. Several musculoskeletal disorders, heart anomalies, and eye diseases are complexly inherited threshold traits.

There are instances when gene expression does not produce the expected phenotype. When an individual has the genotype for a trait or disorder, but does not phenotypically express it, this is referred to as *incomplete penetrance*. This is an all or none phenomenon; you either show the trait or not. The easiest way to remember this concept is that the genotype does not penetrate into the phenotype. If an individual has a certain trait or disorder, but it differs in its severity, age of onset, progression, or form, it is referred to as *variable expressivity*. With this process, all genotypically affected individuals show some aspect of the trait. Polydactyly (extra toes) in cats shows variable expressivity in the number of extra toes present. Many of the inherited disorders listed in the breed chapters show variable expressivity. Penetrance and expressivity may be properties of the mutant gene itself, or can be due to modifying effects of other genes and/or the environment.

Similar genetic conditions can have different genetic causes between breeds, or even within the same breed. If a genetic trait or disorder can be caused by different genes, they are called *genocopies*. In this case, direct genetic tests (of the genotype) in one breed will not work in other breeds. We know that many forms of progressive retinal atrophy (PRA) are genocopies, and expect this to be the case with many other disorders, such as epilepsy and cardiomyopathy. Some breed-related genetic disorders can be related to a sub-population or breed gene pool in a specific country. For this reason, much of the information presented in the breed chapters relates to the breed in the United States in general and may not be applicable to all breed populations worldwide, or possibly all lines within the breed.

Breeding Systems

Mating based on phenotype is called assortative mating. Mating like to like is positive assortative mating. Mating like to unlike (i.e., bringing a new trait in or correcting a fault) is negative assortative mating. Matings based on genotype depend on the relationship between the two individuals being bred. If two parents within a breed are less related than the average relationship within the breed (measured as an inbreeding coefficient), then it is an outbreeding. If the mating of two parents produces an inbreeding coefficient higher than the breed average, it is a linebreeding or inbreeding. Linebreeding concentrates the genes of specific common ancestors behind both parents. Inbreeding is the mating of close relatives, such as parent to offspring, or full brother x sister.

Linebreeding and inbreeding increase homozygosity, or the pairing of like genes (aa or AA) in the offspring. This can increase the expression of both positive and negative recessive traits. Outbreeding increases heterozygosity, or the pairing of unlike genes (Aa). Outbreeding propagates both positive and negative recessive genes in the carrier state. Linebreeding does not create deleterious genes, and outbreeding does not eliminate them. These breeding practices only affect the expression or masking of deleterious genes through homozygosity or heterozygosity. Selection of breeding stock is what affects the increase or decrease in the frequency of desirable and deleterious genes. Inbreeding or tight linebreeding should only be attempted with knowledge of the range of genes that the parents may carry based on prior matings or genetic testing.

Crossbreeding is the production of offspring by mating individuals from two or more breeds. This produces maximum heterozygosity. Designer breeds are created through crossbreeding. Their offspring do not reproduce themselves if bred.

Genetic Diversity

Most breeds have closed gene pools, meaning that breeding individuals must have confirmed pedigrees of ancestry from the existing breed. No new genes can be introduced into the breed, and genes can be lost to the gene pool by selective breeding (or not breeding) of individuals. The problem with limited genetic diversity in purebred populations stems from the effects of deleterious genes. If a breed has a high frequency of a deleterious gene, then the breed will have issues with that disorder. Deleterious genes can cause increased neonatal death and smaller litter size, specific genetic diseases, or impaired immunity. In some cases, selection for a specific phenotype has brought a defective gene along with it at a high frequency. The most extreme example is the linkage of spotting in Dalmatians with the autosomal recessive gene for abnormal purine metabolism (hyperuricosuria). All Dalmatians are homozygous recessive for this defective gene, which can predispose to bladder stones and a skin condition.

Breeds with genetic diversity issues need to determine how they can best improve their situations. Is there enough diversity of normal genes to maintain the health and vitality of the breed? Is there a way to breed away from high frequency defective genes without losing valuable normal genes in the process? Some breeders discourage linebreeding and promote outbreeding in an attempt to protect genetic diversity in their breed. It is not the type of matings utilized (linebreeding or outbreeding) that causes the loss of genes from a breed gene pool. Rather, loss of genes occurs through selection: the use and non-use of offspring. If a breed starts narrowing their focus to breeding stock from a limited number of lines, then a loss of genetic diversity will occur.

The process of maintaining healthy lines, with many breeders crossing between lines and breeding back as they see fit, maintains diversity in the gene pool. If some breeders outbreed, and some linebreed to certain individuals that they favor while others linebreed to others that they favor, then breed-wide genetic diversity is maintained. It is the varied opinion of breeders as to what constitutes the ideal dog or cat, and their selection of breeding stock based on their opinions that maintains breed diversity.

The most important factor for diminished genetic diversity in breeds is the popular sire syndrome. The overuse of a popular sire beyond a reasonable contribution through frequent breedings significantly skews the gene pool in his direction, and reduces the diversity of the gene pool. Any genes that he possesses - whether positive or negative - will increase in frequency. The insidious effect of the popular sire syndrome is the loss of genetic contribution from quality, unrelated males who are not used for breeding. The loss of other quality breeding lines causes a significant loss of breed genetic diversity. The popular sire syndrome is a significant factor in both populous breeds and breeds with small populations.

Genetic Testing

Genetic tests vary on what they are able to identify, and therefore how they can be used in managing genetic disease. Some tests measure the phenotype, or what can be seen in the animal. This may not directly relate to the genotype, or the genes regulating the defect. Screening for cataracts, ausculting for heart murmurs, thyroid autoantibodies, hip and elbow radiographs, urinalysis for crystals or metabolites, skin biopsies, and observation of behavioral traits are all tests of the phenotype. Most *tests of the phenotype* only identify affected individuals, and not carriers.

Direct gene tests utilizing PCR or polymerase chain reaction, are a direct measurement of the genotype. These can be run at any age with a blood sample or cheek swab, regardless of the age of onset of the disorder. With *tests of the genotype*, you can identify affected, carrier, and genetically normal animals.

Some defective genes can be linked to a *genetic marker*, which can be tested for. *Linked-marker based tests* do not identify the defective gene, but a marker that lies close on the chromosome. During the formation of egg or sperm, a *crossover* and trading of genes occurs between paired chromosomes. If a crossover between the marker and the gene occurs, the marker will no longer be linked to the defective gene. False positive and false negative results will occur in the individual, and in all of its descendants. Due to this phenomenon, linkage test results must be compared with results from other family members to determine whether they correlate with the known genotype of relatives. Linked marker tests include those for cerebellar ataxia in Italian Spinone and primary hyperparathyroidism in the Keeshond.

Most tests of the genotype are for genes that are the sole and direct cause of a disease or condition. Others test for *susceptibility genes* that provide liability for the disease. Some of these susceptibility genes are necessary for the animal to be affected, though other yet undiscovered genetic or environmental factors are also necessary. Examples are cord1 PRA in English Springer Spaniels and Miniature Dachshunds, and degenerative myelopathy in several dog breeds. Other susceptibility genes are found to occur at a greater frequency in affected animals, but are not present in all affected animals. An example is the susceptibility gene for perianal fistula/anal furunculosis in German Shepherd Dogs.

Many owners and breeders ask what tests should be done in their cats and dogs. The answer depends on whether the cat or dog is going to be a pet, or be used for breeding. For a pet, it is only important to know that it is not going to be affected by a health-related disorder. For breeding animals, it is important to know if they carry disease liability genes that they can pass on to their offspring. Further information is available in the chapter on Genetic Counseling.

Genetic Registries and Health Surveys

In the United States, several genetic registries have been established to assist breeders with genetic disease control. The Canine Eye Registry Foundation or CERF (http://www.vmdb.org/cerf.html) is a closed database showing only normal eye examination results on dogs examined by ACVO boarded veterinary ophthalmologists. The not-for-profit Orthopedic Foundation for Animals (OFA: www.offa.org) has semi-open registries for phenotypic examinations of hip dysplasia, elbow dysplasia, autoimmune thyroiditis, congenital cardiac disease, and patella luxation, as well as genotypic test results for many inherited disorders. From the OFA web portal you can look up individual animals, and their health testing status. This is Facebook for Animals; each with their own web page and information.

The Canine Health Information Center or CHIC (www.caninehealthinfo.org) is an open health database that has been established by the AKC Canine Health Foundation and the Orthopedic Foundation for Animals. National parent clubs decide to enroll in the CHIC program, and determine the testable genetic disorders for their breed. (For example, hip evaluation, CERF examination, and thyroid testing.) Owners, breeders, and prospective owners can search online for dogs in the OFA/CHIC database, and view their test results. If a dog completes the recommended testing panel, it receives a CHIC number regardless of whether it passes all of the tests. CHIC is about health consciousness, not health perfection. As more testable disorders are identified, few dogs will be normal for all tests. The Kennel Club in the UK has similar Health Breeding Schemes and a searchable Health Tests Results Finder to look up individual dogs. A similar listing of tests is not currently available for cats, however breed-related diseases are found on the Feline Advisory Bureau (FAB-UK) website: www.fabcats.org/breeders/inherited_disorders.

Without data on the occurrence and prevalence of disorders in dog and cat breeds, breeders cannot institute measures to improve them. Breed clubs should routinely perform health surveys (usually every 5 years) to monitor the changing health of the breed. Owners should take the time to fill out surveys, even on healthy animals. Breeders should record the cause and age at death, reproduction rates, dystocia, need for caesarian section, sex of offspring, litter size, number of stillborn offspring, growth rates, and the onset and nature of abnormalities in offspring. Post mortems should be conducted for fading kittens and puppies, and for all deaths. If one does not know why there is loss of cats or dogs, there is loss of ability to improve the welfare and health of the next generation of a breed.

Genetic Counseling and Management of Genetic Disease

The hallmark of genetic disease is our ability to predict its occurrence before its onset, allowing us to alter its morbidity or mortality. The vast majority of dogs and cats are not breeding animals, but they still require genetic counseling for inherited disorders. Owners of large-breed puppies are counseled to feed lower calorie foods to provide for a more uniform growth rate and better joint development. Cats genetically predisposed to FLUTD (Feline Lower Urinary Tract Disorders) and obese "pre-diabetic" cats can receive specific dietary recommendations.

We need to be knowledgeable about what genetic tests are available, and in which individuals they should be run. Dogs from breeds with an incidence of von Willebrand's disease should be tested early in life, so that measures can be taken to prevent excessive hemorrhage during surgery or injury. Dogs at risk of carrying the mdr-1 mutation should be tested early in life, before drug treatment.

In high risk breeds, individual animals should be genetically tested (or verified results documented for parents) before purchase. These include Maine Coon and Ragdoll cats for the autosomal dominant hypertrophic cardiomyopathy gene, Persian and Himalayan cats for autosomal dominant polycystic kidney disease, Boxers for arrythmogenic right ventricular cardiomyopathy, and Doberman Pinschers for dilated cardiomyopathy.

We need to understand the temporal periods when genetic testing will be most accurate, and allow for intervention. Puppy hips should be palpated with a gentle Ortolani procedure at each vaccine visit, and again at spaying or neutering under anesthesia. Juvenile interventional surgery will only benefit those with significant subluxability prior to major growth (for pubic symphysiodesis) or the development of osteoarthritic changes (for triple pelvic osteotomy). Genetic testing for hypothyroidism is based on the presence of thyroglobulin autoantibodies. A dog with normal TgAA levels on two tests at least two years apart between two and six years of age is phenotypically normal. However, TgAA levels should not be measured within 2 to 3 months post-vaccination, as a transient iatrogenic rise can occur during this period.

For most genetic diseases, we know how to either prevent their occurrence, or at least lessen the possibility of producing offspring with genetic disease. This can occur through the genotypic testing of the parents (identification of parents carrying liability genes for genetic disease), phenotypic testing of the parents (identification of parents affected with genetic disease), or pedigree analysis (identification of a carrier and affected risk based on knowledge of the carrier or affected relatives).

The genetic improvement of cats and dogs will only occur through selective breeding. However, improvement will not occur unless we all understand our roles and responsibilities. The responsibility for this improvement lies not just with the breeder; but also with breed organizations, veterinarians, and the general public. Breeders must perform genetic testing on prospective breeding stock before breeding. Breed organizations must identify breed specific health issues through regular breed health surveys, fund research for breed specific disorders, and recommend genetic testing for breeding animals. Veterinarians must counsel prospective owners and breeders on breed specific health issues. They should provide the necessary genetic testing, or direct owners to specialists (ophthalmologists, cardiologists, etc.) that can perform the testing. The general public must become knowledgeable about what genetic tests are needed on parents of prospective kitten and puppy purchases, and how to verify testing status.

Inherent in these responsibilities is the acknowledgement that breeding without genetic testing is irresponsible, and unethical. Genetic testing is health quality control. It is no longer acceptable for a breeder to choose two individuals and breed them together without regard to genetic disease control.

Recommendations for Breeders

What can a breeder, owner, or veterinarian do if it is not known if a condition is inherited? First, a firm veterinary diagnosis needs to be established. This should be done for stillborn or fading puppies and kittens as well. If a disorder is not reported in a breed chapter; is it reported as an inherited condition in other breeds or other species? You should search widely to confirm whether the condition occurs at an increased frequency within a family or within the breed. Even if a mode of inheritance is not determined, knowledge that a condition is genetic allows for specific breeding recommendations.

The best methods for ensuring the health and diversity of any breed's gene pool are to: 1) Avoid the popular sire syndrome. 2) Utilize quality individuals from the breadth of the population to expand the gene pool. 3) Monitor genetic health issues through regular health surveys. 4) Do genetic testing for breed-related disorders. 5) Participate in open health registries.

The most important goal of managing genetic disease is to avoid producing affected individuals. The secondary goal is to reduce the frequency of carriers of defective genes in the population. At the same time, recommendations should allow perpetuation of breeding lines, in order to preserve the genetic diversity of the population. Historically, genetic counseling has ranged from recommendations to not repeat a mating and to outbreed, to recommendations for elimination of all relatives of affected animals from the breeding pool. Neither of these two extremes serves the best long-term interest of specific breeds. Outbreeding may prevent the production of animals affected with rare recessive diseases, but it will propagate and further disperse the detrimental recessive genes.

With widely dispersed or high frequency defective genes, it must be recognized that carriers are spread across the gene pool. Eliminating unique breeding lines because some individuals carry a single defective gene may adversely affect gene pool diversity more than a process that allows a limited number of carriers to reproduce. Conversely, with recently mutated or low frequency defective genes, it is advisable to strictly limit breeding, to avoid dispersion of the defective gene further in the population.

With each new generation, breeders ask, "How can I continue my line and improve it?" Aside from selecting for conformation, behavior and general health, breeders must consider how they are going to reduce the incidence of whichever genetic disorders are present in their breed. There are no answers that will fit every situation. There are, however, guidelines to preserve breeding lines and genetic diversity while reducing the risk of producing animals that carry defective genes, or are affected with genetic defects.

Autosomal Recessive Disorders

In the case of a simple autosomal recessive disorder for which a *direct genetic test for carriers* is available, the recommendation is to test breeding-quality stock, and breed normals to normals, or carriers to normal-testing individuals. This prevents affected offspring from being produced.

Breeders are the custodians of their breed's past and future. "Above all, do no harm" is a primary oath of all medical professionals. Genetic tests are powerful tools, and their use can cause significant positive or negative changes to breed gene pools. Once a genetic test is developed that allows breeders to determine if an animal is a carrier of a defective gene, many owners are likely to simply eliminate carriers from breeding. Although doing so is human nature, this temptation must be overcome. If an owner would breed an individual if it tested normal for a genetic disease, then a carrier result should not change that decision. A direct genetic test should not alter WHO gets bred, only WHO THEY GET BRED TO. One defective gene that can be identified through a genetic test out of tens of thousands of genes is not a reason to stop breeding. A genetic test that should be used to help maintain breed quality and diversity should not result in limiting it.

We know that most individuals carry some unfavorable recessive genes. The more genetic tests that are developed, the greater chance there is of identifying an undesirable gene in a breeding animal. History has shown that breeders can be successful in reducing breed-wide genetic disease through testing and making informed breeding choices. However, there are also examples of breeds that have actually experienced more problems as a result of unwarranted culling and restriction of their gene pools. These problems include: 1) Reducing the incidence of one disease and increasing the incidence of another by repeated use of males known to be clear of the gene that causes the first condition. 2) Creating bottlenecks and diminishing diversity by eliminating all carriers of a gene from the breeding pool, instead of breeding and replacing them. 3) Concentrating on the presence or absence of a single gene and not the quality of the whole animal.

The aim is to replace the carrier breeding-animal with a normal-testing offspring that equals or exceeds it in quality. Additional carrier testing offspring should not be placed in breeding homes; as the goal is to reduce the frequency of the defective gene in the population. As each breeder tests and replaces carrier animals with normal-testing offspring, the problem for the breed as a whole diminishes, while not restricting gene pool diversity.

The problem with a simple autosomal recessive disorder for which *no carrier test exists* is the propagation and dissemination of unapparent carriers in the gene pool. A quality individual that is found to be a carrier of a recessive gene can be retired from breeding and replaced with a quality relative or prior-born offspring. The genes of the retired individual can thus be preserved through the selected relative, but the carrier risk can be cut in half. To further limit the spread of the defective gene, the offspring should be used in only a limited number of carefully planned matings, and then should also be replaced with one or two representative offspring. The rest of the litter should be placed in non-breeding (pet) homes. With this mating scheme, you are maintaining the good genes of the line, reducing the carrier risk with each generation, and replacing, not adding to the overall carrier risk in the breeding population.

Breeders must assess the carrier risk of each individual animal in their breeding program. An open health registry that is supported by the parent club makes it easier for breeders to objectively assess these matters. An example is the genetic disease control program for cerebellar abiotrophy by the Scottish Terrier Club of America (www.stca.biz/health-registries/ca-registry). By determining the average carrier-risk for the breeding population, breeders can select matings that have a projected risk that is lower than the breed average. Relative risk assessments only take into account the identified carrier and affected individuals in the pedigree. Therefore, these estimates determine the minimum risk based on the information available. If additional affected relatives to the pedigree are diagnosed, the computed risk will rise. The relative risk pedigree calculator on the Scottish Terrier website can be used for any breed to compute carrier and affected risk for any simple autosomal recessive disorder.

If a quality breeding animal is at high risk of being a carrier, the best advice is to breed to an individual that has a low risk. Using relative-risk assessment as a tool, breeders should replace higher-risk breeding animals with lower-risk offspring that are equal to or better than their parents in quality. A negative aspect of pedigree analysis is that it selects against families, regardless of an individual's normal or carrier status. On the other hand, it allows for the objective risk assessment and continuation of lines that might otherwise be abandoned due to high carrier-risk.

Autosomal Dominant Disorders

Autosomal dominant genetic disorders are usually easy to manage. Each affected animal has at least one affected parent, but it can be expected that half of the offspring of an affected animal will be free of the defective gene. With disorders that cause death or discomfort, the recommendation is to not breed affected animals. To produce the next generation of a line; a normal full sibling of an affected animal, a normal close relative, or the parent that is normal can be used.

If the defective gene is at a high frequency in the gene pool, eliminating all affected breeding animals in one generation may have a significant negative impact on genetic diversity. When a high frequency autosomal dominant disorder is first identified, some quality, affected animals may have to be bred, and replaced with quality, normal testing offspring. However, once a few generations have gone by and breeders have had the opportunity to replace affected with normal individuals, the continued breeding of affected animals is not ethical.

A problem with some autosomal dominant disorders is incomplete penetrance; where some animals with the defective gene may not show the disorder. Roughly half their offspring, however, may be affected. If a genetic test is available, this is not a problem. Otherwise, pedigree analysis and relative-risk assessment can identify which animals are at risk of carrying incompletely penetrant dominant genes.

Sex-Linked Disorders

For sex-linked (also known as x-linked) recessive defective genes for which carrier tests exist, breeders should follow the same "breed and replace" recommendations as are outlined above in the discussion of autosomal recessive disorders. If there is no test, the defective gene can be traced through the pedigree. Selecting a normal male for breeding loses the defective gene in one generation, regardless of his relationship to affected and carrier relatives. Carrier, affected, or high risk females should not be used, due to the high risk of producing affected male offspring. If a male is affected, he would have received the defective gene from his carrier mother. All of his daughters will be carriers, but none of his sons. Without a test for carriers, you can use relative-risk assessment to breed him to a female that is at low risk of being a carrier. This minimizes the chance of producing affected offspring, and a quality son can be selected for replacement. Rare sex-linked dominant disorders are managed the same way as autosomal dominant disorders. The difference is that affected males will always produce all affected daughters.

Polygenic disorders/Complex Inheritance

Polygenic disorders are those caused by more than one pair of genes. A number of liability genes must combine to cross a threshold and produce an affected individual. Most polygenic disorders have no tests for carriers, but they do have phenotypic tests that can identify affected individuals. Controlling polygenically inherited disorders involves; 1) identifying traits that more closely represent genes being selected against, 2) the standardization of nuisance factors (such as environment) that can limit your selective pressure against the genes and 3) selecting for breadth of pedigree as well as depth of pedigree.

In polygenic disorders, the phenotype of the individual does not directly represent its genotype. If phenotypically normal parents produce affected offspring, both should be considered to carry a genetic load of liability genes that combined to cause the disorder. Breeders must break down affected phenotypes into traits that more directly represent the genes that control them. For example, in hip dysplasia these include clinical signs of lameness, shallow hip sockets, subluxation or remodeling on an extended leg view, and radiographic distractibility on a PennHIP view. If a quality individual is to be bred, but has shallow hip sockets, it should be bred to an individual with deep hip sockets. You need to select for enough genes influencing normal development, to get below the threshold where dysplasia develops.

The environment has a role in the expression of polygenic disorders. Plane of nutrition and environmental stress, especially during critical growth periods can alter the expression of some inherited musculoskeletal disorders. You do not want to overly protect or overly stress the development of prospective breeding animals. Breeders should evaluate prospective breeding individuals raised under fairly uniform conditions, which will not mask or alter the expression of genetic disease.

Polygenic disorders require knowledge of the affected or normal status of full-siblings to prospective breeding animals. Individuals whose siblings are normal and whose parents' sibs are normal have the greatest chance of carrying a low genetic load for the condition. This *breadth of pedigree* analysis is more important than normalcy in the depth of pedigree (parents and grandparents only.) This is why it is important to screen both pet and breeding animals from litters for polygenic disorders, and report the results in open health registries, such as the not-for profit Orthopedic Foundation for Animals (www.offa.org). Affected individuals can be replaced with a normal sib or parent, and bred to a low-liability mate. Breeders can replace the higher risk parent with a quality, lower risk offspring, and repeat the process. In addition, the offspring of breeding dogs should be monitored to see which are passing the disorder with higher frequency.

Undetermined Mode of Inheritance

For disorders without a known mode of inheritance or carrier test, breeders should be counseled to use the same control methods as with polygenic disorders. Animals with a low genetic load for the disorder should be selected for breeding, through the results of examinations of first-degree relatives (littermates, parents, and offspring). If there are multiple generations of normalcy in the breadth of the pedigree, then you can have some confidence that there is less risk that liability genes are being carried.

It is distressing when a genetic disorder is confirmed. Positive and practical genetic counseling recommendations can be made to maintain breed lines and genetic diversity, and improve the overall health of breeds. The total elimination of defective genes will probably be impossible for most breeds. The use of these guidelines can assist breeders in making objective breeding decisions for genetic disease management, while continuing their breeding lines. The individual breeder can use genetic tests to; 1) identify carriers, 2) work to breed away from the defective gene(s), and 3) ensure (through testing) that the defective gene(s) is not reintroduced in future matings. Each breeder will have their own rate of progress, depending on the frequency of the defective gene(s) in their own breeding animals, and which desirable individuals carry liability genes.

Section 2

Introduction

This section contains chapters on 171 dog breeds, including all except the most recent of the AKC breeds at the date of publication. It should be recognized that all mixed-breed and purebred or purposely bred dogs carry detrimental genes and can be affected with genetic disorders. A generally accepted fallacy is that purebred dogs are affected with more genetic disease than mixed-breed dogs. For the most part, this is only true for the rarer breed-specific disorders. The most common canine genetic disorders occur across all breeds, and in practice, we see as much genetic disease in mixed-breed dogs as we do in purebred dogs. These include the most frequent canine genetic disorders reported by the AKC Canine Health Foundation: cancer, inherited eye disease, epilepsy, hip dysplasia, hypothyroidism, heart disease, autoimmune disease, allergies, patella luxation, and renal dysplasia.

There are defective genes that are old in the dog genome, and spread across all dogs regardless of ancestry. The development of pure breeds has compartmentalized genes into breed gene pools. Based on the genetic load of disease causing genes, each breed has different frequencies of common and uncommon genetic disorders. Some defective genes are ancient, and their existence preceded the differentiation of breeds. The autosomal recessive, progressive rod cone degeneration (prcd) form of progressive retinal atrophy (PRA), is caused by the exact same mutation in at least twenty-five different breeds. Other defective mutations occurred more recently, and by propagation through foundation dogs or popular sires, have developed into breed specific genetic disorders.

A recent development in dog breeding is the rise of designer breeds – dogs produced through the purposeful crossbreeding of two different pure breeds. These are not considered specific breeds; because they do not breed true to reproduce themselves if bred together. It is only the original cross, which produces them as the F1 (first filial) generation. There is a general expectation that designer dogs should be healthier, simply because they are crossbred. However, due to the presence of disease liability genes across all breeds, this is not the case. The only way to have a realistic expectation that any purposely bred dog – purebred or crossbred – is going to be healthy is if the breeder is actively testing and screening breeding stock for genetic disease. The purebred parents of designer dogs should be screened for their respective breed-specific screening tests. Prospective owners should ask to see test results on the parents of dogs for sale. Many of these test results are available to the public in online registries from the OFA (Orthopedic Foundation for Animals: www.offa.org), CHIC (Canine Health Information Center: www.caninehealthinfo.org), and CERF (Canine Eye Registry Foundation: www.vmdb.org/cerf.html).

Medical conditions listed in the breed chapters are grouped under the following headers; Inherited Diseases (those with a defined mode of inheritance), and Disease Predispositions (those where a mode of inheritance is not defined). Many texts that report breed related genetic disease do not state the relative frequency of the disorders within the breed. In many instances, a "breed-related disorder" is reported due to a single published case report for a disease in the breed. In this section, the inherited diseases and breed predispositions are ordered based on their perceived incidence in the breed. Reported frequencies are stated based on genetic testing services, published articles, and health surveys. This process is the same as comparing apples to oranges; as the methods, populations, and statistics of each report cannot be adequately compared to each other. However, the disorders are ordered with the most common first, and least common last based on the author's experience.

Recommendations for genetic testing of breeding dogs are based on the breed-specific recommendations of the US parent club through the CHIC program. Where there are additional tests suggested beyond the CHIC recommendations, they are also listed. In all dog breeds, genetic testing of breeding stock for the major common inherited diseases is recommended. These include hip and elbow radiographs for dysplasia (or Legg-Calve-Perthes disease), a CERF eye examination by a board certified veterinary ophthalmologist, a thyroid profile including thyroglobulin autoantibodies, a cardiac evaluation, and a patella evaluation. Most of these are once-in-a-lifetime tests. It is not ethical to breed dogs (either purebred, designer-bred, or purposely bred) without ensuring that both parents are free of testable genetic disease.

Not every dog breed is included in the first edition, and some breed-related disorders may be missing, because there was no published reference at the time of publication. As the book is updated, adjustments and additions will need to be made in order to keep the listings current. Readers are encouraged to send comments to help us update the dog breed section. Use the contact address provided in the book preface. Chapters are in alphabetical order.

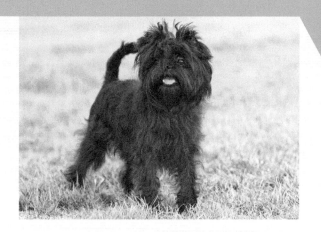

The Breed History

The breed name is a German word for *"Monkey-like terrier"*. The origins of this moniker probably derive from the cute monkey-like expression these dogs possess. Presence of a prominent hairy chin, sweeping moustache and prominent brows gave rise to the unique breed expression.

This ancient breed originated in the Munich area and has contributed to the development of breeds such as the Brussels Griffon (crosses with Pugs may have resulted in the Brussels Griffon).

Other Affenpinscher outcrosses included the smooth haired German Pinscher and German Silky Pinscher. The progenitor genes used in these outcrosses may have derived from a Schnauzer-type Russian ratter.

The ancient core German breed may have branched off into Miniature Schnauzer and Affenpinscher based on size originally. Though first historical records in artwork date to the year 1600, the breed standard was not drawn up until much later and details about the intervening breed development are sketchy. For a while they were termed ratting terriers and were larger in size. AKC first admitted the breed in 1936.

Breeding for Function

These dogs were kept for rat and mice control, and over time they were bred down to a toy size to suit the companionship needs of their owners. They also excelled as watchdogs and rabbit and quail trackers.

Physical Characteristics

Height at Withers: 9-11.5" (23-29 cm).

Weight: 7-8 lb (3.0-3.5 kg).

Coat: The medium-short coat is black, gray, black and tan, or silver with markings, or solid red (some have tan furnishings). They are low shedders. They have low grooming needs except for periodic stripping, and ears need regular plucking. The stiff, dense and wiry-textured coat is about 1" (2.5 cm) in length, and the ear hair is trimmed short. Color is not considered too important, though large white patches are not desirable. In Europe and England, black is the standard breed color.

Longevity: 14-15 years.

Points of Conformation: In the Affenpinscher, high head carriage is seen, eyes are round and dark, palpebral margins are black, ears may be cropped to sit pricked or left naturally (semi-erect on average; though are quite variable). The skull is domed, stop is well-defined, short blunt muzzle narrows to a black nose, lips are black, and a prognathic bite is normal. The neck is short and straight, topline is level, abdomen is slightly tucked up, thorax is broad and deep, they are particularly broad-chested in front; the ribs are moderately sprung. Limbs are straight, dewclaws usually removed, feet are small with thick black pads and nails, high-set tail is carried high and is covered with short hairs.

Recognized Behavior Issues and Traits

Traits ascribed to the Affenpinscher include: Intelligent, low grooming needs, friendly to his master, protective, fearless, alert, curious, loyal, and independent minded. It is suggested that one start earlier for obedience training than with many other breeds. They are quick to learn when focused. In French they are nicknamed "diabolitin moustachu" meaning moustached devil. Some have also referred to them as the *"little ruffian"*.

Can be snappy with children, show terrier tendency to excitement when on alert and can be bold and take on bigger dogs. They enjoy games that require dexterity of forelimbs, and should be introduced early to small pets.

They are very good alert barkers and enjoy close human contact. High-energy dogs, they enjoy games and vigorous runs for 30 minutes or so per day.

Normal Physiologic Variations
None reported

Drug Sensitivities
None reported

Inherited Diseases

Hip Dysplasia: Polygenically inherited trait causing degenerative joint disease and hip arthritis. OFA reports 15.7% affected.[1]

Patella Luxation: Polygenically inherited laxity of patellar ligaments, causing luxation, lameness, and later degenerative joint disease. Treat surgically if causing clinical signs. OFA reports 3.8% affected.[1]

Elbow Dysplasia: Polygenically inherited trait causing elbow arthritis. OFA reports 3.1% affected, but not enough Affenpinschers have been evaluated for statistical confidence.[1]

Legg–Calvé-Perthes Disease: Polygenically inherited aseptic necrosis of the femoral head, resulting in degenerative joint disease of the hip. Can be unilateral or bilateral with onset of degeneration usually between 6-9 months of age. Treat surgically if causing lameness/discomfort. Reported in the breed with a male prevalence on The Affenpinscher Club (UK) website.

Disease Predispositions

Distichiasis: Abnormally placed eyelashes that irritate the cornea and conjunctiva. Can cause secondary corneal ulceration. Identified in 6.38% of Affenpinschers CERF examined by veterinary ophthalmologists between 2000-2005.[2]

Persistent Pupillary Membranes: Strands of fetal remnant connecting; iris to iris, cornea, lens, or involving sheets of tissue. The later three forms can impair vision, and dogs affected with these forms should not be bred. Identified in 6.38% of Affenpinschers CERF examined by veterinary ophthalmologists between 2000-2005.[2]

Retinal Dysplasia: Retinal folds, geographic, and generalized retinal dysplasia with detachment are recognized in the breed. Identified in 4.26% of Affenpinschers CERF examined by veterinary ophthalmologists between 2000-2005.[2]

Cataracts: Anterior or posterior intermediate and punctate cataracts occur in the breed. Unknown mode of inheritance. Identified in 2.13% of Affenpinschers CERF examined by veterinary ophthalmologists between 2000-2005.[2]

Corneal Dystrophy: Affenpinschers can have an epithelial/stromal form of corneal dystrophy. Identified in 2.13% of Affenpinschers CERF examined by veterinary ophthalmologists between 2000-2005.[2]

Hypothyroidism: Inherited autoimmune thyroiditis. Not enough samples have been submitted for thyroid auto-antibodies to Michigan State University to determine an accurate frequency. (Ave. for all breeds is 7.5%).[3,4]

Seasonal Flank Alopecia: Wintertime, bilateral, symmetrical alopecia affecting the flank, dorsum and tail.[5,6]

Anasarca, Cleft Lip/Palate, Cryptorchidism, Dermoid, Elongated Soft Palate, Inhalant Allergies, Keratoconjunctivitis Sicca, Oligodontia, Patent Ductus Arteriosus, Progressive Retinal Atrophy, Retained Primary Teeth, and **Tracheal Collapse** are reported.[7]

Isolated Case Studies

Congenital Hypothyroidism with Epiphyseal Dysplasia: Diagnosed in a 4 year old Affenpinscher presented with a vertebral physeal fracture.[8]

Genetic Tests

Tests of Genotype: none

Tests of Phenotype: CHIC Certification: Required testing includes CERF eye examination at a minimum of 1 year of age, and patella evaluation at a minimum of 1 year of age. Optional testing includes hip radiographs for hip dysplasia and Legg-Calve-Perthes evaluation (See CHIC website; www.caninehealthinfo.org).

Recommend thyroid profile including autoantibodies, elbow radiographs, and cardiac evaluation.

Miscellaneous

- **Breed name synonyms:** Affen
- **Registries:** AKC, UKC, CKC, KCGB (Kennel Club of Great Britain), ANKC (Australian National Kennel Club), NKC (National Kennel Club)
- **AKC rank (year 2008):** 132 (171 dogs registered)
- **Internet resources: Affenpinscher Club of America:** www.affenpinscher.org
  The Affenpinscher Club (UK): www.affenpinscherclubuk.com

References

1. OFA Website breed statistics: www.offa.org Last accessed July. 1, 2010.
2. *Ocular Disorders Presumed to be Inherited in Purebred Dogs.* American College of Veterinary Ophthalmologists. ACVO, 2007.
3. Nachreiner R and Refsal K: Personal communication, Diagnostic Center for Population and Animal Health, Michigan State University. April, 2007
4. Nachreiner RF, Refsal KR, Graham PA, et. al.: Prevalence of serum thyroid hormone autoantibodies in dogs with clinical signs of hypothyroidism. *J Am Vet Med Assoc* 2002 Feb 15;220(4):466-71.
5. Waldman L: Seasonal flank alopecia in affenpinschers. *J Small Anim Pract.* 1995 Jun;36(6):271-3.
6. *White SD: Update on Follicular Alopecias: "Pseudo-Endocrinopathies".* Proceedings, ACVIM Forum, 2005
7. *The Genetic Connection: A Guide to Health Problems in Purebred Dogs.* L Ackerman. p. 193. AAHA Press, 1999.
8. Lieb AS, Grooters AM, Tyler JW, et. al.: Tetraparesis due to vertebral physeal fracture in an adult dog with congenital hypothyroidism. *J Small Anim Pract.* 1997 Aug;38(8):364-7.
9. *The Complete Dog Book, 20th Ed.* The American Kennel Club. Howell Book House, NY 2006. p. 447-449.

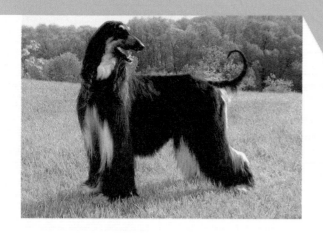

Afghan Hound

Points of Conformation: This breed is noted for the "far-seeing gaze", noble carriage and fine coat. Other key characteristics include prominent hip bones, large feet, and they appear to have an increased stifle angle due to the overlying haircoat. The skull is long and finely chiseled with a slight Roman nose; no pronounced stop is present. The occipital protuberance is prominent, the ears are long and pendulous and covered with long silky hair, and the leather is fine. Eyes are dark, almond-shaped, and almost triangular. The muzzle is very long in this dolichocephalic breed. The nose is moderate in size and black in pigmentation. Neck is long, arched, and the topline is level, though the loin is slightly arched, and there is a marked tuck-up in the abdomen. The thorax is deep, the forelegs straight boned and the radius is very long; tibia is also long, and the feet are well arched with lots of hair covering them, and large toes are present. Their gait is smooth, elastic, and high stepping with strides that cover great distance and seeming effortless. High head and tail carriage is notable. The tail is low set, curled at the end (donut tipped), and has minimal feathering.

The Breed History

The Afghan Hound was first represented in Indian works of art dated 1809. The origin of the breed as the name implies was in Afghanistan and surrounding regions where they were bred for at least a few thousand years by nomadic tribes. Due to the variations of elevation and climate in this harsh wild region, some variation in breed type evolved, distinguishing it from the original Middle Eastern Sight hound. The specimens that became foundation stock for American and European breeding programs arrived in Scotland in 1920 (desert strain), and specimens from the other founding strain (mountain type) arrived in England in 1925. The AKC admitted the breed in 1926.

Breeding for Function

The mountain regions of the north gave rise to Afghans with heavier coats, more compact build and darker coat colors. The arid regions gave rise to a lighter build and color and a less dense coat. Historically this breed was a guard dog, a coursing hound, and even reportedly used for herding. As a coursing sight hound, the dog hunted alongside horsemen. Due to their speed and stamina they often worked ahead of the hunters and due to their agility, they were able to manage hunts over very rough terrain. The quarry varied depending on the locale, and may have included antelope and leopards. More recently, Afghan Hounds have been successfully entered in lure coursing and obedience, but many are now prized solely for their exceptional companionship qualities.

Physical Characteristics

Height at Withers: female 24-26" (61-66 cm), male 26-28" (66-71 cm).

Weight: females 50 lb (23 kg), males 60 lb (27 kg).

Coat: The very fine silky, glossy and long haircoat is shorter on the face, though a long, soft topknot is present. Hair is short also over the topline (the Afghan saddle) in adults. They are shown in a natural unclipped coat. Though all coat colors are accepted except spotted pattern, the presence of white head markings is not encouraged. Puppies have soft fuzzy short hair on their saddles and faces (monkey whiskers) that is replaced by an adult coat at about one year of age.

Longevity: 12-14 years

Recognized Behavior Issues and Traits

Traits ascribed to this breed include: Strong independent streak, strong personality, somewhat difficult to train, and generally aloof with strangers.

These dogs have high grooming needs including daily brushing and regular bathing. They are low shedders. Some resources suggest snoods (hoods) to protect the long hair from soiling or getting in the mouth during mealtime.

These dogs have high exercise needs, and they need to be restricted to fenced enclosures or they will roam. They are very sensitive dogs. Some are good with children, some not. They do best with gentle, quiet children and early socialization is important. It is best to introduce them to other pets and children when the dog is young. Play activities and lots of attention should be provided to alleviate boredom.

Normal Physiologic Variations

Sight hounds have lower normal ranges for T4 and T3 concentrations compared to other breeds.[1]

Echocardiographic Normal Values[2]	
Parameter	Median (Range)
Weight (kg)	23 (17-36)
Heart rate (bpm)	120 (80-140)
LVPWD (mm)	9 (7-11)
LVPWS (mm)	12 (9-18)
LVD (mm)	42 (33-52)
LVS (mm)	28 (20-37)
FS (%)	33 (24-48)
EPSS (mm)	4 (0-10)
RVd (mm)	10 (5-20)
IVSd (mm)	10 (8-12)
IVSs (mm)	13 (8-18)
AOD (mm)	26 (20-34)
LAS (mm)	26 (18-35)
N	20

LVPWD, LV posterior wall dimension at end-diastole; LVPWS, LV posterior wall thickness at end-systole; LVD, LV chamber dimension at end-diastole; LVS, LV chamber dimension at end-systole; FS, percent fractional shortening; EPSS, E-point septal separation; RVD, RV chamber dimension at end-diastole; IVSd, interventricular septal thickness at end-diastole; IVSs, interventricular septal thickness at end-systole; AOD, aortic root at end-diastole; LAS, left atrium at end-systole; N, number of animals.

Drug Sensitivities

Anesthesia: Sight hounds require particular attention during anesthesia. Their lean body conformation with high surface-area-to-volume ratio predisposes them to hypothermia during anesthesia. Impaired biotransformation of drugs by the liver results in prolonged recovery from barbiturate and thiobarbiturate intravenous anesthetics. Propofol, and ketamine/diazepam combination are recommended induction agents.[3]

Inherited Diseases

Elbow Dysplasia: Polygenically inherited trait causing elbow arthritis. OFA reports 6.4% affected.[4]

Hip Dysplasia: Polygenically inherited trait causing degenerative joint disease and hip arthritis. OFA reports 5.8% affected.[4]

Patella Luxation: Polygenically inherited laxity of patellar ligaments, causing luxation, lameness, and later degenerative joint disease. Treat surgically if causing clinical signs. Too few Afghan Hounds have been screened by OFA to determine an accurate frequency.[4]

Afghan Myelopathy (necrotizing myelopathy): Rare, autosomal recessive disorder of spinal cord degeneration. Onset at 3-13 months of age, rapidly progressing from paraparesis to spastic paraplegia. There is no genetic test available.[5,6]

Disease Predispositions

Corneal Dystrophy: A lipid, epithelial/stromal form of corneal dystrophy occurs in the breed. In most cases dystrophic change does not progress to the point of visual impairment. Reported in 9.15% of Afghan Hounds CERF examined by veterinary ophthalmologists 2000-2005.[7]

Hypothyroidism: 7.3% positive for thyroid auto-antibodies based on testing at Michigan State University. (Avg. for all breeds is 7.5%). Dorn reports a 1.8x odds ratio for developing hypothyroidism versus other breeds.[8,9,10]

Persistent Pupillary Membranes: Strands of fetal remnant connecting; iris to iris, cornea, lens, or involving sheets of tissue. The later three forms can impair vision, and dogs affected with these forms should not be bred. Identified in 3.43% of Afghan Hounds CERF examined by veterinary ophthalmologists between 2000-2005.[7]

Cataracts: The breed can develop rapidly progressive juvenile cataracts that begin as equatorial vacuoles between 4 months to 2 years of age and extend into the anterior and posterior cortex. A recessive mode of inheritance is suspected. Identified in 3.20% of Afghan Hounds CERF examined by veterinary ophthalmologists between 2000-2005. CERF does not recommend breeding any Afghan hound with a cataract.[7,11]

Laryngeal Paralysis: The breed is predisposed to acquired laryngeal paralysis due to reduced function of the recurrent laryngeal nerves in older dogs. Arytenoid lateralization achieves the best results as a method of surgical correction in severe cases, though increasing the risk of aspiration pneumonia.[12]

Atrioventricular (Heart) Block: Afghan Hounds are found to be at increased risk of high-grade second- or third-degree atrioventricular block versus other breeds. Treatment is with a pacemaker.[13]

Chylothorax: The Afghan hound is the breed most commonly affected with spontaneous chylous pleural effusion, accounting for 37.5% of all cases. Secondary lung lobe torsion is a frequent complication. There is no age or sex predilection for the condition.[14,15,16]

Lung Lobe Torsion: Lung lobe torsion is rare in dogs and develops most frequently in large deep-chested dogs, particularly Afghan Hounds. Most cases in this breed were secondary to chylothorax. Prognosis after surgery is fair to guarded.[15,16,17]

Demodicosis: Afghan hounds are predisposed to demodex infections. This disorder has an underlying immunodeficiency in its pathogenesis.[18]

Amyloidosis, Brachygnathism, Deafness, Exocrine Pancreatic Insufficiency, Fanconi Syndrome, Gastric Dilatation-Volvulus, Glaucoma, Intervertebral Disk Disease, Megaesophagus, Mitral Valve Disease, Narcolepsy, Shoulder OCD, Oligodontia, Optic Nerve Hypoplasia, Perineal Hernia, Prognathism, Progressive Retinal Atrophy, Pulmonic Stenosis, Retinal Dysplasia, Umbilical Hernia, von Willebrand's Disease, and **Wobbler Syndrome** are reported.[19]

Isolated Case Studies

Arteriosclerosis with Arterial Obstruction: A 13-year-old female Afghan Hound with progressive left hind-limb lameness and absence of a peripheral left hind pulse was found to have advanced arteriosclerosis of the distal aorta, and left external iliac and femoral arteries. Diagnosis was confirmed by ultrasonographic examination of the abdominal aorta and its terminal branches.[20]

Ganglion Cysts: Case study of a 4-month-old male Afghan Hound with subcutaneous ovoid cysts around the caudal right elbow joint and left ischiatic tuberosity. Surgical removal demonstrated abundant mucinous fluid and internal folding, without communication to the joint cavity. These ganglion cysts apparently resulted from the metaplasia of fibroblasts to secreting cells.[21]

D-(+)-glyceric Aciduria: This rare condition was identified in a one year old female Afghan hound with a hepatopathy (increased ALT, bilirubin and bile acids). The hepatopathy resolved with supportive therapy, but the aciduria remained, suggesting that this may be a benign condition.[22]

Congenital Central Diabetes Insipidus: Two Afghan hound sibling puppies showing signs of polyuria and polydipsia were diagnosed with this disorder.[23]

Genetic Tests

Tests of Genotype: Direct test for color and mask alleles is available from HealthGene and VetGen.

Tests of Phenotype: CHIC Certification: Required testing includes hip radiographs, CERF eye examination (minimum of 1 year), and thyroid profile including autoantibodies. (See CHIC website; www.caninehealthinfo.org).

Recommend elbow radiographs, patella evaluation and cardiac evaluation.

Miscellaneous

- **Breed name synonyms:** Tazi, Baluchi hound, Afghan.
- **Registries:** AKC, UKC, CKC, KCGB (Kennel Club of Great Britain), ANKC (Australian National Kennel Club), NKC (National Kennel Club).
- **AKC rank (year 2008):** 93 (631 dogs registered)
- **Internet resources: Afghan Hound Club of America Inc.:** http://clubs.akc.org/ahca/
  Afghan Hound Club of Canada: www.ahcc.ca
  Afghan Hound Association (UK): www.ahaonline.co.uk

References

1. Kintzer PP and Peterson ME: Progress in the Diagnosis and Treatment of Canine Hypothyroidism. 2007. Proceedings, ACVIM 2007.
2. Morrison SA, Moise NS, Scarlett J, et. al.: Effect of breed and body weight on echocardiographic values in four breeds of dogs of differing somatotype. *J Vet Intern Med.* 1992 Jul-Aug;6(4):220-4.
3. Court:MH: Anesthesia of the sighthound. Clin Tech Small Anim Pract 1999 Feb; 14(1):38-43.
4. OFA Website breed statistics: www.offa.org Last accessed July. 1, 2010
5. Averill DR Jr, Bronson RT: Inherited necrotizing myelopathy of Afghan hounds. *J Neuropathol Exp Neurol.* 1977 Jul;36(4):734-47.
6. Cummings JF, de Lahunta A: Hereditary myelopathy of Afghan hounds, a myelinolytic disease. *Acta Neuropathol (Berl).* 1978 Jun 30;42(3):173-81.
7. *Ocular Disorders Presumed to be inherited in Purebred Dogs.* American College of Veterinary Ophthalmologists. ACVO, 2007.
8. Dorn CR: Canine breed-specific risks of frequently diagnosed diseases at veterinary teaching hospitals. Monograph, AKC Caninte Health Foundation. 2000.
9. Nachreiner RF, Refsal KR, Graham PA, et. al.: Prevalence of serum thyroid hormone autoantibodies in dogs with clinical signs of hypothyroidism. J Am Vet Med Assoc 2002 Feb 15;220(4):466-71.
10. Nachreiner R and Refsal K: Personal communication, Diagnostic Center for Population and Animal Health, Michigan State University. April, 2007.
11. Roberts SR, Helper LC: Cataracts in Afghan Hounds. *J Am Vet Med Assoc.* 1972;160:427.
12. Burbidge HM: A review of laryngeal paralysis in dogs. *Br Vet J.* 1995 Jan-Feb;151(1):71-82
13. Schrope DP and Kelch WJ: Signalment, clinical signs, and prognostic indicators associated with high-grade second- or third-degree atrioventricular block in dogs: 124 cases (January 1, 1997-December 31, 1997). J Am Vet Med Assoc. 2006 Jun 1;228(11):1710-7.
14. Fossum TW, Birchard SJ, Jacobs RM: Chylothorax in 34 dogs. J Am Vet Med Assoc. 1986 Jun 1;188(11):1315-8.
15. Gelzer AR, Downs MO, Newell SM, et. al.: Accessory lung lobe torsion and chylothorax in an Afghan hound. *J Am Anim Hosp Assoc.* 1997 Mar-Apr;33(2):171-6.
16. Williams JH, Duncan NM: Chylothorax with concurrent right cardiac lung lobe torsion in an Afghan hound. *J S Afr Vet Assoc.* 1986 Mar;57(1):35-7.
17. Neath PJ, Brockman DJ, King LG: Lung lobe torsion in dogs: 22 cases (1981-1999). *J Am Vet Med Assoc.* 2000 Oct 1;217(7):1041-4.
18. Lemarie SL, Hosgood G, Foil CS: A retrospective study of juvenile- and adult-onset generalized demodicosis in dogs (1986-91). *Veterinary Dermatology.* 1996. 7(1);3-10.
19. *The Genetic Connection: A Guide to Health Problems in Purebred Dogs.* L Ackerman. p. 193-194 AAHA Press, 1999.
20. Zandvliet MM, Stokhof AA, Boroffka S, et. al.: Intermittent claudication in an Afghan hound due to aortic arteriosclerosis. *J Vet Intern Med.* 2005 Mar-Apr;19(2):259-61.
21. Cho KO, Park NY, Kang Mil,et. Al.: Ganglion cysts in a juvenile dog. *Vet Pathol.* 2000 Jul;37(4):340-3.
22. Sewell AC, Moritz A, Duran M: D-(+)-glyceric aciduria in an Afghan hound. *J Inherit Metab Dis.* 1997 Jul;20(3):395-6.
23. Post K, McNeill JR, Clark EG, et. al.: Congenital central diabetes insipidus in two sibling Afghan hound pups. *J Am Vet Med Assoc.* 1989 Apr 15;194(8):1086-8.
24. *The Complete Dog Book, 20th Ed.* The American Kennel Club. Howell Book House, NY 2006. p. 133-137.

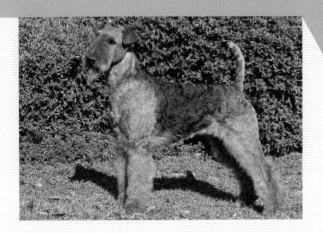

early. The mix of hound and terrier leads to independent thinking traits, and they have high intelligence. They need close human contact, and may chew or dig if left alone for extended periods. The hound component means that they tolerate other dogs much better than typical terriers.

They are low shedders, low allergenic dogs and need regular grooming. They are considered high-energy dogs. They are suitable for both town and country as long as regular exercise is provided.

The Breed History

As with many breeds of dogs, the origins of the Airedale are somewhat obscure. A now-extinct Black and Tan Terrier sometimes called Old English terrier or Broken-haired terrier may have been a progenitor of not only the Airedale, but perhaps also the Fox, Welsh, and Irish terriers. In the latter part of the 1800s, the first show classes for this breed took place. About the same time, a known outcross with the Otterhound breed was carried out to improve the Airedale's capacity for water work and to improve scenting ability.

Breeding for Function

The old terriers were widely used in Yorkshire England for hunting otter, rats, badgers, weasels and other medium game. In Canada, the US, India and Africa they were prized for their bravery in large game hunts. Their utility encompasses police dog work and historically, included service as war dogs. They also perform well in obedience tracking, agility and guarding.

Physical Characteristics

Height at Withers: female 22" (56 cm), male 23" (58.5 cm).

Weight: females 40-48 lb (18-22 kg), males 45-70 lb (20.5-32 kg).

Coat: The dense double coat may have some crimping; the outer layer is wiry while the undercoat is soft. Colors are black and tan with specifically distributed markings. A small white mark on the chest is not penalized.

Longevity: 10-12 years.

Points of Conformation: The head is long with a minor stop, the ears are V-shaped and carried folded. Eyes are dark and small with keen expression, and nose is medium and black. Other points include moderate length neck, chest deep but not broad, topline level and back is short. Legs are straight, tail is carried high, and feet are compact and small. Overall, they are characterized by good bone and athletic appearance, with a solid straight way of going, including good stride length and freedom of movement.

Recognized Behavior Issues and Traits

Breed Traits Ascribed Include: Renowned for being exceptionally loyal devoted companions, good protectors of home and farm, and are noted to be aloof with strangers. Their training should start

Normal Physiologic Variations

None reported

Drug Sensitivities

None reported

Inherited Diseases

Hip Dysplasia: Polygenically inherited trait causing degenerative joint disease and hip arthritis. OFA reports 11.4% affected.[1]

Elbow Dysplasia: Polygenically inherited trait causing elbow arthritis. OFA reports 11% affected.[1]

von Willebrand's Disease (vWD): Autosomal recessive Type I vWD is reported in the Airedale Terrier. This disease causes a mild bleeding disorder. A genetic test has not been developed in this breed.[2]

Hemophilia B (Factor IX Deficiency): Severe, x-linked recessive bleeding disorder documented in this breed. A genetic test is available.[3]

Patella Luxation: Polygenically inherited laxity of patellar ligaments, causing luxation, lameness, and later degenerative joint disease. Treat surgically if causing clinical signs. Too few Airedale Terriers have been OFA evaluated to determine an accurate frequency.[1]

Disease Predispositions

Heart Murmur: Reported at a frequency of 13.3% in the Airedale Terrier Health Survey 2000-2001. Atrial septal defect, pulmonic stenosis, subaortic stenosis, tricuspid valve dysplasia, and ventricular septal defect are reported to occur in the breed.[4,16]

Allergic Dermatitis: Presents with pruritis and pyotraumatic dermatitis (hot spots). The Airedale Terrier Health Survey 2000-2001 reports 11.4% allergic to fleas, 7.7% to inhaled allergens, and 5.0% to food.[4]

Hypothyroidism: Inherited autoimmune thyroiditis. 8.8% positive for thyroid auto-antibodies based on testing at Michigan State University. (Ave. for all breeds is 7.5%). Reported at a frequency of 7.5% in the Airedale Terrier Health Survey 2000-2001.[4,5,6]

Cataracts: Anterior cataracts are the most frequent in the breed. Identified in 6.94% of Airedale Terriers CERF examined by veterinary ophthalmologists between 2000-2005. Reported at a frequency of 8.3% in the Airedale Terrier Health Survey 2000-2001. CERF does not recommend breeding any Airdale Terrier with a cataract.[4,7]

Persistent Pupillary Membranes: Strands of fetal remnant connecting; iris to iris, cornea, lens, or involving sheets of tissue. The later three forms can impair vision, and dogs affected with these forms should not be bred. Identified in 5.78% of Airedale Terriers CERF examined by veterinary ophthalmologists between 2000-2005.[7]

Distichiasis: Abnormally placed eyelashes that irritate the cornea and conjunctiva. Can cause secondary corneal ulceration. Identified in 5.20% of Airedale Terriers CERF examined by veterinary ophthalmologists between 2000-2005.[7]

Cancer: The following frequencies for cancer were reported in the Airedale Terrier Health Survey 2000-2001: Melanoma 4.0%, adenocarcinoma 3.3%, hemangiosarcoma 2.7%, lymphosarcoma 2.5%, osteosarcoma 1.2%, mast cell tumor 1.2%.[4]

Pancreatitis: Inflammation of the pancreas causing vomiting and peritonitis. Can be life threatening if severe. Reported at a frequency of 3.7% in the Airedale Terrier Health Survey 2000-2001.[4]

Corneal Dystrophy: Causes opacities on the surface of the cornea. Age of onset of 9-11 months, which may progress to vision impairment by 3-4 years of age. Sex-linked inheritance suggested in one report. Identified in 3.41% of Airedale Terriers CERF examined by veterinary ophthalmologists between 1991-1999, with none reported between 2000-2005.[7,8,9]

Retinal Dysplasia: Focal folds and geographic retinal dysplasia are seen in the breed. Focal folds were identified in 2.89%, and geographic dysplasia in 0.58% of Airedale Terriers CERF examined by veterinary ophthalmologists between 2000-2005.[7]

Inherited Epilepsy: Grand-mal seizures. Control with anticonvulsant medication. Reported at a frequency of 2.3% in the Airedale Terrier Health Survey 2000-2001. Unknown mode of inheritance.[4]

Autoimmune Hemolytic Anemia (AIHA): Autoimmune destruction of red blood cells. Clinical features include pale mucous membranes, weakness, lethargy and collapse. Treat with immunosuppressive drugs. Reported at a frequency of 2.3% in the Airedale Terrier Health Survey 2000-2001. Reported 45.3x odds ratio versus other breeds. Reported 22.5x odds ratio for concurrent AIHA and ITP.[4,10,11]

Missing Teeth: Reported at a frequency of 2.3% in the Airedale Terrier Health Survey 2000-2001. Unknown mode of inheritance.[4]

Umbilical Hernia: Congenital opening in the body wall from where the umbilical cord was attached. Unknown mode of inheritance. Reported at a frequency of 1.9% in the Airedale Terrier Health Survey 2000-2001.[4]

Progressive Retinal Atrophy (PRA): Inherited degeneration of the retina resulting in blindness. Age of onset around 3 years of age. Mode of inheritance presumed recessive. Reported in 1.83%

of Airedale Terriers CERF examined by veterinary ophthalmologists between 1991-1999, with none reported between 2000-2005.[7]

Entropion: Rolling in of eyelids, often causing corneal irritation or ulceration. Entropion is reported in 1.73% of Airedale Terriers CERF examined by veterinary ophthalmologists between 2000-2005.[7]

Cryptorchidism (Retained Testicles): Can be unilateral or bilateral. Reported at a frequency of 1.7% in the Airedale Terrier Health Survey 2000-2001.[4]

Immune-Mediated Thrombocytopenia (ITP): Autoimmune destruction of blood platelets. Most common presentation is in middle aged females. Reported at a frequency of 1.5% in the Airedale Terrier Health Survey 2000-2001. Reported 22.5x odds ratio for concurrent AIHA and ITP.[4,10]

Dilated Cardiomyopathy: Can present with ventricular arrhythmias, progressing to heart failure. Increased incidence reported in the breed. Two to one ratio of affected males to females. Reported at a frequency of 1.4% in the Airedale Terrier Health Survey 2000-2001.[4,12]

Gastric Dilation/Volvulus (GDV, Bloat): Life-threatening twisting of the stomach within the abdomen. Requires immediate veterinary attention. Reported at a frequency of 1.0% in the Airedale Terrier Health Survey 2000-2001.[4]

Seasonal Flank Alopecia: Bilateral, symmetrical alopecia affecting the flank, dorsum and tail. Affects primarily spayed females, in the Spring or Autumn. Mean age of onset is 3.6 years.[13]

Seborrheic Dermatitis: Skin disorder presenting with greasy skin and haircoat. Dorn reports a 2.06x odds ratio of developing seborrheic dermatitis versus other breeds.[14]

Transitional Cell Carcinoma (TCC, bladder cancer): Increased incidence of this bladder cancer cited in the breed. TCC is a malignant cancer that can be controlled with surgery and piroxicam treatment.[15]

Diskospondylitis: Vertebral bone infection, possibly with an immune component in the breed. There are multiple case reports in related Airedale Terriers. Thought to be due to immunosuppression from decreased immunoglobulin A production.[16,17]

Cerebellar Abiotrophy (CCA, cerebellar ataxia): Disorder causing hypermetria, a high stepping gait, and incoordination. Onset in this breed is 12 weeks of age. Clinical signs usually progress slowly throughout the life of the dog, however some can progress more rapidly to constant stumbling. Occurs at a low frequency in Airedale Terriers.[18]

Chromosomal Intersex, Demodicosis, Exocrine Pancreatic Insufficiency, HyperlipoProteinemia, Hypoadrenocorticism, Intervertrbral Disk Disease, Laryngeal Paralysis, Myasthenia Gravis, Narcolepsy, Panosteitis, Pannus, Polycystic Kidney Disease, Portosystemic Shunt, and Sebaceous Adenitis are reported.[19]

Isolated Case Studies

Pituitary Carcinoma: A 6-year-old Airdale terrier presented with a one month history of progressive behavioral and neurological signs, including proprioceptive deficits, circling, anisocoria, and head pressing. A large, invasive, pituitary carcinoma was diagnosed at post mortem.[20]

Multiple Myeloma: Identified in a 10-year-old neutered male Airedale Terrier with inappetence, weight loss, and lameness. Multiple myeloma was diagnosed based on bone marrow plasmacytosis, multiple lytic bone lesions, and hyperglobulinemia with a clonal gammopathy.[21]

Mixed Germ Cell Tumor: Identified in the lumbar spinal cord of a two-year-old, female Airedale terrier with a history of progressive paraplegia. It was composed of three different types of cells: small round germ cells, large eosinophilic cells, and a rarer differentiated epithelial cell.[22]

Unilateral Horner's Syndrome and Masticatory Muscle Atrophy: Seen in a 9-year-old, spayed female, Airedale Terrier diagnosed with polyradiculoneuritis and ganglionitis that was most severe in the trigeminal nerves.[23]

Genetic Tests

Tests of Genotype: Direct test for Hemophilia B is available from HealthGene.

Tests of Phenotype: CHIC Certification: Required testing includes hip radiographs, congenital cardiac examination, and renal disease testing. Optional recommended testing includes CERF eye examination, thyroid profile including autoantibodies, and elbow radiographs. (See CHIC website; www.caninehealthinfo.org).

Recommend patella evaluation.

Miscellaneous

- **Breed name synonyms:** Airedale, Bingley Terrier (historical), Waterside Terrier (historical), King of Terriers (historical)
- **Registries:** AKC, CKC, UKC, KCGB (Kennel Club of Great Britain), ANKC (Australian National Kennel Club), NKC (National Kennel Club)
- **AKC rank (year 2008):** 58 (1,776 dogs registered)
- **Internet resources: Airedale Terrier Club of America:** www.airedale.org
  National Airedale Terrier Association (UK): http://www.nationalairedale.co.uk/
  Airedale Terrier Club of Canada: www.airedaleterrier.ca

References

1. OFA Website breed statistics: www.offa.org Last accessed July 1, 2010.
2. Brooks M: Transfusion Therapy for Hemostatic Defects. Proceedings, ACVIM Forum, 2003.
3. Gu W, Brooks M, Catalfamo J, et al: Two distinct mutations cause severe hemophilia B in two unrelated canine pedigrees. Thromb Haemost 82:1270-1275, 1999.
4. Glickman L and Glickman N: Airedale Terrier Health Survey 2000-2001. Airedale Terrier Club of America. 2001.
5. Nachreiner R and Refsal K: Personal communication, Diagnostic Center for Population and Animal Health, Michigan State University. Aprial,2007
6. Nachreiner RF, Refsal KR, Graham PA, et. al.: Prevalence of serum thyroid hormone autoantibodies in dogs with clinical signs hypothyroidism. J Am Vet Med Assoc 2002 Feb 15; 220(4):466-71.
7. *Ocular Disorders Presumed to be Inherited in Purebred Dogs.* American College of Veterinary Ophthalmologists. ACVO, 2007
8. Dice PF: Corneal dystrophy in the Airedale. Proc Am Coll Vet Ophthalmol. 1976:7:36.
9. Cooley PL, Dice PF 2nd: Corneal dystrophy in the dog and cat. *Vet Clin North Am Small Anim Pract.* 1990 May;20(3):681-92.
10. Goggs R, Boag AK, & Chan DL: Concurrent immune-mediated haemolytic anaemia and severe thrombocytopenia in 21 dogs. Vet Rec. 2008 Sep 13;163(11):323-7.
11. McAlees TJ: Immune-mediated haemolytic anaemia in 110 dogs in Victoria, Australia. Aust Vet J. 2010 Jan;88(1-2):25-8.
12. Tidholm A, Jonsson L : A retrospective study of canine dilated cardiomyopathy (189 cases). *J Am Anim Hosp Assoc.* 1997 Nov-Dec;33(6):544-50.
13. Miller MA, Dunstan RW: Seasonal flank alopecia in boxers and Airedale terriers: 24 cases (1985-1992). *J Am Vet Med Assoc.* 1993 Dec 1;203(11):1567-72.
14. Dorn CR: Canine breed-specific risks of frequently diagnosed diseases at veterinary teaching hospitals. Monograph. AKC Canine Health Foundation. 2000.
15. Norris AM, Laing EJ, Valli VE, et. al.: Canine bladder and urethral tumors: a retrospective study of 115 cases (1980-1985). *J Vet Intern Med.* 1992 May-Jun;6(3):145-53.
16. Turnwald GH, Shires PK, Turk MA, et. al.: Diskospondylitis in a kennel of dogs: clinicopathologic findings. *J Am Vet Med Assoc.* 1986 Jan 15;188(2):178-83.
17. Barta O, Turnwald GH, Shaffer LM, et. al.: Blastogenesis-suppressing serum factors, decreased immunoglobulin A, and increased beta 1-globulins in Airedale Terriers with diskospondylitis. *Am J Vet Res.* 1985 Jun;46(6):1319-22.
18. Inzana KD: Brain Malformation and Storage Diseases. Proceedings, Western Veterinary Conference, 2002.
19. The Genetic Connection: A Guide To Health Problems in Purebred Dogs. L. Ackerman. P 194, AAHA Press, 1999.
20. Puente S: Pituitary carcinoma in an Airedale terrier. *Can Vet J.* 2003 Mar;44(3):240-2.
21. Ramaiah SK, Seguin MA, Carwile HF, et. al.: Biclonal gammopathy associated with immunoglobulin A in a dog with multiple myeloma. *Vet Clin Pathol.* 2002;31(2):83-9.
22. Ferreira AJ, Peleteiro MC, Carvalho T, et. al.: Mixed germ cell tumour of the spinal cord in a young dog. *J Small Anim Pract.* 2003 Feb;44(2):81-4.
23. Panciera RJ, Ritchey JW, Baker JE, et. al.: Trigeminal and polyradicu-loneuritis in a dog presenting with masticatory muscle atrophy and Homer's Syndrome. Vet Pathol. 2002 Jan;39(1):146-9.
24. *The Complete Dog Book, 20th Ed.* The American Kennel Club. Howell Book House, NY 2006. p 341-344.

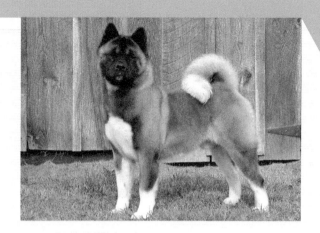

The Breed History

First written records date to the 17th century, where in the Akita Prefecture of Honshu in Northern Japan (Dewa), breeding programs were instituted to produce a sensible hunting dog. At this time, ownership of Akita dogs was restricted to the aristocracy. Their esteem was held so high that in some places they were assigned individually hired caregivers who provided special care. This ancient Japanese dog breed is also cemented in certain spiritual traditions wherein the dog represents good health, and a statue gift of the dog for a new addition to a family represents wishes for health, happiness and a long life for the child. This statue gift is also sent as a get-well message for those ailing. They are of Spitz type, and the ancient progenitor genes came into Japan with migrating Siberian nomads a very long time ago.

Akitas may also include in their heritage crosses of Chow-Chows with Tosa (Shikoku) and Kari dogs. In spite of the special status of this breed, at times, the popularity fell off to the point of near extinction. In 1931, Japan named the breed a national monument. Helen Keller was credited with importing the first specimens of the breed to America. The AKC first registered Akitas in 1972.

Breeding for Function

Their original use was for hunting in rugged territory. Boar and deer were typical game. Alert and possessing good stamina, these dogs were valued hunting companions. They were also reported to have been soft mouthed enough for waterfowl retrieval. Others report their use as pit fighting dogs. They were adapted to a harsh wintry environment, and were renowned for their sturdy, agile, silent work.

Physical Characteristics

Height at Withers: female 24-26" (61-71 cm), male 26-28" (66-71 cm).

Weight: females 75-85lb (34-38.5 kg), males 85-110 lb (38.5-50 kg).

Coat: They have a thick double coat with medium length outer coat hair, and are accepted in many colors including brindle, pinto, or white. The undercoat may be a different color. The outer coat stands up and is harsh and straight while the undercoat is soft, dense and short. Some lines have longer hair than the average, though this variation is not considered correct for show.

Longevity: 11-12 years

Points of Conformation: The full tail held over the back and the alert, pricked ears and bear-like facial expression on the large head characterize this stocky dog. The skull is broad, with broad muzzle and small dark brown eyes, deep set and a triangular shape. A shallow furrow runs in a line up the head extending onto the forehead. Triangular ears are small. Set wide, they are strongly leathered to keep them firmly up. The nose is large and black pigmentation is preferred. The stop is well defined, and both lip and palpebral margins are black. The crested neck is short. The thorax is wide and deep, and ribs are well sprung. The topline is level and the abdomen moderately tucked up. The high set tail is carried over the back curled, and reaches the tarsus. They possess heavily boned and muscled straight limbs, and dewclaws are not generally removed from the forelimbs but from the hind limbs they are. Feet are small, compact and have well knuckled up toes. They move with a moderate stride.

Recognized Behavior Issues and Traits

Traits ascribed to this breed include: Adaptability and intelligence, requires close human companionship, friendly, loyal and docile. They are also described as intelligent, possessing high perseverance; an alert and a faithful companion. Will tend to show aggression towards other dogs so they are best kept solo unless socialized from puppyhood, and even then they may still assert themselves. Needs an experienced owner to perform successful obedience training due to their strong personalities. Dignified carriage, active, independent, aloof with strangers but tend to bark only when a threat is real. Akitas have a strong guarding instinct, and will capably defend home and family. Need plenty of mental stimulation to prevent boredom vices. They have a high shedding tendency. Should be supervised with children and pets, as they can attack members of their own family.

Normal Physiologic Variations

Akitas have a benign autosomal recessive inherited condition of high red blood cell potassium. A survey in Japan showed one-quarter to one-third of Akitas affected.[1,2]

Drug Sensitivities

None reported

Inherited Diseases

Hip Dysplasia: Polygenically inherited trait causing degenerative joint disease and hip arthritis. OFA reports 13.0% affected.[3]

Patella Luxation: Polygenically inherited laxity of patellar ligaments, causing luxation, lameness, and later degenerative joint disease. Treat surgically if causing clinical signs. OFA reports 1.5% affected. Dorn reports a 2.38x odds ratio for developing patella luxation versus other breeds. Another study reports a 6.7x odds ratio versus other breeds.[3,4,5]

Elbow Dysplasia: Polygenically inherited trait causing elbow arthritis. OFA reports 1.3% affected.[3]

Disease Predispositions

Hypothyroidism: Inherited autoimmune thyroiditis. 8.6% positive for thyroid auto-antibodies based on testing at Michigan State University. (Ave. for all breeds is 7.5%). Reported at a frequency of 18.6% in the 2001 ACA Health Survey.[6,7,8]

Gastric Dilation/Volvulus (GDV, Bloat): Life-threatening twisting of the stomach within the abdomen. Requires immediate veterinary attention. Glickman found a 1 in 5 lifetime risk of developing GDV in Akitas. Reported at a frequency of 12.2% in the 2001 ACA Health Survey.[6,9]

Allergic Dermatitis: Inhalant or food allergy. Presents with pruritis and pyotraumatic dermatitis (hot spots). Reported at a frequency of 10.1% in the 2001 ACA Health Survey.[6]

Cranial Cruciate Ligament Rupture (ACL): Traumatic tearing of the anterior cruciate ligament. The breed is found to be one with an increased incidence. Reported at a frequency of 6.6% in the 2001 ACA Health Survey. Treatment is surgery.[6,10]

Sebaceous Adenitis: Disorder of immune mediated sebaceous gland destruction, presenting with hair loss, hyperkeratosis and seborrhoea, usually beginning with the dorsal midline and ears. Diagnosis by skin biopsy. Treat with isotretinoin. An autosomal recessive mode of inheritance is suspected. Reported at a frequency of 3.4% in Sweden.[11,12,13]

Persistent Pupillary Membranes: Strands of fetal remnant connecting; iris to iris, cornea, lens, or involving sheets of tissue. The later three forms can impair vision, and dogs affected with these forms should not be bred. Identified in 2.91% of Akitas CERF examined by veterinary ophthalmologists between 2000-2005.[14]

Retinal Dysplasia: Retinal folds, geographic, and generalized retinal dysplasia with detachment are recognized in the breed. Reported in 1.95% of Akitas CERF examined by veterinary ophthalmologists between 2000-2005.[14]

Uveodermatologic (VKH-like) Syndrome: An autoimmune disease manifested by progressive uveitis and depigmenting dermatitis that closely resembles the human Vogt-Koyanagi-Harada syndrome. Onset 1-1/2 to 4 years of age. Treat with immunosuppressive drugs. One study showed that Akitas with the histocompatability DLA gene DQA1*00201 had a 15.99x odds ratio for developing the syndrome. CERF does not recommend breeding any affected dogs.[14,15,16,17]

Pemphigus Foliaceus: An increased risk of developing immune mediated pemphigus foliaceus was noted in the Akita (Odds ratio = 37.8x). Typical lesions include dorsal muzzle and head symmetric scaling, crusting, and alopecia with peripheral collarettes, characteristic footpad lesions, with erythematous swelling at the pad margins, cracking, and villous hypertrophy. Average age of onset is 4.2 years. Treatment with corticosteroid and cytotoxic medications. One-year survival rate of 53%. Unknown mode of inheritance.[18,19]

Acquired Myasthenia Gravis: Akitas are a breed at increased risk of developing generalized or focal acquired myasthenia gravis. The most common presenting signs were generalized weakness, with or without megaesophagus. Diagnosis is by identifying acetylcholine receptor antibodies.[20]

Juvenile-onset Polyarthritis: Inherited syndrome of cyclic febrile illness and signs of profound joint-related pain. Can also cause concurrent aseptic meningitis. Treatment with immunosuppressive drugs. Unknown mode of inheritance.[21]

Primary (Narrow Angle) Glaucoma: Ocular condition causing increased pressure within the eyeball, and secondary blindness due to damage to the retina. Diagnose with tonometry and gonioscopy. Diagnosed in 1.39% of Akitas presented to veterinary teaching hospitals.[22]

Entropion: Rolling in of eyelids, often causing corneal irritation or ulceration. Entropion is reported in 0.99% of Akitas CERF examined by veterinary ophthalmologists between 2000-2005.[14]

Cataracts: Anterior and posterior cortex punctate cataracts predominate, though posterior nuclear and capsular cataracts also occur in the breed. Identified in 0.85% of Akitas CERF examined by veterinary ophthalmologists between 2000-2005. CERF does not recommend breeding any Akitas with a cataract.[14]

Progressive Retinal Atrophy (PRA): Inherited degeneration of the retina. Onset 1.5 to 3 years of age, initially with night blindness that progresses to day blindness. Form of PRA, and mode of inheritance is not determined in this breed. Reported at a frequency of 0.5% in the 2001 ACA Health Survey. CERF does not recommend breeding any affected Akitas.[6,14, 23,24]

Brachygnathism, Central PRA, Deafness, Epilepsy, Glycogen Storage Disease III, IgA deficiency, Osteochondritis Dissicans (shoulder and stifle), Osteochondrodyplasia, Peripheral Vestibular Disease, Portosystemic Shunt, Prognathism, Renal Dysplasia, and **von Willebrand's Disease** are reported.[25]

Isolated Case Studies

Epidermolysis Bullosa: A 4-year-old female Akita had a 3-year-history of ulcers and scars over the pressure areas on the limbs, and dystrophic nails. The immune mediated disease epidermolysis bullosa was diagnosed based on biopsy, electron microscopy, and special staining.[29]

Multiple Congenital Ocular Defects: Microphthalmia, congenital cataracts, posterior lenticonus, and retinal dysplasia were observed in 6 puppies from 3 litters of Akitas thought to be related to a common male ancestor.[26]

Tracheobronchial Amyloidosis: An 11 year old intact male Akita dog with a chronic non-productive cough was diagnosed with primary diffuse tracheobronchial amyloidosis at necropsy.[27]

Cervical Spinal Arachnoid Cyst: An 18-month-old, intact male Akita presented with a 12-month history of progressive ataxia, hypermetria, and loss of conscious proprioception of all 4 limbs was diagnosed by myelography with an arachnoid cyst between the first two cervical vertebra. Surgery was curative.[28]

Genetic Tests

Tests of Genotype: Direct tests for color and mask alleles are available from VetGen.

Tests of Phenotype: CHIC Certification: Required testing includes hip radiographs, CERF eye examination (annually until year 6, then every other year), and thyroid profile including autoantibodies. Recommended tests include elbow radiographs, and patella evaluation. (See CHIC website; www.caninehealthinfo.org).

Recommend cardiac evaluation.

Miscellaneous

- **Breed name synonyms:** Akita Inu, Shishi Inu, Japanese Akita, Matagiinu (historical name for the breed in Japanese meaning esteemed dog hunter).
- **Registries:** AKC, UKC, CKC, KCGB (Kennel Club of Great Britain), ANKC (Australian National Kennel Club), NKC (National Kennel Club).
- **AKC rank (year 2008):** 52 (3,157 dogs registered)
- **Internet resources: Akita Club of America:** www.akitaclub.org
  Japanese Akita Club of America: www.the-jaca.org
  Akita Club of Canada: www.akitaclub.ca
  Japanese Akita-Inu Club (UK): www.japaneseakita-inu.co.uk

References

1. Fujise H, Higa K, Nakayama T, et. al.: Incidence of dogs possessing red blood cells with high K in Japan and East Asia. *J Vet Med Sci.* 1997 Jun;59(6):495-7

2. Degen M: Pseudohyperkalemia in Akitas. *J Am Vet Med Assoc.* 1987 Mar 1;190(5):541-3.

3. OFA Website breed statistics: www.offa.org Last accessed July 1, 2010.

4. Dorn CR: Canine breed-specific risks of frequently diagnosed diseases at veterinary teaching hospitals. Monograph. AKC Canine Health Foundation. 2000.

5. LaFond E, Breur GJ and Austin CC: Breed susceptibility for developmental orthopedic diseases in dogs. J Am Anim Hosp Assoc. 2002 Sep-Oct;38(5):467-77.

6. Glickman L, Glickman N, and Raghaven M: The Akita Club of America National Health Survey 2000-2001. 2001.

7. Nachreiner R and Refsal K: Personal communication, Diagnostic Center for Population and Animal Health, Michigan State University. April, 2007.

8. Nachreiner RF, Refsal KR, Graham PA, et. al.: Prevalence of serum thyroid hormone autoantibodies in dogs with clinical signs of hypothyroidism. *J Am Vet Med Assoc* 2002 Feb 15;220(4):466-71.

9. Glickman LT, Glickman NW, Schellenberg DB, et. al.: Incidence of and breed-related risk factors for gastric dilatation-volvulus in dogs. *J Am Vet Med Assoc.* 2000 Jan 1;216(1):40-5.

10. Duval JM, Budsberg SC, Flo GL, et. al.: Breed, sex, and body weight as risk factors for rupture of the cranial cruciate ligament in young dogs. *J Am Vet Med Assoc.* 1999 Sep 15;215(6):811-4.

11. Reichler IM, Hauser B, Schiller I, et. al.: Sebaceous adenitis in the Akita: clinical observations, histopathology and heredity. *Vet Dermatol.* 2001 Oct; 12(50:243-53.

12. White SD, Rosychuk RA, Scott KV, et. al.: Sebaceous adenitis in dogs and results of treatment with isotretinoin and etretinate: 30 cases (1990-1994). *J Am Vet Med Assoc.* 1995 Jul 15;207(2):197-200.

13. Hernblad Tevell E, Bergvall K, Egenvall A: Sebaceous adenitis in Swedish dogs, a retrospective study of 104 cases. Acta Vet Scand. 2008 May 25;50(1):11.

14. Ocular Disorders Presumed to be Inherited in Purebred Dogs. American College of Veterinary Ophthalmologists. ACVO, 2007

15. Angles JM, Famula TR, Pedersen NC, et. al.: Uveodermatologic (VKH-like) syndrome in American Akita dogs is associated with an increased frequency of DQA1*00201. *Tissue Antigens.* 2005 Dec;66(6):656-65.

16. Cottrell BD, Barnett KC: Harada disease in the Japanese Akita. J Small Anim Pract 1987;28:517.

17. Murphy CJ, Bellhorn RW: Anti-retinal antibodies associated with Vogt-Koyanagi-Harada-like syndrome in a dog. J Am Anim Hosp Assoc 1991;27:399.

18. Kuhl KA, Shofer FS, Goldschmidt MH: Comparative histopathology of pemphigus foliaceus and superficial folliculitis in the dog. *Vet Pathol.* 1994 Jan;31(1):19-27.

19. Ihrke PJ, Stannard AA, Ardans AA, et. al.: Pemphigus foliaceus in dogs: a review of 37 cases. *J Am Vet Med Assoc.* 1985 Jan 1;186(1):59-66.

20. Shelton GD, Schule A, Kass PH: Risk factors for acquired myasthenia gravis in dogs: 1,154 cases (1991-1995). *J Am Vet Med Assoc.*1997 Dec 1;211(11):1428-31.

21. Dougherty SA, Center SA, Shaw EE, et. al.: Juvenile-onset polyarthritis syndrome in Akitas. *J Am Vet Med Assoc.* 1991 Mar 1;198(5):849-56.

22. Gelatt KN, MacKay EO: Prevalence of the breed-related glaucomas in pure-bred dogs in North America. Vet Ophthalmol. 2004 Mar-Apr;7(2):97-111.

23. O Toole D, Roberts S: Generalized progressive retinal atrophy in two Akita dogs. *Vet Pathol.* 1984 Sep;21(5):457-62.
1997 Dec 1;211(11):1428-31.

24. Paulsen ME, Severin GA, Young S, et al: Progressive retinal atrophy in a colony of Akita dogs. Trans Am Col Vet Ophthalmol 1988;19:1-4.

25. *The Genetic Connection: A Guide to Health Problems in Purebred Dogs.* L Ackerman. p. 195. AAHA Press, 1999.

26. Laratta LJ, Riis RC, Kern TJ, et. al.: Multiple congenital ocular defects in the Akita dog. Cornell Vet. 1985 Jul;75(3):381-92.

27. Labelle P, Roy ME, Mohr FC: Primary diffuse tracheobronchial amyloidosis in a dog. J Comp Pathol. 2004 Nov;131(4):338-40.

28. Hashizume CT: Cervical spinal arachnoid cyst in a dog. Can Vet J. 2000 Mar;41(3):225-7.

29. Nagata M, Shimizu H, Masunaga T, et. al.: Dystrophic form of inherited epidermolysis bullosa in a dog (Akita Inu). *Br J Dermatol.* 1995 Dec;133(6):1000-3.

30. *The Complete Dog Book, 20th Ed.* The American Kennel Club. Howell Book House, NY 2006. P. 228-231.

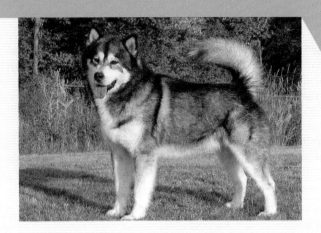

Alaskan Malamute

set high, thickly covered in hair and sits a plume over the topline. Limbs are heavily boned and well muscled, and not bowed. Gait is true and tireless, with long powerful stride and excellent agility. Neck is short, muscular, and has a moderate arch. Topline is straight but slopes down towards the rear of the dog. The feet are large and possess large thick pads, with plenty of hair between the toes. Toes are well arched, and compact. Dewclaws on the rear are removed.

The Breed History

The Malamute is one of the ancient Arctic Sled Dogs, and they are the Native sled dog of Alaska. Their name derives from the Innuit tribe/village (Mahlemuts) that kept them. The Samoyed and Siberian Husky of Russia are cousin breeds. First registration in AKC occurred in 1935. Within the breed are two types based on size and color. M'Loot are larger than the Kotzebue strain, and the Kotzebue consist of dogs with only wolf-gray coat color.

Breeding for Function

Hauling heavy sleds was their primary function. They are still popular as sled racing dogs, and as companion animals. Their forte is in pulling weight, not in their speed, but due to their stamina, they excel at long distance racing.

Physical Characteristics

Height at Withers: female 23" (58.5 cm), male 25" (63.5 cm).

Weight: females 75 lb (34 kg), males 85 lb (38.5 kg).

Coat: They blow their coats twice annually but are relatively low shedding during the rest of the year. They have low bathing and grooming needs since they tend to groom like a cat. They have a very dense double coat with a short (1-2" or 2.5-5 cm) dense wooly soft undercoat and very dense stand out coarse guard hairs in the outer coat that are straight. There are distinct face markings including a face of white or white with a bar or mask. Blue eyes disqualify except in red color dogs, where they are pigmented brown; the palpebral margins, lip margins and nose are black. Coats are commonly gray in different shades, black, red, and sable. All of these have points and markings in a prescribed pattern of a different color. The only solid dog allowed is a white one. Usually most of the underside and the lower limbs of the dog are white.

Longevity: 12 years.

Points of Conformation: The dog is compact, very muscular, with high alert head carriage and possesses a deep thorax (1/2 the height of the dog) with well-sprung ribs. Head is broad, small triangular ears are held erect or pricked up when alert and they are set well back on the skull. Sometimes while running the ears are seen folded back and down. Medium-sized eyes are almond shaped, and dark brown in color. The muzzle gradually tapers. Their tail is

Recognized Behavior Issues and Traits

Terms used to describe this Breed include: active, friendly, and good with children. Also they are loyal, but may fight with other dogs unless socialized, may be strong on the leash, and early obedience training is important since these dogs can be a bit stubborn and are easily bored.

They need a lot of exercise and mental stimulation. They will enjoy gentle children, though early socialization to children is recommended. Other traits include needing lots of human contact, and not considered a good watchdog. They may dig so it is advised to bury fence below grade and make it high (6') and sturdy.

They have low barking tendency but are very vocal with talking noises and may howl.

Tolerate heat OK if given shade and cool water.

Normal Breed Variations

The Alaskan Malamute is a breed with a predisposition to higher eosinophil counts or certain eosinophilic diseases. Two of the more common disease causes of canine hypereosinophilia are pulmonary infiltrates with eosinophils (PIE) and gastrointestinal disease.[1]

If they have snow nose (pink pigment on black nose), they are more prone to skin cancer and sunburn in the low pigment area. Snow nose may disappear in the summer.

Drug Sensitivities

None reported

Inherited Diseases

Hip Dysplasia: Polygenically inherited trait causing degenerative joint disease and hip arthritis. OFA reports 11.5% affected.[2]

Elbow Dysplasia: Polygenically inherited trait causing elbow arthritis. OFA reports 3.2% affected.[2]

Chondrodysplasia with Stomatocytosis (also referred to as Dwarfism or CHD): Autosomal recessive disorder, causing short-limbed dwarfism and hemolytic anemia. Chondrodysplasia Certification Registry of AMCA – examines a 5 generation pedigree – to check for all test-bred normal ancestors.[3,4]

Polyneuropathy: Two forms are reported in the breed. It is unknown if they are related to each other genetically. Hereditary polyneuropathy is an autosomal recessive disorder with an age of onset between 7-18 months of age. It causes progressive posterior ataxia, exercise intolerance, megaesophagus, atrophy of shoulder and thigh muscles, and hyporeflexia. Another form, idiopathic polyneuropathy, causes a distal sensorimotor polyneuropathy in young mature dogs. Mode of inheritance has not been determined. Clinical signs included progressive paraparesis, synchronous pelvic limb gait, exercise intolerance, hyperesthesia, hyporeflexia, muscle atrophy, and tetraplegia. Diagnosis and differentiation between these two disorders is based on electromyography or peripheral nerve biopsy.[5,6]

Cone degeneration (CD): A rare, autosomal recessive condition, causing day blindness. Onset approximately 8 weeks of age. Caused by a mutation in the CNGB3 gene. Affected dogs should not be bred. A direct genetic test is available.[7,8,9,10]

Patella Luxation: Polygenically inherited laxity of patellar ligaments, causing luxation, lameness, and later degenerative joint disease. Treat surgically if causing clinical signs. Too few Alaskan Malamutes have been screened by OFA to determine an accurate frequency.[2]

Disease Predispositions

Hypothyroidism: Inherited autoimmune thyroiditis. 11.1% positive for thyroid auto-antibodies based on testing at Michigan State University. (Ave. for all breeds is 7.5%).[11,12]

Persistent Pupillary Membranes: Strands of fetal remnant connecting; iris to iris, cornea, lens, or involving sheets of tissue. The later three forms can impair vision, and dogs affected with these forms should not be bred. Identified in 8.03% of Alaskan Malamutes CERF examined by veterinary ophthalmologists between 2000-2005.[9]

Posterior Subcapsular Cataracts: Onset around one year of age. Slowly progressive; rarely leading to blindness. CERF does not recommend breeding any Alaskan Malamute with a cataract. Identified in 7.56% of Alaskan Malamutes CERF examined by veterinary ophthalmologists between 2000-2005.[9]

Distichiasis: Abnormally placed eyelashes that irritate the cornea and conjunctiva. Can cause secondary corneal ulceration. Identified in 2.05% of Alaskan Malamutes CERF examined by veterinary ophthalmologists between 2000-2005.[9]

Retinal Dysplasia: Focal folds and geographic retinal dysplasia are seen in the breed. It is questionable whether focal folds can lead to disease, however dogs with the geographic form should not be bred. Identified in 1.17% of Alaskan Malamutes CERF examined by veterinary ophthalmologists between 2000-2005.[9]

Alopecia-X (Coat Funk): Progressive, symmetrical, non-pruritic truncal hair loss usually beginning in early adulthood. ACTH, LDDS, and thyroid panel results are normal. Elevated blood concentrations of 17-hydroxyprogesterone (17-OHP) have been seen post ACTH stimulation. Oral trilostane reversed the condition in some cases. The disorder appears familial.[13]

Glaucoma: An elevation of intraocular pressure (IOP) which, when sustained, causes intraocular damage resulting in blindness. Diagnose with tonometry and gonioscopy. CERF does not recommend breeding any Alaskan Malamute with glaucoma.[9]

Lipid Corneal Stromal Dystrophy: A non-inflammatory corneal opacity (white to gray) present in one or more of the corneal layers; usually inherited and bilateral. Identified in 1.03% of Alaskan Malamutes CERF examined by veterinary ophthalmologists between 2000-2005.[9,14]

Canine Zinc-Responsive Dermatosis: Familial form identified in the breed, characterized by erythema, alopecia, scales, and crusts that primarily affect the head. Diagnosed by skin biopsy. Life-long zinc supplementation is usually necessary.[15]

Isolated Case Studies

Osteochondromatosis (Multiple Cartilaginous Exostoses): Several case reports of young dogs with cervical pain, paresis, and or proprioceptive deficits. Focal lesions may be corrected surgically.[16,17]

Juvenile Nephropathy: Multiple case reports. Kidney disorder identified in 3 littermates. Presented in renal failure between 4-11 months of age.[18,19]

Factor IX Deficiency (Hemophilia B): Identified in a 6 month-old dog with a two week history of bleeding from an oral wound. Factor IX activity was only 1.3% of normal. **Factor VII deficiency** has also been reported in the breed.[20,21]

Myelodysplasia: Case study of weakness of all 4 limbs in an adult dog. No CT or myelographic abnormalities, but diffuse spinal cord myelodysplasia and edema found on necropsy.[22]

Paraoesophageal Hiatal Hernia and Megaoesophagus: Report on a 3 week old dog with regurgitation. An oesophagopexy and a bilateral gastropexy were performed, and the dog gained weight normally.[23]

Maxillary Ameloblastic Carcinoma: A 3-year-old female Alaskan Malamute with a painful, ulcerated mass of the right maxilla was diagnosed with ameloblastic carcinoma. Histologic examination showed a neoplastic proliferation of palisading cells distributed irregularly in cords. The dog was alive 2 years after hemi-maxillec-tomy.[24]

Cryptorchidism, Cutaneous Lupus Erythematosus, Diabetes Mellitus, Epilepsy, Gastric Dilatation-Volvulus, Hemivertebra, Keratoconjunctivitis Sicca, Macrocytosis/stomatocytosis, Muscular Dystrophy, Narcolepsy, OCD-shoulder, Optic nerve hypoplasia, Panosteitis, Patella luxation, Portosystemic shunt, Progressive retinal atrophy, Pulmonic stenosis, Retained teeth, Ulcerative keratitis, Uveal hypopigmentation, Uveodermato-logic syndrome, Ventricular septal defect, and **von Willebrand's disease** are reported.[25]

Genetic Tests

Tests of Genotype: Direct test for color alleles is available from VetGen.

Direct test for CD is available from Optigen.

Tests of Phenotype: CHIC Certification: Required tests are; hip radiograph and CERF eye examination. Optional recommended testing; thyroid profile including auto-antibodies. (See CHIC website: www.caninehealthinfo.org)

Also recommend elbow radiographs, patella evaluation and cardiac evaluation.

Miscellaneous

- **Breed name synonyms:** Malamute, Alaskan Malemute, Malemute
- **Registries:** AKC, UKC, CKC, KCGB (Kennel Club of Great Britain), ANKC (Australian National Kennel Club), NKC (National Kennel Club).
- **AKC rank (year 2008):** 57 (1,737 registered)
- **Internet resources: Alaskan Malamute Club of America Inc.:**
  www.alaskanmalamute.org
  Alaskan Malamute Research Foundation:
  www.malamutehealth.org
  Alaskan Malamute Club of Canada:
  www.quadrant.net/amcc/
  Alaskan Malamute Club of the UK:
  www.alaskanmalamute.org.uk

References

1. Lilliehook I, Tvedten H: Investigation of hypereosinophilia and potential treatments. *Vet Clin North Am Small Anim Pract.* 2003 Nov; 33(6):1359-78, viii
2. OFA Website breed statistics: www.offa.org Last accessed July 1, 2010.
3. Fletch SM, Smart ME, Pennock PW, Subden RE. Clinical and pathologic features of chondrodysplasia (dwarfism) in the Alaskan Malamute. J Am Vet Med Assoc. 1973 Mar 1;162(5):357-61.
4. Subden, RE, Fletch, SM, Smart, MA, et. al.: Genetics of the Alaskan Malamute chondrodysplasia syndrome. Journal of Heredity. 1972:63: 149-152.
5. Braund KG, Shores A, Lowrie CT, Steinberg HS, Moore MP, Bagley RS, Steiss JE. Idiopathic polyneuropathy in Alaskan malamutes. J Vet Intern Med. 1997 Jul-Aug;11(4):243-9.
6. Moe L: Hereditary polyneuropathy of Alaskan malamutes. In: Kirk RW, Bonagura JD (eds). Current Veterinary Therapy XI Small Animal Practice. W.B. Saunders, Philadelphia, PA 1992:1038-1039.
7. Sidjanin DJ, Lowe JK, McElwee JL, Milne BS, Phippen TM, Sargan DR, Aguirre GD, Acland GM, Ostrander EA. Canine CNGB3 mutations establish cone degeneration as orthologous to the human achromatopsia locus ACHM3. Hum Mol Genet. 2002 Aug 1;11(16):1823-33.
8. Rubin, L., Bourns, T.K.R. and Lord, L.H. Hemeralopia in Dogs: Heredity of Hemeralopia in Alaskan Malamutes. American Journal of Veterinary Research, Mar. 1967, pp. 355-357.
9. *Ocular Disorders Presumed to be Inherited in Purebred Dogs.* American College of Veterinary Ophthalmologists. ACVO, 2007
10. Seddon JM, Hampson EC, Smith RI, et. al.: Genetic heterogeneity of day blindness in Alaskan Malamutes. Anim Genet. 2006 Aug;37(4):407-10.
11. Nachreiner R and Refsal K: Personal communication, Diagnostic Center for Population and Animal Health, Michigan State University. April, 2007.
12. Nachreiner RF, Refsal KR, Graham PA, et. al.: Prevalence of serum thyroid hormone autoantibodies in dogs with clinical signs of hypothyroidism. *J Am Vet Med Assoc* 2002 Feb 15;220(4):466-71.
13. Leone F, Cerundolo R, Vercelli A, Lloyd DH: The use of Trilostane for the treatment of Alopecia X in Alaskan Malamutes. *J Am Anim Hosp Assoc.* 2005;41:336-342.
14. Brooks, D. Nonulcerative Keratopathy and Inflammatory Keratitis. Proceedings, Western Veterinary Conference 2002.
15. Colombini, S. Canine zinc-responsive dermatosis. Vet Clin North Am Small Anim Pract 29[6]:1373-83 1999 Nov.
16. Beck JA, Simpson DJ, Tisdall PL. Surgical management of osteochondro-matosis affecting the vertebrae and trachea in an Alaskan Malamute. Aust Vet J. 1999 Jan;77(1):21-3.
17. Caporn TM ; Read RA. Osteochondromatosis of the cervical spine causing compressive myelopathy in a dog. J Small Anim Pract 37[3]:133-7 1996 Mar
18. Vilafranca M ; Ferrer L. Juvenile nephropathy in Alaskan Malamute littermates. Vet Pathol 31[3]:375-7 1994 May
19. Burk RL, Barton CL. Renal failure and hyperparathyroidism in an Alaskan Malamute pup. J Am Vet Med Assoc. 1978 Jan 1;172(1):69-72.
20. Mills JN ; Labuc RH ; Lawley MJ. Factor VII deficiency in an Alaskan malamute. Aust Vet J 75[5]:320-2 1997 May
21. Peterson ME, Dodds WJ. Factor IX deficiency in an Alaskan Malamute. J Am Vet Med Assoc. 1979 Jun 15;174(12):1326-7.
22. Rishniw, M, Wilkerson, MJ, de Lahunta, A. Myelodysplasia in an Alaskan Malamute Dog With Adult Onset of Clinical Signs. Prog Vet Neurol 5[1]:35-38 Spring'94.
23. Kirkby KA, Bright RM, Owen HD: Paraoesophageal hiatal hernia and megaoesophagus in a three-week-old Alaskan malamute. *J Small Anim Pract.* 2005 Aug;46(8):402-5.
24. Jimenez MA, Castejon A, San Roman F, et. al.: Maxillary ameloblastic carcinoma in an Alaskan Malamute. Vet Pathol. 2007 Jan;44(1):84-7.
25. *The Genetic Connection: A Guide to health Problems in Purebred Dogs.* L Ackerman. P. 195-96. AAHA Press.1999.
26. *The Complete Dog Book, 20th Ed.* The American Kennel Club. Howell Book House, NY 2006. P. 232-236.

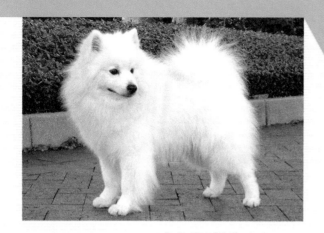

The Breed History

The Spitz family (Nordic type) of dogs includes the American Eskimo Dog, and also the white Keeshond, German Spitz, white Pomeranian, Japanese Spitz, and white Italian Spitz. Some of these other breeds may have contributed to the gene pool of the American Eskimo Dog breed. Early on in America, the breed was referred to as American Spitz. It was in 1995 that the AKC accepted the breed into the registry. The name change to "Eskimo" was done to reflect the Northern origins of the dogs.

Breeding for Function

In the late 19th century in North America they were popular as circus trick dogs. Currently, their primary purpose is as a companion dog.

Physical Characteristics

Toy
Height at Withers: 9-12" (23-30.5 cm)
Weight: 6-10 pounds (2.4-4.5kg)

Miniature
Height at Withers: 12-15" (30.5-38 cm)
Weight: 10-20 pounds (4.5-9kg)

Standard
Height at Withers: 15-19" (38-48 cm)
Weight: 18-35 pounds (8kg-16kg)

UKC recognizes 2 size categories Miniature (males 12-15", females 11-14") Standard (males 15-19", females 14-18")

Coat: Their lip margins, palpebral margins and nose are always black and the double, dense coat is always white or white with biscuit cream tones. The undercoat is dense, short and wooly, the outer coat guard hairs grow straight out through the undercoat and are hard and straight. Breeches and a well-developed ruff are present, particularly in the males. The muzzle hair is short, and the backs of the legs are well feathered.

Longevity: 11-15 years

Points of Conformation: Alert, smooth and quick in action, they possess a compact build; their excellent balance and agility has been carefully selected for. They possess a typical Spitz head with alert, pricked small triangular ears with blunt tips, and ears are thickly covered in fur. The tail is carried over the back and has a well-developed plume. The stop is well defined, the skull is fairly flat and the muzzle is only slightly tapering. The neck is medium in length, and the head is carried high. The topline is level, the thorax is deep with well-sprung ribs, and there is a mild abdominal tuck up. The tail may be dropped off the back at rest in which case it reaches to the level of the tarsus. Dewclaw removal is optional. Feet are compact, toes are well arched, and they have thick hair growth around the toes. The nails are white. Limbs are straight boned with moderate muscling. The eyes are oval and wide-set; a dark brown color is preferred. Note that some tear staining is normal for many dogs.

Recognized Behavior Issues and Traits

Reported breed characteristics include: Agile, very high trainability, affectionate and they like to please. A good alarm barker with high barking tendency, some have tendency to excessive barking. They need close human contact. Early socialization is important so that they are not overly aloof with strangers. Need mental stimulation or will develop boredom vices. Eskie dogs have moderate exercise needs. They do well with other pets if socialized to them early. They have moderate grooming needs. If nervous, they have a tendency to bite.

Normal Physiologic Variations

None reported

Drug Sensitivities

None reported

Inherited Diseases

Progressive Retinal Atrophy (PRA): Autosomal recessive progressive rod cone degeneration (prcd) form. Age of onset is between 3-8 years of age, eventually causing blindness. Optigen testing reports 13% affected, and 57% carriers in American Eskimo Dogs.[1,2,3]

Hip Dysplasia and Legg-Calve Perthes Disease: Polygenically inherited traits causing degenerative hip joint disease and arthritis. OFA reports 9.1% of tested American Eskimo Dogs are affected with hip dysplasia and 2.7% are affected with Legg-Calve Perthes.[4]

Patella Luxation: Polygenically inherited laxity of patellar ligaments, causing luxation, lameness, and later degenerative joint disease. Treat surgically if causing clinical signs. OFA reports 5.4% affected.[4]

Deafness: Congenital deafness can be unilateral or bilateral. Diagnosed by BAER testing.[5]

Elbow Dysplasia: Polygenically inherited trait causing elbow arthritis. OFA reports 0.9% affected.[4]

Pyruvate Kinase Deficiency: Autosomal recessive disorder causing severe hemolytic anemia, progressive osteomyelosclerosis, and hemosiderosis. Death occurs due to anemia or hepatic failure usually at less than 5 years of age. Occurs at a low frequency in the breed. A genetic mutation test is available.[6]

Disease Predispositions

Hypothyroidism: Inherited autoimmune thyroiditis. 7.8% positive for thyroid auto-antibodies based on testing at Michigan State University. (Ave. for all breeds is 7.5%).[7,8]

Hypoadrenocorticism (Addison's Disease): Immune mediated destruction of the adrenal gland. Typical presentation of lethargy, poor appetite, vomiting, weakness, and dehydration can occur from 4 months to several years of age. Treatment with DOCA injections or oral fludrocortisone. Dorn reports a 52.81x odds ratio of developing Addison's disease versus other breeds.[9]

Idiopathic Epilepsy (Inherited Seizures): Control with anti-seizure medication. Dorn reports an 8.75x odds ratio of developing epilepsy versus other breeds.[9]

Cataracts: Anterior cortex cataracts predominate, though posterior intermediate and punctate cataracts also occur in the breed. Unknown mode of inheritance. Identified in 3.56% of American Eskimo Dogs CERF examined by veterinary ophthalmologists between 2000-2005. CERF does not recommend breeding any American Eskimo Dog with a cataract.[1]

Kidney Disease: Dorn reports an 8.28x odds ratio of developing kidney disease versus other breeds. A specific type of kidney disease is not specified. The only reported kidney disease in the breed is a case report of Hereditary Nephropathy (see below).[9]

Alopecia (Endocrine or Hormonal Alopecia): Progressive, symmetrical, non-pruritic, truncal hair loss usually beginning in early adulthood. ACTH, LDDS, and thyroid panel results are normal. Elevated blood concentrations of 17-hydroxyprogesterone (17-OHP) have been seen post ACTH stimulation. Oral trilostane reverses the condition in some cases. The disorder appears familial.[10]

Degenerative Myelopathy (DM): Affected dogs show an insidious onset of upper motor neuron (UMN) paraparesis. The disease eventually progresses to severe tetraparesis. Affected dogs have normal results on myelography, MRI, and CSF analysis. Necropsy confirms the condition. Unknown mode of inheritance. A direct genetic test for an autosomal recessive DM susceptibility gene is available. All affected dogs are homozygous for the gene, however only a small percentage of homozygous dogs develop DM. A genetic test for the susceptibility gene is available.[4,14]

Anasarca, Cryptorchidism, Hemivertebra, Laryngeal Paralysis, Megaesophagus, Methemoglobin Reductase Deficiency, Narcolepsy, Patent Ductus Arteriosus, Prognathism, Sebaceous Adenitis, and **Zinc-Responsive Dermatosis** are reported.[11]

Isolated Case Studies

Hereditary Nephropathy (HN): A 15 month old female American Eskimo Dog from a father-daughter mating was diagnosed with hereditary nephropathy. The clinical and pathologic features of the renal disease identified in the affected dog resembled those of autosomal recessive HN.[12]

Genetic Tests

Tests of Genotype: Direct test for prcd-PRA is available from Optigen.

Direct test for pyruvate kinase deficiency is available from PennGen.

Direct test for a DM susceptability gene is available from the OFA.

Tests of Phenotype: CHIC Certification: Required testing includes hip radiographs, CERF eye examination at a minimum of 2 years of age, and an Optigen prcd-PRA test. Optional testing includes a congenital cardiac evaluation, elbow radiographs, patella evaluation, and a thyroid profile including autoantibodies. (See CHIC website; www.caninehealthinfo.org).

Miscellaneous

- **Breed name synonyms:** Eskie, Spitz, Toy American Eskimo, Miniature American Eskimo, Standard American Eskimo.
- **Registries:** AKC, UKC, NKC (National Kennel Club).
- **AKC rank (year 2008):** 108 (384 dogs registered)
- **Internet resources: American Eskimo Dog Club of America:** www.aedca.org
  The National American Eskimo Dog Association: www.americaneskimo.com/NAEDA/
  The National American Eskimo Dog Association of Canada: www.naedac.ca

References

1. Ocular Disorders Presumed to be Inherited in Purebred Dogs. American College of Veterinary Ophthalmologists. ACVO, 2007
2. Morris Animal Foundation: Morris Animal Foundation Update: Genetic Tests Focus on Breed-Specific Vision Problems. Canine Pract 1999:24[4]:21.
3. Moody JA, Famula TR, et al. Identification of microsatellite markers linked to progressive retinal atrophy in American Eskimo Dogs. AJVR 2005:66(11):1900-1902.
4. OFA Website breed statistics: www.offa.org Last accessed July 1, 2010.
5. Strain GM: Deafness prevalence and pigmentation and gender associations in dog breeds at risk. Vet J. 2004 Jan;167(1):23
6. Giger U: Regenerative anemias caused by blood loss or hemolysis. In: Ettinger, SJ and Feldman EC. (eds.) Textbook of Veterinary Internal Medicine W. B. Saunders, Philadelphia, pp.1784-1804. 2000.
7. Nachreiner R and Refsal K: Personal communication, Diagnostic Center for Population and Animal Health, Michigan State University. April, 2007.
8. Nachreiner RF, Refsal KR, Graham PA, et. al.: Prevalence of serum thyroid hormone autoantibodies in dogs with clinical signs of hypothyroidism. J Am Vet Med Assoc 2002 Feb 15;220(4):466-71.
9. Dorn CR: Canine breed-specific risks of frequently diagnosed diseases at veterinary teaching hospitals. Monograph. AKC Canine Health Foundation. 2000.
10. Chastain CB: Sex Hormone Concentrations in Dogs with Alopecia. Sm Anim Clin Endocrinol 2004:14[1]:37-38.
11. The Genetic Connection: A Guide to Health Problems in Purebred Dogs. L Ackerman. p. 196. AAHA Press, 1999.
12. Lees GE: Update: Inherited Primary Glomerular Diseases in Dogs. Proceedings ACVIM Forum, 2003
13. The Complete Dog Book, 20th Ed. The American Kennel Club. Howell Book House, NY 2006. p. 525-528.
14. Awano T, Johnson GS, Wade CM, et. al.: Genome-wide association analysis reveals a SOD1 mutation in canine degenerative myelopathy that resembles amyotrophic lateral sclerosis. Proc Natl Acad Sci U S A. 2009 Feb 24;106(8):2794-9.

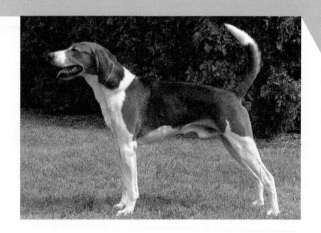

American Foxhound

narrower than the English type, ribs are well sprung and rib cage extends well back. The back is long and level though slightly arched. The limbs are straight, feet are compact with well-arched toes. The tail is carried gaily and curved, with a slight brush at the tip.

The Breed History

Various importations of English Foxhounds took place in the 1700s and these formed the basis for breeding programs in America that gradually changed the original foxhound type to a smaller, finer hound than the English counterpart. Further importations from throughout the British Isles and France occurred during the 1800s, including the importation of English dogs crossed with a Tennessee dog to produce the Walker hound strain.

The Irish imports gave rise to the Trigg and Henry-Birdsong strains. There are a handful of other strains that developed in different regions. Most foxhounds are registered with the International Foxhunter Studbook as opposed to AKC and other breed registries.

Breeding for Function

Over the years, four different hound subtypes were bred to account for differences in their functions in the hunt.

1. Drag hounds that are raced on a drag scent where speed is the sole winning factor
2. Field trial hounds where speed and competitiveness are essential.
3. Fox hunters that work with an on-foot hunter with gun.
4. Pack hounds; the traditional hunt club function.

Even today, only rarely are these dogs kept for companionship or for show purposes.

Physical Characteristics

Height at Withers: female 21-24" (53-61 cm), male 22-25" (56-63.5 cm)

Weight: 65-75 lb (30-34 kg) in the standard, but some are smaller.

Coat: Hard, medium length coat lays flat and any color is accepted. Tricolors (white, tan and black) are the most common.

Longevity: 11-14 years.

Points of Conformation: These dogs typify a dog of moderate proportions. The skull is long and slightly domed, ears are set moderately low, and are long and pendulous with fine leather, and have rounded tips. Wide set eyes are large and brown or hazel in color. The muzzle is square, and a moderate stop is present. The neck is medium in length and not throaty. Thorax is deep and

Recognized Behavior Issues and Traits

Reported breed attributes include: Friendly disposition, very active, low grooming needs. They are not suitable for guarding or watchdog. May run off, so should only be off leash in a fenced enclosure. Gets along well with other dogs and as pets, they are amicable. Good with children and around the house as long as they are raised as house pets; not kenneled.

Not considered an apartment dog. They have high exercise requirements. One needs to start obedience training early because of possible independent streaks.

Normal Physiologic Variations

Pelger-Huet Anomaly: Autosomal recessive inherited blood anomaly causing neutrophils with round, oval, or bean-shaped nuclei and only rare segmented nuclei. No obvious effects of disease seen in affected dogs.[1]

Drug Sensitivities

None reported

Inherited Diseases

Hip Dysplasia: Polygenically inherited trait causing degenerative joint disease and hip arthritis. Too few American Foxhounds have been screened by OFA to determine an accurate frequency.[2]

Elbow Dysplasia: Polygenically inherited trait causing elbow arthritis. Too few American Foxhounds have been screened by OFA to determine an accurate frequency.[2]

Patella Luxation: Polygenically inherited laxity of patellar ligaments, causing luxation, lameness, and later degenerative joint disease. Treat surgically if causing clinical signs. Too few American Foxhounds have been screened by OFA to determine an accurate frequency.[2]

Disease Predispositions

Hypothyroidism: Inherited autoimmune thyroiditis. 9.3% positive for thyroid auto-antibodies based on testing at Michigan State University. (Ave. for all breeds is 7.5%).[3,4]

Leishmaniasis: This infectious disease is primarily only diagnosed in Foxhounds. Research suggests vertical transmission (mother to offspring), though a genetic susceptibility cannot be ruled out.[5,6,7,8]

Deafness: Congenital deafness can be unilateral or bilateral. Diagnosed by BAER testing.[9,10]

Ocular Disorders: Too few American Foxhounds have been CERF examined to determine the frequency of ocular disorders in the breed.[11]

Cricopharyngeal dysphagia, Cryptorchidism, Hound ataxia, and **Thrombopathia** are reported.[12]

Isolated Case Studies
None reported

Genetic Tests
Tests of Genotype: Direct tests for coat color alleles are available from VetGen.

Tests of Phenotype: Recommend hip and elbow radiographs, thyroid profile including autoantibodies, CERF eye examination, patella evaluation and cardiac evaluation

Miscellaneous
- **Breed name synonyms:** Foxhound
- **Registries:** AKC, UKC, CKC, KCGB (Kennel Club of Great Britain), NKC (National Kennel Club)
- **AKC rank (year 2008):** 158 (17 dogs registered)
- **Internet resources: American Foxhound Club Inc.:** www.americanfoxhoundclub.com
  Masters of Foxhounds Association of America: www.mfha.com
  The Foxhound Club of North America: http://fcna.org

References
1. Bowles CA, Alsaker RD, Wolfle TL: Studies of the Pelger-Huet anomaly in foxhounds. *Am J Pathol.* 1979 Jul;96(1):237-47.
2. OFA Website breed statistics: www.offa.org Last accessed July 1, 2010.
3. Nachreiner R and Refsal K: Personal communication, Diagnostic Center for Population and Animal Health, Michigan State University. April, 2007.
4. Nachreiner RF, Refsal KR, Graham PA, et. al.: Prevalence of serum thyroid hormone autoantibodies in dogs with clinical signs of hypothyroidism. J Am Vet Med Assoc 2002 Feb 15;220(4):466-71.
5. Rosypal AC, Troy GC, Zajac AM, et. al.: Emergence of zoonotic canine leishmaniasis in the United States: isolation and immunohistochemical detection of Leishmania infantum from foxhounds from Virginia. *J Eukaryot Microbiol.* 2003;50 Suppl:691-3.
6. Gaskin AA, Schantz P, Jackson J, et. al.: Visceral leishmaniasis in a New York foxhound kennel. *J Vet Intern Med.* 2002 Jan-Feb;16(1):34-44.
7. Grosjean NL, Vrable RA, Murphy AJ, et. al.: Seroprevalence of antibodies against Leishmania spp among dogs in the United States. *J Am Vet Med Assoc.* 2003 Mar 1;222(5):603-6.
8. Petersen CA: New means of canine leishmaniasis transmission in north america: the possibility of transmission to humans still unknown. Interdiscip Perspect Infect Dis. 2009;2009:802712
9. Hiraide F, Paparella MM: Histopathology of the temporal bones of deaf dogs. *Auris Nasus Larynx.* 1988;15(2):97-104.
10. Adams EW: Hereditary deafness in a family of foxhounds. *J Am Vet Med Assoc.* 1956 Mar 15;128(6):302-3.
11. *Ocular Disorders Presumed to be Inherited in Purebred Dogs.* American College of Veterinary Ophthalmologists. ACVO, 2007
12. *The Genetic Connection: A Guide to Health Problems in Purebred Dogs.* L Ackerman. p. 218. AAHA Press, 1999.
13. *The Complete Dog Book, 20th Ed.* The American Kennel Club. Howell Book House, NY 2006. p. 170-172.

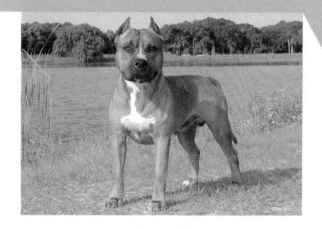

American Staffordshire Terrier

The Breed History

The powerful Greek Mollossian dogs gave rise to the Mastiff strain of dogs. Early Mastiff lines were used to produce fighting dogs. The very early original English Bulldog-type was similar to the modern American Staffordshire Terrier and the Staffordshire Bull Terrier, though the Staffordshire muzzles are longer. It is thought that the English Staffordshire Bull Terrier resulted from a bulldog crossed with Fox Terrier, extinct English White Terrier and/or Manchester terrier.

First AKC registry occurred in 1936, but the American breed had changed in stature (heavier and taller than English version) and those larger dogs were now called American Staffordshire Terrier instead of Staffordshire Bull Terrier. The increased size may have resulted from outcrosses in those lines. There is considerable confusion regarding the American Pit Bull Terrier (American Pit Bull, Pit Bull Terrier) and this breed, the American Staffordshire Terrier. Some registries separate them (such as the UKC); others such as the AKC do not. In stature, the Pit Bull is generally heavier (10-30 lb) and taller (2") than the American Staffordshire Terrier, though since overall body type and temperament are very close, they can be considered a size variant. Those that separate out the Pit Bull point out that additional fighting bulldog outcrosses may have occurred in those lines, and the Pit Bull is not the older, original breed developed for bull baiting as was the Staffordshire, but a fighter dog of more recent origin developed in the US. Facial features vary slightly between Pit Bull and Staffordshire.

Breeding for Function

Hallmark characteristics for the breed fully reflect his original function as a fighting dog and bull baiter, and include exceptional courage, aggressiveness, lightning quickness and agility, remarkable strength, a very strong tenacious bite and powerful head and jaws with a muscular neck to back it up. In America, the breed was helpful around the farm as hunter and guard dog. In recent years, increased companionability has been stressed in breeding programs.

Physical Characteristics

Height at Withers: female 17-18" (43-45.5 cm), male 18-19" (45.5-48 cm).

Weight: 40-50 lb (18-23 kg).

Coat: The short glossy hard coat lays flat and any color or parti-colored is permitted. All-white or all black-and-tan are not favored.

Longevity: 12 years.

Points of Conformation: A stocky, very muscular dog, the head is deep and broad, with a massive masseter muscle bulge. The high set small ears may be held half prick or lightly folded back (rose). They possess a distinct stop. In America, the ears are often cropped to prick up. Round, small, deep-set eyes are low down on the skull, and they have a dark iris and palpebral margins. The nose is black. The muscular heavy-set neck is slightly arched, not throaty. The thorax is broad and deep, and the rib cage stays deep. The topline slopes gradually towards the rear. The powerful tail is short, tapers, and is low set. Limbs are straight-boned, feet are well knuckled, compact and moderate in size. The gait is springy, but moderate in reach.

Recognized Behavior Issues and Traits

Reported breed attributes include: Intelligent, adaptable, and with training, are usually suitable with other dogs. Most have gentle temperaments expressed towards their owners if handled properly and given appropriate obedience training. Children should never tease them and they should not be left alone with children. They should be leashed or exercised in enclosures. Owners should not encourage the defensive or offensive aspect of the dog's temperament. When they bite they hold fast with great crushing power. Small pets and cats should not be raised with this type of dog where possible because of the strong terrier chase and prey instinct. They make good watchdogs. They have low grooming needs and low shedding tendency. They tend to dig if bored. They may snore.

Normal Physiologic Variations

None reported

Drug Sensitivities

None reported

Inherited Diseases

Hip Dysplasia: Polygenically inherited trait causing degenerative joint disease and hip arthritis. OFA reports 25.7% affected.[1]

Elbow Dysplasia: Polygenically inherited trait causing elbow arthritis. OFA reports 18.0% affected.[1]

Patella Luxation: Polygenically inherited laxity of patellar ligaments, causing luxation, lameness, and later degenerative joint disease. Treat surgically if causing clinical signs. OFA reports 1.2% affected.[1]

Cerebellar Cortical Degeneration/Neuronal Ceroid Lipofuscinosis (Ataxia, NCL-A): Autosomal recessive disorder causing hypermetria, a high stepping gait, and incoordination. Onset of clinical signs is usually between 4 to 6 years of age (range of 8 months to 9 years), with the majority of affected dogs surviving from 2 to 4 years. Affected dogs identified world-wide. A direct genetic test is available.[2,3,4,5]

Hyperuricosuria (HUU)/Urate Bladder Stones: An autosomal recessive mutation in the SLC2A9 gene causes urate urolithiasis and can predispose male dogs to urinary obstruction. Estimated at a carrier frequency of 3.17% in the breed. A genetic test is available.[17]

Disease Predispositions

Hypothyroidism: Inherited autoimmune thyroiditis. 14.6% positive for thyroid auto-antibodies based on testing at Michigan State University. (Ave. for all breeds is 7.5%).[6,7]

Distichiasis: Abnormally placed eyelashes that irritate the cornea and conjunctiva. Can cause secondary corneal ulceration. Identified in 5.52% of American Staffordshire Terriers CERF examined by veterinary ophthalmologists between 2000-2005.[8]

Persistent Pupillary Membranes: Strands of fetal remnant connecting; iris to iris, cornea, lens, or involving sheets of tissue. The later three forms can impair vision, and dogs affected with these forms should not be bred. Identified in 4.14% of American Staffordshire Terriers CERF examined by veterinary ophthalmologists between 2000-2005.[8]

Retinal Dysplasia: Focal folds and geographic retinal dysplasia are seen in the breed. It is questionable whether focal folds can lead to disease. Identified in 2.41% of American Staffordshire Terriers CERF examined by veterinary ophthalmologists between 2000-2005.[8]

Cataracts: Location can be anterior, posterior, intermediate or punctate. Cataracts usually develop by one year of age. There is initial opacification of the suture lines progressing to nuclear and cortical cataract formation; complete cataracts and blindness develop by three years of age. A simple autosomal recessive mode of inheritance has been proposed. Identified in 1.39% of American Staffordshire Terriers CERF examined by veterinary ophthalmologists between 2000-2005. CERF does not recommend breeding any American Staffordshire Terrier with a cataract.[8]

Cranial Cruciate Ligament (ACL) Rupture: Traumatic tearing of the ACL in the stifle, causing lameness and secondary arthritis. Treat with surgery. Reported at an increased incidence versus other breeds.[9]

Heart Disease: Several polygenically inherited heart disorders are reported to occur at an increased frequency in American Staffordshire Terriers. Congenital heart disorders include **Pulmonic Stenosis** and **Subvalvular Aortic Stenosis (SAS)**. Later onset disorders include **Mitral Valve Prolapse**. These disorders should be screened for with Doppler echocardiograms. OFA reports 1.4% affected.[1]

Progressive Retinal Atrophy (PRA): Inherited retinal degeneration leading to blindness. Early onset PRA is reported to occur in the breed. Undetermined mode of inheritance.[8,10]

Actinic Keratosis: Affected dogs present with alopecia, erythema, comedones, scales, excoriation, pustules, epidermal collarettes, crusts and scars, with pathologic development of epidermal hyperplasia, parakeratosis, and orthokeratosis. Lesions occur secondary to prolonged UV/sunlight exposure, and may be a precursor to squamous cell carcinoma. Seen at an increased frequency in the breed.[11]

Gastric Carcinoma (Stomach Cancer): Can present with chronic vomiting. Diagnosis by biopsy (endoscopy). Treatment with surgery. Poor long-term survival. Reported to occur at an increased frequency compared to other breeds.[12]

Cleft Lip/Palate, Compulsive Tail Chasing, Cryptorchidism, Cystinuria, Deafness, Demodicosis, Ichthyosis, Patent Ductus Arteriosus, and **Wobblers Syndrome** are reported.[13]

Isolated Case Studies

Sry-negative XX True Hermaphrodite (XX Sex Reversal): Two unrelated male American Staffordshire Terriers were examined. The chromosomal sex was female (XX), and there was an absence of "male" causing SRY or ZFY. XX Sex-reversal is familial in other breeds.[14]

Xanthogranulomatous Inflammation of The Small Bowel: A 12 year old male American Staffordshire Terrier was presented with chronic diarrhea unresponsive to pharmacologic therapy. Disseminated yellow-white nodules 2 to 3 mm in diameter bulging on the serosal surface of the small bowel, as well as on mesenteric tissue, were detected. Lymphangectasia associated with lymphoplasmacytic enteritis was suggested as the cause.[15]

Genetic Tests

Tests of Genotype: Direct test for cerebellar ataxia/NCL-A is available from ANTAGENE and Optigen.

Direct tests for color alleles are available from VetGen.

Direct tests for HUU is available from the UC-Davis VGL and the Animal Health Trust.

Tests of Phenotype: CHIC Certification: Required tests include hip radiographs, cardiac evaluation by a cardiologist, thyroid profile including autoantibodies, and NCL-A genetic test for ataxia. Optional recommended testing includes a CERF eye examination, and elbow radiographs. (See CHIC website; www.caninehealthinfo.org).

Recommend patella evaluation.

Miscellaneous

- **Breed name synonyms:** Pit Bull, American Pit Bull Terrier, AmStaff, Bull-and-Terrier dog (historical). Also historical were street names such as Half and Half, Pit Dog, Yankee Terrier, American Bull Terrier, and Pit Terrier.
- **Registries:** AKC, UKC (registered as American Pit Bull Terrier), CKC, ANKC (Australian National Kennel Club), NKC (National Kennel Club)-here registered as American Pit Bull.
- **AKC rank (year 2008):** 71 (1,236 dogs registered)
- **Internet resources:** Staffordshire Terrier Club of America: www.amstaff.org
American Staffordshire Terrier Club of Canada: www.amstaffclubofcanada.ca

References

1. OFA Website breed statistics: www.offa.org Last accessed July 1, 2010.
2. Olby N, Blot S, Thibaud JL, et. al.: Cerebellar cortical degeneration in adult American Staffordshire Terriers. *J Vet Intern Med.* 2004 Mar-Apr;18(2):201-8.

3. Siso S, Navarro C, Hanzlicek D, et. al.: Adult onset thalamocerebellar degeneration in dogs associated to neuronal storage of ceroid lipopigment. *Acta Neuropathol (Berl)*. 2004 Nov;108(5):386-92.

4. Hanzlicek D, Kathmann I, Bley T, et. al.: Cerebellar cortical abiotrophy in American Staffordshire terriers: clinical and pathological description of 3 cases. *Schweiz Arch Tierheilkd*. 2003 Aug;145(8):369-75.

5. Abitbol M, Thibaud JL, Olby N, et. al.: Identification of a Single Point Mutation Strongly Associated With the Cerebellar Cortical Abiotrophy of the American Staffordshire Terrier. Proceedings, 2009 ACVIM Conference. 2009.

6. Nachreiner R and Refsal K: Personal communication, Diagnostic Center for Population and Animal Health, Michigan State University. April, 2007.

7. Nachreiner RF, Refsal KR, Graham PA, et. al.: Prevalence of serum thyroid hormone autoantibodies in dogs with clinical signs of hypothyroidism. J Am Vet Med Assoc 2002 Feb 15;220(4):466-71.

8. *Ocular Disorders Presumed to be Inherited in Purebred Dogs*. American College of Veterinary Ophthalmologists. ACVO, 2007

9. Duval JM, Budsberg SC, Flo GL, et. al.: Breed, sex, and body weight as risk factors for rupture of the cranial cruciate ligament in young dogs. *J Am Vet Med Assoc*. 1999 Sep 15;215(6):811-4.

10. Akhmedov NB, Baldwin VJ, Zangerl B, et. al.: Cloning and characterization of the canine photoreceptor specific cone-rod homeobox (CRX) gene and evaluation as a candidate for early onset photoreceptor diseases in the dog. *Mol Vis*. 2002 Mar 22;8:79-84.

11. Costa SS, Munhoz TD, Calazans SG, et. al.: Clinical and Epidemiological Evaluation of Actinic Keratosis in Seven Dogs. Proceedings, 2009 WSAVA World Congress. 2009.

12. Gualtieri M, Monzeglio MG, Scanziani E: Gastric neoplasia. Vet Clin North Am Small Anim Pract. 1999 Mar;29(2):415-40.

13. *The Genetic Connection: A Guide to Health Problems in Purebred Dogs*. L Ackerman. p. 196-97. AAHA Press, 1999.

14. Nowacka J, Nizanski W, Klimowicz M, et. al.: Lack of the SOX9 Gene Polymorphism in Sex Reversal Dogs (78, XX; SRY negative). *J Hered*. 2005 Nov-Dec;96(7):797-802.

15. Romanucci M, Malatesta D, Guardiani P, et. al.: Xanthogranu-lomatous inflammation of the small bowel in a dog. Vet Pathol. 2008 Mar;45(2):207-11.

16. *The Complete Dog Book, 20th Ed*. The American Kennel Club. Howell Book House, NY 2006. p. 345-347.

17. Karmi N, Brown EA, Hughes SS, et. al.: Estimated frequency of the canine hyperuricosuria mutation in different dog breeds. J Vet Intern Med. 2010 Nov-Dec;24(6):1337-42.

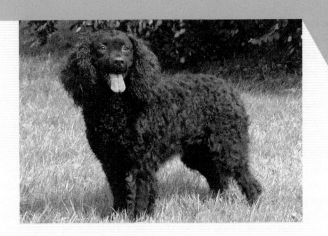

The Breed History

Predominantly found in the US Midwestern states, this dog is thought to have arisen from the Curly-coated Retriever, Tweed and Irish Water Spaniels, and Field Spaniels. The Boykin Spaniel may also be related to this breed. First recognition by the AKC occurred in 1940. The American Water Spaniel is the designated State Dog of Wisconsin and is considered a rare breed.

Breeding for Function

Strictly developed as a dual-purpose gun dog, they are excellent at following scent and flushing the quarry such as birds and rabbits. American Water Spaniels possesses an excellent ability to swim, and thus excel as a water retriever. The heavy tail can help to steady the dog in water like a rudder.

Physical Characteristics

Height at Withers: 15-18" (38-45.5 cm).

Weight: females 25-40 lb (11.5-18 kg), males 30-45 lb (13.5-20.5 kg).

Coat: The haircoat may be wavy or curly and a thick undercoat is present. Colors include liver, chocolate, or brown. Small white markings are accepted on the toes and chest. They are light to moderate shedders and have moderate grooming needs; the haircoat can be a bit oily.

Longevity: 11-12 years

Points of Conformation: Medium size, longer than tall, and solid bone and muscling characterizes this breed. The eyes are light brown, hazel, or dark brown. Eyes are medium-sized, moderately deep set and the palpebral margins are tight. The skull is flat and broad. Ears are long, wide and heavily feathered. The stop is moderate, the muzzle square and fairly long, and the nose is dark brown or black. The neck is short-to-medium, and not throaty. The topline is level, and the thorax moderately deep with well sprung ribs. The tail is carried fairly level, is moderately feathered and tapers at the terminus. Limbs are straight boned, and the feet are webbed and compact. Front dewclaws may be left on. The gait is smooth, powerful and ground covering.

Recognized Behavior Issues and Traits

Reported breed characteristics include: Intelligent, high trainability, loyal, likes to please. He is also considered a good watchdog and has a high barking tendency. They are notable for a high tolerance of pain; a very stoic dog. High activity and exercise needs are evident especially when young. Early obedience training is recommended, as is early socialization; some have a stubborn streak. Can be possessive of toys and food, tending to dominance, and may develop boredom vices if not adequately exercised and challenged mentally. Slow to mature and sensitive; responds well to positive reinforcement in training.

Normal Physiologic Variations

None reported

Drug Sensitivities

None reported

Inherited Diseases

Hip Dysplasia: Polygenically inherited trait causing degenerative joint disease and hip arthritis. OFA reports 7.7% affected.[1]

Elbow Dysplasia: Polygenically inherited trait causing elbow arthritis. Too few American Water Spaniels have been screened by OFA to determine an accurate frequency.[1]

Patella Luxation: Polygenically inherited laxity of patellar ligaments, causing luxation, lameness, and later degenerative joint disease. Treat surgically if causing clinical signs. Too few American Water Spaniels have been screened by OFA to determine an accurate frequency.[1]

Disease Predispositions

Mitral Valve Disease: Mitral valve prolapse and mitral regurgitation was identified in 56% of American Water Spaniels screened with echocardiography at the 2002 AWSC National Specialty. This was identified in dogs both with and without a heart murmur. (See AWSC website)

Distichiasis: Abnormally placed eyelashes that irritate the cornea and conjunctiva. Can cause secondary corneal ulceration. Identified in 30.07% of American Water Spaniels CERF examined by veterinary ophthalmologists between 2000-2005.[2]

Patent Ductus Arteriosus: Polygenically inherited congenital heart disorder, where a fetal vessel remains open after birth, causing a mixing of oxygenated and unoxygenated blood. Affected dogs are usually stunted, and have a loud heart murmur. Diagnosis with Doppler ultrasound. Treat with surgery. Identified in 5% of American Water Spaniels screened with echocardiography at the 2002 AWSC National Specialty. (See AWSC website)

Pulmonic Stenosis: Polygenically inherited congenital heart disorder, where there is a narrowing of the outflow from the pulmonic valve. This can cause exercise intolerance, and right sided heart failure. Diagnosis with Doppler ultrasound. Identified in 5% of American Water Spaniels screened with echocardiography at the 2002 AWSC National Specialty. (See AWSC website)

Hypothyroidism: Inherited autoimmune thyroiditis. 3.7% positive for thyroid auto-antibodies based on testing at Michigan State University. (Ave. for all breeds is 7.5%).[3,4]

Cataracts: Posterior cortex cataracts predominate, although anterior intermediate and punctate cataracts also occur in the breed. Unknown mode of inheritance. Identified in 2.61% of American Water Spaniels CERF examined by veterinary ophthalmologists between 2000-2005. CERF does not recommend breeding any American Water Spaniel with a cataract.[2]

Persistent Pupillary Membranes: Strands of fetal remnant connecting; iris to iris, cornea, lens, or involving sheets of tissue. The later three forms can impair vision, and dogs affected with these forms should not be bred. Identified in 1.63% of American Water Spaniels CERF examined by veterinary ophthalmologists between 2000-2005.[2]

Retinal Dysplasia: Retinal folds, geographic, and generalized retinal dysplasia with detachment are recognized in the breed. Identified in 1.63% of American Water Spaniels CERF examined by veterinary ophthalmologists between 2000-2005.[2]

Idiopathic Epilepsy (Inherited Seizures): Control with anti-seizure medication. Frequency and mode of inheritance not known. Ongoing research in the breed at the University of Missouri.

Degenerative Myelopathy (DM): Affected dogs show an insidious onset of upper motor neuron (UMN) paraparesis at an average age of 11.4 years. The disease eventually progresses to severe tetraparesis. Affected dogs have normal results on myelography, MRI, and CSF analysis. Necropsy confirms the condition. Unknown mode of inheritance. A direct genetic test for an autosomal recessive DM susceptibility gene is available. All affected dogs are homozygous for the gene, however, only a small percentage of homozygous dogs develop DM. The susceptibility allele occurs at a frequency of 46% in the breed.[5]

Allergic Inhalant Dermatitis, Cleft Lip/Palate, Cryptorchidism, Diabetes Mellitus, Follicular Dysplasia, Hermaphrodism, Growth Hormone-Responsive Dermatosis,Inguinal Hernia, Osteochondrodysplasia, and **Progressive Retinal Atrophy** are reported.[6]

Isolated Case Studies
None reported

Genetic Tests

Tests of Genotype: Direct test for DM susceptibility gene is available from OFA.

Tests of Phenotype: CHIC Certification: Required tests include hip radiographs, CERF eye examination (biannually until age 6), and cardiac evaluation. (See CHIC website; www.caninehealthinfo.org). Recommend elbow radiographs, patella evaluation and thyroid profile including autoantibodies.

Miscellaneous
- **Breed name synonyms:** Brown Water Spaniel, AWS.
- **Registries:** AKC, UKC, CKC, NKC (National Kennel Club).
- **AKC rank (year 2008):** 136 (132 dogs registered)
- **Internet resources: American Water Spaniel Club Inc.:** www.americanwaterspanielclub.org
  AWS Partners: http://home.earthlink.net/~awspartners/
  American Water Spaniel Field Association: www.awsfa.org

References

1. OFA Website breed statistics: www.offa.org Last accessed July 1, 2010.
2. *Ocular Disorders Presumed to be Inherited in Purebred Dogs.* American College of Veterinary Ophthalmologists. ACVO, 2007.
3. Nachreiner R and Refsal K: Personal communication, Diagnostic Center for Population and Animal Health, Michigan State University. April, 2007.
4. Nachreiner RF, Refsal KR, Graham PA, et. al.: Prevalence of serum thyroid hormone autoantibodies in dogs with clinical signs of hypothyroidism. J Am Vet Med Assoc 2002 Feb 15;220(4):466-71.
5. Coates JR, Zeng R, Awano T, et. al.: An SOD1 Mutation Associated with Degenerative Myelopathy Occurs in Many Dog Breeds. Proceedings 2009 ACVIM Forum. 2009.
6. *The Genetic Connection: A Guide to Health Problems in Purebred Dogs.* L Ackerman. p. 197. AAHA Press, 1999.
7. *The Complete Dog Book, 20th Ed.* The American Kennel Club. Howell Book House, NY 2006. p. 76-78.

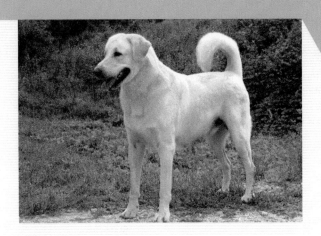

Anatolian Shepherd Dog

The Breed History
An ancient and rare breed, perhaps 6,000 years old, these Central Turkish guard dogs have a commanding presence. In the 1950s first imports to the USA occurred. The AKC registry accepted the breed in 1998.

Breeding for Function
They were resident in a harsh environment, withstanding temperature extremes to carry out flock protection against large predators. This led to a hardy, large working dog that could endure long days of work.

Physical Characteristics
Height at Withers: female 27" (68.5 cm), male 29" (73.5 cm) minimum.

Weight: females 80-120 lb (36.5-54.6 kg), males 110-150 lb (50-68 kg).

Coat: Two coat variants exist; the Short and the Rough. Rough is about 4" (10) cm in length, while Short is 1" (2.54 cm). The undercoat is dense. Some feathering may be present. Color or markings are not limited in this breed, but fawn with a dark mask is common.

Longevity: 12 years.

Points of Conformation: They possess a rugged build, large body frame with heavy muscling and bone, the head is large and the skull has small furrow in the midline. The flews are dry. Eyes are dark brown to amber and almond in shape, palpebral margins dark. Blue or odd irises are not allowed. The ears are triangular, the apex is rounded, and they are folded along the head. The muzzle is square, the nose is dark (brown or black), the neck is moderate in length and musculature, and with a ruff of skin and fur. The topline slopes down towards the croup, Thorax is deep and the ribs are well sprung, and an abdominal tuck up is present. The tail reaches the tarsi, and is high set. At rest, the tail is curved along the back of the legs, and when active it is up high and moves to do a "wheel" movement. Limbs are straight, metacarpals heavy, oval feet have thick pads, and are compact. Some specimens have double dewclaws in back. Dewclaws front and back may be removed. Gait is smooth and long in stride, ground-covering with significant agility.

Recognized Behavior Issues and Traits
Traits ascribed to the breed include: Works well independently, loyal, aloof towards strangers and new territory, calm unless acting in defense of the family or flock, an excellent guard dog but can be fierce in protection. Needs early obedience training to counteract the intelligent self-direction (strong willed) nature it possesses. A reserved attitude is not discouraged. Not considered a companion dog primarily.

Typically a heavy shedder, and they can be a bit clumsy in small areas. Lots of exercise is recommended. Allow them only a free run in enclosed areas. Good with other dogs if raised with them, though they can be territorially aggressive. Tolerate quiet children if socialized to them early.

Normal Physiologic Variations
None reported

Drug Sensitivities
Anatolian Shepherds are reported on the ASDCA website to be sensitive to anesthetics. A reduction in dosage may be required.

Inherited Diseases
Hip Dysplasia: Polygenically inherited trait causing degenerative joint disease and hip arthritis. OFA reports 10.2% affected.[1]

Elbow Dysplasia: Polygenically inherited trait causing elbow arthritis. OFA reports 4.5% affected.[1]

Patella Luxation: Polygenically inherited laxity of patellar ligaments, causing luxation, lameness, and later degenerative joint disease. Treat surgically if causing clinical signs. Too few Anatolian Shepherds have been screened by OFA to determine an accurate frequency.[1]

Disease Predispositions
Hypothyroidism: Inherited autoimmune thyroiditis. 9.5% positive for thyroid autoantibodies based on testing at Michigan State University. (Ave. for all breeds is 7.5%).[2,3]

Ocular Disorders: Too few Anatolian Shepherds have been CERF examined to determine the frequency of ocular disorders in the breed. **Entropion** (rolling in of the eyelids with associated corneal abrasion) is reported to occur at an increased frequency on the ASDCA website.[4]

Osteosarcoma (Bone Cancer): Reported at an increased incidence in the breed on the ASDCA website.

Gastric Dilation/Volvulus (GDV, Bloat): Life-threatening twisting of the stomach within the abdomen. Requires immediate veterinary attention. Reported at an increased incidence on the ASDI website.

Complete Ventral Ankyloglossia (Tongue-tie): Multiple case reports of a complete attachment of the lingual frenulum to the floor of the oral cavity. In one report, three Anatolian Shepherds (two full-brothers and one half-sister) presented at 8 months of age with a history of excessive drooling and poor weight gain. Physical examination revealed that the dogs were unable to protrude their tongues properly, due to a thin tissue band between the sublingual surface of the tongue and the floor of the oral cavity. This tissue band extended from the lingual frenulum to the gingiva of the mandibular incisors. All 3 dogs returned to normal function and weight gain after the tissue band was transected. Unknown mode of inheritance.[5,6]

Distichiasis, Elbow Luxation, and **Renal Dysplasia** are reported.[7]

Isolated Case Studies

Copper Toxicosis (Copper Storage Disease): Identified in a seven year old male Anatolian shepherd with a history of progressive weight loss and vomiting, and a finding of nodular hepatitis with excessive copper accumulation.[8]

Giant Cell Tumor: An eight-year-old female Anatolian Shepherd dog presented with a malignant osteoclast-like giant cell tumor arising from the hilus of the left kidney. Pathologically, the mass was comprised of large osteoclast-like multinucleated giant cells and spindle-spheroidal-shaped cells.[9]

Genetic Tests

Tests of Genotype: none

Tests of Phenotype: Recommend hip and elbow radiographs, CERF eye examination, thyroid profile including autoantibodies, patella evaluation and cardiac evaluation.

Miscellaneous

- **Breed name synonyms:** Anatolian, Anatolian Karabash Dog, Coban Kopegi (Turkish for Shepherd's dog), Karabas, Anatolian Sheperd, Anatolian Shephard, Kangal Dog.
- **Registries:** AKC, UKC, KCGB (Kennel Club of Great Britain), ANKC (Australian National Kennel Club), NKC (National Kennel Club)
- **AKC rank (year 2008):** 110 (373 dogs registered)
- **Internet resources: Anatolian Shepherd Dog Club of America:** www.asdca.org
  Anatolian Shepherd Dogs International: www.anatoliandog.org
  Anatolian Shepherd Dog Club of Great Britain: www.asdc-of-gb.netfirms.com

References

1. OFA Website breed statistics: www.offa.org Last accessed July 1, 2010.
2. Nachreiner R and Refsal K: Personal communication, Diagnostic Center for Population and Animal Health, Michigan State University. April, 2007.
3. Nachreiner RF, Refsal KR, Graham PA, et. al.: Prevalence of serum thyroid hormone autoantibodies in dogs with clinical signs of hypothyroidism. J Am Vet Med Assoc 2002 Feb 15;220(4):466-71.
4. *Ocular Disorders Presumed to be Inherited in Purebred Dogs.* American College of Veterinary Ophthalmologists. ACVO, 2007.
5. Temizsoylu MD, Avki S: Complete ventral ankyloglossia in three related dogs. *J Am Vet Med Assoc.* 2003 Nov 15;223(10):1443-5, 1433.
6. Grundmann S, Hofmann A: Ankyloglossia in an Anatolian Shepherd dog. Schweiz Arch Tierheilkd. 2006 Aug;148(8):417-20
7. *The Genetic Connection: A Guide to Health Problems in Purebred Dogs.* L Ackerman. P. 197. AAHA Press, 1999.
8. Bosje JT, van den Ingh TS, Fennema A, et. al.: Copper-induced hepatitis in an Anatolian shepherd dog. *Vet Rec.* 2003 Jan 18;152(3):84-5.
9. Haziroglu R, Kul O, Tunca R, et. al.: Osteoclast-like giant cell tumour arising from the kidney in a dog. *Acta Vet Hung.* 2005;53(2):225-30.
10. *The Complete Dog Book, 20th Ed.* The American Kennel Club. Howell Book House, NY 2006. p. 237-239.

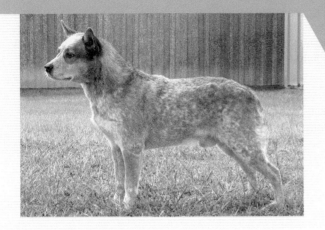

The Breed History

The importation of the Blue Merle Smooth-coated Highland Collie from Scotland crossed with native Dingos produced the required base type for managing feral cattle in large land tracts around Australia. Further crosses with Dalmation (the Bagust's Dog) and Black and Tan Kelpie finalized the current breed type. Breed development progressed throughout the 1800s. First breed standards were drawn up in the year 1902. AKC registry occurred in the year 1980. The older breed names include the word *heeler*, which indicates a dog that works silently at the heels, and crouches low to prevent being kicked after gripping at the coronet or fetlock area of the livestock.

Breeding for Function

These silent durable dogs were highly valued for the protection and herding of large herds of difficult cattle under severe environmental conditions. High efficiency in their work allowed them to last all day in marked temperature extremes. They are also used in field and farm work for sheep, and fowl or hogs.

Physical Characteristics

Height at Withers: female 17-19" (43-48 cm), male 18-20" (45.5-51 cm).

Weight: 35-45 lb (16-20 kg).

Coat: The moderately hard weather resistant coat is double and straight. The undercoat is short and dense. Colors are blue (blue mottled appearance acceptable) or red speckle with or without other markings. Specific markings are set out in the standard. Puppies are born light to white because of the Dalmation breed effect.

Longevity: 12-13 years

Points of Conformation: A sturdy well balanced conformation and highly energized movements characterize this working dog. Utility has dictated points of conformation. They possess a broad skull, a strong profile with definite stop, the muzzle is deep and lips tight, and the nose is always black. They appear dingo-like in many regards. Dark brown eyes are oval, medium-sized, and a sharp stare is normal. Pricked ears are wide set and small to medium in size, and the neck is medium in length and not throaty. The topline is level, thorax deep, ribs well sprung, and the rib cage remains deep caudally. The limbs are straight-boned, feet are round and the toes well arched. The low set tail is slightly curved and reaches to the tarsus. The tail has a brush. A strong smooth gait that appears effortless, and a strong rear quarter driving effort should be apparent.

Recognized Behavior Issues and Traits

Breed attributes ascribed include: Devoted, hard working, aloof and wary with strangers, loyal, intelligent, alert and vested with a high level of courage. Because of their strong protective instincts, these dogs should be introduced to children and small pets when young. They are intricate problem solvers, and work well independently once trained. They have high trainability. They are good watchdogs, but not alarm barkers. They can be aggressive with other dogs and dominant with children. They have high exercise needs and need a rural setting or large fenced enclosure, plus games or jobs to prevent boredom vices. They enjoy human companionship.

Normal Physiologic Variations

None reported

Drug Sensitivities

None reported

Inherited Diseases

Progressive Retinal Atrophy (PRA): Autosomal recessive prcd form. Inherited retinal degeneration leading to blindness. Age of onset between 3-8 years of age. Dorn reports a 12.88x odds ratio for the disease versus other breeds. Optigen prcd testing reports 15.9% affected, and 47.7% carrier in Australian Cattle Dogs. The Australian Cattle Dog Club of America has all Optigen test results posted on the OFA Website. There are some Australian Cattle Dogs diagnosed with a different form of PRA than prcd.[1,2,3]

Hip Dysplasia: Polygenically inherited trait causing degenerative joint disease and hip arthritis. OFA reports 15.3% affected.[1]

Elbow Dysplasia: Polygenically inherited trait causing elbow arthritis. OFA reports 11.6% affected.[1]

Patella Luxation: Polygenically inherited laxity of patellar ligaments, causing luxation, lameness, and later degenerative joint disease. Treat surgically if causing clinical signs. OFA reports 1.6% affected.[1]

Primary Lens Luxation (PLL) and Secondary Glaucoma: An autosomal recessive gene causes primary lens luxation. Homozygous affected dogs usually develop lens luxation between 4-8 years of age. Rarely, heterozygous carriers can develop lens luxation, but at a later age. Lens luxation can lead to secondary glaucoma and blindness. A genetic mutation has been identified, and a genetic test is available. One study reports a 3.1x odds ratio for secondary glaucoma versus other breeds.[4,5]

Spongiform Leukoencephalomyelopathy (Polioencephalomyopathy): Rare maternally (mitochondrial) inherited disorder causing tremors, spastic weakness, ataxia, occasionally seizures, and eventual paralysis beginning at 2-9 weeks of age. Caused by a point mutation in the cytochrome b gene.[6,7,8]

Disease Predispositions

Deafness: Undetermined mode of inheritance though familial pattern. Present at birth. Not associated with a specific color variety in this breed. Strain reports 12.2% unilaterally deaf, and 2.4% bilaterally deaf Australian Cattle Dogs. Diagnosed by BAER testing.[9]

Hypothyroidism: Inherited autoimmune thyroiditis. 7.7% positive for thyroid auto-antibodies based on testing at Michigan State University. (Ave. for all breeds is 7.5%).[10,11]

Cataracts: Anterior and posterior cataracts are equally represented in the breed with intermediate and punctate cataracts. Identified in 4.95% of Australian Cattle Dogs CERF examined by veterinary ophthalmologists between 2000-2005. CERF does not recommend breeding any Australian Cattle Dog with a cataract.[3]

Portosystemic Shunt (PSS, Liver Shunt): Undetermined mode of inheritance but familial pattern. Abnormal blood vessels connecting the systemic and portal blood flow. Vessels are usually intrahepatic in this breed, with a tendency to a right divisional location. Causes stunting, abnormal behavior and possible seizures. Australian studies show significantly higher prevalence in the breed compared to other breeds.[12,13,14]

Primary Glaucoma: Ocular condition causing increased pressure within the eyeball, and secondary blindness due to damage to the retina. United States study of dogs presented to veterinary teaching hospitals showed an increased prevalence in male Australian Cattle Dogs. Dorn reports a 2.07x odds ratio for the disorder versus other breeds. Gelatt reports 1.51% Australian Cattle Dogs affected between 1994-2002. Diagnose with IOP (tonometry) and examination of the iridocorneal angle (gonioscopy).[2,3,15]

Cysinuria and Cystine Bladder Stones: Caused by a metabolic abnormality in cystine metabolism. Australian Cattle Dogs are found to have an increased incidence.[16]

Persistent Pupillary Membranes: Strands of fetal remnant connecting; iris to iris, cornea, lens, or involving sheets of tissue. The later three forms can impair vision, and dogs affected with these forms should not be bred. Identified in 1.03% of Australian Cattle Dogs CERF examined by veterinary ophthalmologists between 2000-2005.[3]

Ceroid Lipofucinosis: Rare storage disease causing progressive blindness and incoordination between 1 and 2 years of age.[17,18]

Isolated Case Studies

Myotonia Hereditaria: An Australian Cattle Dog with generalized muscle stiffness and hypertrophy was examined, and determined to be homozygous recessively affected due to a mutation in the CLCN1 gene. No heterozygous Australian Dogs were identified, and it is not known if this gene is disseminated in the general population. A direct genetic test is available from the University of Guelph AHL.[19]

Achromatopsia (Day Blindness): Observed in a 12-month-old Australian cattle dog.[20]

Dermatomyositis, Osteochondrosis of the Hock, Pelger-Huet Anomaly and **von Willebrand's disease** are reported.[21]

Genetic Tests

Tests of Genotype: Direct test for prcd-PRA is available from Optigen and recommended for all breeding individuals.

Direct test for primary lens luxation is available from OFA and Animal Health Trust.

Direct test for a rare myotonia gene is available from the U-Guelph AHL.

Direct test for black, brown, and yellow colors is available from VetGen.

Tests of Phenotype: CHIC Certification: Required tests include hip and elbow radiographs (2 years of age or older), CERF eye examination (2 years of age or older), gene test for prcd-PRA, and BAER hearing test. Optional tests include patella evaluation (over 1 year of age), cardiac evaluation, and hock radiograph for OCD. (See CHIC website; www.caninehealthinfo.org).

Recommend thyroid profile including autoantibodies.

Bile acids and blood ammonia tests (fasting and post-feeding) if suspect portosystemic shunt.

Miscellaneous

- **Breed name synonyms:** Cattle Dog, ACD, Australian Queensland Heeler, Blue Heeler, Queensland Heeler, Hall's Heelers
- **Registries:** AKC, UKC, CKC, KCGB (Kennel Club of Great Britain), ANKC (Australian National Kennel Club), NKC (National Kennel Club)
- **AKC rank (year 2008):** 68 (1,294 dogs registered)
- **Breed resources: Australian Cattle Dog Club of America:** http://acdca.org/
  Australian Cattle Dog Health, Education and Welfare, Inc, (ACDHEW): www.acdhew.org
  Australian Cattle Dog Club of Canada: www.acdcc.ca
  Australian Cattle Dog Society of Great Britain: www.acdsocietyofgb.com

References

1. OFA Website breed statistics: www.offa.org Last accessed July 1, 2010.
2. Dorn CR: Canine breed-specific risks of frequently diagnosed diseases at veterinary teaching hospitals. Monograph. AKC Canine Health Foundation. 2000.
3. Ocular Disorders Presumed to be Inherited in Purebred Dogs. American College of Veterinary Ophthalmologists. ACVO, 2007.
4. Collier L, McCalla T, Moor CP: Anterior lens luxation in Queensland Heeler (Australian Cattle) dogs. Proc Am Coll Vet Ophthal 1989;20:18.
5. Johnsen DA, Maggs DJ, Kass PH: Evaluation of risk factors for development of secondary glaucoma in dogs: 156 cases (1999-2004). J Am Vet Med Assoc. 2006 Oct 15;229(8):1270-4.
6. Brenner O, de Lahunta A, Summers BA, et. al.: Hereditary polioencephalomyelopathy of the Australian Cattle Dog. Acta Neuropath 1997; Jul;94(1):54-66.
7. Harkin KR, Goggin JM, DeBey BM, et. al.: Magnetic Resonance imaging of

the brain of a dog with hereditary polioencephalomyopathy. *J Am Vet Med Assoc* 1999; May 1; 214(9):1342-44.

8. Li FY, Cuddon PA, Song J, Wood SL, et. al.: Canine spongiform leukoencephalomyelopathy is associated with a missense mutation in cytochrome b. *Neurobiol Dis.* 2005 Jul 15.

9. Strain GM: Deafness prevalence and pigmentation and gender associations in dog breeds at risk. *Vet J* 2004; Jan;167(1):23-32.

10. Nachreiner R and Refsal K: Personal communication, Diagnostic Center for Population and Animal Health, Michigan State University. April, 2007.

11. Nachreiner RF, Refsal KR, Graham PA, et. al.: Prevalence of serum thyroid hormone autoantibodies in dogs with clinical signs of hypothyroidism. J Am Vet Med Assoc 2002 Feb 15;220(4):466-71.

12. Tisdall PL, Hunt GB, Bellenger CR, Malik R: Congenital portosystemic shunts in Maltese and Australian cattle dogs. *Aust Vet J* 1994; Jun; 71(6):174-8.

13. Hunt GB: Effect of breed on anatomy of portosystemic shunts resulting from congenital diseases in dogs and cats: a review of 242 cases. *Aust Vet J* 2004;Dec; 82[12]:746-9.

14. Krotscheck U, Adin CA, Hunt GB, et. al.: Epidemiologic factors associated with the anatomic location of intrahepatic portosystemic shunts in dogs. Vet Surg. 2007 Jan;36(1):31-6.

15. Gelatt KN and MacKay EO: Prevalence of the Breed-Related Glaucomas in Pure-Bred Dogs in North America. *Vet Ophthalmol* Mar-Apr'04; 7[2]:97-111.

16. Case LC, Ling GV, Franti CE, et. al.: Cystine-containing urinary calculi in dogs: 102 cases (1981-1989). *J Am Vet Med Assoc* 1992; Jul 1;201(1):129-33.

17. Sisk DB, Levesque DC, Wood PA, Styer EL: Clinical and pathological features of ceroid lipofucinosis in two Australian cattle dogs. *J Am Vet Med Assoc* 1990; Aug 1; 197(3):361-4.

18. Wood PA, Sisk DB, Styer E, et. al.: Animal model: ceroidosis (ceroid-lipofuscinosis) in Australian cattle dogs. Am J Med Genet. 1987 Apr;26(4):891-8.

19. Finnigan DF, Hanna WJ, Poma R, et. al.: A novel mutation of the CLCN1 gene associated with myotonia hereditaria in an Australian cattle dog. J Vet Intern Med. 2007 May-Jun;21(3):458-63.

20. Hurn SD, Hardman C, Stanley RG: Day-Blindness in Three Dogs: Clinical and Electroretinographic Findings. *Vet Ophthalmol* Jun'03; 6[2]:127-130

21. *The Genetic Connection: A Guide to Health Problems in Purebred Dogs.* L Ackerman. p. 197-8. AAHA Press, 1999.

22. *The Complete Dog Book, 20th Ed.* The American Kennel Club. Howell Book House, NY 2006. p. 607-611.

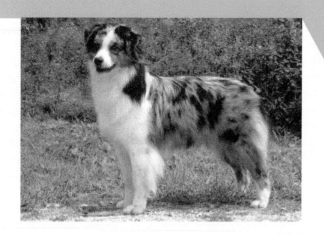

Australian Shepherd

The limbs are straight boned, feet compact and well knuckled up. Rear dewclaws are always removed. Gait is agile, and appearing effortless.

The Breed History

This cattle herding breed was primarily developed in California in the 1900s, but their origins trace back to the immigration of Basque shepherds. In Australia, there are similar dogs called German Coolies, but the Australian Shepherd is considered a separate breed, and was developed in the United States not Australia as the name might imply. Collies and Australian Sheepdogs figure most prominently in the ancestry of the Australian Shepherd. The Australian Shepherd Club of America was established in 1957. First AKC registry dates to 1991.

Breeding for Function

The breed excels at watching large herds. Their "eye" for scanning the herd and reacting only when necessary gives them an edge as the herder's aide. Their sensible herding judgment allows them to manage a herd with a reasonable energy outlay, resulting in the capacity to work long days. Because of their intelligence, their trainability and personality makes them suited for guide dog work, drug detection, for search and rescue missions and as companions.

Physical Characteristics

Height at Withers: female 18-21" (45.5-53 cm), male 20-23" (51-58.5 cm).

Weight: 35-70 lb (16-32 kg).

Coat: The coat is moderate in length and density, wavy or straight and moderate feathering is present on the forelegs and britches; a mane and frill are developed. Colors include red, red merle, blue merle, and black. These may be combined with markings of specified size and distribution including white and copper.

Longevity: 12-13 years

Points of Conformation: These dogs are medium in build and slightly longer than tall. The tail is either naturally bobbed or is docked to about 4" in length. A moderate stop divides the rounded muzzle from skull. An alert expression emanates from almond shaped eyes. Iris pigment is variable and can include brown, blue and amber. Ears are triangular and moderate in size, and break in a fold hanging forward or backwards. The nose is black for all but red or red merle dogs, where a liver nose is evident. Neck is moderate in muscling. The topline is level, ending in a moderately sloping croup. The thorax is deep and the ribs well sprung, and abdomen is moderately tucked up.

Recognized Behavior Issues and Traits

Reported breed attributes include: Affinity for children, loyal, strong guarding and herding instincts, very high intelligence and sound temperament. They are active, tend to get along well with other pets, have high trainability, are aloof with strangers and are good alarm barkers. They are average shedders and best suited to rural living or a home with a large fenced yard. They need mental stimulation to prevent boredom vices. They like to be kept busy with games and social contact.

Normal Physiologic Variations

Merle Coat Color: Caused by a dominant mutation in the SILV gene. Breeding two merle dogs together should be avoided, as homozygous dogs can be born with multiple defects, including blindness, deafness, and heart anomalies.[1,2]

Drug Sensitivities

MDR1/ABCB1 Mutation (Ivermectin/Drug Toxicity): Autosomal recessive disorder in the MDR1/ABCB1 gene allows high CNS drug levels of ivermectin, doramectin, loperamide, vincristine, moxidectin, and other drugs. Causes neurological signs, including tremors, seizures, and coma. A genetic test is available for the mutated gene, showing 10.0% of Australian Shepherds are affected, and 36.9% are carriers. In Germany, 6.9% of Australian Shepherds test homozygous affected, and 25.2% test as carriers.[3,4,5,6,7]

Inherited Disease

Hip Dysplasia: Polygenically inherited trait causing degenerative joint disease and hip arthritis. OFA reports 5.8% affected.[8]

Elbow Dysplasia: Polygenically inherited trait causing elbow arthritis. OFA reports 4.3% affected.[8]

Legg-Calvé-Perthes Disease: Polygenically inherited. Can be unilateral or bilateral, with onset of degeneration usually under 9 months of age. Treat surgically if causing lameness or discomfort. Australian Shepherds found to have a 191.4x odds ratio for developing the disease versus other breeds.[9]

Cataracts: A mutation in the HSF4 gene is associated with co-dominant cataracts in the breed, although other inherited cataracts also occur. Australian Shepherds homozygous for the mutation tend to develop bilateral nuclear cataracts, and dogs with one copy of the defective gene have a 17.7x risk of developing posterior polar subcapsular cataracts. CERF reports anterior and posterior cataracts are equally represented in the breed, and can be intermediate or punctate. Reported in 2.43% of Australian Shepherds CERF examined by veterinary ophthalmologists between 2000-2005. CERF does not recommend breeding any Australian Shepherd with a cataract. A direct genetic test for the HSF4 mutation is available.[10,11,12]

Patella Luxation: Polygenically inherited laxity of patellar ligaments, causing luxation, lameness, and later degenerative joint disease. Treat surgically if causing clinical signs. OFA reports 1.9% affected.[8]

Collie Eye Anomaly/Choroidal Hypoplasia/Coloboma (CEA/CH): Autosomal recessive disorder of eye development that can lead to retinal detachment and blindness. Iris coloboma is reported in 1.45% of Australian Shepherds CERF examined by veterinary ophthalmologists between 2000-2005. A genetic test is available through Optigen, that reports 1% of Australian Shepherds test as affected, and 10% test as carriers. Reported at a frequency of 4.03% affected in an Australian study.[10,13,14]

Hyperuricosuria (HUU)/Urate Bladder Stones: An autosomal recessive mutation in the SLC2A9 gene causes urate urolithiasis and can predispose male dogs to urinary obstruction. Estimated at a carrier frequency of 3.46% in the breed. A genetic test is available.[31]

Multifocal Retinopathy/Retinal Dysplasia: Autosomal recessive retinal pigment epithelial dysplasia causing localized multifocal retinal detachments. Age of onset from 11 to 13 weeks of age. Reported in 0.8% of Australian Shepherds CERF examined by veterinary ophthalmologists between 2000-2005. A genetic test is available.[10]

Progressive Retinal Atrophy (PRA): Autosomal recessive inherited retinal degeneration leading to blindness. Progressive rod cone degeneration (prcd) form occurs at a very low frequency. A genetic test is available.[10]

Disease Predispositions

Hypothyroidism: Inherited autoimmune thyroiditis. 8.6% positive for thyroid auto-antibodies based on testing at Michigan State University. (Ave. for all breeds is 7.5%).[15,16]

Persistent Pupillary Membranes: Strands of fetal remnant connecting; iris to iris, cornea, lens, or involving sheets of tissue. The later three forms can impair vision, and dogs affected with these forms should not be bred. Identified in 4.39% of Australian Shepherds CERF examined by veterinary ophthalmologists between 2000-2005.[10]

Distichiasis: Abnormally placed eyelashes that irritate the cornea and conjunctiva. Can cause secondary corneal ulceration. Identified in 1.44% of Australian Shepherds CERF examined by veterinary ophthalmologists between 2000-2005.[10]

Deafness: Inherited congenital deafness associated with the merle gene. In a multi-breed study; for single merles (Mm), 2.7% were unilaterally deaf and 0.9% were bilaterally deaf. For double merles (MM), 10% were unilaterally deaf and 15% were bilaterally deaf. Diagnosed by BAER testing. Unknown mode of inheritance for deafness, though dominant merle gene must be present.[17,18]

Cryptorchidism (Retained Testicles): Can be unilateral or bilateral. This is a sex-limited disorder with an unknown mode of inheritance. Reported to occur at an increased frequency in the 1999 ASCA Breed Health Survey.[19]

Persistent Hyaloid Artery (PHA): Congenital defect resulting from abnormalities in the development and regression of the hyaloid artery. Does not cause vision problems by itself, but is often associated with other ocular defects. Reported at a frequency of 5.82% in the breed in an Australian study. Identified in 0.61% of Australian Shepherds CERF examined by veterinary ophthalmologists between 2000-2005.[10,14]

Idiopathic Epilepsy (Inherited Seizures): Control with anti-seizure medication. Reported to occur at an increased frequency in the 1999 ASCA Breed Health Survey.[19]

Chronic Superficial Keratitis (CSK)/Pannus: Corneal disease that can cause vision problems due to pigmentation. Treatment with topical ocular lubricants and anti-inflammatory medication. Australian Shepherds are a breed with increased risk of developing CSK. The disorder usually occurs between 4-7 years of age.[20]

Cystine Urinary Calculi: Caused by a metabolic abnormality in cystine metabolism. Australian Shepherds are a breed with increased risk of developing cystine calculi.[21]

Microphthalmia: Microphthalmia with coloboma appears to behave as an incompletely penetrant recessive trait in the merle Australian Shepherd dog. Homozygous merle dogs are usually blind, while heterozygous dogs can be less severely affected.[10,22]

Anterior Crossbite, Brachygnathism, Cerebellar Vermian Hypoplasia, Cutaneous Lupus Erythematosus, Diabetes Mellitus, Factor VIII Deficiency, Osteochondrodysplasia, Panosteitis, Patent Ductus arteriosis, Pelger-Huet Anomaly, Persistent Right Aortic arch, Portosystemic Shunt, Prognathism, Pulmonic Stenosis, and **von Willebrand's Disease** are reported.[23]

Isolated Case Studies

Methylmalonic Aciduria and Cobalamin Malabsorption: Documented in an Australian Shepherd kindred, due to an autosomal recessive mutation in the gene amnionless (AMN).[24]

Neuronal Ceroid Lipofuscinosis: Three 18 month old Australian Shepherd littermates presented with a 1-month history of progressive vision loss, hypermetria, tremors, and personality changes including hyperesthesia. NCL was confirmed on necropsy.[25]

Peripheral Neuroectodermal Tumor: A peripheral primitive neuroectodermal tumor (pPNET), most consistent with a human Ewing's sarcoma, is described in a 5-month-old male Australian Shepherd puppy.[26]

Myofibrillar Myopathy: A 1-year-old male neutered Australian Shepherd dog was evaluated for chronic lameness, contractures, and exercise intolerance. Cardiomyopathy, and myofibrillar myopathy with accumulation of desmin was identified.[27]

Multiple Skeletal Defects: A family of Australian Shepherds was identified with a syndrome including cleft palate, polydactyly, and often syndactyly, shortened tibia-fibula, brachygnathism and scoliosis lethal to males. The disorder may be due to an x-linked gene, or a sex-influenced autosomal gene in conjunction with instability of the merle locus.[28]

Anemia and Osteopetrosis: Case study of a 1-year-old, male Australian Shepherd Dog with severe nonregenerative anemia associated with osteopetrosis. The anemia was attributed to failure to develop normal marrow cavities combined with failure of extramedullary erythropoiesis.[29]

Genetic Tests

Tests of Genotype: Direct tests for CEA/CH, retinal dysplasia, and prcd-PRA are available from Optigen.

Direct test for MDR1 (ivermectin sensitivity) gene is available from Washington State Univ. http://www.vetmed.wsu.edu/depts-VCPL/test.asp

Direct test for increased cataract susceptibility is available from the Animal Health Trust.

Direct test for HUU is available from the UC-Davis VGL and the Animal Health Trust.

Direct test for skin and nose color (black, clear red, brown (red), and dilute colors and black or brown pigmentation on the nose) is available from HealthGene and VetGen.

Tests of Phenotype: CHIC Certification: Required testing includes hip radiographs, elbow radiographs, and CERF eye examination. Optional recommended testing for thyroid profile including autoantibodies, and direct tests for CEA/CH, and MDR1. (See CHIC website; www.caninehealthinfo.org).

Recommend BAER testing for deafness, direct test for cataract succeptability, patella examination, and cardiac evaluation.

Miscellaneous

- **Breed name synonyms:** Aussie, Australian Shepherd, Pastor Dog, Bob-tail, New Mexican Shepherd, California Shepherd, Spanish Shepherd (historical).
- **Registries:** AKC, UKC, CKC, KCGB (Kennel Club of Great Britain), ANKC (Australian National Kennel Club), NKC (National Kennel Club)
- **AKC rank (year 2008):** 29 (6,471 dogs registered)
- **Internet resources: Australian Shepherd Club of America Inc:** www.asca.org
  Australian Shepherd Health and Genetics Institute, Inc. (ASGI): www.ashgi.org
  Canadian National Australian Shepherd Association: www.cnasa.ca
  Australian Shepherd Club of the United Kingdom: www.ascuk.co.uk

References

1. Clark LA, Wahl JM, Rees CA, et. al.: Retrotransposon insertion in SILV is responsible for merle patterning of the domestic dog. Proc Natl Acad Sci U S A. 2006 Jan 31;103(5):1376-81.
2. Hedan B, Corre S, Hitte C, et. al.: Coat colour in dogs: identification of the merle locus in the Australian shepherd breed. BMC Vet Res. 2006 Feb 27;2:9.
3. Geyer J, Doring B, Godoy JR, et. al.: Development of a PCR-based diagnostic test detecting a nt230(del4) MDR1 mutation in dogs: verification in a moxidectin-sensitive Australian Shepherd. J Vet Pharmacol Ther. 2005 Feb;28(1):95-9.
4. Nelson OL, Carsten E, Bentjen SA, et. al.: Ivermectin toxicity in an Australian Shepherd dog with the MDR1 mutation associated with ivermectin sensitivity in Collies. J Vet Intern Med. 2003 May-Jun;17(3):354-6.
5. Geyer J, Doring B, Godoy JR, et. al.: Frequency of the nt230 (del4) MDR1 mutation in Collies and related dog breeds in Germany. J Vet Pharmacol Ther. 2005 Dec;28(6):545-51.
6. Neff MW, Robertson KR, Wong AK, et. al.: Breed distribution and history of canine mdr1-1Delta, a pharmacogenetic mutation that marks the emergence of breeds from the collie lineage. Proc Natl Acad Sci U S A. 2004 Aug 10;101(32):11725-30.
7. Mealey KL and Meurs KM: Breed distribution of the ABCB1-1Delta (multidrug sensitivity) polymorphism among dogs undergoing ABCB1 genotyping. J Am Vet Med Assoc. 2008 Sep 15;233(6):921-4.
8. OFA Website breed statistics: www.offa.org Last accessed July 1, 2010.
9. LaFond E, Breur GJ, Austin CC: Breed susceptibility for developmental orthopedic diseases in dogs. J Am Anim Hosp Assoc. 2002 Sep-Oct;38(5):467-77.
10. *Ocular Disorders Presumed to be Inherited in Purebred Dogs*. American College of Veterinary Ophthalmologists. ACVO, 2007.
11. Mellersh CS, Pettitt L, Forman OP, et. al.: Identification of mutations in HSF4 in dogs of three different breeds with hereditary cataracts. Vet Ophthalmol. 2006 Sep-Oct;9(5):369-78.
12. Mellersh CS, McLaughlin B, Ahonen S, et. al.: Mutation in HSF4 is associated with hereditary cataract in the Australian Shepherd. Vet Ophthalmol. 2009 Nov-Dec;12(6):372-8.
13. Lowe JK, Kukekova AV, Kirkness EF, et. al.: Linkage mapping of the primary disease locus for collie eye anomaly. *Genomics*. 2003 Jul:82(1):86-95.
14. Munyard KA, Sherry CR, Sherry L: A retrospective evaluation of congenital ocular defects in Australian Shepherd dogs in Australia. Vet Ophthalmol. 2007 Jan-Feb;10(1):19-22.
15. Nachreiner R and Refsal K: Personal communication, Diagnostic Center for Population and Animal Health, Michigan State University. April, 2007.
16. Nachreiner RF, Refsal KR, Graham PA, et. al.: Prevalence of serum thyroid hormone autoantibodies in dogs with clinical signs of hypothyroidism. J Am Vet Med Assoc 2002 Feb 15;220(4):466-71.
17. Strain GM: Deafness prevalence and pigmentation and gender associations in dog breeds at risk. *The Veterinary Journal* 2004; 167(1):23-32.
18. Strain GM, Clark LA, Wahl JM, et. al.: Prevalence of deafness in dogs heterozygous or homozygous for the merle allele. J Vet Intern Med. 2009 Mar-Apr;23(2):282-6.
19. Sharp CA and Adolphson P: Results of the 1999 ASCA Breed Health Survey. *Aussie Times*. 2002 Jan-Feb.
20. Chavkin MJ, Roberts SM, Salman MD, et. al.: Risk factors for development of chronic superficial keratitis in dogs. *J Am Vet Med Assoc*. 1994 May 15;204(10):1630-4.
21. Case LC, Ling GV, Franti CE, et. al.: Cystine-containing urinary calculi in dogs: 102 cases (1981-1989). *J Am Vet Med Assoc*. 1992 Jul 1;201(1):129-33.
22. Gelatt KN, Powell NG, Huston K: Inheritance of microphthalmia with coloboma in the Australian shepherd dog. *Am J Vet Res*. 1981 Oct;42(10):1686-90.
23. *The Genetic Connection: A Guide to Health Problems in Purebred Dogs*. L Ackerman. p. 198. AAHA Press, 1999.
24. He Q, Madsen M, Kilkenney A, et. al.: Amnionless function is required for cubilin brush-border expression and intrinsic factor-cobalamin (vitamin B12) absorption in vivo. *Blood*. 2005 Aug 15;106(4):1447-53.
25. O'Brien DP and Katz ML: Neuronal ceroid lipofuscinosis in 3 Australian shepherd littermates. J Vet Intern Med. 2008 Mar-Apr;22(2):472-5.
26. De Cock HE, Busch MD, Fry MM, et. al.: A peripheral primitive neuroectodermal tumor with generalized bone metastases in a puppy. *Vet Pathol*. 2004 Jul;41(4):437-41.
27. Shelton GD, Sammut V, Homma S, et. al.: Myofibrillar myopathy with desmin accumulation in a young Australian Shepherd dog. *Neuromuscul Disord*. 2004 Jul;14(7):399-404.
28. Sponenberg DP, Bowling AT: Heritable syndrome of skeletal defects in a family of Australian shepherd dogs. *J Hered*. 1985 Sep-Oct;76(5):393-4.
29. Lees GE, Sautter JH: Anemia and osteopetrosis in a dog. *J Am Vet Med Assoc*. 1979 Oct 15;175(8):820-4.
30. *The Complete Dog Book, 20th Ed*. The American Kennel Club. Howell Book House, NY 2006. p. 612-615.
31. Karmi N, Brown EA, Hughes SS, et. al.: Estimated frequency of the canine hyperuricosuria mutation in different dog breeds. J Vet Intern Med. 2010 Nov-Dec;24(6):1337-42.

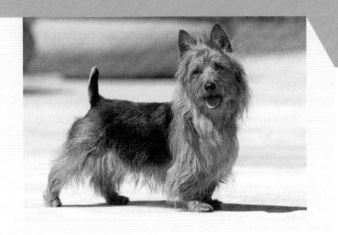

The Breed History

In Australia, the breed was first exhibited in 1899. These terriers were the first of the Aussie breeds, with the breed standard finalized in the year 1896. The AKC registry admitted Australian Terriers in 1960. Breed origins may include the Rough-coated Terrier crossed over many generations with other terriers such as the Skye, Dandie Dinmont, Irish, Cairn, Yorkshire, Black-and-Tan Terrier, and perhaps the Norwich Terrier. They were first brought to North America following the Second World War.

Breeding for Function

This small terrier was bred for both companionship and as a sturdy hunting partner. He also served as protector of sheep flocks and family. Rat and snake control were common tasks for which this terrier was bred.

Physical Characteristics

Height at Withers: 10-11" (25.4-28 cm).

Weight: 12-14 lb (4-7 kg).

Coat: The double coat is water resistant. Outer coat is straight, harsh and broken, and 2-1/2" (6 cm) long except furnishings. Inner coat is dense and short. Colors include blue and tan, sandy, and red. The hairs form a distinct topknot, apron and ruff. White markings on feet and chest are faults.

Longevity: 14 years

Points of Conformation: The Australian Terrier is characterized by a sturdy build, with medium bone and musculature. They possess an alert expression, high head carriage, and the body is a fair bit longer than tall. The gait is smooth and agile. Ears are small, triangular and held pricked up. Oval eyes are small and dark brown, wide-set and palpebral margins are also black. A definite stop is standard. Nose is colored black and the bridge of the nose has a hairless area. Lips are dark, and the neck is long. The thorax has well-sprung ribs and the topline is level. The tail is high-set and carried high; usually docked to about one half of the natural length. Limbs are straight boned, dewclaws are usually removed, feet small and compact, and nails black.

Recognized Behavior Issues and Traits

Reported breed characteristics include: Good in rural and urban environments, courageous, good alarm barkers, low shedding, adaptable, loyal, and intelligent. Can be scrappy with other dogs, enjoys close human companionship, good with other pets if raised with them (except other dogs, especially inter-male), high trainability, very high energy, spirited, like to dig and if off leash, they should be in a securely fenced enclosure; may also jump a fence. Should be socialized to pets and children since the strong chase instinct means that small pets could be viewed as prey.

Normal Physiologic Variations

None reported

Drug Sensitivities

None reported

Inherited Diseases

Patella Luxation: Polygenically inherited laxity of patellar ligaments, causing luxation, lameness, and later degenerative joint disease. Treat surgically if causing clinical signs. Reported 8.0x odds ratio versus other breeds. OFA reports 11.9% affected. Reported at a frequency of 9.0% in the 2002 ATCA Health Survey.[1,2,3]

Hip Dysplasia: Polygenically inherited trait causing degenerative joint disease and hip arthritis. OFA reports 2.4% affected.[1]

Legg-Calvé-Perthes Disease: Polygenically inherited aseptic necrosis of the femoral head, resulting in degenerative joint disease. Can be unilateral or bilateral, with onset of degeneration usually between 6-9 months of age. Treat surgically if causing lameness/discomfort. Reported at a frequency of 1.6% in the 2002 ATCA Health Survey.[2]

Elbow Dysplasia: Polygenically inherited trait causing elbow arthritis. Too few Australian Terriers have been screened by OFA to determine an accurate frequency.[1]

Disease Predispositions

Diabetes Mellitus: Sugar Diabetes. Australian Terriers are the breed with the highest incidence of DM. Caused by a lack of insulin production by the pancreas. Controlled by insulin injections, diet, and glucose monitoring. Reported at a frequency of 9.8% in the 2002 ATCA Health Survey. Unknown mode of inheritance.[2,4,5]

Cataracts: Anterior or posterior intermediate and punctate cataracts occur in the breed. Unknown mode of inheritance. Reported in 4.10% of Australian Terriers presented to veterinary teaching hospitals. Identified in 1.48% of Australian Terriers CERF examined by veterinary ophthalmologists between 2000-2005. Reported at a frequency of 5.1% in the 2002 ATCA Health Survey. CERF does not recommend breeding any Australian Terrier with a cataract.[2,6,7]

Hypothyroidism: Inherited autoimmune thyroiditis. 4.9% positive for thyroid auto-antibodies based on testing at Michigan State University. (Ave. for all breeds is 7.5%). Reported at a frequency of 3.6% in the 2002 ATCA Health Survey.[2,8,9]

Allergic Dermatitis: Presents with pruritis and pyotraumatic dermatitis (hot spots). The 2002 ATCA Health Survey reports 4.7% allergic to fleas, 0.8% to inhaled allergens, and 1.8% to food.[2]

Cranial Cruciate Ligament Rupture (ACL): Traumatic tearing of the anterior cruciate ligament. Treatment is surgery. Reported at a frequency of 4.4% in the 2002 ATCA Health Survey.[2]

Urinary Calculi (Bladder Stones): Mineral content of stones not specified. Reported at a frequency of 4.4% in the 2002 ATCA Health Survey.[2]

Pancreatitis: Inflammation of the pancreas causing vomiting and peritonitis. Can be life threatening if severe. Reported at a frequency of 2.7% in the 2002 ATCA Health Survey.[2]

Deafness: Congenital deafness can be unilateral of bilateral. Diagnosed by BAER testing. Reported at a frequency of 2.3% in the 2002 ATCA Health Survey. Not listed as a breed at risk by Strain.[2,10]

Idiopathic Epilepsy (inherited seizures): Control with anti-seizure medication. Reported at a frequency of 2.1% in the 2002 ATCA Health Survey.[2]

Hyperadrenocorticism (Cushing's disease): Hyperfunction of the adrenal gland caused by a pituitary or adrenal tumor. Clinical signs may include increased thirst and urination, symmetrical truncal alopecia, and abdominal distention. Reported at a frequency of 1.9% in the 2002 ATCA Health Survey.[2]

Cryptorchidism (Retained Testicles): Can be unilateral or bilateral. This is a sex-limited disorder with an unknown mode of inheritance. Reported at a frequency of 1.6% in the 2002 ATCA Health Survey.[2]

Distichiasis: Abnormally placed eyelashes that irritate the cornea and conjunctiva. Can cause secondary corneal ulceration. Identified in 1.48% of Australian Terriers CERF examined by veterinary ophthalmologists between 2000-2005.[6]

Persistent Pupillary Membranes: Strands of fetal remnant connecting; iris to iris, cornea, lens, or involving sheets of tissue. The later three forms can impair vision, and dogs affected with these forms should not be bred. Identified in 1.48% of Australian Terriers CERF examined by veterinary ophthalmologists between 2000-2005.[6]

Mast Cell Tumor (MCT): Skin tumors that can reoccur locally or with distant metastasis. Reported at a frequency of 1.3% in the 2002 ATCA Health Survey.[2]

Keratoconjunctivitis Sicca (KCS, Dry Eye): Ocular condition causing lack of tear production and secondary conjunctivitis, corneal ulcerations, and vision problems. Reported at a frequency of 1.1% in the 2002 ATCA Health Survey.[2]

Allergic Inhalant Dermatitis, Cleft Lip/Palate, Glucocerebrosidosis, Juvenile Cellulitis, Megaesophagus, Patent Ductus Arteriosus, Portosystemic Shunts, Progressive Retinal Atrophy, and **Retinal Dysplasia** are reported.[11]

Isolated Case Studies

Gastrinoma: An 8-year-old, spayed female Australian Terrier was presented with weight loss, inappetence, lethargy and a 2-day history of intermittent vomiting. Fasting serum gastrin levels were markedly elevated. The dog was treated with omeprazole, ranitidine and sucralfate, and remained clinically normal for 26 months. Histopathology and immunocytochemistry confirmed the diagnosis of metastatic gastrinoma.[12]

Ganglioneuroma: An 18-month-old, spayed female Australian Terrier was presented with a 10-month history of chronic large bowel diarrhea. Two rectal masses were removed, and found to be ganglioneuromas on histopathology. There was no recurrence post-surgically.[13]

Primitive Neuroectodermal Tumour: An 18-month-old female Australian terrier that died of central nervous system disease was found to have a large hemorrhagic primitive neuroectodermal tumour with ependymal differentiation replacing the thalamus and part of the hypothalamus of the brain.[14]

Genetic Tests

Tests of Genotype: none

Tests of Phenotype: CHIC Certification: Required testing includes CERF eye examination, patella evaluation, and thyroid profile including autoantibodies. (See CHIC website; www.caninehealthinfo.org). Recommend hip and elbow radiographs, cardiac evaluation, blood and urine glucose tests for diabetes.

Miscellaneous

- **Breed name synonyms:** Aussie, Broken-coated Toy Terrier (Historical).
- **Registries:** AKC, UKC, CKC, KCGB (Kennel Club of Great Britain), ANKC (Australian National Kennel Club), NKC (National Kennel Club).
- **AKC rank (year 2008):** 113 (330 dogs registered)
- **Internet resources:** Australian Terrier Club of America: http://australianterrier.org

References

1. OFA Website breed statistics: www.offa.org Last accessed July. 1, 2010.
2. Australian Terrier Club of America: 2002 ATCA Health Survey. 2002.
3. LaFond E, Breur GJ and Austin CC: Breed susceptibility for developmental orthopedic diseases in dogs. J Am Anim Hosp Assoc. 2002 Sep-Oct;38(5):467-77.
4. Chastain BD and Panciera D: Risk Factors for Diabetes Mellitus in Dogs. *Sm Anim Clin Endocrinol* 2004:14[2]:11.
5. Fall T, Hamlin HH, Hedhammar A, et. al.: Diabetes mellitus in a population of 180,000 insured dogs: incidence, survival, and breed distribution. J Vet Intern Med. 2007 Nov-Dec;21(6):1209-16.
6. *Ocular Disorders Presumed to be Inherited in Purebred Dogs.* American College of Veterinary Ophthalmologists. ACVO, 2007.
7. Gelatt KN, Mackay EO: Prevalence of primary breed-related cataracts in the dog in North America. Vet Ophthalmol. 2005 Mar-Apr;8(2):101-11.
8. Nachreiner R and Refsal K: Personal communication, Diagnostic Center

for Population and Animal Health, Michigan State University. April, 2007.

9. Nachreiner RF, Refsal KR, Graham PA, et. al.: Prevalence of serum thyroid hormone autoantibodies in dogs with clinical signs of hypothyroidism. J Am Vet Med Assoc 2002 Feb 15;220(4):466-71.

10. Strain GM: Deafness prevalence and pigmentation and gender associations in dog breeds at risk. *Vet J.* 2004 Jan;167(1):23-32

11. *The Genetic Connection: A Guide to Health Problems in Purebred Dogs.* L Ackerman. p. 198. AAHA Press, 1999

12. Hughes SM: Canine gastrinoma: a case study and literature review of therapeutic options. N Z Vet J. 2006 Oct;54(5):242-7

13. Reimer ME, Leib MS, Reimer MS, et. al.: Rectal ganglioneuroma in a dog. J Am Anim Hosp Assoc. 1999 Mar-Apr;35(2):107-10

14. Headley SA, Koljonen M, Gomes LA, et. al.: Central primitive neuroectodermal tumour with ependymal differentiation in a dog. J Comp Pathol. 2009 Jan;140(1):80-3.

15. *The Complete Dog Book, 20th Ed.* The American Kennel Club. Howell Book House, NY 2006. p. 348-351.

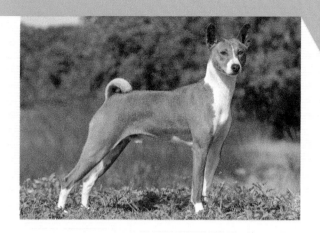

The Breed History

This breed originated in Central Africa, but gained popularity in Egypt—they were given as prized gifts in the times of the Pharaohs. They were exported to the US and Great Britain around 1937, and in 1943 they were first registered in the AKC. Basenjis are well known for the absence of a true bark. They can make noise, but their varied vocalizations are described as yodels, brrs, or roos. The name Basenji probably originates from the African word for "Bush Thing". The BCOA and other clubs worldwide are involved with the *African Stock Project* to bring new Basenjis from Africa to expand the gene pool.

Breeding for Function

The breed was originally developed to point and retrieve, and for hunting reed rats, an indigenous African variety that is particularly large and vicious. They excel both as sight and scent dogs. They are successful in agility competitions and are not now commonly used for hunting.

Physical Characteristics

Height at Withers: female 16 " (40.5 cm), male 17" (43 cm).

Weight: females 22 lb (10 kg), males 24 (11 kg).

Coat: The short, glossy, smooth dense haircoat comes in black, tri-color, brindle, chestnut red—all with white feet, chest and tip of the tail. Distinct borders between colors are desired, and white should never predominate though it can be present elsewhere. They are low shedding dogs, with absent doggie odor and need minimal grooming.

Longevity: 10-12 years.

Points of Conformation: The tail is carried over the straight topline in a curled position, head carriage is high, and the medium-sized ears are carried pricked up, with a furrowed brow. Eyes are hazel to brown. They have short backs, a definite waist and are well muscled with strong bone. They have a horse-like smooth running trot.

Recognized Behavior Issues and Traits

Reported characteristics of these high activity dogs include: Playful, smart, and are known to be courageous hunters. They tend to be fastidious about staying clean, washing themselves with their tongues like a cat. They are independently minded, and cautious around strangers, while being calm and friendly with family, including children. They like to be kept busy, and will do best with a household that provides lots of playtime, exercise and attention.

They are considered a primitive evolved domestic dog.

Normal Physiologic Variations

Females go into heat once a year.

Basenjis have lower resting T_4 thyroid levels, similar to sight hounds. Check thyroid status with thyroid profiles.[1]

Pelger–Huet Anomaly: Basenjis have been diagnosed with this autosomal recessive blood anomaly. Causes neutrophils with round, oval, or bean-shaped nuclei and only rare segmented nuclei. No obvious liability to disease seen in affected dogs.[2]

Drug Sensitivities

None reported

Inherited Diseases

Fanconi Syndrome: Inherited defect in renal tubular transport. Causes glucosuria, hyposthenuria, metabolic acidosis, hyperchloremia, and reduction in glomerular filtration rate. Onset 3-11 years of age. Diagnose by finding glucosuria with normal blood glucose levels. Treat with medications and diet. Seen worldwide. Dorn reports an 11.48x odds ratio in Basenjis versus other breeds. Prevalence of 10% in the United States Basenji population. A linked marker test is offered by the OFA, which suggests an autosomal recessive mode of inheritance. Genetic testing shows 6.3% affected and 41.2% carrier.[3,4,5,6]

Hip Dysplasia: Polygenically inherited trait causing degenerative joint disease and hip arthritis. OFA reports 3.2% affected.[6]

Patella Luxation: Polygenically inherited laxity of patellar ligaments, causing luxation, lameness, and later degenerative joint disease. Treat surgically if causing clinical signs. OFA reports 1.5% affected.[6]

Elbow Dysplasia: Polygenically inherited trait causing elbow arthritis. OFA reports 2.4% affected.[6]

Pyruvate Kinase Deficiency (PK, Basenji Hemolytic Anemia): Autosomal recessive disorder causing severe hemolytic anemia, progressive osteomyelosclerosis, and hemosiderosis. Death occurs due to anemia or hepatic failure usually at less than five years of age. Occurs at a low frequency in the breed. A genetic test is available.[7,8,9]

Disease Predispositions

Persistent Pupillary Membranes: Strands of fetal remnant connecting; iris to iris, cornea, lens, or involving sheets of tissue. The later three forms can impair vision, and dogs affected with these forms should not be bred. PPMs can be associated with corneal opacity or coloboma in this breed. Dorn reports a 110.61x odds ratio in Basenjis versus other breeds. Identified in 47.64% of Basenjis CERF examined by veterinary ophthalmologists between 2000-2005.

Of these, 9.47% were iris to cornea, 3.71% were iris to lens, and 0.47% were iris sheets. PPMs are shown to be inherited in this breed, but the mode of inheritance has not been determined.[3,10,11,12]

Hypothyroidism: Inherited autoimmune thyroiditis. 10.8% positive for thyroid auto-antibodies based on testing at Michigan State University. (Ave. for all breeds is 7.5%).[1,13,14]

Corneal Dystrophy: The endothelial form is associated with persistant papillary membranes in this breed, and can cause edema, keratits, and loss of vision. Basenjis with the endothelial form should not be bred. The epithelial-stromal form causes opacities on the surface of the cornea. Unknown mode of inheritance. The endothelial form is identified in 2.70%, and the epithelial-stromal form is identified in 2.23% of Basenjis CERF examined by veterinary ophthalmologists between 2000-2005.[10]

Cataracts: Posterior and capsular punctate cataracts predominate in the breed. Identified in 2.41% of Basenjis CERF examined by veterinary ophthalmologists between 2000-2005. CERF does not recommend breeding any Basenji with cataracts.[10]

Progressive Retinal Atrophy (PRA): Progressive degeneration of the retina, eventually causing blindness. Typical age of onset between 4 to 10 years, with some reported between ages 3 and 13. Presumed autosomal recessive inheritance. CERF recommends that any Basenji with PRA should not be bred. 1.62% of Basenjis CERF examined by veterinary ophthalmologists between 2000-2005 are labeled suspicious for PRA, and 0.65% are identified with generalized PRA. No genetic test is available.[10]

Demodicosis: Dorn reports a 2.07x odds ratio of developing demodectic mange versus other breeds. This disorder has an underlying immunodeficiency in its pathogenesis.[3]

Optic Nerve Coloboma: Congenital cavity in the optic nerve that can cause blindness or vision impairment. Affected dogs should not be bred. Identified in 0.79% of Basenjis CERF examined by veterinary ophthalmologists between 2000-2005. Can be associated with persistent pupillary membranes in this breed.[10]

Immunoproliferative Enteropathy (IPEB, IPSID, Lymphangiectasia): Inherited disorder causing chronic diarrhea, progressive emaciation, malabsorption and maldigestion. Biopsy findings include villous clubbing and fusion, increased tortuosity of intestinal crypts, and diffuse infiltration of mononuclear inflammatory cells. Lymphangectasia may be secondary. Treatment with immunosuppressive drugs and diet. Unknown mode of inheritance.[15,16]

Cystine Urinary Calculi: Seen at an increased frequency in the breed secondary to cystinuria from Fanconi syndrome.[17]

Epilepsy, Retinal Dysplasia and **Umbilical Hernia** are reported.[18]

Isolated Case Studies

Intrahepatic Venous Obstruction: Intrahepatic post-sinusoidal obstruction, similar to congenital Budd-Chiari syndrome in human patients, was diagnosed in a young Basenji dog.[19]

Genetic Tests

Tests of Genotype: Phenotypic test for Fanconi Syndrome is available from PennGen.

Linked marker test for Fanconi Syndrome is available from the OFA.

Direct test for pyruvate kinase deficiency is available from HealthGene, Optigen, PennGen, University of Missouri, and VetGen.

Direct tests for color alleles is available from VetGen.

Tests of Phenotype: CHIC Certification: Required testing includes hip radiographs, thyroid profile including autoantibodies, CERF eye examination (each year until 6, thereafter every 2 years), and linked marker test for Fanconi syndrome from OFA. (See CHIC website; www.caninehealthinfo.org).

Recommend patella evaluation, elbow radiographs, and cardiac evaluation.

Miscellaneous

- **Breed name synonyms:** Barkless dog, Congo dog, Congo Terrier
- **Registries:** AKC, CKC, UKC (provisional), KCGB (Kennel Club of Great Britain), ANKC (Australian National Kennel Club), NKC (National Kennel Club)
- **AKC rank (year 2008):** 85 (774 dogs registered)
- **Internet resources:** The Basenji Club of America: http://basenji.org
  Basenji Club of Canada: www.basenjiclubofcanada.com
  The Basenji Club of Great Britain: www.basenjiclubofgb.org
  The Basenji Health Endowment: www.basenjihealth.org

References

1. Seavers A, Snow DH, Mason KV, et. al.: Evaluation of the thyroid status of Basenji dogs in Australia. Aust Vet J. 2008 Nov;86(11):429-34.
2. Latimer KS, Prasse KW: Neutrophilic movement of a Basenji with Pelger-Huet anomaly. Am J Vet Res. 1982 Mar;43(3):525-7.
3. Dorn CR: Canine breed-specific risks of frequently diagnosed diseases at veterinary teaching hospitals. Monograph. AKC Canine Health Foundation. 2000.
4. Noonan CH, Kay JM: Prevalence and geographic distribution of Fanconi syndrome in Basenjis in the United States. J Am Vet Med Assoc. 1990 Aug 1;197(3):345-9.
5. Bovee KC, Joyce T, Reynolds R, et. al.: The fanconi syndrome in Basenji dogs: a new model for renal transport defects. Science. 1978 Sep 22;201(4361):1129-31.
6. OFA Website breed statistics: www.offa.org Last accessed July. 1, 2010.
7. Whitney KM, Goodman SA, Bailey EM, et. al.: The molecular basis of canine pyruvate kinase deficiency. Exp Hematol. 1994 Aug;22(9):866-74.
8. Burman SL, Ferrara L, Medhurst CL, et. al.: Pyruvate kinase deficiency anaemia in a Basenji dog. Aust Vet J. 1982 Oct;59(4):118-20.
9. Whitney KM, Lothrop CD Jr: Genetic test for pyruvate kinase deficiency of Basenjis. J Am Vet Med Assoc. 1995 Oct 1;207(7):918-21.
10. Ocular Disorders Presumed to be Inherited in Purebred Dogs. American College of Veterinary Ophthalmologists. ACVO, 2007
11. James RW: Persistent pupillary membrane in basenji dogs. Vet Rec. 1991 Mar 23;128(12):287-8.
12. Mason TA: Persistent pupillary membrane in the Basenji. Aust Vet J. 1976 Aug;52(8):343-4.
13. Nachreiner R and Refsal K: Personal communication, Diagnostic Center for Population and Animal Health, Michigan State University. April, 2007.
14. Nachreiner RF, Refsal KR, Graham PA, et. al.: Prevalence of serum thyroid hormone autoantibodies in dogs with clinical signs of hypothyroidism. J Am Vet Med Assoc 2002 Feb 15;220(4):466-71.

15. Spohr A, Koch J, Jensen AL: Ultrasonographic findings in a basenji with immuno-proliferative enteropathy. *J Small Anim Pract.* 1995 Feb;36(2):79-82.

16. MacLachlan NJ, Breitschwerdt EB, Chambers JM, et. al: Gastroenteritis of basenji dogs. *Vet Pathol.* 1988 Jan;25(1):36-41

17. Case LC, Ling GV, Franti CE, et. al.: Cystine-containing urinary calculi in dogs: 102 cases (1981-1989). *J Am Vet Med Assoc.* 1992 Jul 1;201(1):129-33.

18. *The Genetic Connection: A Guide to Health Problems in Purebred Dogs.* L Ackerman. p. 199, AAHA Press, 1999.

19. Cohn LA, Spaulding KA, Cullen JM, et. al.: Intrahepatic postsinusoidal venous obstruction in a dog. *J Vet Intern Med.* 1991 Nov-Dec;5(6):317-21.

20. *The Complete Dog Book, 20th Ed.* The American Kennel Club. Howell Book House, NY 12006. pp 138-141.

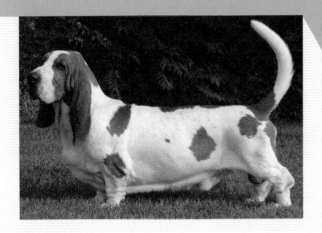

The Breed History

The origins of this breed can be traced back to France and Belgium. The first written documents to record the breed name "Basset Hound" date back to the 1580s. The breed name may derive from the French word for low, **"bas"**. First shown in the late 1800s in England, the breed was registered with AKC in 1884 and soon became popular in the USA.

Breeding for Function

These dogs were used to slow trail game such as rabbit, hare and also sometimes deer. Basset Hounds were prized for their accurate trailing, especially in thick bush. His nose is considered almost as outstanding as a Bloodhound's. Earliest records term the breed "badger hound" indicating their use for badger hunting in the early phases of breed development, and other accounts report them in hunts for wolf and boar. Here they were used in packs. For small game, they were frequently hunted in pairs (termed a brace). They are seen in field trials and tracking, obedience and are popular as well as a companion dog.

Physical Characteristics

Height at Withers: less than 14" (35.5 cm).

Weight: 40-60 lb (18-27 kg).

Coat: The dense, short smooth glossy coat is acceptable in any hound color. Red and white and tricolor are commonly seen.

Longevity: 12 years

Points of Conformation: Their short, very heavily boned legs mean they are slow moving, but agile. The head is large, and the skull has a prominent occipital protuberance. They possess a moderate stop, and skin forms wrinkles on the face when the head is down. The nose is darkly pigmented. Lips are also of dark pigmentation, and end in loose flews. A pronounced dewlap is present. The neck is very muscular and of good length. Eyes are brown and somewhat deep set. This allows the conjunctivae of the lower lids to show. They are said to have a sad expression. The ears are very long, pendulous and low set, with ends curling in. They are deep through the thorax and ribs are well sprung. The skin is significantly loose and wrinkled over the carpal and tarsal areas of the limb. Paws are large, rounded, and slightly deviated laterally from the level of the carpus. Dewclaws

are often removed. The topline is level and tail carriage is typical for hounds— carried high when on a scent. The tail is thick, slightly curved and reaches almost to the ground at rest. The gait is easy, and movement of limbs is parallel.

Recognized Behavior Issues and Traits

Reported breed characteristics include: Gentle, devoted, good for pack or individual hunting or housing, also excellent in the home. Has low grooming requirements, is loyal, active, and independent. The typical mature Basset Hound has moderate exercise needs. They are also described as stubborn, and must be kept on leash. They possess a level temperament, are good with children, and can tend to dig if bored; some are loud alarm barkers. The breed has a problem in some lines with aggressive, uneven tempered dogs. The BHCA recommends that all puppies be temperament tested before placement in homes.

Normal Physiologic Variations

Slow to mature.

They tend to gain weight easily so proper diet and exercise are essential.

Drug Sensitivities

None reported

Inherited Diseases

Hip Dysplasia: Polygenically inherited trait causing degenerative joint disease and hip arthritis. OFA reports 37.4% affected.[1]

Elbow Dysplasia: Polygenically inherited trait causing elbow arthritis. Reported at an increased frequency in the breed, but too few Basset Hounds have been screened by OFA to determine an accurate frequency. Reported 19.5x odds ratio for the fragmented coronoid process form of elbow dysplasia versus other breeds.[1,2]

Patella Luxation (Slipping Kneecaps): Polygenically inherited congenital laxity of patellar ligaments, causing luxation, lameness, and later degenerative joint disease. Treat surgically if causing clinical signs. Too few Basset Hounds have been screened by OFA to determine an accurate frequency.[1]

Basset Hound Hereditary Thrombopathy (BHT): An autosomal recessive bleeding disorder of abnormal platelet function, characterized by a thrombasthenia-like defect in aggregation but normal clot retraction. Glycoprotein IIb-IIIa (GP IIb-IIIa) is detectable in BHT platelets but may be functionally defective. A genetic test is available.[3,4]

von Willebrand's Disease: Autosomal recessive, type I form of this bleeding disorder occurs in the breed. Causes mild, or prolonged bleeding episodes. A genetic test does not exist in this breed.[5]

X-linked Severe Combined Immunodeficiency (XSCID): Rare, X-linked recessive disorder, where affected dogs cannot generate antigen-specific immune responses. A genetic test is available to identify affected males and carrier females.[6]

Disease Predispositions

Ectropion: Rolling out of eyelids, often with a medial canthal pocket. Can be secondary to **macroblepharon**; an abnormally large eyelid opening. Can also cause conjunctivitis. Ectropion is reported in 11.17%, and macroblepharon in 1.52% of Basset Hounds CERF examined by veterinary ophthalmologists between 2000-2005.[7]

Persistent Pupillary Membranes: Strands of fetal remnant connecting; iris to iris, cornea, lens, or involving sheets of tissue. The later three forms can impair vision, and dogs affected with these forms should not be bred. Identified in 5.58% of Basset Hounds CERF examined by veterinary ophthalmologists between 2000-2005.[7]

Primary (Narrow Angle) Glaucoma: Ocular condition causing increased pressure within the eyeball, and secondary blindness due to damage to the retina. Diagnose with tonometry and gonioscopy. Dorn reports an 8.03x odds ratio for developing glaucoma versus other breeds. Diagnosed in 5.44% of Basset Hounds presented to veterinary teaching hospitals.[8,9,10]

Hypothyroidism: Inherited autoimmune thyroiditis. 3.5% positive for thyroid auto-antibodies based on testing at Michigan State University. (Ave. for all breeds is 7.5%).[11,12]

Cataracts: Anterior cortex cataracts predominate, though posterior intermediate and punctate cataracts also occur in the breed. Unknown mode of inheritance. Identified in 3.38% of Basset Hounds CERF examined by veterinary ophthalmologists between 2000-2005. CERF does not recommend breeding any Basset Hound with a cataract.[7]

Distichiasis: Abnormally placed eyelashes that irritate the cornea and conjunctiva. Can cause secondary corneal ulceration. Identified in 1.18% of Basset Hounds CERF examined by veterinary ophthalmologists between 2000-2005.[7]

Gastric Dilation/Volvulus (GDV, Bloat): Life-threatening twisting of the stomach within the abdomen. Requires immediate veterinary attention. Occurs at an increased frequency in the breed.[13]

Intervertebral Disk Disease: The breed is at increased risk for acute paralysis/pain from intervertebral disk extrusion and spinal cord damage. This is an emergency situation that requires immediate veterinary attention.[14]

Idiopathic Seborrhea: Occurs at an increased frequency in the breed, often with concurrent *Malassezia pachydermatis* infection.[15,16]

Temporomandibular Joint (TMJ) Dysplasia: Increased prevalence in the breed of mandibular subluxation when the mouth is opened widely, due to TMJ dysplasia. This results in locking of the coronoid process lateral to the zygomatic arch. Locking can be prevented by osteotomy of a ventral portion of the zygomatic arch.[17]

Retinal Dysplasia: Focal folds are seen in the breed. Focal folds were identified in 1.02% of Basset Hounds CERF examined by veterinary ophthalmologists between 2000-2005.[7]

Persistent Hyaloid Artery: Congenital defect resulting from abnormalities in the development and regression of the hyaloid artery. Identified in 1.02% of Basset Hounds CERF examined by veterinary ophthalmologists between 2000-2005.[7]

Cystinuria/Cystine Bladder Stones: Basset Hounds have an increased risk for developing cystine bladder stones due to a defect in cystine metabolism. Treat with surgical removal and life-long medical therapy. Unknown mode of inheritance in this breed.[18]

Lafora's Disease (Myoclonus Epilepsy): Diagnosed in several Basset hounds with a progressive central nervous system disease culminating in epileptic seizures. Histologically, Lafora bodies are found in neurons and free in the neuropil throughout the cerebrum and cerebellum.[19,20]

Allergic Inhalant Dermatitis, Black Hair Follicular Dysplasia, Brachygnathism, Cervical Vertebral Instability, Corneal Dystrophy, Dermatomyositis, Dilated Cardiomyopathy, Elongated Soft palate, Globoid Cell Leukodystrophy, Hemivertebra, Hypoadrenocorticism, Mycobacterial Susceptibility, Panosteitis, Progressive Retinal Atrophy, Prolapsed Gland of the Nictitans, Pulmonic Stenosis, Sebaceous Adentitis, Subaortic Stenosis, and **Wobbler Syndrome** are reported.[21]

Isolated Case Studies

Sry-negative XX True Hermaphrodite (XX Sex reversal): A phenotypically male 7 month old Basset hound was examined. The chromosomal sex was female (XX), and there was an absence of "male" causing Sry. XX Sex-reversal is familial in other breeds.[22]

Persistent Hyperplastic Tunica Vasculosa Lentis (PHTVL) and Persistent Hyaloid Artery: A 2-year-old Basset hound with unilateral persistent hyperplastic tunica vasculosa lentis and primary vitreous is described. There was leukokoria in the left eye, caused by bluish-white polar densities and hemorrhagic discoloration in the nucleus of the lens.[23]

Persistent Mullerian Duct Syndrome: Diagnosed in a male dog with oviducts, a uterus, and cranial vaginal tract. Usually caused by a defective mullerian inhibiting substance (MIS) receptor.[24]

Congenital Hypotrichosis: Four 4 week-old Basset Hound littermates with predominantly mahogany coats had congenital focal alopecia especially affecting the head and dorsal pelvic region. Histologic diagnosis was hypotrichosis.[25]

Genetic Tests

Tests of Genotype: Direct test for XSCID is available from PennGen.

Direct test for thrombopathia is available from AuburnUniversity:(www.vetmed.auburn.edu/index.pl/boudreaux_mk)

Tests of Phenotype: BHCA recommends hip and elbow radiographs, CERF eye examination (including gonioscopy for glaucoma), thyroid profile including autoantibodies, von Willebrand's factor antigen testing, temperament testing (Puppy Aptitude Testing or American Temperament Test Society certification), and genetic test for thrombopathia.

CHIC Certification: Required testing includes CERF eye examination and gonioscopy (OFA form). Optional testing includes genetic test for thrombopathia. (See CHIC website; www.caninehealthinfo.org).

Recommend patella evaluation and cardiac evaluation.

Miscellaneous

- **Breed name synonyms:** Basset.
- **Registries:** AKC, UKC, CKC, KCGB (Kennel Club of Great Britain), ANKC (Australian National Kennel Club), NKC (National Kennel Club).
- **AKC rank (year 2008):** 33 (5,277 registered)
- **Internet resources: Basset Hound Club of America:**
  www.basset-bhca.org
  The Bassett Hound Club of Canada:
  www.bassethoundclubofcanada.ca
  The Bassett Hound Club (UK): www.bassethoundclub.co.uk

References

1. OFA Website breed statistics: www.offa.org Last accessed July 1, 2010.
2. LaFond E, Breur GJ and Austin CC: Breed susceptibility for developmental orthopedic diseases in dogs. J Am Anim Hosp Assoc. 2002 Sep-Oct;38(5):467-77.
3. Patterson WR, Estry DW, Schwartz KA, et. al.: Absent platelet aggregation with normal fibrinogen binding in basset hound hereditary thrombopathy. *Thromb Haemost.* 1989 Nov 24;62(3):1011-5.
4. Mattson JC, Estry DW, Bell TG, et. al.: Defective contact activation of platelets from dogs with basset hound hereditary thrombopathy. *Thromb Res.* 1986 Oct 1;44(1):23-38.
5. Dodds WJ: Bleeding Disorders in Animals. Proceedings, 2005 World Small Animal Veterinary Association Congress. 2005
6. Perryman LE: Molecular pathology of severe combined immunodeficiency in mice, horses, and dogs. *Vet Pathol.* 2004 Mar;41(2):95-100.
7. *Ocular Disorders Presumed to be Inherited in Purebred Dogs.* American College of Veterinary Ophthalmologists. ACVO, 2007
8. Gelatt KN, MacKay EO: Prevalence of the breed-related glaucomas in pure-bred dogs in North America. *Vet Ophthalmol.* 2004 Mar-Apr;7(2):97-111.
9. Dorn CR: Canine breed-specific risks of frequently diagnosed diseases at veterinary teaching hospitals. Monograph. AKC Canine Health Foundation. 2000.
10. Wyman M, Ketring K: Congenital glaucoma in the basset hound: a biologic model. *Trans Sect Ophthalmol Am Acad Ophthalmol Otolaryngol.* 1976 Jul-Aug;81(4 Pt 1):OP645-52.
11. Nachreiner R and Refsal K: Personal communication, Diagnostic Center for Population and Animal Health, Michigan State University. April, 2007.
12. Nachreiner RF, Refsal KR, Graham PA, et. al.: Prevalence of serum thyroid hormone autoantibodies in dogs with clinical signs of hypothyroidism. J Am Vet Med Assoc 2002 Feb 15;220(4):466-71.
13. Glickman LT, Glickman NW, Perez CM, et. al.: Analysis of risk factors for gastric dilatation and dilatation-volvulus in dogs. *J Am Vet Med Assoc.* 1994 May 1;204(9):1465-71.
14. Dallman MJ, Palettas P, Bojrab MJ: Characteristics of dogs admitted for treatment of cervical intervertebral disk disease: 105 cases (1972-1982). J Am Vet Med Assoc 1992:200[12]:2009-2011.
15. Power HT, Ihrke PJ, Stannard AA, et. al.: Use of etretinate for treatment of primary keratinization disorders (idiopathic seborrhea) in cocker spaniels, west highland white terriers, and basset hounds. J Am Vet Med Assoc. 1992 Aug 1;201(3):419-29.
16. Bond R, Ferguson EA, Curtis CF, et. al.: Factors associated with elevated cutaneous Malassezia pachydermatis populations in dogs with pruritic skin disease. *J Small Anim Pract.* 1996 Mar;37(3):103-7.
17. Robins G, Grandage J: Temporomandibular joint dysplasia and open-mouth jaw locking in the dog. *J Am Vet Med Assoc.* 1977 Nov 15;171(10):1072-6.
18. Hoppe A, Denneberg T: Cystinuria in the dog: clinical studies during 14 years of medical treatment. *J Vet Intern Med.* 2001 Jul-Aug;15(4):361-7.
19. Jian Z, Alley MR, Cayzer J, et. al.: Lafora's disease in an epileptic Basset hound. *N Z Vet J.* 1990 Jun;38(2):75-9.
20. Kaiser E, Krauser K, Schwartz-Porsche D: Lafora disease (progressive myoclonic epilepsy) in the Bassett hound--possibility of early diagnosis using muscle biopsy? *Tierarztl Prax.* 1991 Jun;19(3):290-5.
21. *The Genetic Connection: A Guide to Health Problems in Purebred Dogs.* L Ackerman. p. 199. AAHA Press, 1999.
22. Hubler M, Hauser B, Meyers-Wallen VN, et. al.: Sry-negative XX true hermaphrodite in a Basset hound. *Theriogenology.* 1999 May;51(7):1391-403.
23. Verbruggen AM, Boroffka SA, Boeve MH, et. al.: Persistent hyperplastic tunica vasculosa lentis and persistent hyaloid artery in a 2-year-old basset hound. *Vet Q.* 1999 Apr;21(2):63-5.
24. Nickel RF, Ubbink G, van der Gaag I, et. al.: Persistent mullerian duct syndrome in the basset hound. *Tijdschr Diergeneeskd.* 1992 Apr;117 Suppl 1:31S.
25. Chastain CB, Swayne DE: Congenital hypotrichosis in male basset hound littermates. *J Am Vet Med Assoc.* 1985 Oct 15;187(8):845-6
26. *The Complete Dog Book, 20th Ed.* The American Kennel Club. Howell Book House, NY 2006. p. 142-146.

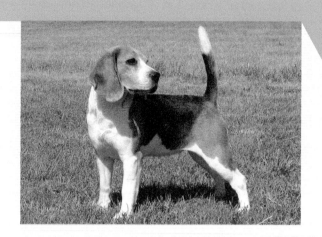

Beagle

Points of Conformation: The skull is broad and slightly domed, ears are long and pendulous with round tips that hang in towards the cheek, the leather is fine, and the ear pinna is broad. Eyes are soft in expression, brown or hazel in color, large and wide-set. Beagles have a moderate stop and square muzzle, minimal flews, large nose and the nostrils start out black but fade with maturity. The neck is medium in length and muscling with no throatiness. The back is short, ribs are well sprung, and forelegs are straight boned. Feet are compact and round. The tail is held high but not over the back, and is shorter than most hound tails and is slightly curved with brush.

The Breed History

Though one of the most popular modern dog breeds, the origins of the Beagle are obscure. Some reports place them in England before Roman times. Many of the early reports date to the 1300s. It is thought that their early lineage included crosses out to other scent hounds, and Foxhounds are variably thought to be derived from the Beagle as a result of those crosses, or perhaps Foxhounds were crossed back to be an early influence on beagle type. The mid 18th century reports indicate two types of hare hunting hounds. The modern beagle apparently derives from the North Country Beagle. The modern American lines were first imported in the 1860s and 1880s. The breed name origins are also obscure, with deviation from Olde English, French or Celtic being cited; the derivative may be from roots such as "begle", "beag", or "begele".

Breeding for Function

As hunters, they are courageous and have a great deal of stamina. They hunt equally well in packs, braced (pairs) or solo, though they are most commonly hunted in packs. They are scent hounds and were bred to hunt hare and rabbit. Today, they are most commonly companion dogs.

Physical Characteristics

Height at Withers: Two distinct varieties:
1. Thirteen Inch: up to 13" high.
2. Fifteen Inch: 13-15" high (maximum height 15" in the United States, 16" in England).

Weight: Thirteen inch variety is generally less than 20 lb (9 kg), Fifteen inch variety is generally 20-30 lb (9-13.5 kg).

Coat: The hard, short-medium outer coat hairs may be of any hound colors. The haircoat is dense. Black, tan and white tri-color is very popular, also common are the red and white. Irish Spotting is a specific spotted marking distribution. Ticking is also accepted; blue tick and red tick being the most common of this pattern. Patch beagle refers to a predominantly white beagle strain (with large black, lemon or red patches generally). Dilutes (e.g., blue) in the coat are also accepted.

Longevity: 13-15 years

Recognized Behavior Issues and Traits

Reported breed characteristics include: Loyal, gentle, trustworthy, playful, adaptable, affectionate, but can be prone to independent thinking and will wander off if not kept on leash or fenced in. The fence needs to be secure to prevent digging and jumping escapes. Considered excellent with children due to a low aggression tendency, assuming they are properly socialized. They possess a moderate to high barking tendency. Not considered a watchdog. Good with other pets, though may chase small ones if not accommodated to their presence.

They have low grooming needs and low to moderate shedding tendency. Good for city or country living. Beagles have low to moderate exercise needs. They need close human companionship or may howl or become destructive. Can be more of a challenge to housebreak than some of the other breeds. Tend to gain weight unless given adequate exercise and dietary intake is controlled.

Normal Physiologic Variations

Echocardiographic Normal Values:[1]	
Parameter	Range
Weight (kg)	5.5-12.0
LVPWD (mm)	6-13
LVPWS (mm)	7-17
LVD (mm)	18-33
LVS (mm)	8-27
FS (%)	20-70
EF (%)	40-100
IVSd (mm)	5-11
IVSs (mm)	6-12
N	50

LVPWD, LV posterior wall dimension at end-diastole; LVPWS, LV posterior wall thickness at end-systole; LVD, LV chamber dimension at end-diastole; LVS, LV chamber dimension at end-systole; FS, percent fractional shortening; EF, ejection fraction; IVSd, interventricular septal thickness at end-diastole; IVSs, interventricular septal thickness at end-systole; N, number of animals.

Drug Sensitivities

None reported

Inherited Diseases

Hip Dysplasia: Polygenically inherited trait causing degenerative joint disease and hip arthritis. OFA reports 17.8% affected.[2]

Patella Luxation: Polygenically inherited trait causing stifle instability and arthritis. OFA reports 1.4% affected.[2]

Elbow Dysplasia: Polygenically inherited trait causing elbow arthritis. Too few Beagles have been evaluated by OFA to determine an accurate frequency.[2]

Primary (Narrow and Open Angle) Glaucoma: Autosomal recessive glaucoma causes bilateral increased pressure within the eyeball between 1-2 years of age. Secondary blindness occurs due to damage to the retina. Diagnose with tonometry and gonioscopy. Diagnosed in 1.10% of Beagles presented to veterinary teaching hospitals. Beagles with open angle glaucoma have increased myocilin protein levels in the aqueous humor, with intermediate levels in heterozygous carriers. A genetic test is not available. CERF does not recommend breeding any Beagle with glaucoma.[3,4,5,6]

Factor VII Deficiency: An autosomal recessive, mild to moderate bleeding disorder occurs in the breed due to a mutation in the cFVII gene. A genetic test is available.[7,8]

Chondrodystrophy (Dwarfism): An autosomal recessive dwarfism occurs in the breed. Affected dogs have a small and disproportionate body size, a shortened neck, curved, deformed legs, a broadened skull, and chronic arthritis. They can be diagnosed by by x-ray stippling (i.e., punctate bright spots) of the wrist bones under 3 months of age, or by a compressed L7 vertebrae at over 6 months. Genetic research is ongoing to identify the defective gene at the Mark Neff lab.

Musladin–Leuke Syndrome (MLS, Chinese Beagle Syndrome): An autosomal recessive disease that affects the development and structure of connective tissue. It is multi-systemic, with involvement of multiple organs, including bone, heart, skin, and muscle. Affected dogs walk up on their toes due to tendon contracture. They often have tighter skin with limited "scruff". They have a flat skull, higher ear set and slanted eyes. The disease shows variable expressivity, and affected dogs live a normal lifespan. See the National Beagle Club and UV-Davis VGL websites for more information. A genetic test is available.

Pyruvate Kinase Deficiency (PK): A rare, autosomal recessive disease of red blood cells causing exercise intolerance with a persistent, severe, and highly regenerative anemia, splenomegaly, and progressive osteosclerosis. A genetic test is available.[9,10]

Tapetal Degeneration: A rare, autosomal recessive degeneration of the tapetum occurs as a result of abnormal postnatal melanosome development. The degeneration of the tapetum does not affect vision and does not result in functional or structural damage to the retina.[3,11]

Disease Predispositions

Periodontal Disease: Beagles are predisposed to periodontal disease, with 44% by two years of age, and up to 81% of older dogs affected. The maxillary premolars are most frequently affected. Few affected Beagles are clinically impaired, though halitosis and gingivitis are usually present.[12,13]

Distichiasis: Abnormally placed eyelashes that irritate the cornea and conjunctiva. Can cause secondary corneal ulceration. Identified in 17.30% of Beagles CERF examined by veterinary ophthalmologists between 2000-2005.[3]

Hypothyroidism: Inherited autoimmune thyroiditis. 16.5% positive for thyroid autoantibodies based on testing at Michigan State University. (Ave. for all breeds is 7.5).[14,15,16]

Retinal Dysplasia: Focal folds are seen in the breed. Identified in 2.70% of Beagles CERF examined by veterinary ophthalmologists between 2000-2005.[3]

Cataracts: Anterior and posterior cataracts are equally represented in the breed, and can be intermediate or punctate. Reported in 2.16% of Beagles CERF examined by veterinary ophthalmologists between 2000-2005. CERF does not recommend breeding any Beagle with a cataract.[3]

Intervertebral Disc Disease (IVDD): Spinal cord disease due to prolapsed disk material. Clinical signs include back pain, scuffing of paws, spinal ataxia, limb weakness, and paralysis. Almost all dogs with IVDD have calcified disk material. Beagles are significantly over-represented with cervical IVDD. Dorn reports a 1.39x odds ratio versus other breeds.[17,18]

Cryptorchidism (Retained Testicles): Can be unilateral or bilateral. This is a sex-limited disorder with an unknown mode of inheritance. Reported as a breed issue on the National Beagle Club website.

Diabetes Mellitus (Sugar Diabetes): Almost exclusively female Beagles are at increased risk of developing diabetes due to immune mediated destruction of the pancreatic beta cells. Treat with insulin injections, dietary management, and glucose monitoring.[19]

Corneal Dystrophy: The breed can form oval epithelial corneal opacities that can progressively block vision. They do not lead to corneal edema.[3,20]

Persistent Pupillary Membranes: Strands of fetal remnant connecting; iris to iris, cornea, lens, or involving sheets of tissue. The later three forms can impair vision, and dogs affected with these forms should not be bred. Identified in 1.62% of Beagles CERF examined by veterinary ophthalmologists between 2000-2005.[3]

Prolapsed Gland of the Nictitans (Cherry Eye): This condition occurs secondary to inflammation of the gland. Identified in 1.35% of Beagles CERF examined by veterinary ophthalmologists between 2000-2005.[3]

Idiopathic Epilepsy (Inherited Seizures): Control with anti-seizure medication. Seizures generally start under one year of age. Reported as a breed issue on the National Beagle Club website.[21]

Pulmonic Stenosis: Narrowing of the right ventricular outflow tract/pulmonary artery. Clinical signs in severely affected dogs include exercise intolerance, stunting, dyspnea, syncope and ascites. A left systolic murmur is present on auscultation. Beagles are over-represented.[22,23]

Juvenile Polyarteritis (Beagle Pain Syndrome): A naturally occurring vasculitis and perivasculitis of unknown etiology occurs in 6-40 month old Beagles, presenting with episodes of fever and neck pain that last 3-7 days. Histologically, the small-to-medium-sized muscular arteries of the heart, cranial mediastinum, and cervical spinal meninges are consistently involved. Undetermined mode of inheritance.[24]

Bladder and Urethral Tumors: Beagles are over-represented with tumors of the bladder and urethra versus other breeds.[25]

Microphthalmia with Multiple Congenital Ocular Defects: Several congenital unilateral and bilateral microphthalmia syndromes are recognized in the breed with associated corneal, lens, and retinal defects. Reported in 0.54% of Beagles CERF examined by veterinary ophthalmologists between 2000-2005. CERF does not recommend breeding any Beagle with microphthalmia.[3,26]

Deafness: Congenital deafness can be unilateral or bilateral. Associated with extreme piebald pigmentation. Diagnose by BAER testing. Unknown mode of inheritance.[27]

Renal Amyloidosis: Beagles were over-represented in a study of renal amyloidosis. Affected dogs were over 6 years of age, with a female preponderance. Clinical signs were consistent with renal failure. Histopathology showed moderate to severe diffuse global glomerular amyloidosis without tubular or glomerular lesions.[28]

Progressive Myoclonic Epilepsy (Lafora's Disease): Older affected Beagles show progressive, intermittent seizures that can progress to status epilepticus. The seizures are often elicited by external stimuli, especially a change in noise or light in the surroundings. Electroencephalographic findings show myoclonus epilepsy. Postmortem histopathological findings include multiple periodic acid-Schiff-positive inclusion bodies consistent with Lafora's disease.[29,30]

Black Hair Follicular Dysplasia, Brachygnathism, Cervical Vertebral Instability, Cleft Lip/Palate, Copper Hepatopathy, Cutaneous Asthenia, Demodicosis, Dilated Cardiomyopathy, Dysfibrinogenemia, Ectodermal Defect, Elongated Soft Palate, Factor VIII Deficiency, Globoid Cell Leukodystrophy, GM-1 Gangliosidosis, Hyperlipidemia, Hypotrichosis, IgA Deficiency, Lissencephaly, Mitral Valve Disease, Narcolepsy, Non-Sphero-cytic Hemolytic Anemia, Optic Nerve Hypoplasia, Panosteitis, Peripheral Vestibular Disease, Prognathism, Progressive Retinal Atrophy, Shaker Disease, Spina Bifida, Vertebral Stenosis, and **XX Sex Reversal** are reported.[31]

Isolated Case Studies

Cobalamin Malabsorption (Methylmalonic Aciduria): A six-month-old beagle was presented with a three-month history of failure to gain weight, lethargy, intermittent vomiting and seizures. Laboratory results showed low serum cobalamin (Cbl)

concentrations, anaemia, leucopenia and methylmalonic aciduria. The disorder responded to parenteral vitamin B12 therapy. This has been identified as an autosomal recessive disorder in other breeds.[32]

Cerebellar Cortical Abiotrophy/Ataxia: Two of five 4-1/2 month old Beagle littermates (a male and a female) presented with cerebellar ataxia, intension tremor, and nystagmus. Purkinje cell degeneration in the cerebellar cortex was seen on necropsy. This has been identified as an autosomal recessive disorder in other breeds.[33]

Membranoproliferative Glomerulonephropathy: 5 of 7 adult Beagles from the same litter developed polyuria, polydipsia, proteinuria, and azotemia by 8 years of age. Membranoproliferative glomerulonephritis was diagnosed on light and electron microscopy of renal biopsies.[34]

Renal Agenesis: Cases of unilateral kidney agenesis have been documented in the literature. Compensatory renal hyperplasia occurs in the opposite kidney, with normal kidney values.[35,36]

Vetricular Septal/Conotruncal Defect: A family of Beagle dogs was identified with congenital heart disease characterized by ventricular septal defect and ventricular outflow abnormalities. Breeding studies suggested an autosomal recessive mode of inheritance.[37]

Genetic Tests

Tests of Genotype: Direct test for MLS is available from UC-Davis VGL.

Direct tests for PK and Factor VII deficiencies are available from PennGen.

Direct test for Factor VII deficiency is available from VetGen.

Direct test for coat color alleles is available from VetGen.

Tests of Phenotype: CHIC certification: Required testing includes hip radiographs, CERF eye examination a direct test for MLS, and either a cardiac evaluation by a cardiologist, or a thyroid profile including autoantibodies. (See CHIC website; www.caninehealthinfo.org).

Recommend patella evaluation and elbow radiographs.

Urine test for Cobalamine Malabsorption/Methylmalonic Aciduria is available from PennGen.

Miscellaneous

- **Breed name synonyms:** English Beagle, Pocket beagle and Glove beagle are historical nicknames for the smallest of the small variety.
- **Registries:** AKC, UKC, CKC, KCGB (Kennel Club of Great Britain), ANKC (Australian National Kennel Club), NKC (National Kennel Club).
- **AKC rank (year 2008):** 5 (33,722 dogs registered)
- **Internet resources:** The National Beagle Club: http://clubs.akc.org/NBC/
  The Beagle Club (UK): www.thebeagleclub.org

References

1. Crippa L, Ferro E, Melloni E, et. al.: Echocardiographic parameters and indices in the normal beagle dog. Lab Anim. 1992 Jul;26(3):190-5.

2. OFA Website breed statistics: www.offa.org Last accessed July 1, 2010.

3. Ocular Disorders Presumed to be Inherited in Purebred Dogs. American College of Veterinary Ophthalmologists. ACVO, 2007.

4. Gelatt KN, MacKay EO: Prevalence of the breed-related glaucomas in pure-bred dogs in North America. Vet Ophthalmol. 2004 Mar-Apr;7(2):97-111.

5. Mackay EO, Källberg ME, and Gelatt KN: Aqueous humor myocilin protein levels in normal, genetic carriers, and glaucoma Beagles. Vet Ophthalmol. 2008 May-Jun;11(3):177-85.

6. Gelatt KN and Gum GG: Inheritance of primary glaucoma in the beagle. Am J Vet Res. 1981 Oct;42(10):1691-3.

7. Spurling NW, Burton LK, Peacock R, et. al.: Hereditary factor-VII deficiency in the beagle. Br J Haematol. 1972 Jul;23(1):59-67.

8. Callan MB, Aljamali MN, Margaritis P, et. al.: A novel missense mutation responsible for factor VII deficiency in research Beagle colonies. J Thromb Haemost. 2006 Dec;4(12):2616-22.

9. Prasse KW, Crouser D, Beutler E, et. al.: Pyruvate kinase deficiency anemia with terminal myelofibrosis and osteosclerosis in a beagle. J Am Vet Med Assoc. 1975 Jun 15;166(12):1170-5.

10. Giger U, Mason GD, and Wang P: Inherited erythrocyte pyruvate kinase deficiency in a beagle dog. Vet Clin Pathol. 1991;20(3):83-86.

11. Burns MS, Bellhorn RW, Impellizzeri CW, et. al.: Development of hereditary tapetal degeneration in the beagle dog. Curr Eye Res. 1988 Feb;7(2):103-14.

12. Kortegaard HE, Eriksen T, and Baelum V: Periodontal disease in research beagle dogs - an epidemiological study. J Small Anim Pract. 2008 Dec;49(12):610-6.

13. Saxe SR, Greene JC, Bohannan HM, et. al.: Oral debris, calculus, and periodontal disease in the beagle dog. Periodontics. 1967 Sep-Oct;5(5):217-25.

14. Nachreiner RF, Refsal KR, Graham PA, et. al.: Prevalence of serum thyroid hormone autoantibodies in dogs with clinical signs of hypothyroidism. *J Am Vet Med Assoc* 2002 Feb 15;220(4):466-71.

15. Nachreiner R and Refsal K: Personal communication, Diagnostic Center for Population and Animal Health, Michigan State University. April, 2007.

16. Musser E and Graham WR: Familial occurrence of thyroiditis in purebred beagles. Lab Anim Care. 1968 Feb;18(1):58-68.

17. Dorn CR: Canine breed-specific risks of frequently diagnosed diseases at veterinary teaching hospitals. Monograph. AKC Canine Health Foundation. 2000.

18. Dallman MJ, Palettas P, and Bojrab MJ: Characteristics of dogs admitted for treatment of cervical intervertebral disk disease: 105 cases (1972-1982). J Am Vet Med Assoc. 1992 Jun15;200(12):2009-11.

19. Fall T, Hamlin HH, Hedhammar A, et. al.: Diabetes mellitus in a population of 180,000 insured dogs: incidence, survival, and breed distribution. J Vet Intern Med. 2007 Nov-Dec;21(6):1209-16.

20. Ekins MB, Sgoutas DS, Waring GO 3rd, et. al.: Oval lipid corneal opacities in beagles: VI. Quantitation of excess stromal cholesterol and phospholipid. Exp Eye Res. 1983 Feb;36(2):279-86.

21. Morita T, Shimada A, Ohama E, et. al.: Oligodendroglial vacuolar degeneration in the bilateral motor cortices and astrocytosis in epileptic beagle dogs. J Vet Med Sci. 1999 Feb;61(2):107-11.

22. McCaw D and Aronson E: Congenital cardiac disease in dogs. Mod Vet Pract. 1984 Jul;65(7):509-12.

23. Patterson DF, Haskins ME, and Schnarr WR: Hereditary dysplasia of the pulmonary valve in beagle dogs. Pathologic and genetic studies. Am J Cardiol. 1981 Mar;47(3):631-41.

24. Snyder PW, Kazacos EA, Scott-Moncrieff JC, et. al.: Pathologic features of naturally occurring juvenile polyarteritis in beagle dogs. Vet Pathol. 1995 Jul;32(4):337-45.

25. Norris AM, Laing EJ, Valli VE, et. al.: Canine bladder and urethral tumors: a retrospective study of 115 cases (1980-1985). J Vet Intern Med. 1992 May-Jun;6(3):145-53.

26. Rubin LF: Hereditary microphakia and microphthalmia syndrome in the beagle. Trans Am Coll Vet Ophthalmol 1971;2:50.

27. Strain GM: Deafness prevalence and pigmentation and gender associations in dog breeds at risk. Vet J. 2004 Jan;167(1):23-32.

28. DiBartola SP, Tarr MJ, Parker AT, et. al.: Clinicopathologic findings in dogs with renal amyloidosis: 59 cases (1976-1986). J Am Vet Med Assoc. 1989 Aug 1;195(3):358-64.

29. Hegreberg GA and Padgett GA: Inherited progressive epilepsy of the dog with comparisons to Lafora's disease of man. Fed Proc. 1976 Apr;35(5):1202-5.

30. Gredal H, Berendt M, and Leifsson PS: Progressive myoclonus epilepsy in a beagle. J Small Anim Pract. 2003 Nov;44(11):511-4.

31. The Genetic Connection: A Guide to Health Problems in Purebred Dogs. L Ackerman. p. 199-200. AAHA Press, 1999.

32. Fordyce HH, Callan MB, and Giger U: Persistent cobalamin deficiency causing failure to thrive in a juvenile beagle. J Small Anim Pract. 2000 Sep;41(9):407-10.

33. Kent M, Glass E, and deLahunta A: Cerebellar cortical abiotrophy in a beagle. J Small Anim Pract. 2000 Jul;41(7):321-3.

34. Rha JY, Labato MA, Ross LA, et. al.: Familial glomerulonephropathy in a litter of beagles. J Am Vet Med Assoc. 2000 Jan 1;216(1):46-50, 32.

35. Diez-Prieto I, García-Rodríguez MB, Ríos-Granja MA, et. al.: Diagnosis of renal agenesis in a beagle. J Small Anim Pract. 2001 Dec;42(12):599-602.

36. Robbins GR: Unilateral renal agenesis in the beagle. Vet Rec. 1965 Nov 13;77(46):1345-7.

37. Diez-Prieto I, García-Rodríguez B, Ríos-Granja A, et. al.: Cardiac conotruncal malformations in a family of beagle dogs. J Small Anim Pract. 2009 Nov;50(11):597-603.

38. *The Complete Dog Book, 20th Ed.* The American Kennel Club. Howell Book House, NY 2006. p. 147-151.

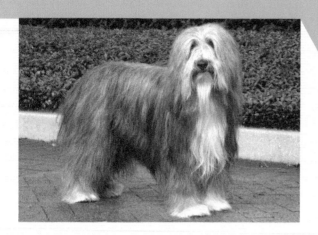

Bearded Collie

can be independent, sometimes a bit stubborn perhaps, but make an exceptional pet for the right owner. They are also reported to be loving, active (bouncy is a word commonly used), and friendly. They have a strong chase instinct, so should not run off-leash out of an enclosure. They like close contact with their family. They are strong alarm barkers and very loyal. Early training and socialization are important. Exercise should include lots of play to help keep them fit and mentally challenged. They may try to herd children by nipping at heels.

The Breed History

An ancient British Isles breed, this Collie may have blood from a variety of stock such as Polish Lowland Sheepdog, Magyar Komondor, and sheep herding dogs of the Isles. Though they do not look like the traditional "collie" image, the name collie merely implies being a sheep dog. Little is in the record until the start of the 1800s for this breed. They came to North America in the 1950s, but were not registered in the AKC until 1976.

Breeding for Function

Bred for herding independently, these dogs also excel at competitive agility and obedience sports. They are excellent drivers and caretakers of livestock. They are particularly suited to working in cold, damp conditions over rough ground. They were also selected for companionship later in breed development.

Physical Characteristics

Height at Withers: female 20-21" (51-53 cm), male 21-22" (53-56 cm).

Weight: females 40-60 lb (18-27 kg), males 40-60 lb (18-27 kg).

Coat: They are double-coated and the outer coat is harsh and flat. No coat trimming is allowed for showing. Black, fawn, blue, brown with or without white markings are the accepted colors, and coats are characteristically thick and shaggy. Coats usually lighten as they mature, then darken and then fade once again as the dog ages.

Longevity: 12-14 years.

Points of Conformation: Medium-sized, they have an athletic build, and their alert inquisitive expression is a feature of the breed. The head is broad with moderate stop, the nose is large and eyes are widely set. Color of nose and eyes are in harmony with the haircoat. Prominent brows frame their large eyes, and their beard is also well developed. Medium-sized ears are pendulous and hairy. The medium neck is slightly arched, topline is level, and the thorax is deep but not broad. The tip of the tail reaches to the tarsus, and is carried low and curved. Feet are oval and toes well arched. Gait is long and straight.

Recognized Behavior Issues and Traits

These dogs are noted for their level temperament and high intelligence. These dogs require a lot of exercise and grooming. They

Normal Physiologic Variations

This breed is slow to mature.

Beardies may be sensitive to loud noises.

Drug Sensitivities

None reported

Inherited Diseases

Hip Dysplasia: Polygenically inherited trait causing degenerative joint disease and hip arthritis. OFA reports 6.1% affected.[1]

Hypoadrenocorticism (Addison's disease): Immune mediated destruction of the adrenal gland. Typical presentation of lethargy, poor appetite, vomiting, weakness, and dehydration can occur from 4 months to several years of age. Controlled by a major recessive gene, but not a simple recessive disorder. Estimated heritability of 0.76. Estimated at a frequency of 2% to 3.4% in the breed. Treatment with DOCA injections or oral fludrocortisone.[2]

Elbow Dysplasia: Polygenically inherited trait causing elbow arthritis. OFA reports 2.6% affected.[1]

Patella Luxation: Polygenically inherited laxity of patellar ligaments, causing luxation, lameness, and later degenerative joint disease. Treat surgically if causing clinical signs. Too few Bearded Collies have been screened by OFA to determine an accurate frequency.[1]

Disease Predispositions

Cataracts: Anterior or posterior punctate cataracts predominate in the breed. Identified in 4.53% of Bearded Collies CERF examined by veterinary ophthalmologists between 2000-2005. CERF does not recommend breeding any Bearded Collie with a cataract.[3]

Persistent Pupillary Membranes: Strands of fetal remnant connecting; iris to iris, cornea, lens, or involving sheets of tissue. The later three forms can impair vision, and dogs affected with these forms should not be bred. Identified in 4.35% of Bearded Collies CERF examined by veterinary ophthalmologists between 2000-2005.[3]

Hypothyroidism: Inherited autoimmune thyroiditis. 4.3% positive for thyroid auto-antibodies based on testing at Michigan State

University. (Ave. for all breeds is 7.5%). Reported at a frequency of 5.9% in the 1996 BCCA Health Survey.[4,5,6]

Retinal Dysplasia: Multifocal and geographic retinal dysplasia. Can cause retinal hemorrhage, retinal detachment, and blindness. Can also be related to subendothelial corneal opacities. Unknown mode of inheritance. Identified in 1.6% of Bearded Collies CERF examined by veterinary ophthalmologists between 2000-2005.[3]

Corneal Dystrophy: A non-inflammatory corneal opacity (white to gray) present in one or more of the corneal layers; usually inherited and bilateral. Unknown mode of inheritance. Identified in 1.33% of Bearded Collies CERF examined by veterinary ophthalmologists between 2000-2005.[3]

Choroidal Hypoplasia: Inadequate development of the choroid present at birth and non-progressive. This condition is more commonly identified in the Collie breed where it is a manifestation of "Collie Eye Anomaly". CERF does not recommend breeding any Bearded Collies affected with the disorder. No genetic test is available in the breed. Identified in 1.15% of Bearded Collies CERF examined by veterinary ophthalmologists between 2000-2005.[3]

Seasonal Flank Alopecia: Seasonal, bilateral, symmetrical alopecia affecting the flank, dorsum and tail.[7]

Primary Lens Luxation: Occurs at an increased frequency in the breed. Often progresses to secondary glaucoma and blindness. Reported relative risk of 4.48x versus other breeds.[8]

Pemphigus Foliaceus: There is a significantly higher risk of developing pemphigus foliaceus versus other breeds. Typical lesions include dorsal muzzle and head symmetric scaling, crusting, and alopecia with peripheral collarettes, characteristic footpad lesions, with erythematous swelling at the pad margins, cracking, and villous hypertrophy. Average age of onset is 4 years. Treatment with corticosteroid and cytotoxic medications. One-year survival rate of 53%. Unknown mode of inheritance.[9]

Symmetrical Lupoid Onychodystrophy: Disorder causing loss of toenails. Onset between 3-8 years of age, affecting 1-2 nails, then progressing to all toenails within 2-9 weeks. Requires lifelong treatment with oral fatty acid supplementation. Multiple affected Bearded Collies have been identified indicating a breed prevalence, but there is no known mode of inheritance.[10]

Brachygnathism, Cleft Lip/Palate, Cryptorchidism, Epilepsy, Oligodontia, Patent Ductus Arteriosus, Prognathism, Progressive Retinal Atrophy, Subaortic Stenosis, Systemic Lupus Erythematosus, and **von Willebrand's Disease** are reported.[11]

Isolated Case Studies

Black Hair Follicular Dysplasia: Identified in one litter of Bearded Collies. Congenital breaking off and loss of black hairs. Total hair loss (of black hairs) by 6-9 months. No treatment is available. Unknown mode of inheritance.[12]

Ectopic Hepatocellular Carcinoma: An ectopic focus of hepatic tissue with associated hepatocellular carcinoma was identified in the greater omentum of a 14-year-old neutered male Bearded Collie.[13]

Genetic Tests

Tests of Genotype: none

Tests of Phenotype: CHIC certification: Required testing includes hip radiographs, CERF eye examination (each year until 5, then every 2 years), and thyroid profile including autoantibodies (each year until 5, then every 2 years). Optional recommended tests include elbow radiographs. (See CHIC website; www.caninehealthinfo.org).

Recommend patella evaluation and cardiac evaluation.

Miscellaneous

- **Breed name synonyms:** Beardie, Highland Collie (historical), Mountain Collie (historical), Hairy Mou'ed Collie (historical) Highland Sheepdog (historical)
- **Registries:** AKC, CKC, UKC, KCGB (Kennel Club of Great Britain), ANKC (Australian National Kennel Club), NKC (National Kennel Club)
- **AKC rank (year 2008):** 109 (383 dogs registered)
- **Internet resources: Bearded Collie Club of America:** www.beardie.net/bcca
  Bearded Collie Club of Canada: http://bccc.pair.com
  Bearded Collie Club (UK): www.beardedcollieclub.co.uk
  BeaCon For Health: Bearded Collie Foundation for Health: www.beaconforhealth.org

References

1. OFA Website breed statistics: www.offa.org Last accessed July 1, 2010.
2. Oberbauer AM, Benemann KS, Belanger JM, et. al.: Inheritance of hypoadrenocorticism in bearded collies. *Am J Vet Res.* 2002 May;63(5):643-7.
3. *Ocular Disorders Presumed to be Inherited in Purebred Dogs.* American College of Veterinary Ophthalmologists. ACVO, 2007.
4. Bearded Collie Club of America: 1996 BCCA Health Survey. 1997.
5. Nachreiner R and Refsal K: Personal communication, Diagnostic Center for Population and Animal Health, Michigan State University. April, 2007.
6. Nachreiner RF, Refsal KR, Graham PA, et. al.: Prevalence of serum thyroid hormone autoantibodies in dogs with clinical signs of hypothyroidism. J Am Vet Med Assoc 2002 Feb 15;220(4):466-71.
7. White SD: Update on Follicular Alopecias: "Pseudo-Endocrinopathies". Proceedings, ACVIM Forum, 2005.
8. Sargan DR, Withers D, Pettitt L, et. al.: Mapping the mutation causing lens luxation in several terrier breeds. J Hered. 2007;98(5):534-8.
9. Ihrke PJ, Stannard AA, Ardans AA, et. al.: Pemphigus foliaceus in dogs: a review of 37 cases. *J Am Vet Med Assoc.* 1985 Jan 1;186(1):59-66.
10. Auxilia ST, Hill PB and Thoday KL: Canine symmetrical lupoid onychodystrophy: a retrospective study with particular reference to management. J Small Anim Pract. 2001 Feb;42(2):82-7.
11. *The Genetic Connection: A Guide to Health Problems in Purebred Dogs.* L Ackerman. P. 200-01, AAHA Press, 2999.
12. Harper RC: Congenital black hair follicular dysplasia in bearded collie puppies. *Vet Rec.* 1978 Jan 28;102(4):87.
13. Burton IR, Limpus K, Thompson KG, et. al.: Ectopic hepatocellular carcinoma in a dog. N Z Vet J. 2005 Dec; 53(6): 466-8.
14. *The Complete Dog Book, 20th Ed.* The American Kennel Club. Howell Book House, NY 2006. p.616-619.

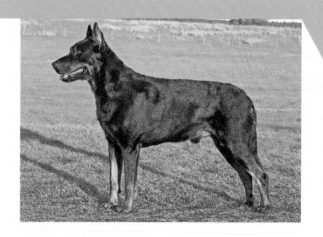

The Breed History

The Beauceron is a distinctly French herding dog, with records going back to 1578. In 1863, Pierre Megnin differentiated, with precision, two types of these sheep dogs: one with a long coat, which became known as the Berger de Brie (Briard), the other with a short coat, which is known as the Berger de Beauce (Beauceron). The bread was accepted for AKC registration in 2007.

Breeding for Function

The Beauceron gives the impression of depth and solidity without bulkiness; exhibiting the strength, endurance and agility required of the herding dog. The whole conformation is a well balanced, solid dog of good height and well muscled without heaviness or coarseness. The dog is alert and energetic with a noble carriage. The Beauceron is the preferred herding dog for sheep and cattle in France.

Physical Characteristics

Height at Withers: female 24 to 26.5" (61-67 cm), male 25.5 to 27.5" (65-70 cm).

Weight: females 80-95 lb (36-43 kg), males 90-110 lb (41-50 kg).

Coat: Outer coat is 1.25" to 1.5", coarse, dense and lying close to the body. It is short and smooth on the head, ears and lower legs. The hair is somewhat longer around the neck. Acceptable coat colors are: Black and Rust, Black and Tan, Grey Black and Tan, and Harlequin.

Longevity: 10-12 years.

Points of Conformation: The Beauceron is medium in all its proportions. The length of body, measured from the point of the shoulder to the point of the buttock, is slightly greater than the height at the withers. The head must be in proportion with the body, measured from the tip of the nose to the occiput it is about 40% of the height at the withers. The eyes are horizontal and slightly oval in shape, and dark brown. The ears are set high, and may be cropped (upright) or natural. The skull is flat or slightly rounded near the sides of the head. The muzzle must not be narrow, pointed, or excessively broad in width. The lips are well pigmented. The teeth meet in a scissors bite. The tail is strong at the base, carried down, descending at least to the point of the hock, forming into a slight J without deviating to the right or to the left. The

feet are large, round, and compact with black nails. Hind double dewclaws form well separated "thumbs" with nails, placed rather close to the foot. Movement is fluid and effortless, covering ground in long reaching strides (extended trot).

Recognized Behavior Issues and Traits

The Beauceron should be discerning and confident. He is a dog with spirit and initiative, wise and fearless with no trace of timidity. Intelligent, easily trained, faithful, gentle and obedient. The Beauceron possesses an excellent memory and an ardent desire to please his master. He retains a high degree of his inherited instinct to guard home and master. Although he can be reserved with strangers, he is loving and loyal to those he knows. Some will display a certain independence. He should be easily approached without showing signs of fear.

Normal Physiologic Variations

Merle Coat Color: Caused by a dominant mutation in the SILV gene. Breeding two merle dogs together should be avoided, as homozygous dogs can be born with multiple defects, including blindness, deafness, and heart anomalies.[1]

Harlequin Coat Color: Genetic studies on the harlequin coat color in Beaucerons have not been carried out. However, the harlequin coat color in Great Danes is due to the combined action of a dominant gene H with the merle gene M in the genotype HhM+. The H gene is a prenatal lethal when homozygous HH, so all Harlequin Great Danes are heterozygous Hh.[2]

Drug Sensitivities

None reported

Inherited Diseases

Hip Dysplasia: Polygenically inherited trait causing degenerative joint disease and hip arthritis. OFA reports 14.7% affected.[3]

Elbow Dysplasia: Polygenically inherited trait causing elbow arthritis. OFA reports 5.5% affected.[3]

Patella Luxation: Polygenically inherited laxity of patellar ligaments, causing luxation, lameness, and later degenerative joint disease. Treat surgically if causing clinical signs. Too few Beaucerons have been screened by OFA to determine an accurate frequency.[3]

Disease Predispositions

Hypothyroidism: Inherited autoimmune thyroiditis. 4.0% positive for thyroid autoantibodies based on testing at Michigan State University. (Ave. for all breeds is 7.5%).[4,5]

Gastric Dilation/Volvulus (GDV, Bloat): Polygenically inherited, life-threatening twisting of the stomach within the abdomen. Requires immediate veterinary attention. Reported as a breed problem on the Beauceron Club of Canada website.

Dermatomyositis–like Disease: Juvenile-onset (usually by 6 months of age) disease that initially presents with papules, pustules, and vesicles eventuating in crusted erosions, ulcers, and alopecia. Chronically affected Beaucerons show scarring, and either hyper or hypopigmentation. Unknown mode of inheritance.[6]

Epidermolysis Bullosa: Cutaneous blistering in response to trauma. Junctional form: Affected Beaucerons show crusted papules and erosions in genital region and at mucocutanoeuos junctions at 6 weeks. Spreads to face, pinnae, medial thighs, perianal regions, feet and tail.[7]

Ocular Disorders: Too few Beaucerons have been CERF examined by veterinary ophthalmologists to determine accurate frequencies for inherited ocular disorders. Entropion, ectropion, and progressive retinal atrophy are reported.[8]

Inhalant Allergies are reported.[9]

Isolated Case Studies

Systemic Lupus Erythematosus (SLE): A six-year-old female Beauceron presented with purulent nasal and ocular discharges, skin lesions (including seborrhea, hyperkeratotic areas, and papules as well as ecchymoses around the eyes, on both sides of the pinnae, and on the vulva), generalized lymph node enlargement, a mitral murmur, and lameness. Serum testing identified antinuclear antibody (ANA) and antidoublestranded-desoxyribonucleic acid (ds-DNA) antibody, confirmed SLE. She had concurrent generalized bacterial infections.[10]

Genetic Tests

Tests of Genotype: None available.

Tests of Phenotype: CHIC Certification: Hip radiographs, CERF eye examination (yearly from age 2 to 8), and echocardiogram by a cardiologist. Recommended tests include elbow radiographs, thyroid profile including autoantibodies (annually until age 5, then every other year), and von Willebrand's disease test. (See CHIC website; www.caninehealthinfo.org).

Recommend patella evaluation.

Miscellaneous

- **Breed name synonyms:** Berger de Beauce, Bas Rouge, Beauce Shepherd.
- **Registries:** AKC, UKC, KCGB (Kennel Club of Great Britain), ANKC (Australian National Kennel Club), NKC (National Kennel Club), FCI.
- **AKC rank (year 2008):** 139 (117 dogs registered.)
- **Internet resources: American Beauceron Club:** www.beauce.org
  Beauceron Club UK: www.beauceronclubuk.com
  The Beauceron Club in Canada: www.beauceronscanada.com

References

1. Clark LA, Wahl JM, Rees CA, et. al.: Retrotransposon insertion in SILV is responsible for merle patterning of the domestic dog. Proc Natl Acad Sci U S A. 2006 Jan 31;103(5):1376-81.
2. O'Sullivan N, Robinson R: Harlequin colour in the Great Dane dog. Genetica. 1988-1989;78(3):215-8.
3. OFA Website breed statistics: www.offa.org Last accessed July. 1, 2010.
4. Nachreiner RF, Refsal KR, Graham PA, et. al.: Prevalence of serum thyroid hormone autoantibodies in dogs with clinical signs of hypothyroidism. *J Am Vet Med Assoc* 2002 Feb 15;220(4):466-71.
5. Nachreiner R and Refsal K: Personal communication, Diagnostic Center for Population and Animal Health, Michigan State University. April, 2007.
6. Ihrke P: Ischemic Skin Disease in the Dog. Proceedings, 2006 World Small Animal Veterinary Association World Congress. 2006.
7. Scott DW, Miller WH and Griffin CE: *Muller and Kirks's Small Animal Dermatology, 5th Ed.,* WB Saunders, p756-757. 1995.
8. *Ocular Disorders Presumed to be Inherited in Purebred Dogs.* American College of Veterinary Ophthalmologists. ACVO, 2007.
9. *The Genetic Connection: A Guide to Health Problems in Purebred Dogs.* L Ackerman. p. 201, AAHA Press, 1999.
10. Clercx C, McEntee K, Gilbert S, et. al.: Nonresponsive generalized bacterial infection associated with systemic lupus erythematosus in a Beauceron. J Am Anim Hosp Assoc. 1999 May-Jun;35(3):220, 222, 224-8.
11. *The Complete Dog Book, 20th Ed.* The American Kennel Club. Howell Book House, NY 2006. p. 695-699.

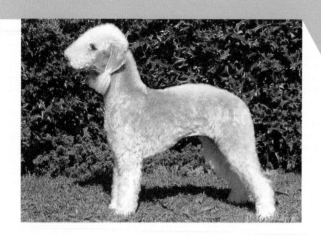

Bedlington Terrier

allergy dogs. Regular exercise is important, and one should introduce other dogs or cats with care when the dog is young. Though a fearless fighter, these dogs are playful and gentle with the family.

Normal Physiologic Variations
None reported

Drug Sensitivities
None reported

Inherited Diseases
Copper Toxicosis (CT): Autosomal recessive disorder causing hepatotoxic levels of copper by 2-4 years of age. Without treatment, affected dogs develop progressive liver disease and die. Acute signs include anorexia, depression, and jaundice. Treat with copper chelating agents and liver support medications. A linkage-based test was previously available that had false positive and negative results. A mutation in exon 2 of the COMMD1 gene (formerly MURR1) has now been identified that provides an accurate direct genetic test. (See genetic tests.) Some reports state that there are phenotypically affected dogs that do not test homozygous recessive for the defective gene, and that a second, undetermined mutated gene may also cause the disease in these dogs. The disease can be diagnosed phenotypically by a liver biopsy after 12 months of age. Worldwide screening for CT in various populations of Bedlington Terriers reveals affected frequencies of 11%-57%, and carrier frequencies of 43%-69%. Molecular genetic diversity studies show reduced diversity in the breed, and a call to use quality carrier Bedlington Terriers in breeding programs (bred to normal mates) to reduce further gene pool loss. Reported at an affected frequency of 12.9% in the BTCA Health Survey 2003-2004.[1,2,3,4,5,6,7,8]

Hip Dysplasia: Polygenically inherited trait causing degenerative joint disease and hip arthritis. OFA reports a high incidence, but very few Bedlington Terriers have been screened to determine an accurate frequency.[9]

Patella Luxation: Polygenically inherited congenital laxity of patellar ligaments, causing medial luxation, lameness, and later degenerative joint disease. Treated surgically if causing clinical signs. OFA reports 12.3% affected. Reported at a frequency of 1.4% in the BTCA Health Survey 2003-2004.[8,9]

Elbow Dysplasia: Polygenically inherited trait causing elbow arthritis. Too few Bedlington Terriers have been screened to determine an accurate frequency.[9]

Retinal Dysplasia: Autosomal recessive disorder, present at birth, with concurrent retinal detachment and cataract. Present at a low frequency in the breed.[10,11,12]

The Breed History
Though the early origins of this breed are somewhat obscure, it is known that the breed was widely used for sporting in Northumberland County in England. The recorded date for the first breeding of a dog referred to as a Bedlington terrier was 1825. The National Bedlington Terrier Club of England was formed in 1877, and the breed was registered in the Kennel Club of England June 1898. Registry in the AKC occurred in 1967.

Breeding for Function
A courageous ratter, pit fighter and vermin eradicator, this breed was renowned for toughness and staying power, and now also enjoys a reputation as an exceptional companion dog.

Physical Characteristics
Height at Withers: female 15.5" (39 cm), male 16.5" (42 cm).

Weight: females 17-20 lb (7.5-9 kg), males 20-23 lb(9-10.5 kg).

Coat: The medium-length haircoat is blue, liver, or sandy; also bi-color such as blue and tan, liver and tan, and sandy and tan. They are trimmed for show to a one-inch coat length on the body. Coat is thick and somewhat curly. Their coat has been called a "lamb's coat"; this is a distinguishing feature of the breed. The coat needs very regular grooming and clipping to prevent matting.

Longevity: 12-14 years.

Points of Conformation: This is a moderately sized dog with an alert demeanor. The head is narrow with no stop, skull is dolichocephalic, and the profile is slightly convex (Roman-nosed). Eyes are almond-shaped, and blue dogs have dark eyes, while others may have a range including hazel. Pendulous ears reach to the lateral commissure of the lips. Nose is pigmented black or brown. They have a long, tapered neck and have a deep thorax, with moderate arch and obvious tuck. Dewclaws are usually removed. The low-set tail reaches to the tarsus. These dogs move straight and true, with a springy gait.

Recognized Behavior Issues and Traits
Reported traits include: Enjoys company, but can be aloof with strangers. The dog will also do alarm barking, and enjoys barking in general. They are average in activity level, and are low shed, low

Disease Predispositions

Hypothyroidism: Inherited autoimmune thyroiditis. 12.7% positive for thyroid auto-antibodies based on testing at Michigan State University. (Ave. for all breeds is 7.5%). Reported at a frequency of 4.3% in the BTCA Health Survey 2003-2004. [8,13,14]

Pancreatic Acinar Atrophy (Exocrine Pancreatic Insufficiency): Immune-mediated pancreatic acinar atrophy. Clinical signs are poor weight gain, and steatorrhea. Treatment is with enzyme supplementation. Reported at a frequency of 8.9% in the BTCA Health Survey 2003-2004.[8]

Cataracts: Anterior, equatorial or posterior intermediate and punctate cataracts occur in the breed. Age of onset 3-24 months. Reported in 8.49% of Bedlington Terriers presented to veterinary teaching hospitals. Identified in 8.41% of Bedlington Terriers CERF examined by veterinary ophthalmologists between 2000-2005. Reported at a frequency of 7.8% in the BTCA Health Survey 2003-2004. CERF Does not recommend breeding any Bedlington Terrier with a cataract.[8,11,15,16]

Persistent Pupillary Membranes: Strands of fetal remnant connecting; iris to iris, cornea, lens, or involving sheets of tissue. The later three forms can impair vision, and dogs affected with these forms should not be bred. Identified in 6.47% of Bedlington Terriers CERF examined by veterinary ophthalmologists between 2000-2005.[11]

Distichiasis: Abnormally placed eyelashes that irritate the cornea and conjunctiva. Can cause secondary corneal ulceration. Identified in 4.96% of Bedlington Terriers CERF examined by veterinary ophthalmologists between 2000-2005. Reported at a frequency of 20.0% in the BTCA Health Survey 2003-2004.[8,11]

Deafness: Congenital deafness can be unilateral of bilateral. Diagnosed by BAER testing. Reported at a frequency of 3.3% in the BTCA Health Survey 2003-2004. Not listed as a breed at risk by Strain.[8,17]

Heart Murmur/Valvular Heart Disease: Reported at a frequency of 3.1% in the BTCA Health Survey 2003-2004. No specific valve involvement reported.[8]

Allergic Dermatitis: Inhalant or food allergy. Presents with pruritis and pyotraumatic dermatitis. Reported at a frequency of 2.7% in the BTCA Health Survey 2003-2004.[8]

Idiopathic Epilepsy (Inherited Seizures): Control with anticonvulsant medication. Reported at a frequency of 2.4% in the BTCA Health Survey 2003-2004.[8]

Dental Issues: The BTCA Health Survey 2003-2004 reports 2.4% of Bedlington Terriers with undershot bites, and 1.2% with missing teeth.[8]

Aggression: Reported at a frequency of 2.3% in the BTCA Health Survey 2003-2004.[8]

Imperforate Nasolacrimal Puncta: Blocked or malformed tear duct. This defect usually results in excessive tearing. Reported at a frequency of 2.1% in the BTCA Health Survey 2003-2004.[8,11]

Hyperadrenocorticism (Cushing's Disease): Hyperfunction of the adrenal gland caused by a pituitary or adrenal tumor. Clinical signs may include increased thirst and urination, symmetrical truncal alopecia, and abdominal distention. Reported at a frequency of 1.6% in the BTCA Health Survey 2003-2004.[8]

Keratoconjunctivitis Sicca (KCS, Dry Eye): Ocular condition causing lack of tear production and secondary conjunctivitis, corneal ulcerations, and vision problems. Age of onset 2-5 years. Reported at an increased frequency verses other breeds. Reported at a frequency of 1.1% in the BTCA Health Survey 2003-2004.[8,18]

Cryptorchidism (Retained Testicles): Can be unilateral or bilateral. This is a sex-limited disorder with an unknown mode of inheritance. Reported at a frequency of 1.1% in the BTCA Health Survey 2003-2004.[8]

Entropion: Rolling in of eyelids, often causing corneal irritation or ulceration. Reported at a frequency of 1.1% in the BTCA Health Survey 2003-2004.[8]

Corneal Dystrophy: Causes opacities on the surface of the cornea. Identified in 1.08% of Belington Terriers CERF examined by veterinary ophthalmologists between 2000-2005.[11]

Glaucoma, Microphthalmia, Osteogenesis Imperfecta, Progressive Retinal Atrophy, and **Renal Dysplasia** are reported.[19]

Isolated Case Studies

None reported

Genetic Tests

Tests of Genotype: Direct test for Copper Toxicosis is available from VetGen and the Animal Health Trust.

Direct test for the brown color allele is available from VetGen.

Tests of Phenotype: CHIC Certification: Required testing includes patella evaluation, CERF eye examination at a minimum of 1 year of age. and genetic test for copper toxicosis. (See CHIC website; www.caninehealthinfo.org).

Recommend hip and elbow radiographs, thyroid profile including autoantibodies, and cardiac evaluation.

Miscellaneous

- **Breed name synonyms:** Rothbury Terrier (historical)
- **Registries:** CKC, AKC, UKC, KCGB (Kennel Club of Great Britain), ANKC (Australian National Kennel Club), NKC (National Kennel Club)
- **AKC rank (year 2008):** 126 (226 dogs registered)
- **Internet resources: Bedlington Terrier Club of America:** http://bedlingtonamerica.com/
  The National Bedlington Terrier Club of England: www.bedlingtons.org.uk
  The Bedlington Terrier Association (UK): www.thebta.info/
  The Bedlington Terrier Health Group (UK): www.bedlingtonterrierhealthgroup.org.uk

References

1. Forman OP, Boursnell ME, Dunmorec BJ: Characterization of the *COMMD1* (*MURR1*) mutation causing copper toxicosis in Bedlington terriers. Anim Genet. 2005 Dec; 36(6); 497-501.

2. Coronado VA, Damaraju D, Kohijoki R, et. al.: New haplotypes in the Bedlington terrier indicate complexity in copper toxicosis. *Mamm Genome*. 2003 Jul;14(7):483-91.

3. van de Sluis B, Peter AT, Wijmenga C: Indirect molecular diagnosis of copper toxicosis in Bedlington terriers is complicated by haplotype diversity. *J Hered*. 2003 May-Jun;94(3):256-9.

4. Koskinen MT, Bredbacka P: Assessment of the population structure of five Finnish dog breeds with microsatellites. *Anim Genet*. 2000 Oct;31(5):310-7.

5. Hultgren BD, Stevens JB, Hardy RM: Inherited, chronic, progressive hepatic degeneration in Bedlington terriers with increased liver copper concentrations: clinical and pathologic observations and comparison with other copper-associated liver diseases. *Am J Vet Res*. 1986 Feb;47(2):365-77.

6. Ubbink GJ, Van den Ingh TS, Yuzbasiyan-Gurkan V, et. al.: Population dynamics of inherited copper toxicosis in Dutch Bedlington terriers (1977-1997). *J Vet Intern Med*. 2000 Mar-Apr;14(2):172-6.

7. Haywood S: Copper toxicosis in Bedlington terriers. Vet Rec. 2006 Nov 11;159(20):687.

8. Bedlington Terrier Club of America: Bedlington Terrier Club of America Health Survey 2003-2004. 2004.

9. OFA Website breed statistics: www.offa.org Last accessed July 1, 2010.

10. Dietz HH: Retinal dysplasia in dogs--a review. *Nord Vet Med*. 1985 Jan-Feb;37(1):1-9.

11. *Ocular Disorders Presumed to be Inherited in Purebred Dogs*. American College of Veterinary Ophthalmologists. ACVO, 2007.

12. Rubin LF: Heredity of retinal dysplasia in the Bedlington terrier. Journal of the American Veterinary Medical Association 1968;152:260-262.

13. Nachreiner R and Refsal K: Personal communication, Diagnostic Center for Population and Animal Health, Michigan State University. April, 2007.

14. Nachreiner RF, Refsal KR, Graham PA, et. al.: Prevalence of serum thyroid hormone autoantibodies in dogs with clinical signs of hypothyroidism. J Am Vet Med Assoc 2002 Feb 15;220(4):466-71.

15. Gelatt KN, Mackay EO: Prevalence of primary breed-related cataracts in the dog in North America. Vet Ophthalmol. 2005 Mar-Apr;8(2):101-11.

16. Nasisse MP: Diseases of the Lens and Cataract Surgery. Proceedings Waltham/OSU Symposium, Small Animal Ophthalmology, 2001.

17. Strain GM: Deafness prevalence and pigmentation and gender associations in dog breeds at risk. Vet J. 2004 Jan;167(1):23-32.

18. Westermeyer HD, Ward DA, Abrams K: Breed predisposition to congenital alacrima in dogs. Vet Ophthalmol. 2009 Jan-Feb;12(1):1-5.

19. *The Genetic Connection: A Guide to Health Problems in Purebred Dogs*. L Ackerman. p. 203. AAHA Press, 1999.

20. *The Complete Dog Book, 20th Ed*. The American Kennel Club. Howell Book House, NY 2006. p. 352-354.

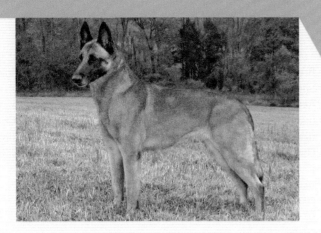

The Breed History

This is one of four subtypes of the Belgian Shepherd dog, this one being primarily developed around the city of Malines (Mechelar), Belgium and is considered to be the original Belgian shepherd type (records date to the 1200s). The other types, divided based on their coat type are Tervuren, Groenendael, and Laekenois. Their common ancestor is the Belgian Sheepdog. The Malinois are the shorthaired black and fawn variety that resemble German Shepherds in general type. Though these coat types share a common breed standard outside the USA, the types are split into separate breeds in America and the AKC, with minor distinguishing characteristics.

Breeding for Function

The very high intelligence and trainability of these dogs are a hallmark of the breed. Obedience, herding, tracking, and Schutzhund round out their talents. Historically, herding was their primary purpose. The breed is recognized for utility in police work and agility, flyball and obedience. They are also popular today as a companion dog.

Physical Characteristics

Height at Withers: female 22-24" (56-61 cm), male 24-26" (61-66 cm).

Weight: 62-75 lb (28-34 kg).

Coat: The coat is similar to the smooth-coated Dutch Shepherd. The weather resistant coat is short and hairs are hard in texture, and fawn hairs are tipped black; undercoat is dense and short, the color is a standard distribution of black and tan (tan ranging from fawn to mahogany). Black ears, mask, muzzle, and points on feet and tail are preferred.

Longevity: 12-14 years

Points of Conformation: High head carriage, chiseled face, alert expression, and a muscular conformation characterize the Malinois. Slightly almond shaped eyes are brown, with black palpebral rims, are medium sized and moderately deep set. Ears are triangular, pricked and the tips pointed. Skull is flattened, and stop is moderate. The muzzle is pointed but not snippy, nose and lips black, neck medium in thickness and length and well muscled. The topline is level, though a mild slope down to the rear is accepted, especially through the croup. The thorax is deep, abdomen is moderately

tucked up, and the tail reaches the tarsus and is carried below horizontal in a curve. Limbs are straight with an oval cross section; dewclaws may be removed in front, and on the hind limbs are usually removed. Foreleg feet are compact and possess strong black nails, though a white nail may accompany a white toe marking. Rear feet may be a bit more elongated. The gait is long, ground covering and smooth. In the breed standard, reference is made to the fact that the breed likes to circle rather than move in a straight line. This is likely a characteristic that derives from their herding behavior.

Recognized Behavior Issues and Traits

Reported breed characteristics include: Highly trainable, intelligent, confident though aloof with strangers, protective without undue aggression, and a high activity level. They are reported to be less likely to bite than Tervuren or Groenendael dogs. This type of dog needs an experienced owner because it is a sensitive dog by nature. Early focused socialization and obedience training is important. Needs human companionship and should be supervised with small children due to high activity and large size. They may try to herd humans by nipping at the heels.

Normal Physiologic Variations

None reported

Drug Sensitivities

None reported

Inherited Diseases

Elbow Dysplasia: Polygenically inherited trait causing elbow arthritis. OFA reports 10.1% affected.[1]

Hip Dysplasia: Polygenically inherited trait causing degenerative joint disease and hip arthritis. OFA reports 5.5% affected.[1]

Patella Luxation: Polygenically inherited laxity of patellar ligaments, causing luxation, lameness, and later degenerative joint disease. Treat surgically if causing clinical signs. Too few Belgian Malinois have been screened by OFA to determine an accurate frequency.[1]

Disease Predispositions

Hypothyroidism: Inherited autoimmune thyroiditis. 8.4% positive for thyroid auto-antibodies based on testing at Michigan State University. (Ave. for all breeds is 7.5%).[2,3]

Cataracts: A nonprogressive, triangular opacity in the posterior cortex is most common in the breed, although anterior, nuclear, and capsular cataracts also occur. Identified in 3.42% of Belgian Malinois CERF examined by veterinary ophthalmologists between 2000-2005. CERF does not recommend breeding any Belgian Malinois with a cataract.[4]

Persistent Pupillary Membranes: Strands of fetal remnant connecting; iris to iris, cornea, lens, or involving sheets of tissue. The later three forms can impair vision, and dogs affected with these forms should not be bred. Identified in 1.04% of Belgian Malinois CERF examined by veterinary ophthalmologists between 2000-2005.[4]

Heat Stroke: In an Israeli study, Belgian Malinois had the highest risk (Odds Ratio of 24x) of developing heat stroke versus other breeds. Thrombocytopenia, disseminated intravascular coagulation and acute renal failure usually resulted in death in affected dogs.[5]

Chronic Superficial Keratitis (Pannus): Corneal disease that can cause vision problems due to pigmentation. Treatment with topical ocular lubricants and anti-inflammatory medication. Identified in 0.15% of Belgian Malinois CERF examined by veterinary ophthalmologists between 2000-2005. CERF does not recommend breeding any Belgian Malinois with pannus.[4]

Retinal Degeneration: A unilateral or bilateral retinal disease which can be progressive. When bilateral, the ophthalmoscopic lesions are sometimes asymmetrical, particularly in the early stages of the disease. Fundus examination shows initially single or multiple focal retinal lesions that appear active (local infiltrative inflammation or granulation) or inactive. The lesions can progress resulting in widespread retinal atrophy. Unknown mode of inheritance, however, males predominate. CERF recommends that affected dogs should not be bred.[4]

Lumbosacral Transitional Vertebrae/Lumbosacral Stenosis: Belgian Malinois have been documented with lumbosacral transitional vertebrae and lumbosacral stenosis. These can be incidental, or cause pain, intermittent rear leg lameness, muscle atrophy, ataxia, and increasingly severe neurologic impairment.[6,7]

Epilepsy, Exertional Myositis, Gastric Dilatation–Volvulus, Prognathism, and **Progressive Retinal Atrophy** are reported.[8]

Isolated Case Studies

Polycystic Kidney Disease: Glomerulocystic kidney disease was identified in a juvenile Belgian Malinois dog with acute renal failure.[9]

Osteosarcoma: An 8-year-old male Belgian Malinois showed progressive caudal paresis of 2 to 3 weeks' duration. Radiography revealed a mottled appearance to the body of L4 and misshapen intervertebral foramen at L4-L5. Computed tomography revealed a soft tissue mass adjacent to or involving the spinal cord and L4, with complete destruction of a portion of the floor of the vertebral foramen. Necropsy examination revealed osteosarcoma, with lesions in L3 to L7, the sacrum, and the lungs.[10]

Genetic Tests

Tests of Genotype: Direct tests are available for presence of black-and-tan and sable coat colors from HealthGene and VetGen.

Tests of Phenotype: CHIC Certification: Required testing includes hip and elbow radiographs, and CERF eye examination. (See CHIC website; www.caninehealthinfo.org).

Recommend thyroid profile including autoantibodies, patella evaluation and cardiac evaluation.

Miscellaneous

- **Breed name synonyms:** Belgian Shepherd Dog, Malinois, Belgian Sheepdog, Chien de Berger Belge
- **Registries:** AKC, UKC [as Belgian Shepherd dog, Malinois coat (along with Tervuren, Groenendael, Laekenois coats)], CKC, KCGB (Kennel Club of Great Britain) as Belgian Shepherd dog, Malinois coat (along with Tervuren, Groenendael, Laekenois coats), ANKC (Australian National Kennel Club) as Belgian Shepherd dog, Malinois coat (along with Tervuren, Groenendael, Laekenois coats), NKC (National Kennel Club) as Belgian Shepherd dog, Malinois coat (along with Tervuren, Groenendael, Laekenois coats).
- **AKC rank (year 2008):** 79 (901 dogs registered)
- **Internet resources:** The Belgian Malinois Club of America: www.malinoisclub.com
  Belgian Shepherd Dog Club of Canada: www.bsdcc.org
  Belgian Shepherd Dog Association of Great Britain: www.bsdaofgb.co.uk

References

1. OFA Website breed statistics: www.offa.org Last accessed July 1, 2010.
2. Nachreiner R and Refsal K: Personal communication, Diagnostic Center for Population and Animal Health, Michigan State University. April, 2007.
3. Nachreiner RF, Refsal KR, Graham PA, et. al.: Prevalence of serum thyroid hormone autoantibodies in dogs with clinical signs of hypothyroidism. J Am Vet Med Assoc 2002 Feb 15;220(4):466-71.
4. Ocular Disorders Presumed to be Inherited in Purebred Dogs. American College of Veterinary Ophthalmologists. ACVO, 2007.
5. Bruchim Y, Klement E, Saragusty J, et. al.: Heat stroke in dogs: A retrospective study of 54 cases (1999-2004) and analysis of risk factors for death. J Vet Intern Med. 2006 Jan-Feb;20(1):38-46.
6. Lang J: Diagnostic Imaging in Lumbosacras Stenosis in Dogs. Proceedings, World Small Animal Veterinary Association World Congress Proceedings, 2005.
7. Carpenter L G, Taylor B., Nye R: Treatment of Degenerative Lumbosacral Stenosis in Military Working Dogs with Dorsal Laminectomy and Pedicle Screw and Rod Fixation. Proceedings, 2003 ACVIM Forum. 2003.
8. The Genetic Connection: A Guide to Health Problems in Purebred Dogs. L Ackerman. p. 201. AAHA Press, 1999.
9. Ramos-Vara JA, Miller MA, Ojeda JL, et. al.: Glomerulocystic kidney disease in a Belgian Malinois dog: an ultrastructural, immunohistochemical, and lectin-binding study. Ultrastruct Pathol. 2004 Jan-Feb;28(1):33-42.
10. Moore GE, Mathey WS, Eggers JS, et. al.: Osteosarcoma in adjacent lumbar vertebrae in a dog. J Am Vet Med Assoc. 2000 Oct 1;217(7):1038-40, 1008.
11. The Complete Dog Book, 20th Ed. The American Kennel Club. Howell Book House, NY 2006. p. 620-623.

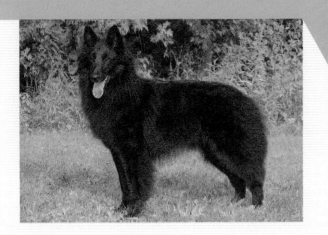

Belgian Sheepdog

reaches the tarsus at rest, and is held low. Limbs are straight boned, with oval cross section, the feet are small, round, toes well knuckled up and well padded, though the rear feet are longer. Nails are black, unless a white toe marking is adjacent in which case they are white. Rear dewclaws should be removed. The gait is springy and low, and ground covering. The breed standard describes a tendency to circle rather than move in a straight line, perhaps referring to the natural herding movements.

The Breed History

In 1891 in the Brabant province, Belgian Sheepdogs were lined up by breed fanciers and divided along coat type. Tervuren, Malinois and Laekenois were the other three Belgian Shepherd coat types. Other provinces followed suit and from then on the breeds were distinguished by these new coat designations. The Groenendael designation reflects the origin (Chateau of Groenendael) of the kennel that first bred this coat type as a distinct type. In some countries and registries, this breed is considered one of the varieties of the Belgian Shepherd, but in America and the AKC, it represents a separate breed.

Breeding for Function

The Belgian Sheepdog has served in many capacities including roles as police dogs, Schutzhund, obedience dogs, tracking, as sled dogs, guide and therapy dogs and for search and rescue. Their original function was for sheep herding. Belgian Sheepdogs have also been used as border patrol dogs, watchdogs, guard dogs, field trial dogs and as war dogs. Some are strictly companion dogs.

Physical Characteristics

Height at Withers: female 22-24" (56-61cm), male 24-26" (61-66 cm).

Weight: 61-63 lb (27.5-28.5 kg).

Coat: Longhaired and black coat are the distinguishing characteristics for this breed. Very small amounts, and specifically distributed white or gray hairs are allowed. The well-developed outer coat is straight and hard, the undercoat is dense, and furnishings include collarets, breeches, and upper limb and tail feathering.

Longevity: 12-14 years

Points of Conformation: The breed is noted for a high head carriage, solid square conformation, and an alert expression. Eyes are brown to dark brown, moderately deep set and medium-sized, ears are erect and triangular in shape, with pointed tips. The skull is flat on top with a moderate stop, and a long narrow muzzle is moderately tapered. The nose is black, lips are black, and the muscular neck is tapered. The topline slopes down gradually to the rear, though in the middle it is level, and the deep thorax is not broad. The abdomen is moderately tucked up. The tapering tail

Recognized Behavior Issues and Traits

Reported breed characteristics include: Intelligent, high trainability but need to start early obedience lessons, and does best with experienced dog owners because of a range of temperaments and degrees of aggression. Versatile, devoted, protective of family and home, aloof with strangers, possessive of master and territorial. They need early socialization.

This type of dog has average grooming needs and has shedding phases twice yearly. They have moderate exercise needs. This sheepdog may try to herd children, nipping at their heels.

Normal Physiologic Variations

None reported

Drug Sensitivities

None reported

Inherited Diseases

Elbow Dysplasia: Polygenically inherited trait causing elbow arthritis. OFA reports 4.7% affected.[1]

Hip Dysplasia: Polygenically inherited trait causing degenerative joint disease and hip arthritis. OFA reports 2.9% affected.[1]

Patella Luxation: Polygenically inherited laxity of patellar ligaments, causing luxation, lameness, and later degenerative joint disease. Treat surgically if causing clinical signs. Too few Belgian Sheepdogs have been screened by OFA to determine an accurate frequency.[1]

Progressive Retinal Atrophy (PRA): Progressive degeneration of the retina, eventually causing blindness. Limited breeding studies suggest autosomal recessive inheritance. Reported to occur at a low frequency in the breed. CERF does not recommend breeding any Belgian Sheepdog with PRA.[2,3,4]

Congenital Nystagmus: An autosomal recessive, spontaneously occurring animal model of human congenital nystagmus (CN) and see-saw nystagmus (SSN) is identified in the Belgian Sheepdog. It is caused by achiasma or uniocular decussation of the optic chiasma. All retinal ganglion cell axons extend directly into the ipsilateral optic tract. CERF does not recommend breeding any affected Belgian Sheepdog.[2,5,6,7]

Disease Predispositions

Idiopathic Epilepsy (inherited seizures): Control with anti-seizure medication. In the Belgian Sheepdog, seizures can be partial or generalized. Prevalence of 9.5% in Denmark with an average age of onset of 3.3 years. Epilepsy has a high heritability in the breed of 0.76 with a polygenic mode of inheritance, though influenced by a single autosomal recessive gene of large effect. Genome-wide linkage scan identifies multiple chromosomal locations for possible epilepsy liability genes.[8,9,10,11]

Persistent Pupillary Membranes: Strands of fetal remnant connecting; iris to iris, cornea, lens, or involving sheets of tissue. The later three forms can impair vision, and dogs affected with these forms should not be bred. Identified in 6.34% of Belgian Sheepdogs CERF examined by veterinary ophthalmologists between 2000-2005.[2]

Hypothyroidism: Inherited autoimmune thyroiditis. 3.1% positive for thyroid auto-antibodies based on testing at Michigan State University. (Ave. for all breeds is 7.5%).[12,13]

Cataracts: Anterior and posterior cortex cataracts predominate, though intermediate and punctate cataracts also occur in the breed. Unknown mode of inheritance. Identified in 2.75% of Belgian Sheepdogs CERF examined by veterinary ophthalmologists between 2000-2005. CERF does not recommend breeding any Belgian Sheepdog with a cataract.[2]

Retinal Dysplasia: Focal folds are seen in the breed. Identified in 1.60% of Belgian Sheepdogs CERF examined by veterinary ophthalmologists between 2000-2005.[2]

Gastric Carcinoma: Diagnosis by contrast radiographic examination, endoscopy, and biopsy. Surgery is the only potentially curative modality for localized gastric carcinoma. Though the prognosis is poor, prolonged survival times in individual animals are possible. Reported at a frequency of 1.13% in Tervurens in Holland, with a mean age of 9.5 years at diagnosis. Computed heritability was 0.09 with a male predominance.[14,15]

Chronic Superficial Keratitis (Pannus): Corneal disease that can cause vision problems due to pigmentation. Age of onset 2-5 years. Treatment with topical ocular lubricants and anti-inflammatory medication. Identified in 0.51% of Belgian Sheepdogs CERF examined by veterinary ophthalmologists between 2000-2005. CERF does not recommend breeding any Belgian Sheepdog with pannus.[2]

Ectodermal Defect, Gracilis or Semitendinosus Myopathy, Hypotrichosis, Micropapilla, Muscular Dystrophy, Prognathism, Subaortic Stenosis, and **Vitiligo** are reported.[16]

Isolated Case Studies

Meningioma: A 15-year-old Belgian Sheepdog presented with ventro-lateral strabismus of the left eye, ptosis of the left upper eyelid and anisocoria with the left pupil fixed and dilated. MRI and necropsy revealed a meningioma to the left of midline and lateral to the sella turcica.[17]

Malignant Fibrous Histiocytoma: A 4 years and 9 months old Belgian Shepherd dog was presented with an acute onset of non-weight bearing lameness and stifle effusion. Rapid progression produced marked periosteal new bone formation. Cytology of a stifle joint aspirate revealed numerous large polygonal neoplastic cells with considerable anisocytosis and anisokaryosis. The deep form of malignant fibrous histiocytoma was diagnosed at necropsy.[18]

Eosinophilic Myositis: A 2-year-old male Belgian sheepdog with eosinophilic myositis, which particularly affects the masticatory muscles, tested positive for the presence of muscle-specific auto-antibodies. Treatment with immunosuppressive drugs.[19]

Synovial hemangioma: An 8-year-old castrated male Belgian Sheepdog with lameness of 3 months' duration was diagnosed with synovial hemangioma. Pain, soft-tissue swelling, and hemarthrosis were localized to the left stifle joint. The dog was free of detectable neoplasia 6 months after amputation of the affected hind leg.[20]

Genetic Tests

Tests of Genotype: Direct test is available for presence of black-and-tan and sable coat colors from HealthGene and VetGen.

Tests of Phenotype: CHIC Certification: Required testing includes hip and elbow radiographs, and CERF eye examination. (See CHIC website; www.caninehealthinfo.org).

Recommend thyroid profile including autoantibodies, patella evaluation and cardiac evaluation.

Miscellaneous

- **Breed name synonyms:** Chien de Berger Belge, Belgian Shepherd, Groenendael.
- **Registries:** AKC, CKC, (in UKC all of the shepherd varieties are together: Groenendael, Malinois, Tervuren, Laekenois), KCGB (Kennel Club of Great Britain)
- **AKC rank (year 2008):** 116 (285 dogs registered)
- **Internet resources:** Belgian Sheepdog Club of America: http://www.bsca.info/home.html
  Belgian Shepherd Dog Club of Canada: www.bsdcc.org
  Belgian Shepherd Dog Association of Great Britain: www.bsdaofgb.co.uk

References

1. OFA Website breed statistics: www.offa.org Last accessed July 1, 2010.
2. *Ocular Disorders Presumed to be Inherited in Purebred Dogs.* American College of Veterinary Ophthalmologists. ACVO, 2007.
3. Miller TR: Generalized Retinopathy in the Belgian Sheepdog. *Invest Ophthalmol Vis Sci.* 1986 :27(suppl.):310.
4. Wolf ED, Samuelson D: Retinopathy in a family of Belgium shepherds. Proc American College of Veterinary Ophthalmologists. 1981 :12: supplement, 1981.
5. Dell'Osso LF, Hertle RW, Williams RW, et. al.: A new surgery for congenital nystagmus: effects of tenotomy on an achiasmatic canine and the role of extraocular proprioception. *J AAPOS.* 1999
6. Dell'Osso LF, Williams RW, Jacobs JB, et. al.: The congenital and see-saw nystagmus in the prototypical achiasma of canines: comparison to the human achiasmatic prototype. *Vision Res.* 1998 Jun;38(11):1629-41.
7. Hogan D, Williams RW: Analysis of the retinas and optic nerves of achiasmatic Belgian sheepdogs. *J Comp Neurol.* 1995 Feb
8. Oberbauer AM, Grossman DI, Irion DN, et. al.: The genetics of epilepsy in the Belgian tervuren and sheepdog. *J Hered.* 2003 Jan-Feb;94(1):57-63.

9. Berendt M, Gulløv CH, & Fredholm M: Focal epilepsy in the Belgian shepherd: evidence for simple Mendelian inheritance. J Small Anim Pract. 2009 Dec;50(12):655-61.

10. Berendt M, Gulløv CH, Christensen SL, et. al.: Prevalence and characteristics of epilepsy in the Belgian shepherd variants Groenendael and Tervueren born in Denmark 1995-2004. Acta Vet Scand. 2008 Dec 22;50:51.

11. Oberbauer AM, Belanger JM, Grossman DI, et. al.: Genome-wide linkage scan for loci associated with epilepsy in Belgian shepherd dogs. BMC Genet. 2010 May 4;11:35.

12. Nachreiner R and Refsal K: Personal communication, Diagnostic Center for Population and Animal Health, Michigan State University. April, 2007.

13. Nachreiner RF, Refsal KR, Graham PA, et. al.: Prevalence of serum thyroid hormone autoantibodies in dogs with clinical signs of hypothyroidism. J Am Vet Med Assoc 2002 Feb 15;220(4):466-71.

14. Gualtieri M, Monzeglio MG, Scanziani E: Gastric neoplasia. *Vet Clin North Am Small Anim Pract.* 1999 Mar;29(2):415-40.

15. Lubbes D, Mandigers PJ, Heuven HC, et. al.: Incidence of gastric carcinoma in Dutch Tervueren shepherd dogs born between 1991 and 2002. Tijdschr Diergeneeskd. 2009 Jul 15-Aug 1;134(14-15):606-10.

16. *The Genetic Connection: A Guide to Health Problems in Purebred Dogs.* L Ackerman. p. 201-02. AAHA Press, 1999.

17. Larocca RD: Unilateral external and internal ophthalmoplegia caused by intracranial meningioma in a dog. *Vet Ophthalmol.* 2000;3(1):3-9.

18. Booth MJ, Bastianello SS, Jiminez M, et. al.: Malignant fibrous histiocytoma of the deep peri-articular tissue of the stifle in a dog. *J S Afr Vet Assoc.* 1998 Dec;69(4):163-8.

19. Shelton GD, Cardinet GH 3rd, Bandman E, et. al.: Fiber type-specific autoantibodies in a dog with eosinophilic myositis. *Muscle Nerve.* 1985 Nov-Dec;8(9):783-90.

20. Miller MA, Pool RR, Coolman BR : Synovial hemangioma in the stifle joint of a dog. Vet Pathol. 2007 Mar;44(2):240-3.

21. *The Complete Dog Book, 20th Ed.* The American Kennel Club. Howell Book House, NY 2006. p. 624-628.

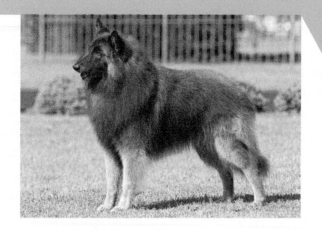

The Breed History

This is one of four coat types of the Belgian Shepherd type dog. This breed originated in the town of Tervuren, Belgium. The other haircoat types are Malinois, Groenendael, and Laekenois. Their common ancestor is the Belgian Sheepdog. The Tervuren are the longhaired, colored other than black variety, though hairs are black tipped. The Tervuren is considered a later variety that the Malinois, and may be derived from the Groenendaels since matings of the latter can produce the Tervuren coat type. Though these coat types share a single breed standard outside the AKC and America, the types are split into separate breeds here, with minor distinguishing characteristics. The first breed standard for the Tervuren was drawn up in 1893. The AKC registered these dogs first in 1959.

Breeding for Function

Very high intelligence and trainability are a breed hallmark. Obedience, herding, tracking, sledding, drug detection, and Schutzhund represent some of their talents. Historically, herding was their primary purpose, with farm protection running second. Currently, they serve as service dogs, police and security dogs, and are widely used in agility trials. Many are also companion dogs.

Physical Characteristics

Height at Withers: female 22-24" (56-61 cm), male 24-26" (61-66 cm).

Weight: Average 62 lb (28 kg).

Coat: The outer coat is long, dense and straight. Hairs are hard but not wiry. The undercoat is dense and soft. Furnishings are more developed in males. Facial hair is short. A non-black longhaired Belgian Shepherd-type dog is the distinguishing characteristic of a Tervuren. Black masking and a fawn to mahogany base color with black tipping is the preferred combination, but other non-black colors are accepted. The dogs tend to get darker with age. A small white chest patch is accepted.

Longevity: 12-14 years

Points of Conformation: These dogs have a strong constitution, square in conformation (females may be a bit longer), lithe and well balanced. Tervurens are solid without being coarse, the head is long, well chiseled, and the eyes are medium sized, almond-shaped, and dark brown in color. The ears are stiff, erect and triangular, the muzzle is pointed, the stop is moderately well defined, and the nose is black. The neck is long, well muscled, and not throaty. The topline is level, the thorax deep, and the abdomen moderately tucked up. The tail is high set and reaches to the tarsus at rest; in action it may be held horizontal to the topline. Limbs are straight boned, and the bone is oval in cross section. Dewclaws may be removed in front, and are usually removed in the rear. Feet are small, compact and well knuckled up with strong nails. The gait is springy and ground covering. As for the Malinois, the standard stipulates a preference to move in a circle over a straight line. This may reflect the herding heritage of this breed.

Recognized Behavior Issues and Traits

Reported breed characteristics include: Defensive-protective, devoted (even possessive), courageous, may be snappy, and has high exercise needs and a high base activity level. Grooming needs are low, and moderate shedding occurs. They are generally good with other dogs in the household, and have variable tolerance to other smaller pets. Not the best choice of dog for a household with a child; they do best with experienced owners.

Normal Physiologic Variations

Leukopenia: Physiologic leukopenia, resulting from low numbers of neutrophils, lymphocytes, and monocytes, may be a typical finding in a large percentage of healthy Belgian Tervuren and is not of clinical importance in otherwise healthy dogs. Healthy Belgian Tervuren may also have RBC counts and hematocrits higher than expected for healthy dogs. In one study of 180 healthy Belgian Tervuren in the United States, total WBC counts ranged from 2,610 to 16,900. All dogs were otherwise clinically normal. In a study in Belgium, only 1 of 94 Tervuren was identified with the condition. Reported at a frequency of 1.3% in the 2003 American Belgian Tervuren Club Health Survey.[1,2,3,4]

Drug Sensitivities

None reported

Inherited Diseases

Elbow Dysplasia: Polygenically inherited trait causing elbow arthritis. OFA reports 4.4% affected.[5]

Hip Dysplasia: Polygenically inherited trait causing degenerative joint disease and hip arthritis. OFA reports 3.6% affected. Reported at a frequency of 2.2% in the 2003 American Belgian Tervuren Club Health Survey.[4,5]

Patella Luxation: Polygenically inherited laxity of patellar ligaments, causing luxation, lameness, and later degenerative joint disease. Treat surgically if causing clinical signs. Too few Belgian Tervurens have been screened by OFA to determine an accurate frequency.[5]

Disease Predispositions

Idiopathic Epilepsy (Inherited Seizures): Control with anti-seizure medication. In the Belgian Tervuren, seizures can be partial or generalized. In the Belgian Tervuren, epilepsy has a high heritability of 0.77 to 0.83 with a polygenic mode of inheritance, though influenced by a single autosomal recessive gene of large effect. Genome-wide linkage scan identifies multiple chromosomal locations for possible epilepsy liability genes. Epilepsy may afflict as much as 17% of the breed. Reported in 8.9% of dogs in the 1998 Tervuren Health Survey, and 8.5% in the 2003 American Belgian Tervuren Club Health Survey. Prevalence of 9.5% in Denmark with an average age of onset of 3.3 years.[4,6,7,8,9,10]

Allergic Dermatitis (Atopy): Inhalant or food allergy. Presents with pruritis and pyotraumatic dermatitis (hot spots). Reported in 7.3% of dogs in the 1998 Tervuren Health Survey, and 7.3% in the 2003 American Belgian Tervuren Club Health Survey.[4,11]

Persistent Pupillary Membranes: Strands of fetal remnant connecting; iris to iris, cornea, lens, or involving sheets of tissue. The later three forms can impair vision, and dogs affected with these forms should not be bred. Identified in 6.88% of Belgian Tervuren CERF examined by veterinary ophthalmologists between 2000-2005. Reported in 2.0% of dogs in the 1998 Tervuren Health Survey, and 3.8% in the 2003 American Belgian Tervuren Club Health Survey.[4,11,12]

Cryptorchidism: Unilateral or bilateral undescended testicles. Reported in 5.1% of males in the 1998 Tervuren Health Survey, and 3.3% in the 2003 American Belgian Tervuren Club Health Survey. This is a sex-limited disorder with an unknown mode of inheritance.[4,11]

Cataracts: Anterior cortex punctate cataracts predominate, though posterior nuclear and capsular cataracts also occur in the breed. Identified in 2.44% of Belgian Tervuren CERF examined by veterinary ophthalmologists between 2000-2005. Reported in 3.4% of dogs in the 1998 Tervuren Health Survey, and 6.2% in the 2003 American Belgian Tervuren Club Health Survey. CERF does not recommend breeding any Belgian Tervuren with a cataract.[4,11,12]

Hypothyroidism: Inherited autoimmune thyroiditis. 3.0% positive for thyroid auto-antibodies based on testing at Michigan State University. (Ave. for all breeds is 7.5%). Reported at a frequency of 6.6% in the 2003 American Belgian Tervuren Club Health Survey.[4,13,14]

Gastric Carcinoma: Diagnosis by contrast radiographic examination, endoscopy, and biopsy. Surgery is the only potentially curative modality for localized gastric carcinoma. Though the prognosis is poor, prolonged survival times in individual animals are possible. Reported at a frequency of 1.13% in Tervurens in Holland, with a mean age of 9.5 years at diagnosis. Computed heritability was 0.09 with a male predominance.[15]

Optic Nerve Hypoplasia/Micropapilla: Congenital defect of optic nerve development affecting vision, or a small optic disc. Identified in 1.05% of Belgian Tervuren CERF examined by veterinary ophthalmologists between 2000-2005.[12]

Demodicosis: Demodectic mange has an underlying immunodeficiency in its pathogenesis. Reported in 2.1% of dogs in the 1998 Tervuren Health Survey, and 2.7% in the 2003 American Belgian Tervuren Club Health Survey.[4,11]

Cancer: Mammary (breast) cancer is reported at a frequency of 1.6%, Lymphoma 1.3%, and Osteosarcoma 1.3% in the 2003 American Belgian Tervuren Club Health Survey.[4]

Vitiligo: Pigment loss most commonly affecting the face and mouth in young adult Belgian Tervurens is due to a regression of melanocytes in the epidermis. Although there is partial repigmentation in some dogs, complete repigmentation does not occur. Unknown mode of inheritance.[16]

Retinal Dysplasia: Focal folds and geographic retinal dysplasia are seen in the breed. Dogs with the geographic form should not be bred. Identified in 0.58% of Belgian Tervuren CERF examined by veterinary ophthalmologists between 2000-2005.[12]

Chronic Superficial Keratitis (Pannus): Belgian Tervuren dogs are more predisposed toward this condition than other breeds. It can cause vision problems due to corneal pigmentation. Age of onset 2-5 years. Treatment with topical ocular lubricants and anti-inflammatory medication. Identified in 0.56% of Belgian Tervuren CERF examined by veterinary ophthalmologists between 2000-2005. CERF does not recommend breeding any affected Belgian Tervuren.[12,17]

Progressive Retinal Atrophy (PRA): Progressive degeneration of the retina, eventually causing blindness. Age of onset 4-5 years. Reported to occur at a low frequency in the breed. CERF does not recommend breeding any Belgian Tervuren with PRA. Mode of inheritance presumed to be autosomal recessive.[12]

Anasarca, Anterior Crossbite, Atrial Septal Defect, Level Bite, Lymphedema, Oligodontia, Prognathism, and **Wry Mouth** are reported.[18]

Isolated Case Studies
None reported

Genetic Tests

Tests of Genotype: Direct tests are available for presence of black-and-tan and sable coat colors from HealthGene and VedtGen.

Tests of Phenotype: CHIC Certification: Required testing includes hip and elbow radiographs, CERF eye examination, and thyroid profile including autoantibodies. (See CHIC website; www. caninehealthinfo.org).

Recommend patella evaluation and cardiac evaluation.

Miscellaneous

- **Breed name synonyms:** Chien de Berger Belge, Tervueren, Terve, Belgian Sheepdog, Belgian Shepherd.
- **Registries:** AKC, UKC (under Belgian Shepherd), CKC, KCGB (Kennel Club of Great Britain), under Belgian Shepherd, ANKC (Australian National Kennel Club), under Belgian Shepherd, NKC (National Kennel Club), under Belgian Shepherd.
- **AKC rank (year 2008):** 103 (452 dogs registered)

- Internet resources: American Belgian Tervuren Club Inc.:
www.abtc.org

Belgian Shepherd Dog Club of Canada: www.bsdcc.org

Belgian Shepherd Dog Association of Great Britain:
www.bsdaofgb.co.uk

References

1. Greenfield CL, Messick JB, Solter PF, et. al.: Leukopenia in six healthy Belgian Tervuren. *J Am Vet Med Assoc.* 1999 Oct 15;215(8):1121-2.

2. Greenfield CL, Messick JB, Solter PE: Results of Hematologic Analyses and Prevalence of Physiologic Leukopenia in Belgian Tervuren. *J Am Vet Med Assoc* 2000:216[6]:866-871.

3. Gommeren K, Duchateau L, Paepe D, et. al.: Investigation of physiologic leukopenia in Belgian Tervuren dogs. J Vet Intern Med. 2006 Nov-Dec;20(6):1340-3.

4. Evans, R and ABTC: 2003 American Belgian Tervuren Club Health Survey. 2004.

5. OFA Website breed statistics: www.offa.org Last accessed July 1, 2010.

6. Oberbauer AM, Grossman DI, Irion DN, et. al.: The genetics of epilepsy in the Belgian tervuren and sheepdog. *J Hered.* 2003 Jan-Feb;94(1):57-63.

7. Famula TR, Oberbauer AM: Reducing the incidence of epileptic seizures in the Belgian Tervuren through selection. *Prev Vet Med.* 1998 Jan;33(1-4):251-9.

8. Berendt M, Gulløv CH, & Fredholm M: Focal epilepsy in the Belgian shepherd: evidence for simple Mendelian inheritance. J Small Anim Pract. 2009 Dec;50(12):655-61.

9. Berendt M, Gulløv CH, Christensen SL, et. al.: Prevalence and characteristics of epilepsy in the Belgian shepherd variants Groenendael and Tervueren born in Denmark 1995-2004. Acta Vet Scand. 2008 Dec 22;50:51.

10. Oberbauer AM, Belanger JM, Grossman DI, et. al.: Genome-wide linkage scan for loci associated with epilepsy in Belgian shepherd dogs. BMC Genet. 2010 May 4;11:35.

11. MacManus D: 1998 Tervuren Health Survey. 1998.

12. *Ocular Disorders Presumed to be Inherited in Purebred Dogs.* American College of Veterinary Ophthalmologists. ACVO, 2007.

13. Nachreiner R and Refsal K: Personal communication, Diagnostic Center for Population and Animal Health, Michigan State University. April, 2007.

14. Nachreiner R and Refsal K: Personal communication, Diagnostic Center for Population and Animal Health, Michigan State University. April, 2007.

15. Lubbes D, Mandigers PJ, Heuven HC, et. al.: Incidence of gastric carcinoma in Dutch Tervueren shepherd dogs born between 1991 and 2002. Tijdschr Diergeneeskd. 2009 Jul 15-Aug 1;134(14-15):606-10.

16. Mahaffey MB, Yarbrough KM, Munnell JF: Focal loss of pigment in the Belgian Tervuren dog. J Am Vet Med Assoc. 1978 Aug 15;173(4):390-6.

17. Chavkin MJ, Roberts SM, Salman MD, et. al.: Risk factors for development of chronic superficial keratitis in dogs. *J Am Vet Med Assoc.* 1994 May 15;204(10):1630-4.

18. *The Genetic Connection: A Guide to Health Problems in Purebred Dogs.* L Ackerman. p. 202. AAHA Press, 1999.

19. *The Complete Dog Book, 20th Ed.* The American Kennel Club. Howell Book House, NY 2006. p. 629-634.

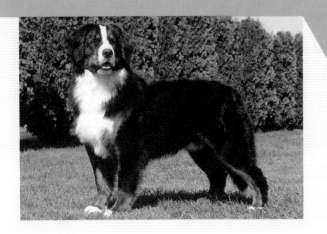

Bernese Mountain Dog

ribs. The tail is carried low when resting and is heavily haired. It reaches to the tarsus or a bit lower. Legs are straight boned, and dewclaws may be removed. Feet are compact and the toes are well arched. Rear dewclaws are removed.

The Breed History

Originating in the middle cantons of Switzerland (Berne region), this hardy dog was likely brought to the Alps by the Romans. These dogs derive from ancient Mastiff-type dogs. Almost lost to extinction, rejuvenation of the breed began in the 1900s. Out-crossing to Newfoundland dogs was one of the steps taken to infuse fresh genes. The first dogs were brought to America in 1926, and first AKC recognition was in the year 1937.

Breeding for Function

The Bernese Mountain dog acted as a drover and guarding dog and also for draft; pulling carts. They are unusually hardy and can live in environments with extremes of temperature and terrain. Today, they are seen in obedience, tracking, agility, and as therapy dogs. They are valued companions.

Physical Characteristics

Height at Withers: female 23-26" (58.5-66 cm), male 25-27.7" (63.5-70 cm).

Weight: females 75-95 lb (34-43 kg), males 80-115 lb (36-52 kg).

Coat: The silky, glossy, thick, straight to slightly wavy and moderately long coat distinguishes this breed from the other Swiss Mountain Dogs. Color is a jet black background with well defined rust markings and white highlight markings for the standard; the tri-color pattern has established marking distribution. Notably, the chest markings in white forms the Swiss cross and a white blaze is usually present. White is also found on the paws and tail tip. When they blow the coat twice per year, heavy shedding occurs; some dogs are low-level shedders year-round.

Longevity: 7-9 years

Points of Conformation: Sturdily built, large, but agility has not been compromised. Heavy bone and musculature are bred into these dogs. The eyes have a gentle expression and are a dark brown, oval shaped and have tight fitting eyelids. Ears are high set, triangular and hang close to the cheek. The skull has a moderate stop and a slight furrow runs up along the midline. The square muzzle ends in a large black nose. Lips are free of flews; they are a dry-mouthed breed. Neck is of medium length, well muscled and the topline is level. The thorax is deep and possesses well-sprung

Recognized Behavior Issues and Traits

Reported breed characteristics include: Faithful, gentle, affectionate, quick learner, hardy, needs close human companionship, may be aloof with strangers, need adequate exercise. Some lines may have temperament quirks. Good with other children and animals. Low barking, though will alarm bark. They need early socialization and obedience training, and are moderately active. Bernese are sensitive dogs; they respond best to gentle firm correction.

Normal Physiologic Variations

Mountain dogs are slow to mature, so should not be asked to do strenuous activity or pull heavy loads before they reach 2-3 years of age.

According to the 2005 BMDCA Health Survey, 59% of breeding females have had at least one **C-section**, and 32% have had difficulty whelping a litter.[1]

A Danish study of Bernese Mountain Dogs suggests that the breed may have higher normal ranges for biochemical values, including: Alkaline Phosphatase/AlkP (0-464), g-glutamyltransferase (0-12.2), amylase (285-1255), and cholesterol (5.29-10.08).[2]

Drug Sensitivities

None reported

Inherited Diseases

Elbow Dysplasia: Polygenically inherited trait causing elbow arthritis. Studies have shown that a significant portion of Bernese Mountain Dogs with elbow dysplasia have fragmented medial coronoid process. Males have a 3.1x risk over females in the breed. Breeding studies show a heritability of 20%, and that dogs with all grades of elbow dysplasia have the same liability for producing the disease in offspring. OFA reports 29.0% affected. Reported at a frequency of 24.5% in the 2005 BMDCA Health Survey. Reported 140.1x odds ratio for fragmented coronoid process, and 50.5x odds ratio for ununited anconeal process forms of elbow dysplasia versus other breeds.[1,3,4,5,6]

Hip Dysplasia: Polygenically inherited trait causing degenerative joint disease and hip arthritis. Reported 7.2x odds ratio versus other breeds. OFA reports 16.0% affected. Reported at a frequency of 14.0% in the 2005 BMDCA Health Survey.[1,3,6]

Patella Luxation: Polygenically inherited laxity of patellar ligaments, causing luxation, lameness, and later degenerative joint disease. Treat surgically if causing clinical signs. OFA reports 3.2% affected.[2]

von Willebrand's Disease Type 1 (vWD): Autosomal recessive genetic disorder causing a mild bleeding syndrome. A direct genetic test is available from VetGen, reporting 1% affected, and 16% carrier in the breed.

Progressive Retinal Atrophy (PRA): An autosomal recessive early retinal degeneration is identified in the breed, with an onset of night blindness around one year of age. Identified in 0.12% of Bernese Mountain Dogs CERF examined by veterinary ophthalmologists between 2000-2005, with an additional 0.24% labeled suspicious for PRA. Confirm with an electroretinogram. A genetic test is not available. CERF does not recommend breeding any Bernese Mountain Dog with PRA.[7,8]

Juvenile Renal Dysplasia: Rare, membranoproliferative glomerulonephritis with concomitant interstitial nephritis. Affected dogs present initially with polyuria and polydipsia, which progresses to clinical renal failure. Affected dogs are identified from months of age to 2-7 years of age. The renal expression of megalin is reduced or completely absent. One study suggests an inherited susceptibility to Borrelia infection as a precipitating factor. The mode of inheritance is polygenic, with a major autosomal recessive gene, and possibly an additional sex-linked gene influencing its expression.[9,10,11,12,13]

Hepatocerebellar Degeneration: A rare, autosomal recessive disease seen in 4-6 week old Bernese Mountain Dogs characterized by progressive cerebellar and hepatic disease. Histologically, degeneration and depletion of Purkinje's cells and vacuolation, degeneration, and nodular regeneration of hepatic tissues are evident.[14]

Disease Predispositions

Mortality/Longevity: Bernese Mountain Dogs are found to have diminished longevity, with a yearly breed-specific mortality risk of 6.5%. The probability for survival by 5 years of age is 83%, and by ten years of age is 30%. The 2005 BMDCA Health Survey found an average age at death of 7.8 years. A danish study showed an average life span of 7.1 years. Mortality studies in Sweden show a significantly increased risk of death due to tumors, especially in male dogs, versus other breeds.[1,15,16,17]

Umbilical Hernia: Congenital umbilical hernias are reported at a frequency of 24.0% in the 2005 BMDCA Health Survey.[1]

Osteoarthritis: Bernese Mountain Dogs have an increased incidence of arthritis. Dorn reports a 1.58x odds ratio versus other breeds. Reported at a frequency of 17.0% in the BMDCA 2005 Health Survey, with an average age of onset of 5.5 years.[1,18]

Allergic Dermatitis (Atopy): Inhalant or food allergy. Presents with pruritis and pyotraumatic dermatitis (hot spots). Reported at a frequency of 16.0% in the 2005 BMDCA Health Survey.[1]

Panosteitis: A self-limiting disease of young, large breed dogs involving the diaphyseal and metaphyseal areas of the tubular long bones, characterized by medullary fibrosis and both endosteal and subperiosteal new bone deposition. Affected dogs show intermittent lameness. Treatment is with non-steroidal anti-inflammatory drugs and rest. Reported at a frequency of 7.3% in the 2005 BMDCA Health Survey, with an average age of onset of 1.1 years.[1]

Cranial Cruciate Ligament Rupture (ACL): Traumatic tearing of the anterior cruciate ligament. Treatment is surgery. Reported at a frequency of 7.3% in the 2005 BMDCA Health Survey. Unknown mode of inheritance.[1]

Malignant Histiocytosis: The breed is predisposed to develop malignant histiocytomas in any area of the body. The most common clinical signs are anorexia, weight loss, lethargy, anemia, and dyspnea and/or coughing. Radiographs in affected dogs usually reveal either pulmonary nodules or consolidation, mediastinal mass, pleural effusion, or hepatomegaly and splenomegaly. The average age of diagnosis is 6.5 years, with an average life expectancy post-diagnosis of 49 days. Dorn reports a 15.07x odds ratio for the disorder versus other breeds. The trait appears to have a major Mendelian gene in its transmission, with a heritability of 0.298. One study in France reported an affected frequency of up to 25%. Reported as the cause of death of 10.7% of Bernese Mountain Dogs in Denmark at an average age of 6.9 years. Reported at a frequency of 4.0% in the 2005 BMDCA Health Survey, though listed as the #1 cause of death.[1,16,17,18,19,20,21,22,23]

Hypothyroidism: Inherited autoimmune thyroiditis. 4.8% positive for thyroid auto-antibodies based on testing at Michigan State University. (Ave. for all breeds is 7.5%). Reported at a frequency of 7.0% in the 2005 BMDCA Health Survey.[1,24,25]

Cataracts: Anterior cortex punctate cataracts predominate, through posterior, nuclear, and capsular cataracts also occur in the breed. Age of onset at 1 year. Identified in 4.03% of Bernese Mountain Dogs CERF examined by veterinary ophthalmologists between 2000-2005. Reported at a frequency of 4.7% in the 2005 BMDCA Health Survey. CERF does not recommend breeding any Bernese Mountain Dog with a cataract.[1,7]

Idiopathic Epilepsy: Grand-mal or petit-mal (partial) seizures are seen in this breed, with an average onset of 1-3 years of age. There is a male predominance. Treat with anticonvulsant medication. Pedigree studies in the breed indicate a polygenic mode of inheritance for grand-mal seizures, with the influence of a major recessive gene. Fly-Biting Petit-Mal Seizures are reported at a frequency of 4.0%, and Grand-mal seizures are reported at a frequency of 1.9% in the 2005 BMDCA Health Survey.[1,26]

Gastric Dilatation-Volvulus (Bloat, GDV): Polygenically inherited, life-threatening twisting of the stomach within the abdomen. Requires immediate veterinary attention. Reported at a frequency of 4.0% in the 2005 BMDCA Health Survey, with an average age of 5 years, and a 23% fatality.[1]

Persistent Pupillary Membranes: Strands of fetal remnant connecting; iris to iris, cornea, lens, or involving sheets of tissue. The later three forms can impair vision, and dogs affected with these forms should not be bred. Identified in 3.49% of Bernese Mountain Dogs CERF examined by veterinary ophthalmologists between 2000-2005.[8]

Mast Cell Tumor (MCT): Skin tumors that can reoccur locally or with distant metastasis. Mast cell tumors produce histamine, which can cause inflammation and ulceration. Reported at a frequency of 3.0% in the 2005 BMDCA Health Survey.[1]

Lymphoma/Lymphosarcoma: Malignant lymphatic cancer that most commonly presents in the lymph nodes, spleen, liver, or heart. Reported at a frequency of 3.0% in the 2005 BMDCA Health Survey.[1]

Humeral Osteochondritis Dissecans (OCD): Polygenically inherited cartilage defect of the humeral head. Causes shoulder joint pain and lameness in young growing dogs. Mild cases can resolve with rest, while more severe cases require surgery. 2.24:1 male to female ratio in the breed. Age of onset usually 2-4 months. 50% of cases are bilateral. Reported 47.1x odds ratio versus other breeds. Dorn reports a 4.40x odds ratio for OCD versus other breeds. Reported at a frequency of 2.9% in the 2005 BMDCA Health Survey. Unknown mode of inheritance.[1,6,18]

Entropion: Rolling in of eyelids, often causing corneal irritation or ulceration. Entropion is reported in 1.89% of Bernese Mountain Dogs CERF examined by veterinary ophthalmologists between 2000-2005. Reported at a frequency of 2.4% in the 2005 BMDCA Health Survey.[1,8]

Cleft Palate: Congenital disorder of incomplete closure of the maxillary processes to form the roof of the mouth. Reported as the #1 most frequent birth defect in the 2005 BMDCA Health Survey.[1]

Susceptability to Borrelia (Lyme disease) Infection: European studies have shown a higher frequency of either clinical Borreliosis or high Borrelia antibodies in Bernese Mountain Dogs compared with other breeds, suggesting an inherited increased susceptibility to infection.[13,27]

Portosystemic Shunt (PSS, lLiver Shunt): Congenital abnormal blood vessel connecting the portal and systemic circulation. More frequently intrahepatic in this breed versus extrahepatic. Causes stunting, abnormal behavior, possible seizures, and secondary ammonium urate urinary calculi in the breed. Treatment of PSS includes partial ligation and/or medical and dietary control of symptoms. Tobias reports a 15.1x odds ratio versus other breeds.[28]

Necrotizing Vasculitis/Sterile Meningitis: Affected dogs present with apathy, fever and increased head and cervical pain. Histopathology shows necrotizing vasculitis in the CNS, with perivascular granulomatous inflammation. Treat with steroids. Unknown mode of inheritance.[29]

Degenerative Myelopathy (DM): Affected dogs show an insidious onset of upper motor neuron (UMN) paraparesis. The disease eventually progresses to severe tetraparesis. Affected dogs have normal results on myelography, MRI, and CSF analysis. Necropsy confirms the condition. Reported at a 4x odds ratio versus other breeds. Unknown mode of inheritance. A direct genetic test for an autosomal recessive DM susceptibility gene is available. All affected dogs are homozygous for the gene, however only a small percentage of homozygous dogs develop DM. OFA reports DM susceptibility gene frequencies of 49% carrier, and 11% homozygous "at-risk".[30]

Hypomyelination of the Spinal Cord (Trembler): The condition is manifested clinically as a tremor of the limbs and head which becomes more intense with excitement or stress and which disappears with sleep. The tremor, which is first noticeable between two and eight weeks old, may persist throughout life but decline with age. An autosomal recessive mode of inheritance is suggested.[31]

Cervical Vertebral Instability (Wobbler Syndrome): Presents with UMN spasticity and ataxia. Imaging studies suggest that the primary lesion is foramenal stenosis and intervertebral instability at C3-7. MRI is superior to myelography in determining site, severity, and nature of the spinal cord compression. Treatment is with surgery. Undetermined mode of inheritance. Reported as a sporadic finding in the breed.[32]

Rosenthal Fiber Encephalopathy (Alexander's Disease): Fatal, neonatal degenerative neurological disease presenting with rapidly progressive nonambulatory tetraparesis, generalized tremors, and depressed mental status. Macroscopically the brain shows moderate enlargement of the lateral ventricles. Histologically there are GFAP positive staining eosinophilic deposits consistent with Rosenthal fibers (RFs) throughout the white matter of the central nervous system, and a marked proliferation of abnormally large astrocytes.[33,34]

Color Dilution Alopecia, Fibrinoid Leukodystrophy, Hypertrophic Osteodystrophy, Hypoadrenocorticism, and **Sebaceous Adenitis** are reported.[35]

Isolated Case Studies

Cervical Cartilaginous Exostosis: A 3-1/2 year old Bernese Mountain Dog exhibited ataxia in the hind limbs and flailing movements in the forelimbs. On survey radiographs of the cervical spine there was a focal calcified mass between the dorsal arch of the atlas and the spinous process of the axis with severe dorsal spinal cord compression. The mass was removed surgically and the dog made a complete recovery. Histopathology of the excised mass was consistent with a diagnosis of cartilaginous exostosis.[36]

Circumcaval Ureter and Intrahepatic Portosystemic Shunt: A 4-month-old Bernese Mountain Dog had an intrahepatic shunt, and hydronephrosis and hydroureter due to the left ureter passing dorsal to the caudal vena cava. The shunt was partially closed with a cellophane band, and the ureter repositioned ventral to the vena cava, and anastomosed.[37]

Nephroblastoma: A 4-month-old female Bernese Mountain Dog examined for abdominal distention was found to have a nephroblastoma. The dog was euthanized due to widespread metastasis.[38]

Fibromatosis: A young, male Bernese Mountain Dog with lameness and diffuse thickening of the soft tissue in the right hind limb, was found to have multilobular, space-occupying lesions within and between the muscles of the right femur. Pathology identified collagen fibers and fibroblasts, and a diagnosis of fibromatosis.[39]

Genetic Tests

Tests of Genotype: Direct test for vWD is available from VetGen.

Direct test for a DM susceptability gene is available from the OFA.

Tests of Phenotype: CHIC Certification: Required testing includes AKC DNA profile, vWD test from VetGen, hip and elbow radiographs, CERF eye examination, and cardiac evaluation by a cardiologist. (See CHIC website; www.caninehealthinfo.org).

Recommend thyroid profile including autoantibodies, patella evaluation and bile acids or blood ammonia for liver shunt.

Miscellaneous

- **Breed name synonyms:** Berner Sennenhund, Berner, Bernese Cattle Dog, Durrbachler (historical).
- **Registries:** AKC, UKC, CKC, KCGB (Kennel Club of Great Britain), ANKC (Australian National Kennel Club), NKC (National Kennel Club).
- **AKC rank (year 2008):** 40 (3,338 dogs registered)
- **Internet resources: Bernese Mountain Dog Club of America**: www.bmdca.org
  Bernese Mountain Dog Club of Canada: www.bmdcc.ca
  Bernese Mountain Dog Club of Great Britain: www.bernese.co.uk
  Berner-Garde Foundation: www.bernergarde.org

References

1. Bernese Mountain Dog Club of America: 2005 BMDCA Health Survey. 2005.
2. Nielsen L, Kjelgaard-Hansen M, Jensen AL, et. al.: Breed-specific variation of hematologic and biochemical analytes in healthy adult Bernese Mountain dogs. Vet Clin Pathol. 2010 Mar;39(1):20-8.
3. OFA Website breed statistics: www.offa.org Last accessed July 1, 2010.
4. Meyer-Lindenberg A, Langhann A, Fehr M, et. al.: Prevalence of fragmented medial coronoid process of the ulna in lame adult dogs. Vet Rec. 2002 Aug 24;151(8):230-4.
5. Beuing R, Janssen N, Wurster H, et. al: The significance of elbow dysplasia (ED) for breeding in Bernese Mountain Dogs in Germany. Schweiz Arch Tierheilkd. 2005 Nov;147(11):491-7.
6. LaFond E, Breur GJ and Austin CC: Breed susceptibility for developmental orthopedic diseases in dogs. J Am Anim Hosp Assoc. 2002 Sep-Oct;38(5):467-77.
7. Chaudieu G, Molon-Noblot S: Early retinopathy in the Bernese Mountain Dog in France: preliminary observations. Vet Ophthalmol. 2004 May-Jun;7(3):175-84.
8. Ocular Disorders Presumed to be Inherited in Purebred Dogs. American College of Veterinary Ophthalmologists. ACVO, 2007.
9. Olenick CL: Congenital renal dysplasia and psychogenic polydipsia in a Bernese mountain dog. Can Vet J. 1999 Jun;40(6):425-6.
10. Minkus G, Breuer W, Wanke R, et. al.: Familial nephropathy in Bernese mountain dogs. Vet Pathol. 1994 Jul;31(4):421-8.
11. Reusch C, Hoerauf A, Lechner J, et. al.: A new familial glomerulonephropathy in Bernese mountain dogs. Vet Rec. 1994 Apr 16;134(16):411-5.
12. Raila J, Aupperle H, Raila G, et. al.: Renal pathology and urinary protein excretion in a 14-month-old bernese mountain dog with chronic renal failure. J Vet Med A Physiol Pathol Clin Med. 2007 Apr;54(3):131-5.
13. Gerber B, Eichenberger S, Wittenbrink MM, et. al.: Increased prevalence of Borrelia burgdorferi infections in Bernese Mountain Dogs: a possible breed predisposition. BMC Vet Res. 2007 Jul 12;3:15.
14. Carmichael KP, Miller M, Rawlings CA, et. al.: Clinical, hematologic, and biochemical features of a syndrome in Bernese mountain dogs characterized by hepatocerebellar degeneration. J Am Vet Med Assoc. 1996 Apr 15;208(8):1277-9.
15. Egenvall A, Bonnett BN, Shoukri M, et. al.: Age pattern of mortality in eight breeds of insured dogs in Sweden. Prev Vet Med. 2000 Jul 3;46(1):1-14.
16. Egenvall A, Bonnett BN, Hedhammar A, et. al.: Mortality in over 350,000 insured Swedish dogs from 1995-2000: II. Breed-specific age and survival patterns and relative risk for causes of death. Acta Vet Scand. 2005;46(3):121-36.
17. Nielsen L, Andreasen SN, Andersen SD, et. al.: Malignant histiocytosis and other causes of death in Bernese mountain dogs in Denmark. Vet Rec. 2010 Feb 13;166(7):199-202.
18. Dorn CR: Canine breed-specific risks of frequently diagnosed diseases at veterinary teaching hospitals. Monograph. AKC Canine Health Foundation. 2000.
19. Paterson S, Boydell P, Pike R: Systemic histiocytosis in the Bernese mountain dog. J Small Anim Pract. 1995 May;36(5):233-6.
20. Schmidt ML, Rutteman GR, van Niel MH, et. al.: Clinical and radiographic manifestations of canine malignant histiocytosis. Vet Q. 1993 Sep;15(3):117-20.
21. Affolter VK, Moore PF:Localized and desiminated histiocytic sarcoma of dendritic cell origin in dogs. Vet Pathol. 2002. Jan;39(1):74-83.
22. Padgett GA, Madewell BR, Keller ET,et. Al,: Inheritance of histiocytosis in Bernese mountain dogs. J Small Anim Pract. 1995 Mar;36(3):93-8.
23. Abadie J, Hédan B, Cadieu E, et. al.: Epidemiology, pathology, and genetics of histiocytic sarcoma in the Bernese mountain dog breed. J Hered. 2009 Jul-Aug;100 Suppl 1:S19-27.
24. Nachreiner R and Refsal K: Personal communication, Diagnostic Center for Population and Animal Health, Michigan State University. April, 2007.
25. Nachreiner RF, Refsal KR, Graham PA, et. al.: Prevalence of serum thyroid hormone autoantibodies in dogs with clinical signs of hypothyroidism. J Am Vet Med Assoc 2002 Feb 15;220(4):466-71.
26. Kathmann I, Jaggy A, Busato A, et. al.: Clinical and genetic investigations of idiopathic epilepsy in the Bernese mountain dog. J Small Anim Pract. 1999 Jul;40(7):319-25.
27. Hovius KE and Houwers DJ: Diagnostic aspects of Borrelia-infections in dogs. Tijdschr Diergeneeskd. 2007 Aug 15;132(16):612-6.
28. Tobias KM, Rohrbach BW: Association of breed with the diagnosis of congenital portosystemic shunts in dogs: 2,400 cases (1980-2002). J Am Vet Med Assoc. 2003 Dec 1;223(11):1636-9.
29. Gerhardt A, Risse R, Meyer-Lindenberg A: Necrotizing vasculitis of the cerebral and spinal leptomeninges in a Bernese mountain dog. Dtsch Tierarztl Wochenschr. 1998 Apr;105(4):139-41.
30. Kathman I,Cizinauskas S, Doherr MG, et. Al,: Daily controlled physiotherapy increases survival time in dogs with suspected degenerative myelopath. J Vet Intern Med. 2006 Jul-Aug;20(4):927-32.
31. Palmer AC, Blakemore WF, Wallace ME, et. al.: Recognition of "trembler", a hypomyelinating condition in the Bernese mountain dog. Vet Rec. 1987 Jun 27;120(26):609-12.
32. Eagleson JS, Diaz J, Platt SR, et. al.: Cervical vertebral malformation-malarticulation syndrome in the Bernese mountain dog: clinical and magnetic resonance imaging features. J Small Anim Pract. 2009 Apr;50(4):186-93.
33. Weissenbock H, Obermaier G, Dahme E: Alexander's disease in a Bernese mountain dog. Acta Neuropathol (Berl). 1996;91(2):200-4.
34. Aleman N, Marcaccini A, Espino L, et. al.: Rosenthal fiber encephalopathy in a dog resembling Alexander disease in humans. Vet Pathol. 2006 Nov;43(6):1025-8.
35. The Genetic Connection: A Guide to Health Problems in Purebred Dogs. L Ackerman. p. 202. AAHA Press, 1999.
36. Bhatti S, Van Ham L, Putcuyps I, et. al.: Atlantoaxial cartilaginous exostosis causing spinal cord compression in a mature Bernese mountain dog. J Small Anim Pract. 2001 Feb;42(2):79-81.
37. Doust RT, Clarke SP, Hammond G, et.al,: Circumcaval ureter associated with an intrahepatic portosystemic shunt in a dog. J Am Vet Med Assoc. 2006 Feb 1; 228(3):389-91.
38. Frimberger AE, Moore AS, Schelling SH: Treatment of nephroblastoma in a juvenile dog. J Am Vet Med Assoc. 1995 Sep 1;207(5):596-8.
39. Welle MM, Sutter E, Malik Y, et. al.: Fibromatosis in a young Bernese Mountain Dog: clinical, imaging, and histopathological findings. J Vet Diagn Invest. 2009 Nov;21(6):895-900.
40. The Complete Dog Book, 20th Ed. The American Kennel Club. Howell Book House, NY 2006. p. 240-243.

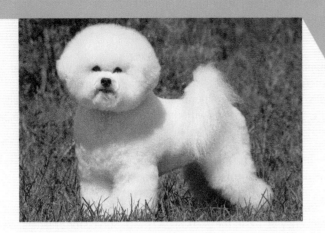

The Breed History

The history of the breed is centered in the Mediterranean. The Barbet Water Spaniel was the chief progenitor of the breed, and the name Bichon evolved from Barbichon, the intermediate ancestor. Four regional varieties (Bichon Havanais, Bolognais, Teneriffe and Maltais) developed. They were favored companions to French and Italian nobility. Frisé is a French term to describe their frizzy, soft hair. They were brought to United States in the mid 1950s, and the first registry in the AKC studbook dates to 1972.

Breeding for Function

This dog was bred for companionship, though their origins from water spaniels give them talents that would be useful for hunting. They were popular in Belgium, but also became a favored trick-performing dog in the late 1800s.

Physical Characteristics

Height at Withers: 9.5-11.5 " (24-29 cm).

Weight: 7-12 lb (3-6 kg).

Coat: Their distinctive white coat is double, with a dense soft inner coat and curly fine outer coat. It is springy and stands up when groomed to give an appearance described as "powder puff". Some dogs have a hint of cream, buff, gray or apricot to the hairs. They have high grooming needs including regular trimming, and are low shedder and low allergen dogs.

Longevity: 14-16 years. Oldest recorded was 21 yrs.

Points of Conformation: This dog is sturdily built and the profuse haircoat is a distinct feature of the breed. The skull is somewhat rounded, a distinct stop is present, and the nose is large and pigmented black. The round eyes are dark brown and palpebral margins and skin around (halo) is black. Ears are pendulous with fine leathers, and the neck is long with a high head carriage. Limbs are straight, and the feet compact. The topline is fairly level, and thorax is deep with moderately sprung ribs; the abdomen has a moderate tuck. Slightly longer than high, they should appear to move effortlessly. Plumed tails are carried over the back, reaching about half way up to withers but the tail bones should not be resting on the back, and a corkscrew tail is considered a serious fault.

Recognized Behavior Issues and Traits

This type of dog is ascribed as: Friendly, with an outgoing temperament. Fear biter or separation anxiety may occur in some shy dogs, but breeding of dogs that deviate from the typical playful Bichon personality is not accepted. They are alarm barkers but not considered watchdogs. They need close human contact, and are considered moderately trainable. They are fine for city life, as they are active dogs with average exercise needs.

Normal Physiologic Variations

None reported

Drug Sensitivities

None reported

Inherited Diseases

Hip Dysplasia and Legg-Calve-Perthes: Polygenically inherited traits causing degenerative joint disease and hip arthritis. OFA reports 6.7% affected with hip dysplasia.[1]

Patella Luxation: Polygenically inherited laxity of patellar ligaments, causing luxation, lameness, and later degenerative joint disease. Treat surgically if causing clinical signs. Reported 4.8x odds ratio versus other breeds. OFA reports 5.5% affected. Reported at a frequency of 12% in the 2007 BFCA Health Survey for Breeders.[1,2,3]

Cataracts: Cataracts appear to be inherited in the Bichon Frise as an autosomal recessive trait. Age at onset of cataract formation ranges from 1.5-13.5 years, with a peak age of 3 years. Posterior cortex cataracts predominate, starting as punctate opacities. One study showed a 5.2x odds ratio in Bichon Frise versus other breeds. Dorn reports a 1.41x odds ratio. The estimated frequency of cataracts in the breed is 11.45%. Affected dogs can develop secondary retinal detachment or glaucoma. Identified in 4.29% of Bichon Frise CERF examined by veterinary ophthalmologists between 2000-2005. Reported at a frequency of 4% in the 2007 BFCA Health Survey for Breeders. CERF does not recommend breeding any Bichon Frise with a cataract.[2,4,5,6,7,8,9,10]

Patent Ductus Arteriosus (PDA): Polygenically inherited congenital heart disorder, where a fetal vessel remains open after birth, causing a mixing of oxygenated and unoxygenated blood. Affected dogs are usually stunted, and have a loud heart murmur. Diagnosis with Doppler ultrasound. Treat with surgery. Dorn reports a 13.35x odds ratio in Bichon Frise versus other breeds.[4]

Elbow Dysplasia: Polygenically inherited trait causing elbow arthritis. OFA reports 0.7% affected.[1]

Disease Predispositions

Lacrimal Gland Hypersecretion: Dorn reports a 171.11x odds ratio in Bichon Frise versus other breeds. Can be associated with entropion, ectopic cilia, blocked tear ducts, allergies, or other causes.[4]

Allergic Dermatitis (Atopy): Inhalant or food allergy. Presents with pruritis and pyotraumatic dermatitis (hot spots). Reported at an increased frequency versus other breeds. Reported at a frequency of 23% in the 2007 BFCA Health Survey for Breeders.[2,11]

Cryptorchidism: Unilateral or bilateral undescended testicles. This is a sex-limited disorder with an unknown mode of inheritance. Reported at a frequency of 11% in the 2007 BFCA Health Survey for Breeders.[2]

Urinary Calculi: The breed is found to be at an increased risk of developing struvite, oxalate, and cystine calculi (due to cystinuria). Dorn reports a 4.68x odds ratio in Bichon Frise versus other breeds. Reported at a frequency of 5% in the 2007 BFCA Health Survey for Breeders.[2,4,12,13,14,15]

Umbilical Hernia: Congenital opening in the body wall from where the umbilical cord was attached. Reported at a frequency of 5% in the 2007 BFCA Health Survey for Breeders. Unknown mode of inheritance.[2]

Distichiasis: Abnormally placed eyelashes that irritate the cornea and conjunctiva. Can cause secondary corneal ulceration. Identified in 3.33% of Bichon Frise CERF examined by veterinary ophthalmologists between 2000-2005.[9]

Corneal Dystrophy: The epithelial/stromal form occurs in the breed, causing opacities on the surface of the cornea. Average age of onset is 2 years. Unknown mode of inheritance. Identified in 2.74% of Bichon Frise CERF examined by veterinary ophthalmologists between 2000-2005.[9]

Ciliary Dyskinesia: Inherited abnormal anatomy and function of cilia. Causes chronic secondary respiratory infections due to abnormal respiratory ciliary clearance, and infertility due to abnormal sperm motility. Unknown mode of inheritance. Reported at a frequency of 2% in the 2007 BFCA Health Survey for Breeders.[2,16]

Persistent Pupillary Membranes: Strands of fetal remnant connecting; iris to iris, cornea, lens, or involving sheets of tissue. The later three forms can impair vision, and dogs affected with these forms should not be bred. Identified in 1.95% of Bichon Frise CERF examined by veterinary ophthalmologists between 2000-2005.[9]

Hypothyroidism: Inherited autoimmune thyroiditis. 1.7% positive for thyroid auto-antibodies based on testing at Michigan State University. (Ave. for all breeds is 7.5%).[17,18]

Primary (Narrow Angle) Glaucoma: Ocular condition causing increased pressure within the eyeball, and secondary blindness due to damage to the retina. Diagnose with tonometry and gonioscopy. Diagnosed in 1.59% of Bichon Frises presented to veterinary teaching hospitals.[19]

Portosystemic Shunt (PSS, Liver Shunt): Congenital disorder, where abnormal blood vessels connecting the systemic and portal blood flow. Vessels can be intrahepatic or extrahepatic. Causes stunting, abnormal behavior and possible seizures. A case study documented secondary pruritis that resolved with surgical correction of the shunt. One study showed a significantly higher prevalence versus other breeds, and a 12:2 female to male ratio in the Bichon Frise. Tobias reports a 13.3x odds ratio versus other breeds. Undetermined mode of inheritance.[20,21,22]

Immune-Mediated Hemolytic Anemia: Auto-immune disorder where the body produces antibodies against its own red blood cells. Treatment with immunosuppressive drugs. There is generally a female preponderance with this disorder. One study found a 5.3x odds ratio in Bichon Frise versus other breeds.[23]

Diabetes Mellitus: Caused by a lack of insulin production by the pancreas. Controlled by insulin injections, diet, and glucose monitoring. Dorn reports a 3.24x odds ratio in Bichon Frise versus other breeds. Unknown mode of inheritance. Reported at a frequency of 1% in the 2007 BFCA Health Survey for Breeders.[2,4]

Motor Dyskinesia: A rare disorder presenting with episodic involuntary skeletal muscle activity with normal levels of consciousness, similar to paroxysmal dystonic choreoathetosis. The disorder is differentiated from partial motor seizure activity by the character of the episodes, absence of identifiable preceding aura, absence of autonomic signs and the fact that multiple limbs are affected in a varying pattern without generalization and loss of consciousness.[24]

Brachygnathism, Deafness, Entropion, Epilepsy, Factor IX Deficiency, Prognathism, Progressive Retinal Atrophy, Retinal Dysplasia, Shaker Syndrome, Ventricular Septal Defect, and **von Willebrand's Disease** are reported.[25]

Isolated Case Studies

Congenital Alopecia: A Bichon Frise puppy was born with an absence of hair follicles, erector pili muscles, sebaceous glands, and sweat glands. This defect was not associated with abnormal pigmentation, normal black and brown pigmentation developed independently of the alopecic pattern.[26]

Hydrocephalus and Antidiuretic Hormone Deficiency: A 13-month-old male bichon frise with a domed skull was examined for the investigation of intermittent seizures, ataxia, abnormal behavior, polyuria, and polydipsia. Severe hyponatremia and hypoosmolality were identified, and diagnostic testing indicated inappropriate antidiuretic hormone secretion. MRI revealed severe hydrocephalus.[27]

Episodic Ataxia/Ion Channelopathy: A four-year-old neutered male Bichon Frise developed chronic, progressive, episodic cerebellar ataxia. All testing was normal. Treatment with 4-aminopyridine resolved all signs, suggesting an ion channelopathy.[28]

Genetic Tests

Tests of Genotype: none

Tests of Phenotype: CHIC Certification: Required testing includes hip radiographs, patella evaluation (after 12 months, and then annually), and CERF eye examination (annually). Optional testing includes congenital cardiac evaluation, and bile acids for liver shunt. (See CHIC website; www.caninehealthinfo.org).

Recommend thyroid profile including autoantibodies and elbow radiographs.

Miscellaneous

- **Breed name synonyms:** Bichon, Bichon Teneriffe, Teneriffe (historical), Bichon a Poil Frise
- **Registries:** AKC, CKC, UKC, KCGB (Kennel Club of Great Britain), ANKC (Australian National Kennel Club), NKC (National Kennel Club)
- **AKC rank (year 2008):** 35 (4,675 dogs registered)
- **Internet resources:** Bichon Frise Club of America:
  www.bichon.org
  Bichon Frise Club of Canada: www.bichonfriseclubofcanada.com
  Bichon Frise Club of Great Britain:
  www.bichonfriseclubofgb.info/

References

1. OFA Website breed statistics: www.offa.org Last accessed July 1, 2010.
2. BFCA Health Committee: 2007 BFCA Health Survey for Breeders. 2008.
3. LaFond E, Breur GJ and Austin CC: Breed susceptibility for developmental orthopedic diseases in dogs. J Am Anim Hosp Assoc. 2002 Sep-Oct;38(5):467-77.
4. Dorn CR: Canine breed-specific risks of frequently diagnosed diseases at veterinary teaching hospitals. Monograph. AKC Canine Health Foundation. 2000.
5. Adkins EA, Hendrix DV: Outcomes of dogs presented for cataract evaluation: a retrospective study. J Am Anim Hosp Assoc. 2005 Jul-Aug;41(4):235-40.
6. Wallace MR, MacKay EO, Gelatt KN, et. al.: Inheritance of cataract in the Bichon Frise. Vet Ophthalmol. 2005 May-Jun;8(3):203-5.
7. Gelatt KN, Mackay EO: Prevalence of primary breed-related cataracts in the dog in North America. Vet Ophthalmol. 2005 Mar-Apr;8(2):101-11.
8. Gelatt KN, MacKay EO: Secondary glaucomas in the dog in North America. Vet Ophthalmol. 2004 Jul-Aug;7(4):245-59.
9. Ocular Disorders Presumed to be Inherited in Purebred Dogs. American College of Veterinary Ophthalmologists. ACVO, 2007.
10. Gelatt, KN, Wallace MR. Andrew SE, et. al: Cataracts in the Bichon Frise: Vet Ophthalmol:2003;6;1;3-9.
11. White SD: Update on Allergies: Atopic Dermatitis. Proceedings, Northeast Veterinary Conference 2004.
12. Jones BR, Kirkman JH, Hogan J, et. al.: Analysis of uroliths from cats and dogs in New Zealand, 1993-96. N Z Vet J. 1998 Dec;46(6):233-6.
13. Case LC, Ling GV, Franti CE, et. al.: Cystine-containing urinary calculi in dogs: 102 cases (1981-1989). J Am Vet Med Assoc. 1992 Jul 1;201(1):129-33.
14. Houston DM, Moore AE, Favrin MG, et. al.: Canine urolithiasis: a look at over 16 000 urolith submissions to the Canadian Veterinary Urolith Centre from February 1998 to April 2003. Can Vet J. 2004 Mar;45(3):225-30.
15. Houston DM & Moore AE: Canine and feline urolithiasis: examination of over 50 000 urolith submissions to the Canadian veterinary urolith centre from 1998 to 2008. Can Vet J. 2009 Dec;50(12):1263-8.
16. Maddux JM, Edwards DF, Barnhill MA, et. al.: Neutrophil function in dogs with congenital ciliary dyskinesia. Vet Pathol. 1991 Sep;28(5):347-53.
17. Nachreiner R and Refsal K: Personal communication, Diagnostic Center for Population and Animal Health, Michigan State University. April, 2007.
18. Nachreiner RF, Refsal KR, Graham PA, et. al.: Prevalence of serum thyroid hormone autoantibodies in dogs with clinical signs of hypothyroidism. J Am Vet Med Assoc 2002 Feb 15;220(4):466-71.
19. Gelatt KN, MacKay EO: Prevalence of the breed-related glaucomas in pure-bred dogs in North America. Vet Ophthalmol. 2004 Mar-Apr;7(2):97-111.
20. Hunt GB: Effect of breed on anatomy of portosystemic shunts resulting from congenital diseases in dogs and cats: a review of 242 cases. Aust Vet J. 2004 Dec;82(12):746-9.
21. Waisglass SE, Gillick A, Cockshutt J, et. al.: Pruritus possibly associated with a portosystemic shunt in a bichon frise puppy. Can Vet J. 2006 Nov;47(11):1109-11.
22. Tobias KM & Rohrbach BW: Association of breed with the diagnosis of congenital portosystemic shunts in dogs: 2,400 cases (1980-2002). J Am Vet Med Assoc. 2003 Dec 1;223(11):1636-9.
23. Miller SA, Hohenhaus AE, Hale AS: Case-control study of blood type, breed, sex, and bacteremia in dogs with immune-mediated hemolytic anemia. J Am Vet Med Assoc. 2004 Jan 15;224(2):232-5.
24. Penderis J, Franklin RJ: Dyskinesia in an adult bichon frise. J Small Anim Pract. 2001 Jan;42(1):24-5.
25. The Genetic Connection: A Guide to Health Problems in Purebred Dogs. L Ackerman. p.202-3, AAHA Press, 1999.
26. Grieshaber TL, Blakemore JC, Yaskulski S: Congenital alopecia in a Bichon Frise. J Am Vet Med Assoc. 1986 May 1;188(9):1053-4
27. Shiel RE, Pinilla M, & Mooney CT: Syndrome of inappropriate antidiuretic hormone secretion associated with congenital hydrocephalus in a dog. J Am Anim Hosp Assoc. 2009 Sep-Oct;45(5):249-52.
28. Hopkins AL & Clarke J: Episodic cerebellar dysfunction in a bichon frise: a canine case of episodic ataxia? J Small Anim Pract. 2010 Aug;51(8):444-6.
29. The Complete Dog Book, 20th Ed. The American Kennel Club. Howell Book House, NY 2006. p. 529-532.

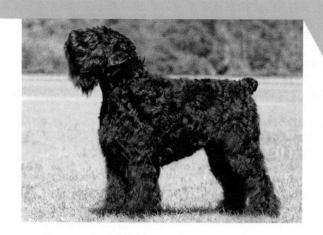

Black Russian Terrier

The palpebral margins are tight and black, as are the lips. No flews. Small triangular ears are high set, and just reach the lateral canthus. Gingival surface is pigmented, and spots of pigment may occur on the tongue. Neck thick, well muscled, the thorax is wide and deep with oval cross section, pronounced withers merge with level topline. The abdomen is well tucked up, loin is short. Limbs are straight, with very short straight metacarpals/metatarsals, and large rounded feet. Nails dark and rear dewclaws often removed. The thick tail is high set, and usually docked to the length of 3-5 vertebrae. Gait is springy, smooth and long.

The Breed History

Following WW II, a kennel in the Soviet Union worked to develop a hardy working dog from resident breeds of the time. The 1950s saw serious breed development using 17 breeds in the initial breeding pool, including Rottweilers, Giant Schnauzers, Airedale, Moscow Diver, Newfoundland and Caucasian Ovcharka dogs. The first breeding crossed Roy, a Giant Schnauzer with a female Rottweiler. By 1981 they were granted official breed status. Of the two subtypes, the more massive constitution is preferred over the terrier type, so much so that the breed was moved from terrier to working breed.

Breeding for Function

These dogs were bred to work as guard dogs and protection dogs. The breeders wished to develop a dog that required minimal coat care, was a large size with exceptional strength and excellent trainability and high but controlled aggression. Early in breed development, appearance was sacrificed for good working ability, and heterogeneous appearance was typical. Two subtypes emerged. The first, a terrier type and the second a more massive "bear" dog with coarse build.

Physical Characteristics

Height at Withers: female 26-29" (66-74 cm), male 27-30" (69-76 cm); disqualified if under 26" (66 cm).

Weight: 77-120 lb (32-54 kg).

Coat: Color must be black, or black intermixed with a few other gray hairs. A thick double coat, with a coarse overcoat and undercoat thick and soft in texture. Length of hairs 1.5-4" (4-10 cm) and has a tousled appearance—not wiry, not curly. Hair in and around the ears is trimmed for show. Fairly easy keeping coat.

Longevity: 10-14 years

Points of Conformation: Robust, this heavily boned dog is well muscled and capable of great endurance. Bitches are more refined, but still strongly built. Only very slightly longer than tall, they give an overall impression of great strength. The skull is broad and strong, with a blocky appearance with moderate stop. A prominent occipital protuberance is characteristic. Nose is large, black. The eyes are oval, medium in size and darkly pigmented.

Recognized Behavior Issues and Traits

Breed attributes ascribed include: Excellent protection instinct, reliable, courageous, calm, intelligent, with high trainability. They are stubborn when it comes to retraining though, as they seem to have very long memories. May be somewhat aloof with strangers. The terrier subtype is somewhat high strung, while the massive type is much more settled, even tranquil when not working.

Normal Breed Variations

None reported

Drug Sensitivities

None reported

Inherited Diseases

Hip Dysplasia: Polygenically inherited trait causing degenerative joint disease and hip arthritis. OFA reports 43.0% affected.[1]

Elbow Dysplasia: Polygenically inherited trait causing elbow arthritis. OFA reports 30.2% affected.[1]

Hyperuricosuria/Urate Urolithiasis (Bladder Stones): Autosomal recessive disorder of urate metabolism due to a mutation in the SLC2A9 gene. Urate bladder stone formation is secondary to hyperuricosuria. Affected dogs require lifelong diet and medication to prevent reoccurrence. A genetic test is available.[2,3]

Patella Luxation: Polygenically inherited laxity of patellar ligaments, causing luxation, lameness, and later degenerative joint disease. Treat surgically if causing clinical signs. Too few Black Russian Terriers have been screened by OFA to determine an accurate frequency.[1]

Disease Predispositions

Hypothyroidism: Inherited autoimmune thyroiditis. Identified in the breed, however too few Black Russian Terriers have been thyroid tested at Michigan State University to determine an accurate frequency. (Ave. for all breeds is 7.5%). OFA reports 2.6% of 38 dogs tested were affected. This number may change as more Black Russian Terriers are tested.[1,4,5]

Progressive Retinal Atrophy (PRA): Inherited degeneration of the retina, progressing to blindness. Onset 6 months to as late as 42 months of age. Black Russian Terriers with PRA go blind gradually, first losing their night vision and then their day vision. Many do not go completely blind until they are 8 years old or older. Undetermined mode of inheritance.[6]

Subaortic Stenosis and Mitral Valve Dysplasia: Identified in three 2 month old Black Russian Terrier littermates. In other breeds, subaortic stenosis is inherited as a polygenic trait.[7]

Other Ocular Disorders: Too few Black Russian Terriers have been CERF examined to determine accurate breed frequencies for ocular disorders.[8]

Isolated Case Studies

Extra Molars (Compound Odontomas): A six month-old, male Black Russian terrier dog was presented for oral masses on both sides of the mandible lateral to the first molars, which radiographs revealed to be small teeth (denticles). Treatment consisted of extraction of all denticles.[9]

Congenital Cataract and Microphthalmia: Case study of a litter of Black Russian Terriers born with congenital cataracts and microphthalmia.[10]

Genetic Tests

Tests of Genotype: Direct test for hyperuricosuria is available from the UC-Davis VGL and Animal Health Trust.

Tests of Phenotype: CHIC Certification: Required testing includes hip and elbow radiographs, CERF eye examination, and cardiac evaluation by a cardiologist. (See CHIC website; www.caninehealthinfo.org).

Recommend thyroid profile including autoantibodies, and patella evaluation.

Miscellaneous

- **Breed name synonyms:** Black Terrier, Chornyi, Terrier Noir Russe, Russian Bear Schnauzer, Tchiorny Terrier
- **Registries:** AKC, CKC, FCI, SKC, ANKC (Australian National Kennel Club), NKC (National Kennel Club)
- **AKC rank (year 2008):** 121 (245 dogs registered)
- **Breed resources: Black Russian Terrier Club of America:** www.brtca.org
  Black Russian Terrier Club of Canada: www.brtcc.ca
  Black Russian Terrier Club (UK): www.rbtclub.co.uk

References

1. OFA Website breed statistics: www.offa.org Last accessed July 1, 2010.
2. Bende B, Nemeth T: High prevalence of urate urolithiosis in the Russian black terrier. Vet Rec. 2004 Aug 21;155(8):239-40.
3. Bannasch D, Safra N, Young A, et. al.: Mutations in the SLC2A9 Gene Cause Hyperuricosuria and Hyperuricemia in the Dog. PLoS Genet. 2008. 4(11): e1000246. doi:10.1371/journal.pgen.1000246
4. Nachreiner R and Refsal K: Personal communication, Diagnostic Center for Population and Animal Health, Michigan State University. April, 2007.
5. Nachreiner RF, Refsal KR, Graham PA, et. al.: Prevalence of serum thyroid hormone autoantibodies in dogs with clinical signs of hypothyroidism. J Am Vet Med Assoc 2002 Feb 15;220(4):466-71.
6. Black Russian Terrier Club of America website: www.brtca.org. Last accessed July 1, 2010.
7. Pikula J, Pikulova J, Bandouchova H, et. al.: Subaortic stenosis and mitral dysplasia in three Black Russian Terrier puppies. Vet. Med. – Czech 2005;50(7): 321–326
8. Ocular Disorders Presumed to be Inherited in Purebred Dogs. American College of Veterinary Ophthalmologists. ACVO, 2007
9. Eickhoff M, Seeliger F, Simon D, et. al.: Erupted bilateral compound odontomas in a dog. J Vet Dent. 2002 Sep;19(3):137-43.
10. Lohmann B, Klesen S: Cataract and microphthalmia in a litter of Russian Terriers [German]. Praktische Tierarzt 1997;78: 981.
11. *The Complete Dog Book, 20th Ed.* The American Kennel Club. Howell Book House, NY 2006. p. 244-247.

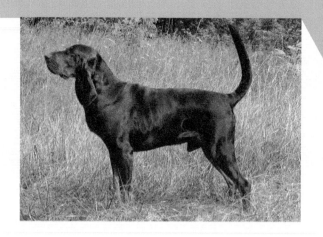

Black and Tan Coonhound

The Breed History
The origins of this breed likely trace back to the Talbot Hound in 11th century England. Later, admixture with American Foxhound and Bloodhound, and the black and tan Virginia Foxhound is likely. The AKC registry admitted the first of this breed in 1945 after a period of breed development in the Southern USA of approximately 200 years.

Breeding for Function
These dogs were bred for hunting raccoons and opossum. Their manner of hunting is similar to the Bloodhound. They move slowly at a determined pace with head down and follow the scent, giving loud voice when ready for the hunter. This signal means the quarry is treed. The dog has also been used for other game such as deer and bear. They are bred to withstand temperature extremes and rough terrain.

Physical Characteristics
Height at Withers: female 23-25" (58.5-63.5 cm), male 25-27" (63.5-68.5 cm).

Weight: 55-75 lb (25-34 kg).

Coat: The coat is glossy, short and dense with a black background highlighted by rich tan markings. This includes a small pumpkin seed sized tan marking above each eye. Any white except a tiny patch of less than 1" (2.5 cm) is a disqualification.

Longevity: 11-12 years

Points of Conformation: An athletic hound with long smooth gait, and moderate musculature and bone, the males are more heavily built. The head is about 9" (23 cm) long, expression is alert, nose is black colored. The flews are well developed. Eyes are brown to hazel, and round. Ears are set low on the head, and are very long and pendulous. They have a medium stop. The neck is medium in length and thickness, and topline is level, the thorax deep and ribs well sprung. The thick tapering tail is carried up when on scent. Feet are compact, and the toes well knuckled up with black nails. The limbs are straight boned.

Recognized Behavior Issues and Traits
Reported breed traits include: Friendly, though some individuals are reserved, watchful, and obedient. Noted to be very intelligent, with an independent streak, and when off leash, need to be restricted to a fenced enclosure. They have high exercise needs, though exhibit low activity levels around the home.

Low grooming needs, and a high drooling tendency also characterizes the breed.

Normal Physiologic Variations
None reported

Drug Sensitivities
None reported

Inherited Diseases
Hip Dysplasia: Polygenically inherited trait causing degenerative joint disease and hip arthritis. OFA reports 14.9% affected.[1]

Elbow Dysplasia: Polygenically inherited trait causing elbow arthritis. OFA reports 1.6% affected.[1]

Patella Luxation: Polygenically inherited laxity of patellar ligaments, causing luxation, lameness, and later degenerative joint disease. Treat surgically if causing clinical signs. Too few Black and Tan Coonhounds have been screened by OFA to determine an accurate frequency.[1]

Hemophilia B (Factor IX Deficiency): Rare, X-linked recessive coagulation disorder causing severe bleeding in this breed.[2]

Disease Predispositions
Hypothyroidism: Inherited autoimmune thyroiditis. 10.0% positive for thyroid auto-antibodies based on testing at Michigan State University. (Ave. for all breeds is 7.5%).[3,4]

Coonhound Paralysis (Polyradiculoneuritis): Disorder of acute paralysis due to transient demyelination, similar to Guillain-Barré syndrome. Caused by exposure to raccoon saliva in genetically susceptible dogs. Affected dogs can recover, but must be supported during remyelinization.[5,6]

Retinal Dysplasia: Focal folds are seen in the breed. Identified in 6.02% of Black and Tan Coonhounds CERF examined by veterinary ophthalmologists between 2000-2005.[7]

Cataracts: Anterior cataracts predominate, although anterior, nuclear, and capsular cataracts also occur in the breed. Unknown mode of inheritance. Identified in 4.22% of Black and Tan Coonhounds CERF examined by veterinary ophthalmologists between 2000-2005. CERF does not recommend breeding any Black and Tan Coonhound with a cataract.[7]

Persistent Pupillary Membranes: Strands of fetal remnant connecting; iris to iris, cornea, lens, or involving sheets of tissue. The later three forms can impair vision, and dogs affected with these forms should not be bred. Identified in 3.01% of Black and Tan Coonhounds CERF examined by veterinary ophthalmologists between 2000-2005.[7]

Ectropion: Rolling out of eyelids, often with a medial canthal pocket. Can also cause conjunctivitis. Ectropion is reported in 1.91% of Black and Tan Coonhounds CERF examined by veterinary ophthalmologists between 1991-1999. None were reported between 2000-2005.[7]

Entropion: Rolling in of eyelids, often causing corneal irritation or ulceration. Entropion is reported in 1.91% of Black and Tan Coonhounds CERF examined by veterinary ophthalmologists between 1991-1999. None were reported between 2000-2005.[7]

Distichiasis: Abnormally placed eyelashes that irritate the cornea and conjunctiva. Can cause secondary corneal ulceration. Identified in 1.20% of Black and Tan Coonhounds CERF examined by veterinary ophthalmologists between 2000-2005.[7]

Progressive Retinal Atrophy (PRA): Inherited degeneration of the retina leading to blindness. Clinically evident by 2 years of age. There may be more than one form of PRA in the breed. Unknown mode of inheritance.[7]

Cryptorchidism, Gastric Dilatation-volvulus, and **Pelger-Huet Anomaly** are reported.[8]

Isolated Case Studies

Disseminated Melanoma: An 11-year-old, Black and Tan Coonhound presented with lameness and osteolysis in the right distal femur and a pulmonary mass. Neoplastic melanocytes were observed from aspirates of the femoral and pulmonary masses. Postmortem examination revealed a disseminated melanoma involving the right femoral bone marrow, lung, multiple lymph nodes, and adrenal gland, with diffuse infiltration of the leptomeninges of the brain and spinal cord.[9]

Genetic Tests

Tests of Genotype: none

Tests of Phenotype: CHIC certification: Required testing includes hip radiographs, CERF eye examination, and congenital cardiac evaluation. Optional testing includes elbow radiographs and thyroid profile including autoantibodies. (See CHIC website; www.caninehealthinfo.org).

Recommend patella evaluation.

Miscellaneous

- **Breed name synonyms:** Coonhound, Black and Tan, American Black and Tan Coonhound.
- **Registries:** AKC, CKC, UKC, (Here known as the American Black and Tan Coonhound), NKC.
- **AKC rank (year 2008):** 42 (3,222 dogs registered)

- Internet resources: **American Black and Tan Coonhound Club:** www.abtcc.com
  American Black and Tan Coonhound Association: www.abtcha.net

References

1. OFA Website breed statistics: www.offa.org Last accessed July 1, 2010.
2. Dodds WJ: Bleeding Disorders in Animals. Proceedings World Small Animal Veterinary Association Congress. 2005
3. Nachreiner R and Refsal K: Personal communication, Diagnostic Center for Population and Animal Health, Michigan State University. April, 2007.
4. Nachreiner RF, Refsal KR, Graham PA, et. al.: Prevalence of serum thyroid hormone autoantibodies in dogs with clinical signs of hypothyroidism. J Am Vet Med Assoc 2002 Feb 15;220(4):466-71.
5. Cummings JF, Haas DC: Coonhound paralysis. An acute idiopathic polyradiculoneuritis in dogs resembling the Landry-Guillain-Barre syndrome. *J Neurol Sci.* 1966 Jan-Feb;4(1):51-81.
6. Holmes DF, Schultz RD, Cummings JF, et. al.: Experimental coonhound paralysis: animal model of Guillain-Barre syndrome. *Neurology.* 1979 Aug;29(8):1186-7.
7. *Ocular Disorders Presumed to be Inherited in Purebred Dogs.* American College of Veterinary Ophthalmologists. ACVO,2007
8. *The Genetic Connection: A Guide to Health Problems in Purebred Dogs.* L Ackerman. p. 203. AAHA Press, 1999.
9. Kim DY, Royal AB, and Villamil JA: Disseminated melanoma in a dog with involvement of leptomeninges and bone marrow. Vet Pathol. 2009 Jan;46(1):80-3.
10. *The Complete Dog Book, 20th Ed.* The American Kennel Club. Howell Book House, NY 2006. p. 152-155.

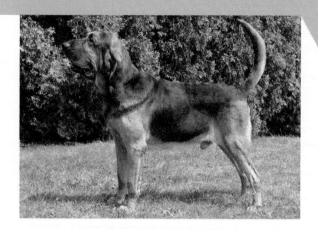

Bloodhound

The Breed History

This breed was renowned as far back as the third century in writings for the ability to track exceptionally well. Characteristically, they were noted for following even a very faint scent until the target or quarry was reached. Thought to originate around the Mediterranean, they were taken to Europe long before the crusades. The black strain was called St. Hubert's, after the Belgian monastery where they were extensively bred in the seventh century, and the white strain was called the Southern, or Talbot hound. By the 1600s this latter strain had died out as a distinct breed. In England, the black strain derivatives were carefully bred in monasteries and by royalty, earning them the nick name "blooded hound"; inferring an aristocratic bloodline of the dog.

Breeding for Function

Bred to follow scent of deer and other large game, their tracking stamina continues to be highly prized. These, the largest of the scent hounds are unlike other military and police dogs; these placid dogs do not attack quarry so their specific working focus is restricted to just trailing. These most famous scent hounds are particularly adept at long distance tracks (one recorded track was 138 miles, 221 km). They are noted for determination and perseverance. Today, they are famous for search and rescue.

Physical Characteristics

Height at Withers: female 23-25" (58.5-63.5 cm), male 25-27" (63.5-68.5 cm).

Weight: females 80-100 lb (36-45 kg), males 90-110 lb (41-50 kg).

Coat: Black and tan, liver and tan, and red are accepted coat colors. Small white areas are permitted on feet, tail tip and chest. Sometimes the above coat colors are flecked with white. Hair is softer textured on the ears, otherwise it is a smooth, short and hard coat.

Longevity: 10-12 years

Points of Conformation: The facial wrinkles and drooping eyes give the dog a somewhat characteristic expression. Their head is long, tapers only slightly and is narrow. The breed standard stipulates a head length of 12" (29.5 cm) or more in males, and 11" (28 cm) or more in females. Their head and neck area is replete with extensive skin folds. The Bloodhound possesses a prominent occipital protuberance, eyes are deep and eyelids droop; the weight

of the flews everts the lower lids. Eye colors match the coat, with hazel and yellow being common pigmentation. Ears are very low set, long and pendulous, but the leather is fairly fine textured. The flews are extensive and merged with neck folds, forming the large dewlap. Body skin is loose. The neck is long, the thorax is rounded and deep, and the loin is mildly arched. The tail is large, long and tapered and carried high. Gait is smooth and elastic on this muscular dog. Legs are straight and solid. Feet are compact and well knuckled.

Recognized Behavior Issues and Traits

Reported breed characteristics include: Docile, placid, well mannered and sometimes shy. They are friendly both with other dogs and with people. They love children and are very patient even with active toddlers. They can be a challenge to obedience train due to a tendency for independent thinking. Young dogs are very boisterous, but though they continue to be high activity dogs outdoors, they are low activity dogs around the home. Puppies are curious, and are known for eating inappropriate objects. They drool, and they may snore. Bloodhounds are not known for alarm barking, but may howl, bay, whine and sing. Provide a well-bedded sleep area to help prevent hygromas. Bloodhounds should not be allowed off leash because they will wander after scents. If bored, they can dig or jump their fences. May tend to pull on leash, so early training is important.

Normal Physiologic Variations

Slow to mature.

Drug Sensitivities

None reported

Inherited Diseases

Hip Dysplasia: Polygenically inherited trait causing degenerative joint disease and hip arthritis. OFA reports 26.1% affected.[1]

Elbow Dysplasia: Polygenically inherited trait causing elbow arthritis. OFA reports 15.4% affected.[1]

Patella Luxation: Polygenically inherited laxity of patellar ligaments, causing luxation, lameness, and later degenerative joint disease. Treat surgically if causing clinical signs. OFA reports 3.4% affected.[1]

Disease Predispositions

Ectropion: Rolling out of eyelids, often with a medial canthal pocket. Can also cause conjunctivitis. Can be secondary to macroblepharon; an abnormally large eyelid opening. Dorn reports a 7.97x odds ratio in Bloodhounds versus other breeds. Ectropion is reported in 30.63% of Bloodhounds CERF examined by veterinary ophthalmologists between 2000-2005.[2,3]

Entropion: Rolling in of eyelids, often causing corneal irritation or ulceration. Dorn reports a 7.97x odds ratio in Bloodhounds versus other breeds. Entropion is reported in 26.25% of Bloodhounds CERF examined by veterinary ophthalmologists between 2000-2005.[2,3]

Retinal Dysplasia: Retinal folds, geographic, and generalized retinal dysplasia with detachment are recognized in the breed. Reported in 8.75% of Bloodhounds CERF examined by veterinary ophthalmologists between 2000-2005.[3]

Gastric Dilation/Volvulus (GDV, Bloat): Life-threatening twisting of the stomach within the abdomen. Requires immediate veterinary attention. Glickman found 8.7% of Bloodhounds developed GDV. Dorn reports an 14.32x odds ratio for GDV versus other breeds.[2,4,5]

Hypothyroidism: Inherited autoimmune thyroiditis. 7.7% positive for thyroid auto-antibodies based on testing at Michigan State University. (Ave. for all breeds is 7.5%).[6,7]

Cataracts: Anterior cortex intermediate cataracts predominate, though posterior, nuclear, and capsular cataracts also occur in the breed. Identified in 6.89% of Bloodhounds CERF examined by veterinary ophthalmologists between 2000-2005. CERF does not recommend breeding any Bloodhound with a cataract.[3]

Persistent Pupillary Membranes: Strands of fetal remnant connecting; iris to iris, cornea, lens, or involving sheets of tissue. The later three forms can impair vision, and dogs affected with these forms should not be bred. Identified in 5.00% of Bloodhounds CERF examined by veterinary ophthalmologists between 2000-2005, with 4.38% involving iris to cornea.[3]

Prolapsed Gland of the Nictitans (Cherry Eye): This condition occurs secondary to inflammation of the gland. Reported in 1.88% of Bloodhounds CERF examined by veterinary ophthalmologists between 2000-2005.[3]

Chronic Superficial Keratitis (Pannus): Inflammation of the cornea, causing vision problems due to corneal pigmentation. Age of onset 2-5 years. Treatment with topical ocular lubricants and anti-inflammatory medication. Identified in 1.88% of Bloodhounds CERF examined by veterinary ophthalmologists between 2000-2005.[3]

Ventricular Septal Defect (VSD): Congenital opening in the interventricular wall causing communication between the left and right ventricles. Often causes a systolic murmur without clinical signs, but can cause tachypnea or exercise intolerance. Reported at a 37x Odds Ratio versus other breeds.[8]

Degenerative Myelopathy (DM): Rare disorder in the breed. Affected dogs show an insidious onset of upper motor neuron (UMN) paraparesis. The disease eventually progresses to severe tetraparesis. Affected dogs have normal results on myelography, MRI, and CSF analysis. Necropsy confirms the condition. Unknown mode of inheritance. A direct genetic test for an autosomal recessive DM susceptibility gene is available. All affected dogs are homozygous for the gene, however only a small percentage of homozygous dogs develop DM. OFA reports DM susceptibility gene frequencies of 39% carrier, and 6% homozygous "at-risk".[9]

Brachygnathism, Cryptorchidism, Keratoconjunctivitis Sicca, and **Spinal Muscular Atrophy** are reported.[10]

Isolated Case Studies

Multiple Congenital Eye Anomalies: Two unrelated Bloodhound puppies were examined for congenital blindness, with microphthalmia, goniodysplasia, cataracts, lenticonus with rupture of the lens capsule, persistent pupillary membranes, persistent hyperplastic tunica vasculosa lentis and persistent hyperplastic primary vitreous (PHTEL/PHPV), and retinal dysplasia.[11]

Persistent Hyperplastic Tunica Vasculosa Lentis/Persistent Hyperplastic Primary Vitreous (PHTVL/PHPV): Case study of a 4 month-old Bloodhound. Presented with posterior polar subcapsular cataracts and pre-retinal glial proliferation.[12]

Genetic Tests

Tests of Genotype: Direct test for a DM susceptability gene is available from the OFA.

Tests of Phenotype: CHIC Certification: Required testing includes hip and elbow radiographs, and cardiac evaluation (recommended by a specialist). Recommended tests include CERF eye examination, patella and PennHIP evaluation. (See CHIC website; www.caninehealthinfo.org).

Recommend thyroid profile including autoantibodies.

Miscellaneous

- **Breed name synonyms:** St. Hubert Hound, St. Hubert's Hound, Chien de St. Hubert, Flemish hound.
- **Registries:** AKC, UKC, CKC, KCGB (Kennel Club of Great Britain), ANKC (Australian National Kennel Club), NKC (National Kennel Club).
- **AKC rank (year 2008):** 43 (3,203 dogs registered)
- **Internet resources: The American Bloodhound Club:** www.bloodhounds.org
  Canadian Bloodhound Club: www.canadianbloodhoundclub.com
  The United Kingdom Bloodhound Club: www.bloodhoundclub.co.uk

References

1. OFA Website breed statistics: www.offa.org Last accessed July 1, 2010.
2. Dorn CR: Canine breed-specific risks of frequently diagnosed diseases at veterinary teaching hospitals. Monograph. AKC Canine Health Foundation. 2000.
3. *Ocular Disorders Presumed to be Inherited in Purebred Dogs.* American College of Veterinary Ophthalmologists. ACVO, 2007.
4. Andrews AH: A study of ten cases of gastric torsion in the bloodhound. *Vet Rec.* 1970 Jun 6;86(23):689-93.
5. Glickman LT, Glickman NW, Schellenberg DB, et. al.: Incidence of and breed-related risk factors for gastric dilatation-volvulus in dogs. *J Am Vet Med Assoc.* 2000 Jan 1;216(1):40-5.
6. Nachreiner R and Refsal K: Personal communication, Diagnostic Center for Population and Animal Health, Michigan State University. April, 2007.
7. Nachreiner RF, Refsal KR, Graham PA, et. al.: Prevalence of serum thyroid hormone autoantibodies in dogs with clinical signs of hypothyroidism. J Am Vet Med Assoc 2002 Feb 15;220(4):466-71.
8. Abbott JA, Hawkes K, Small MT, et. al.: Retrospective Description of Canine Ventricular Septal Defect. Proceedings, 2008 ACVIM Forum. 2008.
9. Awano T, Johnson GS, Wade CM, et. al.: Genome-wide association analysis reveals a SOD1 mutation in canine degenerative myelopathy that resembles amyotrophic lateral sclerosis. Proc Natl Acad Sci U S A. 2009 Feb 24;106(8):2794-9.
10. *The Genetic Connection: A Guide to Health Problems in Purebred Dogs.* L Ackerman. p. 203. AAHA Press, 1999.
11. Venter IJ, van der Lugt JJ, van Rensburg IB, et. al.: Multiple Congenital Eye Anomalies in Bloodhound Puppies. *Vet Comp Ophthalmol* 1996:6[1]:9-13.
12. Gemensky-Metzler AJ, Wilkie DA: Surgical management and histologic and immunohistochemical features of a cataract and retrolental plaque secondary to persistent hyperplastic tunica vasculosa lentis/persistent hyperplastic primary vitreous (PHTVL/PHPV) in a Bloodhound puppy. *Vet Ophthalmol.* 2004 Sep-Oct;7(5):369-75.
13. *The Complete Dog Book, 20th Ed.* The American Kennel Club. Hpwell Book House, NY 2006. P. 156-159.

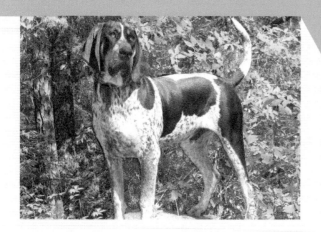

The Breed History

The Bluetick Coonhound's color suggests that it descended from the Grand Bleu de Gascogne (French Staghound) as well as the English Foxhound. In America, Blueticks were referred to as English Coonhounds for many years. In 1945, however, Bluetick breeders broke away from the English breeders because they didn't want to follow the trend toward producing a hot-nosed, faster hunter. Proud of their larger, cold-nosed and resolute, if slower hounds, they re-named their breed and maintained their own hunting style. AKC recognition occurred in 2009.

Breeding for Function

An intelligent, cold-nosed hunter that trees hard and long, the Bluetick has the ability and endurance to stay on the most intricate track. He is a free tonguer on the trail with a medium bawl or bugle voice when striking and trailing. This changes to a steady chop when running and a steady course chop at tree.

Physical Characteristics

Height at withers: males, 22 to 27 inches (56-69 cm), females, 21 to 25 inches (53-64 cm).

Weight: males 55 to 80 pounds (25-36 kg), females 45 to 65 pounds (20.5-29.5 kg).

Coat: Medium coarse and lying close to the body, appearing smooth and glossy. Not rough or too short. Preferred color is a dark blue, thickly mottled body, spotted by various shaped black spots on back, ears and sides. Preference is to more blue than black on body. Head and ears predominately black. With or without tan markings (over eyes, on cheeks, chest and below tail) and red ticking on feet and lower legs.

Longevity: 11 to 12 years.

Points of Conformation: Proportion is square, or slightly longer than tall. The head is 8 to 10 inches long with a prominent stop. The eyes are round and dark brown in color. The ears are set low. The nose is black and large. The neck is muscular, and carried up, with only a slight dewlap. The body should be deep, forechest is moderate, the topline slopes downward slightly from withers to hips. Forelegs are straight from elbows to feet. Rear legs are muscular, and parallel from hip to foot when viewed from behind.

Bluetick Coonhound

Feet are round and well arched. The tail is set slightly below the line of the back, carried high with a forward half-moon curve.

Recognized Behavior Issues and Traits

Reported breed traits include: Friendly, though some individuals are reserved, watchful, and obedient. Noted to be very intelligent, with an independent streak, and when off leash, need to be restricted to a fenced enclosure. They have high exercise needs, though exhibit low activity levels around the home. They need to be socialized to children and other pets early, and may see small pets as prey. Can have a tendency to being dog aggressive. Blueticks have the typical coonhound "bawling" bark.

Low grooming needs, and a high drooling tendency also characterizes the breed.

Normal Physiologic Variations

None reported

Drug Sensitivities

None reported

Inherited Diseases

Hip Dysplasia: Polygenically inherited trait causing degenerative joint disease and hip arthritis. OFA reports 15.8% affected, but too few Bluetick Coonhounds have been evaluated for statistical confidence.[1]

Elbow Dysplasia: Polygenically inherited trait causing elbow arthritis. Too few Bluetick Coonhounds have been screened by OFA to determine an accurate frequency.[1]

Patella Luxation: Polygenically inherited laxity of patellar ligaments, causing luxation, lameness, and later degenerative joint disease. Treat surgically if causing clinical signs. Reported as a breed issue, however too few Bluetick Coonhounds have been screened by OFA to determine an accurate frequency.[1]

Disease Predispositions

Hypothyroidism: Inherited autoimmune thyroiditis. Not enough samples have been submitted for thyroid auto-antibodies to Michigan State University to determine an accurate frequency. (Ave. for all breeds is 7.5%).[2,3]

Coonhound Paralysis (polyradiculoneuritis): Disorder of acute paralysis due to transient demyelination, similar to Guillain-Barré syndrome. Caused by exposure to raccoon saliva in genetically susceptible dogs. Affected dogs can recover, but must be supported during remyelinization.[4,5]

Inherited Ocular Disorders: Too few Bluetick Coonhounds have been CERF examined by veterinary ophthalmologists to determine an accurate frequency of inherited ocular disorders.[6]

Cataracts, Gastric Dilitation–Volvulus, and Hock Luxation are reported.[7]

Isolated Case Studies

Globoid Cell Leukodystrophy (Krabbe disease): An autosomal recessive lysosomal storage disease causing severe neurological symptoms including seizures, hypotonia, blindness, and death in young affected dogs. Three affected males were identified in a litter of Bluetick Coonhounds.[8]

Genetic Tests

Tests of Genotype: None

Tests of Phenotype: Recommend hip and elbow radiographs, CERF eye examination, thyroid profile including autoantibodies, cardiac examination, and patella evaluation.

Miscellaneous

- **Breed name synonyms:** Bluetick
- **Registries:** AKC, UKC, CKC, ANKC (Australian National Kennel Club), NKC (National Kennel Club)
- **AKC rank:** (none) AKC recognized in Dec. 2009. Entire stud book entered.
- **Internet resources:** American Bluetick Hound Association: www.akc.org/akc_clubs/?AmericanBluetickHoundAssociation
  Bluetick Coonhound Breeders of America: www.bluetickbreedersofamerica.com

References

1. OFA Website breed statistics: www.offa.org Last accessed July 1, 2010.
2. Nachreiner R and Refsal K: Personal communication, Diagnostic Center for Population and Animal Health, Michigan State University. April, 2007.
3. Nachreiner RF, Refsal KR, Graham PA, et. al.: Prevalence of serum thyroid hormone autoantibodies in dogs with clinical signs of hypothyroidism. J Am Vet Med Assoc 2002 Feb 15;220(4):466-71.
4. Cummings JF, Haas DC: Coonhound paralysis. An acute idiopathic polyradiculoneuritis in dogs resembling the Landry-Guillain-Barre syndrome. J Neurol Sci. 1966 Jan-Feb;4(1):51-81.
5. Holmes DF, Schultz RD, Cummings JF, et. al.: Experimental coonhound paralysis: animal model of Guillain-Barre syndrome. Neurology. 1979 Aug;29(8):1186-7.
6. Ocular Disorders Presumed to be Inherited in Purebred Dogs. American College of Veterinary Ophthalmologists. ACVO, 2007.
7. The Genetic Connection: A Guide to Health Problems in Purebred Dogs. L Ackerman. p. 203. AAHA Press, 1999.
8. Boysen BG, Tryphonas and L, Harries NW: Globoid cell leukodystrophy in the bluetick hound dog. I. Clinical manifestations. Can Vet J. 1974 Nov;15(11):303-8.
9. AKC Breed Website: www.akc.org/breeds/bluetick_coonhound Last accessed July 1, 2010.

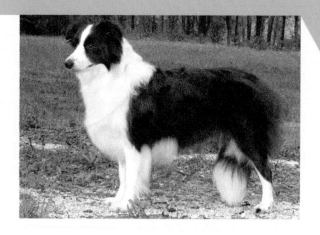

well-sprung ribs characterize these dogs. The tail reaches to at least their tarsus, and though usually carried low, may be held level when excited. The body is a bit longer than high and dewclaws may be removed. Compact feet, straight limbs, and a smooth, long, low, way of going is characteristic.

The Breed History

Scotland and Northern England were the birthplaces of this breed. Many varieties of collies including Scotch Collie, Welsh Sheepdog, and Highland Collies are intermingled in the history of this region and likely contributed to the bloodlines of the Border Collie. This breed received full recognition status in 1995. It is thought to have arisen in the 1700s.

Breeding for Function

Developed primarily for sheep herding but also used for cattle herding, these dogs are often thought to be the "top dog" of sheep herding breeds. They were developed as gatherers not drivers, but they can be trained to do the latter also. Trainability, speed, agility, and livestock sense were key features bred into these dogs. They were also bred to love their work, and so will willingly work all day. So strong is the emphasis on breed functionality that the registries discourage showing for conformation only. Border Collies also excel at obedience and tracking and agility. Other jobs that they excel at include search and rescue, narcotics and bomb sniffing, and guide dog and assistance work.

Physical Characteristics

Height at Withers: female 18-21" (45.5-53 cm), male 19-22" (48-56 cm).

Weight: females 27-42 lb (12-19 kg), males 30-45 lb (13.5-20.5 kg).

Coat: Very dense smooth, rough, or medium coats are found; rough and smooth are the only permitted forms in the AKC standard. Colors include black and tan, tri-color, merle, sable, and black, usually with white markings. Solid white is not accepted. These dogs are average shedders, and should be brushed very regularly. The dense undercoat sheds out in Spring.

Longevity: 12-15 years.

Points of Conformation: The physical characteristics of the Border Collie are not considered a high priority, except how they contribute to their ability to work. These dogs are medium sized, and they possess a very alert expression. Their skull is broad with a moderate stop. Ears are set up and semi-erect, oval eyes are dark brown usually, though blue is acceptable in the merle, and their nose is black. A moderately arched long neck, level topline, deep thorax and

Recognized Behavior Issues and Traits

Reported traits include: If kept as a pet, activities such as obedience or agility are recommended to keep them challenged. They do not do well as sedentary house pets or backyard dogs because they need plenty of mental stimulation, lots of exercise, and human fellowship. They are easy to train, and love to please. If left on their own too much, they may become bored and destructive.

They should not be allowed to run off-leash unless working since they may chase. They should be properly socialized as puppies and may be snappy around children as they try to herd them. They make good alert dogs for home or farm.

Sound sensitivity is reported at a frequency of 28%, and nervousness 13% in the 2007 BCSA Health Survey.[1]

Normal Physiologic Variations

Merle Coat Color: Caused by a dominant mutation in the SILV gene. Breeding two merle dogs together should be avoided, as homozygous dogs can be born with multiple defects, including blindness, deafness, and heart anomalies.[2]

Drug Sensitivities

MDR1 Mutation (Ivermectin/Drug Toxicity): Autosomal recessive disorder in the MDR1 gene allows high CNS drug levels of ivermectin, doramectin, loperamide, vincristine, moxidectin, and other drugs. Causes neurological signs, including tremors, seizures, and coma. A genetic test is available, showing 0.3% affected and 1.3% carrier. In Germany, 0.3% test homozygous affected, and 0.6% test as carriers.[3,4,5]

Inherited Diseases

Hip Dysplasia: Polygenically inherited trait causing degenerative joint disease and hip arthritis. OFA reports 10.9% affected. Reported at a frequency of 7.1% in the 2007 BCSA Health Survey.[1,6]

Collie Eye Anomaly/Choroidal Hypoplasia/Coloboma (CEA/CH): Autosomal recessive disorder of eye development that can lead to retinal detachment and blindness. A genetic test is available through Optigen, that reports 2% of Border Collies test as affected, and 28% test as carriers. Worldwide test results on the Border Collie Health website reports 0.7% affected and 24.8% carrier. Reported 0.7% affected in Switzerland. Reported in 1.64% of Border Collies CERF examined by veterinary ophthalmologists between 2000-2005. CERF does not recommend breeding any Border Collie with CH.[7,8,9,10,11]

Elbow Dysplasia: Polygenically inherited trait causing elbow arthritis. OFA reports 1.4% affected.[6]

Patella Luxation: Polygenically inherited laxity of patellar ligaments, causing luxation, lameness, and later degenerative joint disease. Treat surgically if causing clinical signs. OFA reports 1.1% affected.[6]

Trapped Neutrophil Syndrome (TNS, Static Neutropenia): Congenital autosomal recessive disorder causing mature neutrophils to become trapped in the bone marrow. Affected pups have recurrent infections and fail to thrive. Reported in Border Collies worldwide. This disorder is distinct from cyclic neutropenia. Worldwide test results on the Border Collie Health website reports 0.8% affected and 19.2% carrier. A linked marker genetic test is available.[10,12,13,14]

Progressive Retinal Atrophy (PRA): X-linked recessive mode of inheritance. Age of onset 1-2 years of age. Reported in 0.45% of Border Collies CERF examined by veterinary ophthalmologists between 2000-2005. CERF does not recommend breeding any Border Collie with PRA. The causative mutation is not known, and a genetic test is not available. There may be more than one form of PRA in the breed.[7,15]

Neuronal Ceroid Lipofuscinosis (NCL): Autosomal recessive, degenerative progressive neurological disease causing hyperactivity and later aggression, gait abnormalities, blindness and dementia. Onset between 16 months and 2 years of age. Dogs do not survive more than 6 months from the onset of clinical signs. Worldwide test results on the Border Collie Health website reports 2.6% carriers. A genetic test is available.[10,16,17,18,19,20]

Cobalamin Malabsorption (Methylmalonic Aciduria): Autosomal recessive disorder presenting with chronic, nonregenerative anemia, and methylmalonic aciduria. The disorder responds to parenteral vitamin B12 therapy, and affected animals have a good prognosis with treatment. A phenotypic urine test is available.[21,22]

Disease Predispositions

Hypothyroidism: Inherited autoimmune thyroiditis. 11.2% positive for thyroid auto-antibodies based on testing at Michigan State University. (Ave. for all breeds is 7.5%). Reported at a frequency of 2.9% in the 2007 BCSA Health Survey.[1,23,24]

Persistent Pupillary Membranes: Strands of fetal remnant connecting; iris to iris, cornea, lens, or involving sheets of tissue. The later three forms can impair vision, and dogs affected with these forms should not be bred. Identified in 6.31% of Border Collies CERF examined by veterinary ophthalmologists between 2000-2005.[7]

Epilepsy (Inherited Seizures): Studies show a strong founder effect with a major recessive mode of inheritance. Epilepsy in the Border Collie often has a severe clinical course, with dogs who first seizure under 2 years of age having a diminished life expectancy. Cluster seizures and status epilepticus occur at a higher frequency in the breed. Up to 71% of Border Collies can show anticonvulsant resistance. Dorn reports an 8.79x odds ratio of developing epileptic seizures versus other breeds. Reported at a frequency of 3.3% in the 2007 BCSA Health Survey.[1,25,26]

Lens Luxation: Breed predisposition identified in the Border Collie. Age of onset 3-5 years of age. Often progresses to secondary glaucoma. CERF does not recommend breeding any Border Collie with lens luxation.[7,27,28]

Deafness: Congenital deafness can be unilateral or bilateral. Diagnosed by BAER testing. OFA reports 0.6% of Border Collies BAER test as affected. A study in the United Kingdom showed 2.0% unilaterally deaf, and 0.4% bilaterally deaf. Correlated with blue eyes, with white head pigmentation, and/or the merle gene. In a multi-breed study; for single merles (Mm), 2.7% were unilaterally deaf and 0.9% were bilaterally deaf. For double merles (MM), 10% were unilaterally deaf and 15% were bilaterally deaf.[6,29,30,31,32]

Portosystemic Shunt (PSS, Liver Shunt): Abnormal blood vessels connecting the systemic and portal blood flow. Causes stunting, abnormal behavior and possible seizures. Seen at a higher prevalence in the breed compared to other breeds. Undetermined mode of inheritance.[33]

Osteochondrosis of the Shoulder/Stifle: Age of onset of lameness usually 4-7 months of age. Male predominance. One study identified three affected out of five Border Collie littermates. Reported 15.0x odds ratio for shoulder OCD versus other breeds. Reported at a frequency of 1.9% in the 2007 BCSA Health Survey. Unknown mode of inheritance.[1,34,35]

Cataracts: Anterior or posterior punctate cataracts predominate in the breed. Reported in 1.34% of Border Collies presented to veterinary teaching hospitals. Identified in 1.23% of Border Collies CERF examined by veterinary ophthalmologists between 2000-2005. CERF does not recommend breeding any Border Collie with a cataract.[7,36]

Diabetes Mellitus: Caused by a lack of insulin production by the pancreas. Controlled by insulin injections, diet, and glucose monitoring. Age of onset 6-12 years. A Swedish study showed an increased incidence in the breed, with the majority of affected Border Collies being female. Unknown mode of inheritance.[37]

Separation Anxiety: The breed may have a tendency towards separation anxiety.[38]

Retinal Dysplasia: Focal folds and geographic retinal dysplasia are seen in the breed. Dogs with the geographic form should not be bred. Identified in 0.75% of Border Collies CERF examined by veterinary ophthalmologists between 2000-2005.[7]

Cerebellar Abiotrophy (CA, Ataxia): Identified in multiple siblings of Border Collies presenting with signs of progressive ataxia and hypermetria beginning at 6-8 weeks of age. Pathology demonstrates extensive loss of the cerebellar granular cell layer, with relative sparing of Purkinje cells. Presumptive autosomal recessive mode of inheritance.[39,40]

Ciliary Dyskenesia, Corneal Dystrophy, Cyclic Hematopoiesis, Malignant Hyperthermia, Neuroaxonal Dystrophy, Pannus, Patent Ductus Arteriosis, and **Pelger-Huet Anomaly** are reported.[41]

Isolated Case Studies

Sensory and Motor Neuropathy: A 5-month-old female Border Collie was evaluated because of progressive hind limb ataxia. Sensory nerve conduction velocity was absent in the tibial, common peroneal, and radial nerves and was decreased in the ulnar nerve; motor nerve conduction velocity was decreased in the tibial, common peroneal, and ulnar nerves. Pathology included nerve fiber depletion and axonal degeneration in remaining fibers. A littermate was similarly affected. In another study, two Border Collie littermates were diagnosed with a purely sensory distal peripheral neuropathy.[42,43]

Superficial Necrolytic Dermatitis (Hepatocutaneous Syndrome): Two Border Collies were identified in a study of 36 dogs with diagnoses of superficial necrolytic dermatitis, suggesting a breed prevalence. Affected dogs present with erythema, crusting, exudation, ulceration and alopecia involving footpads, peri-ocular or peri-oral regions, anal–genital regions, and pressure points on the trunk and limbs. Average age of presentation is 10 years. Diagnosis is by biopsy.[44]

Aortic Elastin Dysplasia (Dissecting Hematoma): Two cases of sudden death in a Border Collie and a Border Collie cross. Pathological findings were pericardial tamponade with dissection of the ascending aorta, and unusual splitting of the elastin within the wall of the aorta, as described in Marfan syndrome.[45]

Nemaline Rod Myopathy: Case study of a 10 month old Border Collie with exercise intolerance, abnormal electromyography, and the presence of nemaline rods in fresh, frozen, and glutaraldehyde-fixed biopsies from proximal appendicular limb muscles.[46]

Cervical Syringomyelia and Hydrocephalus with Scoliosis: Case study of a 6-month-old female Border Collie with a 1-month history of progressive curvature of the cervical spine. Suboccipital craniotomy and laminectomy of the first cervical vertebra were performed, improved the scoliosis and syringomyelia.[47]

Myasthenia Gravis and Dysautonomia: A two year old male intact border collie with diarrhea, coughing, vomiting and stranguria had megaoesophagus, flaccid bladder, poor pupillary light reflexes, an absent gag reflex, poor anal tone, and aspiration pneumonia. Testing revealed coexisting autoimmune myasthenia gravis and dysautonomia.[48]

Genetic Tests

Tests of Genotype: Direct test for Collie Eye Anomaly/Choroidal Hypoplasia is available from Optigen. (Recommended for breeding dogs)

Direct test for Neuronal Ceroid Lipofuscinosis (NCL) is available from Optigen and the Animal Health Trust.

Direct test for MDR1 Mutation is available from Washington State Univ. http://www.vetmed.wsu.edu/depts-VCPL/test.aspx. (Recommended for all dogs)

Direct tests for black, brown (red) and true red coat colors, and black and brown nose are available from VetGen and HealthGene.

Linked marker test for Trapped Neutrophil Syndrome (TNS) is available from University of New South Wales http://www.bordercollie.org.au/pdf/TNSsamplinginternational.pdf

Tests of Phenotype: CHIC Certification: Required testing includes hip radiographs, CERF eye examination (annually until age 7), and participation in the CHIC DNA repository. Optional tests include elbow and shoulder radiographs, thyroid profile including autoantibodies, BAER test for deafness, cardiac evaluation, and gene tests for CEA/CH, NCL, and TNS. (See CHIC website; www.caninehealthinfo.org).

Recommend patella evaluation.

Urine test for Methylmalonic Aciduria is available from PennGen.

Miscellaneous

- **Breed name synonyms:** BC
- **Registries:** AKC, CKC, UKC, KCGB (Kennel Club of Great Britain), ANKC (Australian National Kennel Club), NKC (National Kennel Club)
- **AKC rank (year 2008):** 53 (2,104 dogs registered)
- **Internet resources: Border Collie Society of America:** www.bordercolliesociety.com
  American Border Collie Association: www.americanbordercollie.org
  United States Border Collie Club (working collies): www.bordercollie.org
  United States Border Collie Handlers Association: www.usbcha.com
  Canadian Border Collie Association: www.canadianbordercollies.org
  Border Collie Club of Great Britain: www.bordercollieclub.com
  Border Collie Health: www.bordercolliehealth.com

References

1. Border Collie Society of America: 2007 BCSA Health Survey. 2008.
2. Clark LA, Wahl JM, Rees CA, et. al.: Retrotransposon insertion in SILV is responsible for merle patterning of the domestic dog. Proc Natl Acad Sci U S A. 2006 Jan 31;103(5):1376-81.
3. Nelson OL, Carsten E, Bentjen SA, et. al.: Ivermectin toxicity in an Australian Shepherd dog with the MDR1 mutation associated with ivermectin sensitivity in Collies. *J Vet Intern Med.* 2003 May-Jun;17(3):354-6.
4. Geyer J, Doring B, Godoy JR, et. al.: Frequency of the nt230 (del4) MDR1 mutation in Collies and related dog breeds in Germany. J Vet Pharmacol Ther. 2005 Dec;28(6):545-51.
5. Mealey KL & Meurs KM: Breed distribution of the ABCB1-1Delta (multidrug sensitivity) polymorphism among dogs undergoing ABCB1 genotyping. J Am Vet Med Assoc. 2008 Sep 15;233(6):921-4.
6. OFA Website breed statistics: www.offa.org Last accessed July 1, 2010.
7. *Ocular Disorders Presumed to be Inherited in Purebred Dogs.* American College of Veterinary Ophthalmologists. ACVO, 2007
8. Bedford PG: Collie eye anomaly in the border collie. *Vet Rec.* 1982 Jul 10;111(2):34-5.
9. Lowe JK, Kukekova AV, Kirkness EF, et. al.: Linkage mapping of the primary disease locus for collie eye anomaly. *Genomics.* 2003 Jul:82(1):86-95.
10. Border Collie Health website genetic testing statistics. www.bordercolliehealth.com Last accessed July 1, 2010.
11. Walser-Reinhardt L, Hässig M, & Spiess B: Collie eye anomaly in Switzerland. Schweiz Arch Tierheilkd. 2009 Dec;151(12):597-603.
12. Allan FJ, Thompson KG, Jones BR, et. al.: Neutropenia with a probable

hereditary basis in Border Collies. N Z Vet J. 1996 Apr;44(2):67-72.

13. Shearman JR, Zhang QY, Wilton AN: Exclusion of CXCR4 as the cause of Trapped Neutrophil Syndrome in Border Collies using five microsatellites on canine chromosome 19. Animal Genetics 2006;37(1):89.

14. Shearman JR, Wilton AN: Elimination of neutrophil elastase and adaptor protein complex 3 subunit genes as the cause of trapped neutrophil syndrome in Border collies. Animal Genetics 2007;38 (2):188–189.

15. Vilboux T, Chaudieu G, Jeannin P, et. al.: Progressive retinal atrophy in the Border Collie: a new XLPRA. BMC Vet Res. 2008 Mar 3;4:10.

16. Melville SA, Wilson CL, Chiang CS, et. al.: A mutation in canine CLN5 causes neuronal ceroid lipofuscinosis in Border collie dogs. Genomics. 2005 Sep;86(3):287-94.

17. Koie H, Shibuya H, Sato T, et. al.: Magnetic resonance imaging of neuronal ceroid lipofuscinosis in a border collie. J Vet Med Sci. 2004 Nov;66(11):1453-6.

18. Taylor RM, Farrow BR: Ceroid-lipofuscinosis in border collie dogs. Acta Neuropathol (Berl). 1988;75(6):627-31.

19. Studdert VP, Mitten RW: Clinical features of ceroid lipofuscinosis in border collie dogs. Aust Vet J. 1991 Apr;68(4):137-40.

20. Taylor RM, Farrow BR: Ceroid lipofuscinosis in the border collie dog: retinal lesions in an animal model of juvenile Batten disease. Am J Med Genet. 1992 Feb 15;42(4):622-7.

21. Morgan LW, McConnell J: Cobalamin deficiency associated with erythroblastic anemia and methylmalonic aciduria in a border collie. J Am Anim Hosp Assoc. 1999 Sep-Oct;35(5):392-5.

22. Battersby IA, Giger U, Hall EJ: Hyperammonaemic encephalopathy secondary to selective cobalamin deficiency in a juvenile Border collie. J Small Anim Pract. 2005 Jul;46(7):339-4

23. Nachreiner R and Refsal K: Personal communication, Diagnostic Center for Population and Animal Health, Michigan State University. April, 2007.

24. Nachreiner RF, Refsal KR, Graham PA, et. al.: Prevalence of serum thyroid hormone autoantibodies in dogs with clinical signs of hypothyroidism. J Am Vet Med Assoc 2002 Feb 15;220(4):466-71.

25. Dorn CR: Canine breed-specific risks of frequently diagnosed diseases at veterinary teaching hospitals. Monograph. AKC Canine Health Foundation. 2000.

26. Hülsmeyer V, Zimmermann R, Brauer C, et. al.: Epilepsy in Border Collies: clinical manifestation, outcome, and mode of inheritance. J Vet Intern Med. 2010 Jan-Feb;24(1):171-8.

27. Curtis R: Lens luxation in the dog and cat. Vet Clin North Am Small Anim Pract. 1990 May;20(3):755-73.

28. Foster SJ, Curtis R, Barnett KC: Primary lens luxation in the Border collie. J Small Anim Pract 1986;27:1.

29. Platt S, Freeman J, di Stefani A, et. al.: Prevalence of unilateral and bilateral deafness in border collies and association with phenotype. J Vet Intern Med. 2006 Nov-Dec;20(6):1355-62

30. De Risio L, Freeman J, Blott S, et. al.: Prevalence, Heritability and Genetic Correlations of Congenital Sensorineural Deafness and Pigmentation Phenotypes in 4143 Border Collies. Proceedings, 2009 ACVIM Forum. 2009.

31. Strain GM, Clark LA, Wahl JM, et. al.: Prevalence of deafness in dogs heterozygous or homozygous for the merle allele. J Vet Intern Med. 2009 Mar-Apr;23(2):282-6.

32. De Risio L, Lewis T, Freeman J, et. al.: Prevalence, heritability and genetic correlations of congenital sensorineural deafness and pigmentation phenotypes in the Border Collie. Vet J. 2011 Jun;188(3):286-90.

33. Hunt GB: Effect of breed on anatomy of portosystemic shunts resulting from congenital diseases in dogs and cats: a review of 242 cases. Aust Vet J 2004;Dec; 82[12]:746-9.

34. Knecht CD, Van Sickle DC, Blevins WE, et. al.: Osteochondrosis of the shoulder and stifle in 3 of 5 Border Collie littermates. J Am Vet Med Assoc. 1977 Jan 1;170(1):58-60.

35. LaFond E, Breur GJ and Austin CC: Breed susceptibility for developmental orthopedic diseases in dogs. J Am Anim Hosp Assoc. 2002 Sep-Oct;38(5):467-77.

36. Gelatt KN, Mackay EO: Prevalence of primary breed-related cataracts in the dog in North America. Vet Ophthalmol. 2005 Mar-Apr;8(2):101-11.

37. Fall T, Hamlin HH, Hedhammar A, et. al.: Diabetes mellitus in a population of 180,000 insured dogs: incidence, survival, and breed distribution. J Vet Intern Med. 2007 Nov-Dec;21(6):1209-16.

38. Bradshaw JW, McPherson JA, Casey RA, et. al.: Aetiology of separation-related behaviour in domestic dogs. Vet Rec. 2002 Jul 13;151(2):43-6.]

39. Sandy JR, Slocombe RE, Mitten RW, et. al.: Cerebellar abiotrophy in a family of Border Collie dogs. Vet Pathol. 2002 Nov;39(6):736-8.

40. Gill JM, Hewland M: Cerebellar degeneration in the Border collie. N Z Vet J. 1980 Aug;28(8):170.

41. The Genetic Connection: A Guide to Health Problems in Purebred Dogs. L Ackerman. p.203, AAHA Press, 1999.

42. Harkin KR, Cash WC, Shelton GD: Sensory and motor neuropathy in a Border Collie. J Am Vet Med Assoc. 2005 Oct 15;227(8):1263-5, 1250.

43. Vermeersch K, Van Ham L, Braund KG, et. al.: Sensory neuropathy in two Border collie puppies. J Small Anim Pract. 2005 Jun;46(6):295-9.

44. Outerbridge CA, Marks SL, Rogers QR: Plasma amino acid concentrations in 36 dogs with histologically confirmed superficial necrolytic dermatitis. Vet Dermatol. 2002 Aug;13(4):177-86.

45. Boulineau TM, Andrews-Jones L, Van Alstine W: Spontaneous aortic dissecting hematoma in two dogs. J Vet Diagn Invest. 2005 Sep;17(5):492-7.

46. Delauche AJ, Cuddon PA, Podell M, et. al.: Nemaline rods in canine myopathies: 4 case reports and literature review. J Vet Intern Med. 1998 Nov-Dec;12(6):424-30.

47. Takagi S, Kadosawa T, Ohsaki T, et. al.: Hindbrain decompression in a dog with scoliosis associated with syringomyelia. J Am Vet Med Assoc. 2005 Apr 15;226(8):1359-63, 1347.

48. Gajanayake I, Niessen SJ, Cherubini GB, et. al.: Autoimmune myasthenia gravis and dysautonomia in a dog. J Small Anim Pract. 2008 Nov;49(11):593-5.

49. The Complete Dog Book, 20th Ed. The American Kennel Club. Howell Book House, NY 2006. p. 635-639.

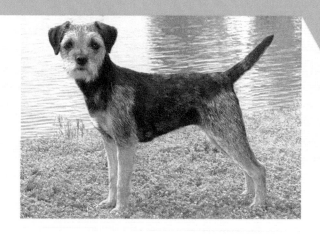

Border Terrier

The Breed History

The name "border" arises from the breed's region of origin, along the border between England and Scotland. They are one of the oldest British terrier breeds, pictured in artwork dating back as far as the year 1869. First AKC registrations occurred in the year 1930.

Breeding for Function

In England, these working terriers helped farmers protect their sheep from predators including foxes. As a valued protector of sheep herds, they were selected for stamina and water resistant coats, which helped them work long days in a harsh environment. They also served as ratters. Today, they are entered in competitions such as flyball, earthdog tests, agility and tracking.

Physical Characteristics

Height at Withers: 10-11" (25.5-28 cm).

Weight: females 11.5-14 lb (5-6 kg), males 13-15.5 lb (6-7 kg).

Coat: The double coat consists of a short dense undercoat and a close, straight wiry topcoat that may have some gaps. Colors accepted include wheaten, red, grizzle and tan, and blue and tan. White is only allowed in a small chest marking. Moderate shedding tendency, and requires stripping twice a year and weekly grooming.

Longevity: 13-15 years

Points of Conformation: Medium in size, the Border Terrier possesses a head described as being like an otter, and the narrow, long body is built to accommodate going to earth, or following the quarry (fox, badger) into the den, but at the same time, his long legs allow him to keep up to horses. The so-called otter head is curved at the stop, eyes are hazel, moderately set apart and moderately sized. The ears are triangular, small, and the leather is moderately thick. They have a wide skull, dark short blocky muzzle and the nose is large and black. The neck is medium in length and muscling; not throaty. The back is level, ribs are flat, and the thorax deep; and stays deep to the back of the chest. The abdomen is not tucked up. The tail is short and tapers from a thick base to end above the tarsus when resting; it is carried high when alert. Limbs are straight boned, feet compact with moderate arch of toes, and the pads thick. The gait is fast, long and smooth.

Recognized Behavior Issues and Traits

Reported breed characteristics include: Friendly, good family dog, high trainability, good natured, high energy and activity levels, and game in the field when hunting (showing perseverance, tenacity, courageous). Should not be off leash unless in a fenced enclosure. May exhibit inter-male aggression but considered less scrappy than most other terriers. Introduce early to children and cats. The Border Terrier will view small pets as prey. Good alarm barkers but may bark excessively, chew, or dig if bored. Likes close human contact. Adaptable to city or country living.

Normal Physiologic Variations

None reported

Drug Sensitivities

None reported

Inherited Disease

Elbow Dysplasia: Polygenically inherited trait causing elbow arthritis. OFA reports 4.5% affected.[1]

Hip Dysplasia and **Legg-Calve Perthes Disease:** Polygenically inherited traits causing degenerative joint disease and hip arthritis. OFA reports 3.6% affected.[1]

Patella Luxation: Polygenically inherited congenital laxity of patellar ligaments causing medial luxation, lameness, and later degenerative joint disease. Treat surgically if causing clinical signs. OFA reports 3.3% of screened Border Terriers affected.[1]

Disease Predispositions

Heart Murmurs: Forty-one percent of Border Terriers screened for heart murmurs at the 2005 BTCA National Specialty by Dr. Deborah Fine were found to have a Grade 2 out of 6 heart murmur on auscultation. Auscultation is not diagnostic for a specific cardiac disorder, and any dog with a murmur should have an echocardiogram.[2]

Cataracts: Anterior cortex punctate cataracts predominate, though posterior, nuclear, and capsular cataracts also occur in the breed. Identified in 3.26% of Border Terriers CERF examined by veterinary ophthalmologists between 2000-2005. CERF does not recommend breeding any Border Terrier with a cataract.[3]

Hypothyroidism: Inherited autoimmune thyroiditis. 2.4% positive for thyroid auto-antibodies based on testing at Michigan State University. (Ave. for all breeds is 7.5%).[4,5]

Persistent Pupillary Membranes: Strands of fetal remnant connecting; iris to iris, cornea, lens, or involving sheets of tissue. The later three forms can impair vision, and dogs affected with these forms should not be bred. Identified in 2.07% of Border Terriers CERF examined by veterinary ophthalmologists between 2000-2005.[3]

Diabetes Mellitus: Caused by immune mediated destruction of the pancreatic beta cells. Treat with insulin, dietary management, and glucose monitoring. Border terriers were found to have a 2.4x odds ratio of developing diabetes versus other breeds. Genetic predisposition is linked to mutations in the CTLA4 gene.[6,7]

Sebaceous Gland Hyperplasia: Border Terriers have a genetic predisposition for generalized sebaceous gland hyperplasia, characterized by greasy skin and hair coat with possible clumping of the hairs but with no concomitant systemic or cutaneous disease. It is caused by an increase in the number of sebaceous gland lobules in the skin. Age of onset is 5 months to 6 years, with a median age of 2 years.[8]

Conotruncal Defect: A syndrome of inherited congenital cardiac disorders is identified in the breed, including **ventricular septal defect (VSD), mitral valve dysplasia (MVD), pulmonic stenosis (PS), aortic stenosis (AS),** and **Tetralogy of Fallot (ToF).** These affected dogs have common ancestors, but a mode of inheritance has not been established. While this is occurring at a low frequency, the BTCA recommends all puppies undergo cardiac screening prior to placement (see genetic tests below).[7]

Canine Epileptoid Cramping Syndrome (CECS, Spike's Disease): Border Terriers worldwide have been identified with this episodic neuromuscular condition, which can easily be confused with epilepsy. In early stages, affected dogs can demonstrate severe trembling, or staggering. Eventually, affected dogs exhibit episodes of cramping of the rear end and back legs, or in the head and neck. Episodes can last from seconds to several minutes. The frequency of CECS episodes can range from once or twice during the animal's lifetime to several times per week. The average age of onset for this disorder is 2-6 years. Pedigree analysis suggests an autosomal recessive mode of inheritance, but this has not been proven. Clinical and molecular genetic research is being conducted at the University of Missouri. A website (www.borderterrier-cecs.com) provides more information on the disorder.

Brachury, Craniomandibular Osteopathy, Cryptorchidism, Oligodontia, Persistent Atrial Standstill, Prognathism, Progressive Axonopathy, Progressive Retinal Atrophy, Retinal Dysplasia, and **Thrombopathia** are reported.[8]

Isolated Case Studies

Renal Dysplasia with Urolithiasis or Fanconi Syndrome: Case study of an 8 week-old Border Terrier with a history of urine dribbling since birth. Calcium phosphate uroliths were removed surgically. A concomitant hypercalcemia was not detected. Despite bilateral renal dysplasia, there was no evidence of renal failure, and the dog remained clinically normal. In another study, two Border Terrier littermates were identified with renal dysplasia and Fanconi syndrome.[9,10]

Ectopic Ureterocele: A 16-week-old, male border terrier was presented for urinary incontinence. Intravenous urography demonstrated a right-sided, extravesical ectopic ureterocele. Neoureterocystostomy and ureterocele omentalization were performed.[11]

Genetic Tests

Tests of Genotype: none

Tests of Phenotype: CHIC Certification: Required tests are; CERF eye examination (recommended annually until 8 years of age), patella evalaution, hip radiograph and congenital cardiac disease certification (by a specialist).

An OFA Pediatric Cardiac Pilot Study requests veterinary cardiac evaluation for murmurs due to congenital heart defects between 6-9 weeks of age (at no charge for OFA submission). (See CHIC website: www.caninehealthinfo.org)

Recommend elbow radiographs, and thyroid profile including autoantibodies.

Miscellaneous

- **Breed name synonyms:** none
- **Registries:** AKC, UKC, CKC, KCGB (Kennel Club of Great Britain), ANKC (Australian National Kennel Club), NKC (National Kennel Club).
- **AKC rank (year 2008):** 80 (899 dogs registered)
- **Internet resources: Border Terrier Club of America:** www.btcoa.org
  The Border Terrier Club (UK): www.theborderterrierclub.co.uk
  Border Terrier Canada: www.borderterriercanada.ca

References

1. OFA Website breed statistics: www.offa.org Last accessed July 1, 2010.
2. Fine DM: Prevalence of Asymptomatic Murmurs in Healthy Border Terriers. http://www.btcoa.org/health/2005CardiacClinic-Stats.pdf Last accessed July 1, 2010.
3. *Ocular Disorders Presumed to be Inherited in Purebred Dogs.* American College of Veterinary Ophthalmologists. ACVO, 2007
4. Nachreiner R and Refsal K: Personal communication, Diagnostic Center for Population and Animal Health, Michigan State University. April, 2007.
5. Nachreiner RF, Refsal KR, Graham PA, et. al.: Prevalence of serum thyroid hormone autoantibodies in dogs with clinical signs of hypothyroidism. J Am Vet Med Assoc 2002 Feb 15;220(4):466-71.
6. Catchpole B, Kennedy LJ, Davison LJ, et. al.: Canine diabetes mellitus: from phenotype to genotype. J Small Anim Pract. 2008 Jan;49(1):4-10.
7. Short AD, Saleh NM, Catchpole B, et. al.: CTLA4 promoter polymorphisms are associated with canine diabetes mellitus. Tissue Antigens. 2010 Mar;75(3):242-52.
8. Dedola C, Ressel L, Hill PB, et. al.: Idiopathic generalized sebaceous gland hyperplasia of the Border terrier: a morphometric study. Vet Dermatol. 2010 Oct;21(5):494-502.
9. Boddy KN, Werner P, 7.Henthorn P, et. al.: Conotruncal Defects in the Border Terrier. *Proceedings ACVIM Forum.* 2004.
10. *The Genetic Connection: A Guide to Health Problems in Purebred Dogs.* L Ackerman. p. 204. AAHA Press, 1999.
11. Clark TP, Panciera R: Calcium phosphate urolithiasis and renal dysplasia in a young dog. *J Am Vet Med Assoc.* 1992 May 15;200(10):1509-11.
12. Darrigrand-Haag RA, Center SA, Randolph JF, Lewis RM, Wood PA. Congenital Fanconi syndrome associated with renal dysplasia in 2 Border Terriers. J Vet Intern Med. 1996;10(6):412-9.
13. Tattersall JA, Welsh E: Ectopic ureterocele in a male dog: a case report and review of surgical management. J Am Anim Hosp Assoc. 2006 Sep-Oct;42(5):395-400.
14. *The Complete Dog Book, 20th Ed.* The American Kennel Club. Howell Book House, NY 2006. p. 355-357.

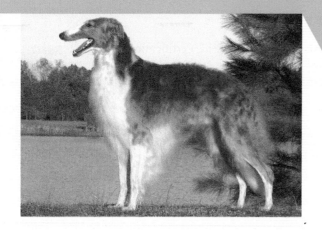

The Breed History

Perhaps as early as the 1200s, Russian aristocrats bred fast sight hounds for hunting and the breed started to take form. Dogs such as the Bearhound, southern coursing hounds of the Tartars, and Owtchar sheepdogs were reported as progenitor breeds. Some also report Saluki and Greyhound as part of the mix. The first breed standard dates back to 1650. Aristocrats used to carry out elaborate wolf hunts, using pairs or trios of Borzois, one horsemen and foxhounds to flush quarry. The first specimen may have been sent to England in 1842. The importation to America began in earnest in the 1890s. The name in Russian is "borzii," meaning swift.

Breeding for Function

Historically, they functioned in the hunt to pin down the quarry (usually wolves) until the horsemen arrived. They were also successfully used to hunt fox and hare. Today they are popular in lure coursing events, obedience, and as valued companions due to their gentle nature and trainability.

Physical Characteristics

Height at Withers: female 26" minimum (66 cm), male 28" minimum (71 cm).

Weight: females 75-90 lb (34-41 kg), males 75-105 lb (34-48 kg).

Coat: The coat is variably curly but long and silky. Short hair is present over the head, and long feathers are found on tail and hindquarters. They possess a prominent neck frill. Any color or color combination is acceptable. Daily brushing and regular bathing are recommended. They have a moderate shedding tendency.

Longevity: 9-13 years

Points of Conformation: Graceful movement and lithe conformation characterize the Borzoi. Males are noticeably heavier set than the females. The skull is very long and narrow, slightly domed and somewhat Roman-nosed in profile. The stop is not prominent, ears are small and obliquely set, eyes are dark with dark palpebral rims. The nose is large and pigmented black. The thorax is very deep and narrow, and neck slightly arched and muscular. The topline is slightly curved, back is short, and abdomen is tucked up. Long bones of the limbs appear oval; narrow when viewed

Borzoi

from the front, but are straight. The feet are well knuckled up and the dewclaws are generally removed. Hindquarters are wider than forequarters. Their long tail is set low and carried low in a curve. A powerful springy gait is desired.

Recognized Behavior Issues and Traits

Reported breed characteristics include: Courageous in the hunt, protective of their owners, tractable, intelligent, affectionate with owners, sensitive, some are aloof, faithful, good with children (best if raised with children); may chase cats or small dogs if not brought up with them. Is active outdoors but quiet in the house, has moderate to high exercise needs, and early training is needed. They can sometimes be independent and a bit stubborn. If off leash, the Borzoi should be in a fenced enclosure. Can be destructive if bored. Considered alarm barkers not guard dogs.

Normal Physiologic Variations

Sight hounds have lower normal ranges for T4 and T3 concentrations compared to other breeds.[1]

Drug Sensitivities

Anesthesia: Sight hounds require particular attention during anesthesia. Their lean body conformation with high surface-area-to-volume ratio predisposes them to hypothermia during anesthesia. Impaired biotransformation of drugs by the liver results in prolonged recovery from barbiturate and thiobarbiturate intravenous anesthetics. Propofol, and ketamine/diazepam combination are recommended induction agents.[2]

Inherited Diseases

Hypothyroidism: Breeding studies of autoimmune thyroiditis in the breed suggest an autosomal recessive inheritance. Thyroid auto-antibodies are usually present by 2.5 years of age. 11.5% positive for thyroid autoantibodies based on testing at Michigan State University. (Ave. for all breeds is 7.5%).[3,4,5,6]

Elbow Dysplasia: Polygenically inherited trait causing elbow arthritis. OFA reports 2.9% affected.[8]

Hip Dysplasia: Polygenically inherited trait causing degenerative joint disease and hip arthritis. The breed has uniformly tight hips, and is used as the gold standard by PennHIP for judging joint laxity (all have a DI < 0.32). OFA reports 1.8% affected with hip dysplasia.[7,8]

Patella Luxation: Polygenically inherited laxity of patellar ligaments, causing luxation, lameness, and later degenerative joint disease. Treat surgically if causing clinical signs. Too few Borzois have been screened by OFA to determine an accurate frequency.[8]

Cervical Malformation/Malarticulation (Wobblers Disease): A congenital anatomical disorder that causes compression of the cervical spinal cord. Clinical signs include limb weakness, proprioceptive deficits, and paralysis. Evidence of an autosomal recessive trait was found in this breed.[9]

Disease Predispositions

Multifocal Chorioretinopathy: Borzoi's can develop a retinopathy that does not progress once developed, and does not cause visual abnormalities. Various studies have found 5.6% to 12% of adult dogs with this lesion. Pedigree analysis and breeding studies rule out a sex-linked or autosomal dominant mode of inheritance, although male dogs predominate. CERF does not recommend breeding any Borzoi with chorioretinopathy.[10,11]

Mammary Cancer: Dorn reports a 17.06x odds ratio of developing mammary cancer versus other breeds.[12]

Gastric Dilation/Volvulus (Bloat): Life-threatening twisting of the stomach within the abdomen. Requires immediate veterinary attention. Dorn reports a 13.47x odds ratio of developing GDV versus other breeds.[12]

Cataracts: Anterior cortex punctate, and capsular cataracts predominate in the breed. Unknown mode of inheritance. Identified in 3.40% of Borzois CERF examined by veterinary ophthalmologists between 2000-2005. CERF does not recommend breeding any Borzoi with a cataract.[11]

Persistent Pupillary Membranes: Strands of fetal remnant connecting; iris to iris, cornea, lens, or involving sheets of tissue. The later three forms can impair vision, and dogs affected with these forms should not be bred. Identified in 1.44% of Borzois CERF examined by veterinary ophthalmologists between 2000-2005.[11]

Progressive Retinal Atrophy (PRA): Inherited degeneration of the retina. Autosomal recessive inheritance in most breeds. 1.03% of Borzois CERF examined by veterinary ophthalmologists between 2000-2005 are labeled suspicious for PRA.[11]

Congenital Malformation of the Canine Tricuspid Valve: Affected Borzois have a mild right-sided heart murmer with this congenital condition. It is inherited as an autosomal dominant trait with reduced penetrance in the Labrador Retriever. OFA reports 0.8% of Borzois have heart disease through cardiac evaluation.[8,13]

Dilated Cardiomyopathy: Primary disease of heart muscle causing arrythmias and heart failure. Unknown mode of inheritance. Reported at an increase frequency in the breed. OFA reports 0.8% of Borzois have heart disease through cardiac evaluation.[8]

Degenerative Myelopathy (DM): Affected dogs show an insidious onset of upper motor neuron (UMN) paraparesis. The disease eventually progresses to severe tetraparesis. Affected dogs have normal results on myelography, MRI, and CSF analysis. Necropsy confirms the condition. Unknown mode of inheritance. A direct genetic test for an autosomal recessive DM susceptibility gene is available. All affected dogs are homozygous for the gene, however only a small percentage of homozygous dogs develop DM. OFA reports DM susceptibility gene frequencies of 25% carrier, and 2% homozygous "at-risk".[8,18]

Microphthalmia, Optic Nerve Hypoplasia, Stifle OCD, Dysfibrinogenemia, Hypertrophic Osteodystrophy, Lymphedema, Methemoglobin Reductase Deficiency, and **Oligodontia** are reported.[14]

Isolated Case Studies

Multisystemic Inflammatory Disease: Report of a 6 week-old dog developing anorexia, temporary intention tremor, seizures, episodic pyrexia, tachypnea, conjunctivitis, otitis and neck pain. Hematological abnormalities included an inflammatory leukogram and regenerative anemia. Post mortem examination revealed a multisystemic inflammatory disease involving thyroids, lymph nodes, spleen, pancreas, bladder and lung, but no lesions to account for the neurological signs.[15]

Cutaneous Malignant Histiocytosis: Report of a 4 year-old dog. This is a multi-system, rapidly progressive disease in which there is simultaneous involvement of multiple organs such as spleen, lymph nodes, lung, bone marrow, skin and subcutis. The disease is poorly responsive to treatment. A canine cell line (CCT) was established from this dog.[16]

Genetic Tests

Tests of Genotype: Direct test of K coat color alleles is available from VetGen.

Direct tests for a DM susceptability gene is available from the OFA.

Tests of Phenotype: CHIC Certification: Required tests are; CERF eye examination, thyroid profile including autoantibodies, cardiac certification, and direct gene test for DM. Optional recommended tests are; hip and elbow radiographs. (See CHIC website: www.caninehealthinfo.org)

Recommend patella evaluation.

Miscellaneous

- **Breed name synonyms:** Russian wolfhound, Psowaya Barsaya.
- **Registries:** AKC, UKC, CKC, KCGB (Kennel Club of Great Britain), ANKC (Australian National Kennel Club), NKC (National Kennel Club).
- **AKC rank (year 2008):** 94 (630 dogs registered)
- **Internet resources: Borzoi Club of America:** www.borzoiclubofamerica.org
  Borzoi Canada: www.borzoicanada.ca
  The Borzoi Club UK: www.theborzoiclub.org.uk

References

1. Kintzer PP and Peterson ME: Progress in the Diagnosis and Treatment of Canine Hypothyroidism. 2007. Proceedings, ACVIM 2007.
2. Court MH: Anesthesia of the sighthound. Clin Tech Small Anim Pract 1999 Feb;14(1):38-43.
3. Conaway DH, Padgett GA, Nachreiner RF. The familial occurrence of lymphocytic thyroiditis in borzoi dogs. Am J Med Genet. 1985 Oct;22(2):409-14.
4. Conaway DH, Padgett GA, Bunton TE, et al. Clinical and histological features of primary progressive, familial thyroiditis in a colony of Borzoi dogs. Vet Path 1985;22: 439-446.
5. Nachreiner R and Refsal K: Personal communication, Diagnostic Center for Population and Animal Health, Michigan State University. April, 2007.
6. Nachreiner RF, Refsal KR, Graham PA, et. al.: Prevalence of serum thyroid

hormone autoantibodies in dogs with clinical signs of hypothyroidism. J Am Vet Med Assoc 2002 Feb 15;220(4):466-71.

7. Kapatkin AS, Gregor TP, Hearon K, Richardson RW, McKelvie PJ, Fordyce HH, Smith GK. Comparison of Two Radiographic Techniques for Evaluation of Hip Joint Laxity in 10 Breeds of Dogs. J Am Vet Med Assoc 224[4]:542-543 Feb 15'04

8. OFA Website breed statistics: www.offa.org Last accessed July. 1, 2010.

9. Olby, N. Update on Canine Wobbler Surgery. Proceedings ACVIM 2003.

10. Storey ES, Grahn BH, Alcorn J: Multifocal chorioretinal lesions in Borzoi dogs. *Vet Ophthalmol.* 2005 Sep-Oct;8(5):337-47.

11. *Ocular Disorders Presumed to be Inherited in Purebred Dogs.* American College of Veterinary Ophthalmologists. ACVO, 2007.

12. Dorn CR: Canine breed-specific risks of frequently diagnosed diseases at veterinary teaching hospitals. Monograph. AKC Canine Health Foundation. 2000.

13. Wright, KN. New Findings in Congenital Malformation of the Canine Tricuspid Valve. Proceedings: ACVIM 2003

14. *The Genetic Connection: A Guide to Health Problems in Purebred Dogs.* L Ackerman. p. 204. AAHA Press, 1999.

15. Cheeseman MT, Kelly DF, Horsfall KL. Multisystemic inflammatory disease in a borzoi dog. J Small Anim Pract. 1995 Jan;36(1):22-4.

16. Sakai H, Nakano H, Yamaguchi R, Yonemaru K, Yanai T, Masegi T. Establishment of a new canine cell line (CCT) originated from a cutaneous malignant histiocytosis. \J Vet Med Sci. 2003 Jun;65(6):731-5.

17. *The Complete Dog Book, 20th Ed.* The American Kennel Club. Howell Book House, NY 2006. p. 160-163.

18. Awano T, Johnson GS, Wade CM, et. al.: Genome-wide association analysis reveals a SOD1 mutation in canine degenerative myelopathy that resembles amyotrophic lateral sclerosis. Proc Natl Acad Sci U S A. 2009 Feb 24;106(8):2794-9.

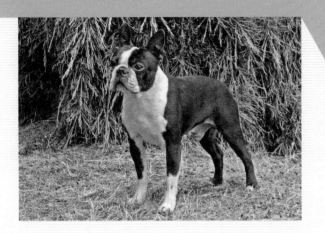

The Breed History

The Boston terrier arose from crosses between white English terriers and English bulldogs; first offspring trace back to the year 1870. Hooper's Judge was the foundation stud. The original crosses were considerably larger than today's standard. Since the breed originated in Boston, this name was chosen to identify this terrier breed. The first AKC registry entries occurred in 1893.

Breeding for Function

This dog was bred as a companion dog, though his origins provide him with capacity for a plucky terrier's courage and defense.

Physical Characteristics

Height at Withers: 15-17" (38-43 cm)

Weight: 3 size types within the breed:
Up to 15 lb (< 7 kg), 15-19 lb (7-8.5 kg), 20-25 lb (9-11 kg)

Coat: Short, fine, flat glossy coat is black, brindle or seal with well demarcated and specifically distributed striking white markings. Seal is a black appearance with a red tone in bright light. Brindle is preferred as the base color.

Longevity: 13-14 years.

Points of Conformation: The compact, sturdy, squarely built body is broad in front across the chest. Boston terriers possess a short body and brachycephalic head with a pronounced stop. The expression is gentle but alert, skull is broad between the ears and without wrinkles, eyes are very wide set with a dark brown color, and the small erect ears are sometimes cropped. Ear leather is fine and hair covering is minimal. The short blocky muzzle is wider than long, the nose is black. Bite is square to mildly undershot. Nictitans should not be visible, and palpebral margins should be dark, the neck is slightly arched, head carriage is high. The topline is level, thorax moderately deep with ribs well sprung, and the tail is short (less than 1/4 of the distance to the tarsus) and tapers with straight or screw ending, and is carried low. The limbs are straight, dewclaws may be taken off, and feet have well knuckled toes, are compact and are small. Gait is agile and straight with good rear driving power.

Boston Terrier

Recognized Behavior Issues and Traits

Boston terriers are described as being of high intelligence with a stubborn streak, alert, very active, playful, and having a very gentle disposition. Moderate exercise requirements, low grooming needs, ability to get along with gentle children and other pets are hallmarks of the breed. Will alarm bark, but they are not considered protectors. Boston terriers are suitable for home and apartment living, and they do not tolerate temperature extremes. They may snore and snort. Some may be picky eaters. They are minimal shedders.

Normal Physiologic Variations

The breed tends to have small litters, with three considered normal.

In Great Britain, 92.3% of Boston Terrier litters are delivered via **C-section.**[1]

Drug Sensitivities

None reported

Inherited Diseases

Hip Dysplasia and Legg-Calve Perthes Disease: Polygenically inherited traits causing degenerative hip joint disease and arthritis. OFA reports 13.5% affected with hip dysplasia.[2]

Cataracts: Two types of cataracts are identified in the breed: An autosomal recessive early-onset hereditary cataract (EHC) has an onset before 6 months and complete opacity by 2 years of age. A genetic test is available for EHC. A late-onset hereditary cataract (LHC) has an onset after 4-5 years of age with a variable progression, and an unknown mode of inheritance. Anterior or posterior intermediate and punctate cataracts occur in the breed. In one large study, 11.11% of Boston terriers had cataracts. Identified in 8.66% of Boston terriers CERF examined by veterinary ophthalmologists between 2000-2005. Dorn reports a 2.14x odds ratio versus other breeds. One study showed a 4.2x odds ratio versus other breeds. CERF does not recommend breeding any Boston Terrier with a cataract.[3,4,5,6,7]

Patella Luxation: Polygenically inherited laxity of patellar ligaments, causing luxation, lameness, and later degenerative joint disease. Treat surgically if causing clinical signs. OFA reports 5.6% affected. Dorn reports a 2.14x odds ratio versus other breeds. Another study reports a 4.2x odds ratio versus other breeds.[2,3,8]

Elbow Dysplasia: Polygenically inherited trait causing elbow arthritis. Too few Boston Terriers have been screened by OFA to determine an accurate frequency.[2]

Disease Predispositions

Brachycephalic Complex: The brachycephalic complex includes stenotic nares, elongated soft palate, everted laryngeal saccules, laryngeal collapse, and occasionally hypoplastic trachea. Boston terriers comprise 15% of all dogs diagnosed with hypoplasia of the trachea. Dorn reports a 10.68x odds ratio for elongated soft palate versus other breeds. Unknown mode of inheritance.[3,9,10,11]

Dystocia: Boston terriers are prone to difficult birthing, due to both a dorsoventrally flattened pelvic canal and large fetuses with big heads.[12]

Distichiasis: Abnormally placed eyelashes that irritate the cornea and conjunctiva. Can cause secondary corneal ulceration. Identified in 3.82% of Boston terriers CERF examined by veterinary ophthalmologists between 2000-2005.[6]

Persistent Pupillary Membranes: Strands of fetal remnant connecting; iris to iris, cornea, lens, or involving sheets of tissue. The later three forms can impair vision, and dogs affected with these forms should not be bred. Identified in 3.61% of Boston Terriers CERF examined by veterinary ophthalmologists between 2000-2005.[6]

Glaucoma: Ocular condition causing increased pressure within the eyeball, and secondary blindness due to damage to the retina. Diagnose with tonometry and gonioscopy. Can be a primary condition or secondary to cataract or lens luxation. Dorn reports a 2.12x odds ratio for developing glaucoma versus other breeds. Another report found a 4.1x odds ratio for secondary glaucoma versus other breeds. Diagnosed in 2.88% of Boston terriers presented to veterinary teaching hospitals. CERF does not recommend breeding any Boston Terrier with glaucoma.[3,6,13,14,15]

Allergic Dermatitis: Inhalant or food allergy. Presents with pruritis and pyotraumatic dermatitis. Reported at an increased frequency in Boston terriers.[16]

Corneal Dystrophy: Epithelial-stromal, and endothelial forms occur in the breed. Endothelial form is associated with progressive corneal edema, which can lead to bullous keratopathy and corneal erosions. Age of onset 6-13 years. Treatment is symptomatic and palliative. Epithelial-stromal form is identified in 2.63% of Boston terriers, and endothelial form in 0.21% of Boston Terriers CERF examined by veterinary ophthalmologists between 2000-2005. CERF does not recommend breeding any Boston Terrier with endothelial corneal dystrophy.[6,17]

Hypothyroidism: Inherited autoimmune thyroiditis. 1.9% positive for thyroid auto-antibodies based on testing at Michigan State University. (Ave. for all breeds is 7.5%).[18,19]

Hyperadrenocorticism (Cushing's Disease): Caused by a functional adrenal or pituitary tumor. Clinical signs may include increased thirst and urination, symmetrical truncal alopecia, and abdominal distention. Dorn reports a 5.60x odds ratio versus other breeds.[3,20,21]

Deafness: Congenital deafness can be unilateral or bilateral. Associated with Irish pattern and piebald pigmentation. Diagnose by BAER testing. Unknown mode of inheritance. OFA reports 1.9% affected.[2,22]

Vitreous Degeneration: Liquefication of the vitreous gel which may predispose to retinal detachment, glaucoma, and blindness. Identified in 1.22% of Boston Terriers CERF examined by veterinary ophthalmologists between 2000-2005.[6]

Hypospadias: Almost 25% of all diagnoses of hypospadias (an abnormal opening of the urethra) occur in Boston terriers. There is a 15:1 male to female prevalence. Cryptorchidism or intersexuality can also accompany the condition.[23]

Atresia Ani (Imperforate Anus): An increased incidence of this congenital condition is reported in the breed, with a frequency of 0.07%, and an odds ratio of 13.77x. Treatment is surgery.[24]

Cleft Lip and Palate: Boston terriers may have an increased frequency of cleft lip and palate versus other breeds.[25]

Hemivertebra and Butterfly Vertebra: May cause scoliosis, pain or spinal cord compression if severe. Unknown mode of inheritance.[26]

Perineal Hernia: Boston terriers have a predisposition to developing perineal hernias. Treatment is surgery.[27,28]

Uveal Cysts: Boston terriers have a higher frequency of uveal cysts than other breeds, with a mean age of cyst development of 6.8 years.[29]

Cataract Resorption-induced Uveitis: Spontaneous cataract resorption, and associated lens-induced uveitis primarily occurs in young Boston Terriers. Medical control of the lens-induced uveitis by use of mydriatics and, infrequently, topical and systemic corticosteroids is essential.[30]

Vascular Ring Anomaly: Reported at an increased frequency in the breed. Causes regurgitation and megaesophagus when solid food is first fed. Correct with surgery.[31]

Glial Tumors: Boston terriers may have a predisposition to nervous tissue tumors of glial origin.[32]

Anasarca, Calcinosis Circumscripta, Cerebellar Vermian Hypoplasia, Craniomandibular Osteopathy, Cryptorchidism, Demodicosis, Entropion, Hydrocephalus, Keratoconjunctivitis Sicca, Mitral valve Disease, Pelger-Huet Anomaly, Progressive Retinal Atrophy, Prolapsed Gland of Nictitans, Pyloric Stenosis, Sacrocaudal Dysgenesis, Spina Bifida, Ulcerative Keratitis, and **Wry Mouth** are reported.[33]

Isolated Case Studies

Muscular Dystrophy: Sarcoglycan-deficient muscular dystrophy has been reported in several young, male and female Boston Terriers. Affected dogs present with muscle atrophy or hypertrophy, gait abnormalities, dysphagia, and dramatically increased CK, AST, and ALT activities.[34]

Dandy-Walker-Like Syndrome: Case report of an affected Boston terrier puppy. Congenital disorder causing cerebellar ataxia and other CNS signs due to cysts arising from the 4th ventricle, dysgenesis of the cerebellar vermis, and hydrocephalus of the 3rd and lateral ventricles. A previous report of this syndrome in Boston terriers suggests the problem may be inherited in this breed.[35]

Tubular Colonic Duplication: A six-month-old, intact female Boston terrier presented with clinical signs of increased frequency of defecation, tenesmus, and constipation, which had been present since birth. A diagnosis of tubular colonic duplication was made via contrast radiography and colonoscopy. The condition was corrected surgically.[36]

Choroid Plexus Carcinoma and Meningeal Carcinomatosis: A 6-year-old neutered female Boston terrier had a slow onset of bilateral visual loss. On magnetic resonance imaging (MRI) there were multiple cyst-like structures found in the parenchyma of the cerebrum, cerebellum and brainstem. Histopathologically the diagnosis was a choroid plexus carcinoma with meningeal carcinomatosis.[37]

Neuroblastoma: A mediastinal neuroblastoma was found in a 15-mth-old Boston terrier with dyspnea. The tumor compressed adjacent lung and invaded the cervical spinal cord.[38]

Genetic Tests

Tests of Genotype: Direct test for early-onset hereditary cataract (EHC) is available from the Animal Health Trust (UK) and VetGen.

Direct test for coat color alleles is available from VetGen.

Tests of Phenotype: CHIC Certification: Required testing includes CERF eye examination, patella examination, and BAER test for deafness. See CHIC website (www.caninehealthinfo.org).

Recommended tests include hip and elbow radiographs, thyroid profile including autoantibodies, and cardiac evaluation.

Miscellaneous

- **Breed Name Synonyms:** Boston, Boston Bulldog, Boston Bull, American Bull Terrier (historical name before 1891). The American Gentleman (nickname)
- **Registries:** AKC, UKC, CKC, KCGB (Kennel Club of Great Britain), ANKC (Australian National Kennel Club), NKC (National Kennel Club)
- **AKC rank (year 2008):** 17 (10,930 dogs registered)
- **Internet resources: Boston Terrier Club of America:** www.bostonterrierclubofamerica.org
  Boston Terrier Club of Canada: www.bostonterrierclubofcanada.com

References

1. Evans KM & Adams VJ: Proportion of litters of purebred dogs born by caesarean section. J Small Anim Pract. 2010 Feb;51(2):113-8.
2. OFA Website breed statistics: www.offa.org Last accessed July 1, 2010.
3. Dorn CR: Canine breed-specific risks of frequently diagnosed diseases at veterinary teaching hospitals. Monograph. AKC Canine Health Foundation. 2000.
4. Adkins EA, Hendrix DV: Outcomes of dogs presented for cataract evaluation: a retrospective study. J Am Anim Hosp Assoc. 2005 Jul-Aug;41(4):235-40.
5. Gelatt KN, Mackay EO: Prevalence of primary breed-related cataracts in the dog in North America. Vet Ophthalmol. 2005 Mar-Apr;8(2):101-11.
6. Ocular Disorders Presumed to be Inherited in Purebred Dogs. American College of Veterinary Ophthalmologists. ACVO, 2007
7. Mellersh CS, Graves KT, McLaughlin B, et. al.: Mutation in HSF4 associated with early but not late-onset hereditary cataract in the Boston Terrier. J Hered. 2007;98(5):531-3.
8. LaFond E, Breur GJ and Austin CC: Breed susceptibility for developmental orthopedic diseases in dogs. J Am Anim Hosp Assoc. 2002 Sep-Oct;38(5):467-77.
9. Coyne BE, Fingland RB: Hypoplasia of the trachea in dogs: 103 cases (1974-1990). J Am Vet Med Assoc. 1992 Sep 1;201(5):768-72.
10. Monnet M: Brachycephalic Airway Syndrome. Proceedings, 2004 World Small Animal Veterinary Association Congress. 2004.
11. Lorinson D, Bright RM, White RAS: Brachycephalic Airway Obstruction Syndrome - A Review of 118 Cases. Canine Pract 1997: 22(5/6):18-21.

12. Eneroth A, Linde-Forsberg C, Uhlhorn M, et. al.: Radiographic pelvimetry for assessment of dystocia in bitches: a clinical study in two terrier breeds. J Small Anim Pract. 1999 Jun;40(6):257-64.
13. Gelatt KN, MacKay EO: Secondary glaucomas in the dog in North America. Vet Ophthalmol. 2004 Jul-Aug;7(4):245-59.
14. Gelatt KN, MacKay EO: Prevalence of the breed-related glaucomas in pure-bred dogs in North America. Vet Ophthalmol. 2004 Mar-Apr;7(2):97-111.
15. Johnsen DA, Maggs DJ, Kass PH, et. al.: Evaluation of risk factors for development of secondary glaucoma in dogs: 156 cases (1999-2004). J Am Vet Med Assoc. 2006 Oct 15;229(8):1270-4.
16. Ackerman, L: Managing Inhalant Allergies I: Proceedings, 2004 Atlantic Coast Veterinary Conference. 2004.
17. Cooley PL, Dice PF 2nd: Corneal dystrophy in the dog and cat. Vet Clin North Am Small Anim Pract. 1990 May;20(3):681-92.
18. Nachreiner R and Refsal K: Personal communication, Diagnostic Center for Population and Animal Health, Michigan State University. April, 2007.
19. Nachreiner RF, Refsal KR, Graham PA, et. al.: Prevalence of serum thyroid hormone autoantibodies in dogs with clinical signs of hypothyroidism. J Am Vet Med Assoc. 2002 Feb 15;220(4):466-71.
20. McManus JL, Nimmons GB, Buchta W: Case report. Surgical and medical management of hyperadrenocorticalism in a Boston Terrier. Can Vet J. 1970 Apr;11(4):78-80.
21. Kaufman J: Diseases of the adrenal cortex of dogs and cats. Mod Vet Pract. 1984 Jun;65(6):429-34.
22. Strain GM: Deafness prevalence and pigmentation and gender associations in dog breeds at risk. Vet J 2004; Jan;167(1):23-32.
23. Hayes HM Jr, Wilson GP: Hospital incidence of hypospadias in dogs in North America. Vet Rec. 1986 May 31;118(22):605-7.
24. Vianna ML, Tobias KM: Atresia ani in the dog: a retrospective study. J Am Anim Hosp Assoc. 2005 Sep-Oct;41(5):317-22.
25. Edmonds L, Stewart RW, Selby L: Cleft lip and palate in Boston terrier pups. Vet Med Small Anim Clin. 1972 Nov;67(11):1219
26. Done SH, Drew RA, Robins GM, et. al: Hemivertebra in the dog: clinical and pathological observations. Vet Rec. 1975 Apr 5;96(14):313-7.
27. Hosgood G, Hedlund CS, Pechman RD, et. al.: Perineal herniorrhaphy: perioperative data from 100 dogs. J Am Anim Hosp Assoc. 1995 Jul-Aug;31(4):331-42.
28. Robertson JJ: Perineal hernia repair in dogs. Mod Vet Pract. 1984 May;65(5):365-8.
29. Corcoran KA, Koch SA: Uveal cysts in dogs: 28 cases (1989-1991). J Am Vet Med Assoc. 1993 Aug 15;203(4):545-6.
30. Gelatt KN: Spontaneous cataract resorption and lens-induced uveitis in the dog. Mod Vet Pract. 1975 May;56(5):331-5.
31. Fossum TW: Surgery of Cardiac Disease. Proceedings, 2009 WSAVA World Congress. 2009.
32. Hayes HM, Priester WA Jr, Pendergrass TW: Occurrence of nervous-tissue tumors in cattle, horses, cats and dogs. Int J Cancer. 1975 Jan 15;15(1):39-47.
33. The Genetic Connection: A Guide to Health Problems in Purebred Dogs. L Ackerman. p. 204-05 AAHA Press, 1999.
34. Deitz K, Morrison JA, Kline K, et. al.: Sarcoglycan-deficient muscular dystrophy in a Boston Terrier. J Vet Intern Med. 2008 Mar-Apr;22(2):476-80.
35. Noureddine C, Harder R, Olby NJ, et. al.: Ultrasonographic appearance of Dandy Walker-like Syndrome in a Boston Terrier. Vet Radiol Ultrasound. 2004 Jul-Aug;45(4):336-9.
36. Shinozaki JK, Sellon RK, Tobias KM, et. al.: Tubular colonic duplication in a dog. J Am Anim Hosp Assoc. 2000 May-Jun;36(3):209-13.
37. Lipsitz D, Levitski RE, Chauvet AE: Magnetic resonance imaging of a choroid plexus carcinoma and meningeal carcinomatosis in a dog. Vet Radiol Ultrasound. 1999 May-Jun;40(3):246-50.
38. Kelly DF: Neuroblastoma in the dog. J Pathol. 1975 Aug;116(4):209-12.
39. The Complete Dog Book, 20th Ed. The American Kennel Club. Howell Book House, NY 2006. p. 533-537.

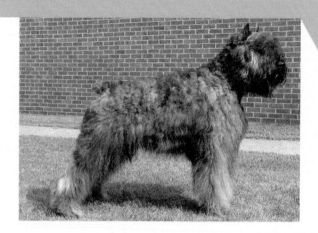

The Breed History

In the region of Flandres in Belgium, and perhaps in Northern France also, this dog was bred strictly as a working dog. Though not well documented, the old Beauceron and Griffons may have contributed to breed genesis. Though records of a dog of this type date back to the 1600s, the first breed standard was drawn up in 1912. Their numbers were decimated during WW1, but the breed was carefully regenerated from a sire, Ch. Nic de Sottegem. The first recognition of the breed by the AKC occurred in 1929.

Breeding for Function

Driving cattle and pulling carts on the farm were their original purposes and now they serve as companion dogs and watchdog (or guard dogs). They require a working award as a defense or police/army working dog before being awarded championship status in their native Belgium, which attests to the continued emphasis of the breed as a working dog. They have also proved well suited to tracking, as war messenger dogs, and as guide dogs for the blind.

Physical Characteristics

Height at Withers: female 23.5-26.5" (59.5-67 cm), male 24.5-27.5" (62-70 cm).

Weight: 60-88 lb (27-40 kg).

Coat: The rugged double coat consists of very harsh hard matte wavy hairs of about 2.5" (6 cm) length, standing out. The undercoat is dense, soft and wooly. Colors include salt and pepper, black, brindle, and gray. Only a small white marking on the chest is accepted (star). Grooming needs are moderate, shedding is average.

Longevity: 10-11 years.

Points of Conformation: The large, square and powerful dog is noted for the shaggy unkempt appearance and large head held in high head carriage. The gait is smooth, agile, and ground covering, The expression is intense, and eyes are colored dark brown and are oval. Palpebral margins are dark and bushy brows are prominent. The nose is large and black. Ears are high set and triangular, rounded at the tips and are sometimes cropped. Large moustache and beard sit at the end of a long slightly tapered muzzle. The skull is flat and wide, and the stop is slight. Neck is muscular and arched, and topline is level, thorax is deep and ribs are well sprung. Though

substantial in the middle, there is a slightly tucked up abdomen. The high set tail is usually docked to leave only 2-3 vertebrae. Limbs are straight and fairly heavily boned and well muscled, they have short metacarpals and metatarsals. Feet are compact and the toes are well knuckled up, nails are black and the pads are thick. Dewclaws may be taken off.

Recognized Behavior Issues and Traits

Descriptions of the breed include traits such as: Bold, fearless, gentle disposition, moderately active, good with children, and a loyal guardian. Good with other dogs if raised with them, good trainability.

They can adapt to urban life if given regular exercise, but are best suited to farm and country. Early socialization and obedience is important to prevent inappropriate protectiveness.

Normal Physiologic Variations

Slow to mature

Drug Sensitivities

None reported

Inherited Diseases

Hip Dysplasia: Polygenically inherited trait causing degenerative joint disease and hip arthritis. OFA reports 15.1% affected.[1]

Elbow Dysplasia: Polygenically inherited trait causing elbow arthritis. OFA reports 9.1% affected. Reported 19.5x odds ratio for the fragmented coronoid process form of elbow dysplasia versus other breeds.[1,2]

Goniodysplasia/Dysplasia of the Pectinate Ligament: Ophthalmologic examination of 72 Bouvier des Flandres dogs revealed 37.5% with variable degrees of goniodysgenesis. All dogs examined had normotensive eyes, and were asymptomatic. Pedigree analysis demonstrated a recessive inheritance. Dysplasia of the pectinate ligament occurs at a high frequency in normal and glaucomatous Bouvier des Flandres dogs, and is severe in glaucomatous eyes. These are considered predisposing factors for the development of glaucoma.[3,4]

Diffuse Polyneuropathy: Rare disease, with affected dogs presenting between 1-3 years of age with tetraparesis without ataxia, delayed proprioceptive positioning in all limbs, incomplete palpebral closure bilaterally, reduced muscle tone and muscle mass in the distal muscles, absent patellar and cutaneous trunci reflexes, decreased flexor reflexes in all limbs and intact nociception. There is no evidence of laryngeal paresis. Histopathology reveals an axonopathy affecting the large caliber myelinated fibers. Preliminary genetic studies indicate an autosomal recessive mode of inheritance.[5]

Patella Luxation: Polygenically inherited laxity of patellar ligaments, causing luxation, lameness, and later degenerative joint disease. Treat surgically if causing clinical signs. Limited OFA evaluations report a low frequency in the breed.[1]

Disease Predispositions

Sebaceous Cysts: The 2004 Bouvier Health Survey reports 15.71% of Bouvier des Flandres dogs develop benign sebaceous cysts.[6]

Allergic Dermatitis: Inhalant or food allergy. Presents with pruritis and pyotraumatic dermatitis (hot spots). Reported at a frequency of 15.68% in the 2004 Bouvier Health Survey.[6]

Arthritis: At some point in their lives, 11.07% of Bouvier des Flandres dogs suffer from arthritis, according to the 2004 Bouvier Health Survey. Dorn reports a 2.81x odds ratio for developing arthritis versus other breeds.[6,7]

Persistent Pupillary Membranes: Strands of fetal remnant connecting; iris to iris, cornea, lens, or involving sheets of tissue. The later three forms can impair vision, and dogs affected with these forms should not be bred. Identified in 7.49% of Bouvier des Flandres dogs CERF examined by veterinary ophthalmologists between 2000-2005.[8]

Cataracts: Anterior, posterior, and capsular cataracts predominate in the breed. Reported at a frequency of 3.71% in the 2004 Bouvier Health Survey. Identified in 5.23% of Bouvier des Flandres dogs CERF examined by veterinary ophthalmologists between 2000-2005. CERF does not recommend breeding any Bouvier des Flandres dog with a cataract.[6,8]

Hypothyroidism: Inherited autoimmune thyroiditis. 4.3% positive for thyroid auto-antibodies based on testing at Michigan State University (Ave. for all breeds is 7.5%), although Dorn reports a 1.42x odds ratio for hypothyroidism versus other breeds.[7,9,10]

Gastric Dilatation-Volvulus (bloat, GDV): Polygenically inherited, life-threatening twisting of the stomach within the abdomen. Requires immediate treatment. Reported at an increased frequency in the breed.[11]

Primary Glaucoma: Causes increased ocular pressure and blindness due to retinal deterioration. Caused by inherited goniodysplasia and dysplasia of the pectinate ligament. Test with gonioscopy and tonometry. Diagnosed in 1.31% of Bouviers presented to veterinary teaching hospitals. Reported at a frequency of 1.71% in the 2004 Bouvier Health Survey. CERF does not recommend breeding any Bouvier des Flandres with glaucoma.[6,8,12,13]

Subaortic Stenosis (SAS): Affected dogs present with a left heart base murmur, aortic velocities greater than 1.5 m/second on Doppler echocardiography, aortic regurgitation, and mitral regurgitation. Can cause exercise intolerance, syncope, and progress to heart failure. Diagnose by auscultation and echocardiography. The breed is one predisposed to subaortic stenosis. Reported at a frequency of 1.30% in the 2004 Bouvier Health Survey. Considered polygenically inherited.[6,14]

Humeral Osteochondritis Dissecans (OCD): Inherited cartilage defect of the humeral head. Causes shoulder joint pain and lameness in young growing dogs. Mild cases can resolve with rest, while more severe cases require surgery. 50% of cases are bilateral. Reported 12.1x odds ratio versus other breeds.[2]

Digital Squamous Cell Carcinoma: The breed is one predisposed to digital squamous cell carcinoma. Treat with toe amputation.[15]

Perineal Hernia: A Dutch study found Bouvier des Flandres a breed predisposed to developing perineal hernias. Treat with surgery.[16]

Villous Atrophy and Enteritis: A Dutch study found Bouvier des Flandres a breed predisposed to developing chronic diarrhea due to intestinal villous atrophy.[17]

Prostate Carcinoma: One study found an increased (8.44x odds ratio) risk for developing prostate carcinoma versus other breeds.[18]

Persistent Hyperplastic Primary Vitreous (PHPV): A congenital defect resulting from abnormalities in the development and regression of the hyaloid artery (the primary vitreous) during embryogenesis. In the Bouvier des Flandres, the condition is associated with retinal dysplasia and detachment, optic nerve hypoplasia, lenticonus, cataract and congenital blindness. CERF does not recommend breeding any Bouvier des Flandres with PHPV.[19]

Muscular Dystrophy: A rare, inherited form of congenital muscular dystrophy occurs in the breed. Affected dogs present with megaesophagus, regurgitation, and weakness. Affected dogs can also show exercise intolerance, muscle atrophy, and overextension of the paws. Histopathological changes occur in all skeletal muscles, but the pharyngeal, laryngeal and esophageal muscles are most severely affected. The mode of inheritance is not determined.[20,21,22]

Congenital Laryngeal Paralysis: A rare inherited disorder in Bouvier des Flandres dogs. Affected dogs present with inspiratory obstructive dyspnea or stridor. Unknown mode of inheritance.[23,24,25,26]

Brachygnathism, Cleft Lip/Palate, Degenerative Myopathy, Entropion, Prognathism, Portosystemic Shunting, and **Seasonal Flank Alopecia** are reported.[27]

Isolated Case Studies

Atresia of the External Acoustic Meatus: A five-year-old male Bouvier des Flandres was presented with chronic ear pain (otalgia) of approximately four and a half years duration. Clinical examination revealed a missing bony ear canal. A total ear canal ablation and bulla osteotomy resolved the otalgia.[28]

Eosinophilic Granulomatous Colitis with Ulceration: A 3-year-old Bouvier de Flandres dog was identified with hemorrhagic diarrhea, anorexia, weight loss and anemia. Abdominal palpation revealed a palpable thickened large intestine. Histopathology revealed eosinophilic granulomatous colitis with ulceration.[29]

Primary Lymphedema and Lymphangiosarcoma: A 4-year-old, spayed female fawn Bouvier des Flandres presented to the Ontario Veterinary College Veterinary Teaching Hospital with a lifelong history of bilateral hind limb edema, and a recently discovered inguinal mass. Based on history, clinical, and histopathological findings, the dog was diagnosed with primary lymphedema and secondary lymphangiosarcoma.[30]

Genetic Tests

Tests of Genotype: Direct test for K allele color genes is available from VetGen.

Tests of Phenotype: CHIC Certification: Required testing includes hip and elbow radiographs, congenital cardiac evaluation, and CERF eye examination. (See CHIC website;www.caninehealthinfo.org).

Recommend thyroid profile including autoantibodies and patella evaluation.

Miscellaneous

- **Breed Name Synonyms:** Bouvier, Belgian Cattle Dog, and historically, toucheur de boeuf, Viulbaard, or koehond.
- **Registries:** AKC, UKC, CKC, KCGB (Kennel Club of Great Britain), ANKC (Australian National Kennel Club), NKC (National Kennel Club)
- **AKC Rank (Year 2008):** 83 (821 dogs registered)
- **Internet resources: The American Bouvier des Flandres Club:** www.bouvier.org
  Bouvier des Flandres Club of Canada: www.bouviercanada.com
  Bouvier Des Flandres Club of Great Britain: www.bouvierclub.co.uk
  Bouvier Health Foundation: www.bouvierhealthfoundation.org

References

1. OFA Website breed statistics: www.offa.org Last accessed July 1, 2010.
2. LaFond E, Breur GJ and Austin CC: Breed susceptibility for developmental orthopedic diseases in dogs. J Am Anim Hosp Assoc. 2002 Sep-Oct;38(5):467-77.
3. Ruhli MB, Spiess BM: Goniodysplasia in the Bouvier des Flandres. Schweiz Arch Tierheilkd. 1996;138(6):307-11.
4. van der Linde-Sipman JS: Dysplasia of the pectinate ligament and primary glaucoma in the Bouvier des Flandres dog. Vet Pathol. 1987 May;24(3):201-6.
5. da Costa RC, Parent J, Poma R: Adult-Onset Distal Sensorimotor Polyneuropathy in Bouvier des Flandres Dogs. Proceedings, 2005 ACVIM Forum. 2005.
6. The Bouvier Health Foundation, Slater M: The 2004 Bouvier Health Survey. 2005.
7. Dorn CR: Canine breed-specific risks of frequently diagnosed diseases at veterinary teaching hospitals. Monograph. AKC Canine Health Foundation. 2000.
8. Ocular Disorders Presumed to be Inherited in Purebred Dogs. American College of Veterinary Ophthalmologists. ACVO, 2007
9. Nachreiner R and Refsal K: Personal communication, Diagnostic Center for Population and Animal Health, Michigan State University. April, 2007.
10. Nachreiner RF, Refsal KR, Graham PA, et. al.: Prevalence of serum thyroid hormone autoantibodies in dogs with clinical signs of hypothyroidism. J Am Vet Med Assoc 2002 Feb 15;220(4):466-71
11. Glickman LT, Glickman NW, Schellenberg DB, et. al.: Incidence of and breed-related risk factors for gastric dilatation-volvulus in dogs. J Am Vet Med Assoc. 2000 Jan 1;216(1):40-5.
12. Wilkie DA: Glaucoma in the Dog I. Proceedings, Western Veterinary Conference 2003.
13. Gelatt KN, MacKay EO: Prevalence of the breed-related glaucomas in pure-bred dogs in North America. Vet Ophthalmol. 2004 Mar-Apr;7(2):97-111.
14. Fuentes VL: Methods Of Screening for Subaortic Stenosis. Proceedings, 14th ECVIM-CA Congress. 2004.
15. Breton K: Death and Derm: Deadly Dermatologic Diseases. Proceedings, 2004 ACVIM Forum. 2004.
16. Sjollema BE, van Sluijs FJ: Perineal hernia in the dog: developments in its treatment and retrospective study in 197 patients. Tijdschr Diergeneeskd. 1991 Feb 1;116(3):142-7.
17. van der Gaag I, Happe RP: The histological appearance of peroral small intestinal biopsies in clinically healthy dogs and dogs with chronic diarrhea. Zentralbl Veterinarmed A. 1990 Jul;37(6):401-16.
18. Teske E, Naan EC, van Dijk EM, et. al.: Canine prostate carcinoma: epidemiological evidence of an increased risk in castrated dogs. Mol Cell Endocrinol. 2002 Nov 29;197(1-2):251-5.
19. Van Rensburg IBJ, Petrick S, Van der Lagt J, Smit M: Multiple inherited eye anomalies including persistent hyperplastic tunica vasculosa lentis in the Bouvier des Flandres. Prog Vet Comp Ophthal 1992;2:143,.
20. Peeters ME, Ubbink GJ: Dysphagia-associated muscular dystrophy: a familial trait in the bouvier des Flandres. Vet Rec. 1994 Apr 23;134(17):444-6.
21. Braund KG, Steinberg HS, Mehta JR: Investigating a degenerative polymyopathy in four related Bouvier des Flandres dogs. Vet Med1990:85(6):558,562-566,568-570.
22. Poncelet L, Gilbert S, Jauniaux T, Balligand M: Swimming Puppy Syndrome in a Litter of Bouvier-Des-Flandres. Annales de
23. Braund KG, Steinberg HS, Shores A, et. al.: Laryngeal paralysis in immature and mature dogs as one sign of a more diffuse polyneuropathy. J Am Vet Med Assoc. 1989 Jun 15;194(12):1735-40.
24. O'Brien J: Spontaneous laryngeal disease in the canine. Laryngoscope. 1975 Dec;85(12 pt 1):2023-5.
25. Venker-Van Haagen AJ, Bouw J, Hartmann W: Hereditary transmission of laryngeal paralysis in Bouviers. Journal of the American Animal Hospital Association 1981;17: 75-76.
26. Venker-van Hagen AJ: Laryngeal paralysis in Bouvier dogs and breeding advice to prevent this condition. Tijdschrift voor Diergeneeskunde 1981;107: 21-22.
27. The Genetic Connection: A Guide to Health Problems in Purebred Dogs. L Ackerman. p. 205. AAHA Press, 1999.
28. House A: Atresia of the distal external acoustic meatus in a Bouvier des Flandres. J Small Anim Pract. 2001 Feb;42(2):88-9.
29. van der Gaag I, van der Linde-Sipman JS:Eosinophilic granulomatous colitis with ulceration in a dog. J Comp Pathol. 1987 Mar;97(2): 179-85.
30. Webb JA, Boston SE, Armstrong J, et.al: Lymphangiosarcoma in a Bouvier des Flandres. J Vet Intern Med. 2004 Jan-Feb; 18(1): 122-4.
31. The Complete Dog Book, 20th Ed. The American Kennel Club. Howell Book House, NY 2006. P. 640-644.

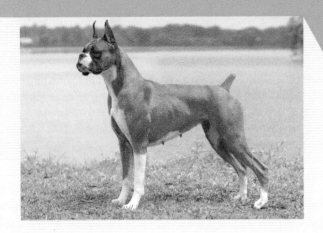

Boxer

The Breed History

This breed originates from Tibetan lines of mastiff dogs; progressive development of the modern breed type has occurred since the 16th century, primarily in Germany. A breed club established the first breed standard in Munich in the late 1800s. The breed is a bulldog type, and these trace back to Molossus bloodlines. Other bloodlines bred into the boxer include terrier and perhaps English Bulldogs. The boxer is thought to get his name from the way he used his front paws during fights since it resembled a human boxing action. Others feel the name is a derivative of the Germanic word *boxl*. The year 1904 marked the first AKC registry.

Breeding for Function

In Germany, the boxer was a top choice for police work. Before fighting and baiting were outlawed, this breed was also used for these old sports. In Germany, the breed was used for hunting large game such as boars or bears and their powerful jaws were used to secure the catch. They were also used in theater and circus. The boxer was also used as a watchdog, assistance dog, and has become a very popular companion and obedience dog.

Physical Characteristics

Height at Withers: female 21-23.5" (53.5-60 cm), male 22.5-25" (57-63.5 cm).

Weight: females 55-65 lb (25-29.5 kg), males 65-80 lb (29.5-36.5 kg). Males are heavier boned.

Coat: The short glossy coat is brindle or fawn. White marking ("flash") is allowed over up to one third of the coat. All-white pups can be born, but are not used for breeding. The mask is usually black.

Longevity: 11-13 years.

Points of Conformation: This dog is a medium-built athletic dog with well-developed musculature, and a springy stride. The brachycephalic head is broad and the muzzle is blunt and broad. Eyes are dark brown, and the forehead wrinkles when ears are pricked. Ears are usually cropped and the nose is black, a distinct stop is present, and a slight prognathism is the standard. The topline slopes slightly down towards the back end, they have a deep thorax with a short back and a slight tuck-up is standard. Dewclaws may be removed and tails are generally docked. Feet are compact, with well-knuckled toes.

Recognized Behavior Issues and Traits

Boxer breed characteristics reported include: A dog with high intelligence, independent minded, and possessing excellent strength and stamina. He is a watchdog and a good defender and loves to be around children. This breed is sometimes aloof with strangers, but enjoys close human contact. They are bred for a stable temperament and can be very playful, even boisterous. They are considered high-energy dogs and should be given daily exercise and play sessions to help them keep fit and mentally challenged. Training and socialization should be consistent and start early. These dogs may snore and can drool. They have low grooming needs, and are low shedders. They tolerate temperature extremes poorly. They should not be off-leash because of their well developed chase and fight instincts.

Normal Physiologic Variations

Heart size, based on the vertebral heart scale is normally larger than other breeds.[1]

Boxer dogs may have an increased relative thickness of the LVW and IVS that is independent of aortic size, aortic velocity, or arterial blood pressure, and this morphology should be taken into consideration when screening Boxers by echocardiography.[2]

A natural bob-tail Boxer line has been developed due to the heterozygous dominant expression of the *T* gene. Homozygous dominant individuals are pre-natally lethal.[3]

Drug Sensitivities

Boxers have reportedly had severe reactions to injectable (IV or IM) acepromazine, including profound hypotension, collapse, respiratory arrest, and profound bradycardia.

Inherited Diseases

Boxer Cardiomyopathy (Arrhythmogenic Right Ventricular Cardiomyopathy, ARVC): Autosomal dominant disorder with incomplete penetrance, characterized by sudden death, ventricular premature complexes (VPCs), ventricular tachycardia, syncope, dilated cardiomyopathy, and heart failure. The primary disease process is ventricular arrhythmia, which is reported in over 30% of all Boxers. Diagnose with 24 hour Holter ECG. Greater than 100 VPCs in 24 hours is abnormal for this breed. VPCs are generally positive in Lead II, suggesting a right ventricular origin. Echocardiogram is generally normal until heart failure/cardiomyopathy develops. Treat with anti-arrhythmic drugs. One study showed that fish oils (omega 3 fatty acids) reduced arrhythmias in affected Boxers. A direct genetic test is available showing homozygous affected dogs more severely affected than heterozygotes. Genetic testing shows 41% heterozygotes and 6% homozygous for the gene.[4,5,6,7,8,9]

Hip Dysplasia: Polygenically inherited trait causing degenerative joint disease and hip arthritis. OFA reports 11.1% affected.[10]

Elbow Dysplasia: Polygenically inherited trait causing elbow arthritis. One study found Boxers to be one of the most commonly affected breeds with the fragmented medial coronoid process form of elbow dysplasia. OFA reports 0.7% affected.[10,11,12]

Patella Luxation: Polygenically inherited laxity of patellar ligaments, causing luxation, lameness, and later degenerative joint disease. Treat surgically if causing clinical signs. Too few Boxers have been screened by OFA to determine an accurate frequency.[10]

Progressive Axonopathy (Boxer Axonopathy): Rare, autosomal recessive disorder presenting with a slowly progressive weakness and incoordination of the hind limbs. Age of onset 2-3 months. Progresses to all four limbs, eventually causing severe paresis and ataxia. No genetic test is available.[13]

Disease Predispositions

Dystocia (Difficult Whelpings): Dystocia presents more commonly in Boxers than other breeds. In a Swedish study, 27.7% of whelpings developed dystocia, with the majority requiring caesarian section. The most common reasons for dystocia were **primary uterine inertia** (60%) and **malpresentation of the fetus** (26%).[14]

Hypothyroidism: Inherited autoimmune thyroiditis. 18.0% positive for thyroid auto-antibodies based on testing at Michigan State University. (Ave. for all breeds is 7.5%).[15,16]

Distichiasis: Abnormally placed eyelashes that irritate the cornea and conjunctiva. Can cause secondary corneal ulceration. Identified in 12.90% of Boxers CERF examined by veterinary ophthalmologists between 2000-2005. Because the condition causes significant corneal disease in the Boxer, CERF discourages breeding affected dogs.[17]

Aortic Stenosis (Subaortic Stenosis, SAS): Affected dogs present with a left heart base murmur, and aortic velocities greater than 1.5 m/second on Doppler echocardiography, aortic regurgitation, and mitral regurgitation. Can cause exercise intolerance, syncope, and progress to heart failure. Occurring in 10% of Boxers screened in one study. Identified in 8.50% of screened Boxers in Italy. Reported at a frequency of 8.1% in Switzerland. Odds ratio of 8.6x versus other breeds. Unknown mode of inheritance – considered polygenic.[18,19,20,21,22,23,24]

Cryptorchidism (Retained Testicles): Can be unilateral or bilateral. Boxers have an increased prevalence of the disorder. Found to be moderately (24%) heritable in the breed in a Danish study. Identified in 9.8% of male pups in a Swedish study. Reported at a frequency of 10.7% with a heritability of 0.24 in a Dutch study.[14,25,26,27]

Persistent Corneal Erosion/Corneal Dystrophy (Ulcerative Keratitis, Indolent Ulcer, Boxer Ulcer): Inherited breed prevalence. Treat with topical medications, keratectomy, flap +/- contact lens. Reported in 9.05% of Boxers CERF examined by veterinary ophthalmologists between 2000-2005.[17,28,29]

Cancer/Neoplasia: A Danish study shows a higher standard morbidity rate (SMR) for both malignant and benign cancers in Boxers versus other breeds.[30]

Mast Cell Tumor (MCT): Boxers are a predisposed breed for developing cutaneous mast cell tumors. Mast cell tumors produce histamine, and can cause inflammation and ulceration. These are typically more benign in Boxers, but they are at higher risk to develop additional MCTs at distant sites (outside the surgical margins).[31,32]

Histiocytic Ulcerative Colitis (Boxer Colitis): Inflammatory bowel disease (IBD) that occurs predominantly in Boxers. The lesions are characterized by mucosal ulceration and a mixed inflammatory cell infiltrate. Treatment is with medication and diet. Enrofloxacin therapy against intramucosal E. coli improves clinical signs in some cases, reflecting an infectious role in the pathogenesis. Some severe cases cannot be controlled. Unknown mode of inheritance.[33,34,35,36]

Gingival Hypertrophy: Older Boxers can develop a proliferative gingival hypertrophy affecting all gum surfaces. Treat with gingivectomy.[37]

Atopic Dermatitis/Inhalant Allergies: Presents with pruritis, pyotraumatic dermatitis (hot spots), and often hives. Reported at an increased frequency in the breed versus other breeds. White Boxers have a higher risk.[38]

Cranial Cruciate Ligament Rupture (ACL): Traumatic tearing of the anterior cruciate ligament. The breed is found to have an increased incidence versus other breeds. Treatment is surgery. Found to be moderately (28%) heritable, with a frequency of 5.7% in the breed in a Danish study.[25,27]

Stifle Osteochondritis Dessicans (OCD): Polygenically inherited cartilage defect. Causes stifle joint pain and lameness in young growing dogs. Mild cases can resolve with rest, while more severe cases require surgery. Reported 56.3x odds ratio versus other breeds.[12]

Ectropion: Rolling out of eyelids, often with a medial canthal pocket. Can also cause conjunctivitis. Dorn reports a 7.97X odds ratio in Boxers versus other breeds. Ectropion is reported in 4.52% of Boxers CERF-examined by veterinary ophthalmologists between 2000-2005.[17]

Pulmonic Stenosis (PS): Congenital cardiac disorder of restricted pulmonic outflow. Echocardiogram findings of restriction of right ventricular outflow tract, pulmonic valve and/or main pulmonary artery on transthoracic imaging from the right parasternal and left cranial parasternal short-axis views. Identified in 3.12% of screened Boxers in Italy. Reported at a frequency of 3.3% in Switzerland. Unknown mode of inheritance.[20,21,23,24]

Cataracts: Anterior cortex intermediate and nuclear punctate cataracts predominate in the breed. Identified in 2.71% of Boxers CERF examined by veterinary ophthalmologists between 2000-2005. CERF does not recommend breeding any Boxer with a cataract.[17]

Epilepsy: Inherited seizures. Can be generalized or partial. Treat with anticonvulsants. Dorn reports a 7.17x odds ratio in Boxers versus other breeds. Found to be moderately (36%) heritable in a Danish study, with a frequency of 2.4%.[25,27,39]

Chronic Pancreatitis: Often subclinical inflammation of the pancreas that can cause intermittent discomfort and gastrointestinal upsets. Can possibly lead to pancreatic insufficiency or diabetes mellitus. Boxers have a 3.0x relative risk versus other breeds.[40]

Demodicosis: Dorn reports a 2.66x odds ratio of developing demodectic mange versus other breeds. This disorder has an underlying immunodeficiency in its pathogenesis. One study shows that a DLA haplotype imparts a 5x odds ratio for the disorder.[39,41]

Follicular Dysplasia: Alopecia primarily to the flank region, beginning at 2-4 years of age. Melatonin may help alleviate clinical signs. Unknown mode of inheritance.[42]

Osteosarcoma (Bone Cancer): Boxers have an increased incidence of developing malignant osteosarcoma versus other breeds. Occurs primarily in the extremities.[43]

Inflammatory Myopathies: Boxers are a breed at increased risk of developing inflammatory myopathies, including polymyositis, masticatory muscle myositis, dermatomyositis-like myopathy, and extraocular myositis. A high proportion of affected Boxers have muscle-specific circulating autoantibodies against sarcolemma antigens. A serum antigen assay can be used as a diagnostic test.[44,45]

Seasonal Flank Alopecia: Bilateral, symmetrical alopecia affecting the flank, dorsum and tail. Affects primarily spayed females in the Spring or Autumn. Mean age of onset is 3.6 years.[46]

Spondylosis Deformans: A study of spondylosis deformans and osteophyte development in Boxers showed that it is a heritable condition, especially at specific vertebral sites. Spondylosis deformans does not usually cause spinal problems for the dog.[47]

Atrial Septal Defect (ASD): Congenital cardiac disorder of the wall between the left and right atria. Causes a left heart base systolic murmur that must be differentiated from subaortic stenosis by echocardiography. Affected dogs show exercise intolerance, syncope, dyspnea, and/or a cough. Reported at a frequency of 0.16% in a Swedish study, but identified at a much higher frequency in a French study.[2,48]

Degenerative Myelopathy: Degenerative condition of the spinal cord in older Boxers presenting with progressive weakness and incoordination of the hind limbs. No treatments have been found to be effective. Unknown mode of inheritance. A direct genetic test for an autosomal recessive DM susceptibility gene is available. All affected dogs are homozygous for the gene, however, only a small percentage of homozygous dogs develop DM. OFA reports DM susceptibility gene frequencies of 38% carrier and 45% homozygous "at risk".[10,49,50,51]

Cleft Lip/Palate: Congenital disorder of facial formation. Found to be moderately (27%) heritable, with a frequency of 2.3% in the breed in a Danish study.[25,27]

Juvenile Nephropathy: Rare disorder in young Boxers presenting with severe polyuria and polydipsia, and progressing to chronic renal failure. Histopathology includes immature glomeruli and/or tubules, and persistent mesenchyme. A reflux nephropathy may be involved in the disease process.[52,53,54,55]

T-Cell Lymphoma (Mycosis Fungoides): Boxers have an increased incidence of developing this more malignant form of cutaneous lymphoma versus other breeds.[56,57]

Oral Cancer: One study found that Boxers were a breed with a significantly higher risk of developing oral and pharyngeal tumors, as compared with all breeds combined.[58]

Intracranial Meningioma: One study found that Boxers are overrepresented compared to other breeds for intracranial meningiomas. These are the most common brain tumor in dogs, and can be benign, or malignant.[59]

Juvenile Necrotizing Vasculitis/Sterile Meningitis: Affected Boxers are all under 2 years of age, presenting with apathy, fever, delayed proprioception, ataxia, and increased head and cervical pain. Histopathology shows necrotizing vasculitis in the CNS, with perivascular granulomatous inflammation. 40% of all dogs with this diagnosis are Boxers. Treat with steroids. Unknown mode of inheritance.[60]

Calcinosis Circumspecta, Central PRA, Cervical Vertebral Instability, Cutaneous Asthenia, Cystinuria, Deafness, Dermoid Sinus, Elongated Soft Palate, Factor II Deficiency, Factor VII Deficiency, Gastric Dilatation-Volvulus, Hyperadrenocorticism, Hypoplastic Trachea, Lupoid Onychopathy, Nodular Dermatofibrosis, Polydontia, Progressive Retinal Atrophy, Prolapsed Gland of Nictitans, Pyloric Stenosis, Sphingomyelinosis, Spina Bifida, Supernumerary Teeth, Tricuspid Valve Dysplasia, and **von Willebrand's Disease** are reported.[61]

Isolated Case Studies

Neuroblastoma: A 2 year old Boxer presenting renal disease and a palpable abdominal mass was diagnosed with a peripheral neuroblastoma.[62]

Polyglandular Syndrome: An 8-year-old spayed female boxer dog, presented because of progressive symmetrical truncal alopecia, lethargy, and intolerance to cold. Pathological findings were immune thyroiditis and lymphocytic adrenalitis.[63]

Type C Niemann-Pick Disease (Lipid Storage Disease): A 9-month-old boxer dog was presented with progressive neurological deterioration. The brain showed increased levels of lactosylceramide and two gangliosides, GM3 and GM2.[64]

Neuronal Vacuolation: Two 6-month-old Boxer littermates presented with progressive pelvic limb paresis and ataxia, upper airway stridor, and visual deficits. Pathology revealed neuronal vacuolation and spinocerebellar degeneration, analogous to the syndrome reported in Rottweilers.[65]

Genetic Tests

Tests of Genotype: Direct test for ARVC is available from North Carolina State University - Meurs Lab.

A direct genetic test for an autosomal recessive DM susceptibility gene is available from the OFA.

Direct test for coat color alleles is available from VetGen.

Tests of Phenotype: Recommend hip and elbow radiographs, CERF eye examination, cardiac evaluation (echocardiogram +/- 24 hour Holter ECG), patella evaluation, and thyroid profile including autoantibodies.

Miscellaneous

- **Breed name synonyms:** Bullenbeisser (historical)
- **Registries:** CKC, AKC, UKC, KCGB (Kennel Club of Great Britain), ANKC(Australian National Kennel Club), NKC (National Kennel Club.
- **AKC rank (year 2008):** 6 (29,705 dogs registered)
- **Internet resources: The American Boxer Club:**
  http://americanboxerclub.org
  Boxer Club of Canada: http://boxerclubofcanada.com
  The British Boxer Club: www.thebritishboxerclub.co.uk

References

1. Lamb CR, Wikeley H, Boswood A, et. al.: Use of breed-specific ranges for the vertebral heart scale as an aid to the radiographic diagnosis of cardiac disease in dogs. *Vet Rec.* 2001 Jun 9;148(23):707-11.

2. Cunningham SM, Rush JE, Freeman LM, et. al.: Echocardiographic ratio indices in overtly healthy Boxer dogs screened for heart disease. J Vet Intern Med. 2008 Jul-Aug;22(4):924-30.

3. Haworth K, Putt W, Cattanach B, et. al.: Canine homolog of the T-box transcription factor T; failure of the protein to bind to its DNA target leads to a short-tail phenotype. Mamm Genome. 2001 Mar;12(3):212-8.

4. Meurs KM: Boxer dog cardiomyopathy: an update. *Vet Clin North Am Small Anim Pract.* 2004 Sep;34(5):1235-44, viii.

5. Spier AW, Meurs KM: Assessment of heart rate variability in Boxers with arrhythmogenic right ventricular cardiomyopathy. *J Am Vet Med Assoc.* 2004 Feb 15;224(4):534-7.

6. Smith CE, Freeman LM, Rush JE, et. al.: Omega-3 fatty acids in Boxer dogs with arrhythmogenic right ventricular cardiomyopathy. J Vet Intern Med. 2007 Mar-Apr;21(2):265-73.

7. Meurs KM, Spier AW, Miller MW, et. al.: Familial ventricular arrhythmias in boxers. J Vet Intern Med. 1999 Sep-Oct;13(5):437-9.

8. Meurs KM, Spier AW, Wright NA, et. al.: Comparison of in-hospital versus 24-hour ambulatory electrocardiography for detection of ventricular premature complexes in mature Boxers. J Am Vet Med Assoc. 2001 Jan 15;218(2):222-4.

9. Meurs KM, Mauceli E, Acland G, et. al.: Genome-Wide Association Identifies a Mutation for Arrhythmogenic Right Ventricular Cardiomyopathy in the Boxer Dog. Proceedings, 2009 ACVIM Conference. 2009.

10. OFA Website breed statistics: www.offa.org Last accessed July 1, 2010.

11. Meyer-Lindenberg A, Langhann A, Fehr M, et. al.: Prevalence of fragmented medial coronoid process of the ulna in lame adult dogs. *Vet Rec.* 2002 Aug 24;151(8):230-4.

12. LaFond E, Breur GJ & Austin CC: Breed susceptibility for developmental orthopedic diseases in dogs. J Am Anim Hosp Assoc. 2002 Sep-Oct;38(5):467-77.

13. Griffiths IR, Duncan ID, Barker J: A progressive axonopathy of Boxer dogs affecting the central and peripheral nervous systems. *J Small Anim Pract.* 1980 Jan;21(1):29-43.

14. Linde Forsberg C and Persson G: A survey of dystocia in the Boxer breed. Acta Vet Scand. 2007 Mar 21;49:8.

15. Nachreiner RF, Refsal KR, Graham PA, et. al.: Prevalence of serum thyroid hormone autoantibodies in dogs with clinical signs of hypothyroidism. J Am Vet Med Assoc 2002 Feb 15;220(4):466-71.

16. Nachreiner R & Refsal K: Personal communication, Diagnostic Center for Population and Animal Health, Michigan State University. April, 2007.

17. *Ocular Disorders Presumed to be Inherited in Purebred Dogs.* American College of Veterinary Ophthalmologists. ACVO, 2007.

18. French A, Luis Fuentes V, Dukes-McEwan J, et. al.: Progression of aortic stenosis in the boxer. *J Small Anim Pract.* 2000 Oct;41(10):451-6.

19. Heiene R, Indrebo A, Kvart C, et. al.: Prevalence of murmurs consistent with aortic stenosis among boxer dogs in Norway and Sweden. *Vet Rec.* 2000 Aug 5;147(6):152-6.

20. Vollmar AC, Fox PR: Assessment of Cardiovascular Disease in 527 Boxers. Proceedings, 2005 ACVIM Forum. 2005.

21. Bussadori C, Pradelli D, Borgarelli M, et. al.: Congenital heart disease in boxer dogs: Results of 6years of breed screening Vet J. 2009 Aug;181(2):187-92.

22. Kienle RD, Thomas WP & Pion PD: The natural clinical history of canine congenital subaortic stenosis. J Vet Intern Med. 1994 Nov-Dec;8(6):423-31.

23. Jenni S, Gardelle O, Zini E, et. al.: Use of auscultation and Doppler echocardiography in Boxer puppies to predict development of subaortic or pulmonary stenosis. J Vet Intern Med. 2009 Jan-Feb;23(1):81-6.

24. Höpfner R, Glaus T, Gardelle O, et. al.: Prevalence of heart murmurs, aortic and pulmonic stenosis in boxers presented for pre-breeding exams in Switzerland. Schweiz Arch Tierheilkd. 2010 Jul;152(7):319-24.

25. Nielen AL, Knol BW, van Hagen MA, et. al.: Genetic and epidemiological investigation of a birth cohort of boxers. *Tijdschr Diergeneeskd.* 2003 Oct 1;128(19):586-90.

26. Yates D, Hayes G, Heffernan M, et. al: Incidence of cryptorchidism in dogs and cats. *Vet Rec.* 2003 Apr 19;152(16):502-4.

27. van Hagen MA, Janss LL, van den Broek J, et. al.: The use of a genetic-counselling program by Dutch breeders for four hereditary health problems in boxer dogs. Prev Vet Med. 2004 Apr 30;63(1-2):39-50.

28. Chavkin MJ, Riis RC, Scherlie PH: Management of a persistent corneal erosion in a boxer dog. *Cornell Vet.* 1990 Oct;80(4):347-56.

29. Cooley PL, Dice PF 2nd: Corneal dystrophy in the dog and cat. *Vet Clin North Am Small Anim Pract.* 1990 May;20(3):681-92.

30. Brønden LB, Nielsen SS, Toft N, et. al.: Data from the Danish veterinary cancer registry on the occurrence and distribution of neoplasms in dogs in Denmark. Vet Rec. 2010 May 8;166(19):586-90.

31. Kiupel M, Webster JD, Miller RA, et. al.: Impact of tumour depth, tumour location and multiple synchronous masses on the prognosis of canine cutaneous mast cell tumours. *J Vet Med A Physiol Pathol Clin Med.* 2005 Aug;52(6):280-6.

32. Misdorp W: Mast cells and canine mast cell tumours. A review. Vet Q. 2004 Dec;26(4):156-69.

33. German AJ, Hall EJ, Kelly DF, et. al.: An immunohistochemical study of histiocytic ulcerative colitis in boxer dogs. J Comp Pathol. 2000 Feb-Apr;122(2-3):163-75.

34. Churcher RK, Watson AD: Canine histiocytic ulcerative colitis. *Aust Vet J.* 1997 Oct;75(10):710-3.

35. Hostutler RA, Luria BJ, Johnson SE, et. al.: Antibiotic-responsive histiocytic ulcerative colitis in 9 dogs. J Vet Intern Med. 2004 Jul-Aug;18(4):499-504.

36. Mansfield CS, James FE, Craven M, et. al.: Remission of histiocytic ulcerative colitis in Boxer dogs correlates with eradication of invasive intramucosal Escherichia coli. J Vet Intern Med. 2009 Sep-Oct;23(5):964-9.

37. Burstone MS, Bond E, Litt R: Familial gingival hypertrophy in the dog (boxer breed). AMA Arch Pathol. 1952 Aug;54(2):208-12.

38. Nødtvedt A, Egenvall A, Bergvall K, et. al.: Incidence of and risk factors for atopic dermatitis in a Swedish population of insured dogs. Vet Rec. 2006 Aug 19;159(8):241-6.

39. Dorn CR: Canine breed-specific risks of frequently diagnosed diseases at veterinary teaching hospitals. Monograph. AKC Canine Health Foundation. 2000.

40. Watson PJ, Roulois AJ, Scase T, et. al.: Prevalence and breed distribution of chronic pancreatitis at post-mortem examination in first-opinion dogs. J Small Anim Pract. 2007 Nov;48(11):609-18.

41. It V, Barrientos L, López Gappa J, et. al.: Association of canine juvenile generalized demodicosis with the dog leukocyte antigen system. Tissue Antigens. 2010 Jul;76(1):67-70.

42. Rachid MA, Demaula CD, Scott DW, et. al.: Concurrent follicular dysplasia and interface dermatitis in Boxer dogs. *Vet Dermatol.* 2003 Jun;14(3):159-66.

43. Misdorp W, Hart AA: Some prognostic and epidemiologic factors in canine osteosarcoma. *J Natl Cancer Inst.* 1979 Mar;62(3):537-45.

44. Evans J, Levesque D, Shelton GD: Canine Inflammatory Myopathies: A Review of 200 Cases. Proceedings, 2003 ACVIM Forum. 2003.

45. Hankel S, Shelton GD, Engvall E, et. al.: Sarcolemma-specific autoantibodies in canine inflammatory myopathy. Vet Immunol Immunopathol. 2006 Sep 15;113(1-2):1-10.

46. Miller MA, Dunstan RW: Seasonal flank alopecia in boxers and Airedale terriers: 24 cases (1985-1992). *J Am Vet Med Assoc.* 1993 Dec 1;203(11):1567-72.

47. Carnier P, Gallo L, Sturaro E, et. al: Prevalence of spondylosis deformans and estimates of genetic parameters for the degree of osteophytes development in Italian Boxer dogs. *J Anim Sci.* 2004 Jan;82(1):85-92.

48. Chetbuul V, Trolle JM, Nicolle A, et. al,:Congenital heart diseases in the boxer dog: A retrospective study of 105 cases (1998-2005). J Vet Med A Physiol Pathol Clin Med. 2006 Sept; 53(7): 346-51.

49. Olby NJ: Decreased Mobility in Old Dogs: Causes and Treatment. Proceedings, 2004 ACVIM Forum. 2004.

50. Miller AD, Barber R, Porter BF, et. al.: Degenerative myelopathy in two Boxer dogs. Vet Pathol. 2009 Jul;46(4):684-7.

51. Awano T, Johnson GS, Wade CM, et. al.: Genome-wide association analysis reveals a SOD1 mutation in canine degenerative myelopathy that resembles amyotrophic lateral sclerosis. Proc Natl Acad Sci U S A. 2009 Feb 24;106(8):2794-9.

52. Peeters D, Clercx C, Michiels L, et. al.: Juvenile nephropathy in a boxer, a rottweiler, a collie and an Irish wolfhound. *Aust Vet J.* 2000 Mar;78(3):162-5.

53. Hoppe A, Karlstam E: Renal dysplasia in boxers and Finnish harriers. J Small Anim Pract. 2000 Sep;41(9):422-6.

54. Kolbjornsen O, Heggelund M, Jansen JH, et. al,: End-stage kidney disease probably due to reflux nephropathy with segmental hypoplasia (Ask-Upmark kidney) in young boxer dogs in Norway.A retrospective study. Vet Pathol. 2008 Jul;45(4)::467-74.

55. Chandler ML, Elwood C, Murphy KF, et. al.: Juvenile nephropathy in 37 boxer dogs. J Small Anim Pract. 2007 Dec;48(12):690-4.

56. Lurie DM, Lucroy MD, Griffey SM: T-Cell-Derived Malignant Lymphoma in the Boxer Breed. *Vet Comp Oncol* 2004: 2[3]:171-175.

57. Pastor M, Chalvet-Monfray K, Marchal T, et. al.: Genetic and environmental risk indicators in canine non-Hodgkin's lymphomas: breed associations and geographic distribution of 608 cases diagnosed throughout France over 1 year. J Vet Intern Med. 2009 Mar-Apr;23(2):301-10.

58. Dorn CR, Priester WA: Epidemiologic analysis of oral and pharyngeal cancer in dogs, cats, horses, and cattle. *J Am Vet Med Assoc.* 1976 Dec 1;169(11):1202-6.

59. Sturges BK, Dickinson PJ, Bollen AW, et. al.: Magnetic resonance imaging and histological classification of intracranial meningiomas in 112 dogs. J Vet Intern Med. 2008 May-Jun;22(3):586-95

60. Behr S & Cauzinille L: Aseptic suppurative meningitis in juvenile boxer dogs: retrospective study of 12 cases. J Am Anim Hosp Assoc. 2006 Jul-Aug;42(4):277-82.

61. *The Genetic Connection: A Guide to Health Problems in Purebred Dogs.* L Ackerman. p 205, AAHA Press, 1999.

62. Forrest LJ,, Galbreath EJ, Dubielzig RR,et. Al,:Peripheral neuroblastoma in a dog. *Vet Radiol Ultrasound.* 1997 Nov-Dec;38(6):457-60.

63. Kooistra HS, Rijnberk A, van den Ingh TS, et. al.: Polyglandular deficiency syndrome in a boxer dog: thyroid hormone and glucocorticoid deficiency. Vet Q. 1995 Jun;17(2):59-63.

64. Kuwamura M, Awakura T, Shimada A, et. al.: Type C Niemann-Pick disease in a boxer dog. *Acta Neuropathol (Berl).* 1993;85(3):345-8.

65. Geiger DA, Miller AD, Cutter-Schatzberg K, et. al.: Encephalomyelopathy and polyneuropathy associated with neuronal vacuolation in two Boxer littermates. Vet Pathol. 2009 Nov;46(6):1160-5.

66. *The Complete Dog Book, 20th Ed.* The American Kennel Club. Howell Book House, NY 2006. p. 248-253.

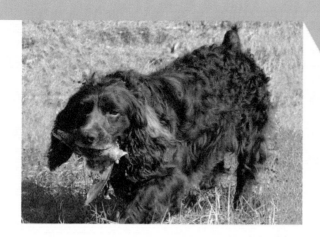

The Breed History

Originally developed from a small stray dog in the early 1900s by Mr. L. Whitaker outside Camden, South Carolina. Initially developed for hunting wild turkeys in the Wateree River and now the dove fields, the duck marshes and as a companion dog. Early ancestors of the Boykin are reported to be the Chesapeake Bay Retriever, Springer Spaniel, Cocker Spaniel, and the American Water Spaniel. AKC recognition occurred in 2009.

Breeding for Function

The Boykin Spaniel is a medium-sized, flushing and retrieving hunting dog, with moderate speed and agility. A favorite of hunters due to its willingness to work all day, as well as its smaller size, which allows the hunter to lift both dog and duck into the boat at the same time.

Physical Characteristics

Height at withers: Males 15.5-18 inches (39.5-46 cm), Females 14-16.5 inches (35.5-42 cm).

Weight: 25-40 pounds (11-18 kg).

Coat: Both an undercoat and an outer coat are present. The coat can range from flat to slightly wavy, with medium length, on the outer coat. The undercoat is short, and dense. The ears, chest, legs and belly are equipped with light fringe or feathering. The color is solid - rich liver, brown or dark chocolate. A small amount of white on chest or toes is permitted.

Longevity: 14-16 years.

Points of Conformation: The Boykin's Expression is alert, self-confident, attractive and intelligent. Eyes are varying shades of brown, set well apart, medium size and oval shaped. Ears are set slightly above or even with the line of the eye. The Skull is fairly broad and flat on top. The stop is moderate. Nose is dark liver with well opened nostrils. The Lips are close fitting and clean. The Bite should be scissors (preferred) or level. Back is straight, strong and essentially level. Loins are short, strong with a slight tuck up. The shoulders are sloping. The croup slopes gently to the tail-set in a natural line. Tail is docked to 3-5 inches. Legs are medium in length, strong, straight and well boned. The gait is effortless with good reach and a long stride that is in balance with the rear quarters for strong driving power. As speed increases it is natural for the legs to fall to a center line of travel.

Recognized Behavior Issues and Traits

The typical Boykin is friendly, a willing worker, intelligent and easy to train. The Boykin Spaniel thrives on human companionship and gets along well with other dogs and children. He shows great eagerness and energy for the hunt yet controllable in the field. He has an active nose, which may lead to a tendency to wander.

Normal Physiologic Variations

None reported

Drug Sensitivities

None reported

Inherited Diseases

Hip Dysplasia: Polygenically inherited trait causing degenerative joint disease and hip arthritis. OFA reports 34.3% affected. Correlated to hip joint laxity in a study in the breed.[1,2]

Patella Luxation: Polygenically inherited laxity of patellar ligaments, causing luxation, lameness, and later degenerative joint disease. Treat surgically if causing clinical signs. OFA reports 21.3% affected.[1]

Elbow Dysplasia: Polygenically inherited trait causing elbow arthritis. OFA reports 4.1% affected.[1]

Exercise Induced Collapse (EIC, Dynamin 1 Mutation): An autosomal recessive disorder of muscle weakness, incoordination and life threatening collapse accompanied by hyperthermia after just five to fifteen minutes of intense exercise or excitement. After 10 to 30 minutes of rest, most dogs return to normal. Undetermined frequency in the breed. A genetic test is available.[3,4]

Disease Predispositions

Distichiasis: Abnormally placed eyelashes that irritate the cornea and conjunctiva. Can cause secondary corneal ulceration. Identified in 10.43% of Boykin Spaniels CERF examined by veterinary ophthalmologists between 2000-2005.[5]

Otitis Externa: Boykin Spaniels are prone to chronic ear infections.[6]

Cataracts: Capsular and anterior and posterior cortex cataracts predominate in the breed. Identified in 4.29% of Boykin Spaniels CERF examined by veterinary ophthalmologists between 2000-2005. CERF does not recommend breeding any Boykin Spaniel with a cataract.[5]

Hypothyroidism: Inherited autoimmune thyroiditis. 3.9% positive for thyroid auto-antibodies based on testing at Michigan State University. (Ave. for all breeds is 7.5%).[7,8]

Retinal Dysplasia: Focal retinal dysplasia and retinal folds are recognized in the breed. Severe cases can progress to retinal detachment. Reported in 2.57% of Boykin Spaniels CERF examined by veterinary ophthalmologists between 2000-2005.[5]

Corneal Dystrophy: The breed can develop an epithelial or stromal non-inflammatory, white to grey corneal opacity. Identified in 2.57% of Boykin Spaniels CERF examined by veterinary ophthalmologists between 2000-2005.[5]

Persistent Pupillary Membranes: Strands of fetal remnant connecting; iris to iris, cornea, lens, or involving sheets of tissue. The later three forms can impair vision, and dogs affected with these forms should not be bred. Identified in 1.57% of Boykin Spaniels CERF examined by veterinary ophthalmologists between 2000-2005.[5]

Persistent Hyaloid Artery (PHA): Congenital defect resulting from abnormalities in the development and regression of the hyaloid artery. Identified in 1.14% Boykin Spaniels CERF-examined by veterinary ophthalmologists between 2000-2005.[5]

Progressive Retinal Atrophy (PRA): Inherited degeneration of the retina. Presumed autosomal recessive inheritance. 0.9% of Boykin Spaniels CERF examined by veterinary ophthalmologists between 2000-2005 are identified as affected or suspicious for PRA. CERF does not recommend breeding any Boykin Spaniel with PRA.[5]

Pulmonic Stenosis is reported.[9]

Isolated Case Studies
None Reported

Genetic Tests
Tests of Genotype: Direct test for exercise induced collapse (EIC) is available from the University of Minnesota Veterinary Diagnostic Lab.

Tests of Phenotype: CHIC Certification: Required testing includes CERF eye examination, patella evaluation, and hip radiographs. Optional testing includes elbow radiographs and a cardiac evaluation for congenital disease. (See CHIC website; www.caninehealthinfo.org).

Recommended testing: Thyroid profile including autoantibodies.

Miscellaneous
- **Breed name synonyms:** Boykin
- **Registries:** AKC, UKC, CKC, FCI, NKC (National Kennel Club)
- **AKC rank (none):** AKC Recognized in December, 2009. Entire stud book entered.
- **Internet resources: Boykin Spaniel Club and Breeders Association of America:** www.boykinspanielclub.org
  Boykin Spaniel Society: www.boykinspaniel.org

References
1. OFA Website breed statistics: www.offa.org Last accessed July 1, 2010.
2. Tsai KL & Murphy KE: Clinical and genetic assessments of hip joint laxity in the Boykin spaniel. Can J Vet Res. 2006 Apr;70(2):148-50.
3. Minor KM, Patterson EE, Gross SD, et. al.: Frequency of the Canine Exercise Induced Collapse Gene in Diverse Breeds. Proceedings, 2009 ACVIM Forum. 2009.
4. Patterson EE, Minor KM, Tchernatynskaia AV, et. al.: A canine DNM1 mutation is highly associated with the syndrome of exercise-induced collapse. Nat Genet. 2008 Oct;40(10):1235-9.
5. Ocular Disorders Presumed to be Inherited in Purebred Dogs. American College of Veterinary Ophthalmologists. ACVO, 2007.
6. Saridomichelakis MN, Farmaki R, Leontides LS, et. al.: Aetiology of canine otitis externa: a retrospective study of 100 cases. Vet Dermatol. 2007 Oct;18(5):341-7.
7. Nachreiner R & Refsal K: Personal communication, Diagnostic Center for Population and Animal Health, Michigan State University. April, 2007.
8. Nachreiner RF, Refsal KR, Graham PA, et. al.: Prevalence of serum thyroid hormone autoantibodies in dogs with clinical signs of hypothyroidism. J Am Vet Med Assoc 2002 Feb 15;220(4):466-71.
9. The Genetic Connection: A Guide to Health Problems in Purebred Dogs. L Ackerman. p. 206, AAHA Press, 1999.
10. AKC Breed Website: www.akc.org/breeds/boykin_spaniel Last accessed July 1, 2010.

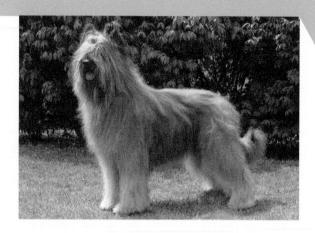

The Breed History

The first written records of this breed originated in the 12th century in France. Napoleon and Charlemagne are reported to have kept Briards. The first breed standard was laid out in 1897. Often referred to as a "heart wrapped in fur", both the Marquis de Lafayette and Thomas Jefferson are credited with bringing the breed to America, and first AKC registrations occurred in 1922. UKC registration occurred in 1948.

Breeding for Function

They were originally used to defend home and farm, but later they became widely used as sheep herding dogs. They have also been used for tracking and hunting, and have served in times of war.

Physical Characteristics

Height at Withers: female 22-25.5" (56-65 cm), male 23 to 27" (58.5-68.5 cm).

Weight: females 50-80 lb. (22.5-36.5 kg), males 60-100 lb. (27.5-45.5 kg).

Coat: The long (6") wavy double coat is solid colored. All colors are accepted except white. Black, gray and shades of tawny are common. The coat requires frequent grooming; they are moderate shedders.

Longevity: 10-12 years.

Points of Conformation: The Briard is a large solidly built powerful dog, with distinctive eyebrows and beard. Their ears are high set and pendulous. Each rear limb carries double dewclaws. The tail has a distinctive tip called a crochet, which is a small hook. The tail is carried low and reaches to the tarsus. Eyes are black or brown with dark palpebral margins; lips and nose are pigmented black. Topline is slightly inclined down towards the croup. They have a deep thorax.

Recognized Behavior Issues and Traits

This dog is reported to be characterized by: High intelligence, bravery, excellent herding instinct, independence, enthusiasm to learn, loyalty, and is reserved with strangers. Training should begin when they are very young to encourage good socialization. Obedience training is encouraged. They need a knowledgeable owner that can invest time to keep the dog challenged. Despite their guarding and watchdog talents, they are considered a gentle dog. They require lots of exercise.

Normal Physiologic Variations

Hypercholesterolemia: Identified in clinically healthy Briards. Affected dogs have normal triglyceride concentrations and no other major abnormalities. Possibly caused by a primary abnormality in cholesterol metabolism. Unknown mode of inheritance.[1,2]

Drug Sensitivities

None reported

Inherited Diseases

Hip Dysplasia: Polygenically inherited trait causing degenerative joint disease and hip arthritis. OFA reports 14.5% affected. Reported at a frequency of 19.4% in France. Reported at a frequency of 14.14% in the BCA Health Survey.[3,4,5]

Congenital Stationary Night Blindness/Retinal dysplasia (CSNB, RPE65 Mutation): Autosomal recessive disorder causing night blindness and varying degrees of day blindness from birth. A mutation test is available from Optigen, that reports 1% affected, and 10% carrier in the breed. CERF does not recommend breeding any Briard affected with CSNB.[6,7,8,9]

Central Progressive Retinal Atrophy (CPRA): Autosomal recessive disease of slowly progressive retinal degeneration, caused by a defect in Vitamin E metabolism. Used to be seen in high numbers of Briards, especially in Europe when on Vitamin E poor diets. Now seen infrequently as diets have improved. CERF does not recommend breeding any Briard with RPED/CPRA.[9,10]

Elbow Dysplasia: Polygenically inherited trait causing elbow arthritis. OFA reports 0.2% affected.[3]

Patella Luxation: Polygenically inherited laxity of patellar ligaments, causing luxation, lameness, and later degenerative joint disease. Treat surgically if causing clinical signs. Too few Briards have been screened by OFA to determine an accurate frequency.[3]

Disease Predispositions

Gastric Dilation/Volvulus (GDV, Bloat): Life-threatening twisting of the stomach within the abdomen. Requires immediate veterinary attention. Reported at a frequency of 11.69% in the BCA Health Survey.[4]

Allergic Dermatitis: Inhalant or food allergy. Presents with pruritis and pyotraumatic dermatitis (hot spots). Reported at a frequency of 6.81% in the BCA Health Survey.[4]

Lymphoma/Lymphosarcoma: Malignant cancer of lymphoid tissue. Reported at a frequency of 6.81% in the BCA Health Survey. There is ongoing research in many breeds into the genetic factors involved in the development of lymphoma.[4]

Hypothyroidism: Inherited autoimmune thyroiditis. 2.8% positive for thyroid auto-antibodies based on testing at Michigan State University. (Ave. for all breeds is 7.5%). Reported at a frequency of 4.89% in the BCA Health Survey.[4,11,12]

Persistent Pupillary Membranes: Strands of fetal remnant connecting; iris to iris, cornea, lens, or involving sheets of tissue. The later three forms can impair vision, and dogs affected with these forms should not be bred. Identified in 2.58% of Briards CERF examined by veterinary ophthalmologists between 2000-2005.[9]

Cataracts: Posterior cortex intermediate and capsular cataracts predominate, though anterior and nuclear cataracts also occur in the breed. Identified in 2.35% of Briards CERF examined by veterinary ophthalmologists between 2000-2005. CERF does not recommend breeding any Briard with a cataract.[9]

Corneal Dystrophy: Briards can have an epithelial/stromal form of corneal dystrophy. Identified in 1.41% of Briards CERF examined by veterinary ophthalmologists between 2000-2005.[9]

Progressive Retinal Atrophy (PRA): Inherited degeneration of the retina progressing to blindness. A late onset PRA is identified in the breed. Early fundus abnormalities usually appear after 4 years of age. Mode of inheritance has not been determined.[9]

Digital Squamous Cell Carcinoma: Toe cancer seen at an increased frequency in black Briards. Treatment is digital amputation.[13]

Open Bite, and Seasonal Flank Alopecia are reported.[14]

Isolated Case Studies

Dandy-Walker-Like syndrome: Congenital disorder causing cerebellar ataxia and other CNS signs due to cysts arising from the 4th ventricle, dysgenesis of the cerebellar vermis, and hydrocephalus of the 3rd and lateral ventricles. Reported in one Briard.[15]

Genetic Tests

Tests of Genotype: Direct test for CSNB is available from Optigen and the Animal Health Trust.

Direct test for black and tawny is available from Health Gene and VetGen.

Tests of Phenotype: CHIC Certification: Required testing includes hip radiographs (at a minimum of 24 months of age), CERF eye examination (at least once between 6 months and 8 years of age), and CSNB genetic test. Optional recommended tests include thyroid profile including autoantibodies, and elbow radiographs. (See CHIC website; www.caninehealthinfo.org).

Recommend patella evaluation and cardiac evaluation.

Miscellaneous

- **Breed name synonyms:** Chien Berger de Brie, Chien d'Aubry (historical).
- **Registries:** CKC, AKC, UKC, KCGB (Kennel Club of Great Britain), ANKC(Australian National Kennel Club), NKC (National Kennel Club)
- **AKC rank in year 2008:** 123 (237 dogs registered)

- **Internet resources: The Briard Club of America** www.BriardClubOfAmerica.org
  The Briard Club of England: www.briards.co.uk/
  Briard Medical Trust: www.briardmedicaltrust.org

References

1. Watson P, Simpson KW, Bedford PG: Hypercholesterolaemia in briards in the United Kingdom. Res Vet Sci. 1993 Jan;54(1):80-5.
2. Johnson MC: Hyperlipidemia Disorders in Dogs. *Compend Contin Educ Pract Vet* 2005:27[5]:361-370.
3. OFA Website breed statistics: www.offa.org Last accessed July 1, 2010.
4. Briard Club of America: BCA Health Survey. 2003.
5. Genevois JP, Remy D, Viguier E, et. al.: Prevalence of hip dysplasia according to official radiographic screening, among 31 breeds of dogs in France. Vet Comp Orthop Traumatol. 2008;21(1):21-4.
6. Aguirre GD, Baldwin V, Pearce-Kelling S, et. al.: Congenital stationary night blindness in the dog: common mutation in the RPE65 gene indicates founder effect. *Mol Vis.* 1998 Oct 30;4:23.
7. Narfstrom K, Wrigstad A, Nilsson SE: The Briard dog: a new animal model of congenital stationary night blindness. *Br J Ophthalmol.* 1989 Sep;73(9):750-6.
8. Narfstrom K: Retinal dystrophy or "congenital stationary night blindness" in the Briard dog. *Vet Ophthalmol.* 1999;2(1):75-76.
9. *Ocular Disorders Presumed to be Inherited in Purebred Dogs.* American College of Veterinary Ophthalmologists. ACVO, 2007
10. Bedford PG: Retinal pigment epithelial dystrophy in the Briard. Vet Rec. 2009 Mar 21;164(12):377.
11. Nachreiner R and Refsal K: Personal communication, Diagnostic Center for Population and Animal Health, Michigan State University. April, 2007.
12. Nachreiner RF, Refsal KR, Graham PA, et. al.: Prevalence of serum thyroid hormone autoantibodies in dogs with clinical signs of hypothyroidism. J Am Vet Med Assoc 2002 Feb 15;220(4):466-71.
13. Wobeser BK, Kidney BA, Powers BE, et. al.: Diagnoses and clinical outcomes associated with surgically amputated canine digits submitted to multiple veterinary diagnostic laboratories. Vet Pathol. 2007 May;44(3):355-61.
14. *The Genetic Connection: A Guide to Health Problems in Purebred Dogs.* L Ackerman. p. 206, AAHA Press, 1999.
15. Schmid V, Lang J, Wolf M: Dandy-Walker-Like syndrome in four dogs: Cisternography as a diagnostic aid. *J Am Anim Hosp Assoc* 1992;28[4]:355-360.
16. *The Complete Dog Book, 20th Ed.* The American Kennel Club. Howell Book House, NY 2006. p 645-649.

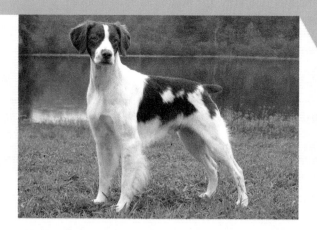

Brittany

The Breed History

In the French province of Brittany, a hunting dog was developed starting in the early 1700s that was intermediate in size between Setters and Spaniels. From these dogs, the Brittany arose. The Brittany may have contributed to the development of the Wachtelhund of Germany. The taillessness and bobtail trait was not introduced to the breed until an outcross in the mid 1800s. They are similar to the Welsh Spaniel in type and may share common ancestors. The first breed standard was developed in the year 1907. First AKC registry was in 1934 and the breed was originally registered as the Brittany Spaniel. The name was shortened to Brittany in 1982.

Breeding for Function

The primary purpose for which this breed was developed was for hunting, as a bird dog. They are known for their exceptional ability to follow scent, and have working habits that are similar to setters. They are versatile, being adept at tracking, setting, flushing or pointing, and retrieving.

Physical Characteristics

Height at Withers: 17.5-20.5" (44.5-52 cm).

Weight: 28-40 lb (13-18 kg).

Coat: The liver and white, and orange and white color patterns are standard. They may be roan also, and some ticking is preferred. Black is not allowed. Bi-color is preferred to tri-color. The coat is flat or wavy, has minimal feathering, and hairs are firm but not silky or wiry.

Longevity: 13-14 years.

Points of Conformation: Brittany Spaniels are compact, square, medium-sized dogs. Some are tailless and if not, sometimes the high set tail is docked to a bobtail of about 4" (10 cm) in length. They possess an alert expression, are medium boned and muscled, eyes are fairly deep set under prominent brows, the eye color varies from dark to amber, short ears are high set, and triangular with slightly rounded tips, and lie flat. Ear leather is fine. The stop is well defined, the muzzle is medium in size and width with a gradual tapering to the nose. The nose may be many shades but not black or two-toned. The lips are dry. Their neck is not throaty, and it is medium in length and muscling. The topline slightly descends over its length towards the rear. They possess a deep thorax with well-sprung ribs, and rib cage stays deep well back. They have a slight abdominal tuck up. Dewclaws may be taken off. Feet are intermediate in size and shape, and limbs are straight. Gait is smooth, low and elastic, with minimal apparent effort.

Recognized Behavior Issues and Traits

Traits ascribed to the breed include: A gay, friendly temperament, alert, lively, loyal, trustworthy, have excellent trainability, are good watchdogs, good in country or city settings, good with children. Early obedience training and socialization are important. They have a high barking tendency, and should only be let out in a fenced enclosure off leash. They also do best with close human contact.

They have significant exercise needs. The Brittany has low grooming needs, and tends to have moderate shedding.

Normal Physiologic Variations

None reported

Drug Sensitivities

None reported

Inherited Diseases

Hip Dysplasia: Polygenically inherited trait causing degenerative joint disease and hip arthritis. OFA reports 14.9% affected.[1]

Patella Luxation: Polygenically inherited laxity of patellar ligaments, causing luxation, lameness, and later degenerative joint disease. Treat surgically if causing clinical signs. OFA reports a high frequency, but too few Brittanys have been screened by OFA to determine an accurate frequency.[1]

Elbow Dysplasia: Polygenically inherited trait causing elbow arthritis. OFA reports 1.9% affected.[1]

Spinal Muscular Atrophy: Autosomal dominant disorder characterized by progressive muscle weakness leading to paralysis. The disease develops in dogs less than 1 year of age and results in paraspinal and proximal pelvic limb muscular atrophy.[2,3]

Cleft Palate: Rare autosomal recessive complete cleft palate identified in a research breeding colony. Affected pups aspirate milk when attempting to nurse.[4]

Compliment Deficiency: Rare autosomal recessive defect clinically characterized by an increased susceptibility to infection and membranoproliferative glomerulonephritis.[5,6]

Disease Predispositions

Hypothyroidism: Inherited autoimmune thyroiditis. 12.0% positive for thyroid autoantibodies based on testing at Michigan State University. (Ave. for all breeds is 7.5%).[7,8]

Mammary Gland Cancer: Dorn reports a 28.43x odds ratio for the disorder versus other breeds. Occurs primarily in unspayed females, especially those who have whelped at least one litter.[9]

Cataracts: Anterior cortex punctate, and posterior cortex intermediate cataracts predominate, though nuclear and capsular cataracts also occur in the breed. Identified in 4.27% of Brittanys CERF examined by veterinary ophthalmologists between 2000-2005. CERF does not recommend breeding any Brittanys with a cataract.[10]

Otitis Externa (Chronic Ear Infection): Brittanys are prone to chronic ear infections according to a Greek study, with a 3.39x odds ratio versus other breeds.[11]

Inherited Epilepsy: Generalized or partial seizures. Control with anticonvulsant medication. Reported as a problem in the breed.[12]

Persistent Pupillary Membranes: Strands of fetal remnant connecting; iris to iris, cornea, lens, or involving sheets of tissue. The later three forms can impair vision, and dogs affected with these forms should not be bred. Identified in 2.04% of Brittanys CERF examined by veterinary ophthalmologists between 2000-2005.[10]

Distichiasis: Abnormally placed eyelashes that irritate the cornea and conjunctiva. Can cause secondary corneal ulceration. Identified in 1.86% of Brittanys CERF examined by veterinary ophthalmologists between 2000-2005.[10]

Primary Lens Luxation: Occurs at an increased frequency in the breed. Often progresses to secondary **glaucoma** and blindness. Reported relative risk of 4.23x versus other breeds. CERF does not recommend breeding any Brittany with lens luxation.[10,13]

Incomplete Ossification of the Humeral Condyle: Brittany spaniels have a high prevalence of humeral condylar fractures due to an inherited incomplete ossification of the humeral condyle. Unknown mode of inheritance.[14]

Cutaneous Lupus Erythematosus (nasal solar dermatitis): Adult onset vesicular form of lupus that causes annular, polycyclic and serpiginous ulcerations distributed over sparsely haired areas of the body. These especially occur during the summer months due to ultraviolet exposure. Treatment is with immunosuppressive drugs and sunscreen.[15]

Spinocerebellar Degeneration: Affected adult Brittany Spaniels present with clinical neurological signs of spinocerebellar disease. Clinically the dogs had a dramatic forward "saluting" movement of the thoracic limbs, hypermetria of the pelvic limbs, cerebellar ataxia and intention tremors. Terminally, dogs crawled in a crouched thoracic posture with neck extension. Lesions were confined to cerebellum, medulla oblongata and spinal cord, consisting of diffuse Purkinje cell loss with massive neurofilament accumulation. The etiology of this syndrome is not determined.[16,17]

Brachygnathism, Cryptorchidism, Factor VIII Deficiency, Hyperlipidemia, Oligodontia, Osteochondritis Dessicans-Shoulder, Prognathism, Progressive Retinal Atrophy, Retinal Dysplasia, Ventricular Septal Defect, and **Wry Mouth** are reported.[18]

Isolated Case Studies

Patent Ductus Arteriosus (PDA): An 11-month-old female Brittany spaniel had a grade IV/IV cardiac murmur, and was diagnosed with a PDA.[19]

Aorticopulmonary Septal Defect: A 2-year-old Brittany Spaniel with pulmonary hypertension, a cardiac murmur and congestive heart failure was diagnosed with aorticopulmonary septal defect. Attempted surgical correction was unsuccessful.[20]

Persistent Left Cranial Vena Cava with Megaesophagus: A 2-month-old Brittany spaniel dog was presented for persistent regurgitation, first observed soon after weaning. Clinical examination and diagnostic imaging showed a vascular ring anomaly due to a persistent left cranial vena cava enclosing the esophagus and trachea, and causing constriction of the esophagus.[21]

Nasal Dermoid Sinus Cyst: A Brittany spaniel had a discharging sinus in the midline of the nose removed surgically. Histopathologic diagnosis was a nasal dermoid sinus cyst.[22]

Linear Papular-pustular Dermatosis: Two separate cases of young Brittany Spaniels developed a unilateral dermatosis extending from the inguinal region to the medial aspect of the metatarsal area. Histology identified an eosinophilic and neutrophilic pustular mural folliculitis with prominent acantholysis of infundibular epithelium. The condition resolved with oral methylprednisolone administration.[23]

Zollinger-Ellison Syndrome and **Myelofibrosis:** Zollinger-Ellison syndrome and myelofibrosis were diagnosed concurrently in a 10-year-old neutered female Brittany Spaniel. She had gastric ulceration, hypergastrinemia, and a gastrin-secreting islet cell tumor with splenic metastases, as well as patchy long-bone medullary sclerosis, nonregenerative anemia and thrombocytopenia. A diagnosis of Zollinger-Ellison syndrome and myelofibrosis was made based on pathology.[24]

Genetic Tests

Tests of Genotype: Direct tests for black, brown (red) and true red coat colors, and black and brown nose are available from HealthGene and VetGen.

Tests of Phenotype: Recommend hip and elbow radiographs, patella examination, CERF eye examination, thyroid profile including autoantibodies and cardiac evaluation.

Miscellaneous

- **Breed name synonyms:** Brittany, Épagneul Breton
- **Registries:** AKC, UKC, CKC, KCGB (Kennel Club of Great Britain), ANKC (Australian National Kennel Club), NKC (National Kennel Club)
- **AKC rank (year 2008):** 30 (6,270 dogs registered)
- **Internet resources: American Brittany Club:** http://clubs.akc.org/brit/
  Brittany Spaniel Club of Great Britain: www.brittanyclub.co.uk
  The Brittany Spaniel Club of Canada: www.members.shaw.ca/brittanyclubofcanada/

References

1. OFA Website breed statistics: www.offa.org Last accessed July 1, 2010.

2. Cork LC, Price DL, Griffin JW, et. al.: Hereditary canine spinal muscular atrophy: canine motor neuron disease. *Can J Vet Res.* 1990 Jan;54(1):77-82.

3. Sack GH Jr, Cork LC, Morris JM, et. al.: Autosomal dominant inheritance of hereditary canine spinal muscular atrophy. *Ann Neurol.* 1984 Apr; 15(4):369-73.

4. Richtsmeier JT, Sack GH Jr, Grausz HM, et. al.: Cleft palate with autosomal recessive transmission in Brittany spaniels. Cleft palate with Craniofacial J. 1994 Sep; 31(5):364-71.

5. Johnson JP, McLean RH, Cork LC, et. al.: Genetic analysis of an inherited deficiency of the third component of complement in Brittany spaniel dogs. *Am J Med Genet.* 1986 Nov;25(3):557-62.

6. Cork LC, Morris JM, Olson JL, et. al.: Membranoproliferative Glomerulone-phritis in Dogs with a Genetically Determined Deficiency of the Third Component of Complement. Clinical Immunology and Immunopathology 1991;60: 455-470.

7. Nachreiner R and Refsal K: Personal communication, Diagnostic Center for Population and Animal Health, Michigan State University. April, 2007.

8. Nachreiner RF, Refsal KR, Graham PA, et. al.: Prevalence of serum thyroid hormone autoantibodies in dogs with clinical signs of hypothyroidism. J Am Vet Med Assoc 2002 Feb 15;220(4):466-71.

9. Dorn CR: Canine breed-specific risks of frequently diagnosed diseases at veterinary teaching hospitals. Monograph. AKC Canine Health Foundation. 2000.

10. *Ocular Disorders Presumed to be Inherited in Purebred Dogs.* American College of Veterinary Ophthalmologists. ACVO, 2007.

11. Saridomichelakis MN, Farmaki R, Leontides LS, et. al.: Aetiology of canine otitis externa: a retrospective study of 100 cases. Vet Dermatol. 2007 Oct;18(5):341-7.

12. Patterson EN: Clinical Characteristics and Inheritance of Idiopathic Epilepsy.Proceedings, Tufts' Canine and Feline Breeding and Genetics Conference. 2007.

13. Sargan DR, Withers D, Pettitt L, et. al.: Mapping the mutation causing lens luxation in several terrier breeds. J Hered. 2007;98(5):534-8.

14. Marcellin-Little DJ, DeYoung DJ, Ferris KK, et. al.: Incomplete ossification of the humeral condyle in spaniels. *Vet Surg.* 1994 Nov-Dec;23(6):475-87.

15. Scott DW: Cutaneous Lupus Erythematosus 2008: Presentation & Management. Proceedings, 2008 ACVIM Forum. 2008.

16. Higgins RJ, LeCouteur RA, Kornegay JN , et. al.: Late-onset progressive spinocerebellar degeneration in Brittany Spaniel dogs. *Acta Neuropathol (Berl).* 1998 Jul;96(1):97-101.

17. Tatalick LM, Marks SL, Baszler TV: Cerebellar abiotrophy characterized by granular cell loss in a Brittany. Veterinary Pathology 1993;30(4):385-8.

18. *The Genetic Connection: A Guide to Health Problems in Purebred Dogs.* L Ackerman. p. 206. AAHA Press, 1999.

19. Olsen D, Harkin KR, Banwell MN, et. al.: Postoperative rupture of an aortic aneurysmal dilation associated with a patent ductus arteriosus in a dog. *Vet Surg.* 2002 May-Jun;31(3):259-65.

20. Eyster GE, Dalley JB, Chaffee A, et. al.: Aorticopulmonary septal defect in a dog. *J Am Vet Med Assoc.* 1975 Dec 15;167(12):1094-6.

21. Larcher T, Abadie J, Roux FA, et. al.: Persistent left cranial vena cava causing oesophageal obstruction and consequent megaoesophagus in a dog. J Comp Pathol. 2006 Aug-Oct;135(2-3):150-2.

22. Anderson DM, White RA: Nasal dermoid sinus cysts in the dog. *Vet Surg.* 2002 Jul-Aug;31(4):303-8.

23. Beningo KE, Scott DW: Idiopathic linear pustular acantholytic dermatosis in a young Brittany Spaniel dog. *Vet Dermatol.* 2001 Aug;12(4):209-13.

24. English RV, Breitschwerdt EB, Grindem CB, et. al.: Zollinger-Ellison syndrome and myelofibrosis in a dog. *J Am Vet Med Assoc.* 1988 May 15;192(10):1430-4.

25. *The Complete Dog Book, 20th Ed.* The American Kennel Club. Howell Book House, NY 2006. p. 15-19.

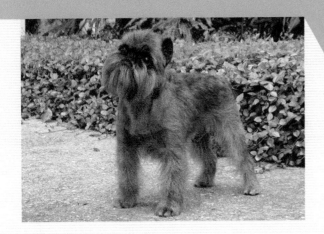

The Breed History

Arising from Afffenpinscher and Belgian street dogs *(chiens barbus)*, the Brussels Griffon is packed with personality plus. Later on in the breed development, first Pug then Ruby Spaniel crosses occurred. It was likely from the Pug crosses that the smooth coated variety arose. Some also place Yorkshire terriers and French Barbet in the breed development tree. Some confusion exists regarding Belgian vs. Brussels Griffons as they are classified differently in Belgium than elsewhere. The AKC first registered the breed in 1910.

Breeding for Function

Bred early on for ratting, the recent focus of breeders was for a companion dog.

Physical Characteristics

Height at Withers: 7-8" (18-20 cm).

Weight: 8-10 lb (3.5-4.5 kg).

Coat: There are two distinct coats—Wirehaired and Smooth-coated *(Brabancon)* types. The rough coat is about 3-4" (7.5-10 cm) in length, dense, with emphasis on maximum wire texture. The Brabancon coat is smooth, short and glossy. Colors include black and tan, black, belge (a mix of black and ruddy brown) with black whiskers and mask, and red.

Longevity: 13-14 years

Points of Conformation: Though toy in size, these dogs are built with a square, sturdy compact conformation and are quick and agile. High head carriage with a very alert expression. Wide set, large, dark, and rimmed with dark palpebral margins and thick lashes, the eyes are quite prominent in the socket. Ears are small, high-set and semi-erect, though if cropped, pricked. They have a pronounced stop, a domed skull and the nose is set back right at the stop, is large and pigmented black. Lip margins are black, and they possess prognathism, and a prominent beard. The neck is medium in length and muscling, with some arching. The short topline is level, thorax is deep, and the ribs well sprung. The high set tail is usually docked to about one-third of the length and usually is held erect. Limbs are straight boned, metacarpals and metatarsals are short and thick, the feet are small and round in shape and the toes are well arched.

Brussels Griffon

Recognized Behavior Issues and Traits

Reported breed characteristics include: Requires early leash and obedience training. The Brussels Griffon has a plucky but sensitive nature and is somewhat shy with strangers. The wire coats need hand stripping but on a maintenance basis, these dogs have average grooming needs. This breed is considered to be a bit slower to housetrain than some other breeds. Intelligent but easily bored, they respond best to positive reinforcement and a patient approach. Good alarm barkers; high barking tendency. Some do not recommend these dogs for those with children under 5 years of age; they can be quite assertive. Brussels Griffon dogs have low to moderate exercise requirements. These little dogs are fearless if threatened. They require close human contact.

Normal Physiologic Variations

Cesarean Section: According to a British study, 39% of Brussels Griffon litters are delivered via **C-section.**[1]

Drug Sensitivities

None reported

Inherited Diseases

Patella Luxation: Polygenically inherited laxity of patellar ligaments, causing luxation, lameness, and later degenerative joint disease. Treat surgically if causing clinical signs. Reported in 7.0% of dogs in the 2004 ABGA Health Survey. Average age of onset 2.3 years. OFA reports a high incidence, but too few Brussels Griffon have been screened to determine an accurate frequency.[2,3]

Hip Dysplasia and Legg-Calve-Perthes Disease: Polygenically inherited traits causing degenerative joint disease and hip arthritis. OFA reports a high incidence, but too few Brussels Griffon have been screened to determine accurate frequencies.[2]

Elbow Dysplasia: Polygenically inherited trait causing elbow arthritis. OFA reports a high incidence, but too few Brussels Griffon have been screened to determine accurate frequency.[2]

Disease Predispositions

Cataracts: Anterior and equatorial cortex intermediate cataracts predominate, though posterior and capsular cataracts also occur in the breed. Reported in 5.41% of Brussels Griffon presented to veterinary teaching hospitals. Reported in 6.7% of dogs in the 2004 ABGA Health Survey (3.5% at less than seven years of age). Identified in 14.84% of Brussels Griffon CERF examined by veterinary ophthalmologists between 2000-2005. CERF does not recommend breeding any Brussels Griffon with a cataract.[3,4,5]

Chiari-like Malformation (Occipital Bone Hypoplasia): This condition is characterized by a shortening of the basicranium and supra-occipital bone with a compensatory lengthening of the cranial vault, especially the parietal bone. CM can be diagnosed with MRI, or with 87% sensitivity from radiographic measurements. In a study skewed toward affected families, CM was observed in 60.7% of Brussels Griffon. CM can predispose, but is not necessary for the brain disease syringomyelia.[6]

Syringomyelia (SM): Syringomyelia is a condition where fluid filled cavities develop within the spinal cord. The majority of affected dogs do not show clinical signs. Clinical signs of SM can present usually between 5 months and 3 years of age, and include persistent scratching at the shoulder region with apparent neck, thoracic limb, or ear pain and thoracic limb lower motor neuron deficits. Diagnosis is by MRI. In a study skewed toward affected families, SM was diagnosed in 37.5% of Brussels Griffon, with 5.8% showing clinical signs. Chiari-like malformation (CM) is a predisposing factor for SM (61.7% with CM had SM, though 22.7% of dogs without CM had SM in this study).[6]

Vitreous Degeneration: Liquefaction of the vitreous gel which may predispose to retinal detachment occurs in the breed. Identified in 14.49% of Brussels Griffon CERF examined by veterinary ophthalmologists between 2000-2005.[4]

Persistent Pupillary Membranes: Strands of fetal remnant connecting; iris to iris, cornea, lens, or involving sheets of tissue. The later three forms can impair vision, and dogs affected with these forms should not be bred. Identified in 5.65% of Brussels Griffon CERF examined by veterinary ophthalmologists between 2000-2005.[4]

Cleft Palate: Congenital disorder of midline closure of palate. Reported in 5% of puppies born in the 2003 ABGA Puppy Mortality Survey.[7]

Allergic Dermatitis: Presents with pruritis and pyotraumatic dermatitis (hot spots). Reported in 3.9% of dogs in the 2004 ABGA Health Survey. Average age of onset 3.6 years.[3]

Epilepsy: Inherited seizures. Can be generalized or partial. Seizures are reported in 2.9% of dogs in the 2004 ABGA Health Survey. The cause of the seizures was not defined.[3]

Cryptorchidism: Unilateral or bilateral undescended testicles. Reported in 2.8% of dogs in the 2004 ABGA Health Survey. This is a sex-limited disorder with an undetermined mode of inheritance.[3]

Persistent Hyaloid Artery (PHA): Congenital defect resulting from abnormalities in the development and regression of the hyaloid artery. Does not cause vision problems by itself, but is often associated with other ocular defects. Identified in 2.47% of Brussels Griffon CERF examined by veterinary ophthalmologists between 2000-2005.[4]

Heart Murmur: Reported in 2.1% of dogs in the 2004 ABGA Health Survey. Average age of onset 5.0 years. The anatomical cause of the heart murmur was not defined, though **mitral valvular disease** is reported in the breed.[3]

Bladder Stones: Reported in 2.1% of dogs in the 2004 ABGA Health Survey. Average age of onset 5.4 years. The mineral content (type) of the bladder stone was not defined.[3]

Distichiasis: Abnormally placed eyelashes that irritate the cornea and conjunctiva. Can cause secondary corneal ulceration. Identified in 1.77% of Brussels Griffon CERF examined by veterinary ophthalmologists between 2000-2005.[4]

Hypothyroidism: Inherited autoimmune thyroiditis. 1.7% positive for thyroid auto-antibodies based on testing at Michigan State University. (Ave. for all breeds is 7.5%).[8,9]

Progressive Retinal Atrophy (PRA): Inherited degeneration of the retina progressing to blindness. Autosomal recessive inheritance in most breeds. Identified in 1.41% of Brussels Griffon CERF examined by veterinary ophthalmologists between 2000-2005. CERF does not recommend breeding any Brussels Griffon with PRA.[4]

Corneal Dystrophy: Brussels Griffon can have an epithelial/stromal form of corneal dystrophy. Identified in 1.41% of Brussels Griffon CERF examined by veterinary ophthalmologists between 2000-2005.[4]

Optic Nerve Coloboma: A congenital cavity in the optic nerve which, if large, may cause blindness or vision impairment. Identified in 0.71% of Brussels Griffon CERF examined by veterinary ophthalmologists between 2000-2005. CERF does not recommend breeding any Brussels Griffon with a coloboma.[4]

Cleft Lip, Retained Primary Teeth, and **Ulcerative Keratitis** are reported.[10]

Isolated Case Studies

Sry-negative XX Sex Reversal (Hermaphrodism): A Brussels Griffon is documented with this autosomal recessive disorder, where outwardly male dogs are chromosomal females (XX), and there is an absence of "male" causing SRY.[11]

Genetic Tests

Tests of Genotype: Direct test for rough or smooth coat is available from VetGen.

Tests of Phenotype: CHIC Certification: Required testing includes CERF eye examination and patella evaluation (after age 2). Optional recommended testing includes hip radiographs, thyroid profile including autoantibodies, electroretinogram for PRA, and MRI for syringomyelia. (See CHIC website; www.caninehealthinfo.org)

American Brussels Griffon Association "Champions For Health" program recommends Patella and Hip radiographs, CERF eye exam and ERG for PRA, thyroid profile including autoantibodies, and MRI for SM.

Recommend elbow radiographs and cardiac evauation.

Miscellaneous
- **Breed name synonyms:** Griffon Bruxellois, Griffon Belge, Belgian Griffon, or Griffons d'Ecurie (historical).
- **Registries:** AKC, UKC, CKC, KCGB (Kennel Club of Great Britain), ANKC (Australian National Kennel Club), NKC (National Kennel Club).
- **AKC rank (year 2008):** 67 (1,320 dogs registered)
- **Internet resources: American Brussels Griffon Association:** www.brussels-griffon.info/

The Griffon Bruxellois Club (UK): www.griffonclub1897.co.uk
National Brussels Griffon Club: www.brussels-griffon.net

References

1. Evans KM & Adams VJ: Proportion of litters of purebred dogs born by caesarean section. J Small Anim Pract. 2010 Feb;51(2):113-8.

2. OFA Website breed statistics: www.offa.org Last accessed July 1, 2010.

3. American Brussels Griffon Association: 2004 ABGA Health Survey. 2004.

4. *Ocular Disorders Presumed to be Inherited in Purebred Dogs.* American College of Veterinary Ophthalmologists. ACVO, 2007.

5. Gelatt KN, Mackay EO: Prevalence of primary breed-related cataracts in the dog in North America. Vet Ophthalmol. 2005 Mar-Apr;8(2):101-11.

6. Rusbridge C, Knowler SP, Pieterse, et. al.: Chiari-like malformation in the Griffon Bruxellois. J Small Anim Pract. 2009 Aug;50(8):386-93.

7. American Brussels Griffon Association: 2003 ABGA Puppy Mortality Survey 2003.

8. Nachreiner R and Refsal K: Personal communication, Diagnostic Center for Population and Animal Health, Michigan State University. April, 2007.

9. Nachreiner RF, Refsal KR, Graham PA, et. al,: Prevalence of serum thyroid hormaone autoantibodies in dogs with clinical signs of hypothyroidism, J Am Vet Med Assoc 2002 Feb 15;220(4): 466-71.

10. *The Genetic Connection: A Guide to Health Problems in Purebred Dogs.* L Ackerman. p. 206 , AAHA Press, 1999.

11. Meyers-Wallen VN: Inherited Disorders of Sexual Development in Dogs and Cats. Proceedings, 2007 Tufts' Canine and Feline Breeding and Genetics Conference. 2007.

12. *The Complete Dog Book, 20th Ed.* The American Kennel Club. Howell Book House, NY 2006. p. 450-453.

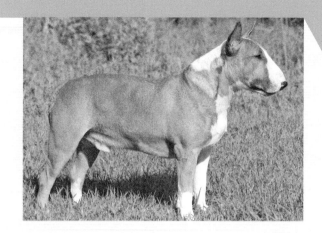

Bull Terrier

The Breed History

First records for the Bull Terrier date back to 1835 in Britain. Crossing a Bulldog with a White English Terrier (now extinct) is thought to have provided the foundation for the breed. Later, a documented outcross to Spanish Pointer was done to increase size. The white variety was first bred around 1860, and the breed was formally split into the white and colored in 1936. The bull terrier in AKC is registered as the standard size breed, (Bull Terrier) and a miniature size, the Miniature Bull Terrier.

Breeding for Function

This breed was valued as a pit fighter. A very strong constitution, agility and tenacity were bred into them. Over the years, the breeders have worked to make the dog more companionable.

Physical Characteristics

Height at Withers: 21-22" (53-56 cm).

Weight: 52-62 lb (24-28 kg).

Coat: The breed is divided into white and colored types. Hairs are short and hard, lie flat, and have good sheen. For white variety: all white or white with limited markings on the head. For colored variety: other base colors than white, may have white markings; brindle is preferred. They are moderate shedders and have low grooming needs.

Longevity: 11-13 years

Points of Conformation: The distinctive head is long, and the face is full and a curve over the top of the skull to the tip of the nose is present. Ears are close set and small, the leather is thin, and they prick erect when dog is alert. Small dark eyes are deep-set, close-set, and piercing in expression. Oblique in shape, blue eyes disqualify. The nose is black, and the neck is very muscular, long, and not throaty. The thorax is round and deep with very well sprung ribs. The back is short and only slightly arched at the loins. Limbs are straight boned, and moderately long. The feet are compact and well-knuckled. The tapering tail is low set, short, and carried parallel to the topline. The gait is smooth and ground covering.

Recognized Behavior Issues and Traits

Reported breed attributes include: Playful, friendly, active. If they bite, they are reluctant to let go and so must never be teased. Dominant personalities are common. Bull Terriers were bred for fighting so will ably defend and may not get along with all dogs (watch especially for inter-male aggression). They are generally deeply attached to their human family. High activity and exercise needs must be met. If left alone without companionship and mental exercise, they may develop boredom vices. Need to be socialized well to children, and also socialized so that they do not become possessive. They are alarm barkers, not nuisance barkers generally. If off leash, they must be in a fenced enclosure. They may consider small pets as prey. Obedience training is important but keep sessions short to prevent boredom.

Normal Physiologic Variations

May vocalize in grumbles and groans and this is distinct from growling.

Echocardiography: In 14 normal bull terriers, the left ventricular wall thickness was greater and the aortic root diameter smaller than those reported as normal for other breeds of comparable body size. Left atrial dimensions were also larger, however this may have been due to the "maximizing" method of measurement. These dogs also had higher aortic velocities than those reported for other breeds. While these dogs were selected to be as close to normal as possible, the breed may have a particular anatomy that produces abnormal left ventricular echocardiographic parameters. Inaccurate diagnoses of left ventricular hypertrophy and left ventricular outflow tract obstruction may result if breed-specific values are not used.[1]

Echocardiographic Normal Values:[1]			
Parameter	Mean	SD	95% CI
Ao l/a (cm)	1.9	0.3	1.3-2.5
Ao s/a (cm)	2	0.2	1.6-2.4
LVld (cm)	3.8	0.3	3.2-4.4
IVSa (cm)	1.3	0.2	0.9-1.7
IVSd (cm)	1	0.2	0.6-1.4
LVFWa (cm)	1.2	0.1	1.0-1.4
LFVWd (cm)	1	0.1	0.8-1.2
FS%	32.5	4.5	24-41
SV (mL)	38.2	7.3	24-53
HR (beats/min)	130.9	22.5	86-176
Weight (kg)	22.9	3.7	*
AoV (m/s)	1.9	0.2	1.5-2.3

SD standard deviation, CI confidence interval, Ao aortic annular diameter, l/a long axis, s/a short axis, LVl left ventricular internal dimension, d diastolic, IVS interventricular septum, s systolic, LVFW left ventricular free wall thickness, FS% fractional shortening, SV stroke volume, HR heart rate, AoV aortic velocity

Parameter	Weight (kg)		
	20	25	30
LA l/a (cm)	2.5-3.4	2.8-3.7	3.1-4.0
LA s/a (cm)	2.2-3.5	2.5-3.8	2.8-4.1
LVIs (cm)	1.9-3.0	2.2-3.2	2.4-3.5

LA is left atrium diameter, l/a is long axis view, s/a is short axis view, LVIs is left ventricular internal dimension during systole

Drug Sensitivities
None reported

Inherited Diseases

Hip Dysplasia: Polygenically inherited trait causing degenerative joint disease and hip arthritis. OFA reports 6.7% affected.[2]

Patella Luxation: Polygenically inherited laxity of patellar ligaments, causing luxation, lameness, and later degenerative joint disease. Treat surgically if causing clinical signs. OFA reports 2.1% affected. Reported at a frequency of 2.84% in the 1997 BTCA Health Survey.[2,3]

Hereditary Nephritis: Autosomal dominant disorder causing renal failure at variable ages in affected dogs due to abnormal kidney basement membrane protein and structure. Dorn reports a 8.16x odds ratio for kidney disease versus other breeds. No genetic test is available.[4,5]

Polycystic Kidney Disease (PKD): Autosomal dominant caused by an undetermined mutation in the PKD 1 gene. Renal cysts are diagnosed by ultrasound. They are usually bilateral, from less than 1 mm to over 2.5 cm in diameter, and occur in the cortex and medulla. Causes chronic renal failure. Dorn reports a 8.16x odds ratio for kidney disease versus other breeds. No genetic test is available.[4,6,7,8,9]

Elbow Dysplasia: Polygenically inherited trait causing elbow arthritis. Too few Bull Terriers have been screened by OFA to determine an accurate frequency.[2]

Lethal Acrodermatitis: An autosomal recessive disease. Affected dogs present with stunting, splayed digits, eating difficulties, skin disease of the face and feet, and increased susceptibility to microbial infections. In older dogs, paronychia, nail disease and hyperkeratosis of the footpads develops, becoming severe in dogs over six months of age. Median survival time is 7 months. Although many of the clinical signs and the pathology of this condition suggest zinc deficiency, the measurement of blood zinc levels as a diagnostic aid is of limited value, and the dogs do not respond to zinc treatment. Reported at a frequency of 0.81% in the 1997 BTCA Health Survey. No genetic test is available.[3,10,11]

Disease Predispositions

Allergic Dermatitis: Inhalant or food allergy. Presents with pruritis and pyotraumatic dermatitis (hot spots). Bull Terriers are at an increased risk versus other breeds, especially white Bull Terriers. Reported at a frequency of 25.56% in the 1997 BTCA Health Survey.[3,12]

Compulsive Tail Chasing and Spinning: Disorder of persistent spinning observed in the breed. Possibly a behavioral compulsion, as 75% of affected dogs respond to clomipramine administration.

However a neurological partial seizure disorder cannot be ruled out, as some dogs have abnormal electroencephalograms and respond to anticonvulsants. Compulsion was reported at a frequency of 18.05%, and spinning 17.65% in the 1997 BTCA Health Survey. Unknown mode of inheritance.[3,13,14]

Deafness: Congenital deafness can be unilateral or bilateral. Diagnosed by BAER testing: Strain reports total (uni or bilateral) deafness frequency of 19.9% in white Bull Terriers, and 1.3% in colored Bull Terriers based on BAER testing. 9.9% of all Bull Terriers test unilaterally deaf, and 1.1% test bilaterally deaf.[15]

Persistent Pupillary Membranes: Strands of fetal remnant connecting; iris to iris, cornea, lens, or involving sheets of tissue. The later three forms can impair vision, and dogs affected with these forms should not be bred. Identified in 7.84% of Bull Terriers CERF examined by veterinary ophthalmologists between 2000-2005.[16]

Hypothyroidism: Inherited autoimmune thyroiditis. 7.0% positive for thyroid autoantibodies based on testing at Michigan State University. (Ave. for all breeds is 7.5%).[17,18]

Primary Lens Luxation: Occurs in the breed due to abnormalities of the suspensory apparatus of the lens (zonule). Often progresses to secondary glaucoma. Relative risk of 65.88x versus other breeds. Identified in 5.88% of Bull Terriers CERF examined by veterinary ophthalmologists between 2000-2005. Unknown mode of inheritance. CERF does not recommend breeding any Bull Terrier with lens luxation.[16,19]

Cataracts: Anterior, posterior, intermediate and punctate cataracts occur in the breed. Identified in 3.92% of Bull Terriers CERF examined by veterinary ophthalmologists between 2000-2005. CERF does not recommend breeding any Bull Terrier with a cataract.[16]

Mitral Valvular Stenosis/Left Ventricular Outflow Tract Obstruction (LVOTO): Found at an increased frequency in Bull Terriers. Echocardiography is a much more sensitive test than auscultation for murmurs. Pathological findings can include thickened, nodular, and stiff mitral valves with short, thickened, and fused chordae tendineae. Myxomatous valvular degeneration, small vessel arteriosclerosis in the myocardium and fibrosis of cardiac conduction tissue were common histologic findings in Bull Terriers with clinical cardiac disease. An increased incidence was found in Bull Terriers affected with PKD, though it could not be identified if there is a direct genetic correlation between the two disorders.[20,21,22]

Aortic Stenosis: Found at an increased frequency in Bull Terriers. Clinical signs can include syncope, exercise intolerance/fatigue, or heart murmur. Cardiac ultrasound shows thickened and/or poorly opening aortic valve leaflets, and an elevated blood flow velocity through the aortic valve annulus (mean v=5.2m/s; range=4.8-5.9). Varying degrees of concentric LVH and mitral valve thickening can be seen. Many affected bull terriers have concurrent severe mitral valve stenosis.[23]

Demodicosis: Demodectic mange dermatitis has an underlying immunodeficiency in its pathogenesis. Dorn reports a 2.14x odds ratio versus other breeds. Unknown mode of inheritance.[9]

Actinic Keratosis: Affected dogs present with alopecia, erythema, comedones, scales, excoriation, pustules, epidermal collarettes, crusts and scars, with pathologic development of epidermal hyperplasia, parakeratosis, and orthokeratosis. Lesions occur secondary to prolonged UV/sunlight exposure, and may be a precursor to squamous cell carcinoma. Seen at an increased frequency in the breed.[24]

Retinal Dysplasia: Focal dysplasia and retinal folds are recognized in the breed, which can lead to retinal detachment. Reported in 1.96% of Bull Terriers CERF-examined by veterinary ophthalmologists between 2000-2005.[16]

Vitreous Degeneration: Liquefaction of the vitreous gel which may predispose to retinal detachment. Identified in 1.96% of Bull Terriers CERF examined by veterinary ophthalmologists between 2000-2005.[16]

Inverted Canines: In affected Bull Terriers, the mandibular canine teeth are tipped (curved) caudally and impact at the mesio-palatal gingival margin of the maxillary canine teeth.[25]

Cerebellar Abiotrophy, Cerebellar Vermian Hypoplasia, Cleft Lip/ Palate, Deep Pyoderma, Ectropion, Entropion, Inguinal Hernia, Keratoconjunctivitis Sicca, Laryngeal Paralysis, Osteochondritis Dessicans–Hock and Stifle, Progressive Retinal Atrophy, Prognathism, Prolapsed Nictitans, Retained Primary Teeth, and **Wry Mouth** are reported.[26]

Isolated Case Studies

Sick Sinus Syndrome: A 6.5-year-old, spayed female bull terrier was investigated for episodic weakness and a syncopal episode. Resting ECG revealed bradycardia (40 to 60 bpm), sinus pauses of typically 2-4s, atrial premature contractions (APCs), and junctional escape beats. Vagal maneuvers did not result in significant sinus pauses, and atropine response was normal in rate but not rhythm, implying a conduction disturbance rather than excessive parasympathetic tone.[27]

Genetic Tests

Tests of Genotype: Direct test for color alleles is avaiable from VetGen.

Tests of Phenotype: CHIC certification: Required testing includes patella examination, cardiac evaluation (recommend echocardiogram), BAER test for deafness, and kidney disease screening with urine protein:creatinine ratio. (See CHIC website; www.caninehealthinfo.org).

Recommended tests include CERF eye examination, hip and elbow radiographs, and thyroid profile including autoantibodies.

Miscellaneous

- **Breed name synonyms:** English Bull Terrier, White Cavalier (for white variety)
- **Registries:** AKC, UKC, CKC, KCGB (Kennel Club of Great Britain), ANKC (Australian National Kennel Club), NKC (National Kennel Club)
- **AKC rank (year 2008):** 57 (1,900 dogs registered)
- **Internet resources: Bull Terrier Club of America:** www.btca.com
  The Bull Terrier Club of Canada: http://thebullterrierclub.ca
  The Bull Terrier Club (UK): www.thebullterrierclub.com

References

1. O'Leary CA, Mackay BM, Taplin RH, et. al.: Echocardiographic parameters in 14 healthy English Bull Terriers. *Aust Vet J.* 2003 Sep;81(9):535-42.
2. OFA Website breed statistics: www.offa.org Last accessed July. 1, 2010.
3. Bull Terrier Club of America & Slater M: 1997 BTCA Health Survey. 1997.
4. O'Leary CA, Ghoddusi M, Huxtable CR: Renal pathology of polycystic kidney disease and concurrent hereditary nephritis in Bull Terriers. *Aust Vet J.* 2002 Jun;80(6):353-61.
5. Hood JC, Dowling J, Bertram JF, et. al.: Correlation of histopathological features and renal impairment in autosomal dominant Alport syndrome in Bull terriers. *Nephrol Dial Transplant.* 2002 Nov;17(11):1897-908.
6. O'Leary CA, Turner S: Chronic renal failure in an English bull terrier with polycystic kidney disease. *J Small Anim Pract.* 2004 Nov;45(11):563-7.
7. O'Leary CA, Mackay BM, Malik R, et. al.: Polycystic kidney disease in bull terriers: an autosomal dominant inherited disorder. *Aust Vet J.* 1999 Jun;77(6):361-6.
8. O'Leary CA, Duffy D, Biros I, et. al.: Linkage confirms canine pkd1 orthologue as a candidate for bull terrier polycystic kidney disease. Anim Genet. 2009 Aug;40(4):543-6.
9. Dorn CR: Canine breed-specific risks of frequently diagnosed diseases at veterinary teaching hospitals. Monograph. AKC Canine Health Foundation. 2000.
10. McEwan NA, McNeil PE, Thompson H, et. al.: Diagnostic features, confirmation and disease progression in 28 cases of lethal acrodermatitis of bull terriers. *J Small Anim Pract.* 2000 Nov;41(11):501-7.
11. Jezyk PF, Haskins ME, MacKay-Smith WE, et. al.: Lethal acrodermatitis in bull terriers. *J Am Vet Med Assoc.* 1986 Apr 15;188(8):833-9.
12. Nødtvedt A, Egenvall A, Bergvall K, et. al.: Incidence of and risk factors for atopic dermatitis in a Swedish population of insured dogs. Vet Rec. 2006 Aug 19;159(8):241-6.
13. Moon-Fanelli AA, Dodman NH: Description and development of compulsive tail chasing in terriers and response to clomipramine treatment. *J Am Vet Med Assoc.* 1998 Apr 15;212(8):1252-7.
14. Dodman NH, Knowles KE, Shuster L, et. al.: Behavioral changes associated with suspected complex partial seizures in bull terriers. *J Am Vet Med Assoc.* 1996 Mar 1;208(5):688-091.
15. Strain GM: Deafness prevalence and pigmentation and gender associations in dog breeds at risk. *Vet J.* 2004 Jan;167(1):23-32.
16. *Ocular Disorders Presumed to be Inherited in Purebred Dogs.* American College of Veterinary Ophthalmologists. ACVO, 2007.
17. Nachreiner RF, Refsal KR, Graham PA, et. al.: Prevalence of serum thyroid hormone autoantibodies in dogs with clinical signs of hypothyroidism. *J Am Vet Med Assoc* 2002 Feb 15;220(4):466-71.
18. Nachreiner R and Refsal K: Personal communication, Diagnostic Center for Population and Animal Health, Michigan State University. April, 2007.
19. Sargan DR, Withers D, Pettitt L, et. al.: Mapping the mutation causing lens luxation in several terrier breeds. J Hered. 2007;98(5):534-8.
20. O'Leary CA, Mackay BM, Taplin RH, et. al.: Auscultation and echocardiographic findings in Bull Terriers with and without polycystic kidney disease. *Aust Vet J.* 2005 May;83(5):270-5.
21. Lehmkuhl LB, Ware WA, Bonagura JD: Mitral stenosis in 15 dogs. *J Vet Intern Med.* 1994 Jan-Feb;8(1):2-17.
22. O'Leary CA & Wilkie I: Cardiac valvular and vascular disease in Bull Terriers. Vet Pathol. 2009 Nov;46(6):1149-55.
23. Oyama MA, Sisson DD, Behr MJ, et. al.: Severe Valvular Aortic Stenosis in Bull Terriers: Clinical, Anatomic and Histopathologic Characteristics. Proceedings, 2003 ACVIM Forum. 2003.
24. Costa SS, Munhoz TD, Calazans SG, et. al.: Clinical and Epidemiological Evaluation of Actinic Keratosis in Seven Dogs. Proceedings, 2009 WSAVA World Congress. 2009.
25. Pavlica Z, Cestnik V: Management of lingually displaced mandibular canine teeth in five bull terrier dogs. J Vet Dent 1995: 12[4]:127-9.
26. *The Genetic Connection: A Guide to Health Problems in Purebred Dogs.* L Ackerman. p. 206-07. AAHA Press, 1999.
27. Kavanagh K: Sick sinus syndrome in a bull terrier. *Can Vet J.* 2002 Jan;43(1):46-8.
28. *The Complete Dog Book, 20th Ed.* The American Kennel Club. Howell Book House, NY 2006. p. 358-361.

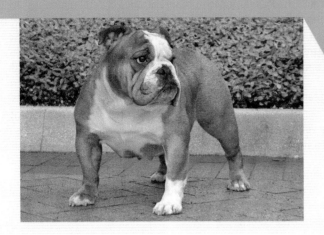

and well arched. The back is somewhat roached (wheel-backed). The thorax is deep with rounded ribs. The abdomen is moderately tucked up. A low set tail is carried low, and the tail tapers and is straight or screwed, but a curly tail is a fault. Limbs are stout and short but fairly straight boned. The elbows stand away from the chest wall. The feet are moderate in size and compact, and are straight ahead but especially the metatarsals deviate outward. This is due to so-called cow hocked conformation. Toes are well knuckled and nails are stubby and strong. The loins sit higher than the shoulder. The rolling gait is loose-jointed and ambling.

The Breed History

Many years ago in the British Isles, a tough dog was developed whose purpose was bull baiting and it is thought that from this stock the modern bulldog arose. The first breed standard was drawn up in 1964.

Breeding for Function

As bull baiters, the breed ancestors possessed the unusual courage and ferocity needed to pursue bulls, but once fighting sports were outlawed in the British Isles in 1835, fanciers sought to continue the breed. In modern days, the breed is widely kept as a companion dog, having had a gentle temperament successfully selected for.

Physical Characteristics

Height at Withers: 12-14" (30.5-35.5 cm)

Weight: 50 lb (22.5 kg), female 40 lb (18 kg)

Coat: The short, flat glossy coat is straight, the hairs are fine, and the skin is quite loose especially around the neck area. Colors include brindle, white, red, fawn, and piebald. A small white chest patch is accepted.

Longevity: 10-12 years

Points of Conformation: These dogs are medium-sized, massive both across the chest and throughout the body. The dark eyes are front facing, set low in the skull, are wide set and round, and moderate in size, the palpebral margins are dark and no nictitans or sclera should show. The ears are very high and wide set, small and thin in leather; termed a rose ear in shape and carriage, which means the folded portion is splayed so that the front is further from the head than the back. This feature helps distinguish the English Bulldog from the French Bulldog because the latter has erect bat ears, and is also smaller in stature.

The head is massive, being both broad and square with a pronounced stop forming a hollow between the eyes. The muzzle is very short, upturned, and the nose is broad and colored black. The flews are very well developed and overhang the lower jaws. A dewlap is well developed, and the head and face are heavily wrinkled. The lower jaw is considerably prognathic and prominent (referred to as chops). The neck is very short and thick, muscular

Recognized Behavior Issues and Traits

Reported breed attributes include: Resolute in a confrontation but kind and gentle with family, children and other pets. Easy to groom, has a moderate shedding tendency, stable temperament, good for town and country; even apartments. Low to moderate exercise needs. Does not tolerate temperature extremes, so needs to be a housedog. Snoring is common and may also drool. The facial wrinkles need daily hygiene.

Normal Physiologic Variations

Bulldogs often have to deliver by **cesarean section.** 8% of all C-sections in a large study were bulldogs. In Great Britain, 86.1% of Bulldog litters are c-sections.[1,2]

Drug Sensitivities

None reported

Inherited Diseases

Hip Dysplasia: Polygenically inherited trait causing degenerative joint disease and hip arthritis. OFA reports 73.2% affected.[3]

Elbow Dysplasia: Polygenically inherited trait causing elbow arthritis. OFA reports a high incidence, but too few Bulldogs have been screened to determine an accurate frequency.[3]

Patella Luxation: Polygenically inherited laxity of patellar ligaments, causing luxation, lameness, and later degenerative joint disease. Treat surgically if causing clinical signs. OFA reports 6.2% affected. Reported 6.1x odds ratio versus other breeds.[3,4]

Hyperuricosuria (HUU)/Urate Urolithiasis: An autosomal recessive disease caused by a mutation in the SLC2A9 gene causes hyperuricosuria and predisposes to urate bladder stones. Stone formation is predominantly seen in males. Bulldogs have a 7.9x Odds Ratio of forming urate bladder stones versus other breeds. A direct genetic test is available.[5,6,7]

Anasarca (Lethal Congenital Edema): Anasarca occurs in the breed. Puppies are born dead and edematous. Can also be associated with cleft palate. Segregation analysis indicates an autosomal recessive mode of inheritance.[8]

Disease Predispositions

Brachycephalic Complex: Stenotic nares, elongated soft palate, everted laryngeal saccules, laryngeal collapse, and occasionally **hypoplastic trachea.** Reported to cause obstructive sleep apnea in the breed. Can cause secondary bronchial collapse. Dorn reports a 29.27x odds ratio for elongated soft palate versus other breeds. Identified in 19.2% of Bulldogs in an Australian study. One study showed the Bulldog as the most frequently affected breed, and an overall surgical curative rate of 94.2%.[9,10,11,12,13,14,15]

Distichiasis: Abnormally placed eyelashes that can cause secondary corneal ulceration. Identified in 15.74% of Bulldogs CERF examined by veterinary ophthalmologists between 2000-2005. CERF states that breeding of affected animals should be discouraged. Dorn reports a 1.48x odds ratio versus other breeds.[9,16]

Entropion: Rolling in of the eyelids, which can predispose to corneal irritation and ulceration. Reported in 14.43% of Bulldogs CERF examined by veterinary ophthalmologists between 2000-2005. Dorn reports a 4.37x odds ratio versus other breeds.[9,16]

Ectropion: A rolling out of the eyelids, that can cause tear pooling, conjunctivitis, and frequent infection. Reported in 8.85% of Bulldogs CERF examined by veterinary ophthalmologists between 2000-2005. Dorn reports a 4.37x odds ratio versus other breeds.[9,16]

Retinal Dysplasia: Focal folds and geographic retinal dysplasia are seen in the breed. Dogs with the geographic form should not be bred. Reported in 7.54% of Bulldogs CERF examined by veterinary ophthalmologists between 2000-2005.[16]

Prolapsed Gland of the Nictitans (Cherry Eye): Occurs at a high frequency in the breed. This condition is secondary to chronic conjunctivitis, usually of an allergic nature.[17]

Hypothyroidism: Inherited autoimmune thyroiditis. 4.2% positive for thyroid auto-antibodies based on testing at Michigan State University. (Ave. for all breeds is 7.5%.).[18,19]

Stifle Osteochondritis Dessicans (OCD): Polygenically inherited cartilage defect. Causes stifle joint pain and lameness in young growing dogs. Mild cases can resolve with rest, while more severe cases require surgery. Reported 44.2x odds ratio versus other breeds.[4]

Keratoconjunctivitis Sicca (KCS, Dry Eye): An abnormality of the tear film, resulting in ocular irritation and/or vision impairment. Age of onset 2-5 years. Treatment with topical ocular lubricants and anti-inflammatory medication. CERF does not recommend breeding any Bulldogs with KCS.[16,20]

Cystine Urolithiasis: Bulldogs have a higher incidence of Cystine (32.3x OR) bladder stones compared to other breeds. Cystine stones are due to a defect in cystine metabolism.[5,6]

Chronic Superficial Keratitis (Pannus): Corneal disease that can cause vision problems due to pigmentation. Treatment with topical ocular lubricants and anti-inflammatory medication. Identified in 1.97% of Bulldogs CERF examined by veterinary ophthalmologists between 2000-2005. CERF does not recommend breeding any Bulldogs with pannus.[16]

Persistent Pupillary Membranes: Strands of fetal remnant connecting; iris to iris, cornea, lens, or involving sheets of tissue. The later three forms can impair vision, and dogs affected with these forms should not be bred. Identified in 1.64% of Bulldogs CERF examined by veterinary ophthalmologists between 2000-2005.[16]

Cataracts: Anterior, posterior, equatorial, and capsular cataracts occur in the breed. Identified in 1.31% of Bulldogs CERF examined by veterinary ophthalmologists between 2000-2005. CERF does not recommend breeding any Bulldogs with a cataract.[16]

Pododermatitis/Interdigital Cysts: Affected dogs can present with erythema. thickening of the skin, alopecia, pyoderma, nodules, ulcers haemorrhagic bullae, and draining tracts. Increased risk versus other breeds.[21]

Pulmonic Stenosis: Bulldogs are the most common breed to have pulmonic stenosis, with an odds ratio of 19.2x versus other breeds. This congenital heart abnormality in Bulldogs frequently is caused by a circumpulmonary left coronary artery originating from a single right coronary artery.[22,23]

Demodicosis: Generalized demodicosis has an underlying immunodeficiency in its pathogenesis. Dorn reports a 3.0x odds ratio versus other breeds.[9]

Hiatal Hernia: The Bulldog has the highest incidence of hiatal hernia for all breeds. The most common presentation is reflux esophagitis. Treatment is with surgery.[24]

Spina Bifida: Review of cases to veterinary teaching hospitals suggests a high incidence of spina bifida in the English Bulldog. Urinary and fecal incontinence is the most common clinical sign. Radiographs and myelography confirm the diagnosis.[25]

Urethrorectal Fistula: Several case reports are in the literature of Bulldogs with congenital urethrorectal fistulas. Affected dogs present with urine dribbling the anus, and chronic cystitis. Treatment is with surgery.[26,27,28]

Cryptorchidism, Deafness, Factor VII Deficiency, Factor VIII Deficiency, Fold Dermatitis, Hemivertebra, Hydrocephalus, Laryngeal Paralysis, Myelodysplasia, Sacrocaudal Dysgenesis, Seasonal Flank Alopecia, Subaortic Stenosis, Supernumerary Teeth, Tetralogy of Fallot, Ventricular Septal Defect, von Willebrand's Disease, and **Wry Mouth** are reported.[29]

Isolated Case Studies

Cerebellar Cortical Degeneration: Three young full-sibling Bulldogs presented with a wide-based stance, marked hypermetria, spasticity, and intention tremors of the head and trunk with loss of balance. Pathology showed a loss of cerebellar Purkinje and granule cells.[30]

Acrochordonous Skin Plaques: Clinical report of numerous, closely associated acrochordons forming a plaque, preferentially located at the dorsal neck of two Bulldogs.[31]

Cor Triatriatum Dexter: A 3.5 month old male Bulldog with ascites and a history of respiratory distress was diagnosed at autopsy with the heart anomaly cor triatriatum dexter.[32]

Parotid Duct Sialolithiasis: Two case reports are in the literature; a 7 year old male Bulldog and a 3 year old male Bulldog. Blockage of the parotid duct with a sialolith causes chronic facial swelling. Surgical removal of the sialolith, or of the salivary gland and duct is curative.[33,34]

Sperm Tail Defects: A 2 year old Bulldog was identified with 93.3% of spermatozoa with morphological tail defects, including strong folding, coiling and fracture of sperm midpieces and tails, axonemal defects and the presence of swollen and unevenly distributed mitochondria. The defect was considered to be genetic in origin.[35]

Genetic Tests

Tests of Genotype: Direct test for HUU is available from the UC-Davis VGL and the Animal Health Trust.

Tests of Phenotype: CHIC Certification: Required testing includes patella evaluation (minimum 1 year of age) and congenital cardiac exam (by a cardiologist, preferably by echocardiography). (See CHIC website; www.caninehealthinfo.org).

Recommended: hip and elbow radiographs, CERF eye examination, and thyroid profile including autoantibodies.

Miscellaneous

- **Breed name synonyms:** English Bulldog
- **Registries:** **AKC, UKC, CKC, KCGB (Kennel Club of Great Britain), ANKC (Australian National Kennel Club)-as British bulldog, NKC (National Kennel Club) **Just termed Bulldog in AKC
- **AKC rank (year 2008):** 8 (23,413 dogs registered)
- **Internet resources:** The Bulldog Club of America: http://thebca.org/
  The British Bulldog Club: www.britishbulldogclub.co.uk
  Bulldog Club of Central Canada: www.bulldogclubofcentralcanada.net/

References

1. Moon PF, Erb HN, Ludders JW, et. al.: Perioperative risk factors for puppies delivered by cesarean section in the United States and Canada. J Am Anim Hosp Assoc. 2000 Jul-Aug;36(4):359-68.
2. Evans KM and Adams VJ: Proportion of litters of purebred dogs born by caesarean section. J Small Anim Pract. 2010 Feb;51(2):113-8.
3. OFA Website breed statistics: www.offa.org Last accessed July 1, 2010.
4. LaFond E, Breur GJ & Austin CC: Breed susceptibility for developmental orthopedic diseases in dogs. J Am Anim Hosp Assoc. 2002 Sep-Oct;38(5):467-77.
5. Ling GV, Franti CE, Ruby AL, et. al.: Urolithiasis in dogs. II: Breed prevalence, and interrelations of breed, sex, age, and mineral composition. Am J Vet Res. 1998 May;59(5):630-42.
6. Bartges JW, Osborne CA, Lulich JP, et. al.: Prevalence of cystine and urate uroliths in bulldogs and urate uroliths in dalmatians. J Am Vet Med Assoc. 1994 Jun 15;204(12):1914-8.
7. Bannasch D, Safra N, Young A, et. al.: Mutations in the SLC2A9 Gene Cause Hyperuricosuria and Hyperuricemia in the Dog. PLoS Genet 4(11) 2008: e1000246. doi:10.1371/journal.pgen.1000246.
8. Ladds PW, Dennis SM, Leipold HW: Lethal congenital edema in Bulldog pups. J Am Vet Med Assoc. 1971 Jul 1;159(1):81-6.
9. Dorn CR: Canine breed-specific risks of frequently diagnosed diseases at veterinary teaching hospitals. MonographAKC6.
10. Torres CV, Hunt GB: Results of surgical correction of abnormalities associated with brachycephalic airway obstruction syndrome in dogs in

Australia. J Small Anim Pract. 2006 Mar;47(3):150-4.
11. Veasey SC, Chachkes J, Fenik P, et. al.: The effects of ondansetron on sleep-disordered breathing in the English bulldog. Sleep. 2001 Mar 15;24(2):155-60.
12. Coyne BE, Fingland RB: Hypoplasia of the trachea in dogs: 103 cases (1974-1990). J Am Vet Med Assoc. 1992 Sep 1;201(5):768-72.
13. Riecks TW, Birchard SJ, & Stephens JA: Surgical correction of brachycephalic syndrome in dogs: 62 cases (1991-2004). J Am Vet Med Assoc. 2007 May 1;230(9):1324-8.
14. Torrez CV & Hunt GB: Results of surgical correction of abnormalities associated with brachycephalic airway obstruction syndrome in dogs in Australia. J Small Anim Pract. 2006 Mar;47(3):150-4.
15. De Lorenzi D, Bertoncello D, & Drigo M: Bronchial abnormalities found in a consecutive series of 40 brachycephalic dogs. J Am Vet Med Assoc. 2009 Oct 1;235(7):835-40.
16. Ocular Disorders Presumed to be Inherited in Purebred Dogs. American College of Veterinary Ophthalmologists. ACVO, 2007
17. Abrams K: Selected Adnexal Diseases in the Dog. Proceedings, 2004 Western Veterinary Conference. 2004.
18. Nachreiner R & Refsal K: Personal communication, Diagnostic Center for Population and Animal Health, Michigan State University. April, 2007.
19. Nachreiner RF, Refsal KR, Graham PA, et. al.: Prevalence of serum thyroid hormone autoantibodies in dogs with clinical signs of hypothyroidism. J Am Vet Med Assoc 2002 Feb 15;220(4):466-71.
20. Colitz CMH: Keratoconjunctivitis Sicca: Cause, Effect & Treatment. Proceedings, 2004 Western Veterinary Conference. 2004.
21. Breathnach R: Intractable Pododermatitis. Proceedings, British Small Animal Veterinary Congress 2006.
22. Buchanan JW: Pathogenesis of single right coronary artery and pulmonic stenosis in English Bulldogs. J Vet Intern Med. 2001 Mar-Apr;15(2):101-4.
23. Buchanan JW: Causes and prevalence of cardiovascular diseases. In Kirk RW, Bonagura JD, eds: Current veterinary therapy XI, Philadelphia, 1992, WB Saunders.
24. Lorinson D, Bright RM: Long-term outcome of medical and surgical treatment of hiatal hernias in dogs and cats: 27 cases (1978-1996). J Am Vet Med Assoc. 1998 Aug 1;213(3):381-4.
25. Wilson JW, Kurtz HJ, Leipold HW, et. al.: Spina bifida in the dog. Vet Pathol. 1979 Mar;16(2):165-79
26. Silverstone AM, Adams WM: Radiographic diagnosis of a rectourethral fistula in a dog. J Am Anim Hosp Assoc. 2001 Nov-Dec;37(6):573-6.
27. Ralphs SC, Kramek BA: Novel perineal approach for repair of a urethrorectal fistula in a bulldog. Can Vet J. 2003 Oct;44(10):822-3.
28. Cruse AM, Vaden SL, Mathews KG, et. al.: Use of computed tomography (CT) scanning and colorectal new methylene blue infusion in evaluation of an English Bulldog with a rectourethral fistula. J Vet Intern Med. 2009 Jul-Aug;23(4):931-4.
29. *The Genetic Connection: A Guide to Health Problems in Purebred Dogs.* L. Ackerman. p. 215-16. AAHA Press, 1999.
30. Gandini G, Botteron C, Brini E, et. al.: Cerebellar cortical degeneration in three English bulldogs: clinical and neuropathological findings. J Small Anim Pract. 2005 Jun;46(6):291-4.
31. Bidaut AP, Gross TL, Noli C, et. al.: Acrochordonous plaques in two Bulldogs and a Pug dog. Vet Dermatol. 2003 Jun;14(3):177-9.
32. Duncan RB Jr, Freeman LE, Jones J, et. al.: Cor triatriatum dexter in an English Bulldog puppy: case report and literature review. J Vet Diagn Invest. 1999 Jul;11(4):361-5.
33. Trumpatori BJ, Geissler K, Mathews KG: Parotid duct sialolithiasis in a dog. J Am Anim Hosp Assoc. 2007 Jan-Feb;43(1):45-51.
34. Tivers MS & Moore AH: Surgical treatment of a parotid duct sialolith in a bulldog. Vet Rec. 2007 Aug 25;161(8):271-2.
35. Rota A, Manuali E, Caire S, et. al.: Severe tail defects in the spermatozoa ejaculated by an English bulldog. J Vet Med Sci. 2008 Jan;70(1):123-5.
36. *The Complete Dog Book, 20th Ed.* The American Kennel Club. Howell Book House, NY 2006. p. 538-542.

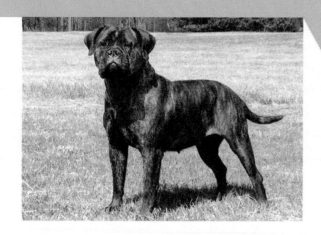

The Breed History

This particular mastiff breed is first recorded in Britain around 1860. Like the Old English Mastiff (*Syn. Mastiff*), it is one of many mastiff-type dogs that originated from ancient Asian stock. The cross of 60% English Mastiff with 40% English Bulldog produced this breed. In 1924, the English Kennel Club first recognized Bullmastiffs as a breed, and in 1933-34, the AKC also recognized this breed.

Breeding for Function

To protect estates from poachers, the bulldog-mastiff type was ideal. They were silent workers, following a human trail by odor, and when pinned down, did not maul their intruders but just held them. Later, they became very popular as guarding and watchdogs.

Physical Characteristics

Height at Withers: female 24-26" (61-66 cm), male 25-27" (63.5-68.5cm).

Weight: females 100-120 lb (45.5-54.5 kg), males 110-130 lb (50-59 kg).

Coat: The short, very dense haircoat is acceptable in fawn, red and brindle. Only a very small white marking on the chest is acceptable.

Longevity: 9-10 years

Points of Conformation: The Bullmastiff is smaller and more compact, with more of a bulldog type head than the English Mastiff. This alert powerful dog is about as long as tall. The skull is large, with a well-wrinkled forehead when alert. Eyes are medium-sized and dark colored, and ears are triangular and carried close to the head; set high. They possess a moderate stop, and the muzzle is deep and broad with dark coloration. Nose is black and large, and the flews moderately pendulous. The neck is moderate in length and arch, with well-developed musculature. The topline is level, and the thorax is wide and deep, with well-sprung ribs. The tail is high set and tapers to end at the tarsus; it is straight/slightly curved. Limbs are heavily boned and straight, feet are medium sized with well-arched toes, black nails and thick pads. The Bullmastiff moves with a ground-covering smooth stride.

Bullmastiff

Recognized Behavior Issues and Traits

Reported breed attributes include: Gentle, self assured, courageous, sensitive to temperature extremes, intelligent, and some are a bit overprotective and may resist obedience training. Very aloof with strangers so early socialization and obedience training is important. Low to moderate exercise needs, good for town or country, low grooming needs, moderate shedders, and have a high drooling and snoring tendency. Good dog for experienced dog handlers.

Normal Physiologic Variations

35% of Bullmastiff litters are delivered by **C-section** according to a UK study.[1]

Drug Sensitivities

None reported

Inherited Diseases

Hip Dysplasia: Polygenically inherited trait causing degenerative joint disease and hip arthritis. OFA reports 24.5% affected.[2]

Elbow Dysplasia: Polygenically inherited trait causing elbow arthritis. OFA reports 13.8% affected. Reported 38.9x odds ratio for the fragmented coronoid process form of elbow dysplasia versus other breeds.[2,3]

Progressive Retinal Atrophy (PRA): An autosomal dominant form of PRA occurs in the breed, with an onset of 6 months to 4 years of age. A genetic test is available.[4,5]

Patella Luxation: Polygenically inherited laxity of patellar ligaments, causing luxation, lameness, and later degenerative joint disease. Treat surgically if causing clinical signs. Too few Bullmastiffs have been screened by OFA to determine an accurate frequency.[2]

Multifocal Retinopathy/Retinal Dysplasia: Autosomal recessive retinal pigment epithelial dysplasia causing localized multifocal retinal detachments. Age of onset from 11 to 13 weeks of age. Reported in 5.26% of Bullmastiffs CERF examined by veterinary ophthalmologists between 2000-2005. A genetic test is available.[4]

Glomerulonephropathy: Rare disorder, where affected dogs present between the ages of 2.5 and 11 years with clinical and laboratory signs of chronic renal failure. Histopathology shows chronic glomerulonephropathy with sclerosis. Pedigree analysis supports an autosomal recessive mode of inheritance.[6]

Cerebellar Ataxia with Hydrocephalus: Rare disorder, where affected puppies have ataxia, hypermetria, conscious proprioceptive deficits, behavioral abnormalities, and a visual deficit. Brain MRI shows symmetric hydrocephalus and focal areas of increased signal intensity within the central nuclei of the cerebellum. Histopathological findings are vacuolation, gliosis and axonal degeneration within the deep cerebellar nuclei. This disorder is most likely inherited in an autosomal recessive manner.[7,8]

Disease Predispositions

Entropion: Rolling in of eyelids, often causing corneal irritation or ulceration. Entropion is reported in 7.12% of Bullmastiffs CERF examined by veterinary ophthalmologists between 2000-2005.[4]

Hypothyroidism: Inherited autoimmune thyroiditis. 5.8% positive for thyroid auto-antibodies based on testing at Michigan State University. (Ave. for all breeds is 7.5%).[9,10]

Distichiasis: Abnormally placed eyelashes that irritate the cornea and conjunctiva. Can cause secondary corneal ulceration. Identified in 4.02% of Bullmastiffs CERF examined by veterinary ophthalmologists between 2000-2005.[4]

Persistent Pupillary Membranes: Strands of fetal remnant connecting; iris to iris, cornea, lens, or involving sheets of tissue. The later three forms can impair vision, and dogs affected with these forms should not be bred. Identified in 3.10% of Bullmastiffs CERF examined by veterinary ophthalmologists between 2000-2005, with 1.55% being iris to cornea.[4]

Ectropion: A rolling out of the eyelids, that can cause tear pooling, conjunctivitis, and frequent infection. Can be secondary to macroblepharon; an abnormally large eyelid opening. Ectropion is reported in 3.10%, and macroblepharon in 2.79% of Bullmastiffs CERF examined by veterinary ophthalmologists between 2000-2005.[4]

Osteochondritis Desicans (OCD): Polygenically inherited joint cartilage defect. Causes joint pain and lameness in young growing dogs. Mild cases can resolve with rest, while more severe cases require surgery. Reported 85.9x odds ratio for hock OCD, and 6.7x odds ratio for shoulder OCD versus other breeds.[3]

Cranial Cruciate Ligament Rupture (ACL): Traumatic tearing of the anterior cruciate ligament. Dorn reports a 2.80x odds ratio in Bullmastiffs versus other breeds. Treatment is surgery.[11]

Cataracts: Capsular cataracts predominate, though anterior, posterior, and nuclear cataracts also occur in the breed. Identified in 2.79% of Bullmastiffs CERF examined by veterinary ophthalmologists between 2000-2005. CERF does not recommend breeding any Bullmastiff with a cataract.[4]

Gastric Dilatation-Volvulus (bloat, GDV): Polygenically inherited, life-threatening twisting of the stomach within the abdomen. Requires immediate treatment. Reported at an increased frequency in the breed.[12]

Dilated Cardiomyopathy (DCM): Dilated cardiomyopathy causing heart failure is identified in the breed. Unknown mode of inheritance.[13]

Cystine Urinary Calculi: Bullmastiffs are a breed with increased risk of developing cystine calculi, due to an abnormality of cystine metabolism.[14]

Lymphoma/Lymphosarcoma: Malignant cancer of lymphoid tissue. An increased prevalence is seen in the breed. In one study, a large family of Bullmastiffs was identified, where 15% of the dogs developed lymphosarcoma over a three year period.[15,16]

Optic Nerve Hypoplasia: A congenital defect of the optic nerve which causes blindness and abnormal pupil response in the affected eye. CERF does not recommend breeding affected dogs. Identified in 1.57% of Bullmastiffs CERF examined by veterinary ophthalmologists between 1991-1999, though none were reported between 2000-2005.[4]

Calvarial Hyperostotic Syndrome (CHS): A clinical syndrome is identified in young male Bullmastiffs of progressive and often asymmetric cortical thickening of the calvaria with irregular, bony proliferation over the frontal, temporal, and occipital bones. Osteopathy is diagnosed based on radiographs and biopsy. In 80% of the cases presented, the lesion is self-limiting.[17]

Oligodendroglial Dysplasia (Spinal Cord Leukodystrophy): Affected Bullmastiffs show a young adult onset, slowly progressive, moderate to severe ataxia of all limbs, spastic tetraparesis that is worse in the pelvic limbs, and a diffuse, action-related, whole-body tremor. Histopathological lesions include white matter myelin plaques, and proliferation of oligodendroglial processes.[18]

Anasarca, Cervical Vertebral Instability, Epilepsy, Panosteitis, Seasonal Flank Alopecia, and **Supernumerary Teeth** are reported.[19]

Isolated Case Studies

Craniomandibular Osteopathy (CMO): A 6-month-old bullmastiff was presented with bilateral painful swellings of the mandible. Craniomandibular osteopathy was diagnosed based on radiographs and biopsy. The condition resolved with palliative care.[20]

Primary Ciliary Dyskinesia: A 2.5-year-old male Bullmastiff with a history of chronic bronchopneumonia and chronic rhinitis was found to have primary ciliary dyskinesia. Diagnostic evaluations included tracheal mucociliary clearance, functional and ultrastructural ciliary examination, induction of ciliogenesis in cell culture, and sperm evaluation.[21]

Juvenile Renal Dysplasia: A 15-week-old female Bull Mastiff which presented with clinical signs of chronic renal failure. Renal dysplasia and concurrent pyelonephritis were diagnosed by ultrasound, clinical pathology, and biopsy.[22]

Muscle Tumors: Primary skeletal muscle lymphoma and muscle hemangiosarcoma have been diagnosed in individual case studies of Bullmastiffs.[23,24]

Medulloepithelioma: A 6-month-old Bullmastiff presented with clinical signs of incomplete upper motor neuron transverse myelopathy involving the hindlimbs. An embryonal medulloepithelioma was found involving the L1 spinal cord.[25]

Lymphangiosarcoma: A 3.5-year-old Bullmastiff presented with vaginal bleeding 3 weeks after cessation of estrus, during which intromission by the male had been unsuccessful. During ovariohysterectomy a large multi-cystic, proliferative, spongy, fluid-filled, brownish-red mass surrounding the cervix and projecting into the abdominal space was removed with the cervix. Histopathology revealed malignant lymphangiosarcoma that had invaded into the surrounding tissues.[26]

Genetic Tests

Tests of Genotype: Direct tests for PRA and Multifocal Retinopathy are available from Optigen.

Tests of Phenotype: CHIC certification: Required testing includes hip and elbow radiographs, CERF eye examination, congenital cardiac evaluation (by a cardiologist or by echocardiography), and thyroid profile including autoantibodies. Optional tests include direct test for PRA, and kidney tests. (See CHIC website; www.caninehealthinfo.org).

Recommend patella evaluation.

Miscellaneous

- **Breed name synonyms:** Gamekeeper's Night Dog (historical).
- **Registries:** AKC, UKC, CKC, KCGB (Kennel Club of Great Britain), ANKC (Australian National Kennel Club), NKC (National Kennel Club).
- **AKC rank (year 2008):** 39 (3,447 dogs registered)
- **Internet resources: American Bullmastiff Association:** http://bullmastiff.us/
  Bullmastiff Fanciers of Canada: www.bmfc.ca
  British Bullmastiff League: www.britishbullmastiffleague.com

References

1. Evans KM & Adams VJ: Proportion of litters of purebred dogs born by caesarean section. J Small Anim Pract. 2010 Feb;51(2):113-8.
2. OFA Website breed statistics: www.offa.org Last accessed July 1, 2010 .
3. LaFond E, Breur GJ & Austin CC: Breed susceptibility for developmental orthopedic diseases in dogs. J Am Anim Hosp Assoc. 2002 Sep-Oct;38(5):467-77.
4. *Ocular Disorders Presumed to be Inherited in Purebred Dogs.* American College of Veterinary Ophthalmologists. ACVO, 2007.
5. Kijas JW, Miller BJ, Pearce-Kelling SE, et. al.: Canine models of ocular disease: outcross breedings define a dominant disorder present in the English mastiff and bull mastiff dog breeds. J Hered. 2003 Jan-Feb;94(1):27-30.
6. Casal ML, Dambach DM, Meister T, et. al.: Familial glomerulonephropathy in the Bullmastiff. *Vet Pathol.* 2004 Jul;41(4):319-25.
7. Johnson RP, Neer TM, Partington BP, et. al.: Familial cerebellar ataxia with hydrocephalus in bull mastiffs. *Vet Radiol Ultrasound.* 2001 May-Jun;42(3):246-9.
8. Carmichael S, Griffiths IR, Harvey MJ: Familial cerebellar ataxia with hydrocephalus in bull mastiffs. *Vet Rec.* 1983 Apr 9;112(15):354-8.
9. Nachreiner R & Refsal K: Personal communication, Diagnostic Center for Population and Animal Health, Michigan State University. April, 2007.
10. Nachreiner RF, Refsal KR, Graham PA, et. al.: Prevalence of serum thyroid hormone autoantibodies in dogs with clinical signs of hypothyroidism. J Am Vet Med Assoc 2002 Feb 15;220(4):466-71.
11. Dorn CR: Canine breed-specific risks of frequently diagnosed diseases at veterinary teaching hospitals. Monograph. AKC Canine Health Foundation. 2000.
12. Glickman LT, Glickman NW, Schellenberg DB, et. al.: Incidence of and breed-related risk factors for gastric dilatation-volvulus in dogs. J Am Vet Med Assoc. 2000 Jan 1;216(1):40-5.
13. Spier AW, Meurs KM, Coovert DD, et. al.: Use of western immunoblot for evaluation of myocardial dystrophin, alpha-sarcoglycan, and beta-dystroglycan in dogs with idiopathic dilated cardiomyopathy. *Am J Vet Res.* 2001 Jan;62(1):67-71.
14. Case LC, Ling GV, Franti CE, et. al.: Cystine-containing urinary calculi in dogs: 102 cases (1981-1989). *J Am Vet Med Assoc.* 1992 Jul 1;201(1):129-33.
15. Onions DE: A prospective survey of familial canine lymphosarcoma. *J Natl Cancer Inst.* 1984 Apr;72(4):909-12.
16. Edwards DS, Henley WE, Harding EF, et. al.: Breed Incidence of Lymphoma in a UK Population of Insured Dogs. *Vet Comp Oncol* 2003: 1[4]:200-206.
17. Pastor KF, Boulay JP, Schelling SH, et. al.: Idiopathic hyperostosis of the calvaria in five young bullmastiffs. *J Am Anim Hosp Assoc.* 2000 Sep-Oct;36(5):439-45.
18. Morrison JP, Schatzberg SJ, De Lahunta A, et. al.: Oligodendroglial dysplasia in two bullmastiff dogs. Vet Pathol. 2006 Jan;43(1):29-35.
19. The Genetic Connection: A Guide to Health Problems in Purebred Dogs. L Ackerman. p. 207-8. AAHA Press, 1999.
20. Huchowski SL: Craniomandibular osteopathy in a bullmastiff. Can Vet J. 2002 Nov; 43(11):883-5.
21. Clercx C, Peeters D, Beths T, et. al.: Use of Ciliogenesis in the Diagnosis of Primary Ciliary Dyskinesia in a Dog. *J Am Vet Med Assoc* 2000: 217[11]:1681-1685.
22. Abraham LA, Beck C, Slocombe RF: Renal dysplasia and urinary tract infection in a Bull Mastiff puppy. Aust Vet J. 2003 Jun; 81(6):336-9.
23. Tucker DW, Olsen D, Kraft SL, et. al.: Primary hemangiosarcoma of the iliopsoas muscle eliciting a peripheral neuropathy. *J Am Anim Hosp Assoc.* 2000 Mar-Apr;36(2):163-7.
24. Harkin KR, Kennedy GA, Moore WE, et. al.: Skeletal muscle lymphoma in a bullmastiff. *J Am Anim Hosp Assoc.* 2000 Jan-Feb;36(1):63-6.
25. Kennedy FA, Indrieri RJ, Koestner A: Spinal cord medulloepithelioma in a dog. *J Am Vet Med Assoc.* 1984 Oct 15;185(8):902-4.
26. Williams JH, Birrell J, Van Wilpe E: Lymphangiosarcoma in a 3.5-year-old Bullmastiff bitch with vaginal prolapse, primary lymph node fibrosis and other congenital defects. *J S Afr Vet Assoc.* 2005 Sep;76(3):165-71.
27. *The Complete Dog Book, 20th Ed.* The American Kennel Club. Howell Book House, NY 2006. p.. 254-257.

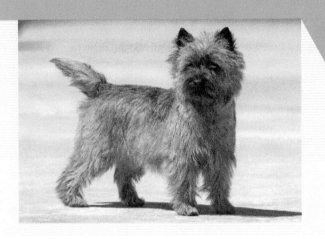

The Breed History

A highly valued working terrier type dog was developed on the Isle of Skye in Scotland that possessed courage fending off unwanted pests, including foxes and otters larger than themselves. In the 1870s, the Dandie Dinmont and Skyes (included Westies, Scotties, and Cairn) were split off into separate types, and by 1912, the Cairns had their own registry and classes. AKC registry began in 1913. From that decade forward, no intermingling of the Westies and Cairns took place. The name cairn means a rock pile used to mark landmarks, and the Cairn terriers would effectively clear these of vermin. As "Toto" in the Wizard of Oz, this likeable dog became a popular pet.

Breeding for Function

A hardy, courageous terrier-type, it was bred to control vermin and this is still emphasized in the breed. They are now valued as a companion dog. The breeding community favors retention of the historical type.

Physical Characteristics

Height at Withers: female 9.5 " (24 cm), male 10" (25.4 cm)

Weight: females 13 lb (6 kg), males 14 lb (6.4kg).

Coat: The double coat may be any color but white, with the outer coat being wiry, and the undercoat soft. Dark points are preferred.

Longevity: 12-15 years.

Points of Conformation: Though short-legged, their movement is free and powerful, and the medium back, deep ribs, and powerful muscles of the hindquarter produce exuberant but balanced activity. A short wide head with black nose, alert deep-set hazel eyes, small pricked up ears, and a tail carried up but not over the back characterize this breed.

Recognized Behavior Issues and Traits

Peppy, spirited, loyal, independent and friendly are some terms used to describe this breed. They are easily trained but need stimulation because if bored, they can chew, bark, or dig. They are low shedders but the coat should be groomed regularly to prevent matting. They have average exercise requirements and do well in city or country. They are good alarm barkers.

Cairn Terrier

Normal Physiologic Variations
None reported

Drug Sensitivities
None reported

Inherited Diseases

Hip Dysplasia and Legg-Calve-Perthes Disease: Polygenically inherited traits causing degenerative hip joint disease and arthritis. Both disorders are reported at high frequencies by OFA, but too few Cairn Terriers are screened to determine accurate frequencies. Reported 17.9x odds ratio for Legg-Calve-Perthes versus other breeds.[1,2]

Patella Luxation: Polygenically inherited laxity of patellar ligaments, causing luxation, lameness, and later degenerative joint disease. Treat surgically if causing clinical signs. Too few Cairn Terriers are screened by OFA to determine accurate frequencies. Padgett reports a frequency of 3.2% in the breed. Reported at a high frequency in the 2005 CTCA Health Survey.[1,3,4]

Ocular Melanosis and Glaucoma: Cairn terriers can have a familial form of ocular melanosis that slowly progresses to melanocytic glaucoma and blindness. The disease is characterized by diffuse intraocular infiltration of heavily pigmented melanocytes. Age of onset 2-14 years. Diagnosed in 1.82% of Cairn terriers presented to veterinary teaching hospitals. Pedigree studies suggest an autosomal dominant mode of inheritance. CERF does not recommend breeding any Cairn Terrier with ocular melanosis.[5,6,7,8,9]

Portosystemic Shunt (PSS, liver shunt)/Hepatoportal Microvascular Dysplasia (MVD): Abnormal blood vessels connecting the systemic and portal blood flow. Vessels can be intra- or extrahepatic, or microvasular. Causes stunting, abnormal behavior and possible seizures. Reported at a frequency of 0.9%. One study reports an odds ratio of 10.7x versus other breeds. Breeding studies show PSS in Cairn terriers is autosomal and most likely polygenic or monogenic with variable expression. Test with bile acids and blood ammonia levels.[10,11,12]

Craniomandibular Osteopathy (CMO): Autosomal recessive, painful non-neoplastic proliferation of bone on the ramus of the mandible and/or the tympanic bulla. Affected dogs present between 3-10 months of age, with varying degrees of difficulty prehending and chewing food, secondary weight loss and atrophy of the temporal and masseter muscles. In most cases, affected dogs are normal after bony remodeling. Padgett reports a frequency of 0.9% in the breed.[3]

Elbow Dysplasia: Polygenically inherited trait causing elbow arthritis. Too few Cairn Terriers are screened by OFA to determine an accurate breed frequency.[1]

Globoid Cell Leukodystrophy (Krabbe disease): A rare autosomal recessive lysosomal storage disease causing severe neurological symptoms including seizures, hypotonia, blindness, and death in young affected dogs. Padgett reports a frequency of 0.1% in the breed. A genetic test is available.[3,13,14]

Pyruvate Kinase Deficiency (PK): A rare, autosomal recessive disease of red blood cells causing exercise intolerance with a persistent, severe, and highly regenerative anemia, splenomegaly, and progressive osteosclerosis. A genetic test is available.[15]

Disease Predispositions

Cryptorchidism (Retained testicles): Can be bilateral or unilateral. Padgett reports a frequency of 9.5% in Cairn terriers. Reported at a high frequency in the 2005 CTCA Health Survey.[3,4]

Persistent Pupillary Membranes: Strands of fetal remnant connecting; iris to iris, cornea, lens, or involving sheets of tissue. The later three forms can impair vision, and dogs affected with these forms should not be bred. Identified in 7.57% of Cairn Terriers CERF examined by veterinary ophthalmologists between 2000-2005.[7]

Cataracts: Posterior and equatorial intermediate cataracts predominate in the breed, though anterior, nuclear, and capsular cataracts also occur. Adult-onset cataracts are reported at a high frequency in the 2005 CTCA Health Survey. Identified in 4.14% of Cairn terriers CERF examined by veterinary ophthalmologists between 2000-2005. CERF does not recommend breeding any Cairn Terrier with a cataract.[4,7]

Temperament Issues: Aggression and shyness are reported at a high frequency in the 2005 CTCA Health Survey.[4]

Heart Murmur: Reported at a high frequency in the 2005 CTCA Health Survey (specific diagnosis not identified).[4]

Kinked Tails (caudal hemivertebra): Congenital disorder reported at a high frequency in the 2005 CTCA Health Survey.[4]

Hernias: Padgett reports 4.1% of Cairn terriers with umbilical hernias and 2.3% with inguinal hernias.[3]

Hypothyroidism: Inherited autoimmune thyroiditis. 3.9% positive for thyroid auto-antibodies based on testing at Michigan State University. (Ave. for all breeds is 7.5%).[16,17]

Dental Issues: Padgett reports 3.0% of Cairn terriers with missing teeth, 1.7% with undershot bites, and 1.3% with overshot bites. Undershot bites are reported at a high frequency in the 2005 CTCA Health Survey.[3,4]

Atopy/Allergic Dermatitis: Presents with pruritis and pyotraumatic dermatitis (hot spots). Cairn terriers have a significantly increased risk for atopy versus other breeds. Dorn reports a 1.67x odds ratio versus other breeds. Padgett reports a frequency of 2.6% in the breed. Reported at a high frequency in the 2005 CTCA Health Survey.[3,4,18,19]

Diabetes Mellitus: Cairn terriers are a breed at increased risk of developing diabetes due to immune mediated destruction of the pancreatic beta cells. Related to immuno-regulatory cytokine gene IL-4. Treat with insulin injections, dietary management, and glucose monitoring. One report showed a 6.5x odds ratio versus other breeds.[20,21,22]

Primary (narrow angle) Glaucoma: Ocular condition causing increased pressure within the eyeball, and secondary blindness due to damage to the retina. Diagnose with tonometry and gonioscopy. Diagnosed in 1.82% of Cairn Terriers presented to veterinary teaching hospitals.[23]

Immune-Mediated Hemolytic Anemia: Autoimmune disorder where the body produces antibodies against its own red blood cells. Treatment with immunosuppressive drugs. There is generally a female preponderance with this disorder. One study found a 5.3x odds ratio in Cairn terriers versus other breeds.[24]

Persistent Hyaloid Artery (PHA): Congenital defect resulting from abnormalities in the development and regression of thehyaloid artery. Does not cause vision problems by itself, but is often associated with other ocular defects. Identified in 1.35% of Cairn Terriers CERF examined by veterinary ophthalmologists between 2000-2005.[7]

Hyperadrenocorticism (Cushing's disease): Caused by a functional adrenal or pituitary tumor. Clinical signs may include increased thirst and urination, symmetrical truncal alopecia, and abdominal distention. Dorn reports a 2.32x odds ratio versus other breeds.[18]

Seborrheic Dermatitis: Skin condition due to overproduction of the sebaceous glands in the skin. Unknown mode of inheritance. Dorn reports a 1.24x odds ratio versus other breeds.[18]

Chronic Hepatitis: Cairn terriers are reported to be overrepresented with a histopathological diagnosis of chronic hepatitis.[25]

Oxalate Urolithiasis: Cairn terriers are a breed with increased risk to develop oxalate-containing bladder stones.[26]

Sertoli Cell Testicular Tumor: Testicular tumor that produces estrogens, causing gynecomastia. Treat with castration. Cairn terrier males have a greater risk of developing sertoli cell tumors than other breeds.[27]

Progressive Neuronopathy: A disorder causing progressive hind limb weakness and ataxia in young (1-1-1/2 year old) Cairn terriers, which deteriorates with exercise. The clinical signs progress over several months to tetraparesis. Histopathology demonstates extensive chromatolytic degeneration of neurons and moderate secondary Wallerian-type degeneration in the spinal cord and brain stem. Can be differentiated clinically from globoid cell leukodystrophy by the exercise-induced deterioration of the neurological signs. Unknown mode of inheritance.[28,29]

Multisystemic Chromatolytic Degeneration: Seven cases have been reported in the published literature. Onset is usually around 3-4 months of age. Clinical signs range from mild episodic paraparesis, to bouts of cataplectic collapse. Pathology reveals widespread chromatolytic degeneration in the brain and spinal cord as well as spinal, autonomic, and enteric ganglia. Unknown mode of inheritance.[30,31]

Base narrow Canines, Cleft Lip/Palate, Factor VIII Deficiency, Factor IX Deficiency, Hydrocephalus, Pancreatitis, Progressive Retinal Atrophy, Retinal Dysplasia, Vitamin A Responsive Dermatosis, von Willebrand's Disease, and Wry Mouth are reported.[32]

Isolated Case Studies

Juvenile Polycystic Kidney and Liver Disease: Three related puppies with abdominal distention caused by nephromegaly and hepatomegaly had gross and histologic polycystic lesions in the kidney and liver.[33]

Pseudohermaphrodite: A 6 1/2-month-old Cairn terrier, considered to be a bilateral cryptorchid male, was presented with dysuria and urinary incontinence. This was found to be due to a congenital communication between the urinary bladder and uterus and resulted in distention of the uterus with urine which could not be voided. An ovariohysterectomy was performed. The dog was found to be a genetic female with what resembled external male genitalia.[34]

Anury (congenital taillessness): Two related Cairn Terriers were born without tails, and abnormality of the sacral and caudal vertebra. Both dogs had fecal incontinence. A mating of the two dogs produced two normal offspring.[35]

Multiple Myeloma/Plasmacytoma: A 13 month old female Cairn terrier was diagnosed with multiple myeloma. Radiographically, pelvic tumor masses and characteristic systemic osteolysis were found.[36]

Bronchoesophageal Fistula: A 1-year-old male Cairn terrier was evaluated for chronic coughing that was aggravated by eating or drinking. Radiography revealed an esophageal diverticulum, regional megaesophagus, and focal interstitial densities in the right caudal and middle lunglobes. Radiographic diagnosis was bronchoesophageal fistula. This report references two other cases of bronchoesophageal fistula in the breed.[37]

Genetic Tests

Tests of Genotype: Direct test for Globoid Leukodystrphy is available from the Jefferson Medical College (215-955-1666) and HealthGene.

Direct test for Pyruvate Kinase Deficiency is available from PennGen.

Tests of Phenotype: Recommend hip and elbow radiographs, patella examination, CERF eye examination, thyroid profile including autoantibodies and cardiac evaluation.

Miscellaneous

- **Breed name synonyms:** Short-Haired Skye (historical), Cairn
- **Registries:** AKC, CKC, UKC, KCGB (Kennel Club of Great Britain), ANKC (Australian National Kennel Club), NKC (National Kennel Club)
- **AKC rank (year 2008):** 51 (2,161 registered)
- **Internet resources: Cairn Terrier Club of America:** www.cairnterrier.org
  Cairn Terrier Club of Canada: www.cairnterrierclub.ca
  The Cairn Terrier Club (UK): www.thecairnterrierclub.co.uk

References

1. OFA Website breed statistics: www.offa.org Last accessed July 1, 2010.
2. LaFond E, Breur GJ & Austin CC: Breed susceptibility for developmental orthopedic diseases in dogs. J Am Anim Hosp Assoc. 2002 Sep-Oct;38(5):467-77.
3. Control of Canine Genetic Diseases. Padgett GA. pp. 164-165. Howell Book House, NY. 1998.
4. Cairn Terrier Club of America: 2005 CTCA Health Survey. 2005.
5. Gelatt KN, MacKay EO: Prevalence of the breed-related glaucomas in pure-bred dogs in North America. Vet Ophthalmol. 2004 Mar-Apr;7(2):97-111.
6. Hanselman BA: Melanocytic glaucoma in a cairn terrier. Can Vet J. 2002 Apr;43(4):296-8.
7. Ocular Disorders Presumed to be Inherited in Purebred Dogs. American College of Veterinary Ophthalmologists. ACVO, 2007.
8. Petersen-Jones SM, Forcier J, & Mentzer AL: Ocular melanosis in the Cairn Terrier: clinical description and investigation of mode of inheritance. Vet Ophthalmol. 2007 Nov-Dec;10 Suppl 1:63-9.
9. Petersen-Jones SM, Mentzer AL, Dubielzig RR, et. al.: Ocular melanosis in the Cairn Terrier: histopathological description of the condition, and immunohistological and ultrastructural characterization of the characteristic pigment-laden cells. Vet Ophthalmol. 2008 Jul-Aug;11(4):260-8.
10. van Straten G, Leegwater PA, de Vries M, et. al.: Inherited congenital extrahepatic portosystemic shunts in Cairn terriers. J Vet Intern Med. 2005 May-Jun;19(3):321-4.
11. Schermerhorn T, Center SA, Dykes NL, et. al: Characterization of hepatoportal microvascular dysplasia in a kindred of cairn terriers. J Vet Intern Med. 1996 Jul-Aug;10(4):219-30.
12. Tobias KM, Rohrbach BW: Association of breed with the diagnosis of congenital portosystemic shunts in dogs: 2,400 cases (1980-2002). J Am Vet Med Assoc. 2003 Dec 1;223(11):1636-9.
13. Wenger DA, Victoria T, Rafi MA, et. al.: Globoid cell leukodystrophy in cairn and West Highland white terriers. J Hered. 1999 Jan-Feb;90(1):138-42.
14. Victoria T, Rafi MA, Wenger DA, et. al.: Cloning of the canine GALC cDNA and identification of the mutation causing globoid cell leukodystrophy in West Highland White and Cairn terriers. Genomics. 1996 May 1;33(3):457-62.
15. Skelly BJ, Wallace M, Rajpurohit YR, et. al.: Identification of a 6 base pair insertion in West Highland White Terriers with erythrocyte pyruvate kinase deficiency. Am J Vet Res. 1999 Sep;60(9):1169-72.
16. Nachreiner R & Refsal K: Personal communication, Diagnostic Center for Population and Animal Health, Michigan State University. April, 2007.
17. Nachreiner RF, Refsal KR, Graham PA, et. al.: Prevalence of serum thyroid hormone autoantibodies in dogs with clinical signs of hypothyroidism. J Am Vet Med Assoc 2002 Feb 15;220(4):466-71.
18. Dorn CR: Canine breed-specific risks of frequently diagnosed diseases at veterinary teaching hospitals. Monograph. AKC Canine Health Foundation. 2000.
19. Schick RO, Fadok VA: Responses of atopic dogs to regional allergens: 268 cases (1981-1984). J Am Vet Med Assoc. 1986 Dec 1;189(11):1493-6.
20. Catchpole B, Ristic JM, Fleeman LM, et. al.: Canine diabetes mellitus: can old dogs teach us new tricks? Diabetologia. 2005 Oct;48(10):1948-56.
21. Catchpole B, Kennedy LJ, Davison LJ, et. al.: Canine diabetes mellitus: from phenotype to genotype. J Small Anim Pract. 2008 Jan;49(1):4-10.
22. Short AD, Catchpole B, Kennedy LJ, et. al.: T cell cytokine gene polymorphisms in canine diabetes mellitus. Vet Immunol
23. Gelatt KN, MacKay EO: Prevalence of the breed-related glaucomas in pure-bred dogs in North America. Vet Ophthalmol. 2004 Mar-Apr;7(2):97-111.
24. Miller SA, Hohenhaus AE, Hale AS: Case-control study of blood type, breed, sex, and bacteremia in dogs with immune-mediated hemolytic anemia. J Am Vet Med Assoc. 2004 Jan 15;224(2):232-5.
25. Watson PJ: Chronic Hepatitis in Dogs. Proceedings, 2009 British Small

Animal Veterinary Congress. 2009.

26. Ling GV, Franti CE, Ruby AL, et. al.: Urolithiasis in dogs. II: Breed prevalence, and interrelations of breed, sex, age, and mineral composition. *Am J Vet Res.* 1998 May;59(5):630-42.

27. Weaver AD: Survey with follow-up of 67 dogs with testicular sertoli cell tumours. *Vet Rec.* 1983 Jul 30;113(5):105-7.

28. Zaal MD, van den Ingh TS, Goedegebuure SA, et. al: Progressive neuronopathy in two Cairn terrier litter mates. *Vet Q.* 1997 Mar;19(1):34-6.

29. Palmer AC, Blakemore WF: Progressive neuronopathy in the cairn terrier. *Vet Rec.* 1988 Jul 2;123(1):39.

30. Cummings JF, De Lahunta A, Moore JJ 3rd: Multisystemic chromatolytic neuronal degeneration in a Cairn terrier pup. *Cornell Vet.* 1988 Jul;78(3):301-14.

31. Cummings JF, de Lahunta A, Gasteiger EL: Multisystemic chromatolytic neuronal degeneration in Cairn terriers. A case with generalized cataplectic episodes. J Vet Intern Med. 1991 Mar-Apr;5(2):91-4.

32. *The Genetic Connection: A Guide to Health Problems in Purebred Dogs.* L Ackerman. p. 208, AAHA Press, 1999.

33. McKenna SC, Carpenter JL: Polycystic disease of the kidney and liver in the Cairn Terrier. *Vet Pathol.* 1980 Jul;17(4):436-42.

34. van Schouwenburg SJ, Louw GJ: A case of dysuria as a result of a communication between the urinary bladder and corpus uteri in a Cairn Terrier. *J S Afr Vet Assoc.* 1982 Mar;53(1):65-6.

35. Hall DS, Amann JF, Constantinescu GM, et. al.: Anury in two Cairn terriers. J Am Vet Med Assoc. 1987 Nov 1;191(9):1113-5.

36. Tuch E, Tuch K: Multiple myeloma/plasmacytoma in a young dog. *Tierarztl Prax.* 1992 Jun;20(3):292-5.

37. Basher AW, Hogan PM, Hanna PE, et. al.: Surgical treatment of a congenital bronchoesophageal fistula in a dog. *J Am Vet Med Assoc.* 1991 Aug 15;199(4):479-82.

38. *The Complete Dog Book, 20th Ed.* The American Kennel Club. Howell Book House, NY 2006. p 362-365.

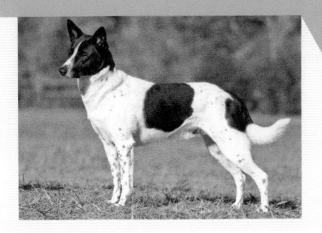

The Breed History

This rare and ancient Israeli breed, which dates back to 2000 BC originates from ancient Pariah dog stock and is named after the Land of Canaan. For many years, the dog apparently ran feral in the Negev desert and the coastal plains. Adoption by some of the Bedouin tribes helped to sustain their numbers. During the Israeli War of Independence and in WWII, a number were located and trained. The first dogs arrived in America in the year 1965. The AKC accepted the breed in 1997.

Breeding for Function

In ancient times, the dogs served as a herding and guard dog for flock and home. During the wars of the 20th century in Israel they served as messengers, mine detectors, trackers, and guard dogs. After WWII, they were further bred and trained for work as service dogs.

Physical Characteristics

Height at Withers: female 19-23" (48-58.5 cm), male 20-24" (51-61 cm).

Weight: females 35-45 lb (16-20.5 kg), males 45-55 lb (20.5-25 kg).

Coat: The flat short (0.5-1.5") harsh outer coat is straight and the inner coat is flat, short and soft. The ruff is more obvious in the male dog. The accepted colors are:
1. Solid (black, brown) with or without specified markings.
2. Mostly solid white, with or without body patches of color, and with a matching symmetrical mask. The mask may contain a small blaze of white only.

Longevity: 12-13 years

Points of Conformation: There are 2 subtypes of dogs, the so –called "stockdog" type and a longer coated, heavier type dog. Overall, the standard requires a medium-sized dog with medium-large erect ears, a long wedge-shaped head and square conformation. Almond-shaped dark colored eyes are slightly slanted up. Palpebral rims are colored liver or black, and the stop is moderate. The neck is moderate in muscling and length and well arched, not throaty. The topline is level except for a slight loin arch. The thorax is moderately deep and ribs are well sprung, and abdomen well tucked up. The "bottle brush" tail may be curled once over the back when excited, and the length of the tail is to

the tarsus at rest. Limbs are straight boned, and dewclaws may be removed. The Canaan dogs have compact feet with well-knuckled toes. Gait is agile, quick, powerful.

Recognized Behavior Issues and Traits

Reported breed characteristics include: Aloof with strangers, loyal, affectionate with owners, high intelligence, sensitive, good trainability. They are considered an easy keeping dog; tolerates warm and cold well. Has moderate shedding tendency, and low grooming needs. The Canaan has moderate exercise needs, and needs thorough and early socialization. Some exhibit inter-dog aggressions, especially inter-male. Canaans are alert alarm barkers, with a moderate to high barking tendency.

Normal Physiologic Variations

None reported

Drug Sensitivities

None reported

Inherited Diseases

Hip Dysplasia: Polygenically inherited trait causing degenerative joint disease and hip arthritis. OFA reports 2.2% affected.[1]

Elbow Dysplasia: Polygenically inherited trait causing elbow arthritis. OFA reports 1.8% affected.[1]

Patella Luxation: Polygenically inherited laxity of patellar ligaments, causing luxation, lameness, and later degenerative joint disease. Treat surgically if causing clinical signs. OFA reports 1.7% affected.[1]

Disease Predispositions

Cataracts: Posterior and nuclear intermediate cataracts predominate in the breed. Identified in 4.35% of Canaan Dogs CERF examined by veterinary ophthalmologists between 2000-2005. CERF does not recommend breeding any Canaan Dog with a cataract.[2]

Persistent Pupillary Membranes: Strands of fetal remnant connecting; iris to iris, cornea, lens, or involving sheets of tissue. The later three forms can impair vision, and dogs affected with these forms should not be bred. Identified in 3.86% of Canaan Dogs CERF examined by veterinary ophthalmologists between 2000-2005.[2]

Distichiasis: Abnormally placed eyelashes that irritate the cornea and conjunctiva. Can cause secondary corneal ulceration. Identified in 2.42% of Canaan Dogs CERF examined by veterinary ophthalmologists between 2000-2005.[2]

Progressive Retinal Atrophy (PRA): Progressive degeneration of the retina, eventually causing blindness. 1.93% of Canaan Dogs CERF examined by veterinary ophthalmologists were diagnosed with generalized PRA, and 1.93% were labeled suspicious for PRA between 2000-2005. Undetermined mode of inheritance. CERF does not recommend breeding any Canaan Dog with PRA.[2,3]

Idiopathic Epilepsy: Generalized or partial seizures. Control with anti-seizure medication. Seen at an increased frequency in the breed. Unknown mode of inheritance.[3]

Cryptorchidism (Retained testicles): Can be bilateral or unilateral. Seen at an increased frequency in the breed.[3]

Hypothyroidism: Inherited autoimmune thyroiditis. 2.1% positive for thyroid auto-antibodies based on testing at Michigan State University. (Ave. for all breeds is 7.5%).[4,5]

Degenerative Myelopathy (DM): Affected dogs show an insidious onset of upper motor neuron (UMN) paraparesis. The disease eventually progresses to severe tetraparesis. Affected dogs have normal results on myelography, MRI, and CSF analysis. Necropsy confirms the condition. A direct genetic test for an autosomal recessive DM susceptibility gene is available. All affected dogs are homozygous for the gene, however only a small percentage of homozygous dogs develop DM. Reported as a clinical disease in the breed. In limited testing, OFA reports a high frequency of Canaan dogs positive for the DM susceptibility gene.[3,6]

Isolated Case Studies
None Reported

Genetic Tests
Tests of Genotype: Direct test for a DM susceptibility gene is available from OFA.

Tests of Phenotype: CHIC Certification: Required tests are; hip and elbow radiographs, patella examination, CERF eye examination, and thyroid profile including autoantibodies. (See CHIC website: www.caninehealthinfo.org)

Recomend cardiac evaluation.

Miscellaneous
- **Breed name synonyms:** Kelef K'naani, Kelev Cana'ani, Canaan.
- **Registries:** AKC, UKC, CKC, KCGB (Kennel Club of Great Britain), ANKC (Australian National Kennel Club), NKC (National Kennel Club).
- **AKC rank (year 2008):** 150 (61 dogs registered)
- **Internet resources:** The Canaan Dog Club of America: www.cdca.org (the AKC parent club)
  The Israel Canaan Dog Club of America: www.itb.it/canaan/icdca/ (UKC parent club)
  British Canaan Dog Society: www.thecanaandog.co.uk

References
1. OFA Website breed statistics: www.offa.org Last accessed July 1, 2010.
2. *Ocular Disorders Presumed to be Inherited in Purebred Dogs.* American College of Veterinary Ophthalmologists. ACVO, 2007.
3. Israel Canaan Dog Club of America: ICDCA Health Database. 2007.
4. Nachreiner R & Refsal K: Personal communication, Diagnostic Center for Population and Animal Health, Michigan State University. April, 2007.
5. Nachreiner RF, Refsal KR, Graham PA, et. al.: Prevalence of serum thyroid hormone autoantibodies in dogs with clinical signs of hypothyroidism. J Am Vet Med Assoc 2002 Feb 15;220(4):466-71.
6. Coates JR, Zeng R, Awano T, et. al.: An SOD1 Mutation Associated with Degenerative Myelopathy Occurs in Many Dog Breeds.Proceedings, 2009 ACVIM Forum. 2009.
7. *The Complete Dog Book, 20th Ed.* The American Kennel Club. Howell Book House, NY 2006. p. 650-653.

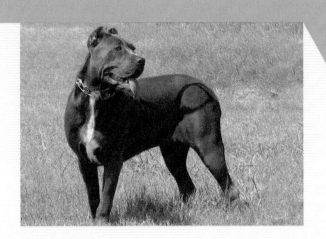

Cane Corso

The Breed History

One of two native Italian "mastiff type" dogs that descended from the Roman canis Pugnaces, the breed's name derives from the Latin "Cohors" which means "Guardian" and "Protector." He was a property watchdog and hunted wild boar. Prior to 1988, the Cane Corso was known only in southern Italy, and was considered very rare, but has still been featured in many paintings throughout Italy's history. AKC recognition occurred in 2010.

Breeding for Function

The Cane was developed to perform multiple tasks from combat to herding of cattle, and guard dog. He was employed in the hunting of large wild animals and also as an "auxiliary warrior" in battles.

Physical Characteristics

Height at withers: Males: 25 to 27.5 inches (63.5-70 cm); Females: 23.5 to 26 inches (60-66 cm).

Weight: Males 99-110 pounds (45-50 kg) Females 88-99 pounds (40-45 kg).

Coat: The breed's coat is short but not smooth, very coarse and thick in order to be perfectly waterproof. It can be black, gray, fawn or red, with brindle variations and a black or gray mask also acceptable.

Longevity: 10-11 years.

Points of Conformation: A muscular, balanced, large-boned dog, rectangular in proportion. The head is molossus type; its total length reaches approximately one third of the height at the withers. Eyes are medium-size, tight, almond-shaped, brown, not round or bulging. Ears are set well above the cheekbones. Nose is large, black or grey, with well-opened nostrils. Lips are firm, with upper lips moderately hanging. The bite is slightly undershot to level. There is only a small amount of dewlap. Depth of the ribcage is equal to half the total height of the dog, descending slightly below the elbow. The rump is round due to muscling. The tail set is an extension of the backline, thick at the root with not much tapering at the tip. The legs are strong and muscular. Elbows are parallel to the ribcage, neither turning in or out. Feet are round and well arched. The gait is free flowing and powerful, effortless, with strong reach and drive, and a single track at full gait.

Recognized Behavior Issues and Traits

The Cane Corso is a protector of his property and owners. Intelligent, the Cane Corso is easily trained. As a large and athletic breed, they need a lot of exercise. They are affectionate to their owner and bond closely with children and family. They can be aggressive to other dogs and to strangers, including other children. Cane Corsos are light shedders, which make grooming simple – all they need is an occasional brushing.

Normal Physiologic Variations

None reported

Drug Sensitivities

None reported

Inherited Diseases

Hip Dysplasia: Polygenically inherited trait causing degenerative joint disease and hip arthritis. OFA reports 40.5% affected. A French study showed 59.7% affected.[1,2]

Elbow Dysplasia: Polygenically inherited trait causing elbow arthritis. OFA reports 10.4% affected.[1]

Patella Luxation: Polygenically inherited laxity of patellar ligaments, causing luxation, lameness, and later degenerative joint disease. Treat surgically if causing clinical signs. Too few Cane Corso have been screened by OFA to determine an accurate frequency.[1]

Multifocal Retinopathy/Retinal Dysplasia: Autosomal recessive retinal pigment epithelial dysplasia causing localized multifocal retinal detachments. Age of onset from 11 to 13 weeks of age. A genetic test is available.

Disease Predispositions

Malassia Otitis: Cane Corso are overrepresented with mycotic otitis. 51.7% of the breed was identified in one study.[3]

Gastric Dilatation–Volvulus (bloat, GDV): Polygenically inherited, life-threatening twisting of the stomach within the abdomen. Requires immediate treatment. Reported as a breed health issue on the CCAA website.

Hypothyroidism: Inherited autoimmune thyroiditis. Not enough samples have been submitted for thyroid auto-antibodies to Michigan State University to determine an accurate frequency. (Ave. for all breeds is 7.5%).[4,5]

Ectropion: Rolling out of eyelids, often with a medial canthal pocket. Can also cause secondary conjunctivitis. Reported as a breed health issue on the CCAA website.

Entropion: A rolling in of the eyelids that can cause corneal irritation and ulceration. Reported as a breed health issue on the CCAA website.

Prolapsed Gland of the Nictitans (Cherry Eye): This condition is secondary to chronic conjunctivitis, usually of an allergic nature. Reported as a breed health issue on the CCAA website.

Demodicosis, generalized: Overgrowth of demodex mites in hair follicles due to an underlying immunodeficiency. Causes hair loss and inflammation. Reported as a breed health issue on the CCAA website.

Idiopathic Epilepsy (inherited seizures): Control with anti-seizure medication. Reported as a breed issue on the Cane Corso Club of Canada website.

Inherited Ocular Disorders: Too few Cane Corsos have been CERF examined by veterinary ophthalmologists to determine an accurate frequency of inherited ocular disorders.[6]

Isolated Case Studies

Primary osseous melanoma: An 18-month-old, female Cane Corso dog was presented with a suspected primary tumor of the tibia. A diagnosis of malignant melanoma was made by cytology. No metastatic lesions were identified. The dog was alive 3-1/2 years after amputation.[7]

Genetic Tests

Tests of Genotype: Direct test for retinal dysplasia is available from Optigen.

Tests of Phenotype: Recommend hip and elbow radiographs, CERF eye examination, thyroid profile including autoantibodies, cardiac evaluation, and patella evaluation.

Miscellaneous

- **Breed name synonyms:** Cane Corso Italiano, Cane di Macellaio, Sicilian Branchiero, Italian Mastiff
- **Registries:** AKC, UKC, FCI, NKC (National Kennel Club)
- **AKC rank:** (none) AKC recognized in June 2010. Entire stud book entered.
- **Internet resources: Cane Corso Association of America:** www.canecorso.org
  Society In America For Cane Corso Italiano: www.thesacci.com
  The British Cane Corso Society: www.canecorso.org.uk
  Cane Corso Club of Canada: www.canecorsoclubofcanada.ca

References

1. OFA Website breed statistics: www.offa.org Last accessed July 1, 2010.
2. Genevois JP, Remy D, Viguier E, et. al.: Prevalence of hip dysplasia according to official radiographic screening, among 31 breeds of dogs in France. Vet Comp Orthop Traumatol. 2008;21(1):21-4.
3. Cristina RT & Dégi J: Studies on Otitis Externa in Dogs. Proceedings, 17th ECVIM-CA Congress. 2007.
4. Nachreiner R & Refsal K: Personal communication, Diagnostic Center for Population and Animal Health, Michigan State University. April, 2007.
5. Nachreiner RF, Refsal KR, Graham PA, et. al.: Prevalence of serum thyroid hormone autoantibodies in dogs with clinical signs of hypothyroidism. J Am Vet Med Assoc 2002 Feb 15;220(4):466-71.
6. Ocular Disorders Presumed to be Inherited in Purebred Dogs. American College of Veterinary Ophthalmologists. ACVO, 2007.
7. Stefanello D, Romussi S, Signorelli P, et. al.: Primary osseous melanoma in the tibia of a dog. J Am Anim Hosp Assoc. 2008 May-Jun;44(3):139-43.
8. AKC Breed Website: www.akc.org/breeds/cane_corso Last accessed July 1, 2010.

Cardigan Welsh Corgi

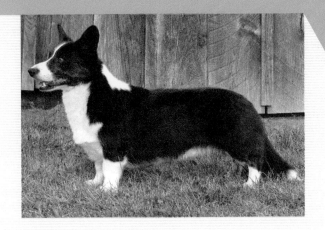

The Breed History

In early history, and arising from the same type of dog that gave rise to the Dachshund, the progenitors of the modern day Cardigan Welsh Corgi were brought to Cardiganshire in Wales around 1200 BC. Other bloodlines that may have contributed to the corgi type include Shipperke, Swedish Valhunds, and Finnish Spitz dogs. Breeders split the breed into Cardigan and Pembroke Corgis around 1934. In 1931, Cardis were first brought to the US, and the AKC registered them in 1935. The name Corgi is thought to be a Celtic word for *dog* or perhaps a Welsh word for *dwarf* dog.

Breeding for Function

These dogs were valued as guarding dogs, and were used to manage cattle by driving and dispersing them on the common pastures. They were also valued as a vermin hunter. They perform well in agility and herding competitions, and have become a popular companion pet.

Physical Characteristics

Height at Withers: female 10.5-12.5 " (26.5-31.5 cm), male 10.5-12.5 " (26.5-31.5 cm).

Weight: females 25-34 lb (11.5-15.5 kg), males 30-38 lb (13.5-17 kg).

Coat: The double coat of medium length should never be primarily white. Blue merle may have pigmented points, and black, red, sable, and brindle coats may have white on chest, legs, neck, face (except around eyes), and tail tip. A tri-color coat is also sometimes seen. They are not clipped for show.

Longevity: 12-15 years.

Points of Conformation: These sturdy, low-set muscular dogs with great agility and intelligence have a very alert expression. Their forefeet normally are displaced laterally and legs bowed due to chondrodystrophic conformation. Their eyes have dark pigmentation at the palpebral margin and the eyes are dark except in the blue merles, where blue eyes are acceptable. The face has a moderate stop, and the muzzle is tapered. Moderate length of neck, and well-sprung ribs with moderate tuck up in loins are evident. The long back has only a slight slope down towards the tail base along the topline. The tail is long and thick and rear dewclaws are generally removed. The Pembroke is shorter, has straighter legs,

ears are smaller and more pointed, and the tail is docked short in comparison.

Recognized Behavior Issues and Traits

Reported breed characteristics include: Loyal, protective intelligent dog, they learn quickly, and are active dogs. They are wary of strangers, and are an excellent alarm barker. Early training and socialization to people and other pets are important for these dogs. They may try to herd children by nipping at the heels, but can be trained away from this behavior. If left alone for long periods, these dogs tend to chew or bark. They benefit from daily moderate exercise, and are generally calmer than Pembrokes. They are high shedders, but require low to moderate grooming.

Normal Physiologic Variations

None reported

Drug Sensitivities

None reported

Inherited Diseases

Hip Dysplasia: Polygenically inherited trait causing degenerative joint disease and hip arthritis. OFA reports 19.1% affected.[1]

Patella Luxation: Polygenically inherited laxity of patellar ligaments, causing luxation, lameness, and later degenerative joint disease. Treat surgically if causing clinical signs. Reported at a high rate, but too few Cardigan Welsh Corgis have been screened by OFA to determine an accurate frequency.[1]

Elbow Dysplasia: Polygenically inherited trait causing elbow arthritis. OFA reports 3.2% affected.[1]

Progressive Retinal Atrophy (PRA): Autosomal recessive rcd3 form of PRA occurs in the breed. Begins with night blindness by 6 months of age, and total blindness by 2-3 years. A genetic test is available, showing 8.5% testing carrier. CERF does not recommend breeding affected dogs.[2,3,4]

Disease Predispositions

Hypothyroidism: Inherited autoimmune thyroiditis. 5.5% positive for thyroid auto-antibodies based on testing at Michigan State University. (Ave. for all breeds is 7.5%).[5,6]

Persistent Pupillary Membranes: Strands of fetal remnant connecting; iris to iris, cornea, lens, or involving sheets of tissue. The later three forms can impair vision, and dogs affected with these forms should not be bred. Identified in 4.71% of Cardigan Welsh Corgis CERF examined by veterinary ophthalmologists between 2000-2007.[7]

Distichiasis: Abnormally placed eyelashes that irritate the cornea and conjunctiva. Can cause secondary corneal ulceration. Identified in 4.20% of Cardigan Welsh Corgis CERF examined by veterinary ophthalmologists between 2000-2005.[7]

Cataracts: Anterior cortex punctate cataracts predominate in the breed. Age of onset 3 years. Reported in 2.53% of Cardigan Welsh Corgis presented to veterinary teaching hospitals. Identified in 1.91% of Cardigan Welsh Corgis CERF examined by veterinary ophthalmologists between 2000-2005. CERF does not recommend breeding any Cardigan Welsh Corgi with a cataract.[7,8]

Degenerative Myelopathy (DM): Affected dogs show an insidious onset of upper motor neuron (UMN) paraparesis at an average age of 11.4 years. The disease eventually progresses to severe tetraparesis. Affected dogs have normal results on myelography, MRI, and CSF analysis. Necropsy confirms the condition. Reported at a frequency of 1.51% in Cardigan Welsh Corgis. Unknown mode of inheritance. A direct genetic test for an autosomal recessive DM susceptibility gene is available. All affected dogs are homozygous for the gene, however, only a small percentage of homozygous dogs develop DM. OFA testing reports 39% carrier and 10% homozygous "at risk" for DM.[9,10]

Retinal Dysplasia: Focal folds and geographic retinal dysplasia are seen in the breed. It is questionable whether focal folds can lead to disease, however dogs with the geographic form should not be bred. Reported in 0.76% of Cardigan Welsh Corgis CERF examined by veterinary ophthalmologists between 2000-2005.[7]

Cystinuria/Cystine Bladder Stones: Caused by a metabolic abnormality in cystine metabolism. Welsh Corgis have an increased risk for developing cystine bladder stones. Treat with surgical removal and life-long medical therapy. Unknown mode of inheritance in this breed. Dorn reports a 4.14x increased odds ratio for bladder stones versus other breeds.[11,12,13,14]

Perineal Hernia: An Australian study identified the Corgi breed as most commonly affected with perineal hernias. The mean age of affected dogs was 9.4 years. Treatment is herniorrhaphy surgery.[15]

Glaucoma: Primary, narrow angle glaucoma occurs in the breed. Can cause blindness due to retinal damage, or secondary lens luxation. Screen with gonioscopy and tonometry. Frequency and mode of inheritance in the breed has not been determined.[16]

Intervertebral Disc Disease (IVDD): Serious neurological condition where disk degeneration and rupture into spinal nerves and the spinal cord causes pain and possible paralysis. Requires immediate veterinary care. Dorn reports a 1.70x increased odds ratio versus other breeds.[14]

Central progressive Retinal Atrophy, Ceroid Lipofuscinosis, and Methemaglobin Reductase Deficiency are reported.[17]

Isolated Case Studies

X-linked Severe Combined Immunodeficiency (XSCID): X-linked recessive disorder was identified in one family of Cardigan Welsh Corgis. Affected dogs cannot generate antigen-specific immune responses. A genetic test was developed to identify carrier females.[18]

Mucopolysaccharidosis VI (MPS VI): PennGen reports MPS VI

identified in the Welsh Corgi. This is an autosomal recessive disorder causing skeletal deformities, including defects in the sternum, vertebrae and particularly the hip joints. To varying degrees they may also experience corneal cloudiness and facial dysmorphia. A genetic test is available.

Genetic Tests

Tests of Genotype: Direct test for rcd3 form of PRA is available from Optigen, Healthgene, VetGen, and the Peterson-Jones Lab. at Michigan State University: http://www.cardigancorgis.com/PRAPressRelease.aspx (517-353-3278)

Direct coat color tests for presence of black, "clear red", chocolate and sable colors, and mask are available from HealthGene and VetGen.

Direct genetic test for an autosomal recessive DM susceptibility gene is available from the OFA.

Direct tests for SCID is available from PennGen.

Phenotypic test for MPS VI is available from PennGen.

Tests of Phenotype: CHIC Certification: Required tests are; CERF eye examination, genetic test for rcd3-PRA, and hip radiographs. (See CHIC website: www.caninehealthinfo.org)

Recommend patella evaluation, elbow radiographs, thyroid profile including autoantibodies, and cardiac evaluation.

Miscellaneous

- **Breed name synonyms:** Cardigan, Corgi, Cardi
- **Registries:** AKC, UKC, CKC , KCGB (Kennel Club of Great Britain), ANKC (Australian National Kennel Club), NKC (National Kennel Club)
- **AKC rank (year 2008):** 82 (845 dogs registered)
- **Internet resources: Cardigan Welsh Corgi Club of America:** www.cardigancorgis.com
  Cardigan Welsh Corgi Association (UK): www.cardiganwelshcorgiassoc.co.uk
  Canadian Cardigan Corgi Club: www.cardigancorgi.ca

References

1. OFA Website breed statistics: www.offa.org Last accessed July 1, 2010.
2. Petersen-Jones SM, Entz DD: An improved DNA-based test for detection of the codon 616 mutation in the alpha cyclic GMP phosphodiesterase gene that causes progressive retinal atrophy in the Cardigan Welsh Corgi. *Vet Ophthalmol.* 2002 Jun;5(2):103-6.
3. Petersen-Jones SM, Entz DD, Sargan DR: cGMP phosphodiesterase-alpha mutation causes progressive retinal atrophy in the Cardigan Welsh corgi dog. *Invest Ophthalmol Vis Sci.* 1999 Jul;40(8):1637-44.
4. Keep JM: Clinical aspects of progressive retinal atrophy in the Cardigan Welsh Corgi. *Aust Vet J.* 1972 Apr;48(4):197-9.
5. Nachreiner R & Refsal K: Personal communication, Diagnostic Center for Population and Animal Health, Michigan State University. April, 2007.
6. Nachreiner RF, Refsal KR, Graham PA, et. al.: Prevalence of serum thyroid hormone autoantibodies in dogs with clinical signs of hypothyroidism. J Am Vet Med Assoc 2002 Feb 15;220(4):466-71.
7. *Ocular Disorders Presumed to be Inherited in Purebred Dogs.* American College of Veterinary Ophthalmologists. ACVO, 2007.
8. Gelatt KN, Mackay EO: Prevalence of primary breed-related cataracts in the dog in North America. Vet Ophthalmol. 2005 Mar-Apr;8(2):101-11.
9. Coates JR, Zeng R, Awano T, et. al.: An SOD1 Mutation Associated with

Degenerative Myelopathy Occurs in Many Dog Breeds.Proceedings, 2009 ACVIM Forum. 2009.

10. Coates JR & Wade C: Update on the Genetic Basis of Canine Degenerative Myelopathy. Proceedings, 2008 ACVIM Forum. 2008.

11. Weichselbaum RC, Feeney DA, Jessen CR, et. al.: Evaluation of the morphologic characteristics and prevalence of canine urocystoliths from a regional urolith center. *Am J Vet Res.* 1998 Apr;59(4):379-87.

12. Bovee KC, McGuire T: Qualitative and quantitative analysis of uroliths in dogs: definitive determination of chemical type. *J Am Vet Med Assoc.* 1984 Nov 1;185(9):983-7.

13. Case LC, Ling GV, Franti CE, et. al.: Cystine-containing urinary calculi in dogs: 102 cases (1981-1989). *J Am Vet Med Assoc.* 1992 Jul 1;201(1):129-33.

14. Dorn CR: Canine breed-specific risks of frequently diagnosed diseases at veterinary teaching hospitals. Monograph. AKC Canine Health Foundation. 2000.

15. Bellenger CR: Perineal hernia in dogs. *Aust Vet J.* 1980 Sep;56(9):434-8.

16. Ketring KL: Schirmer Testing & Tonometry Are "Good Medicine". Proceedings, 2005 Western Veterinary Conference. 2005.

17. *The Genetic Connection: A Guide to Health Problems in Purebred Dogs.* L Ackerman. p. 242-43, AAHA Press, 1999

18. Pullen RP, Somberg RL, Felsburg PJ, et. al.: X-linked severe combined immunodeficiency in a family of Cardigan Welsh corgis. *J Am Anim Hosp Assoc.* 1997 Nov-Dec;33(6):494-9.

19. *The Complete Dog Book, 20th Ed.* The American Kennel Club. Howell Book House, NY 2006. p. 654-658.

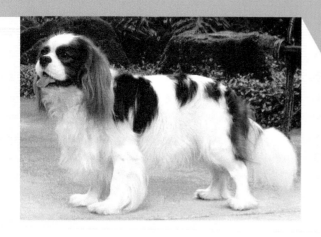

The Breed History

The ancestor of this small spaniel is recorded in tapestry and art in the 15th century; a Toy spaniel was perhaps a luxury item for aristocrats since this was definitely a non-hunting dog. They were the chosen dogs of the Court of King Charles I and II and at this point in this line of dogs, the name was given as King Charles spaniel. In the time of Queen Victoria, a short nosed dome skull type was preferred, and the old type fell out of favor. In the USA, type reflected the old longer-muzzled low stop version of the Toy spaniel of Charles II time, and that variant is now recognized by the old name of English Toy spaniel. In Britain, a return to the long-faced variety that more closely resembled the spaniels in old paintings was bred, and the classic type was accepted into registration as the **Cavalier** King Charles spaniel to distinguish it from the short-nosed King Charles. It was first registered in AKC 1962 in the miscellaneous class, but full recognition occurred in 1996, at which time they were assigned to the Toy group.

Breeding for Function

Bred for companionship. They are suitable for obedience trials as well.

Physical Characteristics

Height at Withers: female 12-13" (30.5-33 cm), male 12-13" (30.5-33 cm).

Weight: females 13-17lb (6-7.5 kg) , males 14-18 lb (6-8 kg).

Coat: The silky, soft, slightly wavy moderately long coat is lightly feathered. *Blenheim* color is a white dog with chestnut markings and a specific chestnut mark on the forehead in a white blaze is favored (Blenheim mark). Other colors include tri-color in red, white and black. Ruby, a red solid, and black and tan are other coat color variants.

Longevity: 9-14 years.

Points of Conformation: They have very soft expressions, and their large dark brown eyes are set wide apart on a broad face. The skull is not domed and a moderate stop is present, the nose is large, square and black. The ears are pendulous and feathering is moderate. Slightly longer than tall, they are moderately boned, and the neck is long and slightly arched. The topline is level and chest is moderately deep with ribs well sprung. Their tail may be docked.

Cavalier King Charles Spaniel

It is held level with the topline or a bit lower. They possess straight legs and compact feet, and dewclaws may be removed. Their movement is smooth and low, and straight with long strides.

Recognized Behavior Issues and Traits

The dog is a devoted, intelligent, playful and friendly dog. They need to be in an environment with lots of human contact. They enjoy the company of children and other pets. They are active and require average exercise. They have a well-developed chase instinct, so must not be off-leash unless in an enclosure. They are moderate shedding dogs and require regular levels of grooming. It is helpful to trim around the paws to help prevent matting. They are known as the perfect lap dog. They are alarm barkers.

Normal Physiologic Variations

AsymptomaticThrombocytopenia/Macrothrombocytopenia: Cavalier King Charles spaniels (CKCS) often have idiopathic asymptomatic thrombocytopenia (< 100,000 platelets/microL). In affected dogs, the thrombocytes are often large. Platelet mass (plateletcrit) is a better measurement of platelet function in the breed. The condition is due to an autosomal recessive mutation in the beta1-tubulin gene. A genetic test is available.[1,2,3,4]

Temporomandibular Joint Dysplasia: Temporomandibular joint dysplasia is a widespread asymptomatic condition in the breed and should be regarded as a normal morphologic variation rather than a pathologic anomaly.[5]

Drug Sensitivities

None reported

Inherited Diseases

Hip Dysplasia and Legg-Calve Perthes Disease: Polygenically inherited traits causing degenerative hip joint disease and arthritis. OFA reports 12.1% affected. Reported at a frequency of 4.2% in the ACKCSC, Inc. Health Survey 2004-2005.[6,7]

Patella Luxation: Polygenically inherited laxity of patellar ligaments, causing luxation, lameness, and later degenerative joint disease. Treat surgically if causing clinical signs. Reported 9.1x odds ratio versus other breeds. OFA reports 2.3% affected. Reported at a frequency of 6.2% in the ACKCSC, Inc. Health Survey 2004-2005.[6,7,8]

Elbow Dysplasia: Polygenically inherited trait causing elbow arthritis. OFA reports 0.7% affected.[6]

Episodic Collapse (Paroxysmal Hypertonicity, Hyperexplexia): Autosomal recessive disorder in the breed. Collapse with increased limb extensor tone triggered by excitement and characterized by a brief period of bunny hopping with the head held down and the rear end raised. Affected dogs may show signs starting at three months of age. Treatment is with clonazepam. The condition resolves over time in some dogs. A genetic test is available.[36,52,53]

Muscular Dystrophy: X-linked recessive muscular dystrophy due to a mutation in the dystrophin gene has been identified in the breed. Affected dogs show clinical signs from a few months of age, including weakness, muscle atrophy, exercise intolerance, dysphagia and macroglossia (enlarged tongue). Serum creatine kinase is usually markedly elevated. Male dogs with the mutation are clinically affected and female dogs with the mutation are silent carriers. Affected males with the same mutation have been identified in the UK and the USA.[9,10]

Congenital Keratoconjunctivitis Sicca (KCS) and Ichthyosiform Dermatosis: Rare autosomal recessive, congenital disorder in the breed of lack of tear production and scaly skin. In affected dogs, the coat appears curly at birth, and the skin deteriorates as the dog matures. The eye condition is treatable with lubricants. A genetic test is available.[58]

Disease Predispositions

Chronic Mitral Valve Disease/Mitral Prolapse: Systolic heart murmurs caused by chronic mitral valve disease are common in the breed, with an average age of diagnosis of 6.25 years. Left atrial enlargement, and not heart enlargement, should be used to evaluate the heart size and indirectly the severity of mitral regurgitation on radiographs. Left atrial enlargement is found to occur only in the last year prior to congestive heart failure. Echocardiographic studies suggest that mitral regurgitation and prolapse may be present in most affected dogs by 5 years of age. Predisposition may be related to serotonin (5HT) metabolism. Heritability estimates of 0.67 for the grade of murmur and 0.33 for the presence/absence of murmur have been calculated in the breed. Heart murmurs are reported at a frequency of 30.7%, and mitral valve disease at 27.0% in the ACKCSC, Inc. Health Survey 2004-2005. Mode of inheritance has not been determined.[7,11,12,13,14,15,16]

Chiari-like Malformation (Occipital Bone Hypoplasia): This condition is characterized by a shortening of the basicranium and supra-occipital bone with a compensatory lengthening of the cranial vault, especially the parietal bone. CM can be diagnosed with MRI. CM can strongly predispose, but is not necessary for the brain disease syringomyelia.[17,18,19,20,21,22,23,24,25,26,27]

Pancreatic Acinar Atrophy (Exocrine Pancreatic Insufficiency): Cavalier King Charles Spaniels are found to have an increased incidence of for immune-mediated pancreatic acinar atrophy. Clinical signs are poor weight gain, and steatorrhea. One study in the UK found a prevalence of 26.3%. Median age of onset is 6 years. Treat with pancreatic enzyme supplementation. Breeding studies suggest an autosomal recessive mode of inheritance in German shepherd dogs, another breed found at risk.[28]

Brachycephalic Complex: Includes **elongated soft palate, stenotic nares, hypoplastic trachea,** and **everted laryngeal saccules.** Causes dyspnea, and can cause collapse and death with extreme stress. Identified in 20.5% of Cavalier King Charles spaniels in an Australian study. Surgery is indicated in severe cases.[29]

Umbilical Hernias: Congenital inherited umbilical hernias are reported at 12.1% in the ACKCSC, Inc. Health Survey 2004-2005.[7]

Retinal Dysplasia: Focal retinal dysplasia with retinal folds is reported in 9.30%, and geographic retinal dysplasia is reported in 3.18% of Cavalier King Charles spaniels CERF examined by veterinary ophthalmologists between 2000-2005. Severe cases can progress to retinal detachment. CERF does not recommend breeding any CKCS with retinal dysplasia. Reported at 3.0% in the ACKCSC, Inc. Health Survey 2004-2005.[7,30]

Distichiasis: Abnormally placed eyelashes that irritate the cornea and conjunctiva. Can cause secondary corneal ulceration. Identified in 9.16% of Cavalier King Charles spaniels CERF examined by veterinary ophthalmologists between 2000-2005. Reported at 2.7% in the ACKCSC, Inc. Health Survey 2004-2005.[7,30]

Corneal Dystrophy: The breed can have an epithelial/stromal form of corneal dystrophy. Age of onset 2-5 years. Identified in 8.24% of Cavalier King Charles spaniels CERF examined by veterinary ophthalmologists between 2000-2005. Reported at 2.7% in the ACKCSC, Inc. Health Survey 2004-2005.[7,30,31]

Deafness: Can be congenital or progressive in the breed, and can be unilateral or bilateral. The progressive form results in deafness by 3-5 years of age. Diagnosed by BAER testing. Reported at 6.2% in the ACKCSC, Inc. Health Survey 2004-2005.[7,32,33]

Cataracts: In the Cavalier King Charles spaniel, onset is at an early age (less than 6 months), affecting the cortex and nucleus with rapid progression to complete cataract, resulting in blindness. Punctate cataracts also occur. Reported in 3.90% of Cavalier King Charles spaniels presented to veterinary teaching hospitals. Identified in 2.98% of Cavalier King Charles spaniels CERF examined by veterinary ophthalmologists between 2000-2005. Reported at 6.0% in the ACKCSC, Inc. Health Survey 2004-2005. CERF does not recommend breeding any CKCS with a cataract.[7,30,34]

Keratoconjunctivitis Sicca (KCS, Dry Eye): Ocular condition causing lack of tear production and secondary conjunctivitis, corneal ulcerations, and vision problems. Age of onset 2-5 years. Treat with topical ocular lubricants and anti-inflammatory medication. Reported at 5.3% in the ACKCSC, Inc. Health Survey 2004-2005.[7,35]

Allergic Dermatitis: Presents with pruritis and pyotraumatic dermatitis (hot spots). Inhalant allergies were identified in 5.0%, Food Allergy was identified in 3.5%, and Hot Sports were identified in 4.8% of Cavalier King Charles spaniels in the ACKCSC, Inc. Health Survey 2004-2005.[7]

Sebaceous Cysts: Benign sebaceous skin cysts are reported at 5.0% in the ACKCSC, Inc. Health Survey 2004-2005.[7]

Syringomyelia (SM): Syringomyelia is a condition where fluid filled cavities develop within the spinal cord. The majority of affected dogs do not show clinical signs. Morphological variation of the atlantoaxial spine found in the breed does not correlate to the occurrence of SM. Chiari-like malformation (CM) is a predisposing factor, but not always present with SM. Crowding of the caudal cranial fossa can be a predisposing factor for developing SM. Ultrasonography through the atlantoccipital junction can identify cerebellar herniation through the foramen magnum, but not a syrinx. Clinical signs of SM can present usually between 5 months and 3 years of age, and include persistent scratching at the shoulder region with apparent neck, thoracic limb, or ear pain and thoracic limb lower motor neuron deficits. Diagnosis is by MRI. The size of the syrinx on MRI, and dorsal horn location are positively correlated to the amount of pain exhibited. Corticosteroid or NSAID treatment can improve, but not resolve the clinical signs. The percentage of Cavalier King Charles Spaniels in the general population with an MRI identified syrinx is not determined, but is expected to be high. Clinical signs of SM are reported at 3.9% in the ACKCSC, Inc. Health Survey 2004-2005. One study computed a heritability of 0.37, with the influence of multiple genes involved.[17,18,19,20,21,22,23,24,25,26,27,36,37,38,39]

Intervertebral Disc Disease (IVDD): Cavalier King Charles spaniels have an increased risk of developing spinal cord disease due to prolapsed disk material. Clinical signs include back pain, scuffing of paws, spinal ataxia, limb weakness, and paralysis. Reported at 3.2% in the ACKCSC, Inc. Health Survey 2004-2005.[7]

Chronic Pancreatitis: Often subclinical inflammation of the pancreas that can cause intermittent discomfort and gastrointestinal upsets, and can possibly lead to pancreatic insufficiency or diabetes mellitus. Cavalier King Charles spaniels have a 3.2x relative risk versus other breeds.[40]

Idiopathic Epilepsy: Generalized or parital seizures. Control with anti-seizure medication. Seizures are reported at a frequency of 3.0% in the ACKCSC, Inc. Health Survey 2004-2005. Unknown mode of inheritance.[6,36]

Femoral Artery Occlusion/Aortic Thromboembolism: Observed in 2.3% Cavalier King Charles spaniels examined. Femoral artery occlusion is not clinically important in dogs because of adequate collateral circulation. The higher frequency in the breed may be due to a primary femoral artery abnormality, or secondary to thrombus formation from heart disease.[41,42]

Hypothyroidism: Inherited autoimmune thyroiditis. 2.2% positive for thyroid auto-antibodies based on testing at Michigan State University. (Ave. for all breeds is 7.5%).[43,44]

Persistent Pupillary Membranes: Strands of fetal remnant connecting; iris to iris, cornea, lens, or involving sheets of tissue. The later three forms can impair vision, and dogs affected with these forms should not be bred. Identified in 1.62% of Cavalier King Charles Spaniels CERF examined by veterinary ophthalmologists between 2000-2005.[30]

Eosinophilic Disease: The breed may have a predisposition to eosinophilic disorders. Several case reports of unrelated Cavalier King Charles spaniels with eosinophilic stomatitis, enteritis, bronchopneumonopathy, or oral granulomas are reported. All responded to corticosteroid therapy.[45,46,47]

Xanthinuria, Xanthine Urolithiasis: Several affected Cavalier King Charles spaniels have been reported with urethral obstruction and renal insufficiency. Xanthinuria is caused by an inherited deficiency of the enzyme xanthine oxidase. An autosomal recessive mode of inheritance is suggested.[48]

Primary Secretory Otitis Media: Affected dogs had moderate to severe head or cervical pain and/or neurological signs. A bulging, but intact, tympanic membrane is found in most cases with a viscous mucus plug filling the middle ear on myringotomy. Treatment consists of repeated removal of the mucus plug, flushing of the middle ear, and local and systemic medical therapy. Tympanostomy tubes may be helpful for chronic recurrent cases. The disorder must be differentiated from syringomyelia in the breed.[49,50]

Fly Catching Behavior: Behavioral disorder identified in the breed with classic clinical signs as if watching, and then catching a fly. Some affected dogs may behave as if their ears or feet are irritated, and some may also chase their tail. Fly catching has previously been classified as a complex partial seizure, however non-responsiveness to anticonvulsants makes it more likely that this is a compulsive disorder.[51]

Diabetes Mellitus: Caused by a lack of insulin production by the pancreas. Controlled by insulin injections, diet, and glucose monitoring. Cavalier King Charles spaniels have a 1.45x risk of developing the disorder. However, members of the breed with a specific IL-10 allele have a 4.05x risk of developing the disorder. Unknown mode of inheritance.[54,55]

Immunoglobulin Deficiency with Pneumocystis Pneumonia: Cavalier King Charles spaniels can have a defect in immunity that makes them susceptible to infection with pneumocystosis. IgG concentrations are lower, and IgM concentrations are significantly higher in the affected dogs.[56]

Microphthalmia: Congenital disorder of a small eye (globe) associated with cataract, and posterior lenticonus. Identified in 0.11% of Cavalier King Charles spaniels CERF examined by veterinary ophthalmologists between 2000-2005. CERF does not recommend breeding any CKCS with this condition.[57]

Brachgnathism, Hydrocephalus, Mitochondrial Myopathy, Prognathism, Progressive Retinal Atrophy, Renal Dysplasia, and **Wry Mouth** are reported.[59]

Isolated Case Studies

Bilateral Renal Agenesis: Two one-day-old littermates were found to have a complete absence of both kidneys. Littermates and the parents had normal kidneys.[60]

Ventricular Septal Defect (VSD): A ventricular septal defect was diagnosed in a 3-month-old male Cavalier King Charles spaniel and corrected surgically.[61]

Juvenile Masticatory Muscle Myositis: Three of four 12-week-old cavalier King Charles spaniel littermates presented with difficulty in opening the mouth. Diagnosis was established immunohistochemistry and histopathology. Corticosteroid treatment resolved the condition in all the affected pups.[62]

Organic Aciduria with Seizures: A 6-month-old, female Cavalier King Charles spaniel exhibited seizures due to an organic aciduria with excessive excretion of hexanoylglycine. Cluster seizures were controlled with anticonvulsants.[63]

Genetic Tests

Tests of Genotype: Direct test for coat color alleles is available from Healthgene and VetGen.

Direct tests for Episodic Collapse and KCS/Ichthyosiform Dermatitis are available from the Animal Health Trust.

Direct test for Macrothrombocytopenia is available from Auburn Univ.-Boudreaux Lab.

Tests of Phenotype: CHIC Certification: Required testing includes hip radiographs, CERF eye examination (at 8-12 weeks, follow up at 12 months, annually until 5 years old, every two years until 9 years old), patella examination, and cardiac evaluation (by a cardiologist, preferably annually). (See CHIC website; www.caninehealthinfo.org.)

CKCSC Clear Heart Recommendations: Only breed dogs without a murmur at 2-1/2 years of age, whose parents both do not have a murmur at 5 years of age. "Heart clear" dogs are listed in the CKCSC Health Registry www.ckcsc.org.

Recommend BAER hearing test, elbow radiographs, thyroid profile including autoantibodies, and MRI for SM.

Miscellaneous

- **Breed name synonyms:** King Charles Spaniel, Cavalier, Cav, Charlies
- **Registries:** AKC, CKC, UKC, KCGB (Kennel Club of Great Britain), ANKC (Australian National Kennel Club), NKC (National Kennel Club)
- **AKC rank (year 2008):** 25 (7,626 dogs registered)
- **Internet resources: American Cavalier King Charles Spaniel Club, Inc.:** www.ackcsc.org
  Cavalier King Charles Spaniel Club–USA: www.ckcsc.org
  Cavalier King Charles Spaniel Club of Canada: www.cavaliercanada.com
  Cavalier King Charles Spaniel Club–UK: www.thecavalierclub.co.uk

References

1. Pedersen HD, Haggstrom J, Olsen LH, et. al.: Idiopathic asymptomatic thrombocytopenia in Cavalier King Charles Spaniels is an autosomal recessive trait. J Vet Intern Med. 2002 Mar-Apr;16(2):169-73.
2. Cowan SM, Bartges JW, Gompf RE, et. al.: Giant platelet disorder in the Cavalier King Charles Spaniel. Exp Hematol. 2004;32(4):344-50.
3. Davis B, Toivio-Kinnucan M, Schuller S, et. al.: Mutation in beta1-tubulin correlates with macrothrombocytopenia in Cavalier King Charles Spaniels. J Vet Intern Med. 2008 May-Jun;22(3):540-5.
4. Tvedten H, Lilliehöök I, Hillström A, et. al.: Plateletcrit is superior to platelet count for assessing platelet status in Cavalier King Charles Spaniels. Vet Clin Pathol. 2008 Sep;37(3):266-71.
5. Dickie AM, Schwarz T, Sullivan M: Temporomandibular joint morphology in Cavalier King Charles Spaniels. Vet Radiol Ultrasound. 2002 May-Jun;43(3):260-6.
6. OFA Website breed statistics: www.offa.org Last accessed July 1, 2010.
7. ACKCSC & Purdue University School of Veterinary Medicine Section of Clinical Epidemiology: American Cavalier King Charles Spaniel Club, Inc. Health Survey 2004-2005. 2006.
8. LaFond E, Breur GJ & Austin CC: Breed susceptibility for developmental orthopedic diseases in dogs. J Am Anim Hosp Assoc. 2002 Sep-Oct;38(5):467-77.
9. Piercy R, and Walmsley G: Muscular dystrophy in Cavalier King Charles spaniels. Vet Rec. 2009 Jul 11;165(2):62.
10. Walmsley GL, Arechavala-Gomeza V, Fernandez-Fuente M, et. al.: Mutational Analysis of Dystrophin-Deficient Muscular Dystrophy in Cavalier King Charles Spaniels. Proceedings, 2009 ACVIM Forum. 2009.
11. Beardow AW, Buchanan JW: Chronic mitral valve disease in cavalier King Charles spaniels: 95 cases (1987-1991). J Am Vet Med Assoc. 1993 Oct 1;203(7):1023-9.
12. Pedersen HD, Lorentzen KA, Kristensen BO: Echocardiographic mitral valve prolapse in cavalier King Charles spaniels: epidemiology and prognostic significance for regurgitation. Vet Rec. 1999 Mar 20;144(12):315-20.
13. Arndt JW, Reynolds CA, Singletary GE, et. al.: Serum serotonin concentrations in dogs with degenerative mitral valve disease. J Vet Intern Med. 2009 Nov-Dec;23(6):1208-13.
14. Hansson K, Häggström J, Kvart C, et. al.: Reader performance in radiographic diagnosis of signs of mitral regurgitation in cavalier King Charles spaniels. J Small Anim Pract. 2009 Sep;50 Suppl 1:44-53.
15. Lewis T, Swift S, Woolliams JA, et. al.: Heritability of premature mitral valve disease in Cavalier King Charles spaniels. Vet J. 2011 Apr;188(1):73-6.
16. Lord P, Hansson K, Kvart C, et. al.: Rate of change of heart size before congestive heart failure in dogs with mitral regurgitation. J Small Anim Pract. 2010 Apr;51(4):210-8.
17. Rusbridge C, Knowler SP: Coexistence of occipital dysplasia and occipital hypoplasia/syringomyelia in the cavalier King Charles spaniel. J Small Anim Pract. 2006 Oct;47(10):603-6.
18. Rusbridge C, Knowler SP: Inheritance of occipital bone hypoplasia (Chiari type I malformation) in Cavalier King Charles Spaniels. J Vet Intern Med. 2004 Sep-Oct;18(5):673-8. Review.
19. Stalin CE, Rusbridge C, Granger N, et. al.: Radiographic morphology of the cranial portion of the cervical vertebral column in Cavalier King Charles Spaniels and its relationship to syringomyelia. Am J Vet Res. 2008 Jan;69(1):89-93.
20. Carruthers H, Rusbridge C, Dubé MP, et. al.: Association between cervical and intracranial dimensions and syringomyelia in the cavalier King Charles spaniel. J Small Anim Pract. 2009 Aug;50(8):394-8.
21. Carrera I, Dennis R, Mellor DJ, et. al.: Use of magnetic resonance imaging for morphometric analysis of the caudal cranial fossa in Cavalier King Charles Spaniels. Am J Vet Res. 2009 Mar;70(3):340-5.
22. Couturier J, Rault D, & Cauzinille L: Chiari-like malformation and syringomyelia in normal cavalier King Charles spaniels: a multiple diagnostic imaging approach. J Small Anim Pract. 2008 Sep;49(9):438-43.
23. Cross HR, Cappello R, Rusbridge C, et. al.: Comparison of cerebral cranium volumes between cavalier King Charles spaniels with Chiari-like malformation, small breed dogs and Labradors. J Small Anim Pract. 2009 Aug;50(8):399-405.
24. Cerda-Gonzalez S, Olby NJ, McCullough S, et. al.: Morphology of the caudal fossa in Cavalier King Charles Spaniels. Vet Radiol Ultrasound. 2009 Jan-Feb;50(1):37-46.
25. Schmidt MJ, Biel M, Klumpp S, et. al.: Evaluation of the volumes of cranial cavities in Cavalier King Charles Spaniels with Chiari-like malformation and other brachycephalic dogs as measured via computed tomography. Am J Vet Res. 2009 Apr;70(4):508-12.
26. Schmidt MJ, Wigger A, Jawinski S, et. al.: Ultrasonographic appearance of the craniocervical junction in normal brachycephalic dogs and dogs with caudal occipital (Chiari-like) malformation. Vet Radiol Ultrasound. 2008 Sep-Oct;49(5):472-6.
27. Driver CJ, Rusbridge C, Cross HR, et. al.: Relationship of brain parenchyma within the caudal cranial fossa and ventricle size to syringomyelia in cavalier King Charles spaniels. J Small Anim Pract. 2010 Jul;51(7):382-6.
28. Batchelor DJ, Noble PJ, Cripps PJ, et. al.: Breed associations for canine exocrine pancreatic insufficiency. J Vet Intern Med. 2007 Mar-Apr;21(2):207-14.
29. Torrez CV & Hunt GB: Results of surgical correction of abnormalities associated with brachycephalic airway obstruction syndrome in dogs in

Australia. J Small Anim Pract. 2006 Mar;47(3):150-4.

30. Ocular Disorders Presumed to be Inherited in Purebred Dogs. American College of Veterinary Ophthalmologists. ACVO, 2007.

31. Crispin SM: Crystalline corneal dystrophy in the dog. Histochemical and ultrastructural study. Cornea. 1988;7(2):149-61.

32. Munro KJ, Cox CL: Investigation of hearing impairment in Cavalier King Charles spaniels using auditory brainstem response audiometry. J Small Anim Pract. 1997 Jan;38(1):2-5.

33. Strain GM: Deafness prevalence and pigmentation and gender associations in dog breeds at risk. Vet J. 2004 Jan;167(1):23-32.

34. Gelatt KN, Mackay EO: Prevalence of primary breed-related cataracts in the dog in North America. Vet Ophthalmol. 2005 Mar-Apr;8(2):101-11.

35. Sanchez RF, Innocent G, Mould J, et. al.: Canine keratoconjunctivitis sicca: disease trends in a review of 229 cases. J Small Anim Pract. 2007 Apr;48(4):211-7.

36. Rusbridge C: Neurological diseases of the Cavalier King Charles spaniel. J Small Anim Pract. 2005 Jun;46(6):265-72. Review

37. Cerda-Gonzalez S, Olby NJ, Broadstone R, et. al.: Characteristics of cerebrospinal fluid flow in Cavalier King Charles Spaniels analyzed using phase velocity cine magnetic resonance imaging. Vet Radiol Ultrasound. 2009 Sep-Oct;50(5):467-76.

38. Rusbridge C, Carruthers H, Dubé MP, et. al.: Syringomyelia in cavalier King Charles spaniels: the relationship between syrinx dimensions and pain. J Small Anim Pract. 2007 Aug;48(8):432-6.

39. Lewis T, Rusbridge C, Knowler P, et. al.: Heritability of syringomyelia in Cavalier King Charles spaniels. Vet J. 2010 Mar;183(3):345-7.

40. Watson PJ, Roulois AJ, Scase T, et. al.: Prevalence and breed distribution of chronic pancreatitis at post-mortem examination in first-opinion dogs. J Small Anim Pract. 2007 Nov;48(11):609-18.

41. Buchanan JW, Beardow AW, Sammarco CD: Femoral artery occlusion in Cavalier King Charles Spaniels. J Am Vet Med Assoc. 1997 Oct 1;211(7):872-4.

42. Gonçalves R, Penderis J, Chang YP, et. al.: Clinical and neurological characteristics of aortic thromboembolism in dogs. J Small Anim Pract. 2008 Apr;49(4):178-84.

43. Nachreiner R & Refsal K: Personal communication, Diagnostic Center for Population and Animal Health, Michigan State University. April, 2007.

44. Nachreiner RF, Refsal KR, Graham PA, et. al.: Prevalence of serum thyroid hormone autoantibodies in dogs with clinical signs of hypothyroidism. J Am Vet Med Assoc 2002 Feb 15;220(4):466-71.

45. Bredal WP, Gunnes G, Vollset I, et. al.: Oral eosinophilic granuloma in three cavalier King Charles spaniels. J Small Anim Pract. 1996 Oct;37(10):499-504.

46. German AJ, Holden DJ, Hall EJ, et. al.: Eosinophilic diseases in two Cavalier King Charles spaniels. J Small Anim Pract. 2002 Dec;43(12):533-8.

47. Joffe DJ, Allen AL: Ulcerative eosinophilic stomatitis in three Cavalier King Charles spaniels. J Am Anim Hosp Assoc. 1995 Jan-Feb;31(1):34-7.

48. van Zuilen CD, Nickel RF, van Dijk TH, et. al.: Xanthinuria in a family of Cavalier King Charles spaniels. Vet Q. 1997 Nov;19(4):172-4.

49. Stern-Bertholtz W, Sjostrom L. Hakanson NW: Primary secretory otitis media in the Cavalier King Charles spaniel: a review of 61 cases. J Small Anim Pract. 2003 Jun;44(6):253-6.

50. Corfield GS, Burrows AK, Imani P, et. al.: The method of application and short term results of tympanostomy tubes for the treatment of primary secretory otitis media in three Cavalier King Charles Spaniel dogs. Aust Vet J. 2008 Mar;86(3):88-94.

51. Brown PR: Fly catching in the cavalier King Charles spaniel. Vet Rec. 1987 Jan 24;120(4):95.

52. Herrtage ME, Palmer AC: Episodic falling in the cavalier King Charles spaniel. Vet Rec. 1983 May 7;112(19):458-9.

53. Wright JA, Smyth JB, Brownlie SE, et. al.: A myopathy associated with muscle hypertonicity in the Cavalier King Charles Spaniel. J Comp Pathol. 1987 Sep;97(5):559-65.

54. Short AD, Catchpole B, Kennedy LJ, et. al.: Analysis of candidate susceptibility genes in canine diabetes. J Hered. 2007;98(5):518-25.

55. Short AD, Catchpole B, Kennedy LJ, et. al.: T cell cytokine gene polymorphisms in canine diabetes mellitus. Vet Immunol Immunopathol. 2009 Mar 15;128(1-3):137-46

56. Watson PJ, Wotton P, Eastwood J, et. al.: Immunoglobulin deficiency in Cavalier King Charles Spaniels with Pneumocystis pneumonia. J Vet Intern Med. 2006 May-Jun;20(3):523-7.

57. Narfstrom K, Dubielzig R: Posterior lenticonus, cataracts and microphthalmia.: congenital defects in the Cavalier King Charles spaniel. Journal of Small Animal Practice 1984;25:669.

58. Barnett KC: Congenital keratoconjunctivitis sicca and ichthyosiform dermatosis in the cavalier King Charles spaniel. J Small Anim Pract. 2006 Sep;47(9):524-8.

59. The Genetic Connection: A Guide to Health Problems in Purebred Dogs. L Ackerman. p.208-9, AAHA Press, 1999.

60. Yates GH, Sanchez-Vazquez MJ, & Dunlop MM: Bilateral renal agenesis in two cavalier King Charles spaniels. Vet Rec. 2007 May 12;160(19):672.

61. Hunt GB, Pearson MR, Bellenger CR, et. al.: Ventricular septal defect repair in a small dog using cross-circulation. Aust Vet J. 1995 Oct;72(10):379-82.

62. Pitcher GD, Hahn CN: Atypical masticatory muscle myositis in three cavalier King Charles spaniel littermates. J Small Anim Pract. 2007 Aprr;48(4):226-8.

63. Platt S, McGrotty YL, Abramson CJ, et. al.: Refractory seizures associated with an organic aciduria in a dog. J Am Anim Hosp Assoc. 2007 May-Jun;43(3):163-7.

64. The Complete Dog Book, 20th Ed. The American Kennel Club. Howell Book House, NY 2006. p. 454-457.

Chesapeake Bay Retriever

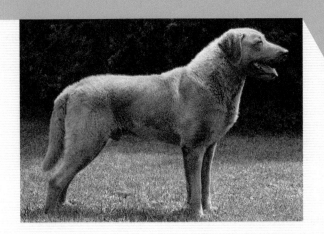

The Breed History

It is thought that early in the 1800s, a shipwreck of a British ship off of Maryland landed the breed progenitors in the US. Some out-crossing to Otterhound, and Curly and Flat-coated Retrievers may have occurred, but because of the exceptional retrieving talent, this line was highly valued. They are thought to have originated in Newfoundland-Labrador from the same stock as the Labrador Retriever. They received AKC recognition in 1885.

Breeding for Function

Bred to fetch ducks from the cold water, this breed is still used for this purpose and Working Dog certificates are awarded to those dogs that continue to show excellent retrieving skills. They are also land retrievers, and are also a popular companion dog. They excel at tracking, obedience, and guarding. They are also being trained as therapy dogs. Their hallmark is exceptional endurance under the most severe conditions (cold water, wind). Some natural haircoat oiliness helps them to repel water away from the skin and undercoat.

Physical Characteristics

Height at Withers: female 21-24" (53-61 cm), male 23-26" (58.5-66 cm).

Weight: females 55-70 lb (25-32 kg), males 65-80 lb (29.5-36.5 kg).

Coat: The double water-resistant coat is brown, sedge grass, or dead grass colored to blend with their surroundings. The outer coat is wavy and dense with coarse, glossy hairs and the inner coat is soft, wooly and oily. Small white spots may be found on some dogs.

Longevity: 10-12 years.

Points of Conformation: A broad skull, large jaws and soft mouth provide the capacity for bird fetching. The face has a moderate stop, and eyes are yellow to amber. The ears are high set, triangular and medium length and pendulous, with medium leather. This medium sized dog has a deep thorax, and is well muscled with strong bones, though not coarsely built. The topline is level or mildly ascending towards the rear. Working dogs would normally have any rear dewclaws removed; fronts as well.

Recognized Behavior Issues and Traits

Reported breed characteristics include: These dogs are noted for their intelligence, alertness, willingness to press on in harsh conditions, and their even-tempered and gently protective natures. The presence of either shyness, or any overly protective tendency is strongly discouraged in the breed. An experienced owner, or one with breeder or other guidance may be best to handle training these somewhat dominant dogs. They may be, on average, more independent, territorial and aggressive than other retrievers. They require regular activity and exercise. They require average grooming, and are low shedders. They do best outside of city.

Normal Physiologic Variations

The coat tends to be oily so bathing 3 or 4 times a year is recommended as a minimum.

Drug Sensitivities

None reported

Inherited Diseases

Hip Dysplasia: Polygenically inherited trait causing degenerative joint disease and hip arthritis. OFA reports 20.8% affected.[1]

Elbow Dysplasia: Polygenically inherited trait causing elbow arthritis. OFA reports 5.6% affected.[1]

Progressive Retinal Atrophy (PRA): Autosomal recessive progressive rod cone degeneration (prcd) form. Age of onset between 4-7 years, eventually causing blindness. Optigen testing reports 4% affected, and 30% carrier in Chesapeake Bay Retrievers. CERF does not recommend breeding any Chesapeake Bay Retriever with PRA. A direct genetic test is available.[2,3]

Exercise Induced Collapse (EIC, Dynamin 1 Mutation): An autosomal recessive disorder of muscle weakness, incoordination and life threatening collapse accompanied by hyperthermia after just five to fifteen minutes of intense exercise or excitement. After 10 to 30 minutes of rest, most dogs return to normal. Limited genetic testing reveals 11% carriers and 1.3% clinically affected homozygous Chesapeake Bay Retrievers. A direct genetic test is available.[4]

von Willebrand's Disease (vWD): Severe, autosomal recessive bleeding disorder, Type III von Willebrand's disease occurs in the breed. A genetic test has not been developed.[5]

Patella Luxation: Polygenically inherited laxity of patellar ligaments, causing luxation, lameness, and later degenerative joint disease. Treat surgically if causing clinical signs. Too few Chesapeake Bay Retrievers have been screened by OFA to determine an accurate frequency.[1]

Disease Predispositions

Hypothyroidism: Inherited autoimmune thyroiditis. 12.9% positive for thyroid auto-antibodies based on testing at Michigan State University. (Ave. for all breeds is 7.5%).[6,7]

Distichiasis: Abnormally placed eyelashes that irritate the cornea and conjunctiva. Can cause secondary corneal ulceration. Dorn reports a 1.53x odds ratio in Chesapeake Bay Retrievers versus other breeds. Identified in 5.98% of Chesapeake Bay Retrievers CERF examined by veterinary ophthalmologists between 2000-2005.[2,8]

Allergic Dermatitis: Inhalant or food allergy. Presents with pruritis and pyotraumatic dermatitis (hot spots). Reported at a frequency of 4.5% in the 2004 ACC Health Survey.[9]

Umbilical Hernia: Congenital opening in the body wall from where the umbilical cord was attached. Reported at a frequency of 4.3% in the 2004 ACC Health Survey. Unknown mode of inheritance.[9]

Cataracts: Posterior cortical, axial, triangular opacities are the major inherited cataract in the breed, though anterior, capsular, and nuclear cataracts also occur. Age of onset around one year of age. Identified in 4.23% of Chesapeake Bay Retrievers CERF examined by veterinary ophthalmologists between 2000-2005. Early reports suggest dominant inheritance with incomplete penetrance. CERF does not recommend breeding any Chesapeake Bay Retriever with a cataract.[2,10]

Idiopathic Epilepsy: Generalized or partial seizures. Control with anti-seizure medication. Reported at a frequency of 3.5% in the 2004 ACC Health Survey. Unknown mode of inheritance.[9]

Humeral Osteochondritis Dissecans (OCD): Polygenically inherited cartilage defect of the humeral head. Causes shoulder joint pain and lameness in young growing dogs. Mild cases can resolve with rest, while more severe cases require surgery. 50% of cases are bilateral. Reported 7.7x odds ratio versus other breeds.[11]

Cranial Cruciate Ligament Rupture (ACL): Traumatic tearing of the anterior cruciate ligament. The breed is found to be one with an increased incidence. Dorn reports a 2.01x odds ratio in Chesapeake Bay Retrievers versus other breeds. Treatment is surgery.[8,12]

Persistent Pupillary Membranes: Strands of fetal remnant connecting; iris to iris, cornea, lens, or involving sheets of tissue. The later three forms can impair vision, and dogs affected with these forms should not be bred. Identified in 1.55% of Chesapeake Bay Retrievers CERF examined by veterinary ophthalmologists between 2000-2005.[2]

Gastric Dilatation-Volvulus (bloat, GDV): Polygenically inherited, life-threatening twisting of the stomach within the abdomen. Requires immediate treatment. Reported at an increased frequency in the breed.[13]

Degenerative Myelopathy (DM): Affected dogs show an insidious onset of upper motor neuron (UMN) paraparesis at an average age of 11.4 years. The disease eventually progresses to severe tetraparesis. Affected dogs have normal results on myelography, MRI, and CSF analysis. Necropsy confirms the condition. Reported at a frequency of 0.83% in Chesapeake Bay Retrievers. Unknown mode of inheritance. A direct genetic test for an autosomal recessive DM susceptibility gene is available. All affected dogs are homozygous for the gene, however, only a small percentage of homozygous dogs develop DM. OFA testing shows 45% carrier and 12% homozygous "at risk" for the DM susceptibility gene.[14,15,16]

Entropion/Ectropion: Rolling in or out of the eyelids. Can cause corneal irritation or conjunctivitis. Dorn reports a 1.40x odds ratio in Chesapeake Bay Retrievers versus other breeds. Entropion is reported in 0.55% and Entropion in 0.09% of Chesapeake Bay Retrievers CERF examined by veterinary ophthalmologists between 2000-2005.[2,8]

Adult-onset Hair Loss (Endocrine Hair Loss): Young adult Chesapeake Bay Retrievers present with nonpruritic, non-inflammatory, hair loss affecting the axillae, latero-ventral thorax, flanks, ventrum, dorsum, rump and/or the caudal part of the thighs in both male and female dogs. Hormonal investigations showed increased adrenal and sex steroid concentration in seven cases. Histopathology revealed follicular hyperkeratosis and plugging, follicular atrophy, and occasional melanin clumping with malformed hair shafts. Unknown mode of inheritance.[17]

Anterior Crossbite, Brachygnathism, Central PRA, Prognathism, Retinal Dysplasia, and **Wry Mouth** are reported.[18]

Isolated Case Studies

Tricuspid Stenosis: A 3-year-old castrated male Chesapeake Bay Retriever was referred for evaluation of tachypnea, exercise intolerance, and cyanosis. On echocardiographs, there was severe tricuspid stenosis and right-to-left atrial-level shunting of blood. Balloon dilation of the stenotic tricuspid valve was palliative.[19]

Lymphangiosarcoma: Case study of a a three-year-old, neutered male Chesapeake Bay Retriever presented for acute swelling of the head, neck, and cranial trunk. Diffuse lymphangiosarcoma involving the superficial and deep dermis and subcutaneous tissue was observed on skin biopsies.[20]

Genetic Tests

Tests of Genotype: Direct test for prcd-PRA is available from Optigen.

Direct test for EIC is available from the University of Minnesota Veterinary Diagnostic Lab.

Direct genetic test for an autosomal recessive DM susceptibility gene is available from the OFA.

Tests of Phenotype: CHIC Certification: Required testing includes hip and elbow radiographs, and CERF eye examination (after 12 months of age). Optional recommended testing for prcd-PRA, thyroid profile including autoantibodies, and congenital cardiac examination. (See CHIC website; www.caninehealthinfo.org).

Recommend patella evaluation.

Miscellaneous

- **Breed name synonyms:** Chessie
- **Registries:** AKC, UKC, CKC, KCGB (Kennel Club of Great Britain), ANKC (Australian National Kennel Club), NKC (National Kennel Club)
- **AKC rank (year 2008):** 48 (2,463 dogs registered)
- **Internet resources: The American Chesapeake Club:**
  www.amchessieclub.org/
  Chesapeake Bay Retriever Club of Canada: www.cbrcc.ca
  Chesapeake Bay Retriever Club (UK):
  www.chesapeakebayretrieverclub.co.uk

References

1. OFA Website breed statistics: www.offa.org Last accessed July 1, 2010.
2. *Ocular Disorders Presumed to be Inherited in Purebred Dogs.* American College of Veterinary Ophthalmologists. ACVO, 2007.
3. Morris Animal Foundation: Morris Animal Foundation Update: Genetic Tests Focus on Breed-Specific Vision Problems. *Canine Pract* 1999:24(4):21.
4. Minor KM, Patterson EE, Gross SD, et. al.: Frequency of the Canine Exercise Induced Collapse Gene in Diverse Breeds. Proceedings, 2009 ACVIM Forum. 2009.
5. Johnson GS, Lees GE, Benson RE, et. al.: A bleeding disease (von Willebrand's disease) in a Chesapeake Bay Retriever. *J Am Vet Med Assoc.* 1980 Jun 1;176(11):1261-3.
6. Nachreiner R & Refsal K: Personal communication, Diagnostic Center for Population and Animal Health, Michigan State University. April, 2007.
7. Nachreiner RF, Refsal KR, Graham PA, et. al.: Prevalence of serum thyroid hormone autoantibodies in dogs with clinical signs of hypothyroidism. J Am Vet Med Assoc 2002 Feb 15;220(4):466-71.
8. Dorn CR: Canine breed-specific risks of frequently diagnosed diseases at veterinary teaching hospitals. Monograph. AKC Canine Health Foundation. 2000.
9. American Chesapeake Club: 2004 American Chesapeake Club Health Survey. 2004.
10. Gelatt KN, Whitley RD, Lavach JD, et. al.: Cataracts in Chesapeake Bay Retrievers. *J Am Vet Med Assoc.* 1979 Dec 1;175(11):1176-8.
11. LaFond E, Breur GJ & Austin CC: Breed susceptibility for developmental orthopedic diseases in dogs. J Am Anim Hosp Assoc. 2002 Sep-Oct;38(5):467-77.
12. Duval JM, Budsberg SC, Flo GL, et. al.: Breed, sex, and body weight as risk factors for rupture of the cranial cruciate ligament in young dogs. J Am Vet Med Assoc. 1999 Sep 15;215(6):811-4.
13. Glickman LT, Glickman NW, Schellenberg DB, et. al.: Incidence of and breed-related risk factors for gastric dilatation-volvulus in dogs. J Am Vet Med Assoc. 2000 Jan 1;216(1):40-5.
14. Coates JR: Degenerative Myelopathy of Pembroke Welsh Corgi Dogs. Proceedings, 2005 ACVIM Forum. 2005.
15. Coates JR & Wade C: Update on the Genetic Basis of Canine Degenerative Myelopathy. Proceedings, 2008 ACVIM Forum. 2008.
16. Awano T, Johnson GS, Wade CM, et. al.: Genome-wide association analysis reveals a SOD1 mutation in canine degenerative myelopathy that resembles amyotrophic lateral sclerosis. Proc Natl Acad Sci U S A. 2009 Feb 24;106(8):2794-9.
17. Cerundolo R, Mauldin EA, Goldschmidt MH, et. al.: Adult-onset hair loss in Chesapeake Bay retrievers: a clinical and histological study. *Vet Dermatol.* 2005 Feb;16(1):39-46.
18. *The Genetic Connection: A Guide to Health Problems in Purebred Dogs.* L Ackerman. p. 209, AAHA Press, 1999.
19. Kunze P, Abbott JA, Hamilton SM, et. al.: Balloon valvuloplasty for palliative treatment of tricuspid stenosis with right-to-left atrial-level shunting in a dog. *J Am Vet Med Assoc.* 2002 Feb 15;220(4):491-6, 464.
20. Fossum TW, Miller MW, Mackie JT: Lymphangiosarcoma in a dog presenting with massive head and neck swelling. *J Am Anim Hosp Assoc.* 1998 Jul-Aug;34(4):301-4.
21. *The Complete Dog Book, 20th Ed.* The American Kennel Club. Howell Book House, NY 2006. p 33-37.

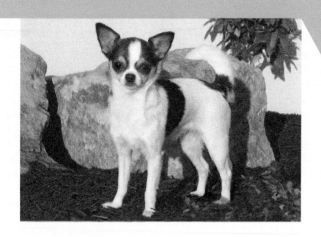

The Breed History

In Mexico an indigenous dog, the *Techichi* was represented in historical records beginning in the 9th century and is considered the primary source of the modern Chihuahua's genes. Some historians believe the dog was crossed with a hairless breed from the Orient at some point. In the travels of Columbus, a similar small mute dog was noted in Cuba. This type of dog was highly treasured in Toltec and Aztec civilizations, so much so that they were often buried with their masters. It is unlikely that the origin of the breed was just in the Chihuahua area of Mexico, but since many of the foundation dogs that were exported in the mid 1800s came from this state, the name was selected. Longhaired varieties may have resulted from Yorkshire Terrier or Papillion crosses. First exports to the US occurred in the early 19th century, and AKC registration began in 1908.

Breeding for Function

The Aztecs used to sometimes sacrifice the red-colored dogs, and the blue ones were considered sacred. Primarily throughout the breed history though, these were highly valued companion dogs.

Physical Characteristics

Height at withers: 6-9" (15-23 cm).

Weight: Under 6 lb (2.5 kg). They are considered the smallest dog breed.

Coat: Two coat varieties exist: smooth and longhaired. Smooth haircoats are glossy, lay close, and are soft textured, and sometimes an undercoat is present. A bit of ruff is preferred. Long coats are soft, flat, and an undercoat is preferred. Some feathering is desirable. Any color is accepted whether solid, solid with markings, or splashed colors.

Longevity: 12-14 years.

Points of Conformation: Their build is compact and well muscled, and they are longer than tall, with fine bones. They have a domed skull, large wide-set dark eyes, though in light dogs, the eye color may match the coat. Domed skulls in some dogs leads to an open fontanelle termed *molera*. Ears are erect when alert, and folded back when resting. They are large and triangular. The muzzle is moderately short and tapers. The nose is black or self-colored, or

Chihuahua

pink in blonde dogs. The neck is short and the topline is level, ribs are well sprung and the thorax is moderate in depth. The tail is sickle shaped and rests out or up over the back (just touching). Limbs are straight, and feet are very small with toes set well apart.

Recognized Behavior Issues and Traits

Breed characteristics reported include: Loyal, alert, and very fast movers. They express many terrier qualities, and have high activity/energy levels. They are noted for poor cold tolerance, and love close human contact and lots of attention. May be snappy with strangers or young children, and can be dominant and aggressive. Medium to high barking tendency, some are picky eaters, good for apartment or house-not for rural outdoors, and have low grooming and exercise needs.

Normal Physiologic Variations

Molera: An open fontanel in the skull (*molera*) is a frequent finding in the breed, and may not always be associated with hydrocephalus.

Infantile Stress Hypoglycemia: Very young Chihuahuas can be vulnerable to stress hypoglycemia once weaned. Treat with oral dextrose and warming.[1]

Merle Coat Color: Caused by a dominant mutation in the SILV gene. Breeding two merle dogs together should be avoided, as homozygous dogs can be born with multiple defects, including blindness, deafness, and heart anomalies.[2]

Cesarean Section/Dystocia: A high percentage of Chihuahua litters show difficult whelping and are delivered by C-section. A study in the UK shows 34.4% of Chihuahua litters are delivered via C-section.[3,4]

Drug Sensitivities

None reported

Inherited Diseases

Patella Luxation: Polygenically inherited laxity of patellar ligaments, causing luxation, lameness, and later degenerative joint disease. Treat surgically if causing clinical signs. Reported 8.9x odds ratio versus other breeds. OFA reports 5.5% affected. Dorn reports a 7.91x odds ratio in Chihuahuas versus other breeds. Reported at an increased fequency in the 2009 CCA Health Survey.[3,5,6,7]

Hip Dysplasia and Legg-Calve Perthes Disease: Polygenically inherited traits causing degenerative hip joint disease and arthritis. Too few Chihuahuas have been screened by OFA to determine an accurate frequency. Reported 26.8x odds ratio for Legg-Calve-Perthes versus other breeds.[5,7]

Elbow Dysplasia: Polygenically inherited trait causing elbow arthritis. Too few Chihuahuas have been screened by OFA to determine an accurate frequency.[5]

Disease Predispositions

Hydrocephalus: Congenital increased volume of cerebrospinal fluid (CSF), with a concurrent dilation of the ventricular system and reduction of brain tissue. Can cause behavior changes, visual defects, impaired motor function, or seizures. Not all Chihuahuas with an open fontanel are hydrocephalic. Dorn reports a 62.63x odds ratio versus other breeds.[6,8]

Dental Issues: A high frequency of undershot bites, overshot bites. and wry mouth are reported in the 2009 CCA Health Survey.[3]

Vitreous Degeneration: Liquefaction of the vitreous gel which may predispose to retinal detachment and blindness. Identified in 5.70% of Chihuahuas CERF examined by veterinary ophthalmologists between 2000-2005.[9]

Collapsing Trachea: Caused by diminished integrity of the cartilage rings in the trachea. Can produce increased coughing, stridor, and respiratory distress. Dorn reports a 5.57x odds ratio versus other breeds.[6]

Persistent Pupillary Membranes: Strands of fetal remnant connecting; iris to iris, cornea, lens, or involving sheets of tissue. The later three forms can impair vision, and dogs affected with these forms should not be bred. Identified in 5.06% of Chihuahuas CERF examined by veterinary ophthalmologists between 2000-2005.[9]

Canine Pattern Baldness: Progressive alopecia developing at the post- and/or pre-auricular regions, along the ventral neck, thorax and abdomen, and on the caudomedial thighs. The hair loss starts around 6 months of age and gradually progresses over the following year, but remains restricted to the described areas.[10]

Umbilical Hernia/Cleft Palate: Both of these congenital anomalies are reported at an increased frequency in the breed.[3]

Cryptorchidism (Retained Testicles): Can be bilateral or unilateral. Chihuahuas have an increased prevalence of the disorder.[3,11]

Cataracts: Anterior and posterior cortex intermediate cataracts predominate in the breed, although nuclear and capsular cataracts also occur. Identified in 4.43% of Chihuahuas CERF examined by veterinary ophthalmologists between 2000-2005. CERF does not recommend breeding any Chihuahua with a cataract.[3,9]

Chronic Valvular Disease/Endocardiosis: Thickening of the heart valves with age, leading to congestive heart disease. Reported increased frequency in the breed. Dorn reports a 3.11x odds ratio versus other breeds.[6,12]

Hypothyroidism: Inherited autoimmune thyroiditis. 2.6% positive for thyroid auto-antibodies based on testing at Michigan State University. (Ave. for all breeds is 7.5%).[13,14]

Portosystemic Shunt (PSS, liver shunt): Congenital disorder, where abnormal blood vessels connecting the systemic and portal blood flow. Vessels can be intrahepatic or extrahepatic. Causes stunting, abnormal behavior and possible seizures. Tobias reports a 4.9x Odds Ratio versus other breeds. Undetermined mode of inheritance.[15]

Progressive Retinal Atrophy (PRA): Inherited degeneration of the retina. Presumed autosomal recessive inheritance. 1.9% of Chihuahuas CERF examined by veterinary ophthalmologists between 2000-2005 are identified as affected, and 1.27% as suspicious for PRA.[9,16]

Urinary Calculi: The breed is found to be at an increased risk of developing oxalate, and cystine bladder stones. Cystine calculi are secondary to a defect in cystine metabolism.[17,18,19]

Corneal Dystrophy: Endothelial form is associated with progressive corneal edema, which can lead to bullous keratopathy and corneal erosions. Onset 6-13 years, with an average of 9.5 years. Treatment is symptomatic and palliative. Identified in 0.63% of Chihuahuas CERF examined by veterinary ophthalmologists between 2000-2005.[9,20]

Pulmonic Stenosis: Inherited congenital malformation of the pulmonic valve. Causes stricture of the right ventricular outflow tract or stricture of the pulmonary artery. The Chihuahua is identified as a breed at increased risk. Undetermined mode of inheritance.[21]

Acquired Myasthenia Gravis: Chihuahuas are a breed at increased risk of developing generalized or focal acquired myasthenia gravis. The most common presenting signs were generalized weakness, with or without megaesophagus. Diagnosis is by identifying serum acetylcholine receptor antibodies.[22]

Necrotizing Meningoencephalitis: A non-suppurative acute to chronic necrotizing meningoencephalitis is identified in Chihuahuas, similar to that seen in the Pug and Maltese breeds. Genetic research suggests different genetic causes between breeds. Affected dogs present with seizures, blindness and mentation changes from 1 to 10 years of age.[23,24,25]

Color Dilution Alopecia, Demodicosis, Factor VIII Deficiency, Glaucoma, Keratoconjunctivitis Sicca, Methemoglobin Reductase Deficiency, Myelodysplasia, Neuroaxonal Dystrophy, Osteochondritis Dessicans–Shoulder, Patent Ductus Arteriosus, Retained Primary Teeth, and **Spina Bifida,** are reported.[26]

Isolated Case Studies

Primary Hypoparathyroidism: Two Chihuahuas were diagnosed in a 15 year study in Australia. Affected dogs presented with Seizures, muscle tremors and fasciculations due to hypocalcemia. Treatment with calcium supplementation.[27]

Leiomyosarcoma: A 2 month-old female Chihuahua had a 3-week history of progressive disorientation, left-sided circling, and incessant whimpering. Necropsy revealed a primary leiomyosarcoma in the midline of the posterior thalamus with secondary obstructive hydrocephalus of the lateral ventricles.[28]

Narcolepsy: A two-year-old male Chihuahua suffered paroxysmal attacks of muscle weakness and immobility elicited by stimulation, such as feeding. Low CSF levels of hypocretin provided a diagnosis of hypocretin-deficient narcolepsy. The dog responded to treatment with imipramine.[29]

Ceroid–Lipofuscinosis: A two-year-old, female chihuahua presented with a six-month history of visual dysfunction. Histologically, swollen neurons possessing yellowish pigment granules in the cytoplasm were observed throughout the CNS. These storage materials stained positively for ceroid-lipofuscinosis. There was a concurrent hydrocephalus.[30]

Esophagobronchial Fistula: A 10-month-old, intact male Chihuahua presented for a 7-month history of regurgitation and coughing. Survey radiographs revealed a soft-tissue opacity within the distal esophagus. A contrast study confirmed the presence of an esophagobronchial fistula.[31]

Cardiac Fibrosarcoma: A 6-year-old Chihuahua dog presented with dyspnea, cyanosis, and pleural effusion. At necropsy, primary cardiac fibrosarcoma of the right atrium was diagnosed.[32]

Absence Seizures with Myoclonus: An eight-month-old Chihuahua was reported with recurrent episodes of head and nose twitching lasting one to two seconds, multiple times per day. EEG confirmed epilepsy.[33]

Genetic Tests

Tests of Genotype: Direct tests for color alleles and coat length are available from VetGen.

Tests of Phenotype: CHIC Certification: Required testing includes congenital cardiac evaluation, CERF eye examination (minimum 1 year of age), and patella evaluation (minimum 1 year of age). (See CHIC website; www.caninehealthinfo.org).

Additional recommended tests are hip and elbow radiographs, and thyroid profile including autoantibodies.

Miscellaneous

- **Breed name synonyms:** Teacup, Chi, Chihauhau
- **Registries:** AKC, UKC, CKC, KCGB (Kennel Club of Great Britain), ANKC (Australian National Kennel Club), NKC (National Kennel Club)
- **AKC rank (year 2008):** 12 (15,985 dogs registered)
- **Internet resources: Chihuahua Club of America:** http://www.chihuahuaclubofamerica.com/ **British Chihuahua Club:** www.the-british-chihuahua-club.org.uk

References

1. Vroom MW, Slappendel RJ: Transient juvenile hypoglycaemia in a Yorkshire terrier and in a Chihuahua. Vet Q. 1987 Apr;9(2):172-6.
2. Clark LA, Wahl JM, Rees CA, et. al.: Retrotransposon insertion in SILV is responsible for merle patterning of the domestic dog. Proc Natl Acad Sci U S A. 2006 Jan 31;103(5):1376-81.
3. Chihuahua Club of America: 2009 Chihuahua Club of America Health Survey. 2009.
4. Evans KM & Adams VJ: Proportion of litters of purebred dogs born by caesarean section. J Small Anim Pract. 2010 Feb;51(2):113-8.
5. OFA Website breed statistics: www.offa.org Last accessed July 1, 2010.
6. Dorn CR: Canine breed-specific risks of frequently diagnosed diseases at veterinary teaching hospitals. Monograph. AKC Canine Health Foundation. 2000.
7. LaFond E, Breur GJ & Austin CC: Breed susceptibility for developmental orthopedic diseases in dogs. J Am Anim Hosp Assoc. 2002 Sep-Oct;38(5):467-77.
8. Axlund TW: Managing the Hydrocephalic Patient: Medical and Surgical Options. Proceedings, 2004 Atlantic Coast Veterinary Conference. 2004.
9. Ocular Disorders Presumed to be Inherited in Purebred Dogs. American College of Veterinary Ophthalmologists. ACVO, 2007.
10. White SD: Update on Follicular Alopecias: 'Pseudo-Endocrinopathies'. Proceedings, 2005 ACVIM Forum. 2005.
11. Yates D, Hayes G, Heffernan M, et. al: Incidence of cryptorchidism in dogs and cats. Vet Rec. 2003 Apr 19;152(16):502-4.
12. Keene BW, Hamlin RL, Rush JE, et. al.: Diagnosis and Management of Canine Chronic Valvular Disease. Proceedings, 2004 Northeast Veterinary Conference. 2004.
13. Nachreiner R & Refsal K: Personal communication, Diagnostic Center for Population and Animal Health, Michigan State University. April, 2007.
14. Nachreiner RF, Refsal KR, Graham PA, et. al.: Prevalence of serum thyroid hormone autoantibodies in dogs with clinical signs of hypothyroidism. J Am Vet Med Assoc 2002 Feb 15;220(4):466-71
15. Tobias KM & Rohrbach BW: Association of breed with the diagnosis of congenital portosystemic shunts in dogs: 2,400 cases (1980-2002). J Am Vet Med Assoc. 2003 Dec 1;223(11):1636-9.
16. Hurn SD, Hardman C, Stanley RG: Day-blindness in three dogs: clinical and electroretinographic findings. Vet Ophthalmol. 2003 Jun;6(2):127-30.
17. Jones BR, Kirkman JH, Hogan J, et. al.: Analysis of uroliths from cats and dogs in New Zealand, 1993-96. N Z Vet J. 1998 Dec;46(6):233-6.
18. Dolinsek D: Calcium oxalate urolithiasis in the canine: surgical management and preventative strategies. Can Vet J. 2004 Jul;45(7):607-9.
17. Ling GV, Franti CE, Ruby AL, et. al.: Urolithiasis in dogs. II: Breed prevalence, and interrelations of breed, sex, age, and mineral composition. Am J Vet Res. 1998 May;59(5):630-42.
20. Cooley PL, Dice PF 2nd: Corneal dystrophy in the dog and cat. Vet Clin North Am Small Anim Pract. 1990 May;20(3):681-92.
21. McCaw D, Aronson E: Congenital cardiac disease in dogs. Mod Vet Pract. 1984 Jul;65(7):509-12.
22. Shelton GD, Schule A, Kass PH: Risk factors for acquired myasthenia gravis in dogs: 1,154 cases (1991-1995). J Am Vet Med Assoc. 1997 Dec 1;211(11):1428-31.
23. Kube SA, Dickinson PJ, Affolter TW, et. al.: Necrotizing Meningoencephalitis in Chihuahua Dogs. Proceedings, 2005 ACVIM Forum. 2005.
24. Pedersen NC, Vernau K, Dickinson P, et. al.: DLA Association in Various Toy Breeds with Immune Mediated Encephalopathies. Proceedings, 4th Tufts' Canine and Feline Breeding and Genetics Conference. 2009.
25. Higgins RJ, Dickinson PJ, Kube SA, et. al.: Necrotizing meningoencephalitis in five Chihuahua dogs. Vet Pathol. 2008 May;45(3):336-46.
26. The Genetic Connection: A Guide to Health Problems in Purebred Dogs. L Ackerman. p. 209. AAHA Press, 1999.
27. Russell NJ, Bond KA, Robertson ID, et. al.: Primary hypoparathyroidism in dogs: a retrospective study of 17 cases. Aust Vet J. 2006 Aug;84(8):285-90.
28. Zabka TS, Lavely JA, Higgins RJ: Primary intra-axial leiomyosarcoma with obstructive hydrocephalus in a young dog. J Comp Pathol. 2004 Nov;131(4):334-7.
29. Tonokura M, Fujita K, Morozumi M, et. al.: Narcolepsy in a hypocretin/orexin-deficient chihuahua. Vet Rec. 2003 Jun 21;152(25):776-9.
30. Kuwamura M, Hattori R, Yamate J, et. al.: Neuronal ceroid-lipofuscinosis and hydrocephalus in a chihuahua. J Small Anim Pract. 2003 May;44(5):227-30.
31. Nawrocki MA, Mackin AJ, McLaughlin R, et. al.: Fluoroscopic and endoscopic localization of an esophagobronchial fistula in a dog. J Am Anim Hosp Assoc. 2003 May-Jun;39(3):257-61.
32. Madarame H, Sato K, Ogihara K, et. al.: Primary cardiac fibrosarcoma in a dog. J Vet Med Sci. 2004 Aug;66(8):979-82.
33. Poma R, Ochi A, & Cortez MA: Absence seizures with myoclonic features in a juvenile Chihuahua dog. Epileptic Disord. 2010 Jun;12(2):138-41.
34. The Complete Dog Book, 20th Ed. The American Kennel Club. Howell Book House, NY 2006. p. 458-461.

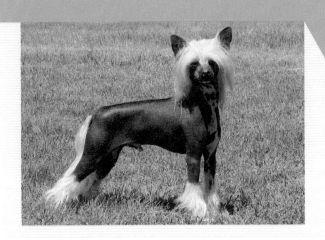

Chinese Crested

at the tip. In action the tail is held high or even over the back. Dewclaws may be removed. The finely boned limbs are straight, the feet are elongated with a "hare" conformation. The gait is quick and agile, but smooth. Skin may have a mottled pigmentation.

The Breed History

In Ancient times, it has been reported that the African hairless dog was taken to China where further breeding reduced the emerging breed to a toy size. Others place hairless South American dogs as distant relatives. First breed records date to the late 1800s. The Chinese crested dogs were left at ports of call around the world when sailors, who used the dogs onboard to control vermin, traded them with local merchants. In Mexico, they may have contributed to the development of the Chihuahua. First AKC registry occurred in 1991.

Breeding for Function

Historically, they were ratters, mousers, and companion dogs.

Physical Characteristics

Height at Withers: 11-13" (28-33 cm)

Weight: 5-12 lb (2-5.5 kg)

Coat: Two coat types exist: Hairless and Powderpuff. Hairless have no body hair. It is present only on the extremities and the head hair is called the crest. From the metacarpals and going distally, and from the tarsus distally they have socks of hair. The tail has a plume of hair as well. In all dogs the hair is silky, but the Powderpuff has a double coat. Any color is accepted, as is any color combination.

Powderpuff is a full-coated variety. Mixed haircoat litters are born to Powderpuff X hairless and hairless X hairless crosses. These two varieties are generally crossed because the hairless dogs are not as vigorous (breeding, integument, missing teeth). The hairless type is AD, and homozygotes are not viable, so hairless dogs are heterozygotes.

Longevity: 12-13 years.

Points of Conformation: A fine-boned toy dog with almost square proportions. Eyes are wide set and nose and eyes are colored to match the coat, and almond shaped. Erect ears are large, the skull is wedge shaped, the stop distinct, and the muzzle tapers. In the hairless variety, missing teeth are not faulted but in Powderpuff they are. The slightly arched neck provides for high head carriage. The topline is level though the croup slopes down slightly. The thorax is moderately shallow and there is a moderate abdominal tuck. The tapered tail reaches the tarsus at rest, and is slender with a curve

Recognized Behavior Issues and Traits

Reported attributes of the breed include: Playful, good for city and apartment living, low grooming needs but high bathing needs, lively, affectionate, does not tolerate temperature extremes well, especially cold.

These dogs are very prone to sunburn and papules. They are low shedders, have a low barking tendency, and need close human companionship.

Normal Physiologic Variations

Hairlessness is caused by a dominant gene that is lethal in utero in the homozygous state. This gene also produces variably expressed missing premolars in the heterozygous state. Because of the lethal homozygous state, breeding two heterozygous hairless dogs together produces a 2:1 ratio of hairless to (homozygous normal) powderpuff dogs. Breeding hairless to powderpuff dogs, produces a 1:1 ratio of hairless to powderpuff offspring.[1,2]

Chinese crested dogs are very sensitive to heat and cold. The skin is thin, and prone to lacerations and dryness. They sweat through their skin so they do not pant as much as other breeds.

Drug Sensitivities

None reported

Inherited Diseases

Incomplete Dentition: It is common to have variable expression of missing premolars with the autosomal dominant hairless phenotype.[1,2]

Patella Luxation: Polygenically inherited laxity of patellar ligaments, causing luxation, lameness, and later degenerative joint disease. Treat surgically if causing clinical signs. OFA reports 4.5% affected.[3]

Primary Lens Luxation (PLL) and Secondary Glaucoma: An autosomal recessive gene causes primary lens luxation. Homozygous affected dogs usually develop lens luxation between 4-8 years of age. Rarely, heterozygous carriers can develop lens luxation, but at a later age. Lens luxation can lead to secondary glaucoma and blindness. A genetic mutation has been identified, and a genetic test is available. OFA testing shows 27% carrier, and 2% affected.[4]

Progressive Retinal Atrophy (PRA): More than one form of PRA occurs in the breed. The autosomal recessive prcd form (age of onset between 3-8 years) occurs, and a genetic test exists but prcd-PRA does NOT appear to be the predominant PRA disease type. (See Optigen website: www.optigen.com) 0.56% of Chinese Crested

Dogs CERF examined by veterinary ophthalmologists between 2000-2005 are identified as affected, and 1.55% as suspicious for PRA. CERF does not recommend breeding Chinese Crested Dogs affected with PRA.[5]

Hip Dysplasia and Legg–Calve Perthes Disease: Polygenically inherited traits causing degenerative hip joint disease and arthritis. Too few Chinese Crested Dogs have been screened by OFA to determine an accurate frequency.[3]

Elbow Dysplasia: Polygenically inherited trait causing elbow arthritis. Too few Chinese Crested Dogs have been screened by OFA to determine an accurate frequency.[3]

Canine Multiple System Degeneration (CMSD): This rare, autosomal recessive disorder causes progressive cerebellar ataxia, with its onset between nine and sixteen weeks of age. Histopathology shows loss of Purkinje's cells, then bilateral symmetric degeneration of the olivary nuclei, followed by degeneration of the substantia nigra and caudate nucleus. Affected dogs do not survive beyond 5-6 months of age.[1]

Disease Predispositions

Vitreous Degeneration: Liquefaction of the vitreous gel which may predispose to retinal detachment and blindness. Vitreous Degeneration is reported in 7.69% of Chinese crested dogs CERF-examined by veterinary ophthalmologists between 2000-2005.[5]

Hypothyroidism: Inherited autoimmune thyroiditis. 7.4% positive for thyroid auto-antibodies based on testing at Michigan State University. (Ave. for all breeds is 7.5%).[6,7]

Sunburn: Chinese crested dogs are very sensitive to sunlight (ultraviolet radiation). Sun block should be used when exposed to direct sunlight.

Cataracts: Anterior and posterior cortex intermediate cataracts predominate in the breed, although nuclear and capsular cataracts also occur. Reported in 5.92% of Chinese Cresteds presented to veterinary teaching hospitals. Identified in 2.02% of Chinese Crested Dogs CERF examined by veterinary ophthalmologists between 2000-2005. CERF does not recommend breeding any Chinese Crested Dogs with a cataract.[5,8]

Persistent Pupillary Membranes: Strands of fetal remnant connecting; iris to iris, cornea, lens, or involving sheets of tissue. The later three forms can impair vision, and dogs affected with these forms should not be bred. Identified in 1.85% of Chinese Crested Dogs CERF examined by veterinary ophthalmologists between 2000-2005.[5]

Comedomes (Blackheads): The skin of Chinese crested dogs are prone to spontaneous comedome formation throughout the dorsal skin, on the limbs and prepuce. Plugged follicles containing abundant sebum and keratic substances resembles human acne.[9]

Deafness: Unilateral or bilateral congenital deafness is reported by Strain. Diagnosed by BAER testing.[10]

Brachygnathism and **Prognathism** are reported.[11]

Isolated Case Studies

None reported

Genetic Tests

Tests of Genotype: Direct test for prcd-PRA test is available from Optigen.

Direct test for PLL is available from the OFA and the Animal Health Trust.

Tests of Phenotype: CHIC Certification: Required testing includes CERF eye examination (annually), patella evaluation (at a minimum of 1 year of age), and a congenital cardiac evaluation. Optional testing includes genetic tests for PLL and prcd-PRA, BAER hearing test, and hip radiographs. (See CHIC website; www.caninehealthinfo.org).

Recommend elbow radiographs and thyroid profile including autoantibodies.

Miscellaneous

- **Breed name synonyms:** Crested, Crestie, Powderpuff, Chinese Edible dog (historical), Chinese Hairless, Chinese Royal Hairless, Chinese Ship Dog (historical), South African Hairless (historical in Africa), Pyramid or Giza Hairless (historical name in Egypt)
- **Registries:** AKC, UKC, CKC, KCGB (Kennel Club of Great Britain), ANKC (Australian National Kennel Club), NKC (National Kennel Club)
- **AKC rank (year 2008):** 54 (2,098 dogs registered)
- **Internet resources: American Chinese Crested Club Inc.:** www.accc.chinesecrestedclub.info/
  Chinese Crested Club of Great Britain: www.thechinesecrestedclubofgb.co.uk
  Chinese Crested Club of Canada: www.chinesecrestedclubcanada.com

References

1. O'brien DP, Johnson GS, Schnabel RD, et. al.: Genetic mapping of canine multiple system degeneration and ectodermal dysplasia Loci. J Hered. 2005 Nov-Dec;96(7):727-34.
2. Drögemüller C, Karlsson EK, Hytönen MK, et. al.: A mutation in hairless dogs implicates FOXI3 in ectodermal development. Science. 2008 Sep 12;321(5895):1462.
3. OFA Website breed statistics: www.offa.org Last accessed July 1, 2010.
4. Sargan DR, Withers D, Pettitt L, et. al.: Mapping the mutation causing lens luxation in several terrier breeds. J Hered. 2007;98(5):534-8.
5. Ocular Disorders Presumed to be Inherited in Purebred Dogs. American College of Veterinary Ophthalmologists. ACVO, 2007.
6. Nachreiner R & Refsal K: Personal communication, Diagnostic Center for Population and Animal Health, Michigan State University. April, 2007.
7. Nachreiner RF, Refsal KR, Graham PA, et. al.: Prevalence of serum thyroid hormone autoantibodies in dogs with clinical signs of hypothyroidism. J Am Vet Med Assoc 2002 Feb 15;220(4):466-71.
8. Gelatt KN, Mackay EO: Prevalence of primary breed-related cataracts in the dog in North America. Vet Ophthalmol. 2005 Mar-Apr;8(2):101-11.
9. Kimura T, Doi K: Spontaneous comedones on the skin of hairless descendants of Mexican hairless dogs. Exp Anim. 1996 Oct;45(4):377-84.
10. Strain GM: Deafness prevalence and pigmentation and gender associations in dog breeds at risk. Vet J 2004; Jan;167(1):23-32.
11. The Genetic Connection: A Guide to Health Problems in Purebred Dogs. L Ackerman. p. 209-10. AAHA Press, 1999.
12. *The Complete Dog Book, 20th Ed.* The American Kennel Club. Howell Book House, NY 2006. p. 462-465.

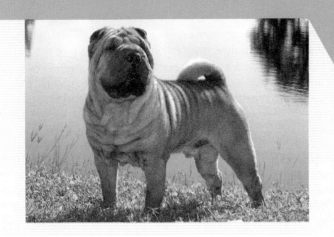

Chinese Shar-pei

broad and flattened, the butterfly nose is black or matching the coat color, nostrils are wide. The tail is thick at its origin, tapers to the tip and is very high set. It curls over the back when the dog is alert. Metatarsals are short, and rear dewclaws are removed. Forelimbs are straight and moderately boned and muscled, feet are medium-sized and toes are arched (not splayed). Their gait is smooth and ground covering.

The Breed History

Dating about 200 BC in the Kwantung province of China, first records of the breed consisted of artwork depictions. The name Shar-Pei means sand skin or sandpaper coat in Chinese. The breed was also found in the province of Guandong. Only this breed and the Chow Chow share the distinctive blue-black tongue. Perhaps Mastiffs and Chow Chows had a role in breed development, though records are not available to confirm this. First exports to the United States occurred in 1973. Full AKC recognition of this breed occurred in 1991.

Breeding for Function

These dogs were originally bred to be fierce fighting dogs, but now are used for companionship.

Physical Characteristics

Height at Withers: 18-20" (45.5-51 cm)

Weight: 45-60 lb (20.5-27 kg)

Coat: The straight, short standoff coat is very unusual in texture, being very short (< 1") and very rough (bristles). Solid colors such as black, cream and red and sable are accepted, but some shading of solids is often present and is acceptable.

Longevity: 11-12 years.

Points of Conformation: Blue-black tongue, palate, gingivae and lips/flews are present. Significant skin wrinkles are also a unique characteristic of this breed. Note that puppies have much more extensive wrinkles than the adult. In the adult the wrinkles may remain on the head, neck, and anterior thorax. Their dark eyes are small, deep set and almond shaped, and the expression is defined as scowling. Irises may be lighter in light coated dogs. The neck is short and strong, with a well-developed dewlap, the topline is fairly level though a dip behind the withers should be present. The thorax has moderate depth. Square, compact conformation, and medium in size, the head is large for the body, and their triangular thick-leathered clamshell ears are small and lying folded flat forward against the head. Prick ears are a disqualification. Their muzzle has a shape described as "hippopotamus" because of its fullness. Soft tissue may even cause a slight bulging or fold of the nose on top of the muzzle. The stop is moderate, and skull is

Recognized Behavior Issues and Traits

Reported breed attributes include: Courageous, alert, intelligent, dignified carriage with scowling visage, aloof with strangers, independent, loyal. Note that some dogs can be aggressive.

Normal Physiologic Variations

Flame follicles in microscopic skin sections are more frequent and found in significantly higher numbers in the Shar-pei breed compared with other breeds. Flame follicles from Shar-pei dogs do not have the same diagnostic significance as in other breeds.[1]

Pseudohyperkalemia, as reported in other breeds of Japanese origin, is a benign condition that has been identified in some Shar Pei.[2]

Drug Sensitivities

None reported

Inherited Diseases

Elbow Dysplasia: Polygenically inherited trait causing elbow arthritis. Reported 4.6x odds ratio for ununited anconeal process form of elbow dysplasia versus other breeds. OFA reports 24.5% affected.[3,4]

Hip Dysplasia: Polygenically inherited trait causing degenerative joint disease and hip arthritis. OFA reports 13.4% affected.[3]

Patella Luxation: Polygenically inherited laxity of patellar ligaments, causing luxation, lameness, and later degenerative joint disease. Treat surgically if causing clinical signs. Reported 11.4x odds ratio versus other breeds. OFA reports 9.9% affected.[3,4]

Primary Lens Luxation: Autosomal recessive inherited disorder in the Shar Pei. The average age of onset of affected dogs is 4.9 years (range 3-6 years). Relative risk of 44.66x versus other breeds. Identified in 1.89% of Shar Peis CERF examined by veterinary ophthalmologists between 2000-2005. CERF does not recommend breeding any Shar Pei with lens luxation. No genetic test is available.[5,6,7]

Disease Predispositions

Entropion: Entropion, a rolling in of the eyelids, can cause corneal irritation and ulceration. It is reported in 38.68% of Shar Peis CERF examined by veterinary phthalmologists between 2000-2005. Reported at a frequency of 34.9% in the CSPCA Health Through Education Health Survey. CERF does not recommend breeding any Shar Pei with entropion.[6,8]

Ear Disease: Bacterial ear infection was identified in 16.0% of Shar Peis, Yeast ear infection was identified in 31.8%, and Stenotic (narrowed) ear canals was identified in 9.2% of Shar Peis in the CSPCA Health Through Education Health Survey.[8]

Shar Pei Fever, Recurrent Fever of Unknown Origin (RFUO): Breed-related disorder causing high fever, swollen joints (especially hocks), and predisposing to renal amyloidosis and renal failure. An epidemiological survey of privately owned dogs indicated a RFUO prevalence of 23% in Shar Pei dogs. Reported at a frequency of 23.0% in the CSPCA Health Through Education Health Survey.[8,9,10]

Allergies: Inhalant allergies were identified in 7.7%, and Food Allergy was identified in 14.1% of Shar Peis in the CSPCA Health Through Education Health Survey.[8]

Cutaneous Mucinosis: Breed-related disorder of dermatitis secondary to mucin accumulation in skin. Studies show a defect in hyaluronic acid metabolism associated with the HAS2 gene. This condition may be related to abnormal mast cell function or accumulation. Treatment is with steroids. Reported at a frequency of 12.1% in the CSPCA Health Through Education Health Survey.[8,11,12,13,14,15,16]

Cobolamin Deficiency: Affected Shar Pei present with signs of chronic small intestinal disease, gastrointestinal protein loss, and possibly exocrine pancreatic insufficiency. Shar Pei have a 55.6x odds ratio versus other breeds. A region of chromosome 13 has been identified that cosegregates with cobalamin deficiency in the Chinese Shar Pei, but the actual gene and mechanism causing the disease has not been identified. Undetermined mode of inheritance. Test with serum cobalamin and B12 levels. Treat with cobalamin supplementation. Affected dogs should not be bred.[17,18]

Persistent Pupillary Membranes: Strands of fetal remnant connecting; iris to iris, cornea, lens, or involving sheets of tissue. The later three forms can impair vision, and dogs affected with these forms should not be bred. Identified in 6.60% of Shar Pei CERF examined by veterinary ophthalmologists between 2000-2005, with 3.77% iris to iris, 1.89% iris to cornea, and 1.89% iris to lens. Dorn reports a 7.47x odds ratio versus other breeds.[6,19]

Aggression: Inter-dog aggression is reported at 15.0%, and aggression toward people reported at 6.4% in the CSPCA Health Through Education Health Survey.[8]

Primary Seborrhea: Abnormality of epidermal differentiation, keratinization and cornification, where the epithelial turnover rate increases to as short as 3-4 days. Characterized by a greasy, flaky, thin haircoat. Dorn reports a 54.36x odds ratio versus other breeds.[20]

Bacterial Skin Infection: Reported at a frequency of 5.0% in the CSPCA Health Through Education Health Survey.[8]

Hypothyroidism: Inherited autoimmune thyroiditis. 4.5% positive for thyroid auto-antibodies based on testing at Michigan State University. (Ave. for all breeds is 7.5%.) Reported at a frequency of 10.6% in the CSPCA Health Through Education Health Survey.[8,21,22]

Renal Amyloidosis (RA): Breed-specific syndrome seen in young Chinese Shar Pei dogs causing renal failure. May be preceded in some dogs by intermittent fever and joint swelling (Shar Pei fever). Pathological findings include deposition of amyloid in the renal medulla, with possible deposition in glomeruli, liver, spleen, stomach, small intestine, myocardium, lymph node, prostate gland, thyroid gland, and pancreas. Shar Pei dogs under 7 years of age have a 10x odds ratio of developing RA. The prevalence of RA among littermates is between 25% and 50%. Reported at a frequency of 4.5% in the CSPCA Health Through Education Health Survey.[8,23,24]

Demodicosis: Focal or generalized demodectic mange has an underlying immunodeficiency in its pathogenesis. Reported at a frequency of 3.5% in the CSPCA Health Through Education Health Survey.[8]

Primary (Narrow Angle) Glaucoma: Ocular condition causing increased pressure within the eyeball, and secondary blindness due to damage to the retina. Diagnose with tonometry and gonioscopy. Diagnosed in 4.40% of Shar Peis presented to veterinary teaching hospitals.[25]

Megaesophagus: Dilated esophagus resulting in regurgitation and possible inhalation pneumonia. Can be secondary to hiatal hernia in this breed. Reported at a frequency of 4.0% in the CSPCA Health Through Education Health Survey.[8]

Cataracts: Capsular and anterior cortex cataracts predominate in the breed, though posterior and nuclear cataracts also occur. Identified in 3.77% of Shar Peis CERF examined by veterinary ophthalmologists between 2000-2005. CERF does not recommend breeding any Shar Pei with a cataract. Reported at a frequency of 3.0% in the CSPCA Health Through Education Health Survey.[6,8]

Chronic Superficial Keratitis (Pannus): Chronic corneal inflammatory process that can cause vision problems due to corneal pigmentation. Treatment with topical ocular lubricants and anti-inflammatory medication. Identified in 2.83% of Shar Peis CERF examined by veterinary ophthalmologists between 2000-2005.[6]

Corneal Dystrophy: The epithelial/stromal form occurs in the breed, causing a bilateral, white to gray, non-inflammatory corneal opacity. Identified in 2.83% of Shar Peis CERF examined by veterinary ophthalmologists between 2000-2005.[6]

Mast Cell Tumors: An increased incidence of mast cell tumors is seen in Shar Peis. In one study, 2.2% of all mast cell tumors submitted for pathology occurred in Shar Peis, despite the breed accounting for only 0.7% of all pathology submissions. In addition, 28% of the mast cell tumors occurred in Shar Peis under 2 years of age. Reported at a frequency of 3.5% in the CSPCA Health Through Education Health Survey.[8,26]

Ectropion: Ectropion, a rolling out of the eyelids, can cause frequent conjunctivitis, and ocular discharge. It is reported in 1.89% of Shar Peis CERF examined by veterinary ophthalmologists between 2000-2005.[6]

Retinal Dysplasia: Focal folds and geographic retinal dysplasia are seen in the breed. Dogs with the geographic form should not be bred. Reported in 1.89% of Shar Pei CERF examined by veterinary ophthalmologists between 2000-2005.[6]

Gastric Dilatation-Volvulus (bloat, GDV): Polygenically inherited, life-threatening twisting of the stomach within the abdomen. Requires immediate treatment. Reported at a frequency of 1.3% in the CSPCA Health Through Education Health Survey.[8,27]

Esophageal Hiatal Hernia: Congenital disorder seen at an increased frequency in the breed. Clinical signs are regurgitation, vomiting, and hypersalivation. Diagnose with survey or barium radiographs showing displacement of the esophagogastric junction and stomach into the thoracic cavity. Affected dogs can also develop secondary megaesophagus, gastroesophageal reflux, esophageal hypomotility, or aspiration pneumonia. Treatment is with surgery.[28,29,30]

Primary Immunodeficiency: Primary immunodeficiency syndromes are described in the breed; including IgA deficiency, and combined IgM, IgA, and IgG deficiency. Clinical signs include frequent recurrent infections (respiratory and skin), and malignancy.[31,32,33]

Pemphigus Foliaceus: The breed has an increased risk (7.9x odds ratio) of developing pemphigus foliaceus. Clinical signs include crusting lesions to the dorsal part of the muzzle and head, progressing to the body. Diagnosis is with biopsy.[34]

Lingual Melanoma: Malignant melanoma of the tongue occurs at increased frequency in Shar Peis compared to other breeds.[35]

Brachycephalic Syndrome, Brachygnathism, Cleft Lip/Palate, Factor XII Deficiency, Fold Dermatitis, Keratoconjunctivitis Sicca, Osteochondritis Dessicans – Shoulder, Prognathism, Progressive Retinal Atrophy, Prolapsed Gland of Nictitans, Seborrhea, and **Subaortic Stenosis** are reported.[36]

Isolated Case Studies

Neutrophilic Vasculitis: Three young Shar-Pei dogs presented with fever, malaise, and widespread cutaneous lesions consisting of skin discolouration, edema, and pus-filled bullae that progressed to ulceration, necrosis, and granulation. Immune-mediated vasculitis was diagnosed, and treatment was with steroids. Two of the three recovered.[37]

Gastrointestinal Epitheliotropic Lymphoma: Three Shar Pei dogs between the ages of 4-8 years were diagnosed with T-cell lymphoma of the gastrointersinal system. Clinical signs were diarrhea, progressive anorexia, weight loss, and vomiting.[38]

Ciliary Dysfunction: A litter of Shar Pei pups was studied with recurrent repiratory infections without immunodeficiency. Absent ciliary function was identified in one of the pups.[39]

Genetic Tests

Tests of Genotype: Direct test for coat and nose color is available from Healthgene and VetGen.

Tests of Phenotype: CHIC Certification: Required tests are; CERF eye examination, hip and elbow radiographs, patella examination, and thyroid profile including autoantibodies. (See CHIC website: www.caninehealthinfo.org)

Recommended cardiac evaluation.

Miscellaneous

- **Breed name synonyms:** Shar-pei, Chinese Fighting Dog
- **Registries:** AKC, UKC, CKC, KCGB (Kennel Club of Great Britain), ANKC (Australian National Kennel Club), NKC (National Kennel Club)
- **AKC rank (year 2008):** 47 (2,583 dogs registered)
- **Internet resources: Chinese Shar-Pei Club of America Inc.:** www.cspca.com
  Shar-Pei Club of Great Britain: www.sharpei-clubofgb.co.uk
  Chinese Shar-pei Club of Canada: www.peiclub.com

References

1. Ordeix L, Fondevila D, Ferrer L, et. al.: Quantitative study of "flame follicles" in skin sections of Shar-pei dogs. Vet Dermatol. 2002 Oct;13(5):261-5.
2. Battison A: Apparent pseudohyperkalemia in a Chinese Shar Pei dog. Vet Clin Pathol. 2007 Mar;36(1):89-93.
3. OFA Website breed statistics: www.offa.org Last accessed July 1, 2010.
4. LaFond E, Breur GJ & Austin CC: Breed susceptibility for developmental orthopedic diseases in dogs. J Am Anim Hosp Assoc. 2002 Sep-Oct;38(5):467-77.
5. Lazarus JA, Pickett JP, Champagne ES: Primary lens luxation in the Chinese Shar Pei: clinical and hereditary characteristics. Vet Ophthalmol. 1998;1(2-3):101-107.
6. Ocular Disorders Presumed to be Inherited in Purebred Dogs. American College of Veterinary Ophthalmologists. ACVO, 2007.
7. Sargan DR, Withers D, Pettitt L, et. al.: Mapping the mutation causing lens luxation in several terrier breeds. J Hered. 2007;98(5):534-8.
8. Chinese Shar Pei Club of America Health Through Education Committee: Health Survey Results. 2007.
9. Rivas AL, Tintle L, Kimball ES, et. al.: A canine febrile disorder associated with elevated interleukin-6. Clin Immunol Immunopathol. 1992 Jul;64(1):36-45.
10. May C, Hammill J, Bennett D: Chinese shar pei fever syndrome: a preliminary report. Vet Rec. 1992 Dec 19-26;131(25-26):586-7.
11. von Bomhard D, Kraft W: Idiopathic mucinosis cutis in Chinese Shar pei dogs: epidemiology, clinical features, histopathologic findings and treatment. Tierarztl Prax Ausg K Klientiere Heimtiere. 1998 May;26(3):189-96.
12. Lopez A, Spracklin D, McConkey S, et. al.: Cutaneous mucinosis and mastocytosis in a shar-pei. Can Vet J. 1999 Dec;40(12):881-3.
13. Welle M, Grimm S, Suter M, et. al.: Mast cell density and subtypes in the skin of Shar Pei dogs with cutaneous mucinosis. Zentralbl Veterinarmed A. 1999 Jul;46(5):309-16.
14. Zanna G, Fondevila D, Bardagí M, et. al.: Cutaneous mucinosis in shar-pei dogs is due to hyaluronic acid deposition and is associated with high levels of hyaluronic acid in serum. Vet Dermatol. 2008 Oct;19(5):314-8.
15. Zanna G, Docampo MJ, Fondevila D, et. al.: Hereditary cutaneous mucinosis in shar pei dogs is associated with increased hyaluronan synthase-2 mRNA transcription by cultured dermal fibroblasts. Vet Dermatol. 2009 Oct;20(5-6):377-82.
16. Akey JM, Ruhe AL, Akey DT, et. al.: Tracking footprints of artificial selection in the dog genome. Proc Natl Acad Sci U S A. 2010 Jan 19;107(3):1160-5.
17. Grützner N, Bishop MA, Suchodolski JS, et. al.: Association Study of Cobalamin Deficiency in the Chinese Shar Pei. J Hered. 2010 Mar-Apr;101(2):211-7.
18. Bishop MA, Xenoulis PG, Suchodolski JS, et. al.: Prevalence of Cobalamin Deficiency in Chinese Shar Peis
19. Dorn CR: Canine breed-specific risks of frequently diagnosed diseases at veterinary teaching hospitals. Monograph. AKC Canine Health Foundation. 2000.
20. Hall JA: Congenital and Hereditary Defects in Skin Disease.2005 Proceedings, Western Veterinary Conference 2005.

21. Nachreiner R & Refsal K: Personal communication, Diagnostic Center for Population and Animal Health, Michigan State University. April, 2007.

22. Nachreiner RF, Refsal KR, Graham PA, et. al.: Prevalence of serum thyroid hormone autoantibodies in dogs with clinical signs of hypothyroidism. J Am Vet Med Assoc 2002 Feb 15;220(4):466-71.

23. DiBartola SP, Tarr MJ, Webb DM, et. al.: Familial renal amyloidosis in Chinese Shar Pei dogs. J Am Vet Med Assoc. 1990 Aug 15;197(4):483-7.

24. Rivas AL, Tintle L, Meyers-Wallen V, et. al.: Inheritance of renal amyloidosis in Chinese Shar-pei dogs. J Hered. 1993 Nov-Dec;84(6):438-42.

25. Gelatt KN, MacKay EO: Prevalence of the breed-related glaucomas in pure-bred dogs in North America. Vet Ophthalmol. 2004 Mar-Apr;7(2):97-111.

26. Miller DM: The occurrence of mast cell tumors in young Shar-Peis. J Vet Diagn Invest. 1995 Jul;7(3):360-3.

27. Glickman LT, Glickman NW, Schellenberg DB, et. al.: Incidence of and breed-related risk factors for gastric dilatation-volvulus in dogs. J Am Vet Med Assoc. 2000 Jan 1;216(1):40-5.

28. Rahal SC, Mamprim MJ, Muniz LM, et. al.: Type-4 esophageal hiatal hernia in a Chinese Shar-pei dog. Vet Radiol Ultrasound. 2003 Nov-Dec;44(6):646-7.

29. Callan MB, Washabau RJ, Saunders HM, et. al.: Congenital esophageal hiatal hernia in the Chinese shar-pei dog. J Vet Intern Med. 1993 Jul-Aug;7(4):210-5.

30. Guiot LP, Lansdowne JL, Rouppert P, et. al.: Hiatal hernia in the dog: a clinical report of four Chinese shar peis. J Am Anim Hosp Assoc. 2008 Nov-Dec;44(6):335-41.

31. Moroff SD, Hurvitz AI, Peterson ME, et. al.: IgA deficiency in shar-pei dogs. Vet Immunol Immunopathol. 1986 Nov;13(3):181-8.

32. Rivas AL, Tintle L, Argentieri D, et. al.: A primary immunodeficiency syndrome in Shar-Pei dogs. Clin Immunol Immunopathol. 1995 Mar;74(3):243-51.

33. Miller WH Jr, Wellington JR, Scott DW: Dermatologic disorders of Chinese Shar Peis: 58 cases (1981-1989). J Am Vet Med Assoc. 1992 Apr 1;200(7):986-90.

34. Kuhl KA, Shofer FS, Goldschmidt MH: Comparative histopathology of pemphigus foliaceus and superficial folliculitis in the dog. Vet Pathol. 1994 Jan;31(1):19-27.

35. Dennis MM, Ehrhart N, Duncan CG, et. al.: Frequency of and risk factors associated with lingual lesions in dogs: 1,196 cases (1995-2004). J Am Vet Med Assoc. 2006 May 15;228(10):1533-7.

36. *The Genetic Connection: A Guide to Health Problems in Purebred Dogs.* L Ackerman. p. 210. AAHA Press, 1999.

37. Malik R, Foster SF, Martin P, et. al.: Acute febrile neutrophilic vasculitis of the skin of young Shar-Pei dogs. Aust Vet J. 2002 Apr;80(4):200-6.

38. Steinberg H, Dubielzig RR, Thomson J, et. al.: Primary gastrointestinal lymphosarcoma with epitheliotropism in three Shar-pei and one boxer dog. Vet Pathol. 1995 Jul;32(4):423-6.

39. Dhein CR, Prieur DJ, Riggs MW, et. al.: Suspected ciliary dysfunction in Chinese Shar Pei pups with pneumonia. Am J Vet Res. 1990 Mar;51(3):439-46

40. *The Complete Dog Book, 20th Ed.* The American Kennel Club. Howell Book House, NY 2006. p. 543-546.

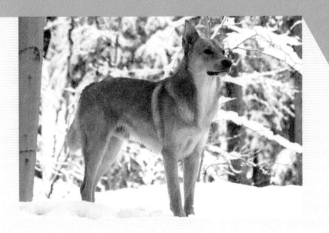

The Breed History

A single dog named Chinook gave rise to this Northern type breed in Wonalancet, New Hampshire. He was born in 1917, the offspring of one of the Peary expedition dog's daughters. Chinook went to the South Pole on the Byrd expedition of 1927. In 1991, the UKC recognized the Chinook as a breed. Breed origins are not documented, though Spitz-type and Mastiff-types are thought to have been included. A very close brush with extinction occurred in the 1970's, but a few dedicated breeders gathered the 12 breeding dogs together in a few homes and by 1990, their numbers had increased to 140, and in '96, 450. A crossbreeding program has been instituted to help increase the gene pool of the dogs. Outcrosses are very selective, with 4 generation pedigree analysis to check for any disorders—only clear dogs are used. Offspring are then crossed with purebred Chinooks and in the fourth generation are considered for registration to register if all health checks and performance meet the breed standard.

Breeding for Function

A sled dog, built for speed and weight pulling, and endurance. They were also carefully selected for a gentle, tractable nature. This gave them a most suitable temperament as a house dog and they have become popular as a companion dog. In modern times, they have also excelled as therapy dogs, in obedience and agility, and carting/pulling.

Physical Characteristics

Height at Withers: female 21- 25" (53-64 cm), male 23-27" (58-69 cm)

Weight: 55-70 lb (25-32 kg)

Coat: Tawny (honey to red-gold) color, dense double coat, of medium length, the low set tail hangs away from the body in a saber shape—has feathers hanging down, and is carried high when active. No white markings are allowed. Black markings at the inner canthus are desirable. No trimming is done at all. Outer hairs are harsh, undercoat is soft. Feet are well-furred and webbed. Ruff present.

Longevity: 12-14 years

Points of Conformation: Broad skull, moderate stop, no wrinkling of the skin on the head, cheeks are chiseled. The muzzle tapering but stays deep, eyes almond shaped and brown in color, though amber accepted but less preferred, nose is large and is set slightly ahead of the front lip line, lip margins and nose black, eyelid rims

dark, slightly pendulous lips. Scissors bite. Ears are wide set, with thick leather and a good cover of fur, and variably set. From drop to prick or helicopter ears are accepted, though both ears should match in setting. Neck is moderately arched. Overall conformation is slightly longer than tall. Ribs well sprung, topline is level though with a curve slightly upwards through the loin. Thorax is deep. Abdomen well tucked up. Feet are oval and toes well knuckled up. Pads are thick and darkly pigmented, and plenty of fur is present around the foot and between toes. Limbs straight, with good bone and well muscled. Dewclaws on the forelimb may be removed, rear dewclaws if present are always removed. Front feet are slightly deviated outward. Gait is characteristically a long fluid trot.

Recognized Behavior Issues and Traits

Breed attributes reported include: Very calm, really friendly, not aggressive—though a reserved attitude to strangers or strange places is not discouraged. As a team dog, their aggressive tendencies to other dogs are not well developed. Shyness/fearfulness is a problem in the breed, with 11% of Chinooks reported in the 2003 COA Chinook health survey.[1]

Normal Breed Variations

None reported

Drug Sensitivities

None reported

Inherited Diseases

Hip Dysplasia: Polygenically inherited trait causing degenerative joint disease and hip arthritis. OFA reports 18.0% affected.[2]

Epilepsy (Chinook Seizures): Both grand-mal and petit-mal seizures are reported in the breed. Breed specific petit-mal seizures are described as an episodic dyskinesia , which can involve just one limb, or a frozen stare. 2003 COA Chinook health survey reported 8% affected with some form of Chinook seizures. This disorder is being studied at the University of Missouri (http://www.canine-epilepsy.net/Chinook/chinook.html). Pedigree indicates an autosomal recessive mode of inheritance.[1,3]

Elbow Dysplasia: Polygenically inherited trait causing elbow arthritis. Too few Chinooks have been screened by OFA to determine an accurate frequency.[2]

Patella Luxation: Polygenically inherited laxity of patellar ligaments, causing luxation, lameness, and later degenerative joint disease. Treat surgically if causing clinical signs. A high frequency is reported by the OFA, but too few Chinooks have been screened to determine an accurate frequency.[2]

Disease Predispositions

Cryptorchidism: Undescended testicles occurs at a high frequency in the breed. 21.5% of males had unilateral cryptorchidism, and

7.7% of males bilateral cryptorchidism in the 2003 COA Chinook health survey. This is a sex-limited disorder with an unknown mode of inheritance.[1]

Hypothyroidism: Inherited autoimmune thyroiditis. 10.0% positive for thyroid auto-antibodies based on testing at Michigan State University. (Ave. for all breeds is 7.5%).[4,5]

Allergic Dermatitis: Presents with pyotraumatic dermatitis (hot spots). Reported in 9.6% of dogs in the 2003 COA Chinook health survey.[1]

Gastrointestinal Disease: Chronic vomiting or colitis was reported in 7.5% of Chinooks in the 2003 COA Chinook health survey.[1]

Persistent Pupillary Membranes: Strands of fetal remnant connecting; iris to iris, cornea, lens, or involving sheets of tissue. The later three forms can impair vision, and dogs affected with these forms should not be bred. Identified in 3.45% of Chinooks CERF examined by veterinary ophthalmologists between 2000-2005.[6]

Retinal Dysplasia: Retinal folds and geographic retinal dysplasia are recognized in the breed. Reported in 3.25% of Chinooks CERF examined by veterinary ophthalmologists between 2000-2005.[6]

Cataracts: Anterior cortex punctate cataracts predominate, though posterior, nuclear, and capsular cataracts also occur in the breed. Identified in 2.92% of Chinooks CERF examined by veterinary ophthalmologists between 2000-2005. CERF does not recommend breeding any Chinook with a cataract.[6]

Isolated Case Studies

Anasarca: Multiple reports of fetal anasarca (hydrops fetalis) are reported in the breed. Affected puppies are born dead and edematous.

Genetic Tests

Tests of Genotype: none

Tests of Phenotype: CHIC Certification: Required testing includes hip radiographs, CERF eye examination, and either cardiac examination, thyroid profile including autoantibodies, patella evaluation or elbow radiographs. Optional recommended tests are; veterinary confirmation of Epilepsy/Chinook Seizures, Cryptorchidism, Dwarfism, or Allergies. (See CHIC website; www. caninehealthinfo.org).

Miscellaneous

- **Breed name synonyms:** none
- **Registries:** UKC, AKC Misc. class, CKC
- **Breed resources: Chinook Club of America (AKC):** www.chinookclubofamerica.org
  Chinook Owners Association (UKC): www.chinook.org
  Chinook Health Fund:
  http://chinookhealthfund.homestead.com/home.html

References

1. Chinook Owners Association, Inc.: 2003 COA Chinook Health Survey. October, 2003.
2. OFA Website breed statistics: www.offa.org Last accessed July 1, 2010.
3. Packer RA, O'Brien DP, Coates JP, et. al.: Characterization and Mode of Inheritance of An Episodic Dyskinesia in The Chinook Dog. Proceedings, 2006 AVIM Forum. 2006.
4. Nachreiner R & Refsal K: Personal communication, Diagnostic Center for Population and Animal Health, Michigan State University. April, 2007.
5. Nachreiner RF, Refsal KR, Graham PA, et. al.: Prevalence of serum thyroid hormone autoantibodies in dogs with clinical signs of hypothyroidism. J Am Vet Med Assoc 2002 Feb 15;220(4):466-71.
6. *Ocular Disorders Presumed to be Inherited in Purebred Dogs.* American College of Veterinary Ophthalmologists. ACVO, 2007.
7. AKC Breed website: www.akc.org/breeds/chinook/ Last accessed Jan, 1 2010.

Chow Chow

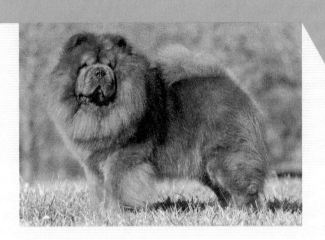

The Breed History

In China about 150 BC, art depicts a Spitz type dog such as this, but it is likely the breed developed earlier in time. History records the presence of these types of dogs during the Tartar invasion of China about 1000 BC. Perhaps the Siberian Husky and Tibetan Mastiff were the breed progenitors or were offshoots from this breed. The name chow chow is a generic shipping term for "such and such" in the cargo hold, also chow may derive from chou, Chinese for edible. Whatever the real meaning, the dogs were given this nickname. They were first brought to England in the year 1880. The AKC admitted the breed in 1903.

Breeding for Function

The Chow has fulfilled many roles over the centuries including hunting by scent for pheasant and other game, companionship, livestock guard dog, pulling loads, producer of fur for clothing, and in China, as a food source.

Physical Characteristics

Height at Withers: 17-20" (43-51 cm)

Weight: 45-70 lb (20-32 kg)

Coat: The double coat is present in two varieties: a short smooth coat and a longer rough coat that stands out. The latter is much more common. Short-coated dogs have a distinct undercoat and the outer coat is dense, hard, and smooth in texture and no feathers or ruff are evident. Colors are solid to solid with shading. Colors accepted include red, black, blue, cinnamon and cream. Whites are very rare.

Longevity: 11-12 years.

Points of Conformation: The Chow has an arctic type with a square strong broad build and compact conformation. The blue tongue and compressed scowling face characterize the breed. The bone is also heavy, muscling moderate and the haircoat is profuse. The head is broad and flat, and the muzzle is blocky. He possesses a high head carriage, and the oblique almond-shaped eyes are deep and wide set with dark brown color. They have tight darkly pigmented palpebral margins. Ears are pricked, small and the leather is moderate in thickness, with slightly rounded tips. On the face, one sees a moderate stop, brows well developed, and the large black nose has well opened nostrils. A slate nose may be present in blue coat colored

chows. Lip margins, and all oral cavity membranes are black and the tongue is blue-black. The neck is full, well muscled and arched, the topline is straight and level, and ribs are well sprung. Limbs are straight, dewclaws may be removed, and feet are compact and sit on well-knuckled toes. A broad pelvis is evident. The tail is well feathered. The long rough coated dogs possess a well-developed ruff, especially in males (sometimes referred to as lion-like). The tapered tail is set high and carried over the back and covered with a profusion of hair. The normal gait is stilted due to the conformation of the rear limbs (straight through both tarsus and stifle).

Recognized Behavior Issues and Traits

Reported attributes of the breed include: Independent, dignified, confident, willful, high intelligence, can be aggressive to other dogs and small pets, aloof with strangers and may attack due to their guarding heritage. Overall, on average have dominant personalities. Their eye placement may trigger defensive responses due to their inability to access the full visual field; may be snappy and will bite if provoked, can tend to be a one-person dog. Early obedience is important, and early socialization is essential to discourage the aforementioned tendencies in some dogs. Should be raised with children or socialized thoroughly and children should be taught how to treat the dog. They need daily grooming to maintain a good coat. These are high shedding dogs. They have moderate exercise needs and are easily housebroken, and have a low doggy odor. They are considered good alarm barkers. They do not tolerate heat and humidity well.

Normal Physiologic Variations

Lip margins, and all oral cavity membranes are black and the tongue is blue-black.

A study in the UK shows 28.1% of litters are born via **C-section**.[1]

Drug Sensitivities

None reported

Inherited Diseases

Elbow Dysplasia: Polygenically inherited trait causing elbow arthritis. OFA reports 47.6% affected. Found at a higher incidence than reported by the OFA in South Africa. Reported 16.6x odds ratio for fragmented coronoid process, 13.3x odds ratio for ununited anconeal process forms of elbow dysplasia, and 108.8x odds ratio for elbow osteochondrosis versus other breeds.[2,3,4]

Hip Dysplasia: Polygenically inherited trait causing degenerative joint disease and hip arthritis. Reported 5.4x odds ratio versus other breeds. OFA reports 19.6% affected.[2,4]

Patella Luxation: Polygenically inherited laxity of patellar ligaments, causing luxation, lameness, and later degenerative joint disease. Treat surgically if causing clinical signs. Reported 6.1x odds ratio versus other breeds. OFA reports 11.4% affected.[2,4]

Congenital Myotonia: Rare, autosomal recessive congenital disorder that causes hindlimb ataxia, a stiff gait, and occasional collapsing. The severe muscle stiffness regresses with exercise. Treatment is with procainamide.[5,6]

Disease Predispositions

Persistent Pupillary Membranes: Strands of fetal remnant connecting; iris to iris, cornea, lens, or involving sheets of tissue. The later three forms can impair vision, and dogs affected with these forms should not be bred. Severely affected Chow Chows can be temporarily or permanently blind due to adherence to the cornea or lens. Dorn reports a 3.89x odds ratio versus other breeds. Identified in 46.45% of Chow Chows CERF examined by veterinary ophthalmologists between 2000-2005, with 45.16% iris to iris, 4.19% iris to cornea, and 1.29% iris to lens. CERF does not recommend breeding any Chow-Chows with the later two categories of PPM.[7,8]

Entropion: A rolling in of the eyelids that can cause corneal irritation and ulceration. It is reported in 39.35% of Chow Chows CERF examined by veterinary ophthalmologists between 2000-2005. Dorn reports a 14.64x odds ratio versus other breeds. CERF does not recommend breeding affected Chow Chows.[7,8]

Hypothyroidism: Inherited autoimmune thyroiditis. 7.4% positive for thyroid auto-antibodies based on testing at Michigan State University. (Ave. for all breeds is 7.5%).[9,10]

Pemphigus Foliaceus: The breed has an increased risk (12.3x odds ratio) of developing pemphigus foliaceus. Clinical signs include crusting lesions to the dorsal part of the muzzle and head, progressing to the body. Diagnosis is with biopsy.[11]

Aggression: Chow Chows are significantly over represented in human bite cases with a 4.0x odds ratio versus other breeds.[12]

Primary (Narrow Angle) Glaucoma: Ocular condition causing increased pressure within the eyeball, and secondary blindness due to damage to the retina. Primary glaucoma in the breed is a bilateral condition due to narrow iridocorneal angles, with an age of onset of 3-6 years. One study shows 4.70% Chow Chows affected. A female preponderance occurs in the breed. Monitor with gonioscopy and tonometry. Dorn reports a 1.35x odds ratio versus other breeds. CERF does not recommend breeding affected Chow Chows.[7,8,13,14]

Cranial Cruciate Ligament Rupture: The Chow Chow has a predisposition for cruciate ligament rupture, due to its straight hind leg conformation. Treatment is with surgery.[15]

Corneal Dystrophy: Chow Chows have been identified with both the epithelial/stromal and endothelial forms of corneal dystrophy. Identified in 1.94% of Chow Chows CERF examined by veterinary ophthalmologists between 2000-2005. CERF does not recommend breeding affected Chow Chows.[7]

Exposure Keratopathy Syndrome: Corneal reactivity and drying from ocular exposure secondary to shallow orbits, exophthalmos, and lagophthalmos. Identified in 1.61% of Chow Chows CERF examined by veterinary ophthalmologists between 2000-2005.[7]

Ectropion: Ectropion, a rolling out of the eyelids, can cause frequent conjunctivitis, and ocular discharge. It is reported in 1.61% of Chow Chows CERF examined by veterinary ophthalmologists between 2000-2005.[7]

Chronic Superficial Keratitis (Pannus): Chronic corneal inflammatory process that can cause vision problems due to corneal pigmentation. Treatment with topical ocular lubricants and anti-inflammatory medication. Identified in 1.29% of Chow Chows CERF examined by veterinary ophthalmologists between 2000-2005.[7]

Cataracts/Congenital Cataracts with Ocular Anomalies: Inherited disorder causing congenital cataracts, sometimes associated with wandering nystagmus, entropion, microphthalmia, persistent pupillary membrane remnants, and multifocal retinal folds. Unknown mode of inheritance. Cataracts are identified in 1.29% of Chow Chows CERF examined by veterinary ophthalmologists between 2000-2005. CERF does not recommend breeding any Chow Chow with a cataract.[7,16]

Alopecia-X (Black Skin Disease, BSD, Coat Funk): Progressive, symmetrical, non-pruritic, truncal hair loss usually beginning in early adulthood. ACTH, LDDS, and thyroid panel results are normal. Oral trilostane reverses the condition in some cases. The disorder appears to be familial.[17,18]

Sebaceous Adenitis: Disorder of immune mediated sebaceous gland destruction, presenting with hair loss, hyperkeratosis and seborrhoea, usually beginning with the dorsal midline and ears. Diagnosis by skin biopsy. Treat with isotretinoin. Reported at an increased frequency in the breed.[19]

Gastric Carcinoma: Chow Chows have the highest frequency of gastric carcinoma compared with other breeds. The most frequent clinical features are vomiting, polydipsia and weight loss, with endoscopic findings of a large deep ulcer with thickened, irregular rims and walls.[20]

Gastric Dilatation-Volvulus (bloat, GDV): Polygenically inherited, life-threatening twisting of the stomach within the abdomen. Requires immediate treatment. Reported at an increased frequency in the breed.[21]

Oral and Lingual Melanoma: Chow Chows have a higher incidence of oral melanomas versus other breeds. One study found a 7.89x relative risk versus other breeds. The gingival, labial mucosa, and tongue are the most common sites. Average age of onset is 11.4 years.[22,23]

Pulmonic Stenosis: Congenital malformation of the pulmonic valve. Causes stricture of the right ventricular outflow tract or stricture of the pulmonary artery. Screen with auscultation and echocardiography. The Chow Chow has a 2.2x odds ratio for the condition versus other breeds. Unknown mode of inheritance.[24]

Atrioventricular Block (AVB): Chow Chows are predisposed to high-grade second- or third-degree AVB. Weakness, lethargy, exercise intolerance, and syncope were the most common clinical signs. Recommended treatment is pacemaker implantation.[25]

Pancreatic Acinar Atrophy (Exocrine pancreatic insufficiency): Chow Chows are a breed at risk for immune-mediated pancreatic acinar atrophy. Clinical signs are poor weight gain, and steatorrhea. Treatment is with enzyme supplementation. Breeding studies suggest an autosomal recessive mode of inheritance in German shepherd dogs, another breed found at risk.[26]

Familial Juvenile Renal Disease: Kidney disorder seen in young Chow Chows causing classical polyuric, azotemic renal failure with anemia. Pathology includes interstitial fibrosis, small glomeruli, and lack of inflammatory cells. Unknown mode of inheritance.[27]

Atresia Ani (Imperforate Anus): An increased incidence of this congenital condition is reported in the breed, with a frequency of 0.043%, and an odds ratio of 8.90x. Treatment is surgery.[28]

Dysmyelination of the Central Nervous System: Rare, inherited congenital disorder causing whole body tremors. Affected dogs can survive with clinical signs. Unknown mode of inheritance.[29,30]

Cervical Vertebral Instability, Color Dilution Alopecia, Dermatomyositis, Diabetes Mellitus, Epilepsy, Hypoadreno-corticism, IgA Deficiency, Keratoconjunctivitis Sicca, Osteocondritis Dessicans – Stifle, Progressive Retinal Atrophy, Tyrosinase Deficiency, Uveodermatological Syndrome, and **Ventricular Septal Defect** are reported.[31]

Isolated Case Studies

Bronchial Cartilage Dysplasia: A 5-month-old Chow Chow that had exercise intolerance, progressive dyspnea, and episodic cough was diagnosed with bronchial cartilage dysplasia and secondary lobar bullous emphysema.[32]

Ciliary Dyskinesia: A Chow Chow was diagnosed with congenital cliliary dyskinesia resembling Kartagener's syndrome. Ciliary ultrastructure was normal, with poor ciliary function. Clinical signs are chronic respiratory infections.[33,34]

Dermoid Sinus: A case report described multiple dermoid sinuses in the dorsal cervical and craniothoracic regions in an adult chow chow dog. One sinus did not open on the skin surface.[35]

Genetic Tests

Tests of Genotype: Direct test for coat color is available from VetGen.

Tests of Phenotype: CHIC Certification: Required tests are; CERF eye examination, hip and elbow radiographs, thyroid profile including autoantibodies, and patella evaluation. (See CHIC website: www.caninehealthinfo.org)

Recommend cardiac evaluation.

Miscellaneous

- **Breed name synonyms:** Chow, Chinese Chow, local nicknames include "Black tongue" and "Black mouth dog" in Chinese. Other Chinese names are lang kou (wolf dog) and hsiung kou (bear dog)
- **Registries:** AKC, UKC, CKC, KCGB (Kennel Club of Great Britain), ANKC (Australian National Kennel Club), NKC (National Kennel Club)

- **AKC rank (year 2008):** 66 (1,359 dogs registered.)
- **Internet resources: Chow Chow Club Inc.:** www.chowclub.org
  Chow Chow Fanciers of Canada: www.chowcanada.ca
  The Chow Chow Club (UK): www.thechowchowclub.co.uk
  Chow Health Website: www.chowhealth.org

References

1. Evans KM & Adams VJ: Proportion of litters of purebred dogs born by caesarean section. J Small Anim Pract. 2010 Feb;51(2):113-8.
2. OFA Website breed statistics: www.offa.org Last accessed July 1, 2010.
3. Kirberger RM & Stander N: Incidence of canine elbow dysplasia in South Africa. J S Afr Vet Assoc. 2007 Jun;78(2):59-62.
4. LaFond E, Breur GJ & Austin CC: Breed susceptibility for developmental orthopedic diseases in dogs. J Am Anim Hosp Assoc. 2002 Sep-Oct;38(5):467-77.
5. Amann JF, Tomlinson J, Hankison JK: Myotonia in a chow chow. J Am Vet Med Assoc. 1985 Aug 15;187(4):415-7.
6. Farrow BR, Malik R: Hereditary myotonia in the chow chow. J Small Anim Pract. 1981 Jul;22(7):451-65.
7. Ocular Disorders Presumed to be Inherited in Purebred Dogs. American College of Veterinary Ophthalmologists. ACVO, 2007.
8. Dorn CR: Canine breed-specific risks of frequently diagnosed diseases at veterinary teaching hospitals. Monograph. AKC Canine Health Foundation. 2000.
9. Nachreiner R & Refsal K: Personal communication, Diagnostic Center for Population and Animal Health, Michigan State University. April, 2007.
10. Nachreiner RF, Refsal KR, Graham PA, et. al.: Prevalence of serum thyroid hormone autoantibodies in dogs with clinical signs of hypothyroidism. J Am Vet Med Assoc 2002 Feb 15;220(4):466-71.
11. Kuhl KA, Shofer FS, Goldschmidt MH: Comparative histopathology of pemphigus foliaceus and superficial folliculitis in the dog. Vet Pathol. 1994 Jan;31(1):19-27.
12. Gershman KA, Sacks JJ, Wright JC: Which dogs bite? A case-control study of risk factors. Pediatrics. 1994 Jun;93(6 Pt 1):913-7.
13. Gelatt KN, MacKay EO: Prevalence of the breed-related glaucomas in pure-bred dogs in North America. Vet Ophthalmol. 2004 Mar-Apr;7(2):97-111.
14. Corcoran KA, Koch SA, Peiffer RL Jr: Primary Glaucoma in the Chow Chow. Progress in Veterinary and Comparative Ophthalmology 1994;4:193.
15. Nieves MA: Cranial Cruciate Ligament Insufficiency. 2006 Proceedings, Western Veterinary Conference 2006.
16. Collins BK, Collier LL, Johnson GS, et. al.: Familial cataracts and concurrent ocular anomalies in chow chows. J Am Vet Med Assoc. 1992 May 15;200(10):1485-91.
17. Frank LA, Hnilica KA, Rohrbach BW, et. al.: Retrospective evaluation of sex hormones and steroid hormone intermediates in dogs with alopecia. Vet Dermatol. 2003 Apr;14(2):91-7.
18. Cerundolo R and Lloyd D: "Alopecia X" in chows, pomeranians and samoyeds.Vet Record 1998;143: 176.
19. Hernblad Tevell E, Bergvall K, et. al.: Sebaceous adenitis in Swedish dogs, a retrospective study of 104 cases. Acta Vet Scand. 2008 May 25;50:11.
20. Penninck DG, Moore AS, Gliatto J: Ultrasonography of canine gastric epithelial neoplasia. Vet Radiol Ultrasound. 1998 Jul-Aug;39(4):342-8.
21. Glickman LT, Glickman NW, Schellenberg DB, et. al.: Incidence of and breed-related risk factors for gastric dilatation-volvulus in dogs. J Am Vet Med Assoc. 2000 Jan 1;216(1):40-5.
22. Ramos-Vara JA, Beissenherz ME, Miller MA, et. al.: Retrospective study of 338 canine oral melanomas with clinical, histologic, and immunohistochemical review of 129 cases. Vet Pathol. 2000 Nov;37(6):597-608.
23. Dennis MM, Ehrhart N, Duncan CG, et. al.: Frequency of and risk factors associated with lingual lesions in dogs: 1,196 cases (1995-2004). J Am Vet Med Assoc. 2006 May 15;228(10):1533-7.

24. Buchanan JW: Causes and prevalence of cardiovascular diseases. In Kirk RW, Bonagura JD, eds: Current veterinary therapy XI, Philadelphia, 1992, WB Saunders.

25. Schrope DP, Kelch WJ: Signalment, clinical signs, and prognostic indicators associated with high-grade second- or third-degree atrioventricular block in dogs: 124 cases (January 1, 1997-December 31, 1997). J Am Vet Med Assoc. 2006 Jun 1;228(11):1710-7.

26. Batchelor DJ, Noble PJ, Cripps PJ, et. al.: Breed associations for canine exocrine pancreatic insufficiency. J Vet Intern Med. 2007 Mar-Apr;21(2):207-14.

27. Brown CA, Crowell WA, Brown SA, et. al.: Suspected familial renal disease in chow chows. J Am Vet Med Assoc. 1990 Apr 15;196(8):1279-84.

28. Vianna ML, Tobias KM: Atresia ani in the dog: a retrospective study. J Am Anim Hosp Assoc. 2005 Sep-Oct;41(5):317-22.

29. Vandevelde M, Braund KG, Walker TL, et. al.: Dysmyelination of the central nervous system in the Chow-Chow dog. Acta Neuropathol (Berl). 1978 Jun 30;42(3):211-5.

30. Vandevelde M, Braund KG, Luttgen PJ, et. al.: Dysmyelination in Chow Chow dogs: further studies in older dogs. Acta Neuropathol (Berl). 1981;55(2):81-7.

31. *The Genetic Connection: A Guide to Health Problems in Purebred Dogs.* L Ackerman. p. 210-211. AAHA Press, 1999.

32. Hoover JP, Henry GA, Panciera RJ: Bronchial cartilage dysplasia with multifocal lobar bullous emphysema and lung torsions in a pup. J Am Vet Med Assoc. 1992 Aug 15;201(4):599-602.

33. Maddux JM, Edwards DF, Barnhill MA, et. al.: Neutrophil function in dogs with congenital ciliary dyskinesia. Vet Pathol. 1991 Sep;28(5):347-53.

34. Edwards DF, Kennedy JR, Toal RL, et. al.: Kartagener's syndrome in a chow chow dog with normal ciliary ultrastructure. Vet Pathol. 1989 Jul;26(4):338-40.

35. Booth MJ: Atypical dermoid sinus in a chow chow dog. J S Afr Vet Assoc. 1998 Sep;69(3):102-4.

36. *The Complete Dog Book, 20th Ed.* The American Kennel Club. Howell Book House, NY 2006. p. 547-552.

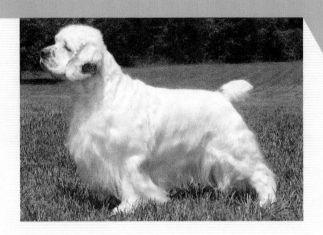

The Breed History

The origins of this breed are obscure. Thought to be French in origin, possible progenitors include the Basset hound and the Alpine Spaniel. Some even place St. Bernard dogs in the gene pool of original contributing breeds. The body type of the Clumber is somewhat different from the rest of the spaniel group. The breed is thought to have gone to England to Clumber Park under the care of the Duke of Newcastle for protection during the French revolution. Even before the AKC was formally established, registries in North America accepted Clumbers (1878).

Breeding for Function

This was a valued hunting dog for French and English nobility, and even some of the British royalty. Though a slow lumbering gait characterizes the breed, this allowed them to work a day in the field without tiring. Preferred as a bird dog, they are quiet and move subtly through dense cover and are used in pack or solo for tracking, flushing and retrieving.

Physical Characteristics

Height at Withers: female 17-19" (43-48 cm), male 19-20" (48-51 cm).

Weight: females 55-70 lb (25-32 kg), males 70-85 lb (32-38.5 kg).

Coat: They are double-coated, colored white, and hairs are dense, straight and soft. Only trimming of the feathering is allowed. Some light markings (termed orange, lemon) and freckles are acceptable, but generally fewer markings are considered better.

Longevity: 10-12 years.

Points of Conformation: A very large square head with prominent forehead and small dorsal furrow, deep stop, fleshy lips with large flews, and a bit of "haw" or third eyelid prominence are specific to this spaniel. This is not a true pathologic eversion of the third gland, but is still referred to as a haw by breeders. Eyes are amber and the ventral eyelid normally droops somewhat, though the standard specifies that full ectropion (or entropion) is penalized. Ears are pendulous and thick leathered with slight feathering. A stocky well-boned low-built breed, thorax is broad, with a thick long neck and deep strong hindquarters. Mild throatiness and dewlap are not faulted. The nose is brown to dark flesh colored. Dewclaws may be removed. In North America, tails are docked. They move with an easy, rolling gait and are designed to move through thick cover. The topline is level and back is long, legs are straight, feet large but not splayed.

Recognized Behavior Issues and Traits

Reported breed characteristics include: This is known to be an easy-going, loyal and pleasant dog that enjoys close human contact. Intelligent and playful, it is of low intrinsic activity when compared with the other spaniels. Clumbers are aloof with strangers, and can be a one-man dog if not socialized early. They are average in trainability and will work hard to please. They tend to drool because of the flews and are known to snore. They are prone to obesity. They require only moderate exercise and like the water. Regular coat grooming is necessary. They are not considered watchdogs.

Normal Physiologic Variations

In Great Britain, 45.2% of Clumber Spaniel litters were delivered by **Cesarean section.**[1]

Drug Sensitivities

None reported

Inherited Diseases

Hip Dysplasia: Polygenically inherited trait causing degenerative joint disease and hip arthritis. OFA reports 45.7% affected. Reported at a frequency of 17.4% in the Clumber Spaniel Club of America Health Survey 2001/2002.[2,3]

Elbow Dysplasia: Polygenically inherited trait causing elbow arthritis. OFA reports 7.6% affected.[2]

Patella Luxation: Polygenically inherited laxity of patellar ligaments, causing luxation, lameness, and later degenerative joint disease. Treat surgically if causing clinical signs. A high incidence is reported, however too few Clumber Spaniels have been screened by OFA to determine an accurate frequency.[2]

Pyruvate Dehydrogenase Deficiency/Mitochondrial Myopathy (PDP1): Autosomal recessive metabolic disorder, where affected dogs show exercise intolerance, collapse, and severe metabolic acidosis. Affected dogs have high serum lactate and pyruvate concentrations and urinary organic acids. Dietary therapy may control clinical signs. Affected dogs have also been treated with human recombinant PDP1. One study reported a worldwide spread of the mutation with a 20% carrier frequency. A genetic test is available.[4,5,6]

Disease Predispositions

Entropion: Rolling in of eyelids, often causing corneal irritation or ulceration. Entropion is reported in 21.55% of Clumber Spaniels CERF examined by veterinary ophthalmologists between 2000-2005. Eyelid problems are reported at a frequency of 33.0% in the Clumber Spaniel Club of America Health Survey 2001/2002.[3,7]

Allergic Dermatitis (Atopy): Inhalant or food allergy. Presents with pruritis and pyotraumatic dermatitis (hot spots). Reported at a frequency of 20.9% in the Clumber Spaniel Club of America Health Survey 2001/2002.[3]

Otitis Externa: Due to their thick and pendulous ears, Clumber Spaniels can have more frequent external ear infections. Reported at a frequency of 20.0% in the Clumber Spaniel Club of America Health Survey 2001/2002.[3]

Ectropion: A rolling out of the eyelids, that can cause tear pooling, conjunctivitis, and frequent infection. Can be secondary to macroblepharon; an abnormally large eyelid opening. Ectropion is reported in 14.41% and macroblepharon in 6.65% of Clumber Spaniels CERF examined by veterinary ophthalmologists between 2000-2005. Eyelid problems are reported at a frequency of 33.0% in the Clumber Spaniel Club of America Health Survey 2001/2002.[3,7]

Intervertebral Disc Disease (IVDD): Serious neurological condition where disk degeneration and rupture into spinal nerves and the spinal cord causes pain and possible paralysis. Requires immediate veterinary care. Reported at a frequency of 13.0% in the Clumber Spaniel Club of America Health Survey 2001/2002.[3]

Retinal Dysplasia: Retinal folds, geographic, and generalized retinal dysplasia with detachment are recognized in the breed. Reported in 7.02% of Clumber Spaniels CERF examined by veterinary ophthalmologists between 2000-2005.[7]

Distichiasis: Abnormally placed eyelashes that irritate the cornea and conjunctiva. Can cause secondary corneal ulceration. Identified in 6.40% of Clumber Spaniels CERF examined by veterinary ophthalmologists between 2000-2005.[7]

Cataracts: Posterior cortex intermediate and anterior cortex punctate cataracts predominate in the breed. Onset 6-18 months of age. Unknown mode of inheritance. Reported in 5.32% of Clumber Spaniels examined at veterinary teaching hospitals. Identified in 4.31% of Clumber Spaniels CERF examined by veterinary ophthalmologists between 2000-2005. Reported at a frequency of 5.2% (mostly punctate) in the Clumber Spaniel Club of America Health Survey 2001/2002. CERF does not recommend breeding any Clumber Spaniel with a cataract.[3,7,8]

Hypothyroidism: Inherited autoimmune thyroiditis. 4.5% positive for thyroid auto-antibodies based on testing at Michigan State University. (Ave. for all breeds is 7.5%). Reported at a frequency of 13.9% in the Clumber Spaniel Club of America Health Survey 2001/2002.[3,9,10]

Anasarca (Lethal Congenital Edema): Puppies are born dead and edematous. Can also be associated with cleft palate. Reported at a frequency of 4.4% in the Clumber Spaniel Club of America Health Survey 2001/2002.[3]

Cryptorchidism (Retained Testicles): Can be unilateral or bilateral. This is a sex-limited disorder with an unknown mode of inheritance. Reported at a frequency of 3.5% in the Clumber Spaniel Club of America Health Survey 2001/2002.[3]

Inflammatory/Irritable Bowel Disease (IBD): Presents with chronic vomiting, diarrhea, and/or weight loss. Affected dogs can usually be controlled with diet and/or medications. Reported at a

frequency of 3.5% in the Clumber Spaniel Club of America Health Survey 2001/2002.[3]

Persistent Pupillary Membranes: Strands of fetal remnant connecting; iris to iris, cornea, lens, or involving sheets of tissue. The later three forms can impair vision, and dogs affected with these forms should not be bred. Identified in 1.85% of Clumber Spaniels CERF examined by veterinary ophthalmologists between 2000-2005.[7]

Cardiomyopathy, Epilepsy, Immune Mediated Hemolytic Anemia, Oligodontia, Panosteitis, Portosystemic Shunt, Prognathism, Progressive Retinal Atrophy and **Wry Mouth** are reported.[3,11]

Isolated Case Studies
None reported

Genetic Tests
Tests of Genotype: Direct genetic test for PDP1 is available at the University of Missouri and the Animal Health Trust.

Tests of Phenotype: CHIC Certification: Required testing includes hip and elbow radiographs, CERF eye examination, and genetic test for PDP1. (See CHIC website; www.caninehealthinfo.org).

Recommend patella examination, thyroid profile including autoantibodies and cardiac evaluation.

Miscellaneous
- **Breed name synonyms:** Clumber
- **Registries:** AKC, CKC, UKC, KCGB (Kennel Club of Great Britain), ANKC (Australian National Kennel Club), NKC (National Kennel Club)
- **AKC rank (year 2008):** 177 (280 dogs registered)
- **Internet resources: Clumber Spaniel Club of America:** www.clumbers.org
  Clumber Spaniel Club of Canada: http://clumbercanada.webs.com/
  The Clumber Spaniel Club (UK): www.clumberspanielclub.co.uk
  Clumber Spaniel Health Foundation: www.clumberhealth.org

References
1. Evans KM & Adams VJ: Proportion of litters of purebred dogs born by caesarean section. J Small Anim Pract. 2010 Feb;51(2):113-8.
2. OFA Website breed statistics: www.offa.org Last accessed July 1, 2010.
3. Froman, R: Clumber Spaniel Club of America Health Survey 2001/2002.
4. Jarvinen AK, Sankari S: Lactic acidosis in a Clumber spaniel. Acta Vet Scand. 1996;37(1):119-21.
5. Shelton GD, Engvall E: Muscular dystrophies and other inherited myopathies. Vet Clin North Am Small Anim Pract 2002: 32 (1):103-124.
6. Cameron JM, Maj MC, Levandovskiy V, et. al.: Identification of a canine model of pyruvate dehydrogenase phosphatase 1 deficiency. Mol Genet Metab. 2007 Jan;90(1):15-23.
7. Ocular Disorders Presumed to be Inherited in Purebred Dogs. American College of Veterinary Ophthalmologists. ACVO, 2007.
8. Gelatt KN, Mackay EO: Prevalence of primary breed-related cataracts in the dog in North America. Vet Ophthalmol. 2005 Mar-Apr;8(2):101-11.
9. Nachreiner R & Refsal K: Personal communication, Diagnostic Center for Population and Animal Health, Michigan State University. April, 2007.
10. Nachreiner RF, Refsal KR, Graham PA, et, al.:Prevalence of serum thyroid hormone autoantibodies in dogs with clinical signs of hypothyroidism. J Am Vet Med Assoc 2002 Feb 15;220(4): 466-71.
11. The Genetic Connection: A Guide to Health Problems in Purebred Dogs. L Ackerman. p.211, AAHA Press, 1999.
12. *The Complete Dog Book, 20th Ed.* The American Kennel Club.Howell Book House, NY 2006. P. 79-82.

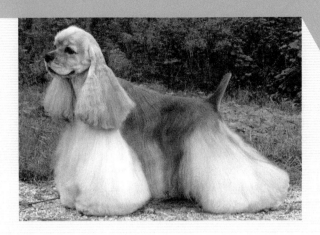

Cocker Spaniel

The Breed History

The Cocker Spaniel is the smallest member of the sporting division, and resulted from the selection of small dogs from the land spaniel group. Breed status was given to this dog in 1892 (England Kennel Club). After import to the USA around 1880, the American type became distinct from the English cocker type, being shorter, heavier coated and having a rounder skull, and now are two quite distinct breeds; American and English Cocker Spaniel. The American cocker is often just termed Cocker Spaniel. The feature role of a cocker type dog in the cartoon "Lady and the Tramp" by Disney resulted in a large sudden surge of the popularity of this breed.

Breeding for Function

This dog was bred to be a hunting dog, and though considered a land spaniel, will work in water readily. The name cocker is thought to derive from "woodcock", game that they were particularly suited for. Today, they commonly serve as a valued home companion, enjoy agility competitions, and still maintain status as one of the most popular AKC breeds.

Physical Characteristics

Height at Withers: female 14" (35.5 cm), male 15" (38 cm)

Weight: females 24-26 lb (11-12 kg), males 26-28 lb (12-13 kg).

Coat: The long silky fine straight to slightly wavy coat is seen in black, cream, red, brown, parti-colored (one color must be white), and a tan point variety (less than 10% coat colored). For solid coats, only small white markings on chest and throat are acceptable. Show divisions by color include solid non-black, black and parti-color. They are well feathered on ears, legs, abdomen and chest.

Longevity: 13-16 years.

Points of Conformation: This is a very balanced, medium length and sized dog, with a refined broad head, large square muzzle and slightly arched long neck. Eyes are large, round and dark brown in color. Ears are long, reaching to the nose and well-feathered, and the leather is thick. The head has a pronounced stop, nose is dark (black, brown, liver). Ribs are well-sprung and the topline slopes slightly downward to a docked tail carried level with the back. Dewclaws may be removed. Their gait is straight and low.

Recognized Behavior Issues and Traits

These dogs are gentle social dogs that are playful and affectionate with family members, and very loyal. They are considered of medium trainability, and are generally good with children. Early socialization and training is very important for these dogs. Those poorly socialized and of timid personality may be snappy, and some lines are known to have temperament changes such as fearful-dominant personalities. These lines may also be dominant-aggressive. For the most part this breed has been carefully selected for gentle, friendly personality. They need plenty of exercise and play time.

They require regular ear hygiene and lots of coat care, with average shedding. They have an average to high barking tendency.

Normal Physiologic Variations
None reported

Drug Sensitivities
None reported

Inherited Diseases

Patella Luxation: Polygenically inherited laxity of patellar ligaments, causing luxation, lameness, and later degenerative joint disease. Treat surgically if causing clinical signs. OFA reports 18.0% affected.[1]

Hip Dysplasia: Polygenically inherited trait causing degenerative joint disease and hip arthritis. OFA reports 6.5% affected.[1]

Progressive Retinal Atrophy (prcd-PRA): Autosomal recessive progressive rod cone degeneration (prcd) form. Age of onset between 3-5 years, eventually causing blindness at 5-7 years. A genetic test is available. CERF does not recommend breeding any Cocker Spaniel with PRA.[2,3]

Elbow Dysplasia: Polygenically inherited trait causing elbow arthritis. OFA reports 1.0% affected.[1]

Sry-negative XX Sex reversal (Hermaphrodism): An autosomal recessive disorder, where outwardly male dogs are chromosomal females (XX), and there is an absence of male causing SRY. A genetic test is not available, however a linked marker has been found.[4,5,6,7,8]

Disease Predispositions

Distichiasis: Abnormally placed eyelashes that irritate the cornea and conjunctiva. Can cause secondary corneal ulceration. Dorn reports a 6.08x odds ratio versus other breeds. Identified in 38.24% of Cocker Spaniels CERF examined by veterinary ophthalmologists between 2000-2005. Reported at a frequency of 5.9% in the 2005 Cocker Spaniel Comprehensive Breed Health Survey.[2,9,10]

Bronchiectasis: Clinical signs of chronic cough with excessive airway mucous. Diagnosis with radiographs. Reported at a frequency of 15.9% and an odds ratio of 4.15x versus other breeds. Treatment is with bronchodilators and possibly corticosteroids.[11]

Hypothyroidism: Inherited autoimmune thyroiditis. 15.7% positive for thyroid auto-antibodies based on testing at Michigan State University. (Ave. for all breeds is 7.5%). Reported at a frequency of 3.8% in the 2005 Cocker Spaniel Comprehensive Breed Health Survey.[10,12,13]

Behavioral Disorders: The 2005 Cocker Spaniel Comprehensive Breed Health Survey reports 10.5% of Cocker Spaniels with behavioral disorders. These include submissive urination (4.7%), separation anxiety (4.4%), and fearfulness towards; people (3.9%), noise (3.9%), children (2.5%), and their environment (2.5%).[10]

Retinal Dysplasia: Focal retinal dysplasia and retinal folds are recognized in the breed. Severe cases can progress to retinal detachment. Reported in 10.04% of Cocker Spaniels CERF examined by veterinary ophthalmologists between 2000-2005.[2]

Chronic Otitis with Ossification of the External Ear Canal: Cocker Spaniels are prone to chronic ear infections, and to dystrophic ossification and closing down of the external ear canal. Dorn reports a 1.45x odds ratio versus other breeds. A Greek study reported a 8.99x odds ratio versus other breeds. Chronic ear infections were reported at a frequency of 9.0% in the 2005 Cocker Spaniel Comprehensive Breed Health Survey.[9,10,14,15]

Cataracts: Anterior and posterior cortex intermediate and punctate cataracts predominate in the breed. Onset of cataracts may occur at less than 2 years, with rapid progression to maturity and associated with significant lens-induced inflammation. Reported at a frequency of 8.77% in one study. Identified in 6.96% of Cocker Spaniels CERF examined by veterinary ophthalmologists between 2000-2005. Reported at a frequency of 5.9% in the 2005 Cocker Spaniel Comprehensive Breed Health Survey. Dorn reports a 2.04x odds ratio versus other breeds. One study showed a 2.6x odds ratio versus other breeds. CERF does not recommend breeding any Cocker Spaniel with a cataract.[2,9,10,16,17]

Glaucoma: Ocular condition causing increased pressure within the eyeball, and secondary blindness due to damage to the retina. Diagnose with tonometry and gonioscopy. One study shows 5.52% Cocker Spaniels affected; the highest frequency of primary glaucoma versus other breeds. A female preponderance occurs in the breed. Secondary glaucoma can also occur after cataract formation in the breed. One report found an odds ratio of 3.7x for secondary glaucoma in Cocker Spaniels. Dorn reports a 5.73x odds ratio for glaucoma versus other breeds. CERF does not recommend breeding any Cocker Spaniel with glaucoma.[2,9,18,19,20,21]

Allergic Dermatitis: Inhalant or food allergy. Presents with pruritis, otitis, and pyotraumatic dermatitis. Reported at a frequency of 5.1% in the 2005 Cocker Spaniel Comprehensive Breed Health Survey.[10]

Prolapsed Gland of the Nictitans (Cherry Eye): This condition is secondary to chronic conjunctivitis, usually of an allergic nature. Reported at a frequency of 4.4% in the 2005 Cocker Spaniel Comprehensive Breed Health Survey. Dorn reports a 2.06x odds ratio for conjunctivitis versus other breeds.[9,10]

Epilepsy: Inherited seizures. Can be generalized or partial seizures. Reported at a frequency of 3.6% in the 2005 Cocker Spaniel Comprehensive Breed Health Survey.[10]

Keratoconjunctivitis Sicca (KCS), Chronic Superficial Keratitis (Pannus), Dry Eye: These ocular conditions can cause conjunctivitis, corneal ulcerations, and vision problems due to corneal pigmentation. Age of onset 2-5 years. Treatment with topical ocular lubricants and anti-inflammatory medication. Pannus was identified in 0.77% of Cocker Spaniels CERF examined by veterinary ophthalmologists between 2000-2005. KCS is reported at a frequency of 3.4% in the 2005 Cocker Spaniel Comprehensive Breed Health Survey. CERF does not recommend breeding any Cocker Spaniel with KCS.[2,10]

Aggression: The breed is one identified with a tendency toward severe dominance aggression. This may be most extreme in intact males, though neutered males and females can also be affected. Reported at a frequency of 3.3% in the 2005 Cocker Spaniel Comprehensive Breed Health Survey.[10,22]

Umbilical Hernia: Reported at a frequency of 2.9% in the 2005 Cocker Spaniel Comprehensive Breed Health Survey.[10]

Deafness: In the Cocker Spaniel, this can be congenital, or secondary to severe, chronic otitis. Can be bilateral or unilateral. Diagnose with BAER testing. Reported at a frequency of 2.8% in the 2005 Cocker Spaniel Comprehensive Breed Health Survey.[10]

Corneal Dystrophy: The breed can develop a posterior polymorphous dystrophy that does not lead to corneal edema. Identified in 2.47% of Cocker Spaniels CERF examined by veterinary ophthalmologists between 2000-2005.[2,23]

Ectropion: Ectropion, a rolling out of the eyelids, can cause frequent conjunctivitis, and ocular discharge. Identified in 1.52% of Cocker Spaniels CERF examined by veterinary ophthalmologists between 2000-2005.[2]

Immune-Mediated Hemolytic Anemia (IMHA) and Idiopathic Thrombocytopenia Purpura (ITP): Autoimmune destruction of blood cells. Cocker Spaniels have a 12.2x odds ratio for IMHA versus other breeds. Females are more frequently affected than males. Unknown mode of inheritance. IMHA is reported at a frequency of 1.0%, and ITP at 0.7% in the 2005 Cocker Spaniel Comprehensive Breed Health Survey.[10,24,25]

Idiopathic Seborrhea: Primary inherited skin disorder presenting with greasy skin and haircoat. Unknown mode of inheritance. The condition responds to treatment with etretinate. Dorn reports a 3.19x odds ratio versus other breeds.[9,26,27]

Dilated Cardiomyopathy: The breed can develop a taurine responsive dilated cardiomyopathy. Affected dogs present in heart failure, and have very low plasma taurine levels. Most affected dogs show a significant (clinical and ECHO) response to taurine supplementation and can usually be weaned off heart medications.[28,29]

Vitamin A responsive Dermatosis: Inherited skin disorder presenting with seborrhea and keratinization. Differentiated from idiopathic seborrhea by skin biopsy and responsiveness to Vitamin A supplementation.[30]

Second and Third Degree Heart Block: Cocker Spaniels are a breed listed as predisposed to high-grade second- or third-degree AVB. The breed is also at risk for sick sinus syndrome. Heavier, older, and sexually intact female dogs were overrepresented in the study group. Weakness, lethargy, exercise intolerance, and syncope were the most common clinical signs. Pacemaker implantation is recommended.[31,32]

Plasmacytoma/Plasma Cell Tumor: Cocker Spaniels were found to have a 10.0x greater risk of developing plasma cell tumors of the tongue than other breeds. Other published case reports document plasmacytoma of the penis, anus and 3rd eyelid. This is a benign tumor, and treatment is with surgery.[33,34,35,36]

Ceroid-Lipofuscinosis: Rare, fatal degenerative neurological disease. Affected Cocker Spaniels have presented between 18 months and 6 years of age with variable signs of progressive hind limb paresis, incoordination, behavior changes, seizures, and/or blindness. Unknown mode of inheritance.[37,38]

Incomplete Ossification of the Humeral Condyle: Cocker Spaniels have an increased incidence of incomplete ossification of the humeral condyle, and associated humeral condylar fractures or degenerative joint disease. There is a male preponderance. A recessive mode of inheritance was suggested based on pedigree analysis.[39]

Episcleritis: Cocker Spaniels are over-represented with a diagnosis of diffuse or nodular episcleritis. Affected dogs can show unilateral or bilateral inflammation and congestion of the scleral vessels with corneal edema and stromal infiltrate of CD3 T-lymphocytes. In one study, 6 of 19 cases were Cocker Spaniels. Treatment is with immunosuppressive medications.[40,41]

Abnormal Platelet Function: Moderate to severe bleeding due to platelet ADP deficiency was identified in 3 families of dogs. Platelet counts, plasma coagulant function and von Willebrand factor are normal, but there is prolonged bleeding time, prolonged platelet aggregation time in response to ADP and collagen.[42]

Oral Malignant Melanoma: Malignant cancer usually involving the gingiva. Can be pigmented or non-pigmented. One study identified a 1.65x relative risk versus other breeds.[43]

Isolated Case Studies

Nasal Dermoid Sinus Cysts: A few cases have been reported in Cocker Spaniels. Affected dogs present with a subcutaneous mass or draining tract over the midline bridge of the nose. Surgical removal is curative. In another case study, an intracranial epidermoid cyst caused syringomyelia.[44,45,46]

Lipid Storage Myopathy: A six-year-old male Cocker Spaniel presented with a three-week history of generalized weakness and muscle pain. Muscle biopsies revealed numerous large lipid droplets within type 1 fibres and to a lesser degree within type 2 fibres. Biochemical testing showed elevated urinary excretion of

lactic, pyruvic and acetoacetic acids, increased urinary excretion of carnitine esters, and increased plasma alanine, consistent with a block in oxidative metabolism.[47]

Progressive Ataxia with Seizures: Case history of a young male Cocker Spaniel with progressive neurological disease evident by 3 months of age, and progressing to uncontrollable seizures by 15 months. Significant lesions were found only in the brain. They consisted of hypoplasia of the cerebellum and the presence of large pale proteinacious inclusions in the perikaryon of neurons in the neocortex and in macrophages.[48]

Congenital Myotonia: A 16-week-old, male Cocker Spaniel suffered from pelvic-limb "bunny hopping" as well as rigidity, spasticity, and ataxia in all limbs. Electrophysiology, and muscle histopathological and histochemical evaluations led to a diagnosis of congenital myotonia.[49]

Focal Myasthenia Gravis: A 10-month-old dog presented with megaesophagus, aspiration pneumonia, no appendicular muscle weakness, but facial muscle weakness. The condition responded to anticholinesterase, and serum antibodies against acetylcholine receptors were documented.[50]

Cerebellar Vermian Hypoplasia: An eight-week-old female Cocker Spaniel was presented with ataxia, dysmetria and intention tremor. Cerebellar hypoplasia with vermal defect was identified on necropsy, comparable to Dandy-Walker syndrome.[51]

Phosphofructokinase Deficiency (PFK): A 3-year-old female American Cocker Spaniel with chronic hemolytic crises was identified with the same mutation found in the autosomal recessive disorder of the English springer spaniel.[52]

Dimelia: A Cocker Spaniel was examined with two left forelimb paws, both originating from the carpus, with symmetrical duplication of metacarpal bones and phalanges. In addition, the left radial head was subluxated and asynchronous growth of the left radius and ulna was noted.[53]

Black hair Follicular Dysplasia, Brachygnathism, Chronic Inflammatory Hepatic Disease, Cleft Lip/Palate, Cryptorchidism, Cyclic Hematopoiesis, Ectodermal Defect, Factor IX Deficiency, Factor X Deficiency, Hypotrichosis, IgA Deficiency, Intervertebral Disc Disease, Malignant Hyperthermia, Microphthalmia, Narcolepsy, Optic Nerve Coloboma and Hypoplasia, Pelger-Huet Anomaly, Portosystemic Shunt, Prognathism, Pulmonic Stenosis, Renal Dysplasia, Sebaceous Adenitis, Vascular ring Anomaly and von Willebrand's Disease are reported.[54]

Genetic Tests

Tests of Genotype: Direct test for prcd-PRA is available from Optigen.

Direct test for Phosphofructokinase deficiency is available from HealthGene, Optigen, PennGen, and VetGen (very rarely seen in the breed).

Direct tests for coat colors (black, brown and buff/red) are available from HealthGene and VetGen.

Tests of Phenotype: CHIC Certification: Required testing includes hip radiographs, and CERF eye examination. (See CHIC website; www.caninehealthinfo.org).

Additional Recommended tests include patella evaluation, thyroid profile including autoantibodies, elbow radiographs, and cardiac evaluation.

Miscellaneous

- **Breed name synonyms:** Cocker, Cocking Spaniel, Cocker Spaniel.
- **Registries:** AKC, UKC, CKC, KCGB (Kennel Club of Great Britain), ANKC (Australian National Kennel Club), NKC (National Kennel Club)
- **AKC rank (year 2008):** 21 (9,481 dogs registered)
- **Internet resources:** American Spaniel Club of America: www.asc-cockerspaniel.org
  American Cocker Spaniel Club of Canada: www.acscc.ca
  American Cocker Spaniel Club of Great Britain: www.acscgb.com

References

1. OFA Website breed statistics: www.offa.org Last accessed July 1, 2010.
2. Ocular Disorders Presumed to be Inherited in Purebred Dogs. American College of Veterinary Ophthalmologists. ACVO, 2007.
3. Aguirre GD, Acland GM: Variation in retinal degeneration phenotype inherited at the prcd locus. Exp Eye Res. 1988 May;46(5):663-87.
4. Kothapalli KS, Kirkness EF, Vanwormer R, Meyers-Wallen VN: Exclusion of DMRT1 as a candidate gene for canine SRY-negative XX sex reversal. Vet J. 2006 May;171(3):559-61.
5. Meyers-Wallen VN: Genetics, genomics, and molecular biology of sex determination in small animals. Theriogenology. 2006 Oct;66(6-7):1655-8.
6. Meyers-Wallen VN, Palmer VL, Acland GM, Hershfield B: Sry-negative XX sex reversal in the American Cocker Spaniel dog. Mol Reprod Dev. 1995 Jul;41(3):300-5.
7. Meyers-Wallen VN, Patterson DF: XX sex reversal in the American Cocker Spaniel dog: phenotypic expression and inheritance. Hum Genet. 1988 Sep;80(1):23-30.
8. Pujar S, Kothapalli KS, Göring HH, et. al.: Linkage to CFA29 detected in a genome-wide linkage screen of a canine pedigree segregating Sry-negative XX sex reversal. J Hered. 2007;98(5):438-44.
9. Dorn CR: Canine breed-specific risks of frequently diagnosed diseases at veterinary teaching hospitals. Monograph. AKC Canine Health Foundation. 2000.
10. American Spaniel Club: 2005 Cocker Spaniel Comprehensive Breed Health Survey. 2006.
11. Hawkins EC, Basseches J, Berry CR, et. al.: Demographic, clinical, and radiographic features of bronchiectasis in dogs: 316 cases (1988-2000). J Am Vet Med Assoc. 2003 Dec 1;223(11):1628-35.
12. Nachreiner R & Refsal K: Personal communication, Diagnostic Center for Population and Animal Health, Michigan State University. April, 2007.
13. Nachreiner RF, Refsal KR, Graham PA, et. al.: Prevalence of serum thyroid hormone autoantibodies in dogs with clinical signs of hypothyroidism. J Am Vet Med Assoc 2002 Feb 15;220(4):466-71.
14. Daniels-McQueen S, Directo AC, Garcia JP: Bilateral ossification of the ear canal in an American Cocker Spaniel. Vet Med Small Anim Clin. 1974 Jun;69(6):747-9.
15. Saridomichelakis MN, Farmaki R, Leontides LS, et. al.: Aetiology of canine otitis externa: a retrospective study of 100 cases. Vet Dermatol. 2007 Oct;18(5):341-7.
16. Adkins EA, Hendrix DV: Outcomes of dogs presented for cataract evaluation: a retrospective study. J Am Anim Hosp Assoc. 2005 Jul-Aug;41(4):235-40.
17. Gelatt KN, Mackay EO: Prevalence of primary breed-related cataracts in the dog in North America. Vet Ophthalmol. 2005 Mar-Apr;8(2):101-11.
18. Sapienza JS, van der Woerdt A: Combined transscleral diode laser cyclophotocoagulation and Ahmed gonioimplantation in dogs with primary glaucoma: 51 cases (1996-2004). Vet Ophthalmol. 2005 Mar-Apr;8(2):121-7.
19. Gelatt KN, MacKay EO: Secondary glaucomas in the dog in North America. Vet Ophthalmol. 2004 Jul-Aug;7(4):245-59.
20. Gelatt KN, MacKay EO: Prevalence of the breed-related glaucomas in pure-bred dogs in North America. Vet Ophthalmol. 2004 Mar-Apr;7(2):97-111.
21. Johnsen DA, Maggs DJ, Kass PH: Evaluation of risk factors for development of secondary glaucoma in dogs: 156 cases (1999-2004). J Am Vet Med Assoc. 2006 Oct 15;229(8):1270-4.
22. Stafford KJ: Opinions of veterinarians regarding aggression in different breeds of dogs. N Z Vet J. 1996 Aug;44(4):138-41.
23. Cooley PL, Dice PF 2nd: Corneal dystrophy in the dog and cat. Vet Clin North Am Small Anim Pract. 1990 May;20(3):681-92.
24. Miller SA, Hohenhaus AE, Hale AS: Case-control study of blood type, breed, sex, and bacteremia in dogs with immune-mediated hemolytic anemia. J Am Vet Med Assoc. 2004 Jan 15;224(2):232-5.
25. Balch A & Mackin A: Canine immune-mediated hemolytic anemia: pathophysiology, clinical signs, and diagnosis. Compend Contin Educ Vet. 2007 Apr;29(4):217-25.
26. Power HT, Lhrke PJ, Stannard AA, Backus KQ: Use of etretinate primary keratinization disorders (idiopathic seborrhea) in Cocker Spaniels, west highland white terriers, and basset hounds. J Am Vet Med Assoc. 1992 Aug 1;201(3):419-29
27. Kwochka KW, Rademakers AM: Cell proliferation kinetics of epidermis, hair follicles, and sebaceous glands of Cocker Spaniels with idiopathic seborrhea. Am J Vet Res. 1989 Nov;50(11):1918-22.
28. Gavaghan BJ, Kittleson MD: Dilated cardiomyopathy in an American Cocker Spaniel with taurine deficiency. Aust Vet J. 1997 Dec;75(12):862-8.
29. Kittleson MD, Keene B, Pion PD, Loyer CG: Results of the multicenter spaniel trial (MUST): taurine- and carnitine-responsive dilated cardiomyopathy in American Cocker Spaniels with decreased plasma taurine concentration. J Vet Intern Med. 1997 Jul-Aug;11(4):204-11.
30. Watson TD: Diet and skin disease in dogs and cats. J Nutr. 1998 Dec;128(12 Suppl):2783S-2789S.
31. Schrope DP, Kelch WJ: Signalment, clinical signs, and prognostic indicators associated with high-grade second- or third-degree atrioventricular block in dogs: 124 cases (January 1, 1997-December 31, 1997). J Am Vet Med Assoc. 2006 Jun 1;228(11):1710-7.
32. Wess G, Thomas WP, Berger DM, et. al.: Applications, complications, and outcomes of transvenous pacemaker implantation in 105 dogs (1997-2002). J Vet Intern Med. 2006 Jul-Aug;20(4):877-84.
33. Dennis MM, Ehrhart N, Duncan CG, et. al.: Frequency of and risk factors associated with lingual lesions in dogs: 1,196 cases (1995-2004). J Am Vet Med Assoc. 2006 May 15;228(10):1533-7.
34. Kim MS, Kim DH, & Choi US: Penile Extramedullary Plasmacytoma in a Dog. Reprod Domest Anim. 2010 Dec;45(6):e454-7.
35. Rannou B, Hélie P, & Bédard C: Rectal plasmacytoma with intracellular hemosiderin in a dog. Vet Pathol. 2009 Nov;46(6):1181-4.
36. Perlmann E, Dagli ML, Martins MC, et. al.: Extramedullary plasmacytoma of the third eyelid gland in a dog. Vet Ophthalmol. 2009 Mar-Apr;12(2):102-5.
37. Minatel L, Underwood SC, Carfagnini JC: Ceroid-lipofuscinosis in a Cocker Spaniel dog. Vet Pathol. 2000 Sep;37(5):488-90.
38. Jolly RD, Hartley WJ, Jones BR, Johnstone AC, Palmer AC, Blakemore WF: Generalized ceroid-lipofuscinosis and brown bowel syndrome in Cocker Spaniel dogs. NZ Vet J 1994; 42:236-239.
39. Marcellin-Little DJ, DeYoung DJ, Ferris KK, Berry CM: Incomplete ossification of the humeral condyle in spaniels. Vet Surg. 1994 Nov-Dec;23(6):475-87.
40. Breaux CB, Sandmeyer LS, Grahn BH: Immunohistochemical investigation of canine episcleritis. Vet Ophthalmol. 2007 May-Jun;10(3):168-72.

41. Andrade AL, Sakamoto SS, Silva CM, et. al.: The Investigation of CD3 Subpopulation of T Lymphocytes in Canine Nodular Granulomatous Episcleritis.Proceedings, 2009 World Small Animal Veterinary Association World Congress. 2009.

42. Callan MB, Bennett JS, Phillips DK, Haskins ME, Hayden JE, Anderson JG, Giger U: Inherited platelet delta-storage pool disease in dogs causing severe bleeding: an animal model for a specific ADP deficiency. Thromb Haemost. 1995 Sep;74(3):949-53.

43. Ramos-Vara JA, Beissenherz ME, Miller MA, et. al.: Retrospective study of 338 canine oral melanomas with clinical, histologic, and immunohistochemical review of 129 cases. Vet Pathol. 2000 Nov;37(6):597-608.

44. Anderson DM, White RA: Nasal dermoid sinus cysts in the dog. Vet Surg. 2002 Jul-Aug;31(4):303-8.

45. Bailey TR, Holmberg DL, Yager JA: Nasal dermoid sinus in an American Cocker Spaniel. Can Vet J. 2001 Mar;42(3):213-5.

46. MacKillop E, Schatzberg SJ, De Lahunta A: Intracranial epidermoid cyst and syringohydromyelia in a dog. Vet Radiol Ultrasound. 2006 Jul-Aug;47(4):339-44.

47. Platt SR, Chrisman CL, Shelton GD: Lipid storage myopathy in a Cocker Spaniel. J Small Anim Pract. 1999 Jan;40(1):31-4.

48. Jolly RD, Schraa I, Halsey TR: Progressive ataxia and seizures in a Cocker Spaniel: a new type of neurodegenerative disease with novel intra-neuronal inclusions. N Z Vet J. 2002 Oct;50(5):203-6.

49. Hill SL, Shelton GD, Lenehan TM: Myotonia in a Cocker Spaniel. J Am Anim Hosp Assoc. 1995 Nov-Dec;31(6):506-9.

50. Webb AA, Taylor SM, McPhee L: Focal myasthenia gravis in a dog. Can Vet J. 1997 Aug;38(8):493-5.

51. Lim JH, Kim DY, Yoon JH, et. al.: Cerebellar vermian hypoplasia in a Cocker Spaniel. J Vet Sci. 2008 Jun;9(2):215-7.

52. Giger U, Smith BF, Woods CB, Patterson DF, Stedman H: Inherited phosphofructokinase deficiency in an American Cocker Spaniel. J Am Vet Med Assoc. 1992 Nov 15;201(10):1569-71.

53. Kim J, Blevins WE, Breur GJ: Morphological and functional evaluation of a dog with dimelia. Vet Comp Orthop Traumatol. 2006;19(4):255-8.

54. *The Genetic Connection: A Guide to Health Problems in Purebred Dogs*. L Ackerman. p. 211-12, AAHA Press, 1999.

55. *The Complete Dog Book, 20th Ed*. The American Kennel Club. Howell Book House, NY 2006. pp 83-88.

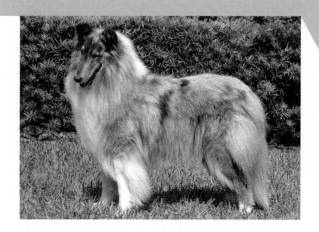

Collie-Rough and Smooth

The Breed History

The rough and smooth Collie can both trace their origins to Scotland and England. In the early 19th century a taller, more refined dog had evolved. A favorite breed of Queen Victoria, and also a star as "Lassie" on television, this breed has maintained popularity for many years. The name may have arisen from the name of the sheep they often guarded in Scotland called the Colley sheep. Others propose the name is Gaelic for "useful".

Breeding for Function

These, the quintessential herding dog were strictly working dogs until about 200 years ago. They have now taken their place as a competition dog, but also are a valued companion. They have also excelled as rescue and guide dogs.

Physical Characteristics

Height at Withers: female 22-24" (56-61 cm), male 24-26" (61-66 cm)

Weight: females 50-65 lb (23-29.5 kg) , males 60-75lb (27-34 kg).

Coat: Rough Collie standard: The thick double haircoat runs over the body except on head and legs; the outer layer is harsh and straight, the inner layer is soft and wooly. Around the neck is a pronounced mane of very thick hair that is more developed in males. Recognized colors include tri-color, blue merle, white and sable and white. Note that the "white" dog has a predominance of white with markings of sable, blue merle or tri-color.
Smooth: A thick undercoat and a short (1"), dense flat coat are the standard.

Longevity: 14-16 years.

Points of Conformation: This breed of dog has a very bright demeanor and their alert "Collie expression" is one of the points of judging. The dog presents a balanced appearance with straight limbs, deep chest, and a smallish head (dolichocephalic skull) with a slight stop and a tapering but blunted muzzle. The eyes are medium sized, almond-shaped and match coat color except in the merle. The ears are normally tipped at the top quarter. Topline is level. Their feet are small, but the toes are well arched. The tail reaches to the tarsal joint or lower.

Recognized Behavior Issues and Traits

Reported breed characteristics include that these dogs are particularly good around children in general. This breed is loyal and makes a good family watchdog—they are vigorous alarm barkers. They have high intelligence and are easy to train. They can be aloof with strangers, and are active outdoors, though less active than border Collies on average. Sometimes, they will nip at children's heels in an attempt to herd them, but training can eliminate this tendency. Regular grooming is necessary; they are considered high shedders. Note that rough and smooth types may occur in the same litter of puppies.

Normal Physiologic Variations

Merle Coat Color: Caused by a dominant mutation in the SILV gene. Breeding two merle dogs together should be avoided, as homozygous dogs can be born with multiple defects, including blindness, deafness, and heart anomalies.[1]

Drug Sensitivities

MDR1 Mutation (Ivermectin/Drug Toxicity): Autosomal recessive disorder in the MDR1 gene allows high CNS drug levels of ivermectin, doramectin, loperamide, vincristine, moxidectin, and other drugs. Causes neurological signs, including tremors, seizures, and coma. A genetic test is available for the mutated gene, showing 35.4% of Collies are affected, and 42.0% are carriers. In Germany, 33.0% test homozygous affected, and 43.1% test as carriers.[2,3,4]

Inherited Diseases

Collie Eye Anomaly/Choroidal Hypoplasia/Coloboma (CEA/CH): Autosomal recessive disorder of eye development that can lead to retinal detachment and blindness. Reported in 67.77% of Collies CERF examined by veterinary ophthalmologists between 2000-2005. CERF does not recommend breeding affected dogs. Reported at a frequency of 24.1% in the Collie Health Foundation Online Health Survey. In switzerland, 8.9% smooth and 36.9% rough collies were affected. Dorn reports a 31.46x odds ratio versus other breeds. A genetic test is available.[5,6,7,8,9,10]

Hip Dysplasia: Polygenically inherited trait causing degenerative joint disease and hip arthritis. OFA reports 2.8% affected. Reported at a frequency of 3.2% in the Collie Health Foundation Online Health Survey.[7,11]

Elbow Dysplasia: Polygenically inherited trait causing elbow arthritis. OFA reports 1.0% affected.[11]

Grey Collie Cyclic Neutropenia: Collies that are homozygous for the dilute (d locus) gene are Grey Collies. Grey Collies can have an autosomal recessive disorder where circulating neutrophil numbers drop every 12 days due to a bone marrow abnormality in blood cell production. Affected dogs are prone to serious infection during episodes of neutropenia, and usually die from chronic infectious insults to the organs. A genetic test is available.[12,13]

Progressive Retinal Atrophy (PRA, rcd-2): An autosomal recessive, early onset rod, cone dysplasia form of PRA can occur in the breed with an onset of 6 weeks of age, and progressing to blindness by 1 year. A genetic test is available.[8,14,15]

von Willebrand's disease (vWD): Type II vWD in the Collie is a serious, sometimes fatal, autosomal recessive bleeding disorder. Cryoprecipitate is more effective, with fewer side effects, than fresh frozen plasma in controlling bleeding episodes. A genetic test is available.

Patella Luxation: Polygenically inherited laxity of patellar ligaments, causing luxation, lameness, and later degenerative joint disease. Treat surgically if causing clinical signs. Too few Collies have been screened by OFA to determine an accurate frequency.[11]

Disease Predispositions

Persistent Pupillary Membranes: Strands of fetal remnant connecting; iris to iris, cornea, lens, or involving sheets of tissue. The later three forms can impair vision, and dogs affected with these forms should not be bred. Identified in 16.31% of Collies CERF examined by veterinary ophthalmologists between 2000-2005. Dorn reports a 4.53x odds ratio versus other breeds.[5,8]

Retinal Dysplasia: Focal retinal dysplasia and retinal folds are recognized in the breed. Severe cases can progress to retinal detachment. Reported in 7.58% of Collies CERF examined by veterinary ophthalmologists between 2000-2005.[8]

Demodicosis, Generalized: Overgrowth of demodex mites in the skin causing hair loss and dermatitis. An immune deficiency underlies the condition. Reported at a frequency of 6.3% in the Collie Health Foundation Online Health Survey.[7]

Gastric Dilation/Volvulus (GDV, Bloat): Life-threatening twisting of the stomach within the abdomen. Requires immediate veterinary attention. Glickman found a 2.1x risk of developing GDV per year of life in Collies. Reported at a frequency of 5.3% in the Collie Health Foundation Online Health Survey.[7,16]

Hypothyroidism: Inherited autoimmune thyroiditis. 4.5% positive for thyroid auto-antibodies based on testing at Michigan State University. (Ave. for all breeds is 7.5%) Reported at a frequency of 5.1% in the Collie Health Foundation Online Health Survey.[7,17,18]

Idiopathic Epilepsy: Inherited seizures. Can be generalized or partial seizures. Collies have an increased incidence versus other breeds. Control with anti-seizure medication. Unknown mode of inheritance. Seizures were reported at a frequency of 5.1%, and epilepsy at 1.6% in the Collie Health Foundation Online Health Survey.[7,19]

Allergic Dermatitis: Inhalant or food allergy. Presents with pruritis and pyotraumatic dermatitis. Reported at a frequency of 4.3% in the Collie Health Foundation Online Health Survey.[7]

Microphthalmia: A congenital defect characterized by a small globes of the eye. Often associated with merle. Identified in 1.56% of Collies CERF examined by veterinary ophthalmologists between 2000-2005. CERF does not recommend breeding affected dogs.[8]

Dermatomyositis: Inherited disorder causing patches of scaling, crusting and alopecia over the muzzle, periorbital skin and distal limbs, and an associated myositis especially affecting the masticatory muscles. Onset between 3-6 months of age. Mode of inheritance is unknown, though some researchers suspect autosomal dominant with incomplete penetrance. Reported at a frequency of 1.5% in the Collie Health Foundation Online Health Survey.[7,20,21]

Distichiasis: Abnormally placed eyelashes that irritate the cornea and conjunctiva. Can cause secondary corneal ulceration. Identified in 1.39% of Collies CERF examined by veterinary ophthalmologists between 2000-2005.[8]

Cataracts: Nuclear cataracts predominate in the breed. Identified in 1.03% of Collies CERF examined by veterinary ophthalmologists between 2000-2005. CERF does not recommend breeding any Collie with a cataract.[8]

Autoimmune Hemolytic Anemia (AIHA): Collies have an increased risk of developing AIHA versus other breeds. Females are more frequently affected than males. Clinical features included pale mucous membranes, weakness, lethargy and collapse. Treatment with prednisone is successful in most cases.[22]

Pemphigus Foliaceus: The breed has an increased risk (3.9x odds ratio) of developing pemphigus foliaceus. Clinical signs include crusting lesions to the dorsal part of the muzzle and head, progressing to the body. Diagnosis is with biopsy.[23]

Chronic Pancreatitis: Often subclinical inflammation of the pancreas that can cause intermittent discomfort and gastrointestinal upsets, and can possibly lead to pancreatic insufficiency or diabetes mellitus. Collies have a 2.0x relative risk versus other breeds.[24]

Corneal Dystrophy: The breed can have an epithelial/stromal form of corneal dystrophy. Age of onset 2-5 years. Identified in 0.56% of Collies CERF examined by veterinary ophthalmologists between 2000-2005.[8,25]

Vesicular Cutaneous Lupus Erythematosus (Nasal Solar Dermatitis): Adult onset vesicular form of lupus that causes annular, polycyclic and serpiginous ulcerations distributed over sparsely haired areas of the body. These especially occur during the summer months due to ultraviolet exposure. Treatment is with immunosuppressive drugs and sunscreen.[26]

Pancreatic Acinar Atrophy (Exocrine pancreatic insufficiency): Collies are a breed at risk for immune-mediated pancreatic acinar atrophy. Clinical signs are poor weight gain, and steatorrhea. Treatment is with enzyme supplementation. Breeding studies suggest an autosomal recessive mode of inheritance in German shepherd dogs, another breed found at risk.[27,28,29]

Proliferative Keratoconjunctivitis (Nodular granulomatous episclerokeratitis): Inflammatory proliferative condition of the conjunctiva, sclera, cornea, or nictitans seen most frequently in the Collie versus other breeds. Average age of onset is 3.8 years. Requires lifelong immunosuppressive therapy.[8,30,31,32]

Gastric Carcinoma: The Collie breed appears to have a higher incidence of gastric carcinoma compared to other breeds. The most frequent clinical features are vomiting, polydipsia and weight loss, with endoscopic findings of a large deep ulcer with thickened, irregular rims and walls.[33]

Perineal Hernia: Older male Collies have a predisposition to developing perineal hernias. Treatment is surgical.[34]

Nasal Adenocarcinoma: Collies have an increased risk versus other breeds of developing nasal adenocarcinoma. Clinical signs include chronic nasal infection, discharge, and epistaxis.[35]

Diabetes Mellitus (Sugar Diabetes): Treat with insulin injections, diet, and glucose monitoring. A British study reported Collies with an increased incidence versus other breeds; however an American study found Collies to have a decreased risk. Unknown mode of inheritance.[36,37]

Colorectal Polyp: The Collie breed is over-represented with diagnoses of colorectal polyps versus other breeds. Clinical signs include dyschezia, periodic intermittent diarrhea and melena, and rectal prolapse of the polyp. Treatment is with surgery. Some polyps can be malignant.[38]

Idiopathic Horner's Syndrome: Collies may be predisposed to the development of Horner's syndrome. Affected dogs have an acute onset of unilateral miosis, ptosis of the upper eyelid, enophthalmos and protrusion of the third eyelid. Most cases resolve without treatment within weeks to months.[39]

Degenerative Myelopathy (DM): Affected dogs show an insidious onset of upper motor neuron (UMN) paraparesis. The disease eventually progresses to severe tetraparesis. Affected dogs have normal results on myelography, MRI, and CSF analysis. Necropsy confirms the condition. A direct genetic test for an autosomal recessive DM susceptibility gene is available. All affected dogs are homozygous for the gene, however only a small percentage of homozygous dogs develop DM. A genetic test for the DM susceptibility gene is available.[40,41]

Brachygnathism, Central Progressive Retinal Atrophy, Cerebellar Abiotrophy, Dysfibrinogenemia, Entropion, Factor VIII Deficiency, Neuroaxonal Dystrophy, Osteochondritis Dessicans–Stifle, Patent Ductus Arteriosis, Posterior Crossbite, Prognathism, Sebaceous Adenitis, and **Supernumerary Teeth** are reported.[42]

Isolated Case Studies

Hypercholesterolemia: Five related rough Collie dogs were diagnosed with corneal lipidosis and hypercholesterolemia. The corneal lipidosis improved with short-chain fructo-oligosaccharide supplementation. However, total cholesterol levels remained high.[43]

Juvenile Nephropathy: Case report of one Collie presenting with severe polyuria and polydipsia, and progressing to chronic renal failure. Histopathology included immature glomeruli and/or tubules, and persistent mesenchyme.[44]

Genetic Tests

Tests of Genotype: Direct tests for CEA/CH and rcd2 (PRA) are available from Optigen.

Direct test for MDR1 is available from Washington State Univ. http://www.vetmed.wsu.edu/depts-VCPL/

Direct test for the cyclic neutropenia is available from HealthGene and VetGen.

Direct test for coat colors sable and tricolor (a locus) is available from HealthGene.

Direct test for von Willebrand's disease is available from VetGen.

Direct test for a DM susceptability gene is available from the OFA.

CHIC Certification: Required testing includes genetic tests for rcd2 and MDR1. (See CHIC website; www.caninehealthinfo.org).

Tests of Phenotype: Recommended tests: hip and elbow radiographs, thyroid profile including autoantibodies, patella evaluation, CERF eye examination, and cardiac evaluation.

Miscellaneous

- **Breed name synonyms:** Old Cockie (historical name for the rough variety), Scottish Collie, Border Collie (historical)
- **Registries:** AKC, CKC, UKC, KCGB (Kennel Club of Great Britain), ANKC (Australian National Kennel Club), NKC (National Kennel Club)
- **AKC rank (year 2008):** 38 (4,016 dogs registered)
- **Internet resources: The Collie Club of America:** www.Collieclubofamerica.org
  Collie Club of Canada: www.Collieclubofcanada.ca
  The Collie Association (UK): www.collie-association.co.uk (Rough)
  Smooth Collie Club of Great Britain: www.smoothcollieclub.com
  Collie Health Foundation: www.Colliehealth.org
  American Working Collie Association: www.awca.net

References

1. Clark LA, Wahl JM, Rees CA, et. al.: Retrotransposon insertion in SILV is responsible for merle patterning of the domestic dog. Proc Natl Acad Sci U S A. 2006 Jan 31;103(5):1376-81.
2. Neff MW, Robertson KR, Wong AK, et. al.: Breed distribution and history of canine mdr1-1Delta, a pharmacogenetic mutation that marks the emergence of breeds from the Collie lineage. Proc Natl Acad Sci U S A. 2004 Aug 10;101(32):11725-30.
3. Geyer J, Doring B, Godoy JR, et. al.: Frequency of the nt230 (del4) MDR1 mutation in Collies and related dog breeds in Germany. J Vet Pharmacol Ther. 2005 Dec;28(6):545-51.
4. Mealey KL & Meurs KM: Breed distribution of the ABCB1-1Delta (multidrug sensitivity) polymorphism among dogs undergoing ABCB1 genotyping. J Am Vet Med Assoc. 2008 Sep 15;233(6):921-4.
5. Dorn CR: Canine breed-specific risks of frequently diagnosed diseases at veterinary teaching hospitals. Monograph. AKC Canine Health Foundation. 2000.
6. Lowe JK, Kukekova AV, Kirkness EF, et. al.: Linkage mapping of the primary disease locus for Collie eye anomaly. Genomics. 2003 Jul;82(1):86-95.
7. Collie Health Foundation: Online Health Survey Results. 2006.
8. *Ocular Disorders Presumed to be Inherited in Purebred Dogs.* American College of Veterinary Ophthalmologists. ACVO, 2007

9. Parker HG, Kukekova AV, Akey DT, et. al.: Breed relationships facilitate fine-mapping studies: a 7.8-kb deletion cosegregates with Collie eye anomaly across multiple dog breeds. Genome Res. 2007 Nov;17(11):1562-71.

10. Walser-Reinhardt L, Hässig M, & Spiess B: Collie eye anomaly in Switzerland. Schweiz Arch Tierheilkd. 2009 Dec;151(12):597-603.

11. OFA Website breed statistics: www.offa.org Last accessed July 1, 2010.

12. Dale DC, Ward SB, Kimball HR, et. al.: Studies of neutrophil production and turnover in grey Collie dogs with cyclic neutropenia. J Clin Invest. 1972 Aug;51(8):2190-6.

13. DiGiacomo RF, Hammond WP, Kunz LL, et. al.: Clinical and pathologic features of cyclic hematopoiesis in grey Collie dogs. Am J Pathol. 1983 May;111(2):224-33.

14. Kukekova AV, Nelson J, Kuchtey RW, et. al.: Linkage mapping of canine rod cone dysplasia type 2 (rcd2) to CFA7, the canine orthologue of human 1q32. Invest Ophthalmol Vis Sci. 2006 Mar;47(3):1210-5.

15. Kukekova AV, Goldstein O, Johnson JL, et. al.: Canine RD3 mutation establishes rod-cone dysplasia type 2 (rcd2) as ortholog of human and murine rd3. Mamm Genome. 2009 Feb;20(2):109-23.

16. Glickman LT, Glickman NW, Schellenberg DB, et. al.: Incidence of and breed-related risk factors for gastric dilatation-volvulus in dogs. J Am Vet Med Assoc. 2000 Jan 1;216(1):40-5.

17. Nachreiner R & Refsal K: Personal communication, Diagnostic Center for Population and Animal Health, Michigan State University. April, 2007.

18. Nachreiner RF, Refsal KR, Graham PA, et. al.: Prevalence of serum thyroid hormone autoantibodies in dogs with clinical signs of hypothyroidism. J Am Vet Med Assoc 2002 Feb 15;220(4):466-71.

19. Loscher W, Schwartz-Porsche D, Frey HH, et. al.: Evaluation of epileptic dogs as an animal model of human epilepsy. Arzneimittelforschung. 1985;35(1):82-7.

20. Hargis AM, Prieur DJ, Haupt KH, et. al.: Prospective study of familial canine dermatomyositis. Correlation of the severity of dermatomyositis and circulating immune complex levels. Am J Pathol. 1986 Jun;123(3):465-79.

21. Haupt KH, Prieur DJ, Moore MP, et. al.: Familial canine dermatomyositis: clinical, electrodiagnostic, and genetic studies. Am J Vet Res. 1985 Sep;46(9):1861-9.

22. Miller SA, Hohenhaus AE, Hale AS: Case-control study of blood type, breed, sex, and bacteremia in dogs with immune-mediated hemolytic anemia. J Am Vet Med Assoc. 2004 Jan 15;224(2):232-5.

23. Kuhl KA, Shofer FS, Goldschmidt MH: Comparative histopathology of pemphigus foliaceus and superficial folliculitis in the dog. Vet Pathol. 1994 Jan;31(1):19-27.

24. Watson PJ, Roulois AJ, Scase T, et. al.: Prevalence and breed distribution of chronic pancreatitis at post-mortem examination in first-opinion dogs. J Small Anim Pract. 2007 Nov;48(11):609-18.

25. Crispin SM: Crystalline corneal dystrophy in the dog. Histochemical and ultrastructural study. Cornea. 1988;7(2):149-61.

26. Jackson HA: Eleven cases of vesicular cutaneous lupus erythematosus in Shetland sheepdogs and rough Collies: clinical management and prognosis. Vet Dermatol. 2004 Feb;15(1):37-41.

27. Westermarck E, Pamilo P, Wiberg M: Pancreatic degenerative atrophy in the Collie breed: a hereditary disease. Zentralbl Veterinarmed A. 1989 Aug;36(7):549-54.

28. Wiberg ME: Pancreatic acinar atrophy in German shepherd dogs and rough-coated Collies. Etiopathogenesis, diagnosis and treatment. A review. Vet Q. 2004 Jun;26(2):61-75.

29. Batchelor DJ, Noble PJ, Cripps PJ, et. al.: Breed associations for canine exocrine pancreatic insufficiency. J Vet Intern Med. 2007 Mar-Apr;21(2):207-14.

30. Paulsen ME, Lavach JD, Snyder SP, et. al.: Nodular granulomatous episclerokeratitis in dogs: 19 cases (1973-1985). J Am Vet Med Assoc. 1987 Jun 15;190(12):1581-7.

31. Breaux CB, Sandmeyer LS, Grahn BH: Immunohistochemical investigation of canine episcleritis. Vet Ophthalmol. 2007 May-Jun;10(3):168-72.

32. Andrade AL, Sakamoto SS, Silva CM, et. al.: The Investigation of CD3 Subpopulation of T Lymphocytes in Canine Nodular Granulomatous Episcleritis.Proceedings, 2009 World Small Animal Veterinary Association World Congress. 2009.

33. Sullivan M, Lee R, Fisher EW: A study of 31 cases of gastric carcinoma in dogs. Vet Rec. 1987 Jan 24;120(4):79-83.

34. Robertson JJ: Perineal hernia repair in dogs. Mod Vet Pract. 1984 May;65(5):365-8.

35. Hayes HM Jr, Wilson GP, Fraumeni HF Jr: Carcinoma of the nasal cavity and paranasal sinuses in dogs: descriptive epidemiology. Cornell Vet. 1982 Apr;72(2):168-79.

36. Davison LJ, Herrtage ME, Catchpole B: Study of 253 dogs in the United Kingdom with diabetes mellitus. Vet Rec 2005 Apr 9; 156[15]:467-71.

37. Marmor M, Willeberg P, Glickman LT, et. al.: Epizootiologic patterns of diabetes mellitus in dogs. Am J Vet Res. 1982 Mar;43(3):465-70.

38. Seiler RJ: Colorectal polyps of the dog: a clinicopathologic study of 17 cases. J Am Vet Med Assoc. 1979 Jan 1;174(1):72-5.

39. Herrera HD, Suranit AP, Kojusner NF, et. al.: Idiopathic Horner's syndrome in Collie dogs. Vet Ophthalmol. 1998;1(1):17-20.

40. Coates JR, Zeng R, Awano T, et. al.: An SOD1 Mutation Associated with Degenerative Myelopathy Occurs in Many Dog Breeds.Proceedings, 2009 ACVIM Forum. 2009.

41. Okada M, Kitagawa M, Kanayama K, et. al.: Negative MRI findings in a case of degenerative myelopathy in a dog. J S Afr Vet Assoc. 2009 Dec;80(4):254-6.

42. *The Genetic Connection: A Guide to Health Problems in Purebred Dogs.* L. Ackerman. p212-13, AAHA Press, 1999.

43. Jeusette I, Grauwels M, Cuvelier C, et. al.: Hypercholesterolaemia in a family of rough Collie dogs. J Small Anim Pract. 2004 Jun;45(6):319-24.

44. Peeters D, Clercx C, Michiels L, et. al.: Juvenile nephropathy in a boxer, a rottweiler, a Collie and an Irish wolfhound. Aust Vet J. 2000 Mar;78(3):162-5.

45. *The Complete Dog Book, 20th Ed.* The American Kennel Club. Howell Book House, NY 2006. p. 659-664.

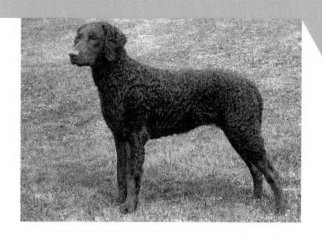

Curly Coated Retriever

The Breed History

The Curly-coated retriever is thought to be derived from Retrieving Setter and English Water Spaniel stock, the St. John's Newfoundland, and perhaps also the Poodle and Irish Water Spaniel. "Curlys" are one of the earliest known breeds of the retriever group, and early breed development occurred in Britain. The breed type was considered set by about 1850. During the two World Wars, and up until the 1960s the breed was close to extinction. The first breed specimens likely arrived in America in 1907. This is still a rare breed.

Breeding for Function

These dual-purpose dogs were particularly effective soft-mouth waterfowl retrievers used for duck, quail and other fowl. The coat was carefully bred for, so that they could withstand cold water hunting and heavy underbrush.

Physical Characteristics

Height at Withers: female 23-25" (58.5-63.5 cm), male 25-27" (63.5-68.5 cm).

Weight: 70-80 lb (32-36 kg).

Coat: The distinctive curly dense coat is made up of an outer coat with discrete short tight curls, though straight shorter hair is found on the face, feet and the pinna hair covering is intermediate in curl. Accepted coat colors are black and liver. Very small white patches are allowed. Black is **dominant**, liver is **recessive** in inheritance. Rare yellows occur but are not an accepted breed color. Has low grooming needs except during shedding times; the coat does not need trimming. Some breeders rarely or never brush these dogs but just periodically bathe them.

Longevity: 10-13 years

Points of Conformation: High head carriage, a distinct, tightly curled water-resistant coat, slightly longer than tall conformation characterize the Curly-coated Retriever. They possess moderate muscling and bone. The wedge-shaped head is more narrow, refined, with the muzzle tapering more than with the other retrievers. The stop is shallow, and the almond shaped eyes are black, brown or amber. The large nose is black or brown. The small ears are folded and close lying, with heavy leather. The neck is moderate in length, and not throaty. The topline is level, with a slight slope downward at the croup. The thorax is deep and moderately sprung ribs stay full towards the rear of the rib cage. The abdomen is moderately tucked up. The tail is straight, thick, tapering and reaches to the tarsus. Limbs are straight boned, and the feet are round with well-knuckled toes. Metacarpals and metatarsals are short. The dewclaws on the forelimb are often removed, and the ones on the hind limbs are usually removed. The dog moves with a long stride, with agility, speed and smoothness.

Recognized Behavior Issues and Traits

Reported breed characteristics include: Willing to please, calm and affectionate, hardy, high trainability, a good guard dog. He is noted to persevere in the field during a hunt. A Curly may be somewhat aloof with strangers. Slow to mature, some also have an independent streak. Early socialization and obedience training is recommended. A low activity level around the home, but typically has high exercise needs. Not recommended for apartment living. The Curly-coated Retriever needs close human companionship.

Normal Physiologic Variations

The coat tends to be oily so bathing 3 or 4 times a year is recommended as a minimum.

Drug Sensitivities

None reported

Inherited Diseases

Hip Dysplasia: Polygenically inherited trait causing degenerative joint disease and hip arthritis. OFA reports 15.3% affected.[1]

Elbow Dysplasia: Polygenically inherited trait causing elbow arthritis. OFA reports 0.5% affected.[1]

Patella Luxation: Polygenically inherited laxity of patellar ligaments, causing luxation, lameness, and later degenerative joint disease. Treat surgically if causing clinical signs. Too few Curly-coated Retrievers have been screened by OFA to determine an accurate frequency.[1]

Glycogenosis Type IIIa (Glycogen Storage Disease, GSD): An autosomal recessive inherited metabolic disorder that causes liver and skeletal muscle disease due to deficiency of the glycogen debranching enzyme (GDE) and tissue storage of abnormally structured glycogen. Clinical signs include episodic exercise intolerance, collapse, and lethargy. This disorder was discovered in an extended family of Curly-coated Retrievers (CCR), with representative cases from USA, Canada, and New Zealand. A genetic test is available and shows 0.5% affected and 8.7% carrier.[2]

Exercise Induced Collapse (EIC, Dynamin 1 Mutation): An autosomal recessive disorder of muscle weakness, incoordination and life threatening collapse accompanied by hyperthermia after just five to fifteen minutes of intense exercise or excitement. After 10 to 30 minutes of rest, most dogs return to normal. Limited genetic testing reveals over 10% carrier Curly Coated Retrievers. A direct genetic test is available.[3]

Disease Predispositions

Hypothyroidism: Inherited autoimmune thyroiditis. 7.3% positive for thyroid auto-antibodies based on testing at Michigan State University. (Ave. for all breeds is 7.5%).[4,5]

Distichiasis: Abnormally placed eyelashes that irritate the cornea and conjunctiva. Can cause secondary corneal ulceration. Identified in 7.64% of Curly Coated Retrievers CERF examined by veterinary ophthalmologists between 2000-2005.[6]

Persistent Pupillary Membranes: Strands of fetal remnant connecting; iris to iris, cornea, lens, or involving sheets of tissue. The later three forms can impair vision, and dogs affected with these forms should not be bred. Identified in 3.82% of Curly Coated Retrievers CERF examined by veterinary ophthalmologists between 2000-2005.[6]

Cataracts: The breed can develop anterior subcapsular striate cortical cataracts between 5-8 years of age, and posterior subcapsular cataracts at 2-4 years of age. Other forms of cataracts also occur in the breed. Identified in 3.64% of Curly Coated Retrievers CERF examined by veterinary ophthalmologists between 2000-2005. CERF does not recommend breeding any Curly Coated Retriever with a cataract.[6]

Follicular Dysplasia (Patterned Baldness): Inherited, non-inflammatory, truncal, symmetrical, cyclic hair loss. Melatonin may allow regrowth. Unknown mode of inheritance.[7]

Vitreous Degeneration: Liquefaction of the vitreous gel which may predispose to retinal detachment. Identified in 2.18% of Curly Coated Retrievers CERF examined by veterinary ophthalmologists between 2000-2005.[6]

Gastric Dilatation-Volvulus (bloat, GDV): Polygenically inherited, life-threatening twisting of the stomach within the abdomen. Requires immediate treatment. Reported at an increased frequency in the breed.[8]

Subaortic Stenosis (SAS) and Tricuspid Valve Dysplasia (TVD): Both polygenically inherited heart disorders have been identified in families of Curly Coated Retrievers. Can lead to congestive heart failure. Diagnose with echocardiography.

Coat dilution alopecia, Corneal Dystrophy, Ectropion, Entropion, Progressive Retinal Atrophy, Retinal Dysplasia, and **von Willebrand's Disease** are reported.[9]

Isolated Case Studies

Mast Cell Leukemia: A seven-year-old female Curly-coated Retriever presented with acute circulatory collapse, emesis, diarrhea, abdominal enlargement, icterus, cyanosis, dyspnea, pulmonary edema, hepatomegaly, ascites, and right ventricular enlargement. Hematologic and biochemical examinations revealed mast cell leukemia, mature neutrophilia, monocytosis, thrombocytopenia,

hemolytic hyperbilirubinemia, hyperhistaminemia, renal and hepatic injuries. Mast cells were distributed systemically, but predominantly in the diaphragm and liver with a large mass among the serosa of ileum, cecum and colon.[10]

Genetic Tests

Tests of Genotype: Direct test for GSD IIIa is available from the Fyfe Lab at Michigan State University http://mmg.msu.edu/faculty/fyfe.htm (517-355-6463x1559).

Direct test for presence of black and liver coat colors, and black and brown nose is available from HealthGene and VetGen.

Tests of Phenotype: CHIC Certification: Required testing includes hip radiographs, congenital cardiac evaluation by a cadiologist, and CERF eye examination. Optional recommended tests are; elbow radiographs, and direct GSD IIIa test. (See CHIC website; www.caninehealthinfo.org).

Recommend thyroid profile, including autoantibodies, and patella evaluation.

Miscellaneous

- **Breed name synonyms:** Curly, Curly-coat Retriever.
- **Registries:** AKC, UKC, CKC, KCGB (Kennel Club of Great Britain), ANKC (Australian National Kennel Club), NKC (National Kennel Club).
- **AKC rank (year 2008):** 138 (129 dogs registered)
- **Internet resources: The Curly Coated Retriever Club of America:** www.ccrca.org
  Curly Coated Retriever Club of Canada: www.angelfire.com/ny/curlycoat/CCRCC.html
  Curly Coated Retriever Club (UK): www.curlycoatedretrieverclub.co.uk

References

1. OFA Website breed statistics: www.offa.org Last accessed July 1, 2010.
2. Gregory BL, Shelton GD, Bali DS, et. al.: Glycogen storage disease type IIIa in curly-coated retrievers. J Vet Intern Med. 2007 Jan-Feb;21(1):40-6.
3. Minor KM, Patterson EE, Gross SD, et. al.: Frequency of the Canine Exercise Induced Collapse Gene in Diverse Breeds. Proceedings, 2009 ACVIM Forum. 2009.
4. Nachreiner R & Refsal K: Personal communication, Diagnostic Center for Population and Animal Health, Michigan State University. April, 2007.
5. Nachreiner RF, Refsal KR, Graham PA, et. al.: Prevalence of serum thyroid hormone autoantibodies in dogs with clinical signs of hypothyroidism. J Am Vet Med Assoc 2002 Feb 15;220(4):466-71.
6. Ocular Disorders Presumed to be Inherited in Purebred Dogs. American College of Veterinary Ophthalmologists. ACVO, 2007.
7. White SD: Update on Follicular Alopecias: "Pseudo-Endocrinopathies". Proceedings, 2005 ACVIM Forum. 2005.
8. Glickman LT, Glickman NW, Schellenberg DB, et. al.: Incidence of and breed-related risk factors for gastric dilatation-volvulus in dogs. J Am Vet Med Assoc. 2000 Jan 1;216(1):40-5.
9. The Genetic Connection: A Guide to Health Problems in Purebred Dogs. L Ackerman. p. 213 AAHA Press, 1999.
10. Hikasa Y, Morita T, Futaoka Y, et. al.: Connective tissue-type mast cell leukemia in a dog. J Vet Med Sci. 2000 Feb;62(2):187-90.
11. The Complete Dog Book, 20th Ed. The American Kennel Club. Howell Book House, NY 2006. p. 38-41.

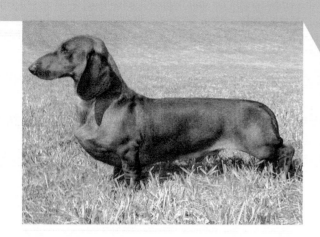

Dachshund

Three haircoat types:

1. Longhaired: Slightly wavy, the haircoat is longer under the body and behind the limbs. The ears particularly, should be endowed with longer silky hair. The tail has the longest hairs of the coat, and is structured to form a flag.
2. Smooth: The shorthaired variety possesses a very flat, glossy short haircoat.
3. Wirehaired: Over the body a thick, rough outer coat and a soft undercoat are interspersed. The ear, brow and jaw are free of the wirehair.

Longevity: 12-15 years

Points of Conformation: A low slung conformation with long back and very short limbs give this dog the appearance of being able to fit down a narrow quarry den. High head carriage and energetic gait provide surprisingly good agility and speed. The head tapers and the eyes are medium sized, almond shaped and have a very darkly pigmented iris. The palpebral margins are pigmented. It is only in dapple coloring that wall eyes are accepted. Ears are pendulous, rounded and of moderate length and set, and they turn inwards towards the tips. Little stop is noted, and the nose is preferred to be pigmented black. The neck is long, slightly arched and muscular without evidence of dewlap. The topline is long and the loin is only slightly arched. The breastbone is prominent, the ribs well sprung, and a characteristic bowing of the legs typical for chondrodystrophic breeds is present. Forelimbs are generally abducted due to carpal deviation. Feet are small, well arched, and possess thick pads. Dewclaws may be removed; rear dewclaws typically are. The tail is slightly curved and carried close to level with topline.

The Breed History

In medieval times, dogs used to hunt badger were termed dachshund; the name means *"badger hound"*. The wirehaired versions were bred in order to protect the dogs from heavy brush. The first definitive records of specific breed type can be traced to the 17th century. By 1900, three varieties; a short, long, and wirehaired were recognized. The first German studbook records date to the mid 1800s. First AKC registry occurred in 1885. Standard and Miniature types are shown in separate class divisions and bred separately.

Breeding for Function

Though bred specifically to take on the tough badger, these standard-sized dogs were also used in packs to hunt wild boar. Stamina and courage were hallmarks of these hunting partners. Smaller versions of the Dachshund were used to hunt fox, and it is this variety that has become most popular. Miniature dachshunds were also in the hunt for hare and rabbit quarry. The typical companion dachshund is a medium-sized smooth coated variety. The breed is noted for below ground work and their scent and vocal skills are well developed.

Physical Characteristics

Height at Withers: no standard, but they are usually under 9" (23 cm).

Weight: Miniature: less than 11 lb (5 kg) at 1 year, Standard: 16-32 lb (7-14.5 kg).

Coat:

1. Solid (self colored): includes red, cream. Nose and nails are black with these dogs.
2. Bi-colored: chocolate, black, Isabella (fawn) and gray (blue), with tan markings. A small white marking is acceptable on the chest. Dark bi-colored dogs have black noses and nails but other colors may have self or brown nose and nail color.
3. Dapple: intermixed light and dark with neither color predominating. In double dapples a larger white chest marking is allowed. Single and double dapple varieties exist. In the latter, white overlays the single dapple coloration.
4. Brindle dogs have a pattern of stripes that are black or dark over the body or within the tan points.

Recognized Behavior Issues and Traits

Reported breed characteristics include: Good in town or country, active outdoors, a gentle companion, a good alert barker, affectionate, and playful. Dachshunds are intelligent, easy to maintain because of low grooming needs, and if properly socialized, good with gentle children. They may have a strong independent, even stubborn streak, may be aggressive with strange dogs and aloof with strangers, and often have high barking and digging tendencies. They will become destructive if bored. Considered an average shedder, the coat care depends on coat type: smooth coats need minimal brushing, wire coats need to be stripped twice per annum, and a long hair coat needs daily grooming. They can tend to be biters, and this should be discouraged when young.

Normal Physiologic Variations

The merle gene produces the dapple coat color in the dachshund. Dapple dachshunds should not be bred together, as homozygous merle (MM) tend to produce microphthalmia, blindness, deafness, and other abnormalities.[1,2,3]

The dilute gene produces the blue coat color in the homozygous state (dd). This can predispose to color dilution alopecia.[4]

In a UK study, 31.2% of Dachund litters were delivered via **C-section**.[5]

Drug Sensitivities
None reported

Inherited Diseases
Patella Luxation: Polygenically inherited laxity of patellar ligaments, causing luxation, lameness, and later degenerative joint disease. Treat surgically if causing clinical signs. OFA reports 7.1% affected.[6]

Hip Dysplasia and Legg-Calve Perthes Disease: Polygenically inherited traits causing degenerative hip joint disease and arthritis. OFA reports 8.1% affected. Reported 4.8x odds ratio for Legg-Calve-Perthes versus other breeds.[6,7]

Progressive Retinal Atrophy (PRA)/Cone-Rod Dystrophy (cord1): Hereditary disorder of retinal degeneration. There are two populations of affected miniature longhaired dachshunds, with one group presenting with night blindness that progresses to total blindness at 4 months to 2 years of age, and another group presenting between 2 years and 15 years of age. Identified in 1.66% of longhaired miniature, 1.30% of longhaired standard, and 1.19% of smooth miniature dachshunds CERF examined by veterinary ophthalmologists between 2000-2005. An autosomal recessive mutation in the RPGRIP1 gene is highly correlated to early age clinical PRA, and slightly less so to the later age presentation. 16% of miniature longhaired dachshunds homozygous for the mutation retain normal sight, and some affected dogs do not carry the RPGRIP1 mutation, demonstrating a more complex etiology for this disease. A second locus had been identified that may modify age of onset of the disorder. A genetic test for the RPGRIP1 mutation is available.[8,9,10,11]

Progressive Retinal Atrophy (PRA)/Cone-Rod Dystrophy (NPHP4): A mutation in the NPHP4 gene is responsible for this autosomal recessive form of cone-rod dysplasia in standard wire-haired Dachshunds. Affected dogs have cone and rod degeneration by 5 weeks of age, and present with pin-point sized pupils. 9.6% of standard wire-haired Dachshunds test carrier in Norway.[12,13,14]

Elbow Dysplasia: Polygenically inherited trait causing elbow arthritis. Too few Dachshunds have been screened by OFA to determine an accurate frequency.[6]

Neuronal Ceroid-Lipofuscinosis (NCL): Dachshunds have two different fatal forms of NCL, that present with ataxia, behavior changes, and seizures. An adult-onset (4.5-6.5 years) form presents between 4.5-6.5 years of age, and a juvenile-onset form presents at 9 months of age. The juvenile-onset form is an autosomal recessive disorder caused by a mutation in the PPT1 gene, and a genetic test is available.[15,16,17,18]

Mucopolysaccharidosis IIIA (MPS IIIA or Sanfilippo A): Autosomal recessive storage disease. Pelvic limb ataxia begins around 3 years of age, progresses gradually within 1-2 y to severe generalized spinocerebellar ataxia. A genetic test is available.[19,20]

Progressive Myoclonic Epilepsy (PME): A fatal autosomal recessive disorder identified in miniature wirehaired dachshunds, causing progressive myoclonic twitching and seizures. The genetic mutation has been identified.[21]

Pyruvate Kinase Deficiency (PK): Autosomal recessive disorder causing severe hemolytic anemia, progressive osteomyelosclerosis, and hemosiderosis. Death occurs due to anemia or hepatic failure usually at less than five years of age. Occurs at a low frequency in the breed. A genetic test is available.[22]

Narcolepsy: Rare, autosomal recessive disorder causing sudden collapse and a sleep-like state elicited by excitement. Identified in a family of dachshunds, and in other sporadic cases. A genetic test is available.[23]

Osteogenesis Imperfecta: Rare, autosomal recessive disease seen in rough-coated juvenile dachshunds. Affected dogs present with pain, spontaneous bone and teeth fractures, joint hyperlaxity, and reduced bone density on radiography. Caused by a mutation in the SERPINH1 gene causing defective collagen synthesis.[24,25]

Disease Predispositions
Intervertebral Disc Disease (IVDD): Spinal cord disease due to prolapsed disk material. Clinical signs include back pain, scuffing of paws, spinal ataxia, limb weakness, and paralysis. Studies have shown that 76% of all dachshunds have radiographically identifiable calcified disk material by 24 months of age. Almost all dogs with IVDD have calcified disk material. Dachshunds with calcified disks had a higher rate of recurrence of IVDD. In a Japanese study, Dachshunds represented 53.3% of dogs with thoracolumbar IVDD at an average age of 5.6 years, and 12.9% of dogs with cervical IVDD at an average age of 7.8 years. Occurs at a frequency of 15.6% in the breed. Dorn reports an 57.01x odds ratio versus other breeds.[26,27,28,29,30]

Persistent Pupillary Membranes: Strands of fetal remnant connecting; iris to iris, cornea, lens, or involving sheets of tissue. The later three forms can impair vision, and dogs affected with these forms should not be bred. Identified in 11.63% of wirehaired miniature, 10.41% of wirehaired standard, 6.22% of longhaired miniature, 4.71% of smooth standard, 3.57% of standard miniature, and 3.03% of longhaired standard Dachshunds CERF-examined by veterinary ophthalmologists between 2000-2005.[10]

Iris Coloboma: A coloboma is a congenital defect which may affect the iris, choroid or optic disc, which may affect vision. Identified in 9.30% of wirehaired miniature, and 4.76% of smooth miniature Dachshunds CERF-examined by veterinary ophthalmologists between 2000-2005. CERF does not recommend breeding affected dogs.[10]

Distichiasis: Abnormally placed eyelashes that irritate the cornea and conjunctiva. Can cause secondary corneal ulceration. Identified in 9.13% of longhaired miniature, 6.93% of longhaired standard, 2.33% of wirehaired miniature and standard, and 1.74% of smooth standard Dachshunds CERF-examined by veterinary ophthalmologists between 2000-2005.[10]

Corneal Dystrophy: Dachshunds can have an epithelial/stromal form of corneal dystrophy. Identified in 4.65% of wirehaired miniature and standard Dachshunds CERF-examined by veterinary ophthalmologists between 2000-2005.[10]

Cataracts: Anterior, posterior, intermediate and punctate cataracts occur in the breed. In a German study of boar-colored wirehaired Dachshunds, primary cataracts were present in 3.83%, and prominent suture lines in 2.76%. Heritabilities ranged from 0.36-0.39, with different forms of cataract positively correlated to each other. Identified in 3.32% of longhaired miniature, 3.23% of smooth standard, 2.60% of wirehaired standard, 2.38% of longhaired standard, and 2.33% of wirehaired miniature Dachshunds CERF-examined by veterinary ophthalmologists between 2000-2005. CERF does not recommend breeding any Dachshund with a cataract.[10,31]

Persistent Hyaloid Artery (PHA): Congenital defect resulting from abnormalities in the development and regression of the hyaloid artery. Identified in 3.35% of wirehaired standard, 1.24% of longhaired miniature, and 1.19% of smooth miniature Dachshunds CERF-examined by veterinary ophthalmologists between 2000-2005.[10]

Hypothyroidism: Inherited autoimmune thyroiditis. 2.8% positive for thyroid auto-antibodies based on testing at Michigan State University. (Ave. for all breeds is 7.5%.)[32,33]

Hyperadrenocorticism (Cushing's Disease): Hyperfunction of the adrenal gland caused by a pituitary or adrenal tumor. Clinical signs may include increased thirst and urination, symmetrical truncal alopecia, and abdominal distention. Dorn reports an 1.80x odds ratio versus other breeds. One study found a high incidence in a family of wire-haired Dachshunds.[26,34,35]

Mitral Valve Disease/Prolapse: Dachshunds are a breed at increased risk of developing mitral regurgitation due to myxomatous changes, and later mitral valve prolapse. Diagnosis by echocardiography. Breeding studies suggest a polygenic mode of inheritance.[36,37]

Chronic Superficial Keratitis/Pannus: A bilateral disease of the cornea which usually starts as a grayish haze to the ventral or ventrolateral cornea, followed by the formation of a vascularized subepithelial growth that begins to spread toward the central cornea; pigmentation follows the vascularization. CERF does not recommend breeding any affected dogs.[10,38]

Punctate Keratitis: Focal circular rings usually affecting the central subepithelial and/or anterior portion of the cornea. There often is an associated dry eye with corneal erosions. The mode of inheritance is unknown. CERF does not recommend breeding any affected dogs.[10,38]

Optic Nerve Coloboma: A congenital cavity in the optic nerve which, if large, may cause blindness or vision impairment. Identified in 2.38% of smooth miniature Dachshunds CERF examined by veterinary ophthalmologists between 2000-2005. CERF does not recommend breeding affected dogs.[10]

Microphthalmia: A congenital defect characterized by small globes of the eye. Often associated with merle. Identified in 2.38% of smooth miniature, 2.33% of wirehaired miniature, and 1.66% of longhaired miniature Dachshunds CERF examined by veterinary ophthalmologists between 2000-2005. CERF does not recommend breeding affected dogs.[10]

Retinal Dysplasia: Focal retinal dysplasia and retinal folds are recognized in the breed. Identified in 2.33% of wirehaired miniature, 1.49% of wirehaired and smooth standard, and 1.08% of longhaired standard Dachshunds CERF examined by veterinary ophthalmologists between 2000-2005.[10]

Color-dilution Alopecia: Condition seen in some blue (dilute) colored Dachshunds. Starts as a gradual onset of dry, dull and poor hair coat quality. Progresses to poor hair regrowth, follicular papules and comedomes. Hair loss and comedome formation are usually most severe on the trunk. Dorn reports an 4.56x odds ratio for developing alopecia versus other breeds. A genetic test is available for the dilute gene.[5,26,39]

Optic Nerve Hypoplasia: Congenital malformation of the optic nerve causing blindness. Identified in 1.24% of smooth standard and 1.19% of smooth miniature Dachshunds CERF examined by veterinary ophthalmologists between 2000-2005. CERF does not recommend breeding any Dachshund with the condition.[10]

Urolithiasis; Xanthine, Cystine: Dachshunds are found to be a breed at increased risk of forming bladder stones. Several cases of xanthine urinary stones have been diagnosed in the breed, suggesting an inherited disorder of xanthine oxidase. The breed also has an increased incidence of Cystinuria and cystine stones versus other breeds.[40,41,42]

Deafness: Dappled dachshunds can have congenital deafness due to the merle gene. Can be unilateral or bilateral. Diagnosed by BAER testing. In a multi-breed study; for single merles (Mm), 2.7% were unilaterally deaf and 0.9% were bilaterally deaf. For double merles (MM), 10% were unilaterally deaf and 15% were bilaterally deaf.[3,43]

Cutaneous Histiocytoma: Benign dermal tumor that usually presents as a single, hairless "button-like" mass in dogs under 3 years of age. The tumor spontaneously regresses over 3 months. Seen at an increased frequency in the breed.[44]

Sudden Acute Retinal Degeneration (SARDS): Degenerative retinal disease causing acute blindness. Age of onset from 1.5 to 15 years, with an average of 8.4 years. In one study, 9% of affected dogs were Dachshunds. Diagnose with ERG.[45,46]

Congenital Myasthenia Gravis: Disorder of exercise induced muscle weakness identified in immature miniature dachshunds. Clinical signs resolve spontaneously by 6 months of age.[47]

Nasopharyngeal Dysgenesis/stenosis: Congenital disorder characterized by expiratory cheek puffing, upper respiratory dyspnea, macroglossia, and dysphagia. Treatment is with surgery. Unknown mode of inheritance.[48]

Sterile Panniculitis: Rare, dermatological disease of subcutaneous fat inflammation characterized by deep cutaneous nodules that often ulcerate and drain pus or oil. Treat with immunosuppressive medications. Miniature Dachshunds represent 51.2% of all cases. Unknown mode of inheritance.[49]

Acanthosis Nigricans, Brachygnathism, Bullous Pemphigoid, Calcinosis Circumscripta, Cleft Lip/Palate, Cryptorchidism, Cutaneous Asthenia, Demodicosis, Dermoid, Entropion,

Glaucoma, Heterochromia Iridis, Juvenile Cellulitis, Keratoconjunctivitis Sicca, Micropapilla, Portosystemic Shunting, Seasonal Flank Alopecia, Sebaceous Adenitis, Sensory Neuropathy, Vasculitis, and von Willebrand's Disease are reported.[50]

Isolated Case Studies

Immunodeficiency and Pneumonocystis Carinii Pneumonia: Seven cases of Dachshunds under one year of age were diagnosed with P. Carinii pneumonia; all had both T-cell and B-cell deficiency. Affected dogs presented with polypnea, tachypnea, and exercise intolerance.[51]

Uveodermatologic (VKH–like) Syndrome: Identified in a female Dachshund. Autoimmune disease manifested by progressive uveitis and depigmenting dermatitis that closely resembles the human Vogt-Koyanagi-Harada syndrome. Treat with immunosuppressive drugs. CERF does not recommend breeding any affected dogs.[10,52]

Genetic Tests

Tests of Genotype: Direct test for PRA/cord1 is available from the University of Missouri and the Animal Health Trust.

Direct test for juvenile Ceroid lipofuscinosis is available from the University of Missouri.

Direct tests for pyruvate kinase deficiency and MPS are available from PennGenn.

Direct test for narcolepsy is available from Optigen.

Direct tests for "true red", black or black and tan or red with dark tips and chocolate or chocolate & tan coat colors, and black or brown nose are available from HealthGene and VetGen.

Direct test for coat length is available from DDC Veterinary and VetGen.

Tests of Phenotype: CHIC Certification: Required testing includes CERF eye examination and patella evaluation. Optional recommended tests are Direct test for PRA/Cord1, thyroid profile including autoantibodies, and BAER test for deafness. (See CHIC website; www.caninehealthinfo.org).

Additional Recommended test: hip and elbow radiographs, and cardiac evaluation.

Miscellaneous

- **Breed name synonyms:** Teckel, Zwergteckel, Normalgrosse Teckel.
- **Registries:** AKC, UKC, CKC, KCGB (Kennel Club of Great Britain), ANKC (Australian National Kennel Club), NKC (National Kennel Club).
- **AKC rank (year 2008):** 7 (26,075 registered)
- **Internet resources: Dachshund Club of America:**
  www.dachshund-dca.org
  National Miniature Dachshund Club, Inc.:
  www.dachshund-nmdc.org
  The Dachshund Club (UK): www.dachshundclub.co.uk

References

1. Dausch D, Wegner W, Michaelis W, et. al.: Eye changes in the merle syndrome in the dog. Albrecht Von Graefes Arch Klin Exp Ophthalmol. 1978 May 2;206(2):135-50.
2. Strain GM: Deafness prevalence and pigmentation and gender associations in dog breeds at risk. Vet J. 2004 Jan;167(1):23-32.
3. Clark LA, Wahl JM, Rees CA, et. al.: Retrotransposon insertion in SILV is responsible for merle patterning of the domestic dog. Proc Natl Acad Sci U S A. 2006 Jan 31;103(5):1376-81.
4. Drögemüller C, Philipp U, Haase B, et. al.: A noncoding melanophilin gene (MLPH) SNP at the splice donor of exon 1 represents a candidate causal mutation for coat color dilution in dogs. J Hered. 2007;98(5):468-73.
5. Evans KM & Adams VJ: Proportion of litters of purebred dogs born by caesarean section. J Small Anim Pract. 2010 Feb;51(2):113-8.
6. OFA Website breed statistics: www.offa.org Last accessed July 1, 2010.
7. LaFond E, Breur GJ & Austin CC: Breed susceptibility for developmental orthopedic diseases in dogs. J Am Anim Hosp Assoc. 2002 Sep-Oct;38(5):467-77.
8. Curtis R, Barnett KC: Progressive retinal atrophy in miniature longhaired dachshund dogs. Br Vet J. 1993 Jan-Feb;149(1):71-85.
9. Mellersh CS, Boursnell ME, Pettitt L, et. al.: Canine RPGRIP1 mutation establishes cone-rod dystrophy in miniature longhaired dachshunds as a homologue of human Leber congenital amaurosis. Genomics. 2006 Sep;88(3):293-301.
10. *Ocular Disorders Presumed to be Inherited in Purebred Dogs.* American College of Veterinary Ophthalmologists. ACVO, 2007.
11. Miyadera K, Kato K, Aguirre-Hernández J, et. al.: Phenotypic variation and genotype-phenotype discordance in canine cone-rod dystrophy with an RPGRIP1 mutation. Mol Vis. 2009 Nov 11;15:2287-305.
12. Wiik AC, Wade C, Biagi T, et. al.: A deletion in nephronophthisis 4 (NPHP4) is associated with recessive cone-rod dystrophy in standard wire-haired dachshund. Genome Res. 2008 Sep;18(9):1415-21.
13. Ropstad EO, Bjerkås E, Narfström K, et. al.: Clinical findings in early onset cone-rod dystrophy in the Standard Wire-haired Dachshund. Vet Ophthalmol. 2007 Mar-Apr;10(2):69-75.
14. Wiik AC, Thoresen SI, Wade C, et. al.: A population study of a mutation allele associated with cone-rod dystrophy in the standard wire-haired dachshund. Anim Genet. 2009 Aug;40(4):572-4.
15. Vandevelde M, Fatzer R: Neuronal ceroid-lipofuscinosis in older dachshunds. Vet Pathol. 1980 Nov;17(6):686-92.
16. Awano T, Katz ML, O'Brien DP, et. al.: A frame shift mutation in canine TPP1 (the ortholog of human CLN2) in a juvenile Dachshund with neuronal ceroid lipofuscinosis. Mol Genet Metab. 2006 Nov;89(3):254-60.
17. Katz ML, Coates JR, Cooper JJ, et. al.: Retinal pathology in a canine model of late infantile neuronal ceroid lipofuscinosis. Invest Ophthalmol Vis Sci. 2008 Jun;49(6):2686-95.
18. Sanders DN, Farias FH, Johnson GS, et. al.: A mutation in canine PPT1 causes early onset neuronal ceroid lipofuscinosis in a Dachshund. Mol Genet Metab. 2010 Aug;100(4):349-56.
19. Fischer A, Carmichael KP, Munnell JF, et. al.: Sulfamidase deficiency in a family of Dachshunds: a canine model of mucopolysaccharidosis IIIA (Sanfilippo A). Pediatr Res. 1998 Jul;44(1):74-82.
20. Aronovich EL, Carmichael KP, Morizono H, et. al.: Canine Heparan Sulfate Sulfamidase and the Molecular Pathology Underlying Sanfilippo Syndrome Type A in Dachshunds. Genomics 2000, 15 Aug;68(1):80-84.
21. Lohi H, Young EJ, Fitzmaurice SN, et. al.: Expanded repeat in canine epilepsy. Science. 2005 Jan 7;307(5706):81.
22. Whitney KM, Goodman SA, Bailey EM, et. al.: The molecular basis of canine pyruvate kinase deficiency. Exp Hematol. 1994 Aug;22(9):866-74.
23. Hungs M, Fan J, Lin L, et. al.: Identification and functional analysis of mutations in the hypocretin (orexin) genes of narcoleptic canines. Genome Res. 2001 Apr;11(4):531-9.
24. Seeliger F, Leeb T, Peters M, et. al.: Osteogenesis imperfecta in two litters of dachshunds. Vet Pathol. 2003 Sep;40(5):530-9.

25. Drögemüller C, Becker D, Brunner A, et. al.: A missense mutation in the SERPINH1 gene in Dachshunds with osteogenesis imperfecta. PLoS Genet. 2009 Jul;5(7):e1000579.

26. Dorn CR: Canine breed-specific risks of frequently diagnosed diseases at veterinary teaching hospitals. Monograph. AKC Canine Health Foundation. 2000.

27. Lappalainen A, Norrgard M, Alm K, et. al.: Calcification of the intervertebral discs and curvature of the radius and ulna: a radiographic survey of Finnish miniature dachshunds. Acta Vet Scand. 2001;42(2):229-36.

28. Jensen VF, Arnbjerg J: Development of intervertebral disk calcification in the dachshund: a prospective longitudinal radiographic study. J Am Anim Hosp Assoc. 2001 May-Jun;37(3):274-82.

29. Mayhew PD, McLear RC, Ziemer LS, et. al.: Risk factors for recurrence of clinical signs associated with thoracolumbar intervertebral disk herniation in dogs: 229 cases (1994-2000). J Am Vet Med Assoc. 2004 Oct 15;225(8):1231-6.

30. Itoh H, Hara Y, Yoshimi N, et. al.: A retrospective study of intervertebral disc herniation in dogs in Japan: 297 cases. J Vet Med Sci. 2008 Jul;70(7):701-6.

31. Müller C, Hamann H, Brahm R, et. al.: Analysis of systematic and genetic effects on the prevalence of different types of primary lens opacifications in the wild-boar-colored wirehaired Dachshund. Berl Munch Tierarztl Wochenschr. 2008 Jul-Aug;121(7-8):286-91.

32. Nachreiner R & Refsal K: Personal communication, Diagnostic Center for Population and Animal Health, Michigan State University. April, 2007.

33. Nachreiner RF, Refsal KR, Graham PA, et. al.: Prevalence of serum thyroid hormone autoantibodies in dogs with clinical signs of hypothyroidism. J Am Vet Med Assoc 2002 Feb 15;220(4):466-71.

34. Ling GV, Stabenfeldt GH, Comer KM, et. al.: Canine hyperadrenocorticism: pretreatment clinical and laboratory evaluation of 117 cases. J Am Vet Med Assoc. 1979 Jun 1;174(11):1211-5.

35. Stritzel S, Mischke R, Philipp U, et. al.: Familial canine pituitary-dependent hyperadrenocorticism in wirehaired Dachshunds. Berl Munch Tierarztl Wochenschr. 2008 Sep-Oct;121(9-10):349-58.

36. Olsen LH, Fredholm M, Pedersen HD, et. al.: Epidemiology and inheritance of mitral valve prolapse in Dachshunds. J Vet Intern Med. 1999 Sep-Oct;13(5):448-56.

37. Olsen LH, Martinussen T, Pedersen HD: Early echocardiographic predictors of myxomatous mitral valve disease in dachshunds. Vet Rec. 2003 Mar 8;152(10):293-7.

38. Brandsch H, Nicodem K: Heredity of keratitis in long-haired dachshunds. Mh Vet-Med 1982;37:216.

39. Kim JH, Kang KI, Sohn HJ, et. al.: Color-dilution alopecia in dogs. J Vet Sci. 2005 Sep;6(3):259-61.

40. Brown NO, Parks JL, Greene RW: Canine urolithiasis: retrospective analysis of 438 cases. J Am Vet Med Assoc. 1977 Feb 15;170(4):414-8.

41. Flegel T, Freistadt R, Haider W: Xanthine urolithiasis in a dachshund. Vet Rec. 1998 Oct 10;143(15):420-3.

42. Hoppe A, Denneberg T: Cystinuria in the dog: clinical studies during 14 years of medical treatment. J Vet Intern Med. 2001 Jul-Aug;15(4):361-7.

43. Strain GM, Clark LA, Wahl JM, et. al.: Prevalence of deafness in dogs heterozygous or homozygous for the merle allele. J Vet Intern Med. 2009 Mar-Apr;23(2):282-6.

44. Skorupski, K: The Histiocytic Diseases: A Clinical Perspective. Proceedings, UC-Davis 2009 Canine Medicine Symposium. 2009.

45. van der Woerdt A, Nasisse MP, Davidson MG. Sudden acquired retinal degeneration in the dog. Progress in Veterinary and Comparative Ophthalmology 1991; 1: 11–18.

46. Montgomery KW, van der Woerdt A, & Cottrill NB: Acute blindness in dogs: sudden acquired retinal degeneration syndrome versus neurological disease (140 cases, 2000-2006). Vet Ophthalmol. 2008 Sep-Oct;11(5):314-20.

47. Dickinson PJ, Sturges BK, Shelton GD, et. al.: Congenital myasthenia gravis in Smooth-Haired Miniature Dachshund dogs. J Vet Intern Med. 2005 Nov-Dec;19(6):920-3.

48. Kirberger RM, Steenkamp G, Spotswood TC, et. al.: Stenotic nasopharyngeal dysgenesis in the dachshund: seven cases (2002-2004). J Am Anim Hosp Assoc. 2006 Jul-Aug;42(4):290-

49. Yamagishi C, Momoi Y, Kobayashi T, et al.: A retrospective study and gene analysis of canine sterile panniculitis. J Vet Med Sci. 2007 Sep;69(9):915-24.

50. *The Genetic Connection: A Guide to Health Problems in Purebred Dogs.* L Ackerman. p. 213-14. AAHA Press, 1999.

51. Lobetti R: Common variable immunodeficiency in miniature dachshunds affected with Pneumonocystis carinii pneumonia. J Vet Diagn Invest. 2000 Jan;12(1):39-45.

52. Herrera HD & Duchene AG: Uveodermatological syndrome (Vogt-Koyan-agi-Harada-like syndrome) with generalized depigmentation in a Dachshund. Vet Ophthalmol. 1998;1(1):47-51.

53. *The Complete Dog Book, 20th Ed.* The American Kennel Club. Howell Book House, NY 2006. p. 164-169.

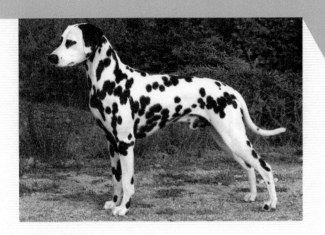

moderate, skull is flat, muzzle blocky, and the nose is black or brown to match the coat. The lips are close and dry. The neck is fairly long, not throaty, and is slightly arched. The topline smoothly descends towards the rear. The thorax is deep, ribs are well sprung, and the abdomen has a moderate tuck up. The curved tail tapers at the tip and reaches the tarsus at rest. Limbs are straight boned, dewclaws may be removed. Feet are very compact with very tough thick pads. Strong nails match the coat color or are white, and the toes are very well arched up.

The Breed History

Artwork depicts a dog of this type back into antiquity in various countries, especially India but the first written records date from the mid 1800s in the region of Dalmatia in western Yugoslavia. Their popularity surged after the Disney movie *One Hundred and One Dalmatians*.

Breeding for Function

Though the breed's utility as a dog accompanying the coach or fire truck of old times is well known, this dog is much more versatile, having been of service in sentry, draft, circus, sheep herding and vermin control. Also less commonly appreciated are the strengths of this breed as a versatile hunter dog performing scenting, bird dog, and retriever functions. Also was used in pack-based hunting for larger game such as wild boar and deer. Today, they serve primarily in companionship roles.

Physical Characteristics

Height at Withers: 19-23" (48-58.5 cm)

Weight: 50-55 lb (23-25 kg)

Coat: Born pure white as puppies, their spots develop as they mature starting at two weeks of age. The flat, short glossy coat consists of fine straight hairs and is black and white or liver and white (the latter is uncommon and is of recessive inheritance). Markings are well demarcated from the white, should not overlap, and should be round with specified minimum and maximum size. If patches of color are present from birth and they have irregular margins—they are a disqualification.

Longevity: 12-14 years

Points of Conformation: As one would expect in a coach dog, a strong, smooth, speedy but effortless ground covering stride and presence of mind and judgment around horses and traffic are paramount. Endurance is a breed hallmark. They are square in conformation and have a muscular, lithe, trim build. They have an alert expression. The skin on the skull is tight (unwrinkled), eyes are deep set and rounded, brown or blue colored and medium-sized. Palpebral margins should be completely pigmented. Ears taper to rounded tips and are moderately sized, pendulous and triangular in shape, lying close to the head. The leather is fine. The stop is

Recognized Behavior Issues and Traits

Reported breed traits include: Highly intelligent, loyal and quick to protect home and family, good watchdog, quick to learn, very high activity levels (exuberant) and high exercise needs, extroverted, playful and sensitive.

They need only low grooming levels and are moderate shedders. Inter-male aggression is sometimes a problem, as can be snippiness and aggression towards people. They can be a bit too lively for very small children but good for older quiet children if socialized. They are generally aloof with strangers and some lines may be a bit high strung. They need human companionship and need activities to keep them busy or they may develop boredom vices.

Normal Physiologic Variations

Hyperuricosuria (Abnormal Purine Metabolism): All Dalmatians are homozygous recessive for a mutation in the SLC2A9 gene causing abnormal purine metabolism and hyperuricosuria. This can predispose to urate bladder stones and Dalmatian bronzing syndrome. A Dalmatian back-cross project begun in 1973 with a breeding between a Dalmatian and an English Pointer reintroduced the normal allele for purine metablism. Repeated matings back to Dalmatians over 13+ generations have produced phenotypically normal Dalamtians that carry the normal allele. These dogs are now registerable as Dalamtians by the UKC, and the AKC.[1]

Dal Red Blood Cell Type: Some Dalmatians lack a red blood cell antigen that causes them to develop novel IgG alloantibodies post-transfusion. These dogs are at risk of delayed and acute hemolytic reactions after subsequent transfusions. Crossmating should be performed for all Dalmatian transfusions.[2]

Drug Sensitivities

None reported

Inherited Diseases

Deafness: Congenital deafness can be unilateral or bilateral. Diagnosed by BAER testing. Strain reports total (uni or bilateral) deafness frequency of 29.9% based on BAER testing. 21.9% of all Dalmatians test unilaterally deaf, and 8.0% test bilaterally deaf. Heritability is estimated at 0.73-0.75 with a polygenic mode of inheritance. Dorn reports a 409.34x odds ratio versus other breeds. Blue eyed Dalmatians (only allowed in the US standard, not internationally) have a much higher incidence of deafness than brown eyed dogs. Deafness and blue eye color are both associated with the MITF gene.[3,4,5,6]

Hip Dysplasia: Polygenically inherited trait causing degenerative joint disease and hip arthritis. OFA reports 4.6% affected.[7]

Elbow Dysplasia: Polygenically inherited trait causing elbow arthritis. OFA reports 0.4% affected.[7]

Patella Luxation: Polygenically inherited laxity of patellar ligaments, causing luxation, lameness, and later degenerative joint disease. Treat surgically if causing clinical signs. Too few Dalmatians have been screened by OFA to determine an accurate frequency.[7]

Disease Predispositions

Urate Urolithiasis: All Dalmatians are affected with hyperurico-suria, and urate crystals are uniformly formed in the breed. Reports show that 34% of male Dalmatians go on to form urate stones. Male Dalmatians have a 14.0x odds ratio for forming urate stones versus female Dalmatians. The heritability of urate bladder stone formation is reported to be 0.87. Dorn reports a 9.03x odds ratio versus other breeds. Treatment is with surgical removal, and prevention with medications. Reported at a frequency of 3.0% in the 2002 Dalmatian Club of America Health Survey.[1,3,8,9,10]

Hypothyroidism: Inherited autoimmune thyroiditis. 16.3% positive for thyroid autoantibodies based on testing at Michigan State University. (Ave. for all breeds is 7.5%) Reported at a frequency of 3.0% in the 2002 Dalmatian Club of America Health Survey.[10,11,12]

Allergic Dermatitis: Inhalant or food allergy. Presents with pruritis and pyotraumatic dermatitis. Dalmatians have a significantly increased risk for atopy versus other breeds. Reported at a frequency of 9.0% in the 2002 Dalmatian Club of America Health Survey.[10,13]

Dalmatian Bronzing Syndrome (Xanthomatosis): Skin condition in dalmatians characterized by a patchy haircoat and bronze hue with folliculitis. This appears to be related to the excessive uric acid excretion that occurs in the Dalmatian. Not all Dalmatians are affected, even though all have elevated uric acid excretion.[14]

Distichiasis: Abnormally placed eyelashes that irritate the cornea and conjunctiva. Can cause secondary corneal ulceration. Identified in 2.37% of Dalmatians CERF-examined by veterinary ophthalmologists between 2000-2005.[15]

Corneal Dystrophy: The breed can have an epithelial/stromal form of corneal dystrophy. Age of onset 2-5 years. Identified in 2.37% of Dalmatians CERF-examined by veterinary ophthalmologists between 2000-2005.[15]

Idiopathic Epilepsy: Inherited seizures. The breed is reported with both generalized and partial-onset seizures. 18.2% start as generalized seizures, and 36.4% begin as partial seizures (with the rest mixed) at a mean age of 3.2 years. 91% of affected Dalmatians progress to generalized seizures. Dorn reports a 4.05x odds ratio versus other breeds. Reported at a frequency of 2.0% in the 2002 Dalmatian Club of America Health Survey. Control with anti-seizure

medication. Unknown mode of inheritance.[3,10,16]

Demodicosis (Generalized): Demodectic mange has an underlying immunodeficiency in its pathogenesis. Dorn reports a 1.42x odds ratio versus other breeds. Reported at a frequency of 2.0% in the 2002 Dalmatian Club of America Health Survey.[3,10]

Behavioral Problems: Dalmatians are over-represented in veterinary behavioral consultations versus other breeds in all categories, including aggression, anxiety, house soiling, and phobias.[17]

Glaucoma: Primary, narrow angle glaucoma occurs in the breed. Can cause blindness due to retinal damage, or secondary lens luxation. Screen with gonioscopy and tonometry. Reported increased incidence in Dalmatians versus other breeds. CERF does not recommend breeding any Dalmatian with glaucoma.[15,18]

Cataracts: Intermediate cataracts predominate in the breed. Reported in 1.69% of Dalmatians CERF examined by veterinary ophthalmologists between 2000-2005. CERF does not recommend breeding any Dalmatian with a cataract.[15]

Iris Coloboma: Developmental defect of the iris. Identified in 1.52% of Dalmatians CERF-examined by veterinary ophthalmologists between 2000-2005. CERF does not recommend breeding any Dalmatian with a coloboma.[15]

Persistent Pupillary Membranes: Strands of fetal remnant connecting; iris to iris, cornea, lens, or involving sheets of tissue. The later three forms can impair vision, and dogs affected with these forms should not be bred. Identified in 1.18% of Dalmatians CERF examined by veterinary ophthalmologists between 2000-2005.[15]

Iris Sphincter Dysplasia (ISD): Abnormality of persistently dilated pupils seen in the breed. The majority of affected dogs are liver spotted, but black spotted dogs with this disorder have also been identified. Slit lamp examination of the eyes by an ophthalmologist reveals dysplasia (abnormal development) or atrophy (degeneration) of the muscles responsible for pupillary contraction. This iris sphincter dysplasia has been noted in puppies as young as 13 weeks of age as well as in adults.[15,19]

Cervical Spondylomyelopathy (Wobbler Syndrome): Presents with neck pain, UMN spasticity and ataxia. Imaging studies suggest that the primary lesion is spinal cord compression at C5-6 or C6-7. MRI is superior to myelography in determining site, severity, and nature of the spinal cord compression. Seen at an increased incidence in the breed. Undetermined mode of inheritance.[20]

Copper-Associated Liver Disease: Copper toxicosis is a documented disorder in Dalmatians. Affected dogs present with gastrointestinal clinical signs, including anorexia and vomiting. All animals have increased ALT and ALP without cholestasis. The mean hepatic copper concentration for nine Dalmatians was 3,197 microg/g dry weight liver (normal, < 450 microg/g) in one report. The findings indicate a primary metabolic defect in hepatic copper metabolism.[21,22]

Actinic Keratosis: Affected dogs present with alopecia, erythema, comedones, scales, excoriation, pustules, epidermal collarettes, crusts and scars, with pathologic development of epidermal hyperplasia, parakeratosis, and orthokeratosis. Lesions occur secondary to prolonged UV/sunlight exposure, and may be a precursor to squamous cell carcinoma. Seen at an increased frequency in the breed.[23]

Laryngeal Paralysis–Polyneuropathy: Rare disorder in young Dalmatians presenting with laryngeal paralysis and megaesophagus. Neurogenic atrophy is present in intrinsic laryngeal and appendicular skeletal muscles. Pathology reveals a diffuse, generalized polyneuropathy, dominated by axonal degeneration. Unknown mode of inheritance.[24,25]

Neuronal Ceroid–Lipofuscinosis (NCL): Rare, fatal inherited degenerative neurological disease. Affected Dalmatians present between 6-12 months of age, and die between 1.5 to 8 years of age. They present with variable signs of blindness, tremor, ataxia, and seizures. Also reported as leucodystrophy in earlier reports. Unknown mode of inheritance. CERF does not recommend breeding any Dalmatian with NCL.[15,26,27]

Brachygnathism, Calcium Oxalate Urolithiasis, Ciliary Dyskinesia, Dermoid, Diabetes Mellitus, Entropion, IgA Deficiency, Microphthalmia, Muscular Dystrophy, Pannus, Prognathism, Progressive Retinal Atrophy, Sebaceous Adenitis, Spina Bifida, Uveal Hypopigmentation, and **Wry Mouth** are reported.[28]

Isolated Case Studies

Dilated Cardiomyopathy (DCM): Identified in eight male Dalmatians fed low protein diets (for prevention of urate uroliths.) All dogs had left-sided heart failure with severe left ventricular dilatation. Mean age of onset was 6.8 years, with a median survival of 10 months. Taurine levels were normal in the affected dogs.[29]

Alport Syndrome: Autosomal dominant Alport Syndrome was identified in a family of Dalmatians in Australia. Affected dogs presented with hematuria, renal failure and deafness at a mean age of 18 months.[30]

Hypertrophic Cardiomyopathy: This heart disease has been reported in the Dalmatian, possibly associated with mitral valve dysplasia.[31]

Acute Respiratory Distress Syndrome (ARDS): Reported in 11 young Dalmatians from four litters. After trauma, tachypnea and noisy respiration progressed to strenuous and rapid respirations, cyanosis, vomiting, and death. Affected dogs had multiple foci of marked atypical hyperplasia and squamous metaplasia of the bronchiolar epithelium, patchy ongoing fibrosis with myofibroblastic metaplasia, smooth muscle hyperplasia and occasional honeycombing of alveolar walls, and hyperplasia of atypical type II pneumocytes. Some affected dogs had renal aplasia and hydrocephalus.[32,33]

Cerebrospinal Hypomyelinogenesis: Identified in a newborn Dalmatian with generalized body tremors, which interfered with the pup's ability to suckle, walk, and maintain sternal recumbency. The pup was euthanatized at eight weeks of age.[34]

Spinal Dysraphism (Syringomyelia, Myelodysplasia): Spinal cord disorder identified in a Dalmatian at 8 weeks of age. Presented as a bunny hopping gait with loss of reciprocal hind limb movement.[35]

Genetic Tests

Tests of Genotype: Direct tests for black and liver (brown) colors, and black or brown nose are available from HealthGene and VetGen.

Direct test for hyperuricosuria is available from UC-Davis VGL and the Animal Health Trust.

Tests of Phenotype: CHIC Certification: Required testing includes hip radiographs and BAER hearing test. Elective tests include CERF eye examination and thyroid profile including autoantibodies. (See CHIC website; www.caninehealthinfo.org).

Additional recommended tests include patella evaluation, elbow radiographs, and cardiac evaluation.

Miscellaneous

- **Breed name synonyms:** Coach Dog, Fire Dog, Fire House Dog, Carriage Dog
- **Registries:** AKC, UKC, CKC, KCGB (Kennel Club of Great Britain), ANKC (Australian National Kennel Club), NKC (National Kennel Club)
- **AKC rank (year 2008):** 76 (983 dogs registered)
- **Internet resources:** The Dalmation Club of America: www.thedca.org
  The Dalmatian Club of Canada: www.dalmatianclubofcanada.ca
  British Dalmatian Club: www.britishdalmatianclub.org.uk
  Dalmatian Club of America Foundation (DCAF): www.dcaf.org

References

1. Bannasch D, Safra N, Young A, et. al.: Mutations in the SLC2A9 gene cause hyperuricosuria and hyperuricemia in the dog. PLoS Genet. 2008 Nov;4(11):e1000246.
2. Blais MC, Berman L, Oakley DA, et. al.: Canine Dal blood type: A red cell antigen lacking in some Dalmatians. J Vet Intern Med. 2007 Mar-Apr;21(2):281-6.
3. Dorn CR: Canine breed-specific risks of frequently diagnosed diseases at veterinary teaching hospitals. Monograph. AKC Canine Health Foundation. 2000.
4. Cargill EJ, Famula TR, Strain GM, et. al.: Heritability and segregation analysis of deafness in U.S. Dalmatians. Genetics. 2004 Mar;166(3):1385-93.
5. Strain GM: Deafness prevalence and pigmentation and gender associations in dog breeds at risk. Vet J. 2004 Jan;167(1):23-32.
6. Stritzel S, Wöhlke A, & Distl O: A role of the microphthalmia-associated transcription factor in congenital sensorineural deafness and eye pigmentation in Dalmatian dogs. J Anim Breed Genet. 2009 Feb;126(1):59-62.
7. OFA Website breed statistics: www.offa.org Last accessed July 1, 2010.
8. Albasan H, Lulich JP, Osborne CA, et. al.: Evaluation of the association between sex and risk of forming urate uroliths in Dalmatians. J Am Vet Med Assoc. 2005 Aug 15;227(4):565-9.
9. Bannasch DL, Ling GV, Bea J, et. al.: Inheritance of urinary calculi in the Dalmatian. J Vet Intern Med. 2004 Jul-Aug;18(4):483-7.
10. Dalmatian Club of America Foundation: The Dalmatian Club of America Health Survey. 2002.
11. Nachreiner R & Refsal K: Personal communication, Diagnostic Center for Population and Animal Health, Michigan State University. April, 2007.
12. Nachreiner RF, Refsal KR, Graham PA, et. al.: Prevalence of

serum thyroid hormone autoantibodies in dogs with clinical signs of hypothyroidism. J Am Vet Med Assoc 2002 Feb 15;220(4):466-71.

13. Schick RO, Fadok VA: Responses of atopic dogs to regional allergens: 268 cases (1981-1984). J Am Vet Med Assoc. 1986 Dec 1;189(11):1493-6.

14. Ackerman L: Pattern Approach to Dermatologic Diagnosis. 2002. Proceedings, Tufts Animal Expo 2002.

15. *Ocular Disorders Presumed to be Inherited in Purebred Dogs.* American College of Veterinary Ophthalmologists. ACVO, 2007.

16. Licht BG, Licht MH, Harper KM, et. al.: Clinical presentations of naturally occurring canine seizures: similarities to human seizures. Epilepsy Behav. 2002 Oct;3(5):460-470.

17. Bamberger M & Houpt KA: Signalment factors, comorbidity, and trends in behavior diagnoses in dogs: 1,644 cases (1991-2001). J Am Vet Med Assoc. 2006 Nov 15;229(10):1591-601.

18. Slater MR, Erb HN: Effects of risk factors and prophylactic treatment on primary glaucoma in the dog.J Am Vet Med Assoc. 1986 May 1;188(9):1028-30.

19. The Dalmatian Club of America Inc. www.thedca.org/eyes.html Last accessed July 1, 2010.

20. da Costa RC & Parent J: Magnetic Resonance Imaging Findings in 60 Dogs with Cervical Spondylomyelopathy. Proceedings, 2009 ACVIM Forum. 2009.

21. Webb CB, Twedt DC, Meyer DJ: Copper-associated liver disease in Dalmatians: a review of 10 dogs (1998-2001). J Vet Intern Med. 2002 Nov-Dec;16(6):665-8.

22. Vannevel JY: Liver disease in young dalmatians. Can Vet J. 1996 Jun;37(6):329.

23. Costa SS, Munhoz TD, Calazans SG, et. al.: Clinical and Epidemiological Evaluation of Actinic Keratosis in Seven Dogs. Proceedings, 2009 WSAVA World Congress. 2009.

24. Braund KG, Shores A, Cochrane S, et. al.: Laryngeal paralysis-polyneuropathy complex in young Dalmatians. Am J Vet Res. 1994 Apr;55(4):534-42.

25. Braund KG, Steinberg HS, Shores A, et. al.: Laryngeal paralysis in immature and mature dogs as one sign of a more diffuse polyneuropathy. J Am Vet Med Assoc. 1989 Jun 15;194(12):1735-40.

26. Goebel HH, Bilzer T, Dahme E, et. al.: Morphological studies in canine (Dalmatian) neuronal ceroid-lipofuscinosis. Am J Med Genet Suppl. 1988;5:127-39.

27. Bjerkas I: Hereditary "cavitating" leucodystrophy in Dalmation dogs. Light and electron microscopic studies. Acta Neuropathol (Berl). 1977 Oct 10;40(2):163-9.

28. *The Genetic Connection: A Guide to Health Problems in Purebred Dogs.* L Ackerman. p. 214. AAHA Press, 1999.

29. Freeman LM, Michel KE, Brown DJ, et. al.: Idiopathic dilated cardiomyopathy in Dalmatians: nine cases (1990-1995). J Am Vet Med Assoc. 1996 Nov 1;209(9):1592-6.

30. Hood JC, Huxtable C, Naito I, et. al.: A novel model of autosomal dominant Alport syndrome in Dalmatian dogs. Nephrol Dial Transplant. 2002 Dec;17(12):2094-8.

31. De Majo M, Britti D, Masucci M, et. al.: Hypertrophic obstructive cardiomyopathy associated to mitral valve dysplasia in the Dalmatian dog: two cases. Vet Res Commun. 2003 Jan;27 Suppl 1:391-3.

32. Jarvinen AK, Saario E, Andresen E, et. al.: Lung injury leading to respiratory distress syndrome in young Dalmatian dogs. J Vet Intern Med. 1995 May-Jun;9(3):162-8.

33. Syrjä P, Saari S, Rajamäki M, et. al.: Pulmonary histopathology in dalmatians with familial acute respiratory distress syndrome (ARDS). J Comp Pathol. 2009 Nov;141(4):254-9.

34. Greene CE, Vandevelde M, Hoff EJ: Congenital cerebrospinal hypomyelinogenesis in a pup. J Am Vet Med Assoc. 1977 Sep 15;171(6):534-6.

35. Neufeld JL, Little PB: Spinal dysraphism in a Dalmatian dog. Can Vet J. 1974 Nov;15(11):335-6.

36. *The Complete Dog Book, 20th Ed.* The American Kennel Club. Howell Book House, NY 2006. p. 553-557.

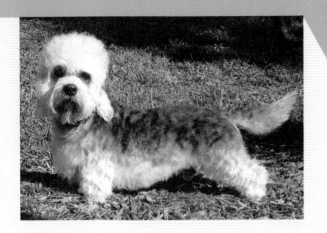

The Breed History

These hardy terriers originated in the hills between England and Scotland and were brought to the public attention in the early 1800's in *Guy Mannering*, a work by Sir Walter Scott. Their breed origins are obscured but the Skye, Cairn and Scotch Terriers may have contributed to their development.

Breeding for Function

These were originally bred as hunting dogs, used particularly in otter tracking, but are now primarily companion dogs. They were also valued as courageous guard dogs.

Physical Characteristics

Height at Withers: 8-11"" (20-28 cm)

Weight: females 18-24 lb (8-11 kg), males 18-24 lb (8-11 kg)

Coat: The dense double coat is about 2" long, and can be either pepper, a blue-gray to silver with tan or silver points, or mustard, a brown-red-cream spectrum with white points. Their topknot is long and the face fully haired; coat hairs are crisp but not wiry, but head hair is silky and soft. Regular grooming is important though they are considered low shedders.

Longevity: 12-15 years.

Points of Conformation: A large head, domed skull, prominent stop, and large eyes with heavy jaw set him apart from other terriers. Dandies are low to the ground and have a broad deep thorax, and scimitar-shaped tail. The ears are small and low and the leather is quite thin. Nose is of moderate size and pigmented dark colored or black. The lips and mouth mucous membranes are also dark. The canine teeth are quite large in this breed. The neck is thick and well muscled, and the topline is low at shoulders and has a mildly arched profile. Feet are round and small, and dewclaws are generally removed on the forelimbs. The dog's gait is straight and low with long strides.

Recognized Behavior Issues and Traits

Reported breed traits include: These dogs are reserved with strangers but affectionate, loyal companions around the home. They are very intelligent, bold, and strong willed, and will adapt to life either in country or city. Training should begin young. Because

Dandie Dinmont Terrier

of their strong chase instinct, they should not be left off-leash unless they are contained in an enclosure. The bark is loud for their size, and they make good alarm bark defenders. They need human contact, and may become one-man dogs. Their overall activity levels are somewhat lower than other terrier breeds.

Normal Physiologic Variations

41.4% of Dandie Dinmont litters are delivered via **cesarean section** in the UK.[1]

Drug Sensitivities

None reported

Inherited Diseases

Hip Dysplasia: Polygenically inherited trait causing degenerative joint disease and hip arthritis. OFA reports a high incidence, but very few Dandie Dinmont Terriers have been screened to determine an accurate frequency.[2]

Patella Luxation: Polygenically inherited laxity of patellar ligaments, causing luxation, lameness, and later degenerative joint disease. Treat surgically if causing clinical signs. Too few Dandie Dinmont Terriers have been screened by OFA to determine an accurate frequency.[2]

Elbow Dysplasia: Polygenically inherited trait causing elbow arthritis. Too few Dandie Dinmont Terriers have been screened by OFA to determine an accurate frequency.[2]

Disease Predispositions

Persistent Pupillary Membranes: Strands of fetal remnant connecting; iris to iris, cornea, lens, or involving sheets of tissue. The later three forms can impair vision, and dogs affected with these forms should not be bred. Identified in 20.75% of Dandie Dinmont Terriers CERF examined by veterinary ophthalmologists between 2000-2005.[3]

Glaucoma: Primary, narrow angle glaucoma occurs in the breed. Can cause blindness due to retinal damage, and secondary lens luxation. Age of onset 6 years and older. Screen with gonioscopy and tonometry. Frequency and mode of inheritance in the breed has not been determined. Dr. Hans Lohi in Finland has discovered a linked marker on chromosome 8 with a proposed autosomal recessive inheritance.[4]

Hypothyroidism: Inherited autoimmune thyroiditis. 8.2% positive for thyroid auto-antibodies based on testing at Michigan State University. (Ave. for all breeds is 7.5%).[5,6]

Distichiasis: Abnormally placed eyelashes that irritate the cornea and conjunctiva. Can cause secondary corneal ulceration. Identified in 5.66% of Dandie Dinmont Terriers CERF examined by veterinary ophthalmologists between 2000-2005.[3]

Cataracts: Anterior, posterior and punctate cataracts occur in the breed. Identified in 5.66% of Dandie Dinmont Terriers CERF examined by veterinary ophthalmologists between 2000-2005. CERF does not recommend breeding any Dandie Dinmont Terrier with a cataract.[3]

Corneal Dystrophy: The breed can have an epithelial/stromal form of corneal dystrophy. Age of onset 2-5 years. Identified in 1.89% of Dandie Dinmont Terriers CERF examined by veterinary ophthalmologists between 2000-2005.[3]

Portosystemic Shunt (PSS, Liver Shunt): Abnormal blood vessels connecting the systemic and portal blood flow. Can be intrahepatic or extrahepatic. Hepatic microvascular dysplasia may also be genetically related to this condition. Causes stunting, abnormal behavior, possible seizures, and can cause secondary ammonium urate urinary calculi. Diagnose with paired fasted and feeding serum bile acid and/or ammonium levels, and abdominal ultrasound. Treatment of PSS includes partial ligation and/or medical and dietary control of symptoms. One survey reported 1.6% of Dandie Dinmont Terriers were affected. Unknown mode of inheritance.[7]

Pituitary-dependent Hyperadrenocorticism (Cushing's Disease): Seven closely related Dandie Dinmont terriers were diagnosed with pituitary-dependent hyperadrenocorticism, suggesting an inherited basis. Caused by a functional pituitary tumor. Clinical signs may include increased thirst and urination, symmetrical truncal alopecia, and abdominal distention. Diagnosis by dexamethasone suppression test and ACTH stimulation test.[8]

Oxalate Urolithiasis (Bladder Stones): The breed may have a predisposition to oxalate bladder stones.[9]

Brachygnathism, Intervertebral Disk Disease, Oligodontia, Prognathism, Progressive Retinal Atrophy, and **Ulcerative Keratitis** are also reported.[10]

Isolated Case Studies

None reported

Genetic Tests

Tests of Genotype: Direct test for mustard and pepper coat color is available from Health Gene.

Tests of Phenotype: Recommend hip and elbow radiographs, CERF eye examination (including gonioscopy), patella evaluation, thyroid profile including autoantibodies and cardiac evaluation.

Miscellaneous

- **Breed name synonyms:** Dandie
- **Registries:** AKC, CKC, UKC, KCGB (Kennel Club of Great Britain), ANKC (Australian National Kennel Club)
- **AKC rank: (year 2008):** 146 (77 dogs registered)
- **Internet resources: Dandie Dinmont Terrier Club of America:** http://clubs.akc.org/ddtca
  Dandie Dinmont Terrier Club of Canada: www.dandiedinmont.org
  The Dandie Dinmont Terrier Club (UK): http://ddtc.co.uk/

References

1. Evans KM & Adams VJ: Proportion of litters of purebred dogs born by caesarean section. J Small Anim Pract. 2010 Feb;51(2):113-8.
2. OFA Website breed statistics: www.offa.org Last accessed July 1, 2010.
3. *Ocular Disorders Presumed to be Inherited in Purebred Dogs.* American College of Veterinary Ophthalmologists. ACVO, 2007.
4. Bedford P: Inherited Disease of the Canine Eye. Proceedings, 2001 WSAVA Congress. 2001.
5. Nachreiner R & Refsal K: Personal communication, Diagnostic Center for Population and Animal Health, Michigan State University. April, 2007.
6. Nachreiner RF, Refsal KR, Graham PA, et. al.: Prevalence of serum thyroid hormone autoantibodies in dogs with clinical signs of hypothyroidism. *J Am Vet Med Assoc* 2002 Feb 15;220(4):466-71.
7. Tobias KM, Rohrbach BW: Association of breed with the diagnosis of congenital portosystemic shunts in dogs: 2,400 cases (1980-2002). J Am Vet Med Assoc. 2003 Dec 1;223(11):1636-9.
8. Scholten-Sloof BE, Knol BW, Rijnberk A, et. al.: Pituitary-dependent hyperadrenocorticism in a family of Dandie Dinmont terriers. *J Endocrinol.* 1992 Dec;135(3):535-42.
9. Shearer AG, Nash AS: Oxalate urolithiasis in Dandie Dinmont terriers. *Vet Rec.* 1992 May 23;130(21):480.
10. *The Genetic Connection: A Guide to Health Problems in Purebred Dogs.* L. Ackerman. p 214, AAHA Press, 1999.
11. *The Complete Dog Book, 20th Ed.* The American Kennel Club. Howell Book House, NY 2006. p. 366-369.

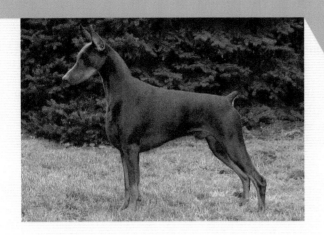

The Breed History

This breed originated in Germany and was recognized in 1900. In the USA, the parent club was formed in 1921. The Doberman originates from a number of breeds including the Rottweiler, German pinscher, and Black and Tan terrier. The name of the breed originates with a German man, Louis Dobermann who was credited for early breed development.

Breeding for Function

Bred for work as a personal protection guard dog, police dog, and war dog, he is now very popular also as a companion. The Dobe is also prized as a police scent-tracking dog. They are also used in Schutzhund, and in search and rescue operations.

Physical Characteristics

Height at Withers: female 24-26" (61-66 cm), male 26-28" (66-71 cm)

Weight: females 66-75 lb (30- 34 kg), males 66-80 lb (30-36.5 kg).

Coat: Breed colors include black, red, fawn and blue with legs, throat and face (muzzle and eye) marked with rusty pigmentation. White spots on chest of less than a half-inch square are allowed. Smooth short and dense hair coat lies close to the skin and is glossy. Black is dominant over red, and non-dilution is dominant over dilution. Albinos may be born, but it is a disqualification.

Longevity: 13 years.

Points of Conformation: Medium sized, powerful, agile, and muscular athletic dog, the Dobermans' way of moving and carriage is proud and springy. The head is long and wedged with almond-shaped brown eyes. In coats other than black, iris pigment may be lighter to match coat, but the darker spectrum of coloration is preferred. The medium length and size ears are usually cropped and carried in a pricked position in North America. They have a slight stop, and flat cheeks taper to a black nose in black dogs and a brown-tan-gray coloration is associated with the other coat colors (red-fawn-blue respectively). A well arched neck that widens at the base, a straight topline, deep-chested with well-sprung ribs, and a tail usually docked short characterize this breed. They possess straight limbs and feet well knuckled and compact. Dewclaws may be removed.

Doberman Pinscher

Recognized Behavior Issues and Traits

This is reported to be a very loyal dog and the Doberman is a natural protector. High intelligence, fearlessness, high activity and alertness, and stamina in service characterize this breed. Dobes are easy to train using positive reinforcement, and starting at a very early age, it is important to include proper socialization to people and other pets. If not properly trained, aggression may develop. This can also happen if Dobes are kenneled or left alone excessively. They need lots of contact with people and frequent exercise and stimulation. They are average shedders and generally need only minimal grooming. This breed is over-represented in flank sucking behavior, a compulsive disorder.[1]

Normal Physiologic Variations

Dilute coat color (d locus) is due to the homozygous recessive expression of a mutation in the melanophilin gene (MLPH). This can predispose to color dilution alopecia. A genetic test is available.[2]

Drug Sensitivities

Doberman pinschers may be predisposed to adverse reactions to potentiated sulfonamides. Non-septic polyarthritis and fever occurring after 8 to 21 days of therapy is the most common sign. Some dogs may develop glomerulonephropathy, focal retinitis, polymyositis, skin rash, fever, anemia, leukopenia, or thrombocytopenia. This may be due to a limited capacity to detoxify the hydroxylamine metabolites of sulphonamides. The reaction may be a type-III hypersensitivity.[3,4]

Inherited Diseases

von Willebrand's Disease Type 1 (vWD): Autosomal recessive genetic disorder causing a mild bleeding syndrome. A genetic test is available from VetGen that reports 25% affected, and 49% carrier in the breed. Dorn reports a 806.44x odds ratio versus other breeds.[5,6]

Dilated Cardiomyopathy (DCM): An autosomal dominant with incomplete penetrance form of heart disease characterized by syncope, dilated cardiomyopathy, sudden death, ventricular tachycardia, and heart failure. Ventricular arrhythmia precedes heart dilation, and may be involved in the cause of DCM in the breed. Diagnose with 24 hour holter ECG and echocardiogram (ECHO). Pimobendan significantly improves the congestive heart failure associated with DCM in Doberman Pinschers. A European study found 50.7% of Dobermans over 8 years of age with an ECHO or holter diagnosis of DCM. A study of cardiac troponin (cTnl) levels showed that levels greater than 0.22 ng/ml could with high sensitivity and specificity identify dogs that will eventually develop DCM prior to any abnormal ECHO or holter changes. An autosomal dominant mutation in a mitochondrial protein gene has been identified. A genetic test for this gene is available.[11,12,13,14,15,16]

Hip Dysplasia: Polygenically inherited trait causing degenerative joint disease and hip arthritis. OFA reports 6.2% affected.[7]

Elbow Dysplasia: Polygenically inherited trait causing elbow arthritis. OFA reports 1.0% affected.[7]

Patella Luxation: Polygenically inherited laxity of patellar ligaments, causing luxation, lameness, and later degenerative joint disease. Treat surgically if causing clinical signs. Too few Doberman Pinschers have been screened by OFA to determine an accurate frequency.[7]

Narcolepsy: Rare, autosomal recessive disorder causing sudden collapse and a sleep-like state elicited by excitement. Clinical episodes begin at four weeks of age, with maximal symptoms by 10-32 weeks of age. A genetic test is available.[8]

Congenital Blindness: A rare autosomal recessive disorder occurs in the breed, presenting with microphthalmia, corneal opacification, absence of the anterior chamber, aphakia, retinal detachment, and dysplasia, and partial depigmentation of the retinal pigment epithelial cells.[9,10]

Disease Predispositions

Hypothyroidism: Inherited autoimmune thyroiditis. 8.4% positive for thyroid auto-antibodies based on testing at Michigan State University. (Ave. for all breeds is 7.5%). May be associated with a DLA class II allele. Dorn reports a 2.51x odds ratio versus other breeds.[5,17,18,19]

Cataracts: Capsular and posterior suture punctate cataracts predominate in the breed. Identified in 4.46% of Doberman Pinschers CERF examined by veterinary ophthalmologists between 2000-2005. CERF does not recommend breeding any Doberman Pinscher with a cataract.[20]

Cervical Vertebral Instability (Wobbler Syndrome): Presents with UMN spasticity and ataxia. Imaging studies suggest that the primary lesion is foramenal stenosis and intervertebral instability at C6-7. MRI is superior to myelography in determining site, severity, and nature of the spinal cord compression. Dorn reports a 94.93x odds ratio versus other breeds. Undetermined mode of inheritance.[5,21,22]

Acral Lick Dermatitis (Lick Granuloma) and Flank Sucking: Behavioral disorders causing skin lesions frequently seen in the Doberman pinscher breed. These may have an obsessive-compulsive component.[1,23]

Prostatic Disease: Doberman pinschers are the most frequently affected breed with prostatic disease. Intact males have the highest risk for bacterial prostatitis, prostate cancer, benign prostatic hyperplasia, and prostatic cysts. Mean age of onset is 8.9 years. Short CAG-1 repeats in the AR-gene are associated with increased risk for prostate cancer.[24,25]

Gastric Dilatation-Volvulus (Bloat, GDV): Polygenically inherited, life-threatening twisting of the stomach within the abdomen. Requires immediate veterinary attention. Doberman pinschers with the deepest thorax relative to width have the greatest risk for GDV.[26]

Demodicosis (Generalized): Doberman pinschers are shown to have a hereditary predisposition for demodectic mange. This

disorder has an underlying immunodeficiency in its pathogenesis. Dorn reports a 3.57x odds ratio versus other breeds.[5,27]

Hormonal Urinary Incontinence: Studies show a breed prevalence for urinary incontinence in spayed female Doberman pinschers.[28]

Persistent Hyperplastic Tunica Vasculosa Lentis and Primary Vitreous (PHTVL/PHPV): Congenital disorder presenting in the breed with variable lesions from spots on the posterior lens to posterior lenticonus, and posterior polar subcapsular cataracts. Reported at a frequency of 6.7% in the Netherlands, and lower frequencies in the US. CERF does not recommend breeding any Doberman Pinscher with PHTVL/PHPV. Inheritance suspected to be autosomal dominant with incomplete penetrance.[20,29]

Persistent Pupillary Membranes: Strands of fetal remnant connecting; iris to iris, cornea, lens, or involving sheets of tissue. The later three forms can impair vision, and dogs affected with these forms should not be bred. Identified in 3.05% of Doberman pinschers CERF-examined by veterinary ophthalmologists between 2000-2005.[20]

Chronic Active Hepatitis (Copper Toxicosis): The disease is predominantly seen in female dogs, usually 4 - 7 years of age. Clinical signs include polyuria/polydipsia, weight loss, anorexia, icterus, and ascites. Affected dogs have increased liver enzymes, bile acids, and hepatic copper concentrations. Pathology shows micronodular cirrhosis, fibrosis, necrosis and lymphocyte and plasma cell infiltration of the portal triads. The disease is strongly linked to a homozygous DLA-MHC haplotype, indicating an immune basis.[30,31,32,33]

Retinal Dysplasia: Retinal folds are recognized in the breed. Can lead to retinal detachment and blindness. Reported in 2.25% of Doberman pinschers CERF-examined by veterinary ophthalmologists between 2000-2005.[20]

Distichiasis: Abnormally placed eyelashes that irritate the cornea and conjunctiva. Can cause secondary corneal ulceration. Identified in 1.44% of Doberman pinschers CERF-examined by veterinary ophthalmologists between 2000-2005.[20]

Follicular dysplasia: Condition causing hair loss in young adult Doberman Pinschers. Most often seen as **Color Dilution Alopecia** in some blue or fawn (dilute)-colored Doberman pinschers, but can also be seen in non-dilute red or black and tan dogs. Starts as a gradual onset of dry, dull and poor hair coat quality. Progresses to poor hair regrowth, follicular papules and comedomes. Hair loss and comedome formation are usually most severe on the trunk. A genetic test is available for the dilute gene.[2,34,35]

Dancing Doberman Disease (Peripheral Neuropathy): Slowly progressive breed-related disorder that develops between six months and seven years of age. Affected dogs have a tendency to flex and straighten one and then both hind limbs while standing. The gait remains normal while walking, but may eventually develop weakness in the hind legs, and be reluctant to stand. Unknown mode of inheritance.[36]

Synovial Myxoma Tumors: Doberman pinschers are overrepresented with synovial myxoma tumors, which offer a much better prognosis (without metastasis) than other synovial cell tumors. The most common sites are stifle and digits.[37,38]

Congenital Deafness and Vestibular Disease: Rare congenital disorder reported in the Doberman pinscher. Affected dogs show early signs of head tilt, lack of coordination, and circling, and become deaf by 3 weeks of age. An autosomal recessive inheritance is proposed.[39]

Juvenile Renal Disease: The disease presents in young Doberman pinschers as anorexia, weight loss, vomiting, lethargy, polydipsia, polyuria, and dehydration. Laboratory findings are azotemia, hyperphosphatemia, lymphopenia, non-regenerative anemia, hypercholesterolemia, and proteinuria.[40,41]

Atherosclerosis: Doberman pinschers have a higher prevalence versus other breeds. Most common clinical signs are lethargy, anorexia, weakness, dyspnea, collapse, and vomiting. Hypercholesterolemia, lipidemia, and hypothyroidism are common in affected dogs. Myocardial fibrosis, infarction, and thickened arteries with narrow lumens are found on necropsy.[42]

Atrial septal defect, Brachygnathism, Bullous Pemphigoid, Chromosomal Intersex, Ciliary Dyskenesis, Diabetes Mellitus, Familial Benign Pemphigus, Fanconi Syndrome, Hemivertebra, Histiocytosis, Hypertrophic Osteodystrophy, Icthyosis, Lupoid Onychopathy, Malignant Hyperthermia, Mucinosis, Osteochondritis Dessicans-Stifle, Oligodontia, Panosteitis, Pemphigus Foliaceus, Prognathism, Progressive Retinal Atrophy, Renal Agenesis, Seasonal Flank Alopecia, Sebaceous Adenitis, Supernumerary Teeth, Vitiligo, Wry Mouth, and **Zinc responsive dermatitis** are reported.[43]

Isolated Case Studies

Chronic Rhinitis and Pneumonia: Eight related Doberman pinschers were identified with chronic rhinitis and pneumonia. A defect in the bactericidal ability of neutrophils was identified.[44]

Congenital Peripheral Vestibular Disease: Individual Doberman pinschers from repeat breedings had unilateral or bilateral congenital peripheral vestibular disease. Clinical pathology was normal. Marked lymphocytic labyrinthitis was discovered microscopically. The occurrence in separate litters suggests an inherited disorder.[45]

Situs Inversus and Diaphragmatic Hernia: A 4 year old female Doberman Pinscher developed dyspnea during sedation. A diaphragmatic hernia was diagnosed, and situs inversus of both the thoracic and abdominal viscera was discovered during surgical repair.[46]

Proximal Femoral Focal Deficiency (PFFD): A 3 month old Doberman Pinscher was identified with a unilateral dysgenesis of the femoral head and neck.[47]

Genetic Tests

Tests of Genotype: Direct test for vWD is available from VetGen.

Direct test for DCM is available from North Carolina State University - Meurs Lab.

Direct test for narcolepsy is available from Optigen and HealthGene.

Direct tests for coat color (black/brown and dilute) are available from HealthGene and VetGen.

Tests of Phenotype: CHIC Certification: Required testing includes hip radiographs, CERF eye examination, thyroid profile including autoantibodies, genetic test for vWD, cardiac evaluation (ECHO and holter), and working dog evaluation (from DPCA). (See CHIC website; www.caninehealthinfo.org).

Recommend elbow radiographs and patella evaluation.

Miscellaneous

- **Breed name synonyms:** Dobe, Doberman, Dobie, Dobermann, Thuringer Pinscher, Plizeilich Soldatenhund.
- **Registries:** AKC, UKC, CKC, KCGB (Kennel Club of Great Britain), ANKC (Australian National Kennel Club), NKC (National Kennel Club)
- **AKC rank (year 2008):** 18 (10,547 dogs registered)
- **Internet resources: Doberman Pinscher Club of America:** www.DPCA.org
  Doberman Pinscher Club of Canada: www.dpcc.ca
  The Doberman Club (UK): www.thedobermannclub.co.uk
  United Doberman Club: www.uniteddobermanclub.com

References

1. Moon-Fanelli AA, Dodman NH & Cottam N: Blanket and flank sucking in Doberman Pinschers. J Am Vet Med Assoc. 2007 Sep 15;231(6):907-12.
2. Philipp U, Hamann H, Mecklenburg L, et. al.: Polymorphisms within the canine MLPH gene are associated with dilute coat color in dogs. BMC Genet. 2005 Jun 16;6:34.
3. Cribb AE, Spielberg SP: An in vitro investigation of predisposition to sulphonamide idiosyncratic toxicity in dogs. Vet Res Commun. 1990;14(3):241-52.
4. Giger U, Werner LL, Millichamp NJ, et. al.: Sulfadiazine-induced allergy in six Doberman pinschers. J Am Vet Med Assoc. 1985 Mar 1;186(5):479-84.
5. Dorn CR: Canine breed-specific risks of frequently diagnosed diseases at veterinary teaching hospitals. Monograph. AKC Canine Health Foundation. 2000.
6. Brooks MB, Erb HN, Foureman PA, et. al.: von Willebrand disease phenotype and von Willebrand factor marker genotype in Doberman Pinschers. Am J Vet Res. 2001 Mar;62(3):364-9.
7. OFA Website breed statistics: www.offa.org Last accessed July 1, 2010.
8. Hungs M, Fan J, Lin L, et. al.: Identification and functional analysis of mutations in the hypocretin (orexin) genes of narcoleptic canines. Genome Res. 2001 Apr;11(4):531-9.
9. Bergsjo T, Arnesen K, Heim P, et. al.: Congenital blindness with ocular developmental anomalies, including retinal dysplasia, in Doberman Pinscher dogs. J Am Vet Med Assoc. 1984 Jun 1;184(11):1383-6.
10. Peiffer RL Jr, Fischer CA: Microphthalmia, retinal dysplasia, and anterior segment dysgenesis in a litter of Doberman Pinschers. J Am Vet Med Assoc. 1983 Oct 15;183(8):875-8.
11. Calvert CA, Wall M: Results of ambulatory electrocardiography in overtly healthy Doberman Pinschers with equivocal echocardiographic evidence of dilated cardiomyopathy. J Am Vet Med Assoc. 2001 Sep 15;219(6):782-4.
12. Calvert CA, Jacobs GJ, Smith DD, et. al.: Association between results of ambulatory electrocardiography and development of cardiomyopathy during long-term follow-up of Doberman pinschers. J Am Vet Med Assoc. 2000 Jan 1;216(1):34-9.
13. Meurs KM, Fox PR, Norgard M, et. al.: A prospective genetic evaluation of familial dilated cardiomyopathy in the Doberman pinscher. J Vet Intern Med. 2007 Sep-Oct;21(5):1016-20.

14. O'Grady MR, Minors SL, O'Sullivan ML, et. al.: Effect of Pimobendan on Case Fatality Rate in Doberman Pinschers with Congestive Heart Failure Caused by Dilated Cardiomyopathy. J Vet Intern Med. 2008 Jun 4.

15. Wess G, Schulze A, Butz V, et. al.: Prevalence of Dilated Cardiomyopathy in Doberman Pinschers in Various Age Groups. J Vet Intern Med. 2010 May-Jun;24(3):533-8.24. Lai CL, L'Eplattenier H, van den Ham R, et. al.: Androgen receptor CAG repeat polymorphisms in canine prostate cancer. J Vet Intern Med. 2008 Nov-Dec;22(6):1380-4.

16. Wess G, Simak J, Mahling M, et. al.: Cardiac Troponin I in Doberman Pinschers with Cardiomyopathy. J Vet Intern Med. 2010 Jul-Aug;24(4):843-9.

17. Kennedy LJ, Quarmby S, Happ GM, et. al.: Association of canine hypothyroidism with a common major histocompatibility complex DLA class II allele. Tissue Antigens. 2006 Jul;68(1):82-6.

18. Nachreiner R & Refsal K: Personal communication, Diagnostic Center for Population and Animal Health, Michigan State University. April, 2007.

19. Nachreiner RF, Refsal KR, Graham PA, et. al.: Prevalence of serum thyroid hormone autoantibodies in dogs with clinical signs of hypothyroidism. J Am Vet Med Assoc. 2002 Feb 15;220(4):466-71.

20. Ocular Disorders Presumed to be Inherited in Purebred Dogs. American College of Veterinary Ophthalmologists. ACVO, 2007

21. da Costa RC, Parent J, Dobson H, et. al.: Comparison of magnetic resonance imaging and myelography in 18 Doberman pinscher dogs with cervical spondylomyelopathy. Vet Radiol Ultrasound. 2006 Oct-Nov;47(6):523-31.

22. Mason TA: Cervical vertebral instability (wobbler syndrome) in the dog. Vet Rec. 1979 Feb 17;104(7):142-5.

23. Virga V: Behavioral Dermatology: Psychogenic Alopecia, ALD and Related Syndromes. Proceedings, 2004 Northeast Veterinary Conference. 2004.

24. Krawiec DR, Heflin D: Study of prostatic disease in dogs: 177 cases (1981-1986). J Am Vet Med Assoc. 1992 Apr 15;200(8):1119-22.

25. Lai CL, L'Eplattenier H, van den Ham R, et. al.: Androgen receptor CAG repeat polymorphisms in canine prostate cancer. J Vet Intern Med. 2008 Nov-Dec;22(6):1380-4.

26. Glickman LT, Glickman NW, Perez CM, et. al.: Analysis of risk factors for gastric dilatation and dilatation-volvulus in dogs. J Am Vet Med Assoc. 1994 May 1;204(9):1465-71.

27. Wilkie BN, Markham RJ, Hazlett C: Deficient cutaneous response to PHA-P in healthy puppies from a kennel with a high prevalence of demodicosis. Can J Comp Med. 1979 Oct;43(4):415-9.

28. Arnold S: Urinary incontinence in castrated bitches. Part 1: Significance, clinical aspects and etiopathogenesis. Schweiz Arch Tierheilkd. 1997;139(6):271-6.

29. Stades FC, Boeve MH, van den Brom WE, et. al.: The incidence of PHTVL/PHPV in Doberman and the results of breeding rules. Vet Q. 1991 Jan;13(1):24-9.

30. Johnson GF, Zawie DA, Gilbertson SR, et. al.: Chronic active hepatitis in Doberman pinschers. J Am Vet Med Assoc. 1982 Jun 15;180(12):1438-42.

31. Mandigers PJ, van den Ingh TS, Spee B, et. al.: Chronic hepatitis in Doberman pinschers. A review. Vet Q. 2004 Sep;26(3):98-106.

32. Crawford MA, Schall WD, Jensen RK, et. al.: Chronic active hepatitis in 26 Doberman pinschers. J Am Vet Med Assoc. 1985 Dec 15;187(12):1343-50.

33. Dyggve H, Kennedy LJ, Meri S, et. al.: Linkage of Doberman Hepatitis to the Canine Major Histocompatibility Complex. Proceedings, 19th ECVIM-CA Congress, 2009.

34. Miller WH Jr.: Follicular dysplasia in adult black and red Doberman pinschers. Vet Dermatol 1990;1:181–187.

35. Moura E & Cirio SM: Follicular dysplasia of the adult doberman pinscher. J Am Anim Hosp Assoc. 2010 Mar-Apr;46(2):143-7.

36. Olby N: Spinal Cord Disease, Neuropathies, and Behavioral Problems. Proceedings, 2004 Western Veterinary Conference. 2004.

37. Craig LE, Julian ME, Ferracone JD: The diagnosis and prognosis of synovial tumors in dogs: 35 cases. Vet Pathol. 2002 Jan;39(1):66-73.

38. Craig LE, Krimer PM, Cooley AJ, et. al.: Canine Synovial Myxoma: 39 Cases. Vet Pathol. 2010 Sep;47(5):931-6.

39. Wilkes MK, Palmer AC: Congenital deafness and vestibular deficit in the doberman. J. of Small Animal Practice. 1992;33: 218-224.

40. Picut CA, Lewis RM: Juvenile renal disease in the Doberman Pinscher: ultrastructural changes of the glomerular basement membrane. J Comp Pathol. 1987 Sep;97(5):587-96.

41. Chew DJ, DiBartola SP, Boyce JT, et. al.: Juvenile renal disease in Doberman Pinscher dogs. J Am Vet Med Assoc. 1983 Mar 1;182(5):481-5.

42. Liu SK, Tilley LP, Tappe JP, et. al.: Clinical and pathologic findings in dogs with atherosclerosis: 21 cases (1970-1983). J Am Vet Med Assoc. 1986 Jul 15;189(2):227-32.

43. *The Genetic Connection: A Guide to Health Problems in Purebred Dogs.* L Ackerman. p 214-15 AAHA Press, 1999.

44. Breitschwerdt EB, Brown TT, De Buysscher EV, et. al.: Rhinitis, pneumonia, and defective neutrophil function in the Doberman pinscher. Am J Vet Res. 1987 Jul;48(7):1054-62.

45. Forbes S, Cook JR Jr: Congenital peripheral vestibular disease attributed to lymphocytic labyrinthitis in two related litters of Doberman pinscher pups. J Am Vet Med Assoc. 1991 Feb 1;198(3):447-9.

46. Witsberger TH, Dismukes DI, Kelmer EY, et. al.: Situs inversus totalis in a dog with a chronic diaphragmatic hernia. J Am Anim Hosp Assoc. 2009 Sep-Oct;45(5):245-8.

47. Salavati M: Proximal femoral focal deficiency (PFFD) in a young Doberman pinscher. J Small Anim Pract. 2008 Sep;49(9):486.

48. *The Complete Dog Book, 20th Ed.* The American Kennel Club. Howell Book House, NY 2006. p. 258-261.

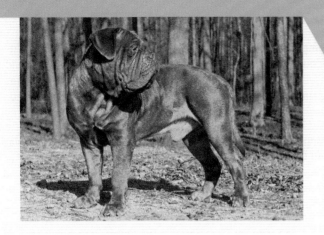

The Breed History

The Dogue de Bordeauxs' is believed to predate the Bullmastiff and the Bulldog. One theory has the breed originating from the Tibetan Mastiff and related to the Greco Roman molossoids used for war at the time of Julius Caesar. Others suggest that the breed existed in ancient France as the Dogues de Bordeaux of Aquitaine. Breed setbacks occurred during the French Revolution (when many of the Dogues de Bordeaux perished with their wealthy masters), and again following World War II. The breed was imported into the United States in the 1890s. During the 1960s, a group of breeders of the Dogue de Bordeaux in France, headed by Raymond Triquet, worked on the rebuilding of the foundation of the breed. In 1970 a new standard was written for the breed, with the most recent update in 1995. This standard is the basis of the standard written for the AKC in 2005.

Breeding for Function

The Dogue de Bordeaux was used as a guardian, a hunter, and a fighter. They were trained to bait bulls, bears, and jaguars, hunt boars, herd cattle, and protect the homes, butcher shops, and vineyards of their masters.

Physical Characteristics

Height at Withers: female 23-26" (58.5-66 cm), male 23.5-27" (60-68.5 cm)

Weight: females at least 99 lb (45 kg) , males at least 110 lb (50 kg).

Coat: All shades of fawn. No mask, or a black or brown mask. Limited white patches are allowed on the chest and paws.

Longevity: Average 5.29 yrs based on the DDBS Longevity Study. Oldest dog was 12 years.[1]

Points of Conformation: The length of the body, measured from the point of the shoulder to the point of the buttock, is greater than the height at the withers, in the proportion of 11/10. The depth of the chest is more than half the height at the withers. The head is large, rather short, and trapezium shaped when viewed from above and in front. The eyes are oval and set wide apart. The ear is small in proportion to the skull and of a slightly darker color than the coat. The cheeks are prominent due to the very strong development of the muscles. The bite is undershot so that there is no contact between the upper and lower incisors. The lower jaw curves upwards. The skin is supple, ample and loose. The tail preferably reaches the hock but not below. the Dogue is well up on his toes despite his weight. The gait is supple and close to the ground, with great reach and drive.

Recognized Behavior Issues and Traits

The Dogue de Bordeaux is gifted for guarding, which he assumes with vigilance and great courage but without aggressiveness. He is a very good companion, being attached to and affectionate toward his master. He is calm and balanced with a high stimulus threshold. The male normally has a dominant character. The breed can be very aggressive with other dogs. Due to their head conformation, they snore and drool.

Normal Physiologic Variations

Heart size and echocardiographic measurements in the breed are more consistent with smaller sized breeds such as the Golden Retriever.[2]

According to a UK study 22.8% of litters are delivered via **C-section**.[3]

Drug Sensitivities

None Reported

Inherited Diseases

Hip Dysplasia: Polygenically inherited trait causing degenerative joint disease and hip arthritis. OFA reports 56% affected.[4]

Elbow Dysplasia: Polygenically inherited trait causing elbow arthritis. OFA reports 21.3% affected.[4]

Multifocal Retinopathy/Retinal Dysplasia: Autosomal recessive retinal pigment epithelial dysplasia causing localized multifocal retinal detachments. Age of onset from 11 to 13 weeks of age. Reported in 3.33% of Dogues de Bordeaux CERF-examined by veterinary ophthalmologists between 2000-2005. CERF does not recommend breeding any Dogue de Bordeaux with retinal dysplasia. A genetic test is available.[5]

Patella Luxation: Polygenically inherited laxity of patellar ligaments, causing luxation, lameness, and later degenerative joint disease. Treat surgically if causing clinical signs. OFA reports 2.2% affected.[4]

Disease Predispositions

Aortic Stenosis (AS): Narrowing of the outflow tract of the heart, causing a murmer and possible later heart disease. 72% of Dogues de Bordeaux have an aortic murmur, with 17% having echocardiographic aortic outflow velocity consistent with aortic stenosis. Undetermined mode of inheritance. An Isreali cohort had concurrent **tricuspid valve dysplasia**.[2,6]

Ectropion: Rolling out of eyelids, often with a medial canthal pocket. Can cause secondary conjunctivitis. Can be secondary to Ectropion is reported in 16.67% of Dogues de Bordeaux CERF examined by veterinary ophthalmologists between 2000-2005.[4]

Distichiasis: Abnormally placed eyelashes that irritate the cornea and conjunctiva. Can cause secondary corneal ulceration. Reported in 6.67% of Dogues de Bordeaux CERF examined by veterinary ophthalmologists between 2000-2005.[5]

Persistent Pupillary Membranes: Strands of fetal remnant connecting; iris to iris, cornea, lens, or involving sheets of tissue. The later three forms can impair vision, and dogs affected with these forms should not be bred. Identified in 6.67% of Dogues de Bordeaux CERF examined by veterinary ophthalmologists between 2000-2005.[5]

Cranial Cruciate Ligament (ACL) Rupture: Traumatic tearing of the ACL in the stifle, causing lameness and secondary arthritis. Treat with surgery. Reported at an increased incidence versus other breeds.[7]

Gastric Dilatation-Volvulus (Bloat, GDV): Polygenically inherited, life-threatening twisting of the stomach within the abdomen. Requires immediate veterinary attention. Reported cause of death of 14.74% of Dogues de Bordeaux.[1]

Lymphoma/Lymphosarcoma: Malignant cancer of the lymphoid tissue. Treatment with chemotherapy. Reported cause of death of 10.4% of Dogues de Bordeaux.[1]

Hypothyroidism: Inherited autoimmune thyroiditis. 3.8% positive for thyroid autoantibodies based on testing at Michigan State University. (Ave. for all breeds is 7.5%). A study in France found 4.5% affected.[8,9,10]

Cataracts: Nuclear and punctate cataracts predominate in the breed. Identified in 3.33% of Dogues de Bordeaux CERF examined by veterinary ophthalmologists between 2000-2005. CERF does not recommend breeding any Dogue de Bordeaux with a cataract.[5]

Corneal Dystrophy: Dogues de Bordeaux can have an epithelial/stromal form of corneal dystrophy. Reported in 2.22% of Dogues de Bordeaux CERF examined by veterinary ophthalmologists between 2000-2005.[5]

Idiopathic Epilepsy (Inherited Seizures): Can be generalized or partial seizures. Treat with anticonvulsant therapy. Reported cause of death of 2.22% of Dogues de Bordeaux.[1]

Palmoplantar Hyperkeratosis (Corny Feet): A disease of abnormal hardening and proliferation of the footpads. Affected dogs develop abnormal footpads around 6 months of age, which then fissure and crack, predisposing them to secondary infection. Undetermined mode of inheritance.[11]

Isolated Case Studies

Suspected Primary Immune Deficiency: A young Dogue de Bordeaux presented with chronic intermittent antibiotic responsive gastrointestinal and respiratory disease, lymphadenitis, tracheitis, hypogammaglobulinaemia, and the absence of B-lymphocytes in lymphoid tissue. A possible B-cell congenital immune deficiency was suspected.[12]

Lymphocytic Insulitis/Juvenile Diabetes Mellitus: A 3-mo-old Dogue de Bordeaux presented with persistent hyperglycemia and insulinopenia. Histological analysis of the pancreas T-cell infiltration of the islets of Langerhans, demonstrating an immune mediated juvenile diabetes.[13]

Congenital Valvular Pulmonic Stenosis, Tricuspid Valve Dysplasia, and Chronic Atrial Fibrillation: A 4-year-old male Dogue de Bordeaux dog with congenital valvular pulmonic stenosis, tricuspid valve dysplasia, and chronic atrial fibrillation had its ventricular heart rate controlled with a novel vagal stimulation system.[14]

Thoracic Stenosis: Two immature Dogues de Bordeaux presented for treatment of paraparesis. Thoracic stenosis was found at T4-6, with lateral compression of the thoracic spinal cord caused by over-sized pedicles. Dorsal laminectomy and partial pediculectomy stabilized their condition.[15]

Genetic Tests

Tests of Genotype: Direct test for Multifocal Retinopathy is available from Optigen.

Tests of Phenotype: CHIC Certification: Cardiac examination by a cardiologist, elbow, hip, and shoulder radiographs. Optional tests include CERF eye examination, thyroid profile including autoantibodies, and patella evaluation. (See CHIC website; www.caninehealthinfo.org).

Miscellaneous

- **Breed name synonyms:** French Mastiff, Bordeaux Bulldog.
- **Registries:** AKC, CKC, ANKC (Australian National Kennel Club), NKC (National Kennel Club), FCI.
- **AKC rank: (year 2008):** 41 (3,223 dogs registered)
- **Internet resources: Dogue de Bordeaux Society of America:** www.ddbs.org
  Canadian Dogue de Bordeaux Club: www.canadiandoguedebordeaxclub.org
  Dogue de Bordeaux Club of Great Britain: www.doguedebordeauxclub.co.uk

References

1. Dogue de Bordeaux Society of America: DDBS Causes of Death in the Dogue de Bordeaux: Survey Results. August 1, 2002.
2. Höllmer M, Willesen JL, Jensen AT, et. al.: Aortic stenosis in the Dogue de Bordeaux. J Small Anim Pract. 2008 Sep;49(9):432-7.
3. Evans KM & Adams VJ: Proportion of litters of purebred dogs born by caesarean section. J Small Anim Pract. 2010 Feb;51(2):113-8.
4. OFA Website breed statistics: www.offa.org Last accessed July 1, 2010.
5. *Ocular Disorders Presumed to be Inherited in Purebred Dogs.* American College of Veterinary Ophthalmologists. ACVO, 2007
6. Ohad DG, Avrahami A, David L, et. al.: Congenital Subaortic Stenosis and Tricuspid Valve Dysplasias in a Cohort of 13 Dogue De Bordeaux Dogs in Israel.Proceedings, 19th ECVIM-CA Congress, 2009.
7. Vezzoni A: Pathogenesis of Spontaneous Failure of Cranial Cruciate Ligament in the Dog. Proceedings, 2004 World Small Animal Veterinary Association World Congress. 2004.
8. Nachreiner RF, Refsal KR, Graham PA, et. al.: Prevalence of serum thyroid

hormone autoantibodies in dogs with clinical signs of hypothyroidism. J Am Vet Med Assoc 2002 Feb 15;220(4):466-71.

9. Nachreiner R & Refsal K: Personal communication, Diagnostic Center for Population and Animal Health, Michigan State University. April, 2007.

10. Segalini V, Hericher T, Grellet A, et. al.: Thyroid function and infertility in the dog: a survey in five breeds. Reprod Domest Anim. 2009 Jul;44 Suppl 2:211-3.

11. Paradis M: Footpad hyperkeratosis in a family of Dogue de Bordeaux. Veterinary Dermatology 1992;3:75-78.

12. Lobetti RG: Suspected primary immune deficiency in a Donge de Bordeaux dog. J S Afr Vet Assoc. 2002 Sep;73(3):133-4.

13. Jouvion G, Abadie J, Bach JM, et. al.: Lymphocytic insulitis in a juvenile dog with diabetes mellitus. Endocr Pathol. 2006 Fall;17(3):283-90.

14. Ohad DG, Sinai Y, Zaretsky A, et. al.: Ventricular rate control using a novel vagus nerve stimulating system in a dog with chronic atrial fibrillation. J Vet Cardiol. 2008 Dec;10(2):147-54.

15. Talbot CE, Pratt J, & Jeffery ND: Imaging Findings and Surgical Treatment of Thoracic Stenosis in Two Dogues de Bordeaux. Proceedings, 2008 British Small Animal Veterinary Congress. 2008.

16. AKC Breed Website: www.akc.org/breeds/dogue_de_bordeaux/ Last accessed July 1, 2010.

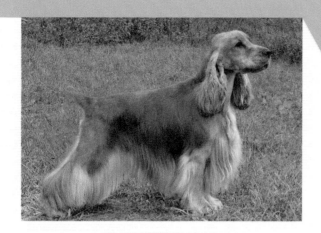

English Cocker Spaniel

The Breed History

Sharing common roots with other spaniels such as English Springers, Irish Water Spaniel, Sussex Spaniel, Field Spaniel and American Cockers, the English Cocker split from the other spaniels when a decision was made to divide land and water spaniels and subsequently, land spaniels into larger (Springer) and smaller (Cocker). In 1892 the Kennel Club of England began registering this breed as the Cocker Spaniel. In the US, the English Cocker Spaniel Club was formed in 1935, and in 1941, lineage studies provided a base to select only non-American cockers for future type development. In the AKC, they formalized standards in 1947, and the CKC registered them starting in 1940.

Breeding for Function

The breed was developed to be a gundog, and is still used for hunting, as well as in showing and companionship. The name *Cocker* derives from this breed's historical focus on hunting woodcock.

Physical Characteristics

Height at Withers: female 15-16" (38-40.5 cm), male 16-17" (40.5-43 cm).

Weight: females 26-32 lb (12-14.5 kg), males 28-34 lb (13-15.5 kg).

Coat: They are well feathered and hair is medium length, with solids (liver, red, black), tan markings, and parti-colors accepted. Field lines have shorter coats. Only a small amount of white marking is acceptable on the chest of solid color dogs.

Longevity: 12-15 years.

Points of Conformation: Of solid stature and good bone, these medium sized hunting dogs are smooth movers, and have a stocky tough appearance, but are never coarse. Alert oval eyes should not show the nictitans and are dark brown or dark hazel. They possess a moderate stop with a slight groove and their nose is colored black or brown. Ears are long, reaching to the nose and leathers are thick. The neck is arching and a moderate length, with a gentle topline sloping downwards to the tail base over a short strong back. They are deep-chested and have a moderate tuck of the abdomen. Limbs are straight and feet are round and compact, with highly arched toes. The tail is carried parallel to the back, and active and is often docked.

Recognized Behavior Issues and Traits

This dog is reported to be: a high energy pet with staying power suited for hunting, and has moderate grooming needs. They are average shedders. They need to be socialized early and training should begin early also. They do well in town or country with regular exercise. They are good alarm barkers. They get along very well with calm children. There is some variability in temperament between different lines of dogs. (See Aggression/Shyness below)

Normal Physiologic Variations

Ear care should be emphasized.

Echocardiography: Seventeen clinically normal adult English Cocker Spaniels from a kennel population with a history of cardiomyopathy were assessed, using M-mode echocardiography, to establish reference values for this breed of dog. Calculation of fractional shortening values identified a group of 5 dogs with reduced fractional shortening (mean +/- SD, 20.97 +/- 3.66%), which indicates that a depression in contractility may be present in some apparently healthy dogs of this kennel population.[1]

Echocardiographic Normal Values:[2]	
Parameter	Mean ± Standard Deviation
Weight (kg)	12.2 ± 2.2
LVPWD (mm)	7.9 ± 1.1
LVD (mm)	33.8 ± 3.3
LVS (mm)	22.2 ± 2.8
FS (%)	34.3 ± 4.5
IVSd (mm)	8.2 ± 1.3
N	12 with normal FS

LVPWD, LV posterior wall dimension at end-diastole; LVD, LV chamber dimension at end-diastole; LVS, LV chamber dimension at end-systole; FS, percent fractional shortening; IVSd, interventricular septal thickness at end-diastole; N, number of animals.

Drug Sensitivities

None Reported

Inherited Diseases

Progressive Retinal Atrophy (PRA): Autosomal recessive progressive rod cone degeneration (prcd) form. Age of onset between 3-8 years of age, eventually causing blindness. Dorn reports a 45.0x odds ratio versus other breeds. Optigen testing reports 11% affected, and 45% carriers in English Cocker Spaniels. CERF does not recommend breeding any English Cocker Spaniel with PRA.[3,4]

Hip Dysplasia: Polygenically inherited trait causing degenerative joint disease and hip arthritis. OFA reports 5.6% affected.[5]

Patella Luxation: Polygenically inherited laxity of patellar ligaments, causing luxation, lameness, and later degenerative joint disease. Treat surgically if causing clinical signs. OFA reports 5.2% affected.[5]

Hereditary Nephropathy/Nephritis (HN): Autosomal recessive disorder causing proteinuria and juvenile-onset chronic renal failure in affected dogs due to abnormal kidney basement membrane protein and structure. A genetic test is available, showing 0.3% affected and 14.6% carrier for the defective gene.[6,7]

Disease Predispositions

Distichiasis: Abnormally placed eyelashes that irritate the cornea and conjunctiva. Can cause secondary corneal ulceration. Dorn reports a 3.99x odds ratio versus other breeds. A heritability of 0.62 was found in a German study. Identified in 15.10% of English Cocker Spaniels CERF examined by veterinary ophthalmologists between 2000-2005.[3,4,8]

Hypothyroidism: Inherited autoimmune thyroiditis. 11.7% positive for thyroid autoantibodies based on testing at Michigan State University. (Ave. for all breeds is 7.5%).[9,10]

Deafness: Congenital deafness can be unilateral or bilateral. Diagnose by BAER testing. Strain reports 5.9% testing unilaterally deaf, and 1.1% bilaterally deaf based on BAER testing, the majority being parti-colored English Cocker Spaniels. Reported at a frequency of 2.86% in the 2002 ECS Health Survey Report.[11,12]

Cataracts: Anterior cortex (intermediate or punctate) and capsular cataracts predominate in the breed. Dorn reports a 1.89x odds ratio versus other breeds. Identified in 14.96% of single-colored and 5.51% of multicolored English Cocker Spaniels in a German study, with a heritability of 0.06 to 0.15. Reported in 8.23% of English Cocker Spaniels presented to veterinary teaching hospitals. Identified in 4.48% of English Cocker Spaniels CERF examined by veterinary ophthalmologists between 2000-2005. Reported at a frequency of 3.31% in the 2002 ECS Health Survey Report. CERF does not recommend breeding any English Cocker Spaniel with a cataract.[3,4,8,12,13,14]

Allergic Dermatitis (Atopy): Inhalant or food allergy. Presents with pruritis and pyotraumatic dermatitis (hot spots). Reported at a frequency of 4.16% in the 2002 ECS Health Survey Report.[12]

Aggression/Shyness: One study showed that owners of aggressive English Cocker Spaniels tended to be more tense, emotionally less stable, shy and undisciplined than owners of low aggression dogs. Aggression toward other dogs was reported at a frequency of 2.80%, and shyness 3.53% in the 2002 ECS Health Survey Report.[12,15]

Persistent Pupillary Membranes: Strands of fetal remnant connecting; iris to iris, cornea, lens, or involving sheets of tissue. The later three forms can impair vision, and dogs affected with these forms should not be bred. Iris to cornea PPMs in this breed cause corneal opacities. A heritability of 0.1 to 0.46 was found in a German study. Identified in 2.80% of English Cocker Spaniels CERF examined by veterinary ophthalmologists between 2000-2005.[4,8]

Inherited Epilepsy: Grand-mal seizures. Control with anticonvulsant medication. Reported at a frequency of 1.92% in the 2002 ECS Health Survey Report. Unknown mode of inheritance.[12]

Glaucoma: Ocular condition causing increased pressure within the eyeball, and secondary blindness due to damage to the retina. Can also predispose to lens luxation. Dorn reports a 1.33x odds ratio versus other breeds. Diagnosed in 1.35% of English Cocker Spaniels presented to veterinary teaching hospitals. A female predominance is seen in English Cocker Spaniels. Screen with gonioscopy and tonometry. Unknown mode of inheritance. CERF does not recommend breeding any English Cocker Spaniel with glaucoma.[3,4,16]

Retinal Dysplasia: Retinal folds, geographic, and generalized retinal dysplasia with detachment are recognized in the breed. Reported in 1.07% of English Cocker Spaniels CERF examined by veterinary ophthalmologists between 2000-2005.[4,17]

Keratoconjunctivitis Sicca (KCS, Dry Eye): Ocular condition causing lack of tear production and secondary conjunctivitis, corneal ulcerations, and vision problems. A later age of onset and female preponderance occurs in English Cocker Spaniels. Treat with topical ocular lubricants and anti-inflammatory medication.[18]

Dilated Cardiomyopathy: Clinical signs include sudden death, dyspnea and other signs of congestive heart failure due to cardiac enlargement and pulmonary edema. Affected dogs develop a progressive left ventricular dilatation. Mean fractional shortening in affected dogs is 25.4 +/- 5.7%. Reported at a frequency of 0.4% in the 2002 ECS Health Survey Report.[1,12,19]

Chronic Hepatitis: Chronic hepatitis without copper storage disease is reported at an increased prevalence in English Cocker Spaniels.[20]

Metabolic Vitamin E Deficiency/Retinal Pigment Epithelial Dystrophy (Central Progressive Retinal Atropy): Syndrome identified in English Cocker Spaniels with clinical signs of neurological dysfunction which can include ataxia, proprioceptive deficits, abnormal spinal reflexes, muscle weakness, retinal pigment epithelial dystrophy, neuroaxonal dystrophy, and intestinal lipofuscinosis. Though to be due to an abnormality in Vitamin E metabolism. Unknown mode of inheritance. CERF does not recommend breeding any affected English Cocker Spaniels.[4,21]

Multiple Ocular Abnormalities: Congenital disorder identified in English Cocker Spaniels in Denmark, characterized by cataracts and microphthalmia. Unknown mode of inheritance.[22]

Brachygnathism, Ceroid Lipofuscinosis, Entropion, Factor II Deficiency, Factor VIII Deficiency, Factor IX Deficiency, Optic Nerve Hypoplasia, Prognathism, Retained Primary Teeth, Struvite Urolithiasis, and **von Willebrand's Disease** are reported.[23]

Isolated Case Studies

Ectopic Ureter and Ureterocele: A 7-month-old, female English cocker spaniel was examined because of a complaint of urinary incontinence. Excretory urography revealed a small right kidney and right-sided hydroureter, ectopic ureter, and ureterocele.[24]

Congenital Vestibular Disease: Reported in a litter of English cocker spaniel puppies, marked by loss of balance and ataxia initially. Subsequent compensation left only one individual with "permanent" head tilt.[25]

Genetic Tests

Tests of Genotype: Direct tests for HN and prcd-PRA are available from Optigen. (Both tests are recommended for breeding dogs.)

Direct tests for black, liver and red colors, and black and brown nose are available from HealthGene and VetGen.

Tests of Phenotype: CHIC Certification: Required tests include hip radiographs, genetic test for prcd-PRA, patella evaluation, and two of the following: thyroid profile including autoantibodies, genetic test for FN, BAER hearing test, or CERF eye examination. (See CHIC website; www.caninehealthinfo.org).

Recommend cardiac evaluation by a cardiologist and elbow radiographs.

Miscellaneous

- **Breed name synonyms:** Cocker, Woodcock spaniel, Cocker Spaniel
- **Registries:** AKC, UKC, CKC, KCGB (Kennel Club of Great Britain), ANKC (Australian National Kennel Club), NKC (National Kennel Club)
- **AKC rank (year 2008):** 70 (1,247 dogs registered)
- **Internet resources: English Cocker Spaniel Club of America:** www.ecsca.org
  English Cocker Spaniel Club of Canada: www.ecscc.ca
  The Cocker Spaniel Club (UK): www.thecockerspanielclub.co.uk

References

1. Gooding JP, Robinson WF, Mews GC: Echocardiographic characterization of dilatation cardiomyopathy in the English cocker spaniel. *Am J Vet Res.* 1986 Sep;47(9):1978-83.
2. Gooding JP, Robinson WF, Mews GC: Echocardiographic assessment of left ventricular dimensions in clinically normal English cocker spaniels. *Am J Vet Res.* 1986 Feb;47(2):296-300.
3. Dorn CR: Canine breed-specific risks of frequently diagnosed diseases at veterinary teaching hospitals. Monograph. AKC Canine Health Foundation. 2000.
4. *Ocular Disorders Presumed to be Inherited in Purebred Dogs.* American College of Veterinary Ophthalmologists. ACVO, 2007.
5. OFA Website breed statistics: www.offa.org Last accessed July 1, 2010.
6. Lees GE, Helman RG, Kashtan CE, et. al.: A model of autosomal recessive Alport syndrome in English cocker spaniel dogs. *Kidney Int.* 1998 Sep;54(3):706-19.
7. Davidson AG, Bell RJ, Lees GE, et. al.: Genetic cause of autosomal recessive hereditary nephropathy in the English Cocker Spaniel. J Vet Intern Med. 2007 May-Jun;21(3):394-401.
8. Engelhardt A, Stock KF, Hamann H, et. al.: Analysis of systematic and genetic effects on the prevalence of primary cataract, persistent pupillary membrane and distichiasis in the two color variants of English Cocker Spaniels in Germany. Berl Munch Tierarztl Wochenschr. 2007 Nov-Dec;120(11-12):490-8.
9. Nachreiner RF, Refsal KR, Graham PA, et. al.: Prevalence of serum thyroid hormone autoantibodies in dogs with clinical signs of hypothyroidism. J Am Vet Med Assoc 2002 Feb 15;220(4):466-71.
10. Nachreiner R & Refsal K: Personal communication, Diagnostic Center for Population and Animal Health, Michigan State University. April, 2007.
11. Strain GM: Deafness prevalence and pigmentation and gender associations in dog breeds at risk. *Vet J.* 2004 Jan;167(1):23-32.
12. English Cocker Spaniel Club of America, Slater MS: 2002 ECS Health Survey Report. 2004.
13. Engelhardt A, Stock KF, Hamann H, et. al.: A retrospective study on the prevalence of primary cataracts in two pedigrees from the German population of English Cocker Spaniels. Vet Ophthalmol. 2008 Jul-Aug;11(4):215-21.
14. Gelatt KN, Mackay EO: Prevalence of primary breed-related cataracts in the dog in North America. Vet Ophthalmol. 2005 Mar-Apr;8(2):101-11.
15. Podberscek AL, Serpell JA: Aggressive behaviour in English cocker spaniels and the personality of their owners. *Vet Rec* 1997: 141[3]:73-6.
16. Gelatt KN, MacKay EO: Prevalence of the breed-related glaucomas in pure-bred dogs in North America. *Vet Ophthalmol.* 2004 Mar-Apr;7(2):97-111.
17. Dietz HH: Retinal dysplasia in dogs--a review. *Nord Vet Med.* 1985 Jan-Feb;37(1):1-9.
18. Sanchez RF, Innocent G, Mould J, et. al.: Canine keratoconjunctivitis sicca: disease trends in a review of 229 cases. J Small Anim Pract. 2007 Apr;48(4):211-7.
19. Staaden RV: Cardiomyopathy of English cocker spaniels. *J Am Vet Med Assoc.* 1981 Jun 15;178(12):1289-92.
20. Watson PJ: Chronic Hepatitis in Dogs. Proceedings, 2009 British Small Animal Veterinary Congress. 2009.
21. McLellan GJ, Cappello R, Mayhew IG, et. al.: Clinical and pathological observations in English cocker spaniels with primary metabolic vitamin E deficiency and retinal pigment epithelial dystrophy. *Vet Rec.* 2003 Sep 6;153(10):287-92.
22. Davidson MG: Congenital cataracts in English cocker spaniels. *Vet Rec.* 1988 Jun 4;122(23):568.
23. *The Genetic Connection: A Guide to Health Problems in Purebred Dogs.* L Ackerman. p. 212, AAHA Press, 1999.
24. Lautzenhiser SJ, Bjorling DE: Urinary incontinence in a dog with an ectopic ureterocele. *J Am Anim Hosp Assoc.* 2002 Jan-Feb;38(1):29-32.
25. Bedford PG: Congenital vestibular disease in the English cocker spaniel. *Vet Rec.* 1979 Dec 8;105(23):530-1.
26. *The Complete Dog Book, 20th Ed.* The American Kennel Club. Howell Book House, NY 2006. p 89-92.

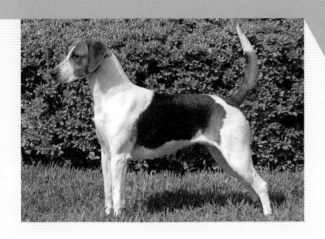

English Foxhound

The Breed History

Careful record keeping by Masters of the Hounds allows the trace back of pedigrees to around 1800. They were first imported to America in 1738. The English foxhound is much larger and heavier than the American counterpart. Breed origins are obscure but may include Fox Terrier and Bloodhound. Many of these dogs are registered in the hunting dog registry, the International Foxhunter Studbook (kept by the British Master of Foxhounds Association) rather than other mainstream registry bodies.

Breeding for Function

The old English tradition of mounted fox hunting led to the breeding of exceptional pack dogs that could sound the scent for the hunt to follow. Foxes were the primary prey.

Physical Characteristics

Height at Withers: female 23-25" (58-63.5 cm), male 25-27" (63.5-69 cm).

Weight: 55-75 lb (25-34 kg).

Coat: The haircoat lays flat and is short and dense with hard hair texture. Colors are black and tan and white, tricolor or white and tan.

Longevity: 11-12 years.

Points of Conformation: The dog is square and moderate in all proportions. The head is of a size to match the dog, with large nose, the ears are set low and pendulous with moderate leather, and often the tips are rounded (the distal segment is trimmed off). The neck is long and not throaty, with slight arch. The thorax is deep and the rib cage does not taper up caudally but extends well back. Feet are round and toes are well knuckled up. Topline is level, and the tail is carried gaily when alert. It tapers at the tip with a fringe of hair (slight brush). Very straight legs, and a low ground-covering gait characterize the breed.

Recognized Behavior Issues and Traits

Reported breed attributes include: Likes to be in a pack, good if raised in a household and good with children if socialized early. High activity, high exercise needs, and thus not well placed in apartments. Low grooming needs, let loose in a fenced area only or may run off after scents.

Needs mental stimulation and human contact if housed solo. Gets along well with other dogs. Moderate barking tendency; also may howl. Has a moderate shedding tendency. Still kept primarily for hunting rather than as a house pet.

Normal Physiologic Variations

Pelger-Huet Anomaly: Autosomal recessive inherited blood disorder causing neutrophils with round, oval, or bean-shaped nuclei and only rare segmented nuclei. No obvious clinical effects in affected dogs.[1]

Drug Sensitivities

None reported

Inherited Diseases

Hip Dysplasia: Polygenically inherited trait causing degenerative joint disease and hip arthritis. OFA reports 2.5% affected.[2]

Elbow Dysplasia: Polygenically inherited trait causing elbow arthritis. OFA reports a high incidence, but too few English Foxhounds have been screened to determine an accurate frequency.[2]

Patella Luxation: Polygenically inherited laxity of patellar ligaments, causing luxation, lameness, and later degenerative joint disease. Treat surgically if causing clinical signs. Too few English Foxhounds have been screened by OFA to determine an accurate frequency.[2]

Disease Predispositions

Hypothyroidism: Inherited autoimmune thyroiditis. 18.2% positive for thyroid auto-antibodies based on testing at Michigan State University. (Ave. for all breeds is 7.5%).[3,4]

Leishmaniasis: This infectious disease is primarily diagnosed in Foxhounds. It is not determined if this is due to a genetic or environmental cause.[5,6]

Deafness: Congenital deafness can be unilateral or bilateral. Diagnosed by BAER testing.[7]

Renal Amyloidosis: Multiple reported cases of kidney failure in related English Foxhounds. Affected dogs have an acute onset of kidney dysfunction, and die within one week. Histological findings in the kidneys show the presence of both glomerular and interstitial amyloid.[8]

Ocular Disorders: Not enough English Foxhounds have had CERF eye examinations to determine accurate frequencies for ocular disorders.[9]

Brachygnathism, Hound Ataxia, Prognathism, and **Thrombopathia** are reported.[10]

Isolated Case Studies
None reported.

Genetic Tests
Tests of Genotype: Direct test for coat color alleles is available from VetGen.

Tests of Phenotype: Recommend hip and elbow radiographs, thyroid profile including autoantibodies, patella evaluation, CERF eye examination and cardiac evaluation.

Miscellaneous
- **Breed name synonyms:** Foxhound
- **Registries:** AKC, UKC, CKC, KCGB (Kennel Club of Great Britain), ANKC (Australian National Kennel Club), NKC (National Kennel Club)
- **AKC rank (year 2008):** 157 (17 dogs registered)
- **Internet resources: English Foxhound Club of America (AKC):**
  13007 Brandywine Rd.
  Brandywine, MD 20613
  Masters of Foxhounds Association of America:
  www.mfha.com

References

1. Bowles CA, Alsaker RD, Wolfle TL: Studies of the Pelger-Huet anomaly in foxhounds. Am J Pathol. 1979 Jul;96(1):237-47.
2. OFA Website breed statistics: www.offa.org Last accessed July 1, 2010.
3. Nachreiner RF, Refsal KR, Graham PA, et. al.: Prevalence of serum thyroid hormone autoantibodies in dogs with clinical signs of hypothyroidism. J Am Vet Med Assoc 2002 Feb 15;220(4):466-71.
4. Nachreiner R & Refsal K: Personal communication, Diagnostic Center for Population and Animal Health, Michigan State University. April, 2007.
5. Swenson CL, Silverman J, Stromberg PC, et. al.: Visceral leishmaniasis in an English foxhound from an Ohio research colony. J Am Vet Med Assoc. 1988 Nov 1;193(9):1089-92.
6. Grosjean NL, Vrable RA, Murphy AJ, et. al.: Seroprevalence of antibodies against Leishmania spp among dogs in the United States. J Am Vet Med Assoc. 2003 Mar 1;222(5):603-6.
7. Strain GM: Deafness prevalence and pigmentation and gender associations in dog breeds at risk. Vet J. 2004 Jan;167(1):23-32
8. Mason NJ, Day MJ: Renal amyloidosis in related English foxhounds. J Small Anim Pract. 1996 Jun;37(6):255-60..
9. *Ocular Disorders Presumed to be Inherited in Purebred Dogs*. American College of Veterinary Ophthalmologists. ACVO, 2007
10. *The Genetic Connection: A Guide to Health Problems in Purebred Dogs*. L Ackerman. P 218. AAHA Press, 1999.
11. *The Complete Dog Book, 20th Ed*. The American Kennel Club. Howell Book House, NY 2006. p. 173-176.

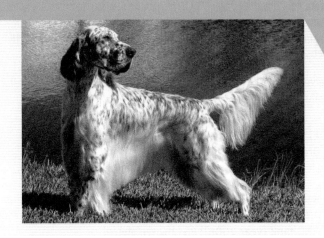

English Setter

The Breed History

As the name implies, they are of English origin, and were renowned bird dogs that first came into the record in the late 1800s. Springer spaniel, Water spaniel and Spanish pointer breeds may have all contributed to this breed's development. The term *setter* relates to the crouching posture (set) the dog originally took when they located the bird.

Breeding for Function

Bred as a bird-hunting dog, to set and retrieve, this dog has established himself as a top field trial performer. They are also prized as companion dogs. The modern field dog has a bit stockier and smaller constitution and less of a coat than the show or companion type. They do well in agility competitions.

Physical Characteristics

Height at Withers: female 24" (61 cm), male 25" (63.5 cm)

Weight: females 60-65 lb (27-29.5 kg), males 65-80 lb (29.5-36.5 kg)

Coat: The flat long and straight to slightly wavy silky coat with feathers may be tri-color, lemon or liver belton, blue (black) or orange (tan) belton. Belton markings are a white background with flecking (speckles) or roan of these colors admixed. Flecking is preferred.

Longevity: 11-12 years.

Points of Conformation: Due to their origins as gundogs for vigorous hunting, this athletic, graceful dog is bred for function. They have mesocephalic skulls, with a well-defined stop and long square muzzle. The occiput is prominent, nose is black or dark brown, pendulous flews are present, and eyes are dark brown and round. Moderate-length ears are of thin leather, pendulous and set low. A long arched fine neck and level topline (can also slightly slope to the rear) are typical. Their deep chest is not broad, and a moderate loin tuck is present. Tapering, the tail finishes at the tarsus joint, and is carried horizontally. Forelegs are strong and straight, the feet are compact and toes are well arched. Dewclaws are often removed. The gait appears effortless, characterized by long, low strides with straight movement.

Recognized Behavior Issues and Traits

Reports of this breed note that they possess an affectionate, docile disposition. They are high activity dogs though, and need regular exercise, and are thus not well placed for city living. They are generally quiet in the house, and are quite placid. Training should start early and they often have a streak of independence. They are alarm barkers.

The coat just needs regular brushing; they are average shedders. They are good with children, and crave close contact with their families. If left alone for extended periods, they may engage in boredom vices such as digging and chewing. Their prominent flews result in some drooling.

Normal Physiologic Variations

English Setters may be more prone to developing eccentrocytes - RBCs that appear in a peripheral blood smear to have their hemoglobin shifted to one side of the cell.[1]

Drug Sensitivities

None reported

Inherited Diseases

Hip Dysplasia: Polygenically inherited trait causing degenerative joint disease and hip arthritis. OFA reports 16.5% affected. Dorn reports a 1.49x odds ratio versus other breeds.[2,3]

Elbow Dysplasia: Polygenically inherited trait causing elbow arthritis. Reported 3.7x odds ratio for ununited anconeal process form of elbow dysplasia versus other breeds. OFA reports 15.1% affected.[2,4]

Patella Luxation: Polygenically inherited laxity of patellar ligaments, causing luxation, lameness, and later degenerative joint disease. Treat surgically if causing clinical signs. Too few English Setters have been screened by OFA to determine an accurate frequency.[2]

Neuronal Ceroid–Lipofuscinosis: Rare, fatal autosomal recessive inherited degenerative neurological disease. Affected English setters present between 6-12 months of age, and die between 20-27 months of age. They present with variable signs of progressive hind limb paresis, incoordination, behavior changes, seizures, and/or blindness. A genetic test is available.[5,6]

Disease Predispositions

Hypothyroidism: Inherited autoimmune thyroiditis. 31.4% positive for thyroid auto-antibodies based on testing at Michigan State University. (Ave. for all breeds is 7.5%) Dorn reports a 1.26x odds ratio versus other breeds.[3,7,8]

Allergic Dermatitis: Inhalant or food allergy. Presents with pruritis and pyotraumatic dermatitis. English setters have a significantly increased risk for atopy versus other breeds. Dorn reports a 1.91x odds ratio versus other breeds.[3,9]

Deafness: Congenital deafness can be unilateral or bilateral. Diagnosed by BAER testing. Strain reports total (uni or bilateral) deafness frequency of 12.4% based on BAER testing. 10.3% of all English setters test unilaterally deaf, and 2.1% test bilaterally deaf. The ESAA maintains a BAER test registry: www.esaa.com/health/Baersearch.asp.[10]

Distichiasis: Abnormally placed eyelashes that irritate the cornea and conjunctiva. Can cause secondary corneal ulceration. Identified in 7.24% of English setters CERF-examined by veterinary ophthalmologists between 2000-2005.[11]

Mammary Cancer: Dorn reports a 36.54x odds ratio for mammary gland cancer versus other breeds.[3]

Osteochondritis Dissecans (OCD), Shoulder: Abnormality of cartilage development causing lameness. Severe cases may require surgery. English setters have a greater than 5x risk of developing shoulder OCD than other breeds. Males are affected more than females. Another study reported a 10.1x odds ratio versus other breeds. Unknown mode of inheritance.[4,12]

Persistent Pupillary Membranes: Strands of fetal remnant connecting; iris to iris, cornea, lens, or involving sheets of tissue. The later three forms can impair vision, and dogs affected with these forms should not be bred. Identified in 1.81% of English Setters CERF examined by veterinary ophthalmologists between 2000-2005.[11]

Cataracts: Anterior or posterior intermediate and punctate cataracts occur in the breed. Identified in 2.71% of English setters CERF-examined by veterinary ophthalmologists between 2000-2005. CERF does not recommend breeding any English Setter with a cataract.[11]

Symmetrical Lupoid Onychodystrophy (SLO): Disorder causing loss of toenails. Onset between 2-8 years of age affecting 1-2 nails, then progressing to all toenails within 2-9 weeks. Requires lifelong treatment with oral fatty acid supplementation +/- prednisone. Kindreds of affected English setters have been identified, but a mode of inheritance is not known.[13]

Brachygnathism, Central PRA, Cutaneous Asthenia, Ectropion, Factor VIII Deficiency, Familial Benign Pemphigus, GM2 gangliosidosis, Keratoconjunctivitis Sicca, Malassezia Dermatitis, Methemoglobin Reductase Deficiency, Prognathism, von Willebrands Disease, and **Wry Mouth** are reported.[14]

Isolated Case Studies

Exocrine Pancreatic Insufficiency: Reported in a family of English setters with juvenile onset chronic inadequate digestion, voluminous foul smelling feces, weight loss with increased appetite, occasional vomiting, and abdominal pain.[15]

Genetic Tests

Tests of Genotype: Direct test for NCL is available from the University of Missouri.

Direct tests for black or black tricolor, liver or liver tricolor and lemon colors, and black or brown nose are available from HealthGene and VetGen.

Tests of Phenotype: CHIC Certification: Required tests are; hip and elbow radiographs, and BAER testing for deafness. Optional recommended thyroid profile including autoantibodies. (See CHIC website: www.caninehealthinfo.org)

Recommend CERF eye examination, patella evaluation, and cardiac evaluation.

Miscellaneous

- **Breed name synonyms:** Llewellin (historical but the term Llewellin Setter is sometimes used today for the field variety), Laverack (historical type), Setting Spaniel (historical)
- **Registries:** AKC, CKC, UKC, KCGB (Kennel Club of Great Britain), ANKC (Australian National Kennel Club), NKC (National Kennel Club)
- **AKC rank (year 2008):** 86 (752 registered)
- **Internet resources: English Setter Association of America:** www.esaa.com
  English Setter Association of England: www.englishsetterassociation.co.uk
  English Setter Club of Canada: www.englishsetterclubofcanada.com

References

1. Caldin M, Carli E, Furlanello T, et. al.: A retrospective study of 60 cases of eccentrocytosis in the dog. Vet Clin Pathol. 2005 Sep;34(3):224-31.
2. OFA Website breed statistics: www.offa.org Last accessed July 1, 2010.
3. Dorn CR: Canine breed-specific risks of frequently diagnosed diseases at veterinary teaching hospitals. Monograph. AKC Canine Health Foundation. 2000.
4. LaFond E, Breur GJ & Austin CC: Breed susceptibility for developmental orthopedic diseases in dogs. J Am Anim Hosp Assoc. 2002 Sep-Oct;38(5):467-77.
5. Katz ML, Khan S, Awano T, et. al.: A mutation in the CLN8 gene in English Setter dogs with neuronal ceroid-lipofuscinosis. Biochem Biophys Res Commun. 2005 Feb 11;327(2):541-7.
6. Koppang N: The English setter with ceroid-lipofuscinosis: a suitable model for the juvenile type of ceroid-lipofuscinosis in humans. Am J Med Genet Suppl. 1988;5:117-25.
7. Nachreiner R & Refsal K: Personal communication, Diagnostic Center for Population and Animal Health, Michigan State University. April, 2007.
8. Nachreiner RF, Refsal KR, Graham PA, et. al.: Prevalence of serum thyroid hormone autoantibodies in dogs with clinical signs of hypothyroidism. J Am Vet Med Assoc. 2002 Feb 15;220(4):466-71.
9. Schick RO, Fadok VA: Responses of atopic dogs to regional allergens: 268 cases (1981-1984). J Am Vet Med Assoc. 1986 Dec 1;189(11):1493-6.
10. Strain GM: Deafness prevalence and pigmentation and gender associations in dog breeds at risk. Vet J. 2004 Jan;167(1):23-32.
11. *Ocular Disorders Presumed to be Inherited in Purebred Dogs.* American College of Veterinary Ophthalmologists. ACVO, 2007.
12. Slater MR, Scarlett JM, Kaderly RE, Bonnett BN: Breed, gender and age as risk factors for canine osteochondritis dissecans. Veterinary and Comparative Orthopaedics and Traumatology 1991; 4:100-106.
13. Ziener ML, Bettenay SV & Mueller RS: Symmetrical onychomadesis in Norwegian Gordon and English setters. Vet Dermatol. 2008 Apr;19(2):88-94.
14. *The Genetic Connection: A Guide to Health Problems in Purebred Dogs.* L Ackerman. p.216 AAHA Press, 1999.
15. Boari A, Williams DA, Famiglibergamini P: Observations on Exocrine Pancreatic Insufficiency in a Family of English Setter Dogs. Journal of Small Animal Practice 1994; 35: 247-250.
16. *The Complete Dog Book, 20th Ed.* The American Kennel Club. Howell Book House, NY 2006. p. 63-66.

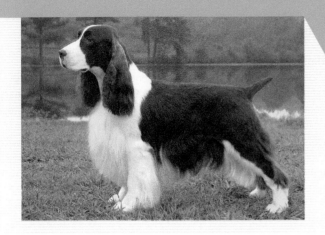

The Breed History

This breed originates from the common springing spaniel stock that gave rise to both small Cocker spaniels and the Field or Springer spaniels. The breed split occurred around 1800. In 1880, the American Spaniel Club was formed. In 1902, the Kennel Club of England accepted the English Springer Spaniel as a breed. The parent club in the US is the English Springer Spaniel Field Trial Association.

Breeding for Function

These dogs excel at gun work and field trials, and are also excellent at flushing game. Their working ability has been emphasized during breed development. They excel in hunt trials, agility and obedience trials. The field spaniel is a little different in type from the "bench" or conformation dog.

Physical Characteristics

Height at Withers: female 19" (48 cm), male 20" (51 cm)

Weight: females 40 lb (18 kg), males 50 lb (23 kg).

Coat: They are double-coated, the hair is medium in length, flat to wavy, and colors include liver and white, black and white, tricolor, and blue or liver roan. They possess feathering on limbs, tail and chest areas.

Longevity: 12-15 years.

Points of Conformation: These are the tallest of the spaniels, but still a medium-sized dog with proud carriage and gentle eyes. Their gait is powerful, agile and enthusiastic. Eyes are oval and set deep and the iris colors are usually hazel to dark brown, with black pigment of the palpebral margins. The nose is liver or black. The ears are long and fine, with moderate leather, muzzle is square, and the gradual stop is grooved. The neck is muscular and lightly arched, the back straight, and the topline slopes only slightly down to the tail base. The chest is deep and the tail is carried close to parallel with the back. They move with a long, low smooth stride.

Recognized Behavior Issues and Traits

Reports characterize the English Springer as a breed of loyal, intelligent dogs. These dogs need close human contact and are considered moderately trainable. They require adequate stimulation and exercise to prevent boredom vices. They should be socialized and trained early and are classed as high-energy dogs. They are solid alarm barkers. They require daily grooming and periodic trimming and clipping, and attention to ear cleanliness is important.

Notable in the literature are reports of "Springer rage syndrome"; this is an older term for aggressive behavioral characteristics seen in some lines of the breed. Nowadays, according to research by Dr. Ilana Riesner, the condition is usually classified as a dominance aggression, possibly related to low serotonin levels.[1] In this breed, the aggression signs bypass intermediate warning cues, and progresses directly from stare to attack. Dr. Bonnie Beaver has also identified mental lapse aggression, a form of sudden, violent aggression with no known treatment.

Normal Physiologic Variations

None Reported

Drug Sensitivities

None Reported

Inherited Diseases

Hip Dysplasia: Polygenically inherited trait causing degenerative joint disease and hip arthritis. OFA reports 13.3% affected.[2]

Elbow Dysplasia: Polygenically inherited trait causing elbow arthritis. OFA reports 13.7% affected.[2]

Patella Luxation: Polygenically inherited laxity of patellar ligaments, causing luxation, lameness, and later degenerative joint disease. Treat surgically if causing clinical signs. OFA reports 2.1% affected.[2]

Retinal Dysplasia: Autosomal recessive, congenital retinal dysplasia is well documented in the breed. Complex linear folds and rosettes occur predominantly in the peripapillary tapetal area of the sensory retina, causing focal retinal detachment. Identified in 5.84% of English Springer Spaniels CERF examined by veterinary ophthalmologists between 2000-2005. CERF does not recommend breeding any English Springer Spaniel with retinal dysplasia.[3,4,5]

Progressive Retinal Atrophy (PRA)/Cone-Rod Dystrophy (cord1): Hereditary disorder causing progressive loss of vision. Onset of clinical signs from 2-9 years of age. Molecular genetic studies show this is not the prcd form of PRA. Identified in 0.6% of English Springer Spaniels CERF examined by veterinary ophthalmologists between 2000-2005. CERF does not recommend breeding any English Springer Spaniel with PRA. An autosomal recessive mutation in the RPGRIP1 gene is highly correlated to clinical PRA, but does not appear to be the sole cause of the disease. In a small study, 7% of English Springer Spaniels homozygous for the mutation retain normal sight, and 40% of affected dogs do not carry the RPGRIP1 mutation, demonstrating a more complex etiology for this disease. A genetic test for the RPGRIP1 mutation is available, which shows 42% of all English Springer Spaniels homozygous for the mutation, and 38% testing as heterozygous carriers. Testing in the UK shows 6% homozygous and 31% heterozygous for the mutation.[3,6]

Phosphofructokinase (PFK) Deficiency: Autosomal recessive disorder causing chronic hemolysis and hemolytic crises, especially with exercise. Muscle wasting and mildly increased serum creatine phosphokinase activity are also found. A genetic test is available, which shows 2.7% carriers. Field trial Springer Spaniels have a higher proportion (4.0%) of carriers versus the conformation (1.2%) group.[7]

Fucosidosis (Storage Disease): Rare, fatal autosomal recessive storage disease causing behavioral changes, progressive ataxia, proprioceptive deficits, dysphagia and wasting between 1-3 years of age. A genetic test is available. Testing in the UK shows 7.4% carrier and 0.9% affected.[8,9]

GM1-Gangliosidosis: Rare, fatal, autosomal recessive lysosomal storage disease, causing dwarfism and neurological impairment by 4-1/2 months of age.[10]

Disease Predispositions

Dominance Aggression: In a large behavioral survey, owner-directed growling or more intense aggression was reported in 48.4% English Springer Spaniels. 26.3% had bitten a human in the past, with two-thirds of these directed at familiar adults and children. Owner-directed aggression in adult English Springer Spaniels was associated with a number of environmental, sex-related, and inherited factors. To reduce the risk of aggression, prospective owners might seek a female, hunting-type English Springer Spaniel from an experienced breeder.[1,11]

Pectinate Ligament Dysplasia (PLD): 25.5% of English Springer Spaniels show PLD via gonioscopic examination. PLD is positively correlated to narrow iridocorneal angle and the development of primary glaucoma.[12]

Persistent Pupillary Membranes: Strands of fetal remnant connecting; iris to iris, cornea, lens, or involving sheets of tissue. The later three forms can impair vision, and dogs affected with these forms should not be bred. Identified in 8.35% of English Springer Spaniels CERF examined by veterinary ophthalmologists between 2000-2005.[3]

Hypothyroidism: Inherited autoimmune thyroiditis. 7.0% positive for thyroid auto-antibodies based on testing at Michigan State University. (Ave. for all breeds is 7.5%).[13,14]

Secondary Glaucoma: Glaucoma causes increased pressure within the eyeball and blindness due to damage to the retina. Secondary glaucoma can occur after cataract formation, lens luxation, uveitis, hyphema, and intraocular neoplasia. The breed is listed as predisposed to secondary glaucoma.[15]

Pemphigus Foliaceus: The breed has an increased risk (20.7x odds ratio) of developing pemphigus foliaceus. Clinical signs include crusting lesions to the dorsal part of the muzzle and head, progressing to the body. Diagnosis is with biopsy.[16]

Idiopathic Epilepsy (Inherited Seizures): In English Springer Spaniels, epilepsy can be generalized (47%) or focal onset (53%).

Average age of onset is 3 years. One study suggests a partially penetrant autosomal recessive, or polygenic mode of inheritance. Control with anticonvulsant medication.[17]

Primary Seborrhea: Inherited predisposition to developing seborrhea. Affected dogs develop a generalized non-pruritic dry scaling which gradually worsens and develops recurrent secondary pyoderma. Some dogs remained in this dry (seborrhoea sicca) stage, but in most cases the dermatosis became greasy and inflamed (seborrhoea oleosa and seborrhoeic dermatitis). Affected dogs with seborrhoea sicca usually respond to topical emollient-humectant agents or oral omega-3/omega-6 fatty acid supplementation. Dorn reports a 1.94x odds ratio versus other breeds.[18,19]

Otitis Externa (Chronic Ear Infection): Ear infections can also be secondary to underlying skin allergies. Bacterial and yeast infections. Dorn reports a 1.94x odds ratio versus other breeds.[18]

Bronchiectasis: Clinical signs of chronic cough with excessive airway mucous. Diagnosis with radiographs. Reported at a frequency of 3.1% and an odds ratio of 2.39x versus other breeds. Treatment is with bronchodilators and possibly corticosteroids.[20]

Lichenoid-Psoriasiform Dermatosis: Breed related skin disorder of chronic dermatitis with an onset between 4-18 months. Affected dogs show erythematous papules and plaques, with corrugated surfaces in the ear canal and in the inguinal area. Later, papules, scale, and adherent keratin mounds developed inside the ear, in the inguinal area, around the mouth, eyes, and anus, and occasionally on the thoracic wall and the limbs. Treatment is with high dose corticosteroids and antibiotics. This disease is differentiated from primary seborrhea by histology and the presence of erythematous papules and plaques.[21]

Mammary Cancer: In Sweden, where female dogs are rarely spayed, 38% of English Springer Spaniels develop breast cancer. The presence of breast cancer liability genes BRCA1 or BRCA2 increase the odds ratio for breast cancer 4x, with BRCA1 strongly associated with malignant cases.[22]

Cataracts: Anterior cortex punctate and posterior subcapsular cataracts predominate in the breed. Identified in 1.66% of English Springer Spaniels CERF examined by veterinary ophthalmologists between 2000-2005. CERF does not recommend breeding any English Springer Spaniel with a cataract.[3]

Sebaceous Adenitis: Disorder of immune mediated sebaceous gland destruction, presenting with hair loss, usually beginning with the dorsal midline and ears. Diagnosis by skin biopsy. Treat with isotretinoin. The English springer spaniel is a breed predisposed to SA, and has more severe clinical signs than other breeds. An autosomal recessive mode of inheritance is suspected. Reported at a frequency of 0.6% in Sweden.[23]

Immune-Mediated Hemolytic Anemia (IMHA): Autoimmune destruction of blood cells. IMHA is reported at an increased frequency versus other breeds. An Australian study showed a 10X odds ratio versus other breeds. There is a female preponderance.[24,25]

Chronic Hepatitis: English Springer Spaniels have a predisposition for a type of chronic hepatitis without copper accumulation which carries a poor prognosis. Mean age of diagnosis of 3.4 years, with an average time to death after diagnosis of 7 months.[26,27]

Bradyarrhythmia: English Springer Spaniels were over represented in a UK study of dogs with slow heart rates requiring pacemaker implantation. English Springer Spaniels presented at a younger age, with a median survival time of 30 months. Diagnoses included **persistent atrial standstill, AV block,** and **sick sinus syndrome.**[28]

Pyothorax: Production and filling of pus in the chest cavity. English Springer Spaniels comprised 6 of 15 reported cases of pyothorax in one study. Treatment is with long-term antibiotics.[29]

Myasthenia Gravis: A rare, congenital form of myasthenia gravis occurs in English Springer Spaniels. Clinical signs are evident from six to eight weeks of age, and include exercise induced weakness without megaesophagus. Raised antibody levels to acetylcholine receptor do not occur.[30]

Congenital Hypomyelinization (Shaking Pups): Rare developmental disorder of lack of myelin in the spinal cord, brainstem and cerebral hemispheres. Affected dogs are reduced size and show gross generalized tremor, particularly when aroused, at about 10-12 days of age. Possible X-linked recessive inheritance.[31,32]

Ciliary Dyskinesia: Inherited abnormal anatomy and function of cilia. Causes chronic secondary rhinitis and bronchopneumonia due to abnormal respiratory ciliary clearance, and infertility due to abnormal sperm motility. Breeding studies suggest an autosomal recessive mode of inheritance.[33,34]

Cerebellar abiotrophy, Cutaneous Asthenia, Deafness, Diabetes Mellitus, Ectropion, Entropion, Factor XI Deficiency, Microphthalmia, Narcolepsy, Patent Ductus Arteriosus, Protein-Losing Enteropathy, Ventricular Septal Defect, von Willebrand's Disease, and **Wooly Syndrome** are reported.[35]

Isolated Case Studies

Dyserythropoiesis, Polymyopathy, and Cardiomegaly: Three related English Springer Spaniels were identified with regurgitation from an early age, slowly progressive temporal muscle atrophy with partial trismus, and mild generalized skeletal muscle atrophy. All dogs exhibited moderate dyserythropoietic anemia, polymyopathy with megaesophagus, and varying degrees of cardiomegaly.[36]

Suspected Mitochondrial Myopathy: A three-year-old, male English Springer Spaniel presented with a three-month history of weakness, incoordination and marked muscle atrophy. Electromyography, nerve-conduction velocity, and muscle biopsy studies were consistent with a mitochondrial myopathy.[37]

Genetic Tests

Tests of Genotype: Direct test for Phosphofructokinase (PFK) deficiency is available from HealthGene, Optigen, PennGen, VetGen, and the Animal Health Trust.

Direct test for PRA risk factor is available from the University of Missouri and the Animal Health Trust.

Direct test for fucosidosis is available from PennGen, and the Animal Health Trust.

Direct tests for black or liver colors, and black or brown nose are available from HealthGene and VetGen.

Tests of Phenotype: Recommended tests include hip and elbow radiographs, CERF eye examination, patella evaluation, thyroid profile including autoantibodies, and cardiac evaluation.

Miscellaneous

- **Breed name synonyms:** Field spaniel (historical), Springer, Springer spaniel
- **Registries:** AKC, UKC, CKC, KCGB (Kennel Club of Great Britain), ANKC (Australian National Kennel Club), NKC (National Kennel Club)
- **AKC rank (year 2008):** 27 (6,690 dogs registered)
- **Internet resources: English Springer Spaniel Field Trial Association Inc.** (parent club in the US): www.essfta.org
  The English Springer Spaniel Club of Great Britain: www.englishspringer.org
  English Springer Spaniel Club of Canada: www.geocities.com/essccanada/

References

1. Reisner IR, Houpt KA, Shofer FS: National survey of owner-directed aggression in English Springer Spaniels. J Am Vet Med Assoc. 2005 Nov 15;227(10):1594-603.
2. OFA Website breed statistics: www.offa.org Last accessed July 1, 2010.
3. Ocular Disorders Presumed to be Inherited in Purebred Dogs. American College of Veterinary Ophthalmologists. ACVO, 2007.
4. Whiteley HE, Young S: The external limiting membrane in developing normal and dysplastic canine retina. Tissue Cell. 1986;18(2):231-9.
5. O'Toole D, Young S, Severin GA, et. al.: Retinal dysplasia of English springer spaniel dogs: light microscopy of the postnatal lesions. Vet Pathol. 1983 May;20(3):298-311.
6. Miyadera K, Kato K, Aguirre-Hernández J, et. al.: Phenotypic variation and genotype-phenotype discordance in canine cone-rod dystrophy with an RPGRIP1 mutation. Mol Vis. 2009 Nov 11;15:2287-305.
7. Giger U, Reilly MP, Asakura T, et. al.: Autosomal recessive inherited phosphofructokinase deficiency in English springer spaniel dogs. Anim Genet. 1986;17(1):15-23.
8. Skelly BJ, Sargan DR, Winchester BG, et. al.: Genomic screening for fucosidosis in English Springer Spaniels. Am J Vet Res. 1999 Jun;60(6):726-9.
9. Smith MO, Wenger DA, Hill SL, et. al.: Fucosidosis in a family of American-bred English Springer Spaniels. J Am Vet Med Assoc. 1996 Dec 15;209(12):2088-90.
10. Alroy J, Orgad U, DeGasperi R, et. al.: Canine GM1-gangliosidosis. A clinical, morphologic, histochemical, and biochemical comparison of two different models. Am J Pathol. 1992 Mar;140(3):675-89.
11. Bamberger M, Houpt KA: Signalment factors, comorbidity, and trends in behavior diagnoses in dogs: 1,644 cases (1991-2001). J Am Vet Med Assoc. 2006 Nov 15;229(10):1591-601.
12. Bjerkas E, Ekesten B, Farstad W: Pectinate ligament dysplasia and narrowing of the iridocorneal angle associated with glaucoma in the English Springer Spaniel. Vet Ophthalmol. 2002 Mar;5(1):49-54.
13. Nachreiner RF, Refsal KR, Graham PA, et. al.: Prevalence of serum thyroid hormone autoantibodies in dogs with clinical signs of hypothyroidism. J Am Vet Med Assoc 2002 Feb 15;220(4):466-71.
14. Nachreiner R & Refsal K: Personal communication, Diagnostic Center for Population and Animal Health, Michigan State University. April, 2007.

15. Gelatt KN, MacKay EO: Secondary glaucomas in the dog in North America. Vet Ophthalmol. 2004 Jul-Aug;7(4):245-59.

16. Kuhl KA, Shofer FS, Goldschmidt MH: Comparative histopathology of pemphigus foliaceus and superficial folliculitis in the dog. Vet Pathol. 1994 Jan;31(1):19-27.

17. Patterson EE, Armstrong PJ, O'Brien DP, et. al.: Clinical description and mode of inheritance of idiopathic epilepsy in English springer spaniels. J Am Vet Med Assoc. 2005 Jan 1;226(1):54-8.

18. Dorn CR: Canine breed-specific risks of frequently diagnosed diseases at veterinary teaching hospitals. Monograph. AKC Canine Health Foundation. 2000.

19. Scott DW, Miller WH: Primary seborrhoea in English springer spaniels: a retrospective study of 14 cases. J Small Anim Pract. 1996 Apr;37(4):173-8.

20. Hawkins EC, Basseches J, Berry CR, et. al.: Demographic, clinical, and radiographic features of bronchiectasis in dogs: 316 cases (1988-2000). J Am Vet Med Assoc. 2003 Dec 1;223(11):1628-35.

21. Mason KV, Halliwell RE, McDougal BJ: Characterization of lichenoid-psoriasiform dermatosis of springer spaniels. J Am Vet Med Assoc. 1986 Oct 15;189(8):897-901.

22. Rivera P, Melin M, Biagi T, et. al.: Mammary tumor development in dogs is associated with BRCA1 and BRCA2. Cancer Res. 2009 Nov 15;69(22):8770-4.

23. Hernblad Tevell E, Bergvall K, & Egenvall A: Sebaceous adenitis in Swedish dogs, a retrospective study of 104 cases. Acta Vet Scand. 2008 May 25;50:11.

24. Macklin, A: Immune-Mediated Hemolytic Anemia: Pathophysiology & Diagnosis. Proceedings, 2009 Western Veterinary Conference. 2009.

25. McAlees TJ: Immune-mediated haemolytic anaemia in 110 dogs in Victoria, Australia. Aust Vet J. 2010 Jan;88(1-2):25-8.

26. Watson PJ, Scase TJ, Roulois AJA, et. al.: Prevalence and Breed Distribution of Hepatic Lesions at Post Mortem in a First Opinion Dog Population and Their Association with Pancreatic Disease. Proceedings, 2009 British Small Animal Veterinary Congress. 2009.

27. Bexfield NH, Scase TJ, Warman SM, et. al.: Chronic Hepatitis in the English Springer Spaniel. Proceedings, 17th ECVIM-CA Congress. 2007.

28. Fonfara S, Loureiro JF, Swift S, et. al.: English springer spaniels with significant bradyarrhythmias--presentation, troponin I and follow-up after pacemaker implantation. J Small Anim Pract. 2010 Mar;51(3):155-61.

29. Johnson MS, Martin MW: Successful medical treatment of 15 dogs with pyothorax. J Small Anim Pract. 2007 Jan;48(1):12-6.

30. Oda K, Lambert EH, Lennon VA, et. al.: Congenital canine myasthenia gravis: I. Deficient junctional acetylcholine receptors. Muscle Nerve. 1984 Nov-Dec;7(9):705-16.

31. Inuzuka T, Duncan ID, Quarles RH: Myelin proteins in the CNS of 'shaking pups'. Brain Res. 1986 Jun;392(1-2):43-50.

32. Griffiths IR, Duncan ID, McCulloch M, et. al.: Shaking pups: a disorder of central myelination in the Spaniel dog. Part 1. Clinical, genetic and light-microscopical observations. J Neurol Sci. 1981 Jun;50(3):423-33.

33. Maddux JM, Edwards DF, Barnhill MA, et. al.: Neutrophil function in dogs with congenital ciliary dyskinesia. Vet Pathol. 1991 Sep;28(5):347-53.

34. Edwards DF, Kennedy JR, Patton CS, et. al.: Familial immotile-cilia syndrome in English springer spaniel dogs. Am J Med Genet. 1989 Jul;33(3):290-8.

35. The Genetic Connection: A Guide to Health Problems in Purebred Dogs. L Ackerman. p. 212, AAHA Press, 1999.

36. Holland CT, Canfield PJ, Watson AD, et. al.: Dyserythropoiesis, polymyopathy, and cardiac disease in three related English springer spaniels. J Vet Intern Med. 1991 May-Jun;5(3):151-9.

37. Tauro A, Talbot CE, Pratt JN, et. al.: Suspected mitochondrial myopathy in a springer spaniel. Vet Rec. 2008 Sep 27;163(13):396-7.

38. *The Complete Dog Book, 20th Ed.* The American Kennel Club. Howell Book House, NY 2006. p 93-98.

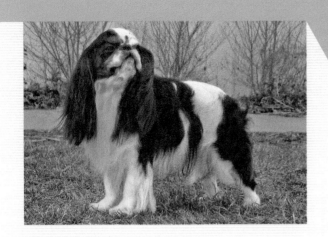

The Breed History

This spaniel was popular in the 17th century with English royalty. The breed was thought to have been in the British Isles for a while before it's popularity peaked. Most agree the root of the breed originally traces back to Japan and China. These original oriental spaniels were probably crossed with Cocker Spaniels, and perhaps Pugs and Springer Spaniels to make up the original progenitor, the Toy Spaniel. The *Blenheim strain*, a chestnut red and white type, was bred for many generations by the Duke of Marlborough. Note that the English Toy Spaniel and the Cavalier King Charles spaniel share close origins (the Toy Spaniel).

Breeding for Function

Toy Spaniels were used for hunting, and this breed was favored for woodcocks. They were also selected for companionship.

Physical Characteristics

Height at Withers: 10" (25.5 cm)

Weight for Females and Males: The ideal is 9-12 lb (4-5.5 kg), but they are accepted up to 14 lb and down to 8 lb.

Coat: The soft coat is long, straight to slightly wavy, with plenty of feathers on limbs. Length varies somewhat between the color varieties. Blenheim dogs have distinct color patches in a specific distribution including a "Blenheim spot", a red marking on top and centered on the skull. Prince Charles dogs are a tri-color of white with patches of black and tan. King Charles dogs are black and tan. Ruby dogs are mahogany red. On the last two color varieties, a very small white chest patch is acceptable.

Longevity: 10-12 years.

Points of Conformation: They possess a square build, with large, dark eyes. The brachycephalic head has a very short muzzle, domed skull, big black nose, prominent stop, and the head is large for the compact body size. The jaw is normally a bit prognathic. They are cobby with good bone but not coarse, and ears are pendulous with thick leather and well feathered. The topline has a moderate arch, back is short and broad and the tail is docked and carried level. Feathering on the tail hangs like a "flag" ~ 3 " long, and some puppies are born with naturally short or screw tails (these are not penalized). The feet are compact and small, fused toes can be seen,

but are not faulted. They have a lively gait that is straight with a good length of stride.

Recognized Behavior Issues and Traits

These dogs are reported to be: very friendly; these make excellent companion dogs. They should be socialized early to discourage timidity. They enjoy close companionship, and are alarm barkers. They are average shedders, and have average grooming needs. They are not particularly active, and do well in town or country, and need only light exercise.

Normal Physiologic Variations

None reported

Drug Sensitivities

None reported

Inherited Diseases

Hip Dysplasia and Legg-Calve Perthes Disease: Polygenically inherited traits causing degenerative hip joint disease and arthritis. Reported at a high frequency, but too few English Toy Spaniels have been screened by OFA to determine an accurate frequency.[1]

Patella Luxation: Polygenically inherited laxity of patellar ligaments, causing luxation, lameness, and later degenerative joint disease. Treat surgically if causing clinical signs. OFA reports 3.0% affected.[1]

Elbow Dysplasia: Polygenically inherited trait causing elbow arthritis. Too few English Toy Spaniels have been screened by OFA to determine an accurate frequency.[1]

Disease Predispositions

Persistent Hyaloid Artery: Congenital defect resulting from abnormalities in the development and regression of the hyaloid artery. Identified in 13.07% of English Toy Spaniels CERF examined by veterinary ophthalmologists between 2000-2005.[2]

Distichiasis: Abnormally placed eyelashes that irritate the cornea and conjunctiva. Can cause secondary corneal ulceration. Identified in 11.36% of English Toy Spaniels CERF examined by veterinary ophthalmologists between 2000-2005.[2]

Retinal Dysplasia: Retinal folds, geographic, and generalized retinal dysplasia with detachment are recognized in the breed. Can lea to retinal detachment and blindness. Reported in 11.36% of English Toy Spaniels CERF examined by veterinary ophthalmologists between 2000-2005. CERF does not recommend breeding any English Toy Spaniel with retinal dysplasia/folds.[2]

Entropion: Rolling in of eyelids, often causing corneal irritation or ulceration. Entropion is reported in 9.66% of English Toy Spaniels CERF examined by veterinary ophthalmologists between 2000-2005.[2]

Corneal Dystrophy: Causes opacities on the surface of the cornea. Average age of onset is 2-5 years. Unknown mode of inheritance. Identified in 9.66% of English Toy Spaniels CERF examined by veterinary ophthalmologists between 2000-2005.[2]

Cataracts: Onset of cataract in the English Toy Spaniel is at an early age (less than 6 months), affecting the cortex and nucleus with rapid progression to complete cataract, resulting in blindness. Capsular and punctate cataracts are also seen. Identified in 5.11% of English Toy Spaniels CERF examined by veterinary ophthalmologists between 2000-2005. CERF does not recommend breeding any English Toy Spaniel with a cataract.[2]

Hypothyroidism: Inherited autoimmune thyroiditis. 3.3% positive for thyroid auto-antibodies based on testing at Michigan State University. (Ave. for all breeds is 7.5%).[3,4]

Chiari type I malformation and Secondary Syringomyelia (SM): Occipital bone hypoplasia with foramen magnum obstruction and secondary syringomyelia occurs in the breed. Clinical signs of SM can present usually between 5 months and 3 years of age, and include persistent scratching at the shoulder region with apparent neck, thoracic limb, or ear pain and thoracic limb lower motor neuron deficits. Diagnosis is by MRI.[5]

Glaucoma, Hydrocephalus, Mitral Valvular Disease, Open Fontanelle, Patent Ductus Arteriosus, and **Umbilical Hernia** are reported on the ETSCA website.

Cleft Palate, Microphthalmia, and **Persistent Primary Vitreous** are reported.[6]

Isolated Case Studies
None reported.

Genetic Tests
Tests of Genotype: None

Tests of Phenotype: Recommend patella evaluation, hip and elbow radiographs, CERF eye examination, cardiac evaluation, and thyroid profile including autoantibodies.

Miscellaneous
- **Breed name synonyms:** King Charles Spaniel, Toy Spaniel, Prince Charles, Blenheim.
- **Registries:** AKC, CKC, UKC, NKC (National Kennel Club)
- **AKC rank (year 2008):** 125 (235 dogs registered)
- **Internet resources: English Toy Spaniel Club of America:** www.englishtoyspanielclubofamerica.org
  King Charles Spaniel Club (UK): www.king-charles-spaniel-club.co.uk

References
1. OFA Website breed statistics: www.offa.org Last accessed July 1, 2010.
2. *Ocular Disorders Presumed to be Inherited in Purebred Dogs.* American College of Veterinary Ophthalmologists. ACVO, 2007.
3. Nachreiner R & Refsal K: Personal communication, Diagnostic Center for Population and Animal Health, Michigan State University. April, 2007.
4. Nachreiner RF, Refsal KR, Graham PA, et. al.: Prevalence of serum thyroid hormone autoantibodies in dogs with clinical signs of hypothyroidism. J Am Vet Med Assoc 2002 Feb 15;220(4):466-71.
5. Churcher RK & Child G: Chiari 1/syringomyelia complex in a King Charles Spaniel. Aust Vet J. 2000 Feb;78(2):92-5.
6. The Genetic Connection: A Guide to Health Problems in Purebred Dogs. L Ackerman. p.216 AAHA Press, 1999.
7. *The Complete Dog Book, 20th Ed.* The American Kennel Club. Howell Book House, NY 2006. p 466-469.

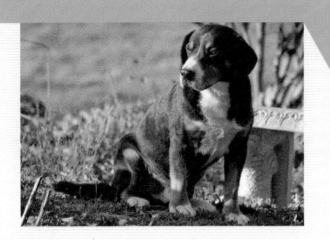

The Breed History

The Swiss Mountain dogs are descended from Molossus type dogs brought by the Romans as they passed through Helvetia over two thousand years ago. The Entlebucher Mountain Dog is the smallest of the four tri-colored Swiss Sennenhund breeds. Originating from Entlebuch, a valley in the district of the Cantons Lucerne and Berne, the first description under the name "Entlebucherhund" dates from the year 1889. The first breed standard was completed in 1927. AKC recognition occurred in 2011.

Breeding for Function

Swiss farmers have historically used the Entlebucher to move cows from pasture to pasture in the Alps. Their keen intelligence, speed and agility also made them useful for the management of other large animals such as horses and hogs.

Physical Characteristics

Height at withers: Males 17 to 21 inches (43-53 cm), Females 16 to 20 inches (40.5-51 cm).

Weight: 55-66 pounds (25-30 kg).

Coat: Double coat. Topcoat short, close fitting, harsh and shiny. Undercoat dense. Tricolor. Basic color must be black with tan (fawn to mahogany) and white markings, which should be as symmetric as possible. The tan markings are placed above the eyes, on cheeks, muzzle, either side of the chest, under the tail, and on all four legs. On legs, the tan is situated between the black and the white. White markings include a distinct small blaze, which runs without interruption from top of head over bridge of nose, and can wholly or partially cover the muzzle. White from chin to chest without interruption. White on all four feet.

Longevity: 11-15 years.

Points of Conformation: Strongly muscled, agile, balanced dog with ample bone; but never overdone. Head is slightly wedged-shaped, clean with parallel lines. Eyes are slightly small, almond shaped, brown with black rims. Ears are high set, nearly level with the topskull, wide, and triangular. Nose and lip margins are black. Teeth are scissors or even. Level topline. Length is elongated in the rib cage and not in loin. Length to height ratio 10 to 8 measured from point of shoulder to point of rump and ground to withers. Tail is natural bob or cropped, with the tail set in continuation of the gently sloping croup. Shoulders are laid back. Upper arm length equal or slightly shorter than shoulder blade. Angle of shoulder blade forming a right angle. Stilfe is well angulated. Legs are short, sturdy, straight and parallel. Paws point straight forward, slightly rounded and well-arched. The gait is ground covering, free, and fluid with good reach and strong drive from rear. As the speed of the gait increases, legs converge – the rear more pronounced.

Recognized Behavior Issues and Traits

The Entlebucher is a confident cattle dog, neither shy nor vicious; may be reserved with strangers. He is lively, active, persistent, self-assured and determined. Cheerful and capable of learning, he is loyal and protective of family, herd and property. He is highly intelligent, versatile and adaptable with a strong willingness to work; is quick and responsive to commands. Entles excel at competitive sports and are willing and enthusiastic partners in any athletic canine activity. The Entlebucher should not be considered a breed for the casual owner. He will remain an active, highly energetic dog for his entire lifetime. Because of the guardian traits of this breed, thorough socialization is required during puppyhood.

Normal Physiologic Variations

None reported

Drug Sensitivities

None reported

Inherited Diseases

Hip Dysplasia: Polygenically inherited trait causing degenerative joint disease and hip arthritis. OFA reports 16.8% affected.[1]

Progressive Retinal Atrophy (prcd-PRA): Autosomal recessive progressive rod cone degeneration (prcd) form. Age of onset between 2-3 years, initially affecting night vision, and eventually causing blindness. 1.9% of Entlebucher Mountain Dogs CERF examined by veterinary ophthalmologists between 2000-2005 are identified as affected, and 1.59% as suspicious for PRA. In a German study, 11.1% of Entlebucher Mountain Dogs were diagnosed with progressive retinal atrophy. A genetic test is available. The frequency of the defective gene in the breed has not been published. CERF does not recommend breeding any Entlebucher Mountain Dog with PRA.[2,3,4]

Elbow Dysplasia: Polygenically inherited trait causing elbow arthritis. Too few Entlebucher Mountain Dogs have been screened by OFA to determine an accurate frequency.[1]

Patella Luxation: Polygenically inherited laxity of patellar ligaments, causing luxation, lameness, and later degenerative joint disease. Treat surgically if causing clinical signs. Too few Entlebucher Mountain Dogs have been screened by OFA to determine an accurate frequency.[1]

Disease Predispositions

Cataracts: Posterior cortex intermediate and diffuse cataracts predominate in the breed. Genomic research identifies a significant marker-trait association to a region on canine chromosome 1. Identified in 8.89% of Entlebucher Mountain Dogs CERF examined by veterinary ophthalmologists between 2000-2005. In a German study, 23.5% of Entlebucher Mountain Dogs were diagnosed with noncongenital cataracts, with a heritability of 0.15 to 0.32. CERF does not recommend breeding any Entlebucher Mountain Dog with a cataract.[2,4,5]

Persistent Pupillary Membranes: Strands of fetal remnant connecting; iris to iris, cornea, lens, or involving sheets of tissue. The later three forms can impair vision, and dogs affected with these forms should not be bred. Identified in 6.35% of Entlebucher Mountain Dogs CERF examined by veterinary ophthalmologists between 2000-2005.[2]

Ureteral Ectopia: Congenital disorder identified in related North American Entlebucher Mountain Dogs. Affected dogs present with varying combinations of urinary incontinence, hydronephrosis, and urinary tract infection. Diagnose with excretory urography, ultrasonography, and urethrocystoscopy. Findings include bilateral intravesicular ectopic ureters (usually associated with hydronephrosis), and bilateral extravesicular ectopic ureters (usually associated with incontinence). Reported at a high frequency. Undetermined mode of inheritance.[6]

Hypothyroidism: Inherited autoimmune thyroiditis. Not enough samples have been submitted for thyroid auto-antibodies to Michigan State University to determine an accurate frequency. (Ave. for all breeds is 7.5%).[7,8]

Glaucoma: Ocular condition causing increased pressure within the eyeball, and secondary blindness due to damage to the retina. Diagnose with tonometry and gonioscopy. In a Swiss study, 3.3% of Entlebucher Mountain Dogs were diagnosed with glaucoma, associated with goniodysgenesis. CERF does not recommend breeding any Entlebucher Mountain Dog with glaucoma.[2,9]

Isolated Case Studies
None Reported

Genetic Tests

Tests of Genotype: Direct test for prcd-PRA is available from Optigen.

Tests of Phenotype: Recommend hip and elbow radiographs, CERF eye examination, thyroid profile including autoantibodies, cardiac examination, and patella evaluation.

Miscellaneous

- **Breed name synonyms:** Entlebucher Sennenhund, Entlebucher Cattle Dog, Entelbuch Mountain Dog, Shepherd Dog from Entlebuch, Dog of the Alpine Herdsman, Entles
- **Registries:** AKC, UKC, CKC, FCI, KCGB (Kennel Club of Great Britain), NKC (National Kennel Club)
- **AKC rank (none):** AKC recognized in January, 2011. Entire stud book entered.

- Internet resources: National Entlebucher Mountain Dog Association: www.nemda.org
  Entlebucher Mountain Dog Club of America: www.emdca.com
  Entlebucher Mountain Dog Club of Great Britain: www.entlebucher.co.uk

References

1. OFA Website breed statistics: www.offa.org Last accessed July 1, 2010.
2. *Ocular Disorders Presumed to be Inherited in Purebred Dogs.* American College of Veterinary Ophthalmologists. ACVO, 2007.
3. Zangerl B, Goldstein O, Philp AR, et. al.: Identical mutation in a novel retinal gene causes progressive rod-cone degeneration in dogs and retinitis pigmentosa in humans. Genomics. 2006 Nov;88(5):551-63.
4. Heitmann M, Hamann H, Brahm R, et. al.: Analysis of prevalence of presumed inherited eye diseases in Entlebucher Mountain Dogs. Vet Ophthalmol. 2005 May-Jun;8(3):145-51.
5. Müller C & Distl O: Association study of candidate genes for primary cataracts and fine-mapping of a candidate region on dog chromosome 1 in Entlebucher mountain dogs. Mol Vis. 2008 May 16;14:883-8.
6. North C, Kruger JM, Venta PJ, et. al.: Congenital Ureteral Ectopia in Continent and Incontinent-Related Entlebucher Mountain Dogs: 13 Cases (2006-2009). J Vet Intern Med. 2010 Sept-Oct;24(5):1055-62.
7. Nachreiner R & Refsal K: Personal communication, Diagnostic Center for Population and Animal Health, Michigan State University. April, 2007.
8. Nachreiner RF, Refsal KR, Graham PA, et. al.: Prevalence of serum thyroid hormone autoantibodies in dogs with clinical signs of hypothyroidism. *J Am Vet Med Assoc* 2002 Feb 15;220(4):466-71
9. Spiess BM: Inherited eye diseases in the Entlebucher mountain dog. Schweiz Arch Tierheilkd. 1994;136(3):105-10.
10. AKC Breed Website: www.akc.org/breeds/entlebucher_mountain_dog Last accessed July 1, 2010.

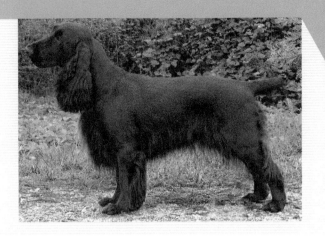

Field Spaniel

muscular with a slight arch. The topline is level. The thorax is deep, the rib cage stays deep caudally and ribs are well sprung. There is little abdominal tuck up, and the low set tail is usually docked. Limbs are straight boned, feet are webbed, large, and round with thick pads. No dewclaws. These dogs are smooth moving with a long low gait and high head carriage.

The Breed History
In the early years of spaniel breed development, the spaniels were divided into water and land spaniels. The land spaniels were generally called Field Spaniels in the 1800s, but in 1892 small spaniels, now termed English Cocker Spaniels were officially split into a new breed based on their lesser weight (< 25 lb). Originally, breeders wished to develop a black spaniel breed. For a while Field Spaniel breeding programs produced a dog of extremely exaggerated type due to repeated outcrosses with Welsh Cocker Spaniel, Basset Hound and Sussex Spaniels. This made them unsuited in conformation for their work. By the 1940s the breed was threatened by extinction. The Field Spaniel breed was recovered by implementing selective breeding practices, and by out-crossing to Cocker Spaniels and English Springer Spaniels. This restored a functional breed type. Field Spaniels are smaller than English Springer Spaniels.

Breeding for Function
Their primary purpose was as a bird dog, particularly for water and heavy cover work. Dogs were selected for good endurance and for tolerance of extreme temperatures.

Physical Characteristics
Height at Withers: female 17" (43 cm), male 18" (45.5 cm)

Weight: 35-50 lb (16-23 kg)

Coat: This single coated dog has colors of liver, black, or roan. The base color may be combined with tan points. Small white chest markings are allowed. The hair is long and lies flat, is straight to slightly wavy, fine and glossy, with feathering as for the setter type.

Longevity: 10-12 years

Points of Conformation: These dogs possess good bone, moderate size and muscling, and are a bit longer than tall. Dark brown to dark hazel moderately deep-set almond shaped eyes are medium in size. Palpebral margins and nose match in pigmentation. No nictitans should be visible. Long, low-set pendulous ears are well feathered, with moderate leather and the tips rounded. There is a distinct occipital protuberance, the muzzle is strong and long, stop is moderate, and the face is well chiseled under the eyes. The nose is large, the nostrils, the lips close and clean, and the neck is long and

Recognized Behavior Issues and Traits
Reported characteristics include: Gentle disposition, high activity levels, need human companionship, independent streak, intelligent, playful though reserved with strangers. Sensitive, friendly, need to have a fence if off leash, high exercise needs, and need early socialization to children. Grooming needs are minimal.

Normal Physiologic Variations
None reported

Drug Sensitivities
None reported

Inherited Diseases
Hip Dysplasia: Polygenically inherited trait causing degenerative joint disease and hip arthritis. OFA reports 18.7% affected. Reported at a frequency of 6.05% in the 2002-2003 Field Spaniel Health Survey.[1,2]

Patella Luxation: Polygenically inherited laxity of patellar ligaments, causing luxation, lameness, and later degenerative joint disease. Treat surgically if causing clinical signs. OFA reports 1.3% affected.[1]

Elbow Dysplasia: Polygenically inherited trait causing elbow arthritis. OFA reports 0.6% affected.[1]

Disease Predispositions
Retinal Dysplasia: Retinal folds, geographic, and generalized retinal dysplasia with detachment are recognized in the breed. Can cause retinal detachment and blindness. Reported in 8.75% of Field Spaniels CERF examined by veterinary ophthalmologists between 2000-2005.[3]

Hypothyroidism: Inherited autoimmune thyroiditis. 6.8% positive for thyroid auto-antibodies based on testing at Michigan State University. (Ave. for all breeds is 7.5%). Reported at a frequency of 8.97% in the 2002-2003 Field Spaniel Health Survey.[1,4,5]

Persistent Pupillary Membranes: Strands of fetal remnant connecting; iris to iris, cornea, lens, or involving sheets of tissue. The later three forms can impair vision, and dogs affected with these forms should not be bred. Identified in 6.69% of Field Spaniels CERF examined by veterinary ophthalmologists between 2000-2005.[4]

Distichiasis: Abnormally placed eyelashes that irritate the cornea and conjunctiva. Can cause secondary corneal ulceration. Identified in 5.15% of Field Spaniels CERF examined by veterinary ophthalmologists between 2000-2005.[3]

Allergic Dermatitis: Inhalant or food allergy. Presents with pruritis and pyotraumatic dermatitis (hot spots). Reported at a frequency of 4.04% in the 2002-2003 Field Spaniel Health Survey.[2]

Cataracts: Anterior cortex punctate, intermediate, and capsular cataracts predominate in the breed. Identified in 3.26% of Field Spaniels CERF examined by veterinary ophthalmologists between 2000-2005. Reported at a frequency of 2.47% in the 2002-2003 Field Spaniel Health Survey. CERF does not recommend breeding any Field Spaniel with a cataract.[2,3]

Idiopathic Epilepsy: Can present with grand-mal or focal seizures. Appears later in the breed, usually between 5-9 years of age. Control with anticonvulsant seizure medication. Unknown mode of inheritance. Reported at a frequency of 1.12% in the 2002-2003 Field Spaniel Health Survey.[2]

Progressive Retinal Atrophy, and Subaortic Stenosis are reported.[6]

Isolated Case Studies

Renal Calculus: Report of a single case of a kidney stone in a Field Spaniel.[7]

Genetic Tests

Tests of Genotype: Direct test for black liver colors, and black or brown nose are available from HealthGene and VetGen.

Tests of Phenotype: CHIC Certification: Required testing includes CERF eye examination (at 2, 4, 6, and 8 years), hip radiograph, and thyroid profile including autoantibodies (at 2 & 6 years) and elbow radiographs. Optional recommended tests include patella examination and cardiac evaluation. (See CHIC website; www.caninehealthinfo.org).

Miscellaneous

- **Breed name synonyms:** none
- **Registries:** AKC, UKC, CKC, KCGB (Kennel Club of Great Britain), ANKC (Australian National Kennel Club), NKC (National Kennel Club)
- **AKC rank (year 2008):** 140 (117 dogs registered)
- **Internet resources: Field Spaniel Society of America:** http://fieldspaniels.org/
  Field Spaniel Society (UK): www.fieldspanielsociety.co.uk

References

1. OFA Website breed statistics: www.offa.org Last accessed July 1, 2010.
2. Field Spaniel Society of America: 2002-2003 Field Spaniel Health Survey. 2003.
3. *Ocular Disorders Presumed to be Inherited in Purebred Dogs.* American College of Veterinary Ophthalmologists. ACVO, 2007.
4. Nachreiner R & Refsal K: Personal communication, Diagnostic Center for Population and Animal Health, Michigan State University. April, 2007.
5. Nachreiner RF, Refsal KR, Graham PA, et. al.: Prevalence of serum thyroid hormone autoantibodies in dogs with clinical signs of hypothyroidism. J Am Vet Med Assoc 2002 Feb 15;220(4):466-71.
6. *The Genetic Connection: A Guide to Health Problems in Purebred Dogs.* L Ackerman. p. 216 AAHA Press, 1999.
7. Ling GV, Ruby AL, Johnson DL, et. al.: Renal calculi in dogs and cats: prevalence, mineral type, breed, age, and gender interrelationships (1981-1993). *J Vet Intern Med.* 1998 Jan-Feb;12(1):11-21.
8. *The Complete Dog Book, 20th Ed.* The American Kennel Club. Howell Book House, NY 2006. p. 99-101.

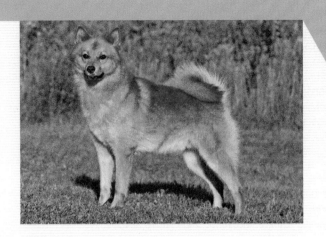

Finnish Spitz

The Breed History

This is the National Dog of Finland. Several thousand years ago in Central Russia, Spitz-type progenitor dogs such as the Russian Laika likely served as the primary gene pool. Due to outcrossing, by the year 1880 The Finnish Spitz dogs were nearly extinct. The final breed standard was drawn up in 1897 (final American standard, 1976). The first specimens arrived in England in 1927, and were exported to the USA in 1959. AKC accepted the Finnish Spitz for registry in the late 1980s.

Breeding for Function

Originally, the breed was a treeing dog (wild turkey, squirrels and martins), though now especially in North America he is primarily a companion dog. In Finland, barking contests are held; this breed possesses other types of vocalizations as well.

Pointing with his head, and tracking using sight, sound, and scent are breed characteristics. In Finland, any champion must prove himself in the field as well as the show ring. King barkers are those dogs that have a distinctive yodel that is judged to be optimal for hunting performance.

Physical Characteristics

Height at Withers: female 15.5-18" (39.5-45.5 cm), male 17.5-20" (44.5-51 cm)

Weight: 31-35 lb (14-16 kg)

Coat: The double coat is dense, outer coat is short (1-2" or 2.5-5 cm) and stands off; it is a very harsh and straight outer coat. The undercoat is lighter in color than the outer coat. Coat color is a red-gold color with a spectrum of a dark, light or in-between shade; coat and ruff is less well developed in the female. Only a few white markings are allowed; tips of toes and chest marks are allowed. Puppies are allowed to have more than what meets the breed standard in dark hairs but they generally fade as the dog matures.

Longevity: 12-15 years

Points of Conformation: A classic foxy "spitz" type is required, with the classic pointed muzzle, erect ears and alert expression. This dog is also characterized by a square conformation, high head carriage and quick gait. The small ears are alertly pricked and triangular, with a sharp point. Dark-rimmed eyes are almond in shape, slanted and moderately wide set; darker colored eyes preferred. There is a pronounced stop, the skull is broad and fairly flat, and the narrow muzzle tapers. The nose and lips are black and lips are tight. The topline is level, and the neck is muscular, not throaty. The thorax is deep with well-sprung ribs, and the abdomen only slightly tucked up. The tail is moderately high set, reaching the tarsus in length, and curls over the topline to rest along the thigh, with a well-developed plume. The limbs are straight boned with moderate muscling and bone, the feet are round, compact, and toes well arched. The dewclaws may be removed in front and in North America, are removed in back also.

Recognized Behavior Issues and Traits

Reported breed characteristics include: Excellent with children, loyal, friendly, courageous, lively with an independent streak, even strong willed. The Finnish Spitz likes cold environments. A well-developed tendency to bark exists due to their history as barking hunting dogs. This type of dog makes a good watchdog. Good with children and other pets, though inter-male dog aggression can be exhibited. High intelligence is characteristic; Finnish Spitz dogs are easily bored, and thus obedience training requires patience. Grooming needs are moderate, except during the heavy shedding season, and they have moderate to high exercise needs.

Normal Physiologic Variations

None reported

Drug Sensitivities

None reported

Inherited Diseases

Hip Dysplasia: Polygenically inherited trait causing degenerative joint disease and hip arthritis. OFA reports 6.1% affected.[1]

Patella Luxation: Polygenically inherited laxity of patellar ligaments, causing luxation, lameness, and later degenerative joint disease. Treat surgically if causing clinical signs. OFA reports 2.9% affected.[1]

Elbow Dysplasia: Polygenically inherited trait causing elbow arthritis. Too few Finnish Spitz have been screened by OFA to determine an accurate frequency.[1]

Disease Predispositions

Hypothyroidism: Inherited autoimmune thyroiditis. Too few Finnish Spitz have been tested for thyroid autoantibodies at Michigan State University to determine an accurate breed frequency. (Ave. for all breeds is 7.5%).[2,3]

Cataracts: Anterior and capsular punctate cataracts predominate in the breed. Identified in 4.35% of Finnish Spitz CERF examined by veterinary ophthalmologists between 2000-2005. CERF does not recommend breeding any Finnish Spitz with a cataract.[4]

Diabetes Mellitus: Sugar diabetes. Caused by a lack of insulin production by the pancreas. Control by insulin injections, diet, and glucose monitoring. Dorn reports an 8.07x odds ratio in Finnish Spitz versus other breeds. Unknown mode of inheritance.[5,6]

Idiopathic Epilepsy (Inherited Seizures): Focal and generalized seizures occur in the breed. Control with anticonvulsant medication. Dorn reports a 7.08x odds ratio in Finnish Spitz versus other breeds. Quantitative EEG analysis can be a useful diagnostic tool in this breed. Unknown mode of inheritance.[5,7]

Immune-Mediated Hemolytic Anemia: Auto-immune disorder where the body produces antibodies against its own red blood cells. Treated with immunosuppressive drugs. There is generally a female preponderance with this disorder. One study found a significantly higher risk in Finnish Spitz versus other breeds. Unknown mode of inheritance.[8]

Alopecia-X (black skin disease, BSD, coat funk): Progressive, symmetrical, non-pruritic, truncal hair loss usually beginning in early adulthood. ACTH, LDDS, and thyroid panel results are normal. Oral trilostane reverses the condition in some cases. The disorder appears to be familial.[9]

Pemphigus Foliaceous: Immune mediated skin disease characterized by crusty eruptions and pustules on the nasal plane, around the eyes and on the footpad. Mean age of onset is 4 years. Diagnosis by biopsy. The Finnish Spitz has a breed predisposition. Unknown mode of inheritance.[10,11]

Atresia Ani (Imperforate Anus): An increased incidence of this congenital condition is reported in the breed, with a frequency of 0.09%, and an odds ratio of 19.40x. Treatment is surgery.[12]

Cleft lip/palate, Glaucoma, Lupus Erythrematosus, Pituitary Dwarfism, Pulmonic Stenosis, Shaker Syndrome, and **Thrombopathia** are reported.[13]

Genetic Tests

Tests of Genotype: none

Tests of Phenotype: Recommend hip and elbow radiographs, patella evaluation, CERF eye examination, thyroid profile including autoantibodies, and cardiac evaluation.

Miscellaneous

- **Breed name synonyms:** Finsk Spets, Suomenpystykorva, Finky, Finkie, Finnish Barking Birddog (historical).
- **Registries:** AKC, UKC, CKC, KCGB (Kennel Club of Great Britain), ANKC (Australian National Kennel Club).
- **AKC rank (year 2008):** 153 (47 dogs registered)
- **Internet resources: Finnish Spitz Club of America:** www.finnishspitzclub.org
  The Finnish Spitz Club (Finland): www.spj.fi

References

1. OFA Website breed statistics: www.offa.org Last accessed July 1, 2010.
2. Nachreiner RF, Refsal KR, Graham PA, et. al.: Prevalence of serum thyroid hormone autoantibodies in dogs with clinical signs of hypothyroidism. J Am Vet Med Assoc 2002 Feb 15;220(4):466-71.
3. Nachreiner R & Refsal K: Personal communication, Diagnostic Center for Population and Animal Health, Michigan State University. April, 2007.
4. *Ocular Disorders Presumed to be Inherited in Purebred Dogs.* American College of Veterinary Ophthalmologists. ACVO, 2007.
5. Dorn CR: Canine breed-specific risks of frequently diagnosed diseases at veterinary teaching hospitals. Monograph. AKC Canine Health Foundation. 2000.
6. Marmor M, Willeberg P, Glickman LT, et. al.: Epizootiologic patterns of diabetes mellitus in dogs. *Am J Vet Res* 1982: 43:465-70.
7. Jeserevics J, Viitmaa R, Cizinauskas S, et. al.: Electroencephalography findings in healthy and Finnish Spitz dogs with epilepsy: visual and background quantitative analysis. J Vet Intern Med. 2007 Nov-Dec;21(6):1299-306.
8. Miller SA, Hohenhaus AE, Hale AS: Case-control study of blood type, breed, sex, and bacteremia in dogs with immune-mediated hemolytic anemia. *J Am Vet Med Assoc.* 2004 Jan 15;224(2):232-5.
9. Rosychuk RAW: Canine Alopecias: What's New? Proceedings, 2008 Western Veterinary Conference. 2008.
10. Breton K: Death & Derm: Deadly Dermatologic Diseases. Proceedings, 2004 ACVIM Forum. 2004.
11. Kuhl KA, Shofer FS, Goldschmidt MH: Comparative histopathology of pemphigus foliaceus and superficial folliculitis in the dog. *Vet Pathol.* 1994 Jan;31(1):19-27.
12. Vianna ML, Tobias KM: Atresia ani in the dog: a retrospective study. J Am Anim Hosp Assoc. 2005 Sep-Oct;41(5):317-22.
13. *The Genetic Connection: A Guide to Health Problems in Purebred Dogs.* L Ackerman. p. 217. AAHA Press, 1999.
14. *The Complete Dog Book, 20th Ed.* The American Kennel Club. Howell Book House, NY 2006. p. 558-562.

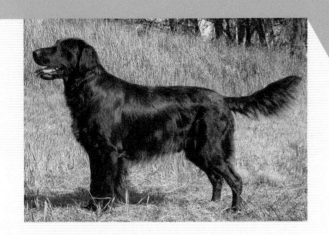

The Breed History

All-purpose retriever dogs were developed by crossing Newfoundland, Spaniel, Setter and Sheepdog type dogs. In the early 19th century, the Black Retriever was found throughout England. Further crosses produced a dog found both in Britain and Newfoundland/Labrador Canada known as the Lesser Newfoundland or St. John's Newfoundland. These dogs subsequently became a source for further crosses with English breeds, resulting in the curly coated retriever from which originated the flat-coated variety. AKC registry began in 1915.

Breeding for Function

At home in cold water, in thick underbrush and field, this has always been a soft-mouthed retriever, and these dogs are still cherished as field trial dogs. Birds, rabbits and hare are common quarry of the hunt. Many are also companions, and the Flat-coated Retriever excels in tracking and agility.

Physical Characteristics

Height at Withers: female 22-23.5" (56-59.5 cm), male 23-24.5" (58.5-62 cm).

Weight: 60-80 lb (27-36.5 kg).

Coat: The thick to slightly wavy flat glossy double coat has well developed feathering. Solid black or liver are accepted colors. Hairs are fine and the undercoat is dense.

Longevity: 12-14 years

Points of Conformation: Bred for function, the conformation is moderate. They are a little longer than high. The distinctive head is smooth and flat with minimal stop, a deep long muzzle, and the neck is moderately long, muscular and slightly arched. No throatiness should be evident. The eyes are dark brown or hazel, wide set and moderate in size, almond-shaped with kind expression. Nose and palpebral margins are black or liver in pigmentation. Lips are tight and dry. Small pendulous ears are thick leathered, well feathered and lie against the head. They possess a level topline, the thorax is deep and the rib cage stays deep well back. The abdomen is moderately tucked up. A wagging tail is characteristic. The gait is emphasized—it must be smooth, long and low. The tail tapers to the tarsus; is carried up but not above topline level, and a slight

bend to the tail is present, but not curled. Limbs are straight boned, moderate in length and front dewclaws may be removed (rear dewclaws are absent), feet are oval to round and toes well arched with thick pads.

Recognized Behavior Issues and Traits

Reported breed characteristics include: High intelligence, enjoys human companionship and has a strong will to work, loyal, playful, happy, active, stable temperament, a wagging tail is highly valued as an indicator of this breed's joyful demeanor. Gets along well with other dogs, is good with children though because of size and activity levels, supervision of young children is important. The Flat coat is good in city or country with adequate exercise. This breed retains vigor into old age. These dogs are considered adequate alarm barkers but not considered a guard dog. They have low grooming needs. Pica, separation anxiety and aggression (inter-dog) are listed behavior problems found in the breed.

Normal Physiologic Variations

None reported

Drug Sensitivities

None reported

Inherited Diseases

Hip Dysplasia: Polygenically inherited trait causing degenerative joint disease and hip arthritis. OFA reports 4.3% affected.[1]

Patella Luxation: Polygenically inherited laxity of patellar ligaments, causing luxation, lameness, and later degenerative joint disease. Treat surgically if causing clinical signs. OFA reports 1.8% affected. Reported at a frequency of 4.2% in males, and 3.2% in females in the 2000 FCRSA Health Survey.[1,2]

Elbow Dysplasia: Polygenically inherited trait causing elbow arthritis. OFA reports 0.8% affected.[1]

Disease Predispositions

Pectinate Ligament Dysplasia (PLD) and Glaucoma: PLD is a significant predisposing factor to the development of glaucoma. Blindness and lens luxation can occur with glaucoma if not treated quickly. PLD occurs in 34.7% of Flat Coated Retrievers, and has an estimated heritability of 0.7. Diagnose with gonioscopy and tonometry. Glaucoma is reported at a frequency of 1.0% in the breed. CERF does not recommend breeding any Flat Coated Retriever with glaucoma.[3,4,5,6]

Distichiasis: Abnormally placed eyelashes that irritate the cornea and conjunctiva. Can cause secondary corneal ulceration. Identified in 11.12% of Flat-coated Retrievers CERF examined by veterinary ophthalmologists between 2000-2005.[5]

Malignant Histiocytosis: Malignant histiocytomas are soft-tissue sarcomas that can occur in the skin, thorax, lungs, liver, spleen, kidneys, adrenal glands and brain. Treatment is palliative, as this malignant disease is fatal. Soft Tissue Sarcomas account for 55% of the malignant samples, and 26% of all tumor samples in a study of 1,023 Flat Coated Retriever tissue samples. 63% of the soft tissue sarcomas were diagnosed as undifferentiated. In a UK study 20.9% of deaths were from soft tissue sarcomas, at a median age of 8 years.[7,8,9,10]

Hypothyroidism: Inherited autoimmune thyroiditis. 5.0% positive for thyroid autoantibodies based on testing at Michigan State University. (Ave. for all breeds is 7.5%).[11,12]

Inherited Epilepsy: Generalized or partial seizures. Control with anticonvulsant medication. Reported at a frequency of 4.1% in males, and 1.5% in females in the 2000 FCRSA Health Survey.[2]

Gastric Dilatation-Volvulus (Bloat, GDV): Polygenically inherited, life-threatening twisting of the stomach. Requires immediate veterinary attention. Reported at a frequency of 3.8% in males, and 3.3% in females in the 2000 FCRSA Health Survey.[2]

Cataracts: Anterior cortex punctate cataracts predominate in the breed. Age of onset 4 years of age and older. Identified in 5.70% of Flat-coated Retrievers CERF examined by veterinary ophthalmologists between 2000-2005. CERF does not recommend breeding any Flat Coated Retriever with a cataract.[5]

Persistent Pupillary Membranes: Strands of fetal remnant connecting; iris to iris, cornea, lens, or involving sheets of tissue. The later three forms can impair vision, and dogs affected with these forms should not be bred. Identified in 2.66% of Flat Coated Retrievers CERF examined by veterinary ophthalmologists between 2000-2005.[5]

Benign Cutaneous Histiocytoma: These account for 48 per cent of the benign tumors, and 25 per cent of all tumor samples in a study of 1,023 Flat-coated Retriever tissue samples.[9]

Corneal Dystrophy, Ectropion, Entropion, Optic Nerve Hypoplasia, and **Progressive Retinal Atrophy** are reported.[13]

Isolated Case Studies

Immune-mediated Hemolytic Anemia with Concurrent Soft-tissue Sarcoma: A seven-year-old flat-coated retriever presenting with immune-mediated hemolytic anemia was also diagnosed a widespread, poorly differentiated sarcoma involving the lungs, pericardium, thoracic lymph nodes and spleen.[14]

Spinal Cord Epidermoid Cyst: Case study of a 1-1/2 year old flat-coated retriever with an intramedullary space-occupying lesion in the form of an epidermoid cyst. Complete excision was not possible, as the cystic tissue was intimately attached to the spinal cord parenchyma.[15]

Genetic Tests

Tests of Genotype: Direct tests for black, liver and yellow coat colors and black and brown nose are available from HeathGene and VetGen.

Tests of Phenotype: Recommend hip and elbow radiographs, patella examination, CERF eye examination, thyroid profile including autoantibodies, and cardiac evaluation.

Miscellaneous

- **Breed name synonyms:** Flat Coat, Flat-coat Retriever.
- **Registries:** AKC, UKC, CKC, KCGB (Kennel Club of Great Britain), ANKC (Australian National Kennel Club).
- **AKC rank (year 2008):** 98 (605 dogs registered)
- **Internet resources: Flat-coated Retriever Society of America Inc.:** www.fcrsainc.org
  Flatcoated Retriever Society (UK): www.flatcoated-retriever-society.org
  Flat-coated Retriever Society of Canada: www.flatcoat.ca
  Flat-Coated Retriever Foundation: www.fcrfoundation.org

References

1. OFA Website breed statistics: www.offa.org Last accessed July 1, 2010.
2. Flat Coated Retriever Society of America: 2000 Sharon Myers Health Survey. 2000.
3. Wood JL, Lakhani KH, Read RA: Pectinate ligament dysplasia and glaucoma in Flat Coated Retrievers. II. Assessment of prevalence and heritability. *Vet Ophthalmol.* 1998;1(2-3):91-99.
4. Read RA, Wood JLN, Lakhani KH: Pectinate ligament dysplasia (PLD) and glaucoma in Flat Coated Retrievers. I. Objectives, technique and results of a PLD survey. *Veterinary Ophthalmology* 1998: 1 (2-3), 85-90.
5. *Ocular Disorders Presumed to be Inherited in Purebred Dogs.* American College of Veterinary Ophthalmologists. ACVO, 2007.
6. Wood JL, Lakhani KH, & Henley WE: An epidemiological approach to prevention and control of three common heritable diseases in canine pedigree breeds in the United Kingdom. Vet J. 2004 Jul;168(1):14-27.
7. Brown DE, Thrall MA, Getzy DM, et. al.: Cytology of canine malignant histiocytosis. *Vet Clin Pathol.* 1994;23(4):118-123.
8. Morris JS, McInnes EF, Bostock DE, et. al: Immunohistochemical and histopathologic features of 14 malignant fibrous histiocytomas from Flat-Coated Retrievers. *Vet Pathol.* 2002 Jul;39(4):473-9.
9. Morris JS, Bostock DE, McInnes EF, et. al.: Histopathological survey of neoplasms in flat-coated retrievers, 1990 to 1998. *Vet Rec.* 2000 Sep 9;147(11):291-5.
10. Dobson J, Hoather T, McKinley TJ, et. al.: Mortality in a cohort of flat-coated retrievers in the UK. Vet Comp Oncol. 2009 Jun;7(2):115-21.
11. Nachreiner RF, Refsal KR, Graham PA, et. al.: Prevalence of serum thyroid hormone autoantibodies in dogs with clinical signs of hypothyroidism. J Am Vet Med Assoc 2002 Feb 15;220(4):466-71.
12. Nachreiner R & Refsal K: Personal communication, Diagnostic Center for Population and Animal Health, Michigan State University. April, 2007
13. *The Genetic Connection: A Guide to Health Problems in Purebred Dogs.* L Ackerman. p 217. AAHA Press, 1999.
14. Mellanby RJ, Holloway A, Chantrey J, et. al.: Immune-mediated haemolytic anaemia associated with a sarcoma in a flat-coated retriever. *J Small Anim Pract.* 2004 Jan;45(1):21-4.
15. Shamir MH, Lichovsky D, Aizenberg I, et. al.: Partial surgical removal of an intramedullary epidermoid cyst from the spinal cord of a dog. *J Small Anim Pract.* 1999 Sep;40(9):439-42.
16. *The Complete Dog Book, 20th Ed.* The American Kennel Club. Howell Book House, NY 2006. p. 42-46.

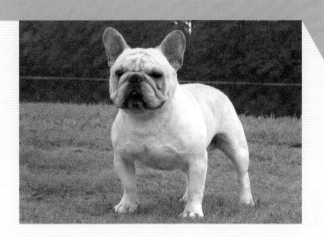

French Bulldog

The Breed History
The French Bulldog was derived from the English Bulldog in the mid 1800s. The French Bulldog is of smaller stature. First specimens reached the United States in 1896.

Breeding for Function
Their primary function has always been as a companion, but perhaps they also functioned in the household as ratters and as watchdogs. Though breeds from which they derive were fighting dogs, "Frenchies" were bred for a calm stable temperament and not viciousness.

Physical Characteristics
Height at Withers: 12" (30.5 cm)

Weight: Less than 28 lb (12.5 kg)

Coat: The very short, fine and flat glossy coat is brindle, white, brindle and white, or fawn. Black is a disqualification, as are liver, or black and tan, black and white, and mouse.

Longevity: 11-12 years

Points of Conformation: They possess a compact square conformation with heavy bone and muscling. The broad-based fine-leathered erect "bat" ears of the French Bulldog distinguish it from the English Bulldog (the latter having rose ears). Another distinguishing feature is the shape of the skull. In the French Bulldog it is flat between the ears but domed over the eyes, producing a strong-browed appearance. The head is large and square. The muzzle is short, broad and blocky, and the stop is well defined such that between the eyes there is a distinct groove. Wrinkles are set on a very short nose. The nose is black except in lighter colored dogs. The moderately deep-set dark eyes are set well apart and low in the skull forward facing, are round and moderate in size and don't show the nictitans. The lower jaw is prognathic with very prominent black flews. The neck is short, thick and arched, and covered with very loose skin. The short back is arched (roach). The abdomen is tucked up and the thorax is deep and broad (barrel-shaped). The tail may be screwed or straight, is low set, short and tapers to a fine tip. Limbs are ideally straight boned, feet are compact, and toes well knuckled up. The nails are stubby. Forelimbs are set wide apart. The gait is somewhat rolling due to the broad thorax.

Recognized Behavior Issues and Traits
Reported breed traits include: Intelligent, affectionate, alert, playful, love human companionship, low barking tendency, low shedding tendency, and low grooming needs. Good for city or country. Considered a good dog for seniors. Needs daily hygiene of facial wrinkles to prevent dermatitis. Tend to snore.

Normal Physiologic Variations
Cesarean Section: In Great Britain, 81.3% of French Bulldog litters are delivered by **C-section**.[1]

Drug Sensitivities
None reported

Inherited Diseases
Hip Dysplasia: Polygenically inherited trait causing degenerative joint disease and hip arthritis. OFA reports 32.6% affected.[2]

Patella Luxation: Polygenically inherited laxity of patellar ligaments, causing luxation, lameness, and later degenerative joint disease. Treat surgically if causing clinical signs. OFA reports 5.2% affected.[2]

Elbow Dysplasia: Polygenically inherited trait causing elbow arthritis. OFA reports 2.9% affected.[2]

Juvenile Cataracts (Hereditary Cataracts, HC): Autosomal recessive disorder causing bilateral nuclear and cortical cataracts with an onset around 3 months of age. Identified in 2.46% of French Bulldogs CERF examined by veterinary ophthalmologists between 2000-2005. CERF does not recommend breeding any French Bulldog with a cataract. A genetic test is available.[3]

Hemophilia B (Factor IX Deficiency): X-linked recessive coagulation disorder causing severe bleeding in this breed. In one family, concurrent Hemophilia A was identified.[4]

Disease Predispositions
Hemivertebra and Butterfly Vertebra: Misshapen or malformed vertebra. May cause scoliosis, pain, or spinal cord compression if severe. In the majority of affected French Bulldogs, the thoracic vertebrae are involved. Reported at a frequency of 35.1% in the FBDCA Health Survey. Unknown mode of inheritance.[5]

Brachycephalic Complex: The brachycephalic complex includes **stenotic nares, elongated soft palate, everted laryngeal saccules, laryngeal collapse,** and occasionally **hypoplastic trachea.** Can also cause bronchial collapse. Can cause difficulty breathing, and collapse if severe, or stressed. The FBDCA Health Survey reports the following frequencies: stenotic nares (21.6%0, elongated soft palate (15.8%), and hypoplastic trachea (4.36%).[5,6,7]

Allergic Dermatitis (Atopy): Inhalant or food allergy. Presents with pruritis and pyotraumatic dermatitis (hot spots). French Bulldogs show an increased prevalence versus other breeds for both inhalant and food allergy. Reported at a frequency of 28.0% in the FBDCA Health Survey, with food allergy reported at 14.2%.[5,8]

Distichiasis: Abnormally placed eyelashes that irritate the cornea and conjunctiva. Can cause secondary corneal ulceration. Identified in 6.96% of French Bulldogs CERF examined by veterinary ophthalmologists between 2000-2005.[3]

Intervertebral Disc Disease (IVDD): Acute spinal cord disease due to prolapsed disk material. Clinical signs include back pain, scuffing of paws, spinal ataxia, limb weakness, and paralysis. Reported at a frequency of 5.5% in the FBDCA Health Survey.[5]

Persistent Pupillary Membranes: Strands of fetal remnant connecting; iris to iris, cornea, lens, or involving sheets of tissue. The later three forms can impair vision, and dogs affected with these forms should not be bred. Identified in 4.50% of French Bulldogs CERF examined by veterinary ophthalmologists between 2000-2005.[3]

Cryptorchidism (Retained Testicles): Can be unilateral or bilateral. Reported at a frequency of 4.2% in the FBDCA Health Survey.[5]

Demodicosis: Generalized demodicosis has an underlying immunodeficiency in its pathogenesis. Reported at a frequency of 4.1% in the FBDCA Health Survey.[5]

Degenerative Myelopathy (DM): Affected dogs show an insidious onset of upper motor neuron (UMN) paraparesis at an average age of 11.4 years. The disease eventually progresses to severe tetraparesis. Affected dogs have normal results on myelography, MRI, and CSF analysis. Necropsy confirms the condition. Unknown mode of inheritance. A direct genetic test for an autosomal recessive DM susceptibility gene is available. All affected dogs are homozygous for the gene, however, only a small percentage of homozygous dogs develop DM. The susceptibility allele occurs at a frequency of 23% in the breed. Clinical DM is reported at a frequency of 2.3% in the FBDCA Health Survey.[5,9]

Retinal Dysplasia: Retinal folds, geographic, and generalized retinal dysplasia with detachment are recognized in the breed. Can cause retinal detachment and blindness. Reported in 2.05% of French Bulldogs CERF examined by veterinary ophthalmologists between 2000-2005.[3]

Entropion: Rolling in of the eyelids, which can predispose to corneal irritation and ulceration. Reported in 1.36% of French Bulldogs CERF examined by veterinary ophthalmologists between 2000-2005.[3]

Hypothyroidism: Inherited autoimmune thyroiditis. 1.1% positive for thyroid autoantibodies based on testing at Michigan State University. (Ave. for all breeds is 7.5%).[10,11]

Histiocytic Ulcerative Colitis: Several case studies are published. Affected dogs present with chronic large bowel diarrhea, tenesmus and hematochezia. Colonic biopsies are characterized by infiltrations of PAS positive histiocytes in the lamina propria. There may only be minimal improvement with nutritional and medical therapy. Unknown mode of inheritance.[12,13,14]

Pulmonic Stenosis (PS): Congenital cardiac disorder of restricted pulmonic outflow. Echocardiogram findings of restriction of right ventricular outflow tract, pulmonic valve and/or main pulmonary artery on transthoracic imaging from the right parasternal and left cranial parasternal short-axis views. Reported at an increased frequency in the breed.[15]

Hiatal Hernia: French Bulldogs have a predisposition to paraesophageal hiatal hernia.[16,17]

Necrotizing Meningoencephalitis: A non-suppurative acute to chronic necrotizing meningoencephalitis is identified in French Bulldogs, similar to that seen in the Pug, Maltese and Yorkshire Terrier breeds. Affected dogs present with seizures, ataxia, blindness and mentation changes from 1 to 10 years of age.[18,19]

Anasarca, Cleft Palate/Lip, Deafness, Fold Dermatitis, Spina Bifida, and **von Willebrand's Disease** are reported.[20]

Isolated Case Studies

Ventricular Septal Defect (VSD): Case report of a 4-month-old male French Bulldog with a left heart base grade 3/6 systolic murmur, and a right heart base grade 4/6 systolic murmur. Doppler ultrasonography and cardiac catheterization revealed a supracristal ventricular septal defect (VSD) with accompanying aortic regurgitation.[21]

Muscular Dystrophy: An 8 month old male French Bull dog was diagnosed with dystrophin deficient muscular dystrophy. Clinical signs included; apathy, muscle weakness, dysphagia, regurgitation and dyspnea.[22]

Fibrinoid Leukodystrophy: A 1 and 1/2 year old French bulldog exhibited megaesophagus, general emaciation and weakness, and died due to aspiration pneumonia. Histopathology revealed discolored foci in the white matter of the cerebellum and brain stem, with Rothenthal fibers and hypertrophic astrocytes in the perivascular, subependymal and subpial area.[23]

Oligodendroglioma: A 5-year-old, male French bulldog presented with bradycardia, dyspnea, and decerebrate rigidity was necropsied. Macroscopic findings were restricted to a brain mass consisting of diffuse proliferated neoplastic oligodendroglial cells characterized by small, round, and hyperchromatic nuclei with clear cytoplasm and the cells aggressively invaded into the adjacent parenchyma. The mass was diagnosed as oligodendroglioma.[24]

XX Sex Reversal: A 3-month-old outwardly female French Bulldog presented with an enlarged clitoris with an os clitoris, and inguinal hernias containing testicles. A diagnosis of SRY-negative XX sex reversal was made based on the gonadal histology and cytogenetic analysis.[25]

Genetic Tests

Tests of Genotype: Direct test for juvenile cataract is available from the Animal Health Trust and VetGen.

Direct test for the DM susceptability gene is available from OFA.

Direct tests for fawn, brindle(black) and liver coat colors, and black or brown nose are available from HealthGene.

Tests of Phenotype: CHIC Certification: Required testing includes hip radiographs, CERF eye examination (recommended annually) and patella evaluation. Recommended tests include thyroid profile including autoantibodies, and congenital cardiac disease evaluation. (See CHIC website; www.caninehealthinfo.org).

Recommend elbow radiographs.

Miscellaneous

- **Breed Name Synonyms:** Frenchie, Boule Dogue Français
- **Registries:** AKC, UKC, CKC, KCGB (Kennel Club of Great Britain), ANKC (Australian National Kennel Club), NKC (National Kennel Club)
- **AKC rank (year 2008):** 26 (6,963 dogs registered)
- **Internet resources: French Bulldog Club of America:**
  www.frenchbulldogclub.org
  French Bulldog Club of England:
  www.frenchbulldogclubofengland.org.uk
  French Bulldog Fanciers of Canada:
  www.frenchbulldogfanciers.com

References

1. Evans KM & Adams VJ: Proportion of litters of purebred dogs born by caesarean section. J Small Anim Pract. 2010 Feb;51(2):113-8.
2. OFA Website breed statistics: www.offa.org Last accessed July 1, 2010.
3. *Ocular Disorders Presumed to be Inherited in Purebred Dogs.* American College of Veterinary Ophthalmologists. ACVO, 2007.
4. Slappendel RJ: Hemophilia A and hemophilia B in a family of French bulldogs. *Tijdschr Diergeneeskd.* 1975 Oct 15;100(20):1075-88.
5. French Bull Dog Club of America: 2009 FBDCA Health Survey. 2009.
6. Monnet M: Brachycephalic Airway Syndrome. Proceedings, 2004 World Small Animal Veterinary Association Congress. 2004.
7. De Lorenzi D, Bertoncello D, & Drigo M: Bronchial abnormalities found in a consecutive series of 40 brachycephalic dogs. J Am Vet Med Assoc. 2009 Oct 1;235(7):835-40
8. Tarpataki N, Pápa K, Reiczigel J, et. al.: Prevalence and features of canine atopic dermatitis in Hungary. Acta Vet Hung. 2006 Sep;54(3):353-66.
9. Coates JR, Zeng R, Awano T, et. al.: An SOD1 Mutation Associated with Degenerative Myelopathy Occurs in Many Dog Breeds. Proceedings 2009 ACVIM Forum. 2009.
10. Nachreiner R & Refsal K: Personal communication, Diagnostic Center for Population and Animal Health, Michigan State University. April, 2007.
11. Nachreiner RF, Refsal KR, Graham PA, et. al.: Prevalence of serum thyroid hormone autoantibodies in dogs with clinical signs of hypothyroidism. J Am Vet Med Assoc. 2002 Feb 15;220(4):466-71.
12. Tanaka H, Nakayama M, Takase K, et. al.: Histiocytic ulcerative colitis in a French bulldog. *J Vet Med Sci.* 2003 Mar;65(3):431-3.
13. Van der Gaag I, Van Toorenburg JV, Voorhout G, et. al.: Histiocytic ulcerative colitis in a French Bulldog. *J Small Anim Pract.* 1978 May;19(5):283-90.
14. Hall EJ: Breed-Specific Intestinal Disease. Proceedings, 2004 World Small Animal Veterinary Association Congress. 2004.
15. Toschi Corneliani R, Locatelli C, Domenech O, et. al.: Retrospective Study of Pulmonic Stenosis in 259 Dogs. Proceedings, 18th ECVIM-CA Congress. 2008.
16. Washabau RJ: Diagnosis and Management of Swallowing Disorders. Proceedings, 2009 WSAVA World Congress. 2009.
17. Teunissen GH, Happe RP, Van Toorenburg J, et. al.: Esophageal hiatal hernia. Case report of a dog and a cheetah. *Tijdschr Diergeneeskd.* 1978 Jul 15;103(14):742-9.
18. Timmann D, Konar M, Howard J, et. al.: Necrotising encephalitis in a French bulldog. J Small Anim Pract. 2007 Jun;48(6):339-42.
19. Spitzbarth I, Schenk HC, Tipold A, et. al.: Immunohistochemical Characterization of Inflammatory and Glial Responses in a Case of Necrotizing Leucoencephalitis in a French Bulldog. J Comp Pathol. 2010 Feb-Apr;142(2-3):235-41.
20. *The Genetic Connection: A Guide to Health Problems in Purebred Dogs.* L Ackerman. p. 207. AAHA Press, 1999.
21. Shimizu M, Tanaka R, Hirao H, et. al.: Percutaneous transcatheter coil embolization of a ventricular septal defect in a dog. *J Am Vet Med Assoc.* 2005 Jan 1;226(1):69-72, 52-3.
22. Gama Filho HAN, Oliveira CM, Dias CTS, et. al.: Muscular Dystrophy in a French Bulldog: First Case Report. Proceedings, 2009 WSAVA World Congress. 2009
23. Ito T, Uchida K, Nakamura M, et. al.: Fibrinoid Leukodystrophy (Alexander's Disease-Like Disorder) in a Young Adult French Bulldog. J Vet Med Sci. 2010 Oct;72(10):1387-90.
24. Park CH: Oligodendroglioma in a French bulldog. *J Vet Sci.* 2003 Aug;4(2):195-7.
25. Campos M, Moreno-Manzano V, García-Roselló M, et. al.: SRY-Negative XX Sex Reversal in a French Bulldog. Reprod Domest Anim. 2011 Feb;46(1):185-8.
26. *The Complete Dog Book, 20th Ed.* The American Kennel Club. Howell Book House, NY 2006. p. 563-566.

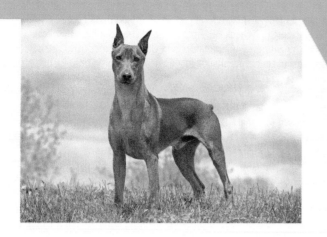

The Breed History

European guarding and herding dogs were used to develop this ancient breed. Originally called Smooth Haired Pinschers, these dogs were involved in German dog breed development for the other Pinschers and the Schnauzers. First records of the German Pinscher were from the mid 1800s. Before the World Wars, the breed contained the Schnauzer colors such as salt and pepper and pure black, colors now extinct and not in the breed standard. One person is credited for single-handedly saving the breed from extinction in the early 1950s. He was required to outcross the remaining few dogs at the start of his efforts in order to regenerate gene diversity. As popularity grew in America in the 1980s, the first national breed club was formed and the AKC accepted the breed.

Breeding for Function

An ancient breed, they are suitable for watchdog and companionship. Considered a very vigilant watch dog, they are suitable for experienced dog owners.

Physical Characteristics

Height at Withers: 17-20" (43-51 cm)

Weight: 25-45 lb (11-20 kg)

Coat: Coat is dense, close lying and short. Texture may be medium to hard, and the hairs should be glossy. Fawn (Isabella) through reds, to reds admixed with black (stag red). Richer full red is preferred in the red coated dogs. Also see black or blue with ideally, sharply demarcated red or tan markings. Marking distribution is specified in the breed standard. Any white is undesirable in this breed.

Longevity: 12-14 years

Points of Conformation: Square in proportion, this medium sized dog is well muscled. They have a blunt wedge-shaped flat skull, cheeks are flat, stop is barely visible. High set ears are sometimes cropped. Uncropped ears are triangular with a fold, though some stand erect. Eyes are oval and do not protrude, and have a piercing expression. Nose and lips are black, bite is a scissors. The neck is arched, and no loose skin should be evident. The topline slopes down slightly towards the rear, with a slight rise over the loin—back is short, abdomen has moderate tuck up. Tail usually docked short and is carried high. Moderately boned long straight limbs, front

dewclaws may be removed, round feet are small, well knuckled up with dark nails and pads. The gait is fluid with good reach, and no rolling.

Recognized Behavior Issues and Traits

Reported breed attributes include: Alert, active, intelligent and loves to learn, loyal, watchful, fearless, determined, high energy. Good endurance and vigilance, courageous when needed. Good alarm barker, but not an excessive barker. Strong chase drive. Obedience training is essential in order to channel a sometimes independent nature and assertive will. Stay playful well into maturity. These dogs may not be suited to be around young children (< 9) without supervision. Moderately active—tend to be dominant. They do best if given activities/work to do.

Normal Physiologic Variations

Dilute coat color is due to the homozygous recessive expression of a mutation in the melanophilin gene (MLPH). This can predispose to color dilution alopecia.[1]

Drug Sensitivities

None reported.

Inherited Diseases

Hip Dysplasia: Polygenically inherited trait causing degenerative joint disease and hip arthritis. OFA reports 0.7% affected.[2]

Elbow Dysplasia: Polygenically inherited trait causing elbow arthritis. OFA shows a high frequency, but too few German Pinschers have been screened to determine an accurate frequency.[2]

Patella Luxation: Congenital laxity of patellar ligaments causing luxation, lameness, and later degenerative joint disease. Treated surgically if causing clinical signs. Too few German Pinschers have been screened to determine an accurate frequency.[2]

von Willebrand's Disease (vWD) Type 1: Autosomal recessive genetic disorder causing a mild bleeding syndrome, usually after trauma or surgery. A genetic test is available, showing 17% testing carrier.

Disease Predispositions

Cataracts: Anterior or posterior intermediate and punctate cataracts occur in the breed. Diagnosed in 6.5% German Pinschers undergoing ophthalmoscopic examination in one survey. Pedigree analysis suggests recessive inheritance. Identified in 13.73% of German Pinschers CERF examined by veterinary ophthalmologists between 2000-2005. CERF does not recommend breeding any German Pinscher with a cataract.[3,4]

Persistent Hyperplastic Tunica Vasculosa Lentis (PHTVL): Presents with posterior polar subcapsular cataracts and pre-retinal glial proliferation. Diagnosed in 8.4% German Pinschers undergoing ophthalmoscopic examination in one survey. Pedigree analysis suggests recessive inheritance. CERF does not recommend breeding any German Pinscher with PHTVL.[3,4]

Optic Nerve Hypoplasia/Micropapilla: A congenital defect of the optic nerve which causes blindness. CERF does not recommend breeding any German Pinscher with the condition.[4]

Hypothyroidism: Inherited autoimmune thyroiditis. 5.3% positive for thyroid auto-antibodies based on testing at Michigan State University. (Ave. for all breeds is 7.5%).[5,6]

Persistent Pupillary Membranes: Strands of fetal remnant connecting; iris to iris, cornea, lens, or involving sheets of tissue. The later three forms can impair vision, and dogs affected with these forms should not be bred. Identified in 3.27% of German Pinschers CERF examined by veterinary ophthalmologists between 2000-2005.[4]

Color Dilution Alopecia (CDA): Hair loss syndrome associated with the dilute coat color. Starts as a gradual onset of dry, dull and poor hair coat quality. Progresses to poor hair regrowth, follicular papules and comedomes. Hair loss and comedome formation are usually most severe on the trunk.[1]

Corneal Dystrophy: Causes opacities on the surface of the cornea. Unknown mode of inheritance. Identified in 1.96% of German Pinschers CERF examined by veterinary ophthalmologists between 2000-2005.[4]

Persistent Right Aortic Arch (PRAA): Eighteen young German Pinschers in 16 litters from Germany and the Netherlands had megaesophagus secondary to PRAA with an aberrant left subclavian artery. Surgery is corrective. A complex mode of inheritance was suggested.[7]

Isolated Case Studies

XX Sex Reversal: A 5 month-old German Pinscher presented with an enlarged clitoris. Surgery revealed a uterus, and two histologically confirmed ovotestes. The dog had an XX karyotype, and tested negative for the SRY gene, so a diagnosis of XX sex reversal was offered.[8]

Genetic Tests

Tests of Genotype: Direct test for von Willebrand's Disease (vWD) is available from VetGen.

Tests of Phenotype: CHIC Certification: Required testing includes CERF eye examination, hip radiographs, and genetic test for vWD. Optional recommended test includes cardiac evaluation (echocardiogram). (See CHIC website; www.caninehealthinfo.org).

Recommend thyroid profile including autoantibodies, elbow radiographs, and patella examination.

Miscellaneous

- **Breed name synonyms:** Standard Pinscher, Historical SYN: Smooth Haired Pinscher.
- **Registries:** AKC, CKC, FCI, KCGB (Kennel Club of Great Britain), ANKC (Australian National Kennel Club), NKC (National Kennel Club)
- **AKC rank (year 2008):** 141 (108 dogs registered)
- **Breed resources: German Pinscher Club of America:** www.german-pinscher.com
  German Pinscher Club (UK): www.germanpinscher.org.uk

References

1. Philipp U, Hamann H, Mecklenburg L, et. al.: Polymorphisms within the canine MLPH gene are associated with dilute coat color in dogs. BMC Genet. 2005 Jun 16;6:34.
2. OFA Website breed statistics: www.offa.org Last accessed July 1, 2010.
3. Leppanen M, Martenson J, Maki K: Results of ophthalmologic screening examinations of German Pinschers in Finland--a retrospective study. Vet Ophthalmol. 2001 Sep;4(3):165-9.
4. *Ocular Disorders Presumed to be Inherited in Purebred Dogs.* American College of Veterinary Ophthalmologists. ACVO, 2007.
5. Nachreiner R & Refsal K: Personal communication, Diagnostic Center for Population and Animal Health, Michigan State University. April, 2007.
6. Nachreiner RF, Refsal KR, Graham PA, et. al.: Prevalence of serum thyroid hormone autoantibodies in dogs with clinical signs of hypothyroidism. J Am Vet Med Assoc 2002 Feb 15;220(4):466-71.
7. Menzel J & Distl O: Unusual vascular ring anomaly associated with a persistent right aortic arch and an aberrant left subclavian artery in German pinschers. Vet J. 2011 Mar;187(3):352-5.
8. Poth T, Breuer W, Walter B, et. al.: Disorders of sex development in the dog-Adoption of a new nomenclature and reclassification of reported cases. Anim Reprod Sci. 2010 Sep;121(3-4):197-207.
9. *The Complete Dog Book, 20th Ed.* The American Kennel Club. Howell Book House, NY 2006. p. 262-265.

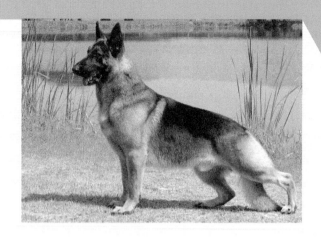

German Shepherd Dog

in size and length; not throaty. The thorax is deep and ribs well sprung, and ribs stay deep far back in the rib cage, resulting in a short loin. The topline is level, but slowly descending, with withers higher than the rear, and the abdomen is moderately tucked up. The tail extends to the tarsus, is low set, and gently curved. The limbs are straight boned, the long bones oval in cross-section. All dewclaws may be removed, but normally are left on in front and removed behind. Feet are compact, toes moderately arched, pads thick, and nails are tough and dark.

The Breed History

Closely related to the Dutch and Belgian Shepherds, the German shepherd has gained unmistakable worldwide popularity. In Germany, particularly in the Bavaria and Wurtemmburg areas where the breed was refined. Due to their massive popularity in the 20th century, some lines have had medical or behavioral disorders introduced. At one point, popularity of the breed surged after the appearance of a German Shepherd in the Rin-Tin-Tin role.

Breeding for Function

Farm dog, gundog, sheep herding, guide dog for blind, tracker, Schutzhund, and search and rescue are some of the functions ably performed by this popular dog. They are also extremely popular as a companion.

Physical Characteristics

Height at Withers: female 22-24" (56-61 cm), male 24-26" (61-66 cm).

Weight: 75-95 lb (34-43 kg).

Coat: The double coat consists of an inner coat of soft, dense short hair, the outer coat is medium in length and dense, straight to slightly wavy, and somewhat harsh or wiry; lying close. Hairs are longer on the tail. Longhaired and shorthaired shepherd varieties exist, and in the past a wirehaired variety also. In the show ring today only the shorthaired variety is shown. Most colors are permitted, but the rich black and tan is the most common. Other colors include gray, and black, and tan. Dilutes and whites are faults and disqualifications respectively. There is a separate white shepherd breed.

Longevity: 12-13 years

Points of Conformation: The image of the breed is of a powerful, rugged, working dog with a long, low, gliding elastic effortless trot and possessing a bright fearless expression. The conformation is longer than tall, the head is chiseled and long, tapering to a wedge-shaped muzzle, the eyes expressive and medium in size and setting and are almond shaped, slightly oblique, and dark brown in color. The ears are erect when alert, moderate in size with broad base, with moderate leather thickness and are moderately low set. The nose is black, lips are tight and pigmented, the neck moderate

Recognized Behavior Issues and Traits

Reported breed characteristics include: Very high trainability, somewhat aloof with strangers, high intelligence, loyal, courageous, around the home possessing a calm demeanor; some lines are timid, shy or aggressive.

Strong guard dog instincts are bred into these dogs and so they should be socialized early to other pets and children. Early obedience training is also important. High exercise and mental stimulation needs are a hallmark. They require a moderate amount of grooming, and will blow their coat twice yearly at which time high shedding occurs.

Normal Physiologic Variations

None Reported

Drug Sensitivities

MDR1 Mutation (Ivermectin/Drug Toxicity): Autosomal recessive disorder in the MDR1 gene allows high CNS drug levels of ivermectin, doramectin, loperamide, vincristine, moxidectin, and other drugs. Causes neurological signs, including tremors, seizures, and coma. A genetic test is available for the mutated gene. In one study, the defective gene was found at a frequency of 6% in white German Shepherds and those carrying white factor.[1,2]

Inherited Diseases

Elbow Dysplasia: Polygenically inherited trait causing elbow arthritis. Reported 43.7x odds ratio for fragmented coronoid process, 8.2x odds ratio for ununited anconeal process forms of elbow dysplasia, and 14.9x odds ratio for elbow osteochondrosis versus other breeds. UAP is reported at a frequency of 4.8% in the AGSDCF 2004 Health Survey. OFA reports 19.3% affected.[3,4,5]

Hip Dysplasia: Polygenically inherited trait causing degenerative joint disease and hip arthritis. Dorn reports 2.20x odds ratio versus other breeds. Another study reports a 5.7x odds ratio versus other breeds. Joint laxity based on a distraction index is more highly correlated to the development of degenerative joint disease than in other breeds. Reported at a frequency of 10.1% in the AGSDCF 2004 Health Survey. OFA reports 19.1% affected.[3,4,5,6,7]

Pancreatic Acinar Atrophy (Exocrine Pancreatic Insufficiency): Most studies show that German Shepherds have an autosomal recessive immune-mediated pancreatic acinar atrophy. One study showed only 2 of 6 dogs from an affected to affected mating developed disease, showing that this is not a simple autosomal recessive disease. Clinical signs are poor weight gain, and steatorrhea. Diagnose with canine trypsin-like immunoreactivity (cTLI) assay. Treatment is with enzyme supplementation. A British study reports an affected frequency of 18% in the breed. A linked marker has been found, but the causative gene has not been identified.[8,9,10,12]

Patella Luxation: Polygenically inherited trait causing stifle instability and arthritis. OFA reports 0.8% affected.[3]

Hereditary Multifocal Renal Cystadenocarcinoma and Nodular Dermatofibrosis: Rare, autosomal recessive kidney cancer characterized by bilateral, multifocal tumors in the kidneys, uterine leiomyomas and nodules in the skin consisting of dense collagen fibers. Mean age of onset is 6.4 years, and mean age of death is 9.3 years. A mutation has been identified in Norwegian and US families of German Shepherd dogs. A genetic test is available.[13,14]

Hemophilia A: Rare, x-linked recessive bleeding disorder. Males are primarily affected. Affected dogs can show bleeding from the mouth, subcutaneous and intramuscular haematomas and lameness due to joint hematomas.[15,16]

von Willebrand's disease (vWD): Rare, autosomal recessive mild bleeding disorder documented in some German Shepherd families in South Africa. No test for carriers is available.[17]

Hyperuricosuria (HUU)/Urate Bladder Stones: An autosomal recessive mutation in the SLC2A9 gene causes urate urolithiasis and can predispose male dogs to urinary obstruction. Estimated at a carrier frequency of 2.60% in the breed. A genetic test is available.[11]

Mucopolysaccharidosis (MPSVII): Rare, autosomal recessive lysosomal storage disorder presenting with progressive juvenile inability to ambulate, skeletal deformities, corneal cloudiness, cytoplasmic granules in the neutrophils and lymphocytes of blood and CSF and urinary glycosaminoglycans. A genetic test is available.[18]

Pituitary Dwarfism: Rare, autosomal recessive disorder of pituitary disfunction. Affected dogs present with growth retardation and stagnant development of the hair coat. The disorder is due to a combined deficiency of GH, TSH, and prolactin together with impaired release of gonadotropins. ACTH secretion is preserved. The combined pituitary hormone deficiency is associated with cyst formation and pituitary hypoplasia.[19,20,21]

Platelet Procoagulant Deficiency: Rare autosomal recessive bleeding disorder of platelet function that diminishes fibrin clot formation. Affected dogs have increased residual serum prothrombin assays. The defective gene is linked to canine chromosome 27.[22]

Disease Predispositions

Behavioral Abnormalities: German Shepherd dogs are overrepresented for aggression behavioral diagnoses in a veterinary school behavior service population. These include interdog aggression and aggression toward humans. The AGSDCF 2004 Health Survey reports 6.7% fearful, 5.0% with separation anxiety, and 4.4% with agreesion.[5,23,24]

Allergic Dermatitis: Inhalant or food allergy. Presents with pruritis and pyotraumatic dermatitis (hot spots). In an Italian study, 20% of German Shepard Dogs with dermatological disease also had an adverse food reaction. Skin allergies are reported at a frequency of 6.4%, inhallent allergies 4.6%, and food allergies 4.4% in the AGSDCF 2004 Health Survey.[5,25]

Hypothyroidism: Inherited autoimmune thyroiditis. Reported at a frequency of 5.5% in the AGSDCF 2004 Health Survey. 6.4% positive for thyroid autoantibodies based on testing at Michigan State University. (Ave. for all breeds is 7.5%).[5,26,27]

Panosteitis: Self-limiting disorder of intermittent lameness involving the diaphyseal and metaphyseal areas of the tubular long bones in young dogs prior to skeletal maturation. Reported 3.3x odds ratio versus other breeds. Reported at a frequency of 10.1% in the AGSDCF 2004 Health Survey.[4,5]

Gastric Dilatation–Volvulus (Bloat, GDV)/Intestinal Volvulus/ Splenic Torsion: German Shepherds are at increased risk for life-threatening twisting of the stomach, intestines, or spleen within the abdomen. Requires immediate veterinary attention. Gastic or intestinal volvulus was the cause of death of 15% of German Shepherds in one teaching hospital study. GDV is reported at a frequency of 8.5% in the AGSDCF 2004 Health Survey.[5,28,29,30,31]

Stifle Osteochondritis Dessicans (OCD): Polygenically inherited cartilage defect. Causes stifle joint pain and lameness in young growing dogs. Mild cases can resolve with rest, while more severe cases require surgery. Reported 17.5x odds ratio versus other breeds.[4]

Perianal Fistula/Furunculosis: Inflammatory disorder creating perianal ulceration and fistulas. Treat with anti-inflammatory medications and tacrolimus. Dorn reports a 14.31x odds ratio versus other breeds. Reported at a frequency of 5.3% with a male preponderance in the AGSDCF 2004 Health Survey. Presence of a specific allele in the major histocompatability complex produces an odds ratio of 3.7x versus German Shepherds without the allele, and dogs homozygous for this allele have an earlier onset. A test for the susceptibility gene is available.[5,6,32,33]

Degenerative Myelopathy (DM): Affected dogs show an insidious onset of upper motor neuron (UMN) paraparesis at an average age of 11.4 years. The disease eventually progresses to severe tetraparesis. Affected dogs have normal results on myelography, MRI, and CSF analysis. Necropsy confirms the condition. Unknown mode of inheritance. A direct genetic test for an autosomal recessive DM susceptibility gene (SOD1 mutation) is available. OFA reports 21% test homozygous, and 30% test heterozygous for the susceptibility gene. All affected dogs are homozygous for the gene, however, only a small percentage of homozygous dogs develop DM. Some studies suggest an immune or inflammatory pathogenesis for DM in German Shepherds. Reported at a frequency of 9.2% in the AGSDCF 2004 Health Survey.[3,5,34,35]

Corneal Dystrophy: Inherited disorder causing epithelial/stromal white to grey oval or ring shaped opacities in the corneas. Reported in 4.88% of German Shepherd dogs CERF-examined by veterinary ophthalmologists between 2000-2005.[36]

Hypertrophic Osteodystrophy (HOD): Immune-mediated disorder causing fever, and painful, swollen joints and bones in young dogs. Occurs mostly within 3-14 days post-vaccination. Age of onset is 8-16 weeks. Reported 9.6x odds ratio versus other breeds. Unknown mode of inheritance.[4]

Hemangiosarcoma: Malignant neoplasm most often presenting in the spleen, heart, or bone marrow. Splenic hemangiosarcoma most often presents due to an acute bleed. Usually metastatic by the time of diagnosis. German Shepherds have a 4.7x odds ratio versus other breeds.[28,37]

Cranial Cruciate Ligament (ACL) Rupture: Traumatic tearing of the ACL in the stifle, causing lameness and secondary arthritis. Treat with surgery. Affected German Shepherd dogs have a significantly greater tibial plateau angle (TPA) versus other breeds. TPA measurements may be helpful to screen prospective breeding dogs.[38,39]

Congential or Juvenile Cataract: German Shepherd dogs can develop bilateral posterior cortical cataracts at 8-12 weeks of age that progress to involve the Y-sutures and nucleus. These juvenile cataracts are thought to be recessively inherited. A rare congenital cataract has been observed in German Shepherd dogs and is thought to be dominantly inherited. Reported at a frequency of 3.4% in the AGSDCF 2004 Health Survey. Cataracts are reported in 4.97% of German Shepherd dogs CERF-examined by veterinary ophthalmologists between 2000-2005. CERF does not recommend breeding any German Shepherd dog with a cataract.[5,36,40,41]

Chronic Superficial Keratitis (Pannus): Chronic corneal inflammatory process that can cause vision problems due to corneal pigmentation. Treatment with topical ocular lubricants and anti-inflammatory medication. German Shepherds are at increased risk. Identified in 3.16% of German Shepherd dogs CERF-examined by veterinary ophthalmologists between 2000-2005. CERF does not recommend breeding any German Shepherd dog with pannus.[36,42]

Persistent Pupillary Membranes: Strands of fetal remnant connecting; iris to iris, cornea, lens, or involving sheets of tissue. The later three forms can impair vision, and dogs affected with these forms should not be bred. Identified in 1.99% of German Shepherd dogs CERF-examined by veterinary ophthalmologists between 2000-2005.[36]

Retinal Dysplasia: Retinal folds, geographic, and generalized retinal dysplasia with detachment are recognized in the breed. Can lead to blindness. Reported in 1.99% of German Shepherd dogs CERF examined by veterinary ophthalmologists between 2000-2005.[36]

Degenerative Lumbosacral Stenosis (DLS)/Cauda Equina Syndrome: Lumbosacral spinal cord compression due to DLS occurs most frequently in German Shepherd dogs (25.6% of cases). Clinical signs of lumbar pain, pelvic limb lameness, urinary and fecal incontinence and self mutilation occur at an average age of 5.4 years. The disorder can present with IV disc degeneration, sacral osteochondrosis, vertebral end plate sclerosis, facet joint tropism, ventral sacral subluxation, ligamentum flavum hypertrophy, and/

or entrapment of cauda equina nerve roots. Survey radiographs are not predictive for the development of DLS. Lumbosacral transitional vertebra can predispose to DLS, and cause an earlier onset. Treatment is by dorsal decompressive laminectomy.[43,44,45,46,47,48]

Immune dysfunction/IgA deficiency: Several disorders seen in the German Shepherd dog appear to be related to a deficiency of IgA function. These include **inflammatory bowel disease, mucocutaneous pyoderma, systemic aspergillosis,** and **leishmaniosis.** See under specific disease headings.

Inflammatory Bowel Disease (IBD): German Shepherds are overrepresented for cases of inflammatory bowel disease and antibiotic responsive diarrhea. It is thought that an immune dysfunction can be the cause, and some researchers propose an intestinal IgA abnormality. Chronic diarrhea is reported at a frequency of 4.2%, and IBD 3.7% in the AGSDCF 2004 Health Survey.[5,49,50]

Aortic Stenosis (Subaortic Stenosis, SAS): Affected dogs present with a left heart base murmur, aortic velocities greater than 1.5 m/second on Doppler echocardiography, aortic regurgitation, and mitral regurgitation. Can cause exercise intolerance, syncope, and progress to heart failure. German Shepherds are reported at an increased frequency versus other breeds. Unknown mode of inheritance–considered polygenic.[51]

Ventricular Arrhythmia/Sudden Cardiac Death: An inherited arrhythmia in young German Shepherd dogs can cause sudden death, usually between 22-26 weeks of age due to ventricular tachycardia (VT). Affected dogs often have no clinical signs prior to a fatal arrhythmia. 24-hour Holter monitoring can identify ventricular premature contractions (VPCs), VPC couplets, and VT. The disorder may be related to abnormalities in calcium cycling between cells. The mode of inheritance is undetermined.[52,53,54,55]

Perineal Hernia: German Shepherds are the most frequent breed diagnosed with perineal hernia. Treat with surgery.[56]

Epilepsy (Inherited Seizures): Inherited seizures can be generalized or partial seizures. A male preponderance is reported in the breed. Control with anticonvulsant medications. Undetermined mode of inheritance.[57]

Aquired Megaesophagus: German Shepherds are overrepresented in diagnoses of acquired megaesophagus. Causes include peripheral neuropathy, laryngeal paralysis, acquired myasthenia gravis, esophagitis, and gastric dilatation. Hypothyroidism is not associated with megaesophagus. Clinical signs include regurgitation, excess salivation, and aspiration pneumonia.[58]

Myesthenia Gravis: An immune-mediated disorder of circulating anti-acetylcholine receptor antibodies cause generalized appendicular muscle weakness with or without **megaesophagus,** or selective esophageal, facial and pharyngeal muscular weakness. German Shepherds are reported with a 4.8x odds ratio versus other breeds.[59,60]

Systemic Lupus Erythematosis (SLE)/Discoid Lupus Erythematosus (DLE): German Shepherds are overrepresented for these immune-mediated diseases. SLE primarily affects male German Shepherds at approximately 5 years of age with polyarthritis, and renal and mucocutaneous disorders. In DLE cases, German Shepherds comprised 44.4% of all cases in one study, and also tend to have more multifocal lesions. Treatment is with immune-modulating drugs.[61,62]

German Shepherd Pyoderma (GSP)/Mucocutaneous Pyoderma: Skin disease caused by immune deficiency, presenting with lesions to the lips, nasal planum, nares, perioral skin and less commonly, the eyelids, vulva, prepuce and anus. Responds to antibiotic therapy.[61,63,64,65]

Congenital Vascular Anomalies: Multiple reports exist of German Shepherd puppies with multiple congenital cardiac anomalies including **patent ductus arteriosus (PDA), persistent right aortic arch (PRAA)**, and secondary **megaesophagus**. German Shepherds are reported with a breed prevalence for PDA and PRAA.[66,67]

Calcinosis Circumscripta: Calcinosis circumscripta is an uncommon syndrome of dystrophic, metastatic or iatrogenic mineralization of calcium salts in soft tissues. Lesions usually occur on the hind feet or tongue in 1-4 year old dogs. 28.6% of canine cases occur in German Shepherd dogs.[68]

Systemic Aspergillosis: Young to middle-age female German Shepherd dogs are over-represented in cases of systemic aspergillosis. Thought to be associated with a **primary IgA abnormality**. Affected dogs present with variable signs of leucocytosis, hyperglobulinemia, diskospondylitis, osteomyelitis and thoracic lymphadenomegaly. The disease is usually fatal, but some dogs can be maintained on antifungal drugs for up to two years.[69,70,71]

Leishmaniosis/Visceral Leishmaniosis: German Shepherd dogs are overrepresented in cases of leishmaniosis. Affected dogs can present with peripheral lymphadenopathy, splenomegaly, and anemia. Susceptability may be due to an **IgA abnormality**.[71,72,73]

Familial Cutaneous Vasculopathy: Affected young puppies present with pyrexia, footpad swelling and depigmentation, crusting and ulceration of ear tips and tail tips, and focal depigmentation of the nasal planum. Biopsies show multifocal nodular dermatitis with neutrophils and mononuclear inflammatory cells surround foci of dermal collagenolysis, and degenerative and inflammatory vessel lesions. The disease is thought to be a immune mediated disease against abnormal collagen. Breeding studies suggest an autosomal recessive mode of inheritance.[74]

Dilated Cardiomyopathy (DCM): A UK study identified 4 German Shepherd dogs under 8 years of age in heart failure due to dilated cardiomyopathy. Other studies have not shown a breed prevalence. In this study, increased expression of the SERCA1 gene in the myocardium is thought to be an adaptive response.[75]

Acral lick Dermatitis, Base-Narrow Canines, Brachygnathism, Central PRA, Cerebellar Abiotrophy, Cervical Vertebral Instability, Cleft Lip/Palate, Cutaneous Asthenia, Deafness, Demodicosis, Dermatomyositis, Dermoid, Ectodermal Dysplasia, Factor IX Deficiency, Giant Axonal Neuropathy, Hyperparathyroidism, Lupoid Onchyopathy, Lymphedema, Masticatory Myositis, Micropapilla, Mitral Valve Disease, Oligodontia, Optic

Nerve Hypoplasia, Osteochondrodysplasia, Pelger–Huet Anomaly, Pemphigus Erythematosus, Peripheral Vestibular Disease, Sebaceous Adenitis, Tricuspid Valve Dysplasia, Uveodermatological Syndrome, Vitiligo, and **Wry Mouth** are reported.[76]

Isolated Case Studies

Primary Hypoparathyroidism: Case studies show German Shepherd dogs overrepresented with a diagnosis of primary hypoparathyroidim. Affected dogs presented with seizures, muscle tremors and fasciculations, stiff gait, tetany, muscle cramping, behavioural change, hyperventilation, and profound hypocalcemia. Treat with calcium supplementation and vitamin D therapy.[77,78]

Laryngeal Paralysis in White German Shepherds: Spontaneous bilateral and unilateral laryngeal paralysis is reported in multiple juvenile white German Shepherds. Clinical signs include respiratory stridor. One dog had concurrent **megaesophagus**.[79]

Mitochondrial Myopathy: A 9 month old male German Shepherd presented with progressive exercise intolerance, a stiff, stilted gait and marked atrophy and hypotonia of skeletal muscle. CK, LDH, and AST were all elevated. Muscle biopsy demonstrated abnormal mitochondria.[80]

Genetic Tests

Tests of Genotype: A direct genetic test for an autosomal recessive DM susceptibility gene is available from the OFA.

Direct test for an anal furunculosis/perianal fistula susceptibility gene is available from Genoscoper: www.genoscoper.com

Direct test for Mucopolysaccharidosis (MPSVII) is available from PennGen.

Direct test for Renal Cystadenocarcinoma Nodular Dermatofibrosis is available from VetGen.

Direct test for HUU is available from the UC-Davis VGL and the Animal Health Trust.

Direct test for coat length is available from the Animal Health Trust, and VetGen.

Direct test for bicolor, solid black and sable colors are available from HealthGene and VetGen.

Direct test for MDR1 (ivermectin sensitivity) gene in white German Shepherds is available from Washington State Univ. http://www.vetmed.wsu.edu/depts-VCPL/test.aspx

Tests of Phenotype: CHIC Certification: Required testing includes hip and elbow radiographs, and temperament test. Optional tests include cardiac evaluation, thyroid profile including autoantibodies, CERF eye examination (annually until 6 years, then every other year), and DM susceptibility test. (See CHIC website; www.caninehealthinfo.org).

Miscellaneous

- **Breed Name Synonyms:** German Shepherd, Deutsche Schäferhund, German Shepard, German Shephard, Alsatian, German Police Dog.
- **Registries:** AKC, UKC, CKC, KCGB (Kennel Club of Great Britain), ANKC (Australian National Kennel Club), NKC (National Kennel Club).
- **AKC rank (year 2008):** 3 (40,909 dogs registered)
- **Internet resources: German Shepherd Dog Club of America:** www.gsdca.org

  German Shepherd Dog Club of Canada Inc.: www.gsdcc.ca

  German Shepherd Dog League of Great Britain: www.gsdleague.co.uk/

  British Association for German Shepherd Dogs: www.bagsd.net

  The American German Shepherd Dog Charitable Foundation, Inc.: www.agsdcf.org

  German Shepherd Dog club of America–Working Dog Association: www.gsdca-wda.org

  The White German Shepherd Dog Club of America: www.wgsdca.org

References

1. Mealey KL, & Meurs KM: Breed distribution of the ABCB1-1Delta (multidrug sensitivity) polymorphism among dogs undergoing ABCB1 genotyping. J Am Vet Med Assoc. 2008 Sep 15;233(6):921-4.
2. Neff MW, Robertson KR, Wong AK, et. al.: Breed distribution and history of canine mdr1-1Delta, a pharmacogenetic mutation that marks the emergence of breeds from the collie lineage. Proc Natl Acad Sci U S A. 2004 Aug 10;101(32):11725-30.
3. OFA Website breed statistics: www.offa.org Last accessed July,1 2010
4. LaFond E, Breur GJ & Austin CC: Breed susceptibility for developmental orthopedic diseases in dogs. J Am Anim Hosp Assoc. 2002 Sep-Oct;38(5):467-77.
5. American German Shepherd Dog Charitable Foundation, Inc.: AGSDCF 2004 Health Survey. 2005.
6. Dorn CR: Canine breed-specific risks of frequently diagnosed diseases at veterinary teaching hospitals. Monograph. AKC Canine Health Foundation. 2000.
7. Smith GK, Mayhew PD, Kapatkin AS, et. al.: Evaluation of risk factors for degenerative joint disease associated with hip dysplasia in German Shepherd Dogs, Golden Retrievers, Labrador Retrievers, and Rottweilers. J Am Vet Med Assoc. 2001 Dec 15;219(12):1719-24.
8. Batchelor DJ, Noble PJ, Cripps PJ, et. al.: Breed associations for canine exocrine pancreatic insufficiency. J Vet Intern Med. 2007 Mar-Apr;21(2):207-14.
9. Clark LA, Wahl JM, Steiner JM, et. al.: Linkage analysis and gene expression profile of pancreatic acinar atrophy in the German Shepherd Dog. Mamm Genome. 2005 Dec;16(12):955-62.
10. Moeller EM, Steiner JM, Clark LA, et. al.: Inheritance of pancreatic acinar atrophy in German Shepherd Dogs. Am J Vet Res. 2002 Oct;63(10):1429-34.
11. Karmi N, Brown EA, Hughes SS, et. al.: Estimated frequency of the canine hyperuricosuria mutation in different dog breeds. J Vet Intern Med. 2010 Nov-Dec;24(6):1337-42.
12. Westermarck E, Saari SA, & Wiberg ME: Heritability of exocrine pancreatic insufficiency in German Shepherd dogs. J Vet Intern Med. 2010 Mar-Apr;24(2):450-2.
13. Lingaas F, Comstock KE, Kirkness EF, et. al.: A mutation in the canine BHD gene is associated with hereditary multifocal renal cystadenocarcinoma and nodular dermatofibrosis in the German Shepherd dog. Hum Mol Genet. 2003 Dec 1;12(23):3043-53.
14. Moe L, & Lium B: Hereditary multifocal renal cystadenocarcinomas and nodular dermatofibrosis in 51 German shepherd dogs. J Small Anim Pract.
1997 Nov;38(11):498-505.
15. Stokol T,& Parry B: Efficacy of fresh-frozen plasma and cryoprecipitate in dogs with von Willebrand's disease or hemophilia A. J Vet Intern Med. 1998 Mar-Apr;12(2):84-92.
16. Parry BW, Howard MA, Mansell PD, et. al.: Haemophilia A in German shepherd dogs. Aust Vet J. 1988 Sep;65(9):276-9.
17. Lobetti RG, & Dippenaar T: Von Willebrand's disease in the German shepherd dog. J S Afr Vet Assoc. 2000 Jun;71(2):118-21.
18. Silverstein Dombrowski DC, Carmichael KP, et. al.: Mucopolysaccharidosis type VII in a German Shepherd Dog. J Am Vet Med Assoc. 2004 Feb 15;224(4):553-7, 532-3.
19. Allan GS, Huxtable CR, Howlett CR, et. al.: Pituitary dwarfism in German Shepherd dogs. J Small Anim Pract. 1978 Dec;19(12):711-27.
20. Andresen E, & Willeberg P: Pituitary dwarfism in German shepherd dogs: additional evidence of simple, autosomal recessive inheritance. Nord Vet Med. 1976 Oct;28(10):481-6.
21. Kooistra HS, Voorhout G, Mol JA, et. al.: Combined pituitary hormone deficiency in german shepherd dogs with dwarfism. Domest Anim Endocrinol. 2000 Oct;19(3):177-90.
22. Brooks M, Etter K, Catalfamo J, et. al.: A genome-wide linkage scan in German shepherd dogs localizes canine platelet procoagulant deficiency (Scott syndrome) to canine chromosome 27. Gene. 2010 Jan 15;450(1-2):70-5.
23. Bamberger M, & Houpt KA: Signalment factors, comorbidity, and trends in behavior diagnoses in dogs: 1,644 cases (1991-2001). J Am Vet Med Assoc. 2006 Nov 15;229(10):1591-601.
24. Rugbjerg H, Proschowsky HF, Ersbøll AK, et. al.: Risk factors associated with interdog aggression and shooting phobias among purebred dogs in Denmark. Prev Vet Med. 2003 Apr 30;58(1-2):85-100.
25. Proverbio D, Perego R, Spada E, et. al.: Prevalence of adverse food reactions in 130 dogs in Italy with dermatological signs: a retrospective study. J Small Anim Pract. 2010 Jul;51(7):370-4.
26. Nachreiner RF, Refsal KR, Graham PA, et. al.: Prevalence of serum thyroid hormone autoantibodies in dogs with clinical signs of hypothyroidism. J Am Vet Med Assoc 2002 Feb 15;220(4):466-71.
27. Nachreiner R & Refsal K: Personal communication, Diagnostic Center for Population and Animal Health, Michigan State University. April, 2007.
28. Craig LE: Cause of death in dogs according to breed: a necropsy survey of five breeds. J Am Anim Hosp Assoc. 2001 Sep-Oct;37(5):438-43.
29. Cairó J, Font J, Gorraiz J, et. al.: Intestinal volvulus in dogs: a study of four clinical cases. J Small Anim Pract. 1999 Mar;40(3):136-40.
30. Brockman DJ, Washabau RJ, Drobatz KJ, et. al.: Canine gastric dilatation/volvulus syndrome in a veterinary critical care unit: 295 cases (1986-1992). J Am Vet Med Assoc. 1995 Aug 15;207(4):460-4.
31. Neath PJ, Brockman DJ, & Saunders HM: Retrospective analysis of 19 cases of isolated torsion of the splenic pedicle in dogs. J Small Anim Pract. 1997 Sep;38(9):387-92.
32. Barnes A, O'Neill T, Kennedy LJ, et. al.: Association of canine anal furunculosis with TNFA is secondary to linkage disequilibrium with DLA-DRB1*. Tissue Antigens. 2009 Mar;73(3):218-24.
33. Kennedy LJ, O'Neill T, House A, et. al.: Risk of anal furunculosis in German shepherd dogs is associated with the major histocompatibility complex. Tissue Antigens. 2008 Jan;71(1):51-6.
34. Awano T, Johnson GS, Wade CM, et. al.: Genome-wide association analysis reveals a SOD1 mutation in canine degenerative myelopathy that resembles amyotrophic lateral sclerosis. Proc Natl Acad Sci U S A. 2009 Feb 24;106(8):2794-9.
35. Kamishina H, Oji T, Cheeseman JA, et. al.: Detection of oligoclonal bands in cerebrospinal fluid from German Shepherd dogs with degenerative myelopathy by isoelectric focusing and immunofixation. Vet Clin Pathol. 2008 Jun;37(2):217-20.
36. Ocular Disorders Presumed to be Inherited in Purebred Dogs. American College of Veterinary Ophthalmologists. ACVO, 2007.
37. Prymak C, McKee LJ, Goldschmidt MH, et. al.: Epidemiologic, clinical, pathologic, and prognostic characteristics of splenic hemangiosarcoma and

splenic hematoma in dogs: 217 cases (1985). J Am Vet Med Assoc. 1988 Sep 15;193(6):706-12.

38. Morris E, Lipowitz AJ: Comparison of tibial plateau angles in dogs with and without cranial cruciate ligament injuries. J Am Vet Med Assoc. 2001 Feb 1;218(3):363-6.

39. Guastella DB, Fox DB, Cook JL: Tibial plateau angle in four common canine breeds with cranial cruciate ligament rupture, and its relationship to meniscal tears. Vet Comp Orthop Traumatol. 2008;21(2):125-8.

40. Barnett KC: Hereditary cataract in the German shepherd dog. J Small Anim Pract 1986: 27:387.

41. von Hippel E: (Embryological investigation of hereditary congenital cataract, of lamellar cataract in dogs as well as a peculiar form of capsular cataract). Graefes Arch Ophthalmol. 1930: 124:300.

42. Rapp E, & Kölbl S: Ultrastructural study of unidentified inclusions in the cornea and iridocorneal angle of dogs with pannus. Am J Vet Res. 1995 Jun;56(6):779-85.

43. Suwankong N, Meij BP, Voorhout G, et. al.: Review and retrospective analysis of degenerative lumbosacral stenosis in 156 dogs treated by dorsal laminectomy. Vet Comp Orthop Traumatol. 2008;21(3):285-93.

44. Steffen F, Hunold K, Scharf G, et. al.: A follow-up study of neurologic and radiographic findings in working German Shepherd Dogs with and without degenerative lumbosacral stenosis. J Am Vet Med Assoc. 2007 Nov 15;231(10):1529-33.

45. Flückiger MA, Damur-Djuric N, Hässig M, et. al.: A lumbosacral transitional vertebra in the dog predisposes to cauda equina syndrome. Vet Radiol Ultrasound. 2006 Jan-Feb;47(1):39-44.

46. Seiler GS, Häni H, Busato AR, et. al.: Facet joint geometry and intervertebral disk degeneration in the L5-S1 region of the vertebral column in German Shepherd dogs. Am J Vet Res. 2002 Jan;63(1):86-90.

47. Morgan JP, Bahr A, Franti CE, et. al.: Lumbosacral transitional vertebrae as a predisposing cause of cauda equina syndrome in German shepherd dogs: 161 cases (1987-1990). J Am Vet Med Assoc. 1993 Jun 1;202(11):1877-82.

48. Mathis KR, Havlicek M, Beck JB, et. al.: Sacral osteochondrosis in two German Shepherd Dogs. Aust Vet J. 2009 Jun;87(6):249-52.

49. Littler RM, Batt RM, & Lloyd DH.: Total and relative deficiency of gut mucosal IgA in German shepherd dogs demonstrated by faecal analysis. Vet Rec. 2006 Mar 11;158(10):334-41.

50. German AJ, Hall EJ, & Day MJ: Relative deficiency in IgA production by duodenal explants from German shepherd dogs with small intestinal disease. Vet Immunol Immunopathol. 2000 Aug 31;76(1-2):25-43.

51. Tidholm A: Retrospective study of congenital heart defects in 151 dogs. J Small Anim Pract. 1997 Mar;38(3):94-8.

52. Cruickshank J, Quaas RL, Li J, et. al.: Genetic Analysis of Ventricular Arrhythmia in Young German Shepherd Dogs. J Vet Intern Med. 2009 Mar-Apr;23(2):264-70.

53. Moïse NS, Riccio ML, Kornreich B, et. al.: Age dependence of the development of ventricular arrhythmias in a canine model of sudden cardiac death. Cardiovasc Res. 1997 Jun;34(3):483-92.

54. Moïse NS, Gilmour RF Jr, Riccio ML, et. al.: Diagnosis of inherited ventricular tachycardia in German shepherd dogs. J Am Vet Med Assoc. 1997 Feb 1;210(3):403-10.

55. Jesty SA, Kornreich BG, Cordeiro J, et. al.: Cardiomyocyte Calcium Transients in German Shepherd Dogs with Inherited Ventricular Arrhythmias. Proceedings, 2008 ACVIM Forum, 2008.

56. Sjollema BE, van Sluijs FJ: Perineal hernia in the dog: developments in its treatment and retrospective study in 197 patients. Tijdschr Diergeneeskd. 1991 Feb 1;116(3):142-7.

57. Falco MJ, Barker J, & Wallace ME: The genetics of epilepsy in the British Alsatian. J Small Anim Pract. 1974 Nov;15(11):685-92.

58. Gaynor AR, Shofer FS, Washabau RJ: Risk factors for acquired megaesophagus in dogs. J Am Vet Med Assoc. 1997 Dec 1;211(11):1406-12.

59. Wray JD & Sparkes AH: Use of radiographic measurements in distinguishing myasthenia gravis from other causes of canine megaoesophagus. J Small Anim Pract. 2006 May;47(5):256-63.

60. Shelton GD, Willard MD, Cardinet GH 3rd, et. al.: Acquired myasthenia gravis. Selective involvement of esophageal, pharyngeal, and facial muscles. J Vet Intern Med. 1990 Nov-Dec;4(6):281-4.

61. Wiemelt SP, Goldschmidt MH, Greek JS, et. al.: A retrospective study comparing the histopathological features and response to treatment in two canine nasal dermatoses, DLE and MCP. Vet Dermatol. 2004 Dec;15(6):341-8.

62. Fournel C, Chabanne L, Caux C, et. al.: Canine systemic lupus erythematosus. I: A study of 75 cases. Lupus. 1992 May;1(3):133-9.

63. Rosser EJ Jr.: German Shepherd Dog pyoderma. Vet Clin North Am Small Anim Pract. 2006 Jan;36(1):203-11, viii.

64. Chabanne L, Marchal T, Denerolle P, et. al.: Lymphocyte subset abnormalities in German shepherd dog pyoderma (GSP). Vet Immunol Immunopathol. 1995 Dec;49(3):189-98.

65. Bassett RJ, Burton GG, & Robson DC: Antibiotic responsive ulcerative dermatoses in German Shepherd Dogs with mucocutaneous pyoderma. Aust Vet J. 2004 Aug;82(8):485-9.

66. Christiansen KJ, Snyder D, Buchanan JW, et. al.: Multiple vascular anomalies in a regurgitating German shepherd puppy. J Small Anim Pract. 2007 Jan;48(1):32-5.

67. Holt D, Heldmann E, Michel K, et. al.: Esophageal obstruction caused by a left aortic arch and an anomalous right patent ductus arteriosus in two German Shepherd littermates. Vet Surg. 2000 May-Jun;29(3):264-70.

68. Tafti AK, Hanna P, Bourque AC: Calcinosis circumscripta in the dog: a retrospective pathological study. J Vet Med A Physiol Pathol Clin Med. 2005 Feb;52(1):13-7.

69. Schultz RM, Johnson EG, Wisner ER, et. al.: Clinicopathologic and diagnostic imaging characteristics of systemic aspergillosis in 30 dogs. J Vet Intern Med. 2008 Jul-Aug;22(4):851-9.

70. Day MJ, Penhale WJ, Eger CE, et. al.: Disseminated aspergillosis in dogs. Aust Vet J. 1986 Feb;63(2):55-9.

71. Day MJ, & Penhale WJ: Serum immunoglobulin A concentrations in normal and diseased dogs. Res Vet Sci. 1988 Nov;45(3):360-3.

72. Miranda S, Roura X, Picado A, et. al.: Characterization of sex, age, and breed for a population of canine leishmaniosis diseased dogs. Res Vet Sci. 2008 Aug;85(1):35-8.

73. Keenan CM, Hendricks LD, Lightner L, et. al.: Visceral leishmaniasis in the German shepherd dog. II. Pathology. Vet Pathol. 1984 Jan;21(1):80-6.

74. Weir JA, Yager JA, Caswell JL, et. al,: Famillial cutaneous vasculopathy of German shepherds: clinical, genetic and preliminary pathological and immunological studies. Can Vet J.1994 Dec;35(12):763-9.

75. Summerfield N, Peters ME, Hercock CA, et. al.: Immunohistochemical evidence for expression of fast-twitch type sarco(endo)plasmic reticulum Ca(2+) ATPase (SERCA1) in German shepherd dogs with dilated cardiomyopathy myocardium. J Vet Cardiol. 2010 Apr;12(1):17-23.

76. *The Genetic Connection: A Guide to Health Problems in Purebred Dogs.* L Ackerman. p. 218-19. AAHA Press, 1999.

77. Russell NJ, Bond KA, Robertson ID, et. al.: Primary hypoparathy-roidism in dogs: a retrospective study of 17 cases. Aust Vet J. 2006 Aug;84(8):285-90.

78. Ramsey IK, Dennis R, & Herrtage ME: Concurrent central diabetes insipidus and panhypopituitarism in a German shepherd dog. J Small Anim Pract. 1999 Jun;40(6):271-4.

79. Ridyard AE, Corcoran BM, Tasker S, et. al.: Spontaneous laryngeal paralysis in four white-coated German shepherd dogs. J Small Anim Pract. 2000 Dec;41(12):558-61.

80. Paciello O, Maiolino P, Fatone G, et. al.: Mitochondrial myopathy in a german shepherd dog. Vet Pathol. 2003 Sep;40(5):507-11.

81. *The Complete Dog Book, 20th Ed.* The American Kennel Club. Howell Book House, NY 2006. p. 665-670.

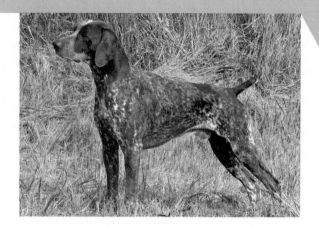

German Shorthaired Pointer

The Breed History

Many breeds have been crossed to produce this elegant hunting dog including the English foxhound, German bird dog, Schweisshunde, Spanish pointer, English pointer and perhaps others. This breed was first exported to North America in the 1920s, and first entered into the AKC registry in 1930.

Breeding for Function

This dog has earned the reputation of being a versatile and obedient all-purpose fur and feather hunting dog. Their keen nose, intelligence and high athleticism combine to produce a dependable hunting companion under harsh conditions. Their utility extends beyond their pointer name to include scent work, water work, retriever, and medium game dog. They are valued as companions, trackers, field trial, obedience, and hunting dogs.

Physical Characteristics

Height at Withers: female 21-23" (53-58.5 cm), male 23-25" (58.5-63.5 cm)

Weight: females 45-60 lb (20.5-27.5 kg), males 55-70 lb (25-32 kg).

Coat: The short glossy, firm hair is colored liver or liver and white in patches, ticking, or liver roan.

Longevity: 12-15 years.

Points of Conformation: This dog is of medium size and athletic build, close to square, with medium bone and muscling, and an alert demeanor. Their skulls are mesocephalic, their almond-shaped eyes are medium-sized and dark brown. The ears lie flat and are pendulous, jaws are powerful, muzzle is square, stop is graduated but not definite (in contrast to a Pointer stop), and the muzzle profile should not be dished. Their brown nose is large and projects out somewhat. The neck is long and slightly arched, chest is deep and ribs well-sprung. They are moderately tucked in the abdomen and the loin is arched. The back is short and tail is set high and generally docked; it's carried low at rest and horizontally when in motion. Dewclaws may be removed, and feet are well arched and toes webbed. Limbs are straight, but the dog will single track at a faster trot. The stride is long and smooth, they possess an elastic agile way of moving. These well-balanced dogs are bred for no extreme points.

Recognized Behavior Issues and Traits

They make good companion dogs as well as hunting companions. Because they are bred to work all day, a dog kept for a companion requires a high level of exercise and mental stimulation to stay healthy both physically and emotionally. They are intelligent and active around the house, and need close human companionship. Their grooming needs are low, and they are average shedders. They are alarm barkers, aloof with strangers, and develop a strong bond with their caregiver. These dogs can dig and jump out of a yard if left unattended. They are not suitable for apartment life.

Normal Physiologic Variations

None reported

Drug Sensitivities

None reported

Inherited Diseases

Hip Dysplasia: Polygenically inherited trait causing degenerative joint disease and hip arthritis. OFA reports 4.4% affected. Reported at a frequency of 1.19% in the 2005 GSP Health Survey.[1,2]

Cone Degeneration (CD): An autosomal recessive disease causing day-blindness, colorblindness, and photophobia between 8 and 12 weeks of age, due to the absence of retinal cone function. Ophthalmoscopic examination remains normal. A genetic test exists, and Optigen testing shows 14% of German Shorthaired Pointers test as carriers. CERF does not recommend breeding any German Shorthaired Pointer affected with CD.[3,4]

von Willebrand's disease (vWD): Type II vWD in the German Shorthaired Pointer is a serious, sometimes fatal, autosomal recessive bleeding disorder. Cryoprecipitate is more effective, with fewer side effects, than fresh frozen plasma in controlling bleeding episodes. A genetic test is available.[5]

Elbow Dysplasia: Polygenically inherited trait causing elbow arthritis. OFA reports 1.2% affected.[1]

Patella Luxation: Polygenically inherited laxity of patellar ligaments, causing luxation, lameness, and later degenerative joint disease. Treat surgically if causing clinical signs. Too few German Shorthaired Pointers have been screened by OFA to determine an accurate frequency.[1]

Sry-Negative XX Sex Reversal (Hermaphrodism): An autosomal recessive disorder, where outwardly male dogs are chromosomal females (XX), and there is an absence of "male" causing SRY. Reported at a frequency of 0.74% in the 2005 GSP Health Survey.[2,6,7]

Disease Predispositions

Hypothyroidism: Inherited autoimmune thyroiditis. 8.1% positive for thyroid auto-antibodies based on testing at Michigan State University. (Ave. for all breeds is 7.5%).[8,9]

Persistent Pupillary Membranes: Strands of fetal remnant connecting; iris to iris, cornea, lens, or involving sheets of tissue. The later three forms can impair vision, and dogs affected with these forms should not be bred. Identified in 6.28% of German Shorthaired Pointers CERF-examined by veterinary ophthalmologists between 2000-2005.[4]

Mammary Tumors: Cancer presenting primarily in unspayed females. Reported at a frequency of 5.55% of females in the 2005 GSP Health Survey.[2]

Behavioral Abnormalities: Noise phobia is reported at a frequency of 5.04% and dog to dog aggression at 4.92% in the 2005 GSP Health Survey.[2]

Umbilical Hernia: Congenital opening of the body wall at the umbilicus. Should be closed surgically if large. Reported at a frequency of 4.06% in the 2005 GSP Health Survey.[2]

Cryptorchidism (Retained Testicles): Can be unilateral or bilateral. Reported at a frequency of 4.04% of males in the 2005 GSP Health Survey.[2]

Distichiasis: Abnormally placed eyelashes that irritate the cornea and conjunctiva. Can cause secondary corneal ulceration. Identified in 3.52% of German Shorthaired Pointers CERF-examined by veterinary ophthalmologists between 2000-2005.[4]

Cataracts: Anterior cortex punctate and posterior cortex intermediate cataracts predominate in the breed. Onset 6-18 months of age. Unknown mode of inheritance. Identified in 3.30% of German Shorthaired Pointers CERF-examined by veterinary ophthalmologists between 2000-2005. Reported at a frequency of 2.72% in the 2005 GSP Health Survey. CERF does not recommend breeding any German Shorthaired Pointer with a cataract.[2,4]

Malocclusion (Overbite, Underbite): In a 1992 Health Survey, bite problems was listed as the most frequent abnormality, with 3.23% affected. One study of severe overbites in a German Shorthaired Pointer kennel suggested an autosomal recessive inheritance. Most experts believe that bites are polygenically inherited, with different sets of genes controlling maxillary and mandibular jaw length, and the number and placement of teeth. Overbite is reported at a frequency of 2.51% in the 2005 GSP Health Survey.[2,10]

Idiopathic Epilepsy: Inherited seizures. Control with anticonvulsant medication. Unknown mode of inheritance. Dorn reports a 16.78x odds ratio in German Shorthaired Pointers versus other breeds. Reported at a frequency of 2.87% in the 2005 GSP Health Survey.[2,11]

Humeral Osteochondritis Dissecans (OCD): Polygenically inherited cartilage defect of the humeral head. Causes shoulder joint pain and lameness in young growing dogs. Mild cases can resolve with rest, while more severe cases require surgery. 50% of cases are bilateral. Reported 5.5x odds ratio versus other breeds.[12]

Demodicosis, Generalized: Dorn reports a 4.77x odds ratio versus other breeds. Demodectic mange has an underlying immunodeficiency in its pathogenesis. Reported at a frequency of 2.61% in the 2005 GSP Health Survey.[2,11]

Gastric Dilatation-Volvulus (Bloat, GDV): Polygenically inherited, life-threatening twisting of the stomach within the abdomen.

Requires immediate veterinary attention. Reported at a frequency of 1.59% in the 2005 GSP Health Survey.[2]

Mast Cell Tumor (MCT): Skin tumors that produce histamine, causing inflammation and ulceration. They can reoccur locally or with distant metastasis. Reported at a frequency of 1.56% in the 2005 GSP Health Survey.[2]

Allergies: Inhalent or food. Presents with pruritis and pyotraumatic dermatitis (hot spots). Inhalent allergy is reported at a frequency of 1.41%, and food allergy at 1.28% in the 2005 GSP Health Survey.[2]

Entropion: A rolling in of the eyelids that can cause corneal irritation and ulceration. Reported at a frequency of 1.25% in the 2005 GSP Health Survey.[2]

Retinal Dysplasia: Retinal folds, geographic, and generalized retinal dysplasia with detachment are recognized in the breed. Reported in 1.23% of German Shorthaired Pointers CERF-examined by veterinary ophthalmologists between 2000-2005. CERF does not recommend breeding any German Shorthaired Pointer with retinal dysplasia.[4]

Cutaneous Lupus Erythematosus/Lupoid Dermatosis: An immune-mediated inflammatory disease presenting with variably painful and itchy scaling and crusting around face, ears, back, hocks and scrotum. Onset between three months to three years of age. Can wax and wane, or be persistent. Diagnosis is by skin biopsy. Treated with immunosuppressive drugs and fatty acid supplements. Usually progressive with a poor long term prognosis. Diagnosed in German Shorthaired Pointers worldwide. Undefined mode of inheritance.[13,14]

Acquired Myasthenia Gravis: German Shorthaired Pointers are a breed at increased risk of developing generalized or focal acquired myasthenia gravis. The most common presenting signs were generalized weakness, with or without megaesophagus. Diagnosis is by identifying acetylcholine receptor antibodies.[15]

Oral Cancer: One study found that German Shorthaired Pointers were a breed with a significantly higher risk of developing oral and pharyngeal tumors, as compared with all breeds combined.[16]

Hemivertebra: Rare inherited disorder of thoracic scoliosis due to hemivertebra. Autosomal recessive inheritance is suggested.[17]

Everted Cartilage of the Third Eyelid: A scroll-like curling of the cartilage of the third eyelid, usually everting the margin. Can be unilateral or bilateral, and cause ocular irritation.[4,18]

Persistent Hyperplastic Tunica Vasculosa Lentis and Primary Vitreous (PHTVL/PHPV): A congenital defect resulting from abnormalities in the development and regression of the embryologic vascular network surrounding the lens. Can cause posterior lenticonus/globus, colobomata, intralenticular hemorrhage and/or secondary cataracts. CERF does not recommend breeding any German Shorthaired Pointer with PHTVL/PHPV. Unknown mode of inheritance.[4,19]

Atresia Ani (Imperforate Anus): An increased incidence of this congenital condition is reported in the breed, with a frequency of 0.028%, and an odds ratio of 5.79x. Treatment is surgery.[20]

Acral Mutilation Syndrome, Brachygnathism, Epidermosis Bullosa, Factor IX Deficiency, Factor XII Deficiency, GM-2

Gangliosidosis, Hypoadrenocorticism, Lymphedema, Seasonal Flank Alopecia, and Subaortic Stenosis are reported.[21]

Isolated Case Studies

Paroxysmal Dyskinesia: A male German Shorthaired Pointer presented with an intermittent gait abnormality initially seen at 1 year of age. With excitement, the dog developed kyphosis, and bilateral hip and stifle flexion with ambulation. The episodes usually lasted up to 30 minutes. The condition was eliminated with anticonvulsant medication, and returned when the medication was stopped.[22]

Hemophilia A: Factor VIII deficiency, was diagnosed in a male German Shorthaired Pointer as a result of testing for a coagulopathy. This is an X-linked recessive genetic disorder.[23]

Branchial Cyst: A 7 year-old spayed German Shorthaired Pointer was determined to have a branchial cyst in the subcutaneous tissues of the cervical/facial area.[24]

Muscular Dystrophy: X-linked recessive muscular dystrophy was identified in a family of German Shorthaired Pointers, due to a large deletion in the dystrophin gene.[25]

Genetic Tests

Tests of Genotype: Direct test for cone degeneration (CD) is available from Optigen.

Direct tests for black, red/orange and brown colors, and black or brown nose are available from HealthGene and VetGen.

Direct test for vWD is available from VetGen.

Tests of Phenotype: CHIC Certification: Cardiac Evaluation by a specialist/cardiologist, hip radiographs, CERF eye evaluation (each year until 6, then every 2 years), and direct genetic test for cone degeneration. Optional tests include elbow radiographs, and thyroid profile including autoantibodies. (See CHIC website; www.caninehealthinfo.org).

Recommend patella evaluation.

Miscellaneous

- **Breed name synonyms:** GSP, Kurzhaar, Deutscher Kurzhaariger Vorstehund, German Shorthair, German Pointer
- **Registries:** AKC, CKC, UKC, KCGB (Kennel Club of Great Britain), ANKC (Australian National Kennel Club), NKC (National Kennel Club)
- **AKC rank (year 2008):** 16 (11,110 dogs registered)
- **Internet resources: German Shorthaired Pointer of America Inc.:** www.gspca.org
  German Shorthaired Pointer Club of Canada: www.gspcanada.com
  The German Shorthaired Pointer Club (UK): www.gsp.org.uk

References

1. OFA Website breed statistics: www.offa.org Last accessed July 1, 2010.
2. Slater MR: 2005 German Shorthaired Pointer Health Survey: Final Report. Jan 29, 2007.
3. Sidjanin DJ, Lowe JK, McElwee JL, et. al.: Canine CNGB3 mutations establish cone degeneration as orthologous to the human achromatopsia locus ACHM3. Hum Mol Genet. 2002 Aug 1;11(16):1823-33.
4. Ocular Disorders Presumed to be Inherited in Purebred Dogs. American College of Veterinary Ophthalmologists. ACVO, 2007.
5. Kramer JW, Venta PJ, Klein SR, et. al.: A von Willebrand's factor genomic nucleotide variant and polymerase chain reaction diagnostic test associated with inheritable type-2 von Willebrand's disease in a line of german Shorthaired Pointer dogs. Vet Pathol. 2004 May;41(3):221-8.
6. Meyers-Wallen VN, Bowman L, Acland GM, et. al.: Sry-negative XX sex reversal in the German Shorthaired Pointer dog. J Hered. 1995 Sep-Oct;86(5):369-74.
7. Sommer MM, Meyers-Wallen VN: XX true hermaphroditism in a dog. J Am Vet Med Assoc. 1991 Feb 1;198(3):435-8.
8. Nachreiner RF, Refsal KR, Graham PA, et. al.: Prevalence of serum thyroid hormone autoantibodies in dogs with clinical signs of hypothyroidism. *J Am Vet Med Assoc* 2002 Feb 15;220(4):466-71.
9. Nachreiner R & Refsal K: Personal communication, Diagnostic Center for Population and Animal Health, Michigan State University. April, 2007.
10. Byrne MJ, Byrne GM: Inheritance of "overshot" malocclusion in German Shorthaired Pointers. Vet Rec. 1992 Apr 25;130(17):375-6.
11. Dorn CR: Canine breed-specific risks of frequently diagnosed diseases at veterinary teaching hospitals. Monograph. AKC Canine Health Foundation. 2000.
12. LaFond E, Breur GJ & Austin CC: Breed susceptibility for developmental orthopedic diseases in dogs. J Am Anim Hosp Assoc. 2002 Sep-Oct;38(5):467-77.
13. Bryden SL, White SD, Dunston SM: Clinical, Histopathological and Immunological Characteristics of Exfoliative Cutaneous Lupus Erythematosus in 25 German Short-Haired Pointers. Vet Dermatol 2005:16[4]:239-252.
14. Mauldin EA, Morris DO, Brown DC, et. al.: Exfoliative cutaneous lupus erythematosus in German shorthaired pointer dogs: disease development, progression and evaluation of three immunomodulatory drugs (ciclosporin, hydroxychloroquine, and adalimumab) in a controlled environment. Vet Dermatol. 2010 Apr 1. [Epub ahead of print]
15. Shelton GD, Schule A, Kass PH: Risk factors for acquired myasthenia gravis in dogs: 1,154 cases (1991-1995). J Am Vet Med Assoc. 1997 Dec 1;211(11):1428-31.
16. Dorn CR, Priester WA: Epidemiologic analysis of oral and pharyngeal cancer in dogs, cats, horses, and cattle. J Am Vet Med Assoc. 1976 Dec 1;169(11):1202-6.
17. Kramer JW, Schiffer SP, Sande RD, et. al.: Characterization of heritable thoracic hemivertebra of the German Shorthaired Pointer. J Am Vet Med Assoc. 1982 Oct 15;181(8):814-5.
18. Martin CL & Leach R: Everted membrane nictitans in German Shorthaired Pointers. J Am Vet Med Assoc 1970; 157:1229.
19. Berger SL: Persistent hyperplastic tunica vasculosa lentis/persistent hyperplastic primary vitreous in the German Shorthaired Pointer. Proc Am Coll Vet Ophthalmol 1995; 26:42.
20. Vianna ML, Tobias KM: Atresia ani in the dog: a retrospective study. J Am Anim Hosp Assoc. 2005 Sep-Oct;41(5):317-22.
21. *The Genetic Connection: A Guide to Health Problems in Purebred Dogs*. L Ackerman. p 219 AAHA Press, 1999.
22. Harcourt-Brown T: Anticonvulsant responsive, episodic movement disorder in a German Shorthaired Pointer. J Small Anim Pract. 2008 Jul 4.
23. Joseph SA, Brooks MB, Coccari PJ, et. al.: Hemophilia A in a German Shorthaired Pointer: clinical presentations and diagnosis. J Am Anim Hosp Assoc. 1996 Jan-Feb;32(1):25-8.
24. Clark DM, Kostolich M, Mosier D: Branchial cyst in a dog. J Am Vet Med Assoc. 1989 Jan 1;194(1):67-8.
25. Schatzberg S, Olby N, Steingold S, et. al.: A polymerase chain reaction screening strategy for the promoter of the canine dystrophin gene. Am J Vet Res. 1999 Sep;60(9):1040-6.
26. *The Complete Dog Book, 20th Ed*. The American Kennel Club. Howell Book House, NY 2006. p 24-28.

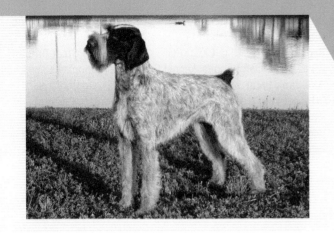

German Wirehaired Pointer

The Breed History

In the 1800s, demand was high for all-purpose hunting dogs. In Germany, the name "retrieving pointer", or "Deutsch-Drahthaar" was applied to all such general purpose wirehaired dogs. The name translates as German (Deutsch) Wire (draht) hair (haar). From this type of wirehaired dog, four subtypes were developed around 1870. In addition to the German Wirehaired pointer, these offshoots also included Pudelpointer, Stichelhaar and Griffon. Wirehaired pointers were general purpose dogs with Poodle, Pointer, and French Wirehaired Pointing Griffon traits. The first breed standard dates to the year 1902. The first German Wirehaired Pointer dogs were exported to America in the 1920s. Initial AKC breed registration occurred in 1959. The German Shorthaired pointer is not just a short haired version of this breed; their origins differ significantly. The Wirehaired Pointer has no direct hound descendents whereas the Shorthaired Pointer does.

Breeding for Function

Bred for both water, and land work, fur and feather, flushing, retrieving and pointing, and with the wire coat, the breed was particularly selected for the ability to work in rough close brush. Endurance and agility were selected for. These dogs have also been used in Shutzhund, tracking, obedience, agility, and for skijoring.

Physical Characteristics

Height at Withers: female 22-24" (56-61cm), male 24-26" (61-66 cm).

Weight: 45-70 lb (20-32 kg).

Coat: Somewhat water repellent, the coat lies flat, with wiry, straight hairs about 1.5-2" (4-5 cm) long, Well developed brows, beard and moustache help to protect the face from underbrush. The dense undercoat is shed during warmer months. Liver and white spotted is the standard color for the breed, with liver roan, ticking and roan in liver and white dogs, or solid liver being other accepted colorations. The face, (though not necessarily muzzle) and ears are liver, sometimes with a white blaze.

Longevity: 12-14 years

Points of Conformation: The German Wirehaired pointer is medium sized, with sturdy constitution, the head is moderately long, eyes are brown, oval, and medium sized. Pendulous ears are moderate in size and rounded, hanging closely alongside the head. The nose is brown, the muzzle is square and the stop moderate. The slightly arched neck is moderately long and clean, the topline gradually descends towards the rear. The thorax is deep and ribs well sprung. Abdominal tuck up is obvious. The high set tail is carried above the topline when alert. The tail if docked is shortened to about 2/5 of the native length. Limbs are straight boned and they are slightly longer than tall. Dewclaws are generally removed. Round feet have webbed toes and possess heavy nails and pads, with well knuckled up toes. The gait is smooth, and long strided.

Recognized Behavior Issues and Traits

Reported breed characteristics include: Stable temperament, active, high exercise needs, low grooming needs, aloof with strangers, intelligent. They have a moderate shedding tendency, and love to please. They may become a one-man dog and are loyal to family. Good with children if they are socialized early, and the children are calm. Will ably defend home or self if threatened. These dogs need mental stimulation or they may become destructive. Early obedience training is important. Typically they have a low tendency to dig, keep leashed unless in a fenced enclosure. This type of dog is generally considered too active for apartment life.

Normal Physiologic Variations

In a survey in Great Brittian, 47.8% of German Wirehaired pointer litters were born via **ceseran section**.[1]

Drug Sensitivities

None reported

Inherited Diseases

Hip Dysplasia: Polygenically inherited trait causing degenerative joint disease and hip arthritis. Reported 7.1x odds ratio versus other breeds. OFA reports 9.1% affected.[2,3]

Elbow Dysplasia: Polygenically inherited trait causing elbow arthritis. OFA reports 3.0% affected.[2]

Patella Luxation: Polygenically inherited laxity of patellar ligaments, causing luxation, lameness, and later degenerative joint disease. Treat surgically if causing clinical signs. Too few German Wirehaired Pointers have been screened by OFA to determine an accurate frequency.[2]

von Willebrand's disease (vWD): Type II vWD in the German Wirehaired Pointer is a serious, sometimes fatal, autosomal recessive bleeding disorder. Cryoprecipitate is more effective, with fewer side effects, than fresh frozen plasma in controlling bleeding episodes. A genetic test is available.[4,5]

Hemophilia B (Factor IX Deficiency): Mild, X-linked recessive bleeding disorder documented in this breed. A genetic test is available.[6]

Disease Predispositions

Hypothyroidism: Inherited autoimmune thyroiditis. 18.6% positive for thyroid auto-antibodies based on testing at Michigan State University. (Ave. for all breeds is 7.5%). One of the ten highest breeds in frequency of the disorder.[7,8]

Humeral Osteochondritis Dissecans (OCD): Polygenically inherited cartilage defect of the humeral head. Causes shoulder joint pain and lameness in young growing dogs. Mild cases can resolve with rest, while more severe cases require surgery. There is a 2.24:1 male to female ratio. 75% of all cases are unilateral. Reported 38.8x odds ratio versus other breeds. Reported at a frequency of 1.36% in the German Wirehaired Pointer.[3,9]

Cataracts: Cataracts occur in the breed. Onset 6-18 months of age. Unknown mode of inheritance. Too few German Wirehaired Pointers have been CERF eye examined to determine an accurate frequency in the breed. CERF does not recommend breeding any German Wirehaired Pointer with a cataract.[10]

Atrioventricular (Heart) Block: German Wirehaired Pointers are found to be at increased risk of high-grade second- or third-degree atrioventricular block versus other breeds. Treatment is with a pacemaker.[11]

Brachygnathism, Entropion, Osteochondritis Dessicans-Shoulder, Prognathism, and **Retinal Dysplasia** are reported.[12]

Isolated Case Studies

Day Blindness: A 5 month old German Wirehaired Pointer presented with day blindness (achromatopsia), consistent with cone degeneration seen in German Shorthaired Pointers.[13]

Diffuse Bronchiolo-alveolar Carcinoma: An eight-year-old female German Wirehaired Pointer was presented with signs of respiratory distress. Radiography indicated the presence of a diffuse interstitial lung disease. A primary lung cancer with an unusually diffuse distribution of miliary/micronodular lesions was found at postmortem examination. Histological diagnosis was bronchiolo-alveolar carcinoma.[14]

Genetic Tests

Tests of Genotype: Direct test for Hemophilia B is available from Cornell Animal Health Diagnostic Center (607.253.3900).

Direct test for vWD is available from VetGen.

Direct test for black, red/orange and brown colors, and black or brown nose is available from HealthGene and VetGen.

Tests of Phenotype: CHIC Certification: Hip and elbow radiographs, thyroid profile including autoantibodies (minimum of 2 years, then annually until 4 years), CERF eye evaluation (annually if breeding), and gene test for vWD. Optional tests include cardiac evaluation (preferably by a cardiologist), and patella evaluation. (See CHIC website; www.caninehealthinfo.org).

Miscellaneous

- **Breed name synonyms:** Deutscher Drahthaariger Vorstehhund, Drahthaar, German Pointer (Wirehaired).
- **Registries:** AKC, UKC, CKC, KCGB (Kennel Club of Great Britain), ANKC (Australian National Kennel Club), NKC (National Kennel Club).
- **AKC rank (year 2008):** 72 (1,213 dogs registered)
- **Internet resources: German Wirehaired Pointer Club of America:** http://www.gwpca.com/
  Verein Deutsch-Drahthaar Group Canada: www.vdd-canada.ca
  German Wirehaired Pointer Club (UK): www.gwpclub.co.uk

References

1. Evans KM & Adams VJ: Proportion of litters of purebred dogs born by caesarean section. J Small Anim Pract. 2010 Feb;51(2):113-8.
2. OFA Website breed statistics: www.offa.org Last accessed July 1, 2010.
3. LaFond E, Breur GJ & Austin CC: Breed susceptibility for developmental orthopedic diseases in dogs. J Am Anim Hosp Assoc. 2002 Sep-Oct;38(5):467-77.
4. Kramer JW, Venta PJ, Klein SR, et. al.: A von Willebrand's factor genomic nucleotide variant and polymerase chain reaction diagnostic test associated with inheritable type-2 von Willebrand's disease in a line of german shorthaired pointer dogs. Vet Pathol. 2004 May;41(3):221-8.
5. Brooks M, Raymond S, Catalfamo J: Severe, recessive von Willebrand's disease in German Wirehaired Pointers. J Am Vet Med Assoc. 1996 Sep 1;209(5):926-9.
6. Brooks MB, Gu W, Barnas JL, et. al.: A Line 1 insertion in the Factor IX gene segregates with mild hemophilia B in dogs. Mamm Genome. 2003 Nov;14(11):788-95.
7. Nachreiner RF, Refsal KR, Graham PA, et. al.: Prevalence of serum thyroid hormone autoantibodies in dogs with clinical signs of hypothyroidism. J Am Vet Med Assoc 2002 Feb 15;220(4):466-71.
8. Nachreiner R & Refsal K: Personal communication, Diagnostic Center for Population and Animal Health, Michigan State University. April, 2007.
9. Rudd RG, Whitehair JG, Margolis JH: Results of management of osteochondritis dissecans of the humeral head in dogs : 44 cases [1982 to 1987]. J Am Anim Hosp Assoc 1990: 26[2]:173-178.
10. Ocular Disorders Presumed to be Inherited in Purebred Dogs. American College of Veterinary Ophthalmologists. ACVO, 2007.
11. Schrope DP & Kelch WJ: Signalment, clinical signs, and prognostic indicators associated with high-grade second- or third-degree atrioventricular block in dogs: 124 cases (January 1, 1997-December 31, 1997). J Am Vet Med Assoc. 2006 Jun 1;228(11):1710-7.
12. The Genetic Connection: A Guide to Health Problems in Purebred Dogs. L Ackerman. p. 219-20. AAHA Press, 1999.
13. McElroy RP: Day blindness in a German wirehaired pointer. Vet Rec. 2006 Feb 4;158(5):175.
14. Bertazzolo W, Zuliani D, Pogliani E, et. al.: Diffuse bronchiolo-alveolar carcinoma in a dog. J Small Anim Pract. 2002 Jun;43(6):265-8.
15. The Complete Dog Book, 20th Ed. The American Kennel Club. Howell Book House, NY 2006. p. 29-32.

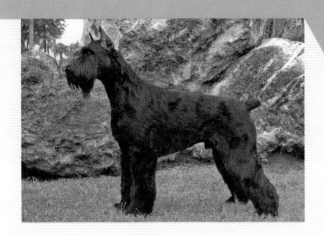

towards the rear quarters. Limbs are straight boned. The tail is carried high when active, and usually docked to be 1.5-3.0" (3.5-7.5 cm). Feet are compact and the toes well arched. Black nails and thick pads are standard. Dewclaws are usually removed from forelimbs; if present on hind limbs, they are removed. The gait is strong, straight, low, and has a spring to the stride.

The Breed History

This breed was derived from the Standard Schnauzer by crossing with the Great Dane, and also the Bouvier des Flandres. First breed records appeared in Southern Germany in the late 1800s. The AKC registered the breed in 1930.

Breeding for Function

The dog was used in the South Bavaria and Wurtemmburg regions of Germany for driving livestock, specifically cattle because of the great size and strength of this type of dog. Other tasks were as a watchdog and butcher's dog. Since the World Wars, this breed has been used extensively in Germany as a guarding and police dog.

Physical Characteristics

Height at Withers: male 25.5-27.5" (65-70 cm), female 23.5-25.5" (59.5-65 cm).

Weight: 70-77 lb (32-35 kg).

Coat: The weather resistant dense double coat consists of soft hair underneath, and a hard, wiry medium length overcoat. Salt and pepper or solid black are the standard colors. Salt and pepper is produced by a mixture of white/black banded hairs mixed with solid black and solid white hairs. A dark face mask is present on both colors. Needs to have the undercoat stripped twice per annum and the beard and moustache area may need to be cleaned after eating; classified in the moderate to high grooming needs category. Low shedding tendency is present if the coat is stripped.

Longevity: 10-12 years

Points of Conformation: A larger version of the Standard Schnauzer type, this breed shares the same basic conformation points. Square conformation, with well muscled straight limbs, a significant brow and beard and wiry haircoat distinguish the Schnauzer type. The head is rectangular, a slight stop is evident, and they possess a flat and moderately wide skull. The large nose is black. Triangular ears are medium in length with fairly thick leathers, and carried high and close to the head. Ears may be cropped. Eyes are deep set and colored dark brown, medium in size and oval. The neck is moderate in length and muscling. Not throaty. The thorax is deep and ribs well sprung. Moderate abdomen tuck up is present. The back is short and straight; gradually lowering

Recognized Behavior Issues and Traits

Reported breed characteristics include: Good endurance, highly intelligent, high trainability, obedient, alert, reliable, loyal and playful. Good guard for home and family, courageous and territorial. Good in city or country settings. Has high exercise and mental stimulation needs, if not fulfilled, will lead to boredom. Early socialization and obedience training are recommended.

Normal Physiologic Variations

Giant Schnauzers have much lower red blood cell thiopurine methyltransferase activity (7.9-20 U of RBC per milliliter; median, 13.1; $P < .001$) than other breeds. This could affect thiopurine (azathioprine) drug toxicity and efficacy in canine patients.[1]

Drug Sensitivities

None reported

Inherited Diseases

Hip Dysplasia: Polygenically inherited trait causing degenerative joint disease and hip arthritis. OFA reports 18.1% affected.[2]

Elbow Dysplasia: Polygenically inherited trait causing elbow arthritis. OFA reports 7.8% affected.[2]

Patella Luxation: Polygenically inherited laxity of patellar ligaments, causing luxation, lameness, and later degenerative joint disease. Treat surgically if causing clinical signs. Too few Giant Schnauzers have been screened by OFA to determine an accurate frequency.[2]

Cobalamin Malabsorption: An autosomal recessive selective intestinal malabsorption of cobalamin (Cbl) occurs in Giant Schnauzers. Affected puppies exhibited chronic inappetence and failure to thrive beginning between 6 and 12 wk of age. Neutropenia with hypersegmentation, anemia with anisocytosis and poikilocytosis, and megaloblastic changes of the bone marrow occur. Serum Cbl concentrations are low, and methylmalonic aciduria and homocysteinemia are present. Treat with vitamin B12 supplementation. A genetic test is available.[3]

Congenital Hypothyroid Dwarfism: Rare inherited disorder, with affected puppies showing dwarfism, lethargy, somnolence, gait abnormalities, and constipation. Laboratory tests show anemia, hypercholesterolemia, and occasional hypercalcemia. Radiographic skeletal surveys disclosed epiphyseal dysgenesis and delayed skeletal maturation. Affected dogs have low basal serum thyroxine concentrations that fail to increase following the administration of TSH, and markedly reduced to absent gamma camera imaging of the thyroid gland. Reported as a secondary or tertiary, rather than primary hypothyroidism. Pedigree analysis suggests an autosomal recessive mode of inheritance.[4]

Hyperuricosuria (HUU)/Urate Bladder Stones: An autosomal recessive mutation in the SLC2A9 gene causes urate urolithiasis and can predispose male dogs to urinary obstruction. Estimated at a carrier frequency of 11.20% in the breed. A genetic test is available.[22]

Disease Predispositions

Hypothyroidism: Inherited autoimmune thyroiditis. 15.5% positive for thyroid auto-antibodies based on testing at Michigan State University. (Ave. for all breeds is 7.5%) Another study found 16% affected in the breed. A specific DLA class II (major histocompatability complex) haplotype produces a 6.5x odds ratio of developing the disorder. Dorn reports a 2.28x odds ratio versus other breeds.[5,6,7,8,9]

Persistent Pupillary Membranes: Strands of fetal remnant connecting; iris to iris, cornea, lens, or involving sheets of tissue. The later three forms can impair vision, and dogs affected with these forms should not be bred. Identified in 5.95% of Giant Schnauzers CERF examined by veterinary ophthalmologists between 2000-2005.[10]

Cataracts: Intermediate and punctate cataracts predominate in the breed. Age of onset from less than a year to 7 years. Identified in 4.46% of Giant Schnauzers CERF examined by veterinary ophthalmologists between 2000-2005.[10]

Inherited Epilepsy: Grand-mal or petit-mal seizures. Control with anticonvulsant medication. Dorn reports a 9.97x odds ratio versus other breeds. 1.23% of first time admissions of Giant Schnauzers to Veterinary Colleges are for epilepsy.[5,11]

Retinal Dysplasia: Retinal folds, geographic, and generalized retinal dysplasia with detachment are recognized in the breed. Reported in 2.60% of Giant Schnauzers CERF examined by veterinary ophthalmologists between 2000-2005.[10]

Hormonal Urinary Incontinence: Multiple studies show a breed prevalence for urinary incontinence in spayed female Giant Schnauzers.[12,13]

Everted Cartilage of the Third Eyelid: Unilateral or bilateral scroll-like curling of the cartilage of the third eyelid, everting the margin. May cause mild ocular irritation. Identified in 1.49% of Giant Schnauzers CERF examined by veterinary ophthalmologists between 2000-2005.[10]

Cranial Cruciate Ligament Rupture (ACL): Traumatic tearing of the anterior cruciate ligament. Treatment is surgery. Dorn reports a 2.44x odds ratio versus other breeds.[5]

Gastric Dilatation-Volvulus (Bloat, GDV): Polygenically inherited, life-threatening twisting of the stomach within the abdomen. Requires immediate veterinary attention. Diagnosed at an increased frequency in the breed. Giant Schnauzers with the deepest thorax relative to width have the greatest risk for GDV.[14]

Digital Squamous Cell Carcinoma: Toe cancer seen at an increased frequency in black Giant Schnauzers. Treatment is digital amputation.[15]

Symmetrical Lupoid Onychodystrophy: Disorder causing loss of toenails. Onset between 3-8 years of age affecting 1-2 nails, then progressing to all toenails within 2-9 weeks. Requires lifelong treatment with oral fatty acid supplementation. Diagnosed at an increased frequency in the breed. (See GSCA website.)

Brachygnathism, Cryptorchidism, Glaucoma, Narcolepsy, Prognathism, Progressive Retinal Atrophy, Tricuspid Valve Dysplasia, and **von Willebrand's Disease** are reported.[16]

Isolated Case Studies

Immune-Mediated Neutropenia and Thrombocytopenia: Neutropenia, thrombocytopenia, and splenomegaly were recognized in 3 unrelated adult female giant schnauzers. Antineutrophil antibodies were demonstrated in 2 dogs. Splenectomy and steroid and azathioprine therapy reversed the condition.[17]

Nasal Philtrum Arteritis: A Giant Schnauzer was identified with a solitary, well-circumscribed, linear ulcer on the nasal philtrum, with repeated episodes of arterial bleeding. Histopathological findings included lymphoplasmacytic dermatitis, proliferating spindle cells of either myofibroblast or smooth muscle origin, and deep dermal arteries and arterioles subjacent to the ulcer. The lesion responded to steroidal treatment.[18]

Lymphocytic Leukemia: A 7-year-old male Giant Schnauzer had a history of severe vomiting, lethargy, weight loss, polydipsia and polyuria. Diagnostics revealed leucocytosis with a marked lymphocytosis, mild non-regenerative anaemia, thrombocytopenia, hypercalcemia and azotemia. Circulating lymphocytes were small and well-differentiated, and the same lymphoid population was present in bone marrow. Chronic lymphocyctic leukemia with associated paraneoplastic hypercalcemia was diagnosed.[19]

Central Diabetes Insipidus: A 9-year-old male giant Schnauzer with polyuria and polydipsia was diagnosed with central diabetes insipidus by vasopressin measurements during hypertonic stimulation. A large pituitary tumor, was visualized by CT scan, and identified as a melanotrophic tumor of the pars intermedia.[20]

Genetic Tests

Tests of Genotype: Direct test for Cobalamin Malabsorption is available from PennGen.

Direct test for HUU is available from the UC-Davis VGL and the Animal Health Trust.

Tests of Phenotype: CHIC Certification: Required testing includes CERF eye examination, thyroid profile including autoantibodies, and hip radiograph. (See CHIC website; www.caninehealthinfo.org).

Recommend elbow radiographs, patella evaluation, and cardiac evaluation.

Miscellaneous

- **Breed name synonyms:** Rieseinschnauzer, MÜnchener (historical), Munich Schnauzer (historical), Russian Bear Schnauzer (historical).
- **Registries:** AKC, UKC, CKC, KCGB (Kennel Club of Great Britain), ANKC (Australian National Kennel Club), NKC (National Kennel Club).
- **AKC rank (year 2008):** 87 (751 dogs registered)
- **Internet resources: The Giant Schnauzer Club of America:** www.giantschnauzerclubofamerica.com
  Giant Schnauzer Club (UK): www.giantschnauzerclub.co.uk
  Giant Schnauzer Club Canada: www.giantschnauzercanada.com

References

1. Kidd LB, Salavaggione OE, Szumlanski CL, et. al.: Thiopurine methyltransferase activity in red blood cells of dogs. *J Vet Intern Med.* 2004 Mar-Apr;18(2):214-8.

2. OFA Website breed statistics: www.offa.org Last accessed July 1, 2010.

3. Fyfe JC, Giger U, Hall CA, et. al.: Inherited selective intestinal cobalamin malabsorption and cobalamin deficiency in dogs. *Pediatr Res.* 1991 Jan;29(1):24-31.

4. Greco DS, Feldman EC, Peterson ME, et. al.: Congenital hypothyroid dwarfism in a family of giant schnauzers. *J Vet Intern Med.* 1991 Mar-Apr;5(2):57-65.

5. Dorn CR: Canine breed-specific risks of frequently diagnosed diseases at veterinary teaching hospitals. Monograph. AKC Canine Health Foundation. 2000.

6. Nachreiner RF, Refsal KR, Graham PA, et. al.: Prevalence of serum thyroid hormone autoantibodies in dogs with clinical signs of hypothyroidism. J Am Vet Med Assoc. 2002 Feb 15;220(4):466-71.

7. Nachreiner R & Refsal K: Personal communication, Diagnostic Center for Population and Animal Health, Michigan State University. April, 2007.

8. Ferm K, Björnerfeldt S, Karlsson A, et. al.: Prevalence of diagnostic characteristics indicating canine autoimmune lymphocytic thyroiditis in giant schnauzer and hovawart dogs. J Small Anim Pract. 2009 Apr;50(4):176-9.

9. Wilbe M, Sundberg K, Hansen IR, et. al.: Increased genetic risk or protection for canine autoimmune lymphocytic thyroiditis in Giant Schnauzers depends on DLA class II genotype. Tissue Antigens. 2010 Jun;75(6):712-9.

10. *Ocular Disorders Presumed to be Inherited in Purebred Dogs.* American College of Veterinary Ophthalmologists. ACVO, 2007.

11. Patterson E: Clinical Characteristics and Inheritance of Idiopathic Epilepsy. Proceedings, 2007 Tufts' Canine and Feline Breeding and Genetics Conference. 2007.

12. Arnold S: Urinary incontinence in castrated bitches. Part 1: Significance, clinical aspects and etiopathogenesis. *Schweiz Arch Tierheilkd.* 1997;139(6):271-6.

13. Blendinger C, Blendinger K, Bostedt H: Urinary incontinence in spayed bitches. 1. Pathogenesis, incidence and disposition. *Tierarztl Prax.* 1995 Jun;23(3):291-9.

14. Glickman LT, Glickman NW, Perez CM, et. al.: Analysis of risk factors for gastric dilatation and dilatation-volvulus in dogs. J Am Vet Med Assoc. 1994 May 1;204(9):1465-71.

15. Paradis M, Scott DW, Breton L: Squamous cell carcinoma of the nail bed in three related giant schnauzers. *Vet Rec.* 1989 Sep 16;125(12):322-4.

16. *The Genetic Connection: A Guide to Health Problems in Purebred Dogs.* L Ackerman. p. 236-37. AAHA Press, 1999.

17. Vargo CL, Taylor SM & Haines DM: Immune mediated neutropenia and thrombocytopenia in 3 giant schnauzers. Can Vet J. 2007 Nov;48(11):1159-63.

18. Torres SM, Brien TO, Scott DW: Dermal arteritis of the nasal philtrum in a Giant Schnauzer and three Saint Bernard dogs. *Vet Dermatol.* 2002 Oct;13(5):275-81.

19. Kleiter M, Hirt R, Kirtz G, et. al.: Hypercalcaemia associated with chronic lymphocytic leukaemia in a Giant Schnauzer. *Aust Vet J.* 2001 May;79(5):335-8.

20. Goossens MM, Rijnberk A, Mol JA, et. al.: Central diabetes insipidus in a dog with a pro-opiomelanocortin-producing pituitary tumor not causing hyperadrenocorticism. *J Vet Intern Med.* 1995 Sep-Oct;9(5):361-5.

21. *The Complete Dog Book, 20th Ed.* The American Kennel Club. Howell Book House, NY 2006. p. 266-271.

22. Karmi N, Brown EA, Hughes SS, et. al.: Estimated frequency of the canine hyperuricosuria mutation in different dog breeds. J Vet Intern Med. 2010 Nov-Dec;24(6):1337-42.

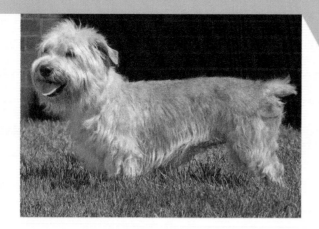

The Breed History

This breed originates in Ireland in County Wicklow. It is still a rare breed—in the USA about 400 terriers are registered with their national breed club. The Irish Kennel Club recognized the breed in 1934, a long time after the genesis of this very old breed. The AKC recognized the breed in the terrier group in October 2004.

Breeding for Function

This is an agile powerful hunting terrier of ancient terrier type. Breeding in ancient times was focused on producing a dog with excellent vermin control skills, and also an aid to the fox and badger hunter. A unique historical task was to be a turnspit dog. This was a wheel that the dog turned which rotated the spit over the fire for roasting pig and other meats. Their deep bark makes them sound like a much larger dog. They excel at obedience.

Physical Characteristics

Height at Withers: 12.5-14" (32-35.5 cm)

Weight: 35 lb (16 kg)

Coat: Medium length, double, with harsh overcoat. Accepted colors include blue, brindle (usually blue) and wheaten. Needs 1-2x weekly brushing, and once to twice annual stripping. Ears need to be plucked. Bathing done on an as-need basis.

Longevity: 10-15 years

Points of Conformation: Head is large, skull broad, eyes are round and wide set. Rose or half prick ears are small and set back and high on the skull. A scissors bite or level bite is accepted. Muzzle tapering to the black nose, and stop is pronounced. The neck is thick, and topline is unique to the breed, with a gentle curve up to the lumbar area. Limbs are short, and have some bowing—the compact front feet turn slightly out while the rear feet are straight. The thorax is deep and full but not barrel shaped. Hindquarters are heavily muscled. Generally the tail is docked to 1/2 length, and is carried high while active. The gait is smooth, flowing and covers a lot of ground with each stride. Is longer than tall in overall proportions.

Recognized Behavior Issues and Traits

Breed attributes reported include: Courageous, stoic, hardy, stubborn, independent, spirited when working, but tame at home.

Glen of Imaal Terrier

Game for a fight with other dogs, but can live fine with other pets if socialized early to them. A little less active than other terrier breeds. Strong chase instinct—need to be loose only in a secured fence enclosure—the fence needs to be designed to counteract their excellent digging skills. They have a low bark tendency. Work silently. Not considered the best of swimmers. Good with older children—can be a bit strong and active for youngsters.

Normal Physiologic Variations
None reported

Drug Sensitivities
None reported

Inherited Diseases

Hip Dysplasia: Polygenically inherited trait causing degenerative joint disease and hip arthritis. OFA reports 30.0% affected.[1]

Elbow Dysplasia: Polygenically inherited trait causing elbow arthritis. OFA reports 16.2% affected.[1]

Patella Luxation: Polygenically inherited laxity of patellar ligaments, causing luxation, lameness, and later degenerative joint disease. Treat surgically if causing clinical signs. Too few Glen of Imaal Terriers have been screened to determine an accurate frequency.[1]

Progressive Retinal Atrophy (PRA)/Cone-Rod Dystrophy (crd3): Autosomal recessive disorder of cone, and then rod retinal degeneration. Clinical signs begin in middle age as night blindness and difficulty in dim light, and progresses to complete blindness. Affected dogs can be identified ophthalmoscopically as young as 3 years of age, with progression over several years. Identified in 4.14% of Glen of Imaal Terriers CERF examined by veterinary ophthalmologists between 2000-2005. CERF does not recommend breeding any Glen of Imaal Terriers with PRA/crd. A direct genetic test is available.[2,3]

Disease Predispositions

Hypothyroidism: Inherited autoimmune thyroiditis. 7.1% positive for thyroid auto-antibodies based on testing at Michigan State University. (Ave. for all breeds is 7.5%).[4,5]

Allergic Skin Disease: Inhalant or food allergies. Causes pruritis and pyotraumatic dermatitis (hot spots). Reported to occur in the breed.

Distichiasis: Abnormally placed eyelashes that irritate the cornea and conjunctiva. Can cause secondary corneal ulceration. Identified in 4.13% of Glen of Imaal Terriers CERF examined by veterinary ophthalmologists between 2000-2005.[2]

Cataracts: Anterior and equatorial cortex cataracts predominate in the breed. Identified in 3.31% of Glen of Imaal Terriers CERF examined by veterinary ophthalmologists between 2000-2005.

CERF does not recommend breeding any Glen of Imaal Terrier with a cataract.[2]

Aortic Stenosis: Affected dogs present with a left heart base murmur, and aortic velocities greater than 1.5 m/second on Doppler echocardiography, aortic regurgitation, and mitral regurgitation. Can cause exercise intolerance, syncope, and progress to heart failure. This congenital heart defect has been diagnosed in Glen of Imaal terriers. Dogs should be screened for heart murmurs.

Entropion, and **Seasonal Flank Alopecia** are reported.[6]

Isolated Case Studies
None reported

Genetic Tests
Tests of Genotype: Direct test for crd3 is available from Optigen.

Tests of Phenotype: CHIC Certification: Required testing includes hip radiographs, CERF eye examination (annually until age 8), and genetic test for crd3 PRA. (See CHIC website; www.caninehealthinfo.org).

Recommend elbow radiographs, thyroid profile including autoantibodies, patella examination, and cardiac examination.

Miscellaneous
- **Breed name synonyms:** none
- **Registries:** AKC, UKC, ANKC (Australian National Kennel Club), NKC (National Kennel Club), KCGB, FCI
- **AKC rank (year 2008):** 156 (32 dogs registered)
- **Breed resources: Glen of Imaal Club of America:** www.glens.org
  The Glen of Imaal Terrier Association (UK): www.goita.co.uk

References
1. OFA Website breed statistics: www.offa.org Last accessed July 1, 2010.
2. Ocular Disorders Presumed to be Inherited in Purebred Dogs. American College of Veterinary Ophthalmologists. ACVO, 2007
3. Goldstein O, Mezey JG, Boyko AR, et. al.: An ADAM9 mutation in canine cone-rod dystrophy 3 establishes homology with human cone-rod dystrophy 9. Mol Vis. 2010 Aug 11;16:1549-69.
4. Nachreiner RF, Refsal KR, Graham PA, et. al.: Prevalence of serum thyroid hormone autoantibodies in dogs with clinical signs of hypothyroidism. J Am Vet Med Assoc. 2002 Feb 15;220(4):466-71.
5. Nachreiner R & Refsal K: Personal communication, Diagnostic Center for Population and Animal Health, Michigan State University. April, 2007.
6. *The Genetic Connection: A Guide to Health Problems in Purebred Dogs.* L Ackerman. p. 220. AAHA Press, 1999.
7. *The Complete Dog Book, 20th Ed.* The American Kennel Club. Howell Book House, NY 2006. p. 378-381.

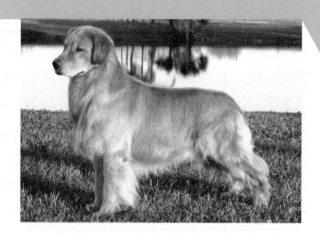

The Breed History

Golden Retrievers are perennial favorites as companion animal dogs, but their origins were in the hunt fields of the British Isles. The hunt was a popular sport, especially fowling. The genealogy of the Golden Retriever breed is thought to include Newfoundland dogs, Tweed Water Spaniels (and other spaniels), Flat-coated Retriever, Bloodhound and Irish Setters. These dogs were first brought to North America in the 1890s. First AKC Golden Retriever breed registration occurred in 1925.

Breeding for Function

Selection was for a versatile breed that could perform well in the hunt of both upland game and waterfowl. Obedience, hunting trials, companion guide dogs for the blind, tracking, and search and rescue are talents possessed by this breed. They are generally considered a gundog.

Physical Characteristics

Height at Withers: female 21.5-22.5" (54.5-57 cm), male 23-24" (58.5-61 cm).

Weight: females 55-65 lb (25-29.5 kg), males 65-75 lb (29.5-34 kg).

Coat: The double coat has a very high hair density, repels water effectively and some feathering of underbody, forelimbs, and back of thigh/underside of the tail is present. The standard color is gold, but this color exists in a spectrum from light-dark-medium-dark, with the latter preferred. Red is not accepted. Some waviness is accepted.

Longevity: 10-15 years

Points of Conformation: This dog is a muscular, powerful, balanced dog, possessing a free smooth gait. The skull is broad, and stop is well defined, the square strong muzzle blends with the skull smoothly, and there is no heaviness in the flews. The deep-set eyes are moderately wide set, and are pigmented brown. The eyelids fit closely and have dark margins. Ears are moderately short, triangular, and the nose is darkly pigmented. The neck is medium in length, and well muscled. The topline is level, and slopes slightly to the croup. The thorax is deep, and ribs well sprung. The abdomen shows little tuck up, and the thick tail is slightly curved and generally carried horizontally. The tail bones reach to the level of the tarsus.

Limbs are straight boned, and the dewclaws are usually left on forelimbs. The feet are round shaped, well knuckled, and compact.

Recognized Behavior Issues and Traits

Reported breed characteristics include: Eager, alert, friendly, trustworthy; this breed is known for the ability to tolerate other pets and children. Needs lots of exercise, easy to train, relaxed, responsive, and they rarely bite because of their waterfowl handling instincts. They have a moderate shedding tendency, and moderate grooming needs. They possess very high trainability; a real willingness to please. Though they may alarm bark, they are not considered watchdogs. Goldens need close human contact, and are not good as kenneled dogs. They need plenty of mental stimulation and play to keep them happy.

Normal Physiologic Variations

Echocardiographic Normal Values:[1]	
Parameter	Mean (Range)
Weight (kg)	32 (23-41)
Heart rate (bpm)	100 (80-140)
LVPWD (mm)	10 (8-12)
LVPWS (mm)	15 (10-19)
LVD (mm)	45 (37-51)
LVS (mm)	27 (18-35)
FS (%)	39 (27-55)
EPSS (mm)	5 (1-10)
RVd (mm)	13 (7-27)
IVSd (mm)	10 (8-13)
IVSs (mm)	14 (10-17)
AOD (mm)	24 (14-27)
LAS (mm)	27 (16-32)
N	20

LVPWD, LV posterior wall dimension at end-diastole; LVPWS, LV posterior wall thickness at end-systole; LVD, LV chamber dimension at end-diastole; LVS, LV chamber dimension at end-systole; FS, percent fractional shortening; EPSS, E-point septal separation; RVD, RV chamber dimension at end-diastole; IVSd, interventricular septal thickness at end-diastole; IVSs, interventricular septal thickness at end-systole; AOD, aortic root at end-diastole; LAS, left atrium at end-systole; N, number of animals.

Drug Sensitivities

None Reported

Inherited Diseases

Hip Dysplasia: Polygenically inherited trait causing degenerative joint disease and hip arthritis. OFA reports 19.9% affected. Reported at a frequency of 18.21% in the 1998 GRCA National Health Survey.[2,3]

Elbow Dysplasia: Polygenically inherited trait causing elbow arthritis. OFA reports 11.2% affected. Reported 5.5x odds ratio for fragmented coronoid process, 4.9x odds ratio for ununited anconeal process forms of elbow dysplasia, and 42.2 odds ratio for elbow osteochondrosis versus other breeds.[2,4]

Patella Luxation: Polygenically inherited laxity of patellar ligaments, causing luxation, lameness, and later degenerative joint disease. Treat surgically if causing clinical signs. OFA reports 2.7% affected.[2]

Progressive Retinal Atrophy (prcd-PRA): Autosomal recessive progressive rod cone degeneration (prcd) form. Age of onset is between 3-8 years of age, eventually causing blindness. Optigen testing reports 1% affected, and 26% carriers in Golden Retrievers. Another autosomal recessive form of **PRA (GR-PRA1)** also occurs in the breed, with an average age of onset of 7 years. Genetic testing shows gene frequencies of 5% (UK), 6% (Sweden) 2% (France), and < 0.5% (US).[5,6]

Hemophilia A (Factor VIII Deficiency): X-linked recessive disorder causing excessive bleeding after trauma or surgery. Affected Golden Retrievers are identified in the US and Canada.[7]

Spectrin Deficiency: Rare, autosomal dominant disorder of erythrocyte osmotic fragility and spherocytosis. Can preclude hemolytic anemia in the breed. Identified in 17% of Dutch Golden Retrievers.[8]

von Willebrand's Disease: Autosomal recessive disorder of mild bleeding, usually associated with surgery, trauma, estrus, or parturition. Reported at a frequency of 18% in a Dutch population of Golden Retrievers, though a similar high frequency is not evident in the US population.[9]

Ichthyosis/Primary Cornification Defect: An autosomal recessive inherited, nonpruritic skin disease affecting young Golden Retrievers of either sex and characterized by symmetrical, predominantly ventro-lateral scaling and hyperpigmentation of the trunk. Pathology reveals moderate to severe laminated or compact orthokeratotic epidermal hyperkeratosis without significant involvement of the stratum granulosum. A genetic test is available.[10,11,12]

Sensorimotor Axonopathy: Rare, maternally (mitochondria) inherited disorder causing a slowly progressive course of ataxia and dysmetria with an insidious onset between 2 and 8 months of age. Necropsy reveals a central and peripheral sensorimotor axonopathy, with the proprioceptive pathways being most severely affected. Caused by a mutation in the mitochondrial tRNA (tyr) gene.[13,14]

Disease Predispositions

Allergic Dermatitis: Inhalant or food allergies. Presents with pruritis and pyotraumatic dermatitis (hot spots). The breed has a significant frequency of allergies, with a computed heritability of 0.47. Hot spots are reported at a frequency of 36.43%, flea allergy at 15.17%, inhalant allergy at 10.18%, and food allergy at 6.37% in the 1998 GRCA National Health Survey.[3,15]

Otitis Externa (Chronic Ear Infections): Can also be secondary to allergic skin disease. Bacterial, yeast, or mixed infection. Reported at a frequency of 20.22% in the 1998 GRCA National Health Survey.[3]

Sebaceous Cysts: Benign skin cysts with accumulation of sebaceous material. Reported at a frequency of 14.75% in the 1998 GRCA National Health Survey.[3]

Hypothyroidism: Inherited autoimmune thyroiditis. 13.2% positive for thyroid autoantibodies based on testing at Michigan State University. (Ave. for all breeds is 7.5%). Dorn reports a 1.86x odds ratio versus other breeds. Reported at a frequency of 23.75% in the 1998 GRCA National Health Survey.[3,16,17,18]

Distichiasis: Abnormally placed eyelashes that irritate the cornea and conjunctiva. Can cause secondary corneal ulceration. Identified in 9.70% of Golden Retrievers CERF examined by veterinary ophthalmologists between 2000-2005. Dorn reports a 1.97x odds ratio versus other breeds. Reported at a frequency of 4.78% in the 1998 GRCA National Health Survey.[3,5,16]

Cataracts: Posterior cortical cataracts predominate in the breed, usually between 9 months to 3 years of age. The breed also can develop Y-suture cataracts. Identified in 5.61% of Golden Retrievers CERF examined by veterinary ophthalmologists between 2000-2005. Reported at a frequency of 12.74% in the 1998 GRCA National Health Survey. CERF does not recommend breeding any Golden Retriever with a cataract.[3,15,19,20]

Epilepsy (Inherited Seizures): Generalized seizures are usually seen in Golden Retrievers with an onset of 1 to 3 years of age. Treat with anticonvulsant medications. Unknown mode of inheritance. Seizures are reported at a frequency of 8.93% in the 1998 GRCA National Health Survey.[3,21]

Hemangiosarcoma: Malignant cancer of red blood cells, usually involving the spleen, liver, heart, or bone marrow. Molecular genetic studies increased expassion of vascular endothelial growth factor reception (VEGFR1) in the breed. Reported at a frequency of 7.34% in the 1998 GRCA National Health Survey.[3,22]

Lymphoma/Lymphosarcoma: Malignant cancer of lymphoid tissue. Both B-cell and T-cell (mycosis fungoides) occur in the breed. Reported at a frequency of 5.06% in the 1998 GRCA National Health Survey.[3,23]

Iris Cysts: Fluid filled sacs arising from the posterior surface of the iris, to which they may remain attached or break free and float into the anterior chamber. Usually occur in mature dogs. Can occasionally block the iridocorneal angle causing uveitis and glaucoma. Identified in 4.33% of Golden Retrievers CERF examined by veterinary ophthalmologists between 2000-2005.[5]

Mast Cell Tumor (MCT): Golden Retrievers are a predisposed breed for developing cutaneous mast cell tumors. These tumors produce histamine, causing inflammation and ulceration. The breed has a 3.8x risk versus other breeds of developing multiple mast cell tumors. Reported at a frequency of 4.64% in the 1998 GRCA National Health Survey.[3,24]

Aortic Stenosis (Subaortic Stenosis, SAS): Affected dogs present with a left heart base murmur, aortic velocities greater than 1.5 m/second on Doppler echocardiography, aortic regurgitation, and mitral regurgitation. Can cause exercise intolerance, syncope, and progress to heart failure. Golden Retrievers represented 30% of cases in one study. Odds ratio of 5.5x versus other breeds. Unknown mode of inheritance–considered polygenic. Heart murmur is reported at a frequency of 5.13%, and SAS at 1.39% in the 1998 GRCA National Health Survey.[25,26]

Seborrhea: Skin disorder presenting with greasy skin and haircoat. Can be primary or secondary to allergies or infection. Reported at a frequency of 3.32% in the 1998 GRCA National Health Survey.[3]

Gastric Dilation/Volvulus (GDV, Bloat): Life-threatening twisting of the stomach within the abdomen. Requires immediate veterinary attention. Reported at a frequency of 2.98% in the 1998 GRCA National Health Survey.[3]

Panosteitis: Affected dogs show intermittent lameness involving the diaphyseal and metaphyseal areas of the tubular long bones prior to skeletal maturation. Reported at a frequency of 2.42% in the 1998 GRCA National Health Survey.[3]

Osteochondritis Dessicans (OCD): Defect in cartilage maturation in young dogs, causing joint lesions and lameness. Treatment with rest, or surgery in severe cases. Severe cases can result in later arthritis and degenerative joint disease. Reported 12.6x odds ratio for shoulder OCD, and 3.9x odds ratio for stifle OCD versus other breeds. Reported at a frequency of 2.42% in the 1998 GRCA National Health Survey.[3,4]

Osteosarcoma: Malignant bone cancer, usually affecting the appendicular skeleton. Cytogenetic studies show recurrent breed-related mutation. Reported at a frequency of 2.28% in the 1998 GRCA National Health Survey.[3,27]

Persistent Pupillary Membranes: Strands of fetal remnant connecting; iris to iris, cornea, lens, or involving sheets of tissue. The later three forms can impair vision, and dogs affected with these forms should not be bred. Identified in 2.19% of Golden Retrievers CERF examined by veterinary ophthalmologists between 2000-2005.[5]

Cranial Cruciate Ligament (ACL) Rupture: Traumatic tearing of the ACL in the stifle, causing lameness and secondary arthritis. Treat with surgery. Reported at an increased incidence versus other breeds. Reported at a frequency of 2.08% in the 1998 GRCA National Health Survey.[3,28]

Uveitis: Inflammation of the uveal tract of the eye. Can progress to cataracts, glaucoma, or blindness. Can be idiopathic, or secondary to neoplasia (lymphoma), infection, or iris cysts. Golden Retrievers are the most commonly reported breed with the disorder.[29,30,31]

Glaucoma: Increased intra-ocular pressure, that can lead to blindmess from retinal death or detachment, uveitis, and corneal lesions. Can be primary or secondary. Golden Retrievers represent 5% of reported cases of glaucoma. Of these, 52% are associated with iris cysts.[31,32]

Retinal Dysplasia: Focal retinal dysplasia and retinal folds are recognized in the breed. Identified in 1.36% of Golden Retrievers CERF-examined by veterinary ophthalmologists between 2000-2005. Suggested autosomal recessive inheritance.[5,33]

Hypertrophic Osteodystrophy (HOD): Immune-mediated disorder causing fever, and painful, swollen joints and bones in young dogs. Occurs mostly within 3-14 days post-vaccination. Age of onset is 8-16 weeks. Reported 5.4x odds ratio versus other breeds.[4]

Histiocytic Sarcoma/Histiocytosis: Malignant cancer of CD11d+ macrophages, producing masses in the spleen, liver, lung, bone marrow, +/or eye. Mean age of diagnosis of 8.61 +/- 2.43 years, with a less than 6 month life expectancy. Golden Retrievers are overrepresented in diagnoses versus other breeds.[34,35,36]

Spontaneous Chronic Corneal Epithelial Defects (SCCED): Golden Retrievers are reported as a breed with an increased prevalence of spontaneous corneal epithelial defects. Research indicates a role of substance P.[37]

Oral Malignant Melanoma: Malignant cancer usually involving the gingiva. Can be pigmented or non-pigmented. One study identified a 1.84x relative risk versus other breeds.[38]

Idiopathic Horner's Syndrome: Horner's syndrome consists of unilateral miosis, ptosis, enophthalmos, and prolapsed nictitans. Male Golden Retrievers are overrepresented in canine cases. Most cases resolve over time.[39]

Juvenile Renal Dysplasia: Affected Golden Retrievers under 3 years of age initially present with polydipsia/polyuria and isosthenuria. With progressive renal failure, vomiting, anorexia, and weight loss develop. Histopathological findings include cystic glomerular atrophy, periglomerular fibrosis, fetal glomeruli, collecting tubule epithelial hyperplasia, and primitive mesenchymal connective tissue. Unknown mode of inheritance.[40,41]

Megaesophagus: Golden Retrievers are overrepresented in diagnoses of acquired megaesophagus. Causes include peripheral neuropathy, laryngeal paralysis, acquired myasthenia gravis, esophagitis, and gastric dilatation. Hypothyroidism is not associated with megaesophagus in the breed. Clinical signs include regurgitation, excess salivation, and aspiration pneumonia.[42]

Myesthenia Gravis: An immune-mediated disorder of circulating anti-acetylcholine receptor antibodies cause generalized appendicular muscle weakness with or without megaesophagus, or selective esophageal, facial and pharyngeal muscular weakness. Golden Retrievers are reported with a 2.2x odds ratio versus other breeds.[43,44]

Cricopharyngeal Dysfunction/Achalasia: Congenital abnormality of the upper esophageal sphincter due to stricture, or abnormal function. Diagnose with video fluoroscopy. Reported as a breed-related disorder, with a major autosomal recessive gene controlling its expression, and a heritability of 0.61.[45]

Idiopathic Pericardial Effusion: Golden Retrievers are overrepresented with this diagnosis, which is not due to tumor, trauma, or infection. Prognosis is good with pericardectomy.[46]

Intracranial Meningioma: One study found that Golden Retrievers are overrepresented compared to other breeds for intracranial meningiomas. These are the most common brain tumor in dogs, and can be benign, or malignant.[47,48]

Choroid Plexus Brain Tumor: Golden Retrievers are overrepresented in reported cases of choroid plexus carcinoma and choroid plexus papilloma. The breed has a 3.7x relative risk versus other breeds.[49]

Lingual Fibrosarcoma: Golden Retrievers have a 3.64x odds ratio versus other breeds of developing this cancer of the tongue.[50]

Limbal Melanoma: Benign eye mass, usually originating from the dorsal limbus. Golden Retrievers have a 5.8x odds ratio of limbal melanomas versus other breeds.[51]

Leukemia: A UK study showed that Golden Retrievers were overrepresented versus other breeds with diagnoses of acute and chronic lymphoid leukaemia (ALL and CLL), and acute and chronic myeloid leukaemia (AML and CML).[52]

Thyroid Cancer: Golden Retrievers have a 2.2 odds ratio versus other breeds of developing thyroid cancer. Affected dogs are usually between 10-15 years of age with a thyroid mass, and a diagnosis of carcinoma, or less frequently adenocarcinoma.[53]

Acral lick Dermatitis, Anasarca, Central Progressive Retinal Atrophy, Cerebellar Abiotrophy, Cervical Vertebral Instability, Degenerative Myelopathy, Entropion, Hypoadrenocorticism, Juvenile Cellulitis, Micropapilla, Nodular Dermatofibrosis, Oligodontia, Optic Nerve Hypoplasia, Proliferative Episcleritis, Seasonal Flank Alopecia, Sebaceous Adenitis, Silica Urolithiasis, Supernumerary Teeth, and **Tetralogy of Fallot** are reported.[54]

Isolated Case Studies

Taurine Deficient Dilated Cardiomyopathy (DCM): A family of Golden Retrievers was identified with taurine deficient DCM. Many individuals were weaned off heart medications and were able to be maintained only on taurine supplementation.[55]

Ciliary Dyskinesia: Several case reports of ciliary dyskinesia are reported in the breed. Affected dogs present with exercise intolerance, recurrent nasal discharge, bronchitis, and situs inversus.[56,57,58]

GM2-Gangliosidosis: Fatal, autosomal recessive lysosomal storage disease causing progressive ataxia and seizures. Identified in a Golden Retriever in Japan.[59]

Hypomyelinating Polyneuropathy: Identified in two Golden Retriever littermates with chronic peripheral neuropathy. Fibers of all calibers were hypomyelinated.[60]

Multisystem Axonopathy: Several young Golden Retriever between 3-5 months of age presented with generalized weakness, tremors, and progressive generalized muscle atrophy. Clinical signs were all lower motor neuron, witout proprioceptive ataxia. Pathology revealed a diffuse spinal cord axonopathy and motor neuron depletion.[61]

Muscular Dystrophy: X-linked recessive fatal disorder of stilted gait, gait restriction and muscle hypertrophy. Identified in a litter of Golden Retrievers in the 1980's, from which numerous research colonies have been developed as a canine form of Duchenne muscular dystrophy. The disorder does not exist in the general Golden Retriever population.[62,63]

Genetic Tests

Tests of Genotype: Direct test for prcd-PRA is available from Optigen. (Recommended for breeding dogs.)

Direct test for GR-PRA1 is available from thje Animal Health Trust and Optigen.

Direct test for Ichthyosis is available from Antagene.

Tests of Phenotype: CHIC Certification: Required testing includes hip and elbow radiographs, CERF eye examination (annually until 8 years), and cardiac evaluation by a cardiologist. (See CHIC website; www.caninehealthinfo.org).

Recommend thyroid profile including autoantibodies, and patella evaluation.

Miscellaneous

- **Breed name synonyms:** Yellow Retriever, Russian Retriever, Golden, Golden Flat-coat (historical).
- **Registries:** AKC, UKC, CKC, KCGB (Kennel Club of Great Britain), ANKC (Australian National Kennel Club), NKC (National Kennel Club).
- **AKC rank (year 2008):** 4 (34,485 dogs registered)
- **Internet resources:** Golden Retriever Club of America: www.grca.org
  Golden Retriever Club of Canada: www.grcc.net
  The Golden Retriever Club (UK): www.thegoldenretrieverclub.co.uk

References

1. Morrison SA, Moise NS, Scarlett JM, et al: Effect of breed and body weight on echocardiographic values of four breeds of dogs of differing weight and somatotype. J Vet Intern Med. 1992; 6:220.
2. OFA Website breed statistics: www.offa.org Last accessed July 1, 2010.
3. Glickman L, Glickman N, & Thorpe R: The Golden Retriever Club of America National Health Survey 1998-1999. Purdue University School of Veterinary Medicine. 1999.
4. LaFond E, Breur GJ & Austin CC: Breed susceptibility for developmental orthopedic diseases in dogs. J Am Anim Hosp Assoc. 2002 Sep-Oct;38(5):467-77.
5. Ocular Disorders Presumed to be Inherited in Purebred Dogs. American College of Veterinary Ophthalmologists. ACVO, 2007.
6. Zangerl B, Goldstein O, Philp AR, et al.: Identical mutation in a novel retinal gene causes progressive rod-cone degeneration in dogs and retinitis pigmentosa in humans. Genomics 2006; 88:551-563.
7. Brooks MB, Barnas JL, Fremont J, et. al.: Cosegregation of a factor VIII microsatellite marker with mild hemophilia A in Golden Retriever dogs. J Vet Intern Med. 2005 Mar-Apr;19(2):205-10.
8. Slappendel RJ, van Zwieten R, van Leeuwen M, et. al.: Hereditary spectrin deficiency in Golden Retriever dogs. J Vet Intern Med. 2005 Mar-Apr;19(2):187-92.
9. Feldman BF & Brummerstedt E: Von Willebrand's factor deficiency in a random population of Danish golden retrievers. Nord Vet Med. 1986 Nov-Dec;38(6):378-82.
10. Cadiergues MC, Patel A, Shearer DH, et. al.: Cornification defect in the golden retriever: clinical, histopathological, ultrastructural and genetic characterisation. Vet Dermatol. 2008 Jun;19(3):120-9.
11. Mauldin EA, Credille KM, Dunstan RW, et. al.: The clinical and morphologic features of nonepidermolytic ichthyosis in the golden retriever. Vet Pathol. 2008 Mar;45(2):174-80.
12. Guaguere E, Bensignor E, Küry S, et. al.: Clinical, histopathological and

genetic data of ichthyosis in the golden retriever: a prospective study. J Small Anim Pract. 2009 May;50(5):227-35.

13. Jäderlund KH, Orvind E, Johnsson E, et. al.: A neurologic syndrome in Golden Retrievers presenting as a sensory ataxic neuropathy. J Vet Intern Med. 2007 Nov-Dec;21(6):1307-15.

14. Baranowska I, Jäderlund KH, Nennesmo I, et. al.: Sensory ataxic neuropathy in golden retriever dogs is caused by a deletion in the mitochondrial tRNATyr gene. PLoS Genet. 2009 May;5(5):e1000499.

15. Shaw SC, Wood JL, Freeman J, et. al.: Estimation of heritability of atopic dermatitis in Labrador and Golden Retrievers. Am J Vet Res. 2004 Jul;65(7):1014-20.

16. Dorn CR: Canine breed-specific risks of frequently diagnosed diseases at veterinary teaching hospitals. Monograph. AKC Canine Health Foundation. 2000.

17. Nachreiner RF, Refsal KR, Graham PA, et. al.: Prevalence of serum thyroid hormone autoantibodies in dogs with clinical signs of hypothyroidism. *J Am Vet Med Assoc* 2002 Feb 15;220(4):466-71.

18. Nachreiner R & Refsal K: Personal communication, Diagnostic Center for Population and Animal Health, Michigan State University. April, 2007.

19. Rubin LF: Cataract in Golden Retrievers. J Am Vet Med Assoc. 1974 Sep 1;165(5):457-8.

20. Gelatt KN: Cataracts in the Golden Retriever dog. Vet Med Small Anim Clin. 1972 Oct;67(10):1113-5.

21. Lengweiler C & Jaggy A: Clinical, epidemiologic and therapeutic aspects of idiopathic epilepsy in 25 golden retrievers: results of a long term study. Schweiz Arch Tierheilkd. 1999;141(5):231-8.

22. Tamburini BA, Trapp S, Phang TL, et. al.: Gene expression profiles of sporadic canine hemangiosarcoma are uniquely associated with breed. PLoS One. 2009 May 20;4(5):e5549.

23. Wilkerson MJ, Dolce K, Koopman T, et. al.: Lineage differentiation of canine lymphoma/leukemias and aberrant expression of CD molecules. Vet Immunol Immunopathol. 2005 Jul 15;106(3-4):179-96.

24. Murphy S, Sparkes AH, Blunden AS, et. al.: Effects of stage and number of tumours on prognosis of dogs with cutaneous mast cell tumours. Vet Rec. 2006 Mar 4;158(9):287-91.

25. Tidholm A: Retrospective study of congenital heart defects in 151 dogs. J Small Anim Pract. 1997 Mar;38(3):94-8.

26. Kienle RD, Thomas WP & Pion PD: The natural clinical history of canine congenital subaortic stenosis. J Vet Intern Med. 1994 Nov-Dec;8(6):423-31.

27. Thomas R, Wang HJ, Tsai PC, et. al.: Influence of genetic background on tumor karyotypes: evidence for breed-associated cytogenetic aberrations in canine appendicular osteosarcoma. Chromosome Res. 2009;17(3):365-77.

28. Morris E & Lipowitz AJ: Comparison of tibial plateau angles in dogs with and without cranial cruciate ligament injuries. J Am Vet Med Assoc. 2001 Feb 1;218(3):363-6.

29. Massa KL, Gilger BC, Miller TL, et. al.: Causes of uveitis in dogs: 102 cases (1989-2000). Vet Ophthalmol. 2002 Jun;5(2):93-8.

30. Sapienza JS, Simó FJ & Prades-Sapienza A: Golden Retriever uveitis: 75 cases (1994-1999). Vet Ophthalmol. 2000;3(4):241-246.

31. Esson D, Armour M, Mundy P, et. al.: The histopathological and immunohistochemical characteristics of pigmentary and cystic glaucoma in the Golden Retriever. Vet Ophthalmol. 2009 Nov-Dec;12(6):361-8.

32. Deehr AJ & Dubielzig RR: A histopathological study of iridociliary cysts and glaucoma in Golden Retrievers. Vet Ophthalmol. 1998;1(2-3):153-158.

33. Long SE & Crispin SM: Inheritance of multifocal retinal dysplasia in the golden retriever in the UK. Vet Rec. 1999 Dec 11;145(24):702-4.

34. Naranjo C, Dubielzig RR, & Friedrichs KR: Canine ocular histiocytic sarcoma. Vet Ophthalmol. 2007 May-Jun;10(3):179-85.

35. Moore PF, Affolter VK, Vernau W, et. al.: Canine hemophagocytic histiocytic sarcoma: a proliferative disorder of CD11d+ macrophages. Vet Pathol. 2006 Sep;43(5):632-45.

36. Schultz RM, Puchalski SM, Kent M, et. al.: Skeletal lesions of histiocytic sarcoma in nineteen dogs. Vet Radiol Ultrasound. 2007 Nov-Dec;48(6):539-43.

37. Murphy CJ, Marfurt CF, McDermott A, et. al.: Spontaneous chronic corneal epithelial defects (SCCED) in dogs: clinical features, innervation, and effect of topical SP, with or without IGF-1. Invest Ophthalmol Vis Sci. 2001 Sep;42(10):2252-61.

38. Ramos-Vara JA, Beissenherz ME, Miller MA, et. al.: Retrospective study of 338 canine oral melanomas with clinical, histologic, and immunohistochemical review of 129 cases. Vet Pathol. 2000 Nov;37(6):597-608.

39. Boydell P: Idiopathic horner syndrome in the golden retriever. J Neuroophthalmol. 2000 Dec;20(4):288-90.

40. de Morais HS, DiBartola SP & Chew DJ: Juvenile renal disease in golden retrievers: 12 cases (1984-1994). J Am Vet Med Assoc. 1996 Aug 15;209(4):792-7.

41. Kerlin RL & Van Winkle TJ: Renal dysplasia in golden retrievers. Vet Pathol. 1995 May;32(3):327-9.

42. Gaynor AR, Shofer FS & Washabau RJ: Risk factors for acquired megaesophagus in dogs. J Am Vet Med Assoc. 1997 Dec 1;211(11):1406-12.

43. Wray JD & Sparkes AH: Use of radiographic measurements in distinguishing myasthenia gravis from other causes of canine megaoesophagus. J Small Anim Pract. 2006 May;47(5):256-63.

44. Shelton GD, Willard MD, Cardinet GH 3rd, et. al.: Acquired myasthenia gravis. Selective involvement of esophageal, pharyngeal, and facial muscles. J Vet Intern Med. 1990 Nov-Dec;4(6):281-4.

45. Davidson AP, Pollard RE, Bannasch DL, et. al.: Inheritance of cricopharyngeal dysfunction in Golden Retrievers. Am J Vet Res. 2004 Mar;65(3):344-9.

46. Aronsohn MG & Carpenter JL: Surgical treatment of idiopathic pericardial effusion in the dog: 25 cases (1978-1993). J Am Anim Hosp Assoc. 1999 Nov-Dec;35(6):521-5.

47. Sturges BK, Dickinson PJ, Bollen AW, et. al.: Magnetic resonance imaging and histological classification of intracranial meningiomas in 112 dogs. J Vet Intern Med. 2008 May-Jun;22(3):586-95.

48. Greco JJ, Aiken SA, Berg JM, et. al.: Evaluation of intracranial meningioma resection with a surgical aspirator in dogs: 17 cases (1996-2004). J Am Vet Med Assoc. 2006 Aug 1;229(3):394-400.

49. Westworth DR, Dickinson PJ, Vernau W, et. al.: Choroid Plexus Tumors in 56 Dogs (1985-2007). J Vet Intern Med. 2008 Sep-Oct;22(5):1157-65.

50. Dennis MM, Ehrhart N, Duncan CG, et. al.: Frequency of and risk factors associated with lingual lesions in dogs: 1,196 cases (1995-2004).

51. Donaldson D, Sansom J, Scase T, et. al.: Canine limbal melanoma: 30 cases (1992-2004). Part 1. Signalment, clinical and histological features and pedigree analysis. Vet Ophthalmol. 2006 Mar-Apr;9(2):115-9.

52. Adam F, Villiers E, Watson S, et. al.: Clinical pathological and epidemiological assessment of morphologically and immunologically confirmed canine leukaemia. Vet Comp Oncol. 2009 Sep;7(3):181-95.

53. Wucherer KL & Wilke V: Thyroid cancer in dogs: an update based on 638 cases (1995-2005). J Am Anim Hosp Assoc. 2010 Jul-Aug;46(4):249-54.

54. *The Genetic Connection: A Guide to Health Problems in Purebred Dogs.* L. Ackerman. p. 220. AAHA Press, 1999.

55. Bélanger MC, Ouellet M, Queney G, et. al.: Taurine-deficient dilated cardiomyopathy in a family of golden retrievers. J Am Anim Hosp Assoc. 2005 Sep-Oct;41(5):284-91.

56. Morrison WB, Wilsman NJ, Fox LE, et. al.: Primary ciliary dyskinesia in the dog. J Vet Intern Med. 1987 Apr-Jun;1(2):67-74

57. Afzelius BA, Carlsten J & Karlsson S: Clinical, pathologic, and ultrastructural features of situs inversus and immotile-cilia syndrome in a dog. J Am Vet Med Assoc. 1984 Mar 1;184(5):560-3.

58. Reichler IM, Hoerauf A, Guscetti F, et. al.: Primary ciliary dyskinesia with situs inversus totalis, hydrocephalus internus and cardiac malformations in a dog. J Small Anim Pract. 2001 Jul;42(7):345-8.

59. Matsuki N, Yamato O, Kusuda M, et. al.: Magnetic resonance imaging of GM2-gangliosidosis in a golden retriever. Can Vet J. 2005 Mar;46(3):275-8.

60. Braund KG, Mehta JR, Toivio-Kinnucan M, et. al.: Congenital hypomyelinating polyneuropathy in two golden retriever littermates. Vet Pathol. 1989 May;26(3):202-8.

61. da Costa RC, Parent JM, Poma R, et. al.: Multisystem axonopathy and neuronopathy in Golden Retriever dogs. J Vet Intern Med. 2009 Jul-Aug;23(4):935-9.

62. Sharp NJ, Kornegay JN, Van Camp SD, et. al.: An error in dystrophin mRNA processing in golden retriever muscular dystrophy, an animal homologue of Duchenne muscular dystrophy. Genomics. 1992 May;13(1):115-21.

63. Kornegay JN, Tuler SM, Miller DM, et. al.: Muscular dystrophy in a litter of golden retriever dogs. Muscle Nerve. 1988 Oct;11(10):1056-64.

64. *The Complete Dog Book, 20th Ed.* The American Kennel Club. Howell Book House, NY 2006. p. 47-51.

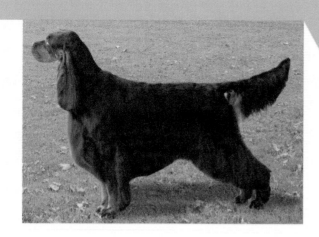

Gordon Setter

They have compact feet with arched toes and straight strong limbs. Their gait is characterized by long easy strides, and it is normal to see the tail flag while going. Legs arc in a straight flowing motion.

The Breed History

Written records originate in the early 1600s when setting dogs of exceptional endurance were described. This type of dog was of Scottish origin, and was bred as a one-man gundog. The word "Setters" was used because these dogs were known to "set" when they had the prey in site. The set was a semi-seated position. The black and tans were a favorite of the Duke of Gordon in the early 1800s and they are thought to take their name from this man. Gordon setters first came to North America in the mid 1800s. They were first registered with the AKC in 1892.

Breeding for Function

They are popular both as a show dog and a reliable hunting dog. Field lines are slightly smaller in stature. Gordons excel at pointing and retrieving birds. They are excellent scent trackers, and are noted to be slow but steady.

Physical Characteristics

Height at Withers: female 23-26" (58.5-66 cm), male 24-27" (61-68.5 cm)

Weight: females 50-70 lb (22.5-32 kg), males 55-80lb (25-36.5 kg). Weights vary widely within the breed.

Coat: All dogs are a glossy black with rich mahogany to chestnut markings. Their hair is slightly wavy or straight, fine-textured with long hairs, and on the tail they have moderate feathers. Junctions of markings with the coat are clearly delineated, not smudgy. Acceptable markings have very specific size and distribution in this breed. Regular grooming is important and they are considered an average shedder. Red coat color: Caused by an autosomal recessive gene (ee). Normally tan markings can be differentiated, especially when viewed in sunlight. Recessive e allele occurs in low frequency in the breed, and can be tested for by VetGen.

Longevity: 10-12 years.

Points of Conformation: The head is chiseled with a strong, square long muzzle and low set, heavy ears. His sturdy bone and robust, athletic build suits his reputation for stamina. The back is strong and short, with a moderately sloping topline. The thorax is deep with moderate girth, and the tail tapers not quite at the level of the tarsus, and is carried close to horizontal. Dewclaws may be removed.

Recognized Behavior Issues and Traits

Reported breed traits include: They are aloof with strangers, but show devoted loyalty to home and family. They are intelligent, alert and fearless and should be socialized early. They are generally good around children. Gordons require plenty of exercise. Training should also start early because like most hunting breeds, they have a streak of independence. They should not be allowed off-leash unless fenced. They have a tendency to bark, and if left alone for extended periods, may resort to boredom digging or chewing.

Normal Physiologic Variations

None reported

Drug Sensitivities

None reported

Inherited Diseases

Hip Dysplasia: Polygenically inherited trait causing degenerative joint disease and hip arthritis. OFA reports 19.5% affected. French Kennel Club screening shows 30.8% affected between 2000-2006.[1,2]

Elbow Dysplasia: Polygenically inherited trait causing elbow arthritis. OFA reports 13.6% affected. Reported 19.8x odds ratio for the fragmented coronoid process form of elbow dysplasia versus other breeds.[1,3]

Patella Luxation: Polygenically inherited laxity of patellar ligaments, causing luxation, lameness, and later degenerative joint disease. Treat surgically if causing clinical signs. Too few Gordon Setters have been screened by OFA to determine an accurate frequency.[1]

Progressive Retinal Atrophy (PM): Two progressive retinal atrophies occur in the breed. An autosomal recessive rcd4 form causes progressive loss of vision at an average of 10 years of age. A genetic test is available for this form of PRA. Testing in the US shows 30% carrier and 3% affected. An earlier onset, presumed autosomal recessive PRA also occurs in the breed with an average age of onset between 3 and 6 years of age. A genetic test is not available for this form. PRA is identified in 0.6% of Gordon Setters CERF examined by veterinary ophthalmologists between 2000-2005.[5,6]

Cerebellar Abiotrophy (CCA, Cerebellar Ataxia): Autosomal recessive disorder causing cerebellar hypermetria, a high stepping gait, and incoordination. Clinical signs usually progress slowly throughout the life of the dog, however some can progress more rapidly to constant stumbling. Diagnose by clinical signs, MRI/CT, or post-mortem examination. Occurs at a low frequency, with a wide pedigree spread worldwide.[4,7]

Lethal Inherited Encephalopathy (LIE, DUNGd): Fatal, autosomal recessive disorder causing gait and postural abnormalities, progressive weakness, and recumbency by 5-6 weeks of age. Puppies develop normally until 3-4 weeks of age, when they begin to cry incessantly, flex their necks, and walk backwards. Caused by an undetermined metabolic abnormality in glycine conjugation resulting in an organic aciduria. Occurs at a low frequency, with a wide pedigree spread.[8,9]

Disease Predispositions

Sebaceous Cysts: GSCA 2004 Gordon Setter Health Survey reports 25.53% of Gordon Setters develop benign sebaceous cysts. Dorn reports a 1.99x odds ratio of developing sebaceous cysts versus other breeds.[10,11]

Hypothyroidism: Inherited autoimmune thyroiditis. 11.6% positive for thyroid auto-antibodies based on testing at Michigan State University. (Ave. for all breeds is 7.5%).[12,13]

Lymphosarcoma: Both B cell (multicentric lymph node cancer) and T cell (cutaneous lymphoma/mycosis fungoides) lymphoma are reported in the breed. The 2004 GSCA Gordon Setter Health Survey reports 3.27% of Gordon Setters affected with lymphosarcoma. Dorn reports a 15.52x odds ratio of developing lymphosarcoma versus other breeds.[10,11]

Persistent Pupillary Membranes: Strands of fetal remnant connecting; iris to iris, cornea, lens, or involving sheets of tissue. The later three forms can impair vision, and dogs affected with these forms should not be bred. Identified in 4.41% of Gordon Setters CERF examined by veterinary ophthalmologists between 2000-2005.[5]

Gastric Dilatation–Volvulus (Bloat, GDV): Polygenically inherited, life-threatening twisting of the stomach within the abdomen. Requires immediate treatment. 2004 GSCA Gordon Setter Health Survey reports a 4.01% affected rate. Dorn reports a 4.74x odds ratio of developing GDV versus other breeds. Glickman reports a 4.1x odds ratio.[10,11,14]

Oral Malignant Melanoma: Malignant cancer usually involving the gingiva in this breed. Can be pigmented or non-pigmented. One study identified a 5.17x relative risk versus other breeds.[15]

Ectropion: Rolling out of eyelids, often with a medial canthal pocket. Can also cause secondary conjunctivitis, which Dorn finds has a 2.49x odds ratio in Gordon Setters versus other breeds. Ectropion is reported in 1.2% of Gordon Setters CERF examined by veterinary ophthalmologists between 2000-2005.[5,10]

Retinal Dysplasia: Retinal folds, geographic, and generalized retinal dysplasia with detachment are recognized in the breed. Can lead to blindness. Reported in 1.6% of Gordon Setters CERF examined by veterinary ophthalmologists between 2000-2005.[5]

Juvenile Renal Disease: Progressive renal dysfunction in young Gordon Setters. Typically presents with increased drinking and urination, weight loss or unthriftiness, consistently dilute urine, and elevated kidney blood tests. Affected dogs do not leak urinary protein until late in the disease. Onset from weeks of age to over a year in age. Some dogs remain with mild signs, while others rapidly progress to kidney failure. Unknown mode of inheritance, with a wide pedigree spread. Diagnosis by kidney biopsy or pathology.[6]

Symmetrical Lupoid Onychodystrophy (SLO): Disorder causing loss of toenails. Onset between 2-8 years of age affecting 1-2 nails, then progressing to all toenails within 2-9 weeks. Requires lifelong treatment with oral fatty acid supplementation +/- prednisone. Kindreds of affected Gordon setters have been identified, but a mode of inheritance is not known. Antinuclear antibodies were identified in some affected dogs.[16,17]

Cataracts, Entropion, Epilepsy, Hypertrophic Osteodystrophy, Juvenile Cellulitis, Keratoconjunctivitis Sicca, and **Micropapilla** are reported.[18]

Isolated Case Studies

Black Hair Follicular Dysplasia: Isolated case reports of affected Gordon Setters. Loss of black hairs beginning around 4 weeks of age. Total loss of all black hair by 6-9 months of age. No treatment. Antinuclear antibodies were identified in some affected dogs.[16]

Vitiligo/Leukotrichia: Isolated case reports of 6-12 year old Gordon Setters with progressively expanding areas of white hair, often beginning on the head or neck. Caused by autoantibodies to pigmented cells. Does not affect the health of the dog. Can affect both black and tan areas, however some cases begin in only the tan areas. Unknown mode of inheritance.[19]

Vitamin A Responsive Dermatosis: Isolated case reports of affected Gordon Setters. Causes pruritis in this breed, especially on top of back with small firm hives. Responds to Vitamin A supplementation. Relapses if treatment is stopped.

Congenital Venous Aneurysm: Unilateral dilatation of the right jugular, maxillary, and linguofacial veins identified in a 5 month old Gordon Setter. The aneurysm was removed surgically.[20]

Reticuloendotheliosis: Seven year old Gordon Setter presented with progressive weakness, debility, and diarrhea with melena. Clinical evaluation revealed splenomegaly, severe nonregenerative anemia, thrombocytopenia and leukopenia with many large blast cells in the peripheral blood.[21]

Genetic Tests

Tests of Genotype: Direct test for black, liver, and red coat color is available from VetGen.

Direct test for rcd4 PRA is available from the Animal Health Trust

Tests of Phenotype: CHIC Certification: Required testing includes hip radiographs, elbow radiographs, and CERF eye examination. (See CHIC website; www.caninehealthinfo.org).

Recommend thyroid profile including autoantibodies, patella evaluation, and heart examination.

Miscellaneous

- **Breed name synonyms:** Gordon, Black and Tan (historical)
- **Registries:** AKC, CKC, UKC, KCGB (Kennel Club of Great Britain), ANKC (Australian National Kennel Club), NKC (National Kennel Club)
- **AKC rank (year 2008):** 92 (636 dogs registered)
- **Internet resources:** Gordon Setter Club of America Inc. www.gsca.org

  British Gordon Setter Club: www.britishgordonsetterclub.org.uk

  Gordon Setter Club of Canada: www.gordensetterclubcanada.com

References

1. OFA Website breed statistics: www.offa.org Last accessed July 1, 2010.
2. Genevois JP, Remy D, Viguier E, et. al.: Prevalence of hip dysplasia according to official radiographic screening, among 31 breeds of dogs in France. Vet Comp Orthop Traumatol. 2008;21(1):21-4.
3. LaFond E, Breur GJ & Austin CC: Breed susceptibility for developmental orthopedic diseases in dogs. J Am Anim Hosp Assoc. 2002 Sep-Oct;38(5):467-77.
4. de Lahunta A, Fenner WR, Indrieri RJ, et. al.: Hereditary cerebellar cortical abiotrophy in the Gordon Setter. *J Am Vet Med Assoc.* 1980 Sep 15;177(6):538-41.
5. *Ocular Disorders Presumed to be Inherited in Purebred Dogs.* American College of Veterinary Ophthalmologists. ACVO, 2007.
6. Bell JS: Health Update on Progressive Retinal Atrophy and Juvenile Renal Dysplasia in the Gordon Setter. Gordon Setter News. Oct 2003.
7. Steinberg HS, Troncoso JC, Cork LC, et. al.: Clinical features of inherited cerebellar degeneration in Gordon setters. *J Am Vet Med Assoc.* 1981 Nov 1;179(9):886-90.
8. Yaeger MJ, Majercik K, Carter M: An autosomal recessive, lethal, neurologic disease of Gordon Setter puppies. *J Vet Diagn Invest.* 2000 Nov;12(6):570-3.
9. Gorgi AA, O'Brien DP, Shelton GD, et. al.: Inborn Error of Metabolism In Gordon Setter Puppies: Organic Acid Profile and Candidate Gene Sequencing.Proceedings, 2008 ACVIM Forum. 2008.
10. Dorn CR: Canine breed-specific risks of frequently diagnosed diseases at veterinary teaching hospitals. Monograph. AKC Canine Health Foundation. 2000.
11. Slater MR: 2004 GSCA Gordon Setter Health Survey: Final Report. December 17, 2004.
12. Nachreiner R & Refsal K: Personal communication, Diagnostic Center for Population and Animal Health, Michigan State University. April, 2007.
13. Nachreiner RF, Refsal KR, Graham PA, et. al.: Prevalence of serum thyroid hormone autoantibodies in dogs with clinical signs of hypothyroidism. J Am Vet Med Assoc. 2002 Feb 15;220(4):466-71.
14. Glickman LT, Glickman NW, Perez CM, et. al.: Analysis of risk factors for gastric dilatation and dilatation-volvulus in dogs. *J Am Vet Med Assoc.* 1994 May 1;204(9):1465-7
15. Ramos-Vara JA, Beissenherz ME, Miller MA, et. al.: Retrospective study of 338 canine oral melanomas with clinical, histologic, and immunohistochemical review of 129 cases. Vet Pathol. 2000 Nov;37(6):597-608.
16. Ovrebo Bohnhorst J, Hanssen I, Moen T: Antinuclear antibodies (ANA) in Gordon setters with symmetrical lupoid onychodystrophy and black hair follicular dysplasia. *Acta Vet Scand.* 2001;42(3):323-9.
17. Ziener ML, Bettenay SV & Mueller RS: Symmetrical onychomadesis in Norwegian Gordon and English setters. Vet Dermatol. 2008 Apr;19(2):88-94.
18. *The Genetic Connection: A Guide to Health Problems in Purebred Dogs.* L Ackerman. p 220-21, AAHA Press, 1999.
19. Naughton GK, Mahaffey M, Bystryn JC, et. al.: Antibodies to surface antigens of pigmented cells in animals with vitiligo. Proc Soc Exp Biol Med. 1986 Mar;181(3):423-6.
20. Salmeri KR, Bellah JR, Ackerman N, et. al.: Unilateral congenital aneurysm of the jugular, linguofacial, and maxillary veins in a dog. J Am Vet Med Assoc. 1991 Feb 15;198(4):651-4.
21. Coons FH, George JW, Appel GO: Reticuloendotheliosis in a dog. *Cornell Vet.* 1976 Apr;66(2):249-57.
22. *The Complete Dog Book, 20th Ed.* The American Kennel Club. Howell Book House, NY 2006. p 67-71.

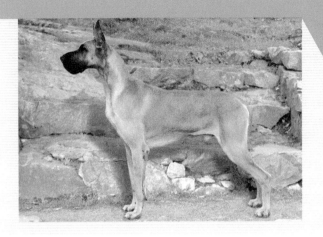

Great Dane

The Breed History

The name "Great Dane" originates in the French language; the meaning is "Big Danish". Proudly termed "King of Dogs", "Gentle Giant" or "Apollo of Dogs" by breed fanciers, this was actually a breed originating in Germany, so it is unclear how it became named "Dane". The Tibetan Mastiff is thought to be a direct ancestor of the Great Dane. Also linked to breed development is the Alaunt from Asian Russia, the English Mastiff and the Irish Wolfhound. Other reports place Greyhound in the mix later in the breed development, a step that may have greatly refined the mastiff type. Distinct Great Dane lineage can be traced back about 400 years. In a meeting that took place about 1880, a resolution was passed to name this breed "Deutsche Dogge" which translates roughly as "German Mastiff," and at that time, it was decreed that the breed name Great Dane should not be applied to this breed, but in spite of this, the name persists today in English-speaking countries. The first breed standard was adopted in 1891.

Breeding for Function

In Germany this breed excelled at wild boar hunting. Because it took great power, courage, and stamina to hunt boar, the focus of breeding programs was to produce a large, courageous, powerful, agile and very fast dog. They were also used as war dogs. Guarding of estates and carriages was also a task the Great Dane excelled at. These days, most dogs are companion dogs.

Physical Characteristics

Height at Withers: female minimum 28" (71 cm), but ideally, 30" (76 cm) or more. Male: minimum is 30" (cm), the ideal is over 32" (81 cm).

Weight: 100-120 lb (45.5-55 kg).

Coat: The very short, thick and glossy coat is accepted in the following colors: Fawn (yellow-gold with black mask), brindle (yellow-gold base with well defined black stripes and usually black masked), blue (steel blue), black, and harlequin (white base with medium-sized irregular patches of black over the haircoat).

Longevity: 7-9 years

Points of Conformation: These dogs possess a large well chiseled head with a flat skull, and the head is rectangular in outline, with a pronounced stop. The nose is ridged but not split. The conformation is well balanced; the build is heavier in males, both in bone and musculature. The gait is a straight, low, elastic long and powerful ground-covering stride. The almond-shaped eyes are usually darkly pigmented, medium-sized and deep-set and the palpebral margins do not evert. Ears are medium sized, high-set and the leather is moderately thick. The folded ears rest close to the cheeks. Ears are sometimes cropped to stay pricked in North America. The nose is large and pigmented black or close to black except in harlequins where a spotted nose is allowed. The neck is long and free of dewlaps, arched, and the topline is short and level. The thorax is very deep and broad, and ribs are well sprung. Abdomen tuck up is pronounced. The tail is set high, is thick at the base, then tapers to reach to the tarsus; is carried level during movement and low when at rest. Limbs are long and straight boned, feet are compact and well knuckled, and dewclaw removal is optional.

Recognized Behavior Issues and Traits

Reported breed characteristics include: Courageous in the hunt, but friendly and gentle in the home—even playful. Good with children, easy to groom, clean but needs lots of space to exercise in a fenced area. Not suitable for an apartment or small homes. Fairly good trainability, some are aggressive with other dogs unless they know them, early obedience training is important, they possess average activity levels, and have moderate to high exercise needs. This is a late maturing breed. Some Great Danes can be shy and people aggressive.

Normal Physiologic Variations

Merle Coat Color: Caused by a dominant mutation in the SILV gene. Breeding two merle dogs together should be avoided, as homozygous dogs can be born with multiple defects, including blindness, deafness, and heart anomalies.[1]

Harlequin Coat Color: Due the combined action of a dominant gene H with the merle gene M in the genotype HhM+. The H gene is a prenatal lethal when homozygous HH, so all Harlequin Danes are heterozygous Hh.[2,3]

Echocardiographic Normal Values:[4]	
Parameter	90% Confidence Interval
AO (cm)	2.8-3.4
AOexc (cm)	0.6-1.3
LA (cm)	2.8-4.6
LA/AO	0.9-1.5
LVd (cm)	4.4-5.9
LVs (cm)	3.4-4.5
%FS	18-36
%EF	33-65
LVET (sec)	0.12-0.18
Vcf (cir/sec)	1.0-2.3
EPSS (cm)	0.5-1.2
VSd (cm)	1.2-1.6
VSs (cm)	1.4-1.9
VS%Δ	6-32
VSexc (cm)	0.2-0.8
LVWd (cm)	1.0-1.6
LVWs (cm)	1.1-1.9
LVW%Δ	-9-29
LVWexc (cm)	0.9-1.5
HR	100-130
Kg	52-75
N	15

AO, aorta; LA, left atrium; LV, left ventricle; FS, fractional shortening; EF, ejection fraction; LVET, left ventricular ejection time; Vcf, velocity of circumferential; EPSS, E-point to septal separation; VS, ventricular septum; VS%Δ, change in VS thickness between diastole and systole; LVW, left ventricular wall; HR, heart rate; N, number of animals.

Drug Sensitivities
None reported

Inherited Diseases

Hip Dysplasia: Polygenically inherited trait causing degenerative joint disease and hip arthritis. OFA reports 12.0% affected.[5]

Dilated Cardiomyopathy (DCM): Affected dogs have reduced shortening fraction (FS) in the presence of clinical and radiographic signs of left-sided or biventricular heart failure. Atrial fibrillation is the most common arrhythmia. Some affected Great Danes may be asymptomatic, with ECHO or Doppler necessary to make the diagnosis. Molecular genetic studies show changes in calstabin and triad in gene expression. Pedigree analysis suggests that DCM in the breed involves a major X-linked recessive gene, although polygenic inheritance cannot be ruled out. Reported at a frequency of 5% in the Great Dane Club Of America National Health Survey.[6,7,8,9]

Elbow Dysplasia: Polygenically inherited trait causing elbow arthritis. OFA reports 3.8% affected.[5]

Patella Luxation: Polygenically inherited laxity of patellar ligaments, causing luxation, lameness, and later degenerative joint disease. Treat surgically if causing clinical signs. OFA reports 1.4% affected.[5]

Disease Predispositions

Gastric Dilation/Volvulus (GDV, Bloat): Life-threatening twisting of the stomach within the abdomen. Requires immediate veterinary attention. There is a 42.4% lifetime risk of developing GDV in Great Danes, with 9.2% of all Great Danes dying from the condition. Risk of death from GDV after prophylactic gastropexy decreased 29.6x fold. Dorn reports a 43.23x odds ratio versus other breeds. Bloat with torsion is reported at a frequency of 11%, and without torsion at 4% in the Great Dane Club Of America National Health Survey.[7,10,11,12]

Hypothyroidism: Inherited autoimmune thyroiditis. 10.1% positive for thyroid auto-antibodies based on testing at Michigan State University. (Ave. for all breeds is 7.5%) Reported at a frequency of 5% in the Great Dane Club Of America National Health Survey.[7,13,14]

Allergic Dermatitis: Inhalant or food allergy. Presents with pruritis and pyotraumatic dermatitis. Reported at a frequency of 10% in the Great Dane Club Of America National Health Survey.[7]

Cataracts: Anterior cortex, posterior cortex, equatorial intermediate and punctate cataracts predominate in the breed. Identified in 6.93% of Great Danes CERF-examined by veterinary ophthalmologists between 2000-2005. Reported at a frequency of 3% in the Great Dane Club Of America National Health Survey. CERF does not recommend breeding any Great Dane with a cataract.[7,15]

Panosteitis: Self-limiting disease of young, large breed dogs involving the diaphyseal and metaphyseal areas of the tubular long bones. Affected dogs show intermittent lameness. Reported at a frequency of 5% in the Great Dane Club Of America National Health Survey.[7]

Ectropion: Rolling out of eyelids, often with a medial canthal pocket. Can cause secondary conjunctivitis. Reported in 4.87% of Great Danes CERF-examined by veterinary ophthalmologists between 2000-2005. Reported at a frequency of 4% in the Great Dane Club Of America National Health Survey.[7,15]

Distichiasis: Abnormally placed eyelashes that irritate the cornea and conjunctiva. Can cause secondary corneal ulceration. Identified in 4.50% of Great Danes CERF-examined by veterinary ophthalmologists between 2000-2005.[15]

Eury/Macroblepharon: An exceptionally large palpebral fissure. With laxity, may lead to lower lid ectropion and upper lid entropion. Either of these conditions may lead to severe ocular irritation. Identified in 4.50% of Great Danes CERF-examined by veterinary ophthalmologists between 2000-2005.[15]

Demodicosis (Generalized): Dorn reports a 1.79x odds ratio for developing demodectic mange versus other breeds. This disorder has an underlying immunodeficiency in its pathogenesis. Reported at a frequency of 4% in the Great Dane Club Of America National Health Survey.[7,10]

Osteosarcoma (OSA): Great Danes are a breed with a predisposition (5x Odds Ratio) for developing malignant osteosarcoma versus other breeds. One study showed a prevalence of 4.4%, and an Odds Ratio of 12.0x versus other breeds. Forelimb OSA was more frequent than hindlimb OSA in Great Danes. Reported at a frequency of 3% in the Great Dane Club Of America National Health Survey.[7,16,17]

Entropion: Rolling in of eyelids, often causing corneal irritation or ulceration. Entropion is reported in 2.31% of Great Danes CERF-examined by veterinary ophthalmologists between 2000-2005. Reported at a frequency of 3% in the Great Dane Club Of America National Health Survey.[7,15]

Cervical Vertebral Instability (Wobbler Syndrome): Vertebral disorder causing spinal cord compression and ataxia. Radiographic examinations suggest that the primary lesion is foramenal stenosis and intervertebral instability at C6-7. Reported at a frequency of 2% in the Great Dane Club Of America National Health Survey.[7,18,19]

Osteochondritis Dissecans (OCD): Abnormality of cartilage development causing lameness in the shoulder, elbow, hock or stifle. Severe cases may require surgery. Dorn reports a 22.26x odds ratio versus other breeds. Reported 87.0x odds ratio for elbow OCD, 32.8x odds ratio for shoulder OCD, and 309.4x odds ratio for stifle OCD versus other breeds. Reported at a frequency of 2% in the Great Dane Club Of America National Health Survey.[7,10,20,21]

Hypertrophic Osteodystrophy (HOD): Immune-mediated disorder causing fever, and painful, swollen joints and bones in young Great Danes. Occurs mostly within 3-14 days post-vaccination. Age of onset is 8-16 weeks. Unknown mode of inheritance. Reported 189.8x odds ratio versus other breeds. Reported at a frequency of 2% in the Great Dane Club Of America National Health Survey.[7,21,22]

Persistent Pupillary Membranes: Strands of fetal remnant connecting; iris to iris, cornea, lens, or involving sheets of tissue. The later three forms can impair vision, and dogs affected with these forms should not be bred. Identified in 1.52% of Great Danes CERF-examined by veterinary ophthalmologists between 2000-2005. Dorn reports a 3.59x odds ratio versus other breeds.[10,15]

Diskospondylitis: Great Danes have a 7.3x odds ratio for developing vertebral infection versus mixed breed dogs. Treatment is with long-term antibiotics.[23]

Eversion of the Cartilage of the Third Eyelid: A scroll-like curling of the cartilage of the third eyelid, usually everting the margin. May cause mild ocular irritation. Identified in 1.22% of Great Danes CERF-examined by veterinary ophthalmologists between 2000-2005.[15]

Iris Ciliary Body Cysts: Pigmented cysts arise from pigmented epithelial cells of the ciliary body. Ciliary body cysts, may predispose to glaucoma. Review of hospital admissions shows a 37.01 odds ratio for ciliary body cysts in Great Danes. Identified in 1.03% of Great Danes CERF-examined by veterinary ophthalmologists between 2000-2005.[15,25]

Primary Glaucoma (Goniodysgenesis): Goniodysgenesis has a heritability of 0.52 in Great Danes, and this is positively correlated to the high incidence of glaucoma in the breed. Reported at a frequency of 0.3% in the Great Dane Club Of America National Health Survey. CERF does not recommend breeding any Great Dane with glaucoma.[7,15,24]

Secondary Glaucoma (with Ciliary Body Cysts): Occurs with cysts in the anterior and posterior chamber. Review of hospital admissions shows a 2.23x odds ratio for glaucoma and 37.01x odds ratio for ciliary body cysts in Great Danes.[25]

Hypoadrenocorticism (Addison's Disease): Immune mediated destruction of the adrenal gland. Typical presentation of lethargy, poor appetite, vomiting, weakness, and dehydration occurring from 4 months to several years of age. Treatment with DOCA injections or oral fludrocortisone. Great Danes are at significantly higher risk versus other breeds. Unknown mode of inheritance. Reported at a frequency of 0.3% in the Great Dane Club Of America National Health Survey.[7,26]

Mitral Valvular Malformation: Great Danes are overrepresented. Affected dogs have mitral regurgitation, which can progress to congestive heart disease. Average age of recognition is 7.3 months. Abnormalities include changes to the annulus, leaflets, chordae tendineae, and papillary muscles. Reported at a frequency of 0.1% in the Great Dane Club Of America National Health Survey.[7,27]

Splenic Torsion: Great Danes are found to be at increased risk for splenic torsion versus other breeds. Treatment is immediate surgery.[28]

Inherited Myopathy: A hereditary, non-inflammatory myopathy occurs in Great Danes of both sexes before one year of age. Clinical signs are exercise intolerance, muscle wasting, and an exercise-induced tremor. Serum creatinine kinase levels are elevated. Affected muscles show slow oxydatine fiber phenotype disrupted sarcomeric architecture and accumulation of mitochondrial organelles. Most dogs are affected severely, though some may survive into adulthood. All have had fawn or brindle coat coloration. An autosomal recessive inheritance is suspected.[29,30]

Megaesophagus: Great Danes are overrepresented in diagnoses of primary megaesophagus. Onset can be at weaning, or in adulthood. Clinical signs include regurgitation, excess salivation, and aspiration pneumonia.[31]

Epidermolysis Bullosa Acquisita (Bullous Pemphigus): Eruptive autoimmune skin disorder characterized by vesicles that rapidly progress to ulcers, typically in the oral cavity, pads and medial pinnae. Seen in young to adolescent Great Danes. Variable response to steroids and immunosuppressive therapy.[32,33]

Acral lick Dermatitis, Brachygnathism, Color Dilution Alopecia, Cystinuria, Hemeralopia, Lymphedema, Oligodontia, Prognathism, Progressive Retinal Atrophy, Retinal Dysplasia, Spinal Muscular Atrophy, Subaortic stenosis, Tricuspid Valve Dysplasia, Uveal Hypopigmentation, Vascular Ring Anomaly, von Willebrand's Disease, Wry Mouth, and **Zinc-Responsive Dermatosis** are reported.[34]

Isolated Case Studies

Cecocolic Volvulus: Two male Great Danes were diagnosed with volvulus of the cecum and large intestines. Clinical signs included peracute to acute onset of vomiting, mild abdominal distention and pain, lack of feces, and tenesmus. Diagnosis by radiography.[35]

Primary Orthostatic Tremors: Two unrelated two year old Great Danes were identified with orthostatic tremors that only occurred when standing at rest. The tremors were controlled with phenobarbitol.[36]

Recurrent Limb Edema: Great Danes have been identified with multiple episodes of cool, pitting edema limited to one or more limbs.

Episodes lasted for several days, and the time between episodes varied from 2 weeks to 1 year. No etiology is identified, and the edema was unresponsive to treatment.[37]

Myasthenia Gravis: A case report identified three Great Dane littermates all developing myasthenia gravis between 2-3 years of age. Acetylcholine receptor auto-antibody titres were positive.[38]

Genetic Tests

Tests of Genotype: Direct tests for coat color (including mask and dilute) are available from HealthGene and VetGen.

Tests of Phenotype: CHIC Certification: Required testing includes hip radiographs, CERF eye examination, thyroid profile including autoantibodies and cardiac evaluation. (See CHIC website; www.caninehealthinfo.org).

Recommend elbow radiographs and patella evaluation.

Miscellaneous

- **Breed name synonyms:** Dane, Deutsche Dogge, German Mastiff, Dogue Allemand (historical).
- **Registries:** AKC, UKC, CKC, KCGB (Kennel Club of Great Britain), ANKC (Australian National Kennel Club), NKC (National Kennel Club).
- **AKC rank (year 2008):** 22 (8,994 dogs registered)
- **Internet resources: Great Dane Club of America:** www.gdca.org
  The Great Dane Club (UK): www.thegreatdaneclub.com
  The Great Dane Club of Canada: www.gdcc.ca

References

1. Clark LA, Wahl JM, Rees CA, et. al.: Retrotransposon insertion in SILV is responsible for merle patterning of the domestic dog. Proc Natl Acad Sci U S A. 2006 Jan 31;103(5):1376-81.
2. O'Sullivan N, Robinson R: Harlequin colour in the Great Dane dog. Genetica. 1988-1989;78(3):215-8.
3. Clark LA, Starr AN, Tsai KL, et. al.: Genome-wide linkage scan localizes the harlequin locus in the Great Dane to chromosome 9. Gene. 2008 Jul 15;418(1-2):49-52.
4. Koch J, Pedersen HD, Jensen AL, et al: M-mode echocardiographic diagnosis of dilated cardiomyopathy in giant breed dogs. J Vet Med A. 1996; 43:297-304.
5. OFA Website breed statistics: www.offa.org Last accessed July 1, 2010.
6. Meurs KM, Miller MW, Wright NA: Clinical features of dilated cardiomyopathy in Great Danes and results of a pedigree analysis: 17 cases (1990-2000). J Am Vet Med Assoc. 2001 Mar 1;218(5):729-32.
7. Slater MR: Great Dane Club Of America National Health Survey. 2004.
8. Chetboul V, Sampedrano CC, Testault I, et. al.: Use of tissue Doppler imaging to confirm the diagnosis of dilated cardiomyopathy in a dog with equivocal echocardiographic findings. J Am Vet Med Assoc. 2004 Dec 15;225(12):1877-80, 1864.
9. Oyama MA, Chittur SV & Reynolds CA: Decreased triadin and increased calstabin2 expression in Great Danes with dilated cardiomyopathy. J Vet Intern Med. 2009 Sep-Oct;23(5):1014-9.
10. Dorn CR: Canine breed-specific risks of frequently diagnosed diseases at veterinary teaching hospitals. Monograph. AKC Canine Health Foundation. 2000.
11. Ward MP, Patronek GJ, Glickman LT: Benefits of prophylactic gastropexy for dogs at risk of gastric dilatation-volvulus. Prev Vet Med. 2003 Sep 12;60(4):319-29.
12. Glickman LT, Glickman NW, Schellenberg DB, et. al.: Incidence of and breed-related risk factors for gastric dilatation-volvulus in dogs. J Am Vet Med Assoc. 2000 Jan 1;216(1):40-5.
13. Nachreiner RF, Refsal KR, Graham PA, et. al.: Prevalence of serum thyroid hormone autoantibodies in dogs with clinical signs of hypothyroidism. J Am Vet Med Assoc 2002 Feb 15;220(4):466-71.
14. Nachreiner R & Refsal K: Personal communication, Diagnostic Center for Population and Animal Health, Michigan State University. April, 2007.
15. Ocular Disorders Presumed to be Inherited in Purebred Dogs. American College of Veterinary Ophthalmologists. ACVO, 2007.
16. Misdorp W, Hart AA: Some prognostic and epidemiologic factors in canine osteosarcoma. J Natl Cancer Inst. 1979 Mar;62(3):537-45.
17. Rosenberger JA, Pablo NV, & Crawford PC: Prevalence of and intrinsic risk factors for appendicular osteosarcoma in dogs: 179 cases (1996-2005). J Am Vet Med Assoc. 2007 Oct 1;231(7):1076-80.
18. Mason TA: Cervical vertebral instability (wobbler syndrome) in the dog. Vet Rec. 1979 Feb 17;104(7):142-5.
19. Drost WT, Lehenbauer TW, Reeves J: Mensuration of cervical vertebral ratios in Doberman pinschers and Great Danes. Vet Radiol Ultrasound. 2002 Mar-Apr;43(2):124-31.
20. Slater MR, Scarlett JM, Kaderly RE, Bonnett BN: Breed, gender and age as risk factors for canine osteochondritis dissecans. Veterinary and Comparative Orthopaedics and Traumatology 1991; 4:100-106.
21. LaFond E, Breur GJ & Austin CC: Breed susceptibility for developmental orthopedic diseases in dogs. J Am Anim Hosp Assoc. 2002 Sep-Oct;38(5):467-77.
22. Miller C: Hypertrophic osteodystrophy in a Great Dane puppy. Can Vet J. 2001 Jan;42(1):63-6.
23. Burkert BA, Kerwin SC, Hosgood GL, et. al.: Signalment and clinical features of diskospondylitis in dogs: 513 cases (1980-2001). J Am Vet Med Assoc. 2005 Jul 15;227(2):268-75.
24. Wood JL, Lakhani KH, Mason IK, et. al.: Relationship of the degree of goniodysgenesis and other ocular measurements to glaucoma in Great Danes. Am J Vet Res. 2001 Sep;62(9):1493-9
25. Spiess BM, Bolliger JO, Guscetti F, et. al.: Multiple ciliary body cysts and secondary glaucoma in the Great Dane: a report of nine cases. Vet Ophthalmol. 1998;1(1):41-45.
26. Peterson ME, Kintzer PP, Kass PH: Pretreatment clinical and laboratory findings in dogs with hypoadrenocorticism: 225 cases (1979-1993). J Am Vet Med Assoc. 1996 Jan 1;208(1):85-91.
27. Litu SK, Tilley LP: Malformation of the canine mitral valve complex. J Am Vet Med Assoc. 1975 Sep 15;167(6):465-71
28. Neath PJ, Brockman DJ, Saunders HM: Retrospective analysis of 19 cases of isolated torsion of the splenic pedicle in dogs. J Small Anim Pract. 1997 Sep;38(9):387-92.
29. Feliu-Pascual AL, Shelton GD, Targett MP, et. al.: Inherited myopathy of great Danes. J Small Anim Pract. 2006 May;47(5):249-54.
30. Chang KC, McCulloch ML, & Anderson TJ: Molecular and cellular insights into a distinct myopathy of Great Dane dogs. Vet J. 2010 Mar;183(3):322-7.
31. Marks, SL: Regurgitation in Dogs--More Common Than You Think! Proceedings, 2009 Western Veterinary Conference. 2009
32. Olivry T, Fine J, Dunston SM, et. al.: Canine epidermolysis bullosa acquisita: circulating autoantibodies target the aminoterminal non-collagenous (NC1) domain of collagen VII in anchoring fibrils. Veterinary Dermatology. 1998; 9: 19-31.
33. Hill PB, Boyer P, Lau P, et. al.: Epidermolysis bullosa acquisita in a great Dane. J Small Anim Pract. 2008 Feb;49(2):89-94.
34. The Genetic Connection: A Guide to Health Problems in Purebred Dogs. L Ackerman. p. 221. AAHA Press, 1999.
35. Carberry CA, Flanders JA: Cecal-colic volvulus in two dogs. Vet Surg. 1993 May-Jun;22(3):225-8.
36. Garosi LS, Rossmeisl JH, de Lahunta A, et. al.: Primary orthostatic tremor in Great Danes. J Vet Intern Med. 2005 Jul-Aug;19(4):606-9.
37. Webb JA, Abrams-Ogg A, Hall JA, et. al.: A Syndrome of Recurrent Limb Edema in Great Danes. Proceedings, 18th ECVIM-CA Congress, 2008.
38. Kent M, Glass EN, Acierno M, et. al.: Adult onset acquired myasthenia gravis in three Great Dane littermates. J Small Anim Pract. 2008 Dec;49(12):647-50.
39. The Complete Dog Book, 20th Ed. The American Kennel Club. Howell Book House, NY 2006. p. 271-275.

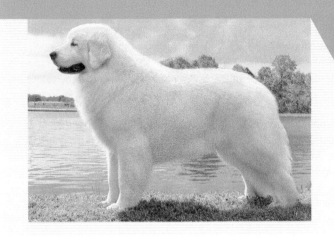

The Breed History

Originally from Siberia or Central Asia, it is thought that this breed entered Europe at least 1000 years BC. The ancient Asiatic mastiff-type is believed to be the primary ancestor. Common lineage may trace to Kuvasz, Kuvac, or Turkish Karabash dogs. As an aside, it is reported that this breed, and/or the Pyrenean Mastiff, when crossed with black English Retrievers may have given rise to the Newfoundland breed. The first formal breed standard was drawn up in 1927. Great Pyrenees were first registered with AKC in 1933. The Pyrenean Mastiff is a much larger breed, though it likely arose from similar ancestors. At one point, the Great Pyrenean dog was close to extinction. They are named after the mountain range in which much of the breed development took place.

Breeding for Function

Originally used for shepherding, the dog also functioned as a guard dog for the nobility. As a shepherd's dog, it was fitted with a spiked collar, and its bravery and long haircoat helped to protect it when it fended off wolves and bears. For the shepherding families, this dog would also serve as a watchdog and a draft dog. During WWI, this breed was put to work as a pack dog. Today, the Great Pyrenees generally functions as a companion breed.

Physical Characteristics

Height at Withers: female 25-29" (63.5-73.5 cm), male 27-32" (68.5-81.5 cm).

Weight: female 85 lb (38.5 kg), male 100 lb (45.5 kg).

Coat: They possess a very thick, full coat of white or almost white color though markings of gray, tan or badger are allowed (up to one third of body). The double coat consists of a fine wooly undercoat and a hard, long, flat and very dense outer coat that is slightly wavy. The ruff is more pronounced in males. Feathers are found on the back of the thighs and front legs. Has moderate grooming needs consisting of a thorough brush twice weekly (hair tends to resist tangling and shed dirt). High shedding occurs during the coat change spring and fall.

Longevity: 10-11 years

Points of Conformation: In general body type, it is said that they are built like a brown bear. They are large but still agile, and their gait is powerful, smooth and covers lots of ground. Their muscling and bone is medium in substance. The skull is wedge-shaped, and almond-shaped eyes are medium in size and pigmented dark brown. Palpebral margins are darkly pigmented. Ears are V-shaped with rounded tips, and small-to-medium sized, set at eye level and rest close to the head. They have a slightly tapering muzzle, no stop, and the nose and lips are pigmented black. The Great Pyrenees has a minimal dewlap, a strong medium length neck, topline is level, thorax is deep and broad, and ribs well sprung. Some abdominal tuck up is present. The bones of the tail reach the tarsus, the heavily plumed tapering tail is carried both over the back and low. Legs are straight boned; the single dewclaw (front) and double dewclaw behind are not removed. Round feet are large and pads are thick.

Recognized Behavior Issues and Traits

Reported breed traits include: Devoted, intelligent, guarding family and home as they would a sheep flock; quite territorial. Loyal and fearless, they are sometimes independent, even strong willed, but known to be gentle and patient with human family members. Need to begin socialization and obedience training early. Slow to mature. Needs open space, has moderate exercise needs but tends to be quiet around the home. Need to keep in a fenced enclosure if off leash. High barking tendency exists in some dogs.

Normal Physiologic Variations

Double hind limb dewclaws are always present. The breed is homozygous for this autosomal dominant condition.

In a UK study, 28.9% of Great Pyrenees litters were born via **Cesarean section.**[1]

Drug Sensitivities

None reported

Inherited Diseases

Hip Dysplasia: Polygenically inherited trait causing degenerative joint disease and hip arthritis. OFA reports 9.2% affected.[2]

Multifocal Retinopathy/Retinal Dysplasia: Autosomal recessive retinal pigment epithelial dysplasia causing localized multifocal retinal detachments. Age of onset from 11 to 13 weeks of age. Identified in 3.22% of Great Pyrenees CERF examined by veterinary ophthalmologists between 2000-2005. CERF does not recommend breeding any Great Pyrenees with retinal dysplasia. A genetic test is available.[3,4,5]

Elbow Dysplasia: Polygenically inherited trait causing elbow arthritis. OFA reports 1.5% affected.[2]

Patella Luxation: Polygenically inherited laxity of patellar ligaments, causing luxation, lameness, and later degenerative joint disease. Treat surgically if causing clinical signs. Dorn reports 2.99x odds ratio versus other breeds. Another study reports a 64.0x odds ratio versus other breeds. Reported at a frequency of 2.88% in the 2004 GPCA Health Survey. OFA reports 1.2% affected.[2,6,7,8]

Glanzmann's Thrombasthenia (GT): This defect causes frequent epistaxis, and gingival bleeding during teething in young dogs. Caused by a defect in intrinsic platelet function involving glycoprotein complex IIb-IIIa. Affected dogs have normal platelet numbers, and normal coagulation panels. Simple autosomal recessive mode of inheritance. A genetic test is available.[9,10]

Chondrodysplasia: Disproportionate dwarfism caused by a simple autosomal recessive gene. Causes short limbs and short trunk. Radiographically, there is metaphyseal flaring of all long bones and costochondral junctions of the ribs. Vertebral bodies are poorly ossified, with thin, concave end plates. Affected dogs can also be deaf. This condition occurs at a low frequency. There is ongoing research at UC-Davis to identify the defective gene.[11]

Disease Predispositions

Otitis Externa: 71.6% of Great Pyrenees have reported an ear infection in the 2004 GPCA Health Survey.[6]

Panosteitis: Self-limiting disease of young, large breed dogs involving the diaphyseal and metaphyseal areas of the tubular long bones. Affected dogs show intermittent lameness. Treat with rest. Reported 5.3x odds ratio versus other breeds. Reported at a frequency of 39.7% in the 2004 GPCA Health Survey.[6,8]

Persistent Pupillary Membranes: Strands of fetal remnant connecting; iris to iris, cornea, lens, or involving sheets of tissue. The later three forms can impair vision, and dogs affected with these forms should not be bred. Identified in 27.48% of Great Pyrenees CERF examined by veterinary ophthalmologists between 2000-2005.[5]

Arthritis: 11.6% of Geat Pyrenees reported arthritis between 4-12.5 years of age in the 2004 GPCA Health Survey.[6]

Allergic Dermatitis: Inhalant or food allergy. Presents with pruritis and pyotraumatic dermatitis (hot spots). Reported at a frequency of 8.7% in the 2004 GPCA Health Survey.[6]

Hypothyroidism: Inherited autoimmune thyroiditis. 6.5% positive for thyroid auto-antibodies based on testing at Michigan State University. (Ave. for all breeds is 7.5%). Reported at a frequency of 6.0% in the 2004 GPCA Health Survey.[6,12,13]

Cataracts: Anterior, posterior, and equatorial intermediate cataracts predominate in the breed. Identified in 5.69% of Great Pyrenees CERF examined by veterinary ophthalmologists between 2000-2005. CERF does not recommend breeding any Great Pyrenees with a cataract.[5]

Osteosarcoma: Malignant long bone cancer. Reported at a frequency of 4.1% in the 2004 GPCA Health Survey.[6]

Osteochondrosis (OCD) of the Shoulder: Inherited cartilage defect of the shoulder joint. Causes lameness in young growing dogs. Male prevalence. Mild cases may heal on own with rest. Severe cases require surgery. Reported 42.7x odds ratio versus other breeds. Dorn reports an 8.95x odds ratio for OCD versus other breeds.[7,8]

Distichiasis: Abnormally placed eyelashes that irritate the cornea and conjunctiva. Can cause secondary corneal ulceration. Identified in 1.98% of Great Pyrenees CERF examined by veterinary ophthalmologists between 2000-2005.[5]

Hypoadrenocorticism (Addison's Disease): Immune mediated destruction of the adrenal gland. Typical presentation of lethargy, poor appetite, vomiting, weakness, and dehydration can occur from 4 months to several years of age. Treatment with DOCA injections or oral fludrocortisone. Reported at a frequency of 1.7% in the 2004 GPCA Health Survey.[6]

Entropion: Entropion, a rolling in of the eyelids, can cause corneal irritation and ulceration. Identified in 1.49% of Great Pyrenees CERF examined by veterinary ophthalmologists between 2000-2005.[5]

Corneal Dystrophy: The epithelial/stromal form occurs in the breed, causing a bilateral, white to gray, non-inflammatory corneal opacity. Identified in 1.24% of Great Pyrenees CERF examined by veterinary ophthalmologists between 2000-2005.[5]

Gastric Dilation/Volvulus (Bloat): Life-threatening twisting of the stomach within the abdomen. Requires immediate veterinary attention. Reported at a frequency of 1.0% in the 2004 GPCA Health Survey.[6]

Deafness: Unilateral or bilateral congenital deafness is reported by Strain. Diagnosed by BAER testing. OFA reports a high frequency, but too few Great Pyrenees have been tested for statistical accuracy.[2,14]

Laryngeal Paralysis-polyneuropathy Complex: Affected Great Pyrenees dogs present at less than 6 months of age with laryngeal paralysis and megaesophagus. Pathology reveals distal axonal degeneration. Prognosis is poor. An autosomal recessive mode of inheritance is suspected.[15]

Isolated Case Studies

Hemophilia A: Reported in a male puppy who developed facial and shoulder hematomas and gingival bleeding. Coagulation studies revealed normal bleeding and prothrombin times, prolonged clotting and activated partial prothrombin times and decreased factor VIII activity. The dam and a female littermate also had decreased factor VIII activity and were probably carriers of the disease.[16]

Factor XI Deficiency: Autosomal recessive bleeding disorder reported to occur in the breed.[17]

Congenital Preputial and Penile Deformity: Report of surgical correction in a puppy, presenting with dysuria and prepuce edema. The dog had a stenotic preputial orifice, and an inability to extend the penis from the prepuce.[18]

Left Ventricular Outflow Tract-Right Atrial Communication (Gerbode Type Defect): Identified in a 6 year old male with associated with bacterial endocarditis. Vegetative mural endocardial lesions were observed grossly, and gram-negative coccobacilli that were consistent with Bordetella avium-like organisms were observed histopathologically. LV-RA shunt (Gerbode defect) is a rare cardiac defect in humans that can be either congenital or, more rarely, secondary to septic endocarditis.[19]

Craniomandibular Osteopathy: Reported two dogs with mandibular swelling, pain, fever and, in dog 1, lameness. Radiographs demonstrated extensive, active new bone formation on the ventral aspect of the mandibular bodies of both dogs.[20]

Cor Triatriatum Dexter: A Young Great Pyrenees with poor growth and ascites was identified with a septum dividing the right atrium into two separate chambers. Surgical correction was successful.[21]

Brachygnathism, Prognathism, Cervical Vertebral Instability, Optic Nerve Hypoplasia, Tricuspid Valve Dysplasia, and **von Willebrand's Disease** are reported.[22]

Genetic Tests

Tests of Genotype: Direct test for Glannzmann's thrombasthenia (GT) is available from the Auburn Univ-Boudreaux Lab.

Direct test for Multifocal Retinopathy is available from Optigen.

Tests of Phenotype: CHIC Certification: Hip radiographs, patella evaluation, and one of the following: thyroid profile including autoantibodies, CERF eye examination, cardiac examination, radiographs for elbow dysplasia or shoulder osteochondrosis (OCD), and brainstem audio-evoked response (BAER) test for deafness. (See CHIC website; www.caninehealthinfo.org).

Miscellaneous

- **Breed name synonyms:** Pyrenean Mountain Dog, Le Chien des Pyrénées, Le Grande Chien des Montagnes, Pyr, historical names: Pyrenean bearhound, Pyrenean wolf dog.
- **Registries:** AKC, UKC, CKC, KCGB (Kennel Club of Great Britain), ANKC (Australian National Kennel Club), NKC (National Kennel Club).
- **AKC rank (year 2008):** 62 (1,444 registered)
- **Internet resources: Great Pyrenees Club of America:** http://clubs.akc.org/gpca/
  The Pyrenean Mountain Dog Club of Great Britain: www.pmdc.org.uk
  Great Pyrenees Club of Canada: http://pyrcanada.com
  Great Pyrenees Club of America's Health Information Center: www.gpcahealth.org

References

1. Evans KM & Adams VJ: Proportion of litters of purebred dogs born by caesarean section. J Small Anim Pract. 2010 Feb;51(2):113-8.
2. OFA Website breed statistics: www.offa.org Last accessed July 1, 2010.
3. Grahn BH, Cullen CL: Retinopathy of Great Pyrenees dogs: fluorescein angiography, light microscopy and transmitting and scanning electron microscopy. Vet Ophthalmol. 2001 Sep;4(3):191-9.
4. B.H. Grahn; H. Philibert; C.L. Cullen; D.M. Houston; H.A. Semple; S.M. Schmutz: Multifocal Retinopathy of Great Pyrenees Dogs. Vet Comp Ophthalmol 1[4]:211-221 Dec'98
5. Ocular Disorders Presumed to be Inherited in Purebred Dogs. American College of Veterinary Ophthalmologists. ACVO, 2007.
6. GPCA Health Committee: 2004 GPCA Health Survey Report. Feb. 2006.
7. Dorn CR: Canine breed-specific risks of frequently diagnosed diseases at veterinary teaching hospitals. Monograph. AKC Canine Health Foundation. 2000.
8. LaFond E, Breur GJ & Austin CC: Breed susceptibility for developmental orthopedic diseases in dogs. J Am Anim Hosp Assoc. 2002 Sep-Oct;38(5):467-77.
9. Boudreaux MK, Lipscomb DL: Clinical, biochemical, and molecular aspects of Glanzmann's thrombasthenia in humans and dogs. Vet Pathol. 2001 May;38(3):249-60.
10. Lipscomb DL, Bourne C, Boudreaux MK: Two genetic defects in alphaIIb are associated with type I Glanzmann's thrombasthenia in a Great Pyrenees dog: a 14-base insertion in exon 13 and a splicing defect of intron 13. Vet Pathol 37[6]:581-8 2000 Nov.
11. Bingel SA, Sande RD: Chondrodysplasia in five Great Pyrenees. J Am Vet Med Assoc. 1994 Sep 15;205(6):845-8.
12. Nachreiner RF, Refsal KR, Graham PA, et. al.: Prevalence of serum thyroid hormone autoantibodies in dogs with clinical signs of hypothyroidism. J Am Vet Med Assoc 2002 Feb 15;220(4):466-71.
13. Nachreiner R & Refsal K: Personal communication, Diagnostic Center for Population and Animal Health, Michigan State University. April, 2007.
14. Strain GM: Deafness prevalence and pigmentation and gender associations in dog breeds at risk. Vet J 2004; Jan;167(1):23-32.
15. Gabriel A, Poncelet L, Van Ham L, et. al.: Laryngeal paralysis-polyneuropathy complex in young related Pyrenean mountain dogs. J Small Anim Pract. 2006 Mar;47(3):144-9.
16. Golden JG, Banknieder AR, Bruestle ME: Hemophilia in a Great Pyrenees. Mod Vet Pract. 1980 Aug;61(8):671-4
17. Fogh JM, Fogh IT: Inherited coagulation disorders. Vet Clin North Am Small Anim Pract. 1988 Jan;18(1):231-43.
18. Olsen, Dennis & Salwei, Rochelle: Surgical Correction of a Congenital Preputial and Penile Deformity in a Dog. J Am Anim Hosp Assoc 37[2]:187-192 Mar-Apr'01
19. Ramirez GA, Espinosa de los Monteros A, Rodriguez F, Weisbrode SE, Jaber JR, Herraez P: Left ventricular outflow tract-right atrial communication (Gerbode type defect) associated with bacterial endocarditis in a dog. Vet Pathol. 2003 Sep;40(5):579-82.
20. Franch J, Cesari JR, Font J: Craniomandibular osteopathy in two Pyrenean mountain dogs. Vet Rec. 1998 Apr 25;142(17):455-9.
21. Mitten RW, Edwards GA & Rishniw M: Diagnosis and management of cor triatriatum dexter in a Pyrenean mountain dog and an Akita Inu. Aust Vet J. 2001 Mar;79(3):177-80.
22. The Genetic Connection: A Guide to Health Problems in Purebred Dogs. L Ackerman. p. 221. AAHA Press, 1999.
23. The Complete Dog Book, 20th Ed. The American Kennel Club. Howell Book House, NY 2006. p. 276-280.

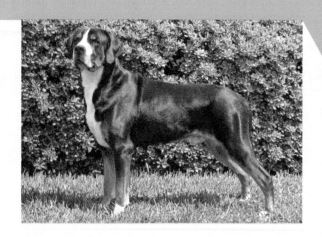

The Breed History

Thought to have been brought by the Romans to the Alps, these dogs and those of the Swiss Sennenhund group derive from Mastiff type dogs (Mollasian or Molloser). The Greater Swiss Mountain dog is the oldest and the largest of the Swiss working dogs. It was not until 1908 that the breed was rescued from a slow decline; first registrations occurred in the Swiss Kennel Club a few years later. Numbers did not rebound until well after the Second World War. This breed contributed to the development of the Rottweiler and Saint Bernard. The Bernese Mountain dog is also related. First specimens were exported to America in 1967. The AKC first accepted Swiss Mountain dogs into the studbook in 1993, with full breed recognition assigned in 1995.

Breeding for Function

This was an all purpose farm dog bred to help with herding, droving, guarding, and draft (cart pulling etc.).

Physical Characteristics

Height at Withers: female 23.5-27" (59.5-68.5 cm), male 25.5-28.5" (65-72.5 cm)

Weight: females 85-110 lb (38.5-50 kg), males 115-140 lb (53.5-63.4 kg).

Coat: Double coated, the inner coat is thick and short, the outer coat is dense and hard (< 2" long). Coat color is a tri-color; a base of black with rust and white markings. Symmetrical rust markings of brows, cheek and chest, on the four legs and tail, with white highlights of muzzle and blaze are standard. On the chest, a cross, and the tail tip and feet white markings are also important; also on the neck a collar marking is permitted.

Longevity: 7-9 years

Points of Conformation: Being a powerful draft dog, the constitution is that of a heavily muscled and boned dog. The skull is broad and flat, and the muzzle is blunt, and there are only minor flews. The medium-sized ears are triangular with rounded tips, and are high-set and folded so that the ears lay close to the head. Eyes are dark brown with a gentle expression, and they are medium in size, with closely fitting black palpebral margins. The nose is also black. The neck is moderate in length and muscularity,

without throatiness. The topline is level, and the thorax is deep with well-sprung ribs. The tail reaches the tarsus and is carried low at rest, though during exercise it is elevated to topline. Legs are straight boned, feet are round and the toes are well arched. Rear dewclaws are generally removed. Gait should reflect power and be ground covering, and for their size this breed is very agile.

Recognized Behavior Issues and Traits

Reported breed characteristics include: Bold, faithful, willing worker, alert, vigilant, can be argumentative with other dogs (especially inter-male aggression) though he is gentle with people. Not suitable for apartment living. During shedding, grooming needs are high, but the rest of the year the Swissy requires brushing only once or twice per week. They are slow to mature and these dogs require close human contact. The Swissy tends to be slow in housetraining. Needs suitable work or play to prevent boredom. He requires early socialization and obedience training and has moderate exercise needs. Low exercise intensity is recommended until skeletal maturity. The Swissy has a well-developed alarm barking tendency (and a very loud, booming bark) and strong guarding instinct. His strong prey drive may mean that small pets are seen as prey. Some dogs have a tendency to dominance. Due to their size and strength, they are generally very strong on the leash and as such, may be best for experienced dog owners, and in homes with older children. Not considered ideal for a seniors due to size and strength. These dogs have poor tolerance of high ambient temperatures.

Normal Physiologic Variations

Breeding females can have difficulty whelping, and may require a Cesarean section.

Drug Sensitivities

None reported

Inherited Diseases

Hip Dysplasia: Polygenically inherited trait causing degenerative joint disease and hip arthritis. OFA reports 19.1% affected.[1]

Elbow Dysplasia: Polygenically inherited trait causing elbow arthritis. OFA reports 11.3% affected.[1]

Patella Luxation: Polygenically inherited laxity of patellar ligaments, causing luxation, lameness, and later degenerative joint disease. Treat surgically if causing clinical signs. OFA reports 0.5% affected.[1]

Disease Predispositions

Distichiasis: Abnormally placed eyelashes that irritate the cornea and conjunctiva. Can cause secondary corneal ulceration. Identified in 31.82% of Greater Swiss Mountain Dogs CERF examined by veterinary ophthalmologists between 2000-2005.[2]

Urinary Incontinence: Greater Swiss Mountain Dogs have increased risk to develop urinary incontinence. Treat with DES (for females) or phenylpropanolamine. Reported at a frequency of 11.0% in the 2000-2001 GSMDCA Health Survey, with a frequency of 20.0% in females.[3]

Humeral Osteochondritis Dissecans: Polygenically inherited cartilage defect of the humeral head. Causes shoulder joint pain and lameness in young growing dogs. Mild cases can resolve with rest, while more severe cases require surgery. Reported at a frequency of 5.4% in the 2000-2001 GSMDCA Health Survey. Diagnosed in 15.3% of Greater Swiss Mountain Dogs who had shoulder radiographs taken. Unknown mode of inheritance.[3]

Umbilical Hernia: Congenital opening in the body wall from where the umbilical cord was attached. Reported at a frequency of 9.6% in the 2000-2001 GSMDCA Health Survey. Unknown mode of inheritance.[3]

Cataracts: Anterior cortex punctate and posterior cortex intermediate cataracts predominate in the breed. Identified in 8.12% of Greater Swiss Mountain Dogs CERF examined by veterinary ophthalmologists between 2000-2005. CERF does not recommend breeding any Greater Swiss Mountain Dog with a cataract.[2]

Gastric Dilation/Volvulus (GDV, Bloat): Life-threatening twisting of the stomach within the abdomen. Requires immediate veterinary attention. Reported at a frequency of 5.3% in the 2000-2001 GSMDCA Health Survey. Unknown mode of inheritance.[3]

Inherited Epilepsy: Grand-mal seizures. Control with anticonvulsant medication. Reported at a frequency of 4.6% in the 2000-2001 GSMDCA Health Survey. Unknown mode of inheritance.[3]

Persistent Pupillary Membranes: Strands of fetal remnant connecting; iris to iris, cornea, lens, or involving sheets of tissue. The later three forms can impair vision, and dogs affected with these forms should not be bred. Identified in 3.97% of Greater Swiss Mountain Dogs CERF examined by veterinary ophthalmologists between 2000-2005.[2]

Hypothyroidism: Inherited autoimmune thyroiditis. 3.7% positive for thyroid autoantibodies based on testing at Michigan State University. (Ave. for all breeds is 7.5%).[4,5]

Fly-biting Seizures/Partial Seizures: Seen at an increased frequency in the breed. Control with anticonvulsant medication. Reported at a frequency of 1.3% in the 2000-2001 GSMDCA Health Survey. Unknown mode of inheritance.[3,6]

Lumbosacral Transitional Vertebra (LTV): The breed has a significantly greater incidence of LTV than other breeds. This can lead to pain and neurological impairment from cauda equina syndrome.[7]

Panosteitis and **von Willebrand's Disease** are reported.[8]

Isolated Case Studies

Pemphigus Vegetans: A 4-year-old male Greater Swiss Mountain Dog presented with multifocal cutaneous verrucous and crusted papules and pustules, as well as skin and mucosal erosions and ulcers. Histopathology revealed hyperplastic intraepidermal pustular and suprabasal acantholytic dermatosis resembling human pemphigus vegetans.[9]

Genetic Tests

Tests of Genotype: none

Tests of Phenotype: CHIC Certification: Required testing includes hip and elbow radiographs, and CERF eye examination. Optional recommended tests include shoulder radiographs, and anecdotal data on epilepsy, splenic torsion, and gastric torsion. (See CHIC website; www.caninehealthinfo.org).

Recommend thyroid profile including autoantibodies, patella evaluation and cardiac evaluation.

Miscellaneous

- **Breed name synonyms:** Swissy, Grosser Schweizer Sennenhund, Swiss Mountain Dog, Great Swiss Cattle Dog, Great Swiss Mountain Dog, Greater Swiss Mountain dog.
- **Registries:** AKC, CKC, NKC (National Kennel Club), FCI.
- **AKC rank (year 2008):** 89 (715 dogs registered)
- **Internet resources: Greater Swiss Mountain Dog Club of America:** www.gsmdca.org
  Great Swiss Mountain Dog Club of Great Britain: www.gsmd.org.uk

References

1. OFA Website breed statistics: www.offa.org Last accessed July 1, 2010.
2. *Ocular Disorders Presumed to be Inherited in Purebred Dogs.* American College of Veterinary Ophthalmologists. ACVO, 2007.
3. Greater Swiss Mountain Dog Club of America: 2000 & 2001 GSMDCA Breed Health Survey. 2002.
4. Nachreiner RF, Refsal KR, Graham PA, et. al.: Prevalence of serum thyroid hormone autoantibodies in dogs with clinical signs of hypothyroidism. *J Am Vet Med Assoc* 2002 Feb 15;220(4):466-71.
5. Nachreiner R & Refsal K: Personal communication, Diagnostic Center for Population and Animal Health, Michigan State University. April, 2007.
6. Thomas WB: Movement Disorders in Small Animals: Shaking, Head Bobbing, Fly Biting, and Dancing Dobermans. Proceedings, 2002 Tufts Animal Expo. 2002.
7. Flückiger M, Damur-Djuric N, Steffen F: Lumbosacral Transitional Vertebra In the Dog: Prevalence in Different Breeds and in Dogs Suffering From Cauda Equina Compression Syndrome. Proceedings, 2004 World Small Animal Veterinary Association Congress. 2004.
8. *The Genetic Connection: A Guide to Health Problems in Purebred Dogs.* L Ackerman. p. 222. AAHA Press, 1999.
9. Heimann M, Beco L, Petein M, et. al.: Canine hyperplastic intraepidermal pustular and suprabasal acantholytic dermatosis with features of human pemphigus vegetans. Vet Pathol. 2007 Jul;44(4):550-5.
10. *The Complete Dog Book, 20th Ed.* The American Kennel Club. Howell Book House, NY 2006. p. 281-283.

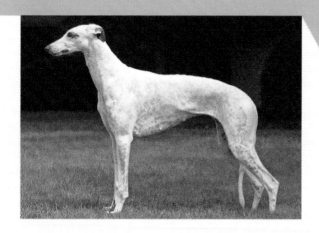

The Breed History

Greyhounds are ancient sight or "gaze" hounds originating from the Egyptian Sloughi lines that were brought to England about 900 AD. Early origins trace back to 3000-5000 BC in the Middle East (Egypt). They are considered both the oldest and fastest breed of dog. They were registered in the AKC by the time of the second breed standards edition in 1855.

Breeding for Function

This breed was originally developed to accompany mounted hunters primarily for coursing hares. They were also used to hunt stag, fox, wild boar and gazelle. Also termed a "gazehound", their keen vision and exceptional speed allowed them to be an effective hunting partner. The most popular use for this dog in modern times is as a racing dog. There are two modern sub-types in the breed; show and racing. The show dog is a slightly heavier conformation, but the temperament is the same.

Physical Characteristics

Height at Withers: female 27-28" (68-71 cm), male 28-30" (70-76 cm)

Weight: females 60-65 lb (27-29 kg), males 65-70 (29-32 kg).

Coat: The short fine haircoat is set close to the skin surface and colors include brindle, fawn, black, white, red, and blue.

Longevity: 10-12 years.

Conformation Points: This muscular, highly athletic dog has a long, flat, medium weight skull with a slight stop (dolichocephalic skull), dark eyes, small fine partially upright ears, a long muscular neck, very deep chest and well-sprung rib cage, with moderately arched loins and a thin waist. They have fine-boned long limbs, with small compact feet well knuckled up, and carry their long tapering thin tail low.

Recognized Behavior Issues and Traits

The greyhound is known to be a very affectionate dog; gentle, but somewhat cautious around strangers. In the home environment, it requires a low to average amount of exercise only, but outdoors enjoys a good free run. It has a strong chase instinct, and this should be kept in mind when around other (smaller) pets and children. The coat needs very little care. They enjoy close human companionship, though they are not known to be one-man dogs. Training progresses quickly, but they are easily bored, so a variety of tasks is important. They think well for themselves and therefore work well independently. They may try to greet friends by jumping up and hugging, and tend to sneak off with favorite household items. Yards should be fenced if they are let outside off leash.

Normal Physiologic Variations

Echocardiographic Normal Values:[1]	
Parameter	Median +/- S.D.
Weight (kg)	20.7-32.5
LVPWD (mm)	12.1 +/- 1.7
LVPWS (mm)	15.2 +/- 2.2
LVD (mm)	44.1 +/- 3.0
LVS (mm)	32.5 +/- 3.5
FS (%)	25.4 +/- 6.3
IVSd (mm)	10.6 +/- 1.7
IVSs (mm)	13.4 +/- 2.5
N	16

LVPWD, LV posterior wall dimension at end-diastole; LVPWS, LV posterior wall thickness at end-systole; LVD, LV chamber dimension at end-diastole; LVS, LV chamber dimension at end-systole; FS, percent fractional shortening; IVSd, interventricular septal thickness at end-diastole; IVSs, interventricular septal thickness at end-systole; N, number of animals.

Another Study (Echocardiographic values without sedation):[2] IVSd (mm): 10-16, LVIDd (mm): 40-50, LVIDs (mm): 28-36, LVWd (mm): 8-13, FS%: 24-37, Vcf (Circ/sec): 1.2-2.2

Vertebral Heart Size (VHS) is larger than in other breeds, with a mean of 10.5 +/- 0.1 on a lateral radiograph.[3]

A soft (1-2/6) **Left Basilar Systolic Murmur** is identified in a majority of Greyhounds. It is associated with an increased aortic velocity, and is not related to heart disease.[4]

Normal **Systemic Blood Pressure Values** are about 20 mmHg higher than other breeds. Normal range for **hematocrit** varies with geographic location, but is generally between 50-65%. This range is higher than for many breeds.[5]

Up to 26% of all Greyhounds with normal blood clotting parameters can show excessive bleeding after injury or surgical procedures. This is due to weaker clot strength (kinetics) and increased fibrinolysis in the breed.[6]

Thyroid Values: Greyhounds, as with all sight hounds, have lower normal ranges for T4 and T3 concentrations compared to other breeds. The following are average values:[7]
T4: 13.9 +/- 6.3 nmol/L
fT4: 11.6 +/- 6.5 pmol/L

cTSH: 0.20 +/- 0.21 ng/ml
T4 after TSH admin: 36.4 +/- 10 nmol/L
fT4 after TSH admin: 16.7 +/- 7.2 pmol/L

Greyhounds have higher normal **creatinine** levels than non-Greyhounds, with a mean of 1.6 mg/dL (range 1.2-1.9 mg/dL).[8]

Drug Sensitivities

Anesthesia: Sight hounds require particular attention during anesthesia. Their lean body conformation with high surface-area-to-volume ratio predisposes them to hypothermia during anesthesia. Impaired biotransformation of drugs by the liver results in prolonged recovery from barbiturate and thiobarbiturate intravenous anesthetics.[9]

Deficient hydroxylation of propofol by hepatic cytochrome P-450 isoforms may contribute to slow clearance of propofol by greyhounds.[10]

Inherited Diseases

Hip Dysplasia: Polygenically inherited trait causing degenerative joint disease and hip arthritis. OFA reports 2.1% affected. Reported at a frequency of 0.6% in a web-based Greyhound health survey.[11,12]

Elbow Dysplasia: Polygenically inherited trait causing elbow arthritis. Too few Greyhounds have been evaluated by OFA to determine an accurate frequency.[11]

Patella Luxation: Polygenically inherited trait causing stifle instability and arthritis. Too few Greyhounds have been evaluated by OFA to determine an accurate frequency.[11]

Polyneuropathy: A rare, autosomal recessive polyneuropathy presenting with progressive weakness and gait abnormalities between 3 and 9 months of age is identified in conformation Greyhounds. Pathology reveals mild to marked reduction in nerve fiber density, axonal swelling, and secondary muscle atrophy. The disease is caused by a mutation in the NDRG1 gene. Limited testing did not reveal the mutation in racing Greyhound lines. A direct genetic test is available.[13]

Disease Predispositions

Supernumerary Teeth: One study found a 36.4% incidence of supernumerary teeth; most often maxillary first premolars.[14]

Periodontal Disease: Dorn reports a 8.95x odds ratio for developing periodontal disease versus other breeds.[15]

Osteoarthritis: Degenerative joint disease accompanied by pain and lameness. Treat with anti-inflammatory drugs. Reported at a frequency of 17.5% in a web-based Greyhound health survey.[12]

Cataracts: Posterior cortex imtermediate and anterior cortex punctate cataracts predominate in the breed. Reported at a frequency of 17% in a survey of retired racing Greyhounds. Identified in 5.43% of Greyhounds CERF-examined by veterinary ophthalmologists between 2000-2005. CERF Does not recommend breeding any Greyhound with a cataract.[16,17]

Thigh Alopecia: As Greyhounds age, they are prone to symmetrical alopecia over their thigh areas. Reported at 20% in a pathological study of Greyhounds. Reported at a frequency of 16.3% in a web-based Greyhound health survey.[12,18]

Endocardiosis (Mitral Valvular Disease): A pathological study of deceased Greyhounds found that 10.4% had signs of endocardiosis or mitral valvular thickening. No correlation to clinical signs or heart disease were available. Heart murmers were reported at a frequency of 5.3% in a web-based Greyhound health survey.[12,18,19]

Vitreous Degeneration: Liquefaction of the vitreous gel which may predispose to retinal detachment. Reported at a frequency of 31% in a survey of retired racing Greyhounds. Identified in 3.42% of Greyhounds CERF-examined by veterinary ophthalmologists between 2000-2005. CERF does not recommend breeding any Greyhound with the condition.[16,17]

Chronic Glomerulonephritis: Chronic kidney diease was identified microscopically on necropsy of 6.9% of Greyhounds in one study, however it was found in 64% of those over 7.5 years of age. No correlation to clinical disease or azotemia was investigated. Dorn reports a 5.42x odds ratio for kidney disease versus other breeds.[15,18]

Osteosarcoma: Malignant bone cancer, usually affecting the limbs. Reported at a frequency of 5.9% in a web-based Greyhound health survey. The proximal humerus was the most frequent location, with the distal radius, proximal tibia, distal tibia, distal femur, and proximal femur the other locations reported. Another study showed a frequency of 6.2% with an average age of 9.9 years.[12,20]

Digital Keratoma (Corns): Greyhounds have a predilection to forming footpad corns, which are painful, hard keratin accumulations in the deep dermis and epidermis. There is a male predilection with over 90% affecting digits 3 or 4 in the thoracic limbs. Remove when identified. Reported at a frequency of 5.9% in a web-based Greyhound health survey.[12,21,22]

Allergic Dermatitis: Inhalant or food allergies. Presents with pruritis and pyotraumatic dermatitis (hot spots). Inhalant allergy was reported at 1.4% and food allergy at 5.5% in a web-based Greyhound health survey.[12]

Cardiac Arrhythmias: In racing Greyhounds, maximal sprinting increases the incidence of cardiac arrhythmias during the early recovery period: mainly sinus tachycardia, ventricular extrasystoles, ventricular tachycardia, and electrical alternans.[23]

Progressive Retinal Atrophy (PRA)/Retinal Degeneration: Undetermined mode of inheritance. PRA in the greyhound may begin as early as 12 months of age, and affected dogs may progress to complete blindness at a relatively young age. Nyctalopia (night blindness) is not an initial finding in affected Greyhounds. Reported at a frequency of 4% in a survey of retired racing Greyhounds. CERF does not recommend breeding any Greyhound with PRA.[16,17,24]

Chronic Superficial Keratitis (Pannus): A chronic corneal inflammatory process that can cause vision problems due to corneal pigmentation. Treatment with topical ocular lubricants and anti-inflammatory medication. One study found Greyhounds to be a breed at increased risk. Reported at a frequency of 4% in a survey of retired racing Greyhounds. Identified in 4.11% of Greyhounds CERF-examined by veterinary ophthalmologists between 2000-2005. CERF does not recommend breeding any Greyhound with pannus.[16,17,25]

Sesamoid Disease: Greyhounds (especially racing Greyhounds) can develop acute to chronic forelimb lameness due to fragmentation of the 2nd and 7th metacarpophalangeal sesamoid bones, with secondary degenerative joint disease. One study showed that a reduction in number of vascular foramina is correlated to increased risk for the disease.[26]

Central Tarsal Bone Fracture: Racing Greyhounds can develop factures of the central tarsal bone secondary to accumulation and coalescence of branching arrays of fatigue microcracks. This may occur more frequently in the right hind limb; the outside limb when racing.[27,28,29]

Otitis Externa (Chronic Ear Infections): Can also be secondary to allergic skin disease. Bacterial, yeast, or mixed infection. Reported at a frequency of 2.5% in a web-based Greyhound health survey.[12]

Inflammatory Bowel Disease (IBD): An immune mediated disorder presenting as gastrointestinal inflammation and irritation. It can present with vomiting, diarrhea, or weight loss. Affected dogs can usually be controlled with diet and/or medications. Reported at a frequency of 2.4% in a web-based Greyhound health survey.[12]

Idiopathic Epilepsy (Inherited Seizures): Can be generalized or partial seizures. Control with anti-seizure medication. Reported at a frequency of 2.4% in a web-based Greyhound health survey.[12]

Lumbosacral Stenosis/Cauda Equina Syndrome: Narrowing of the bony canal at the end of the spinal cord, can cause pain, ataxia, and progressive neurological impairment. Reported at a frequency of 2.0% in a web-based Greyhound health survey.[12]

Intervertebral Disc Disease (IVDD): Spinal cord disease due to prolapsed disk material. Clinical signs include back pain, scuffing of paws, spinal ataxia, limb weakness, and paralysis. Reported at a frequency of 2.0% in a web-based Greyhound health survey.[12]

Symmetrical Lupoid Onychodystrophy (SLO): Disorder causing loss of toenails. Onset between 2-8 years of age affecting 1-2 nails, then progressing to all toenails within 2-9 weeks. Requires lifelong treatment with oral fatty acid supplementation +/- prednisone. Reported at a frequency of 1.8% in a web-based Greyhound health survey.[12]

Hypothyroidism: Inherited autoimmune thyroiditis. 1.7% positive for thyroid autoantibodies based on testing at Michigan State University. (Ave. for all breeds is 7.5). Reported at a frequency of 11% in a web-based Greyhound health survey.[12,30,31,32]

Babesiosis: Greyhounds comprise a significant percentage of dogs seropositive for Babesia canis vogeli. Reported at a frequency of 2.6% in a web-based Greyhound health survey. Greyhounds presenting with **immune-mediated hemolytic anemia** or **thrombocytopenia** should be screened for babesiosis.[12,33,34,35]

Primary Lens Luxation: Often progresses to secondary glaucoma. Identified in 1.37% of Greyhounds CERF examined by veterinary ophthalmologists between 2000-2005. CERF does not recommend breeding any Greyhound with lens luxation.[16]

Cranial Cruciate Ligament (ACL) Rupture: Traumatic tearing of the ACL in the stifle, causing lameness and secondary arthritis. Treat with surgery. Reported at a frequency of 1.1% in a web-based Greyhound health survey.[12]

Lymphoma/Lymphosarcoma: Malignant cancer of lymphoid tissue. Can be B-cell or T-cell (mycosis fungoides) disease. Reported at a frequency of 1.1% in a web-based Greyhound health survey.[12]

Hemangiosarcoma: A malignant cancer of red blood cells, usually involving the spleen, liver, heart, or bone marrow. Greyhounds are found to be at increased risk of developing visceral and non-visceral hemangiosarcomas and hemangiomas versus other breeds. Reported at a frequency of 1.1% in a web-based Greyhound health survey.[12,36]

Cutaneous and Renal Glomerular Vasculopathy (CRGV) (Alabama Rot): A vascular disease of unknown etiology affecting the skin and kidneys of racing Greyhounds. Affected dogs can present with symptoms of cutaneous ulcers of the extremities, thrombocytopenia, and in advanced cases acute renal insufficiency. There is no evidence of infectious or immune-complex disease in the pathogenesis. Prognosis for recovery is poor if azotemia is present.[37,38,39]

Juvenile Endocrine and Exocrine Pancreatic Atrophy: Several cases of Greyhounds with compound failure of the endocrine and exocrine pancreas have been identified. Cases range from 4 weeks to 18 months of age, with a median of 12 weeks. Clinical signs are typical for both endocrine and exocrine diseases. Pathology reveals acinar cell apoptosis, zymogen granule loss, cytoplasmic clearing or vacuolar change, lobular atrophy, islet loss, and lymphocytic or lymphoplasmacytic pancreatitis.[40]

Greyhound Meningoencephalitis: Rare, non-suppurative meningoencephalitis primarily affecting young greyhounds between 4-18 months of age. Affected dogs develop either acute or insidious neurological signs including head tilting, circling, ataxia, recumbency and blindness. Pathological changes include cerebral cortex perivascular cuffing and gliosis. Gene expression studies identify an autoimmune pathogenesis. There is no treatment.[41,42,43]

Malignant Hyperthermia: Exercise and anesthesia induced malignant hyperthermia is reported in isolated Greyhound cases.[44,45,46,47]

Renal Arteriosclerosis: Endothelial damage to the renal arteries due to hemodynamic forces of sheer stress and pressure pulse velocity is identified in young, race-trained Greyhounds. Correlation to later kidney disease is not determined.[48]

Brachygnathism, Cryptorchidism, Factor VIII Deficiency, Gastric Dilation/Volvulus, Megaesophagus, Optic Nerve Hypoplasia, Osteochondritis Dessicans of the stifle and shoulder, Spina Bifida, and **von Willebrand's disease** are reported.[49]

Isolated Case Studies

Acute B cell Lymphoblastic Leukaemia: A 12 week old Greyhound with lethargy, inappetence, shifting lameness, pyrexia and hepatosplenomegaly had anaemia, thrombocytopenla, neutropenia and large numbers of atypical mononuclear leucocytes. The pup died 4 days after presentation.[50]

Persistent Right Aortic Arch (PRAA): Repeat matings between two Greyhounds produced puppies with regurgitation and secondary megaesophagus due to PRAA. Surgery is curative. Greyhounds are not a breed reported with an increased incidence of this inherited congenital disorder.[51]

Avulsion of the Tibial Tubercle: Isolated cases are reported. In one report, six of seven Greyhound pups aged 5-1/2 months old avulsed their tibial tubercle. Avulsion was bilateral in four of the dogs. Osteochondrosis of the cranioproximal tibial physis was identified pathologically.[52,53]

Genetic Tests

Tests of Genotype: Direct test for polyneuropathy is available from Optigen.

Direct test for black mask is available from HealthGene and VetGen.

Tests of Phenotype: CHIC Certification: Cardiac evaluation by a cardiologist, and blood sample donation to the CHIC DNA repository. (See CHIC website: www.caninehealthinfo.com)

Recommend hip and elbow radiographs, CERF eye examination, patella evaluation, and thyroid profile including autoantibodies.

Miscellaneous

- **Breed Name Synonyms:** none
- **Registries:** AKC, CKC, UKC, KCGB (Kennel Club of Great Britain), ANKC (Australian National Kennel Club), NKC (National Kennel Club)
- **AKC Rank (Year 2008):** 129 (183 dogs registered)
- **Internet resources: Greyhound Club of America:** www.greyhoundclubofamerica.org
  National Greyhound Association (Racing Association, the sole registry for racing greyhounds): www.ngagreyhounds.com
  Greyhound Rescue Adoption Service directory of Adoption Agencies: www.greyhound.org

References

1. Page A, Edmunds G, & Atwell RB: Echocardiographic values in the greyhound. Aust Vet J. 1993 Oct;70(10):361-4.
2. Snyder PS, Sato T, Atkins CE. A comparison of echocardiographic indices of the nonracing, healthy greyhound to reference values for other breeds. Vet Radiol Ultrasound 1995;36:387-392
3. Marin LM, Brown J, McBrien C, et. al.: Vertebral heart size in retired racing Greyhounds. Vet Radiol Ultrasound. 2007 Jul-Aug;48(4):332-4.
4. Fabrizio F, Baumwart R, Iazbik MC, et. al.: Left basilar systolic murmur in retired racing greyhounds. J Vet Intern Med. 2006 Jan-Feb;20(1):78-82.
5. Steiss JE, Brewer WG, Welles E, Wright JC: Hematologic and serum biochemical reference values in retired Greyhounds. Compend Cont Educ 2000;22:243-248.
6. Vilar P, Couto CG, Westendorf N, et. al.: Thromboelastographic tracings in retired racing greyhounds and in non-greyhound dogs. J Vet Intern Med. 2008 Mar-Apr;22(2):374-9.
7. Gaughan KR, Bruyette DS: Thyroid function testing in Greyhounds. Am J Vet Res 2001;62:1130–1133.
8. Feeman WE 3rd, Couto CG, & Gray TL: Serum creatinine concentrations in retired racing Greyhounds. Vet Clin Pathol. 2003;32(1):40-2.
9. Court MH: Anesthesia of the sighthound. Clin Tech Small Anim Pract 1999 Feb;14(1):38-43.
10. Court MH, Hay-Kraus BL, Hill DW, Kind AJ, Greenblatt DJ. Propofol hydroxylation by dog liver microsomes: assay development and dog breed differences. Drug Metab Dispos 1999 Nov;27(11):1293-9
11. OFA Website breed statistics: www.offa.org Last accessed July 1, 2010.
12. Lord LK, Yaissle JE, Marin L, et. al.: Results of a web-based health survey of retired racing Greyhounds. J Vet Intern Med. 2007 Nov-Dec;21(6):1243-50.
13. Drögemüller C, Becker D, Kessler B, et. al.: A deletion in the N-myc downstream regulated gene 1 (NDRG1) gene in Greyhounds with polyneuropathy. PLoS One. 2010 Jun 22;5(6):e11258.
14. Dole RS, Spurgeon TL. Frequency of supernumerary teeth in a dolichocephalic canine breed, the greyhound. Am J Vet Res 1998 Jan;59(1):16-7
15. Dorn CR: Canine breed-specific risks of frequently diagnosed diseases at veterinary teaching hospitals. Monograph. AKC Canine Health Foundation. 2000.
16. *Ocular Disorders Presumed to be Inherited in Purebred Dogs.* American College of Veterinary Ophthalmologists. ACVO, 2007.
17. Lynch GL: Ophthalmic examination findings in a group of retired racing Greyhounds. Vet Ophthalmol. 2007 Nov-Dec;10(6):363-7.
18. Schoning P & Cowan LA: Gross and microscopic lesions of 230 Kansas greyhounds. J Vet Diagn Invest. 1993 Jul;5(3):392-7.
19. Schoning PR: Endocardiosis and other heart disease in greyhounds. Zentralbl Veterinarmed A. 1995 Apr;42(2):99-104.
20. Rosenberger JA, Pablo NV, Crawford PC, et. al.: Prevalence of and intrinsic risk factors for appendicular osteosarcoma in dogs: 179 cases (1996-2005). J Am Vet Med Assoc. 2007 Oct 1;231(7):1076-80.
21. Guilliard MJ, Segboer I & Shearer DH: Corns in dogs; signalment, possible aetiology and response to surgical treatment. J Small Anim Pract. 2010 Mar;51(3):162-8.
22. Balara JM, McCarthy RJ, Kiupel M, et. al.: Clinical, histologic, and immunohistochemical characterization of wart-like lesions on the paw pads of dogs: 24 cases (2000-2007). J Am Vet Med Assoc. 2009 Jun 15;234(12):1555-8.
23. Ponce Vazquez J, Pascual Gomez F, Alvarez Badillo A, Dolz Luna JF, Rodriguez Rodriguez LP. Cardiac arrhythmias induced by short-time maximal dynamic exercise (sprint): a study in greyhounds. Rev Esp Cardiol 1998 Jul;51(7):559-65
24. Slatter DH, Blogg JR, & Constable IJ: Retinal degeneration in Greyhounds. Aust Vet J. 1980 Mar;56(3):106-15.
25. Chavkin MJ, Roberts SM, Salman MD, et. al.: Risk factors for development of chronic superficial keratitis in dogs. J Am Vet Med Assoc. 1994 May 15;204(10):1630-4.
26. Daniel A, Read RA & Cake MA: Vascular foramina of the metacarpopha-langeal sesamoid bones of Greyhounds and their relationship to sesamoid disease. Am J Vet Res. 2008 Jun;69(6):716-21.
27. Tomlin JL, Lawes TJ, Blunn GW, et. al.: Fractographic examination of racing greyhound central (navicular) tarsal bone failure surfaces using scanning electron microscopy. Calcif Tissue Int. 2000 Sep;67(3):260-6.
28. Johnson KA, Muir P, Nicoll RG, et. al.: Asymmetric adaptive modeling of central tarsal bones in racing greyhounds. Bone. 2000 Aug;27(2):257-63.
29. Boudrieau RJ, Dee JF, & Dee LG: Central tarsal bone fractures in the racing Greyhound: a review of 114 cases. J Am Vet Med Assoc. 1984 Jun 15;184(12):1486-91.
30. Nachreiner RF, Refsal KR, Graham PA, et. al.: Prevalence of serum thyroid hormone autoantibodies in dogs with clinical signs of hypothyroidism. *J Am Vet Med Assoc* 2002 Feb 15;220(4):466-71.
31. Nachreiner R & Refsal K: Personal communication, Diagnostic Center for Population and Animal Health, Michigan State University. April, 2007.

32. Sist MD, Refsal KR & Nachreiner RF: A Laboratory Survey of Autoimmune Thyroiditis and Hypothyroidism in Selected Sight Hound Breeds. Proceedings of the 2009 Tufts' Canine and Feline Breeding and Genetics Conference. 2009.

33. Taboada J, Harvey JW, Levy MG, Breitschwerdt EB. Seroprevalence of babesiosis in Greyhounds in Florida. J Am Vet Med Assoc 1992 Jan 1;200(1):47-50

34. Birkenheuer AJ, Correa MT, Levy MG, et. al.: Geographic distribution of babesiosis among dogs in the United States and association with dog bites: 150 cases (2000-2003). J Am Vet Med Assoc. 2005 Sep 15;227(6):942-7.

35. Breitschwerdt EB, Malone JB, MacWilliams P, et. al.: Babesiosis in the Greyhound. J Am Vet Med Assoc. 1983 May 1;182(9):978-82.

36. Schultheiss PC: A retrospective study of visceral and nonvisceral hemangiosarcoma and hemangiomas in domestic animals. J Vet Diagn Invest. 2004 Nov;16(6):522-6.

37. Hertzke DM, Cowan LA, Schoning P, et. al.: Glomerular ultrastructural lesions of idiopathic cutaneous and renal glomerular vasculopathy of greyhounds. Vet Pathol. 1995 Sep;32(5):451-9.

38. Cowan LA, Hertzke DM, Fenwick BW, et. al.: Clinical and clinicopathologic abnormalities in greyhounds with cutaneous and renal glomerular vasculopathy: 18 cases (1992-1994). J Am Vet Med Assoc. 1997 Mar 15;210(6):789-93.

39. Carpenter JL, Andelman NC, Moore FM, et. al.: Idiopathic cutaneous and renal glomerular vasculopathy of greyhounds. Vet Pathol. 1988 Nov;25(6):401-7.

40. Brenner K, Harkin KR, Andrews GA, et. al.: Juvenile pancreatic atrophy in Greyhounds: 12 cases (1995-2000). J Vet Intern Med. 2009 Jan-Feb;23(1):67-71.

41. Daly P, Drudy D, Chalmers WS, et. al.: Greyhound meningoencephalitis: PCR-based detection methods highlight an absence of the most likely primary inducing agents. Vet Microbiol. 2006 Dec 20;118(3-4):189-200.

42. Callanan JJ, Mooney CT, Mulcahy G, et. al.: A novel nonsuppurative meningoencephalitis in young greyhounds in Ireland. Vet Pathol. 2002 Jan;39(1):56-65.

43. Greer KA, Daly P, Murphy KE, et. al.: Analysis of gene expression in brain tissue from Greyhounds with meningoencephalitis. Am J Vet Res. 2010 May;71(5):547-54.

44. Kirmayer AH, Klide AM, & Purvance JE: Malignant hyperthermia in a dog: case report and review of the syndrome. J Am Vet Med Assoc. 1984 Nov 1;185(9):978-82.

45. Dickinson PJ & Sullivan M: Exercise induced hyperthermia in a racing greyhound. Vet Rec. 1994 Nov 19;135(21):508.

46. Leary SL, Anderson LC, Manning PJ, et. al.: Recurrent malignant hyperthermia in a Greyhound. J Am Vet Med Assoc. 1983 Mar 1;182(5):521-2.

47. Bagshaw RJ, Cox RH & Knight DH: Malignant hyperthermia in a Greyhound. J Am Vet Med Assoc. 1978 Jan 1;172(1):61-2.

48. Bjotvedt G, Hendricks GM, & Brandon TA: Hemodynamic basis of renal arteriosclerosis in young greyhounds. Lab Anim Sci. 1988 Feb;38(1):62-7.

49. *The Genetic Connection: A Guide to Health Problems in Purebred Dogs*. L Ackerman. p. 222, AAHA Press, 1999.

50. Adams J, Mellanby RJ, Villiers E, et. al.: Acute B cell lymphoblastic leukaemia in a 12-week-old greyhound. J Small Anim Pract. 2004 Nov;45(11):553-7.

51. Gunby JM, Hardie RJ, & Bjorling DE: Investigation of the potential heritability of persistent right aortic arch in Greyhounds. J Am Vet Med Assoc. 2004 Apr 1;224(7):1120-2, 1111.

52. Skelly CM, McAllister H, & Donnelly WJ: Avulsion of the tibial tuberosity in a litter of greyhound puppies. J Small Anim Pract. 1997 Oct;38(10):445-9.

53. Power JW: Avulsion of the tibial tuberosity in the greyhound. Aust Vet J. 1976 Nov;52(11):491-5.

54. *The Complete Dog Book, 20th Ed*. The American Kennel Club. Howell Book House, NY 2006. pp 177-179.

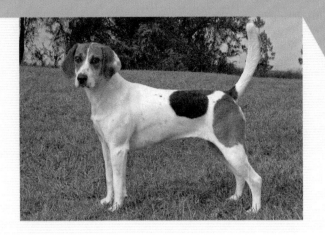

The Breed History

Records going back to the 1260s in England show them to have been hunting dogs, and over time, the primary records tracing their development rested with the registered packs of the AMHB. Their development is not well documented prior to that time, but their progenitors are thought to have arisen in ancient times (BC). Foundation dogs were derived from the smaller stature Foxhounds in part. Early on, Harriers were more popular than Beagles. The last pack in the US was lost in 1970.

Breeding for Function

Scent hounds bred for versatility, pack compatibility, and working ability both with an on-foot or mounted hunter. Used to be a pack hunter, accompanying the mounted hunt. Hare was the primary target, though fox, rabbits and other quarry were often included in their hunt. The HCA continues to offer a Hunting Certificate in order to maintain the competence of the working ability of this ancient breed. They must seek the quarry, mark their find with voice, and pursue the quarry as needed.

Physical Characteristics

Height at Withers: 19-21" (48-53 cm)

Weight: 35-45 lb (16-20 kg)

Coat: A dense short glossy, hard coat and color is not considered a limiting feature, though many are tricolor. Low grooming needs are a feature of this breed. Ears need to be checked regularly.

Longevity: 12-15 years

Points of Conformation: Sturdy conformation, with good bone and muscling—they appear similar to a smaller Foxhound. Almost as tall as they are long, they are quiet while resting, but really intense while working. Eyes are pigmented brown through hazel, depending on the coat color, are wide set and medium sized. Ears are rounded, low set and hang close to the head. Skull shows a prominent forehead, with moderate stop and a squarish muzzle. Lips clean and tight, nose is large and teeth may be scissors or level bite. The neck is long and not throaty, topline level and thorax is deep and the ribs are well sprung. Loin is short and strong, tail is high set, and carried gaily with a taper to a brushed point. Carriage over the back is not accepted. Limbs are straight and well boned without being coarse

or heavy, feet are round, well knuckled up and pads are tough and thick. Gait is low, forward and looks effortless.

Recognized Behavior Issues and Traits

Breed attributes ascribed include: Strong willed, intelligent, affectionate, independent, tend to wander off following a scent, needs to be kept in a fenced enclosure. One may need to bury wire underground so they do not dig out! Early obedience training is a must. They need contact with people and do well with other dogs. Need stimulation to prevent boredom vices; are active, tireless dogs. Vocal dogs, playful, adaptable, and good alert barkers.

Normal Physiologic Variations

Tend to gain weight easily.

Drug Sensitivities

None reported

Inherited Diseases

Hip Dysplasia: Polygenically inherited trait causing degenerative joint disease and hip arthritis. OFA reports 14.5% affected.[1]

Patella Luxation: Polygenically inherited laxity of patellar ligaments, causing luxation, lameness, and later degenerative joint disease. Treat surgically if causing clinical signs. Too few Harriers have been screened to determine an accurate frequency.[1]

Elbow Dysplasia: Polygenically inherited trait causing elbow arthritis. Too few Harriers have been screened to determine an accurate frequency.[1]

Disease Predispositions

Persistent Pupillary Membranes: Strands of fetal remnant connecting; iris to iris, cornea, lens, or involving sheets of tissue. The later three forms can impair vision, and dogs affected with these forms should not be bred. Identified in 2.7% of Harriers CERF examined by veterinary ophthalmologists between 2000-2005.[2]

Cataracts: Anterior and posterior intermediate cataracts predominate in the breed. Identified in 2.03% of Harriers CERF examined by veterinary ophthalmologists between 2000-2005.[2]

Progressive Retinal Atrophy (PRA): Degenerative disorder of the retina causing blindness. Harriers suspicious for PRA have been identified in CERF examinations by veterinary ophthalmologists between 2000-2005.[2]

Cerebellar Abiotrophy (Cerebellar Ataxia): Progressive neurological disorder causing cerebellar hypermetria, a high stepping gait, and incoordination. Age of onset 2-7 years. Diagnosis by clinical signs, MRI/CT, or post-mortem.[3]

Epilepsy and **Inguinal Hernia** are reported.[4]

Isolated Case Studies

Juvenile Renal Dysplasia: Puppies from one litter of Harriers showed polyuria and polydipsia that progressed to kidney failure. Pathologically diagnosed, with renal dysplasia.[5]

Genetic Tests

Tests of Genotype: none

Tests of Phenotype: Recommend hip and elbow radiographs, CERF eye examination, patella evaluation, thyroid profile including autoantibodies, and cardiac evaluation.

Miscellaneous

- **Breed name synonyms:** none
- **Registries:** AKC, FCI, CKC, UKC, ARHA, SKC, AMHB (Association of Masters of Harriers and Beagles)
- **AKC rank (year 2008):** 155 (35 dogs registered)
- **Breed resources: Harrier Club of America:** www.harrierclubofamerica.com

References

1. OFA Website breed statistics: www.offa.org Last accessed July 1, 2010.
2. *Ocular Disorders Presumed to be Inherited in Purebred Dogs.* American College of Veterinary Ophthalmologists. ACVO, 2007.
3. Bagley RS: Differential Diagnosis of Animals with Intracranial Disease, Part 2: Diseases of the Brain Stem, Cranial Nerves, and Cerebellum. Proceedings, Atlantic Coast Veterinary Conference 2002.
4. *The Genetic Connection: A Guide to Health Problems in Purebred Dogs.* L Ackerman. p. 203. AAHA Press, 1999.
5. Hoppe A, Karlstam E: Renal dysplasia in boxers and Finnish harriers. J Small Anim Pract. 2000 Sep;41(9):422-6.
6. *The Complete Dog Book, 20th Ed.* The American Kennel Club. Howell Book House, NY 2006. p. 180-183.

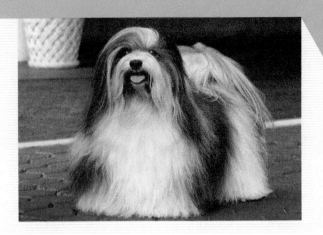

The Breed History

The Havanese dog is thought to have originated on the Isle of Malta two thousand years ago. Tenerife dogs were the ancestors of the Bichon family of dogs. Those dogs that were later exported to Cuba were the seed stock for the modern Havanese breed. These dogs are designated "National Dog of Cuba". Queen Victoria and Charles Dickens owned Havanese dogs. The modern breed that is distributed outside of Cuba derives from just eleven dogs that served as foundation stock. The Havanese is considered a rare breed.

Breeding for Function

Companionship has been their primary purpose, though because of their willingness to please and their intelligence, these dogs have been applied to obedience work.

Physical Characteristics

Height at Withers: 9-10.5" (23-26.5 cm).

Weight: 8-11 lb (3.5-5 kg).

Coat: The silky double coat consists of soft short undercoat hairs covered by a profusion of long (6-8" or 15-20 cm) soft hairs. The outer coat hairs may be straight, curly or wavy. The waviest coats cord naturally. Only foot hair trimming is allowed for showing. Many colors are acceptable including black, blue, silver, gold, cream, white, champagne and chocolate or these in bi- or tri-color combinations. The hair over the eyes is very long, covering them fully if not combed back.

Longevity: 12-15 years

Points of Conformation: The Havanese dog is similar to the Bichon in build with long back, short legs and a profuse soft haircoat. Their gait is characteristically springy and the plumed tail is curled over the back. Eyes are almond shaped, dark brown, large and have darkly pigmented palpebral rims. Ears have long feathers and are medium in size and folded, with moderately pointed tips. The skull is broad, slightly rounded, the stop is moderate, and the muzzle tapers. The button nose is very large and black, though in chocolates, the nose is self. The neck is moderate in length and muscling, and the topline is level, though over the croup it rises slightly to the high set tail. The tail may drop off the back when resting. The thorax is of moderate depth, with well-sprung ribs.

Front and rear dewclaws may be removed, limbs are straight boned, and the feet have well developed pads; toes are well arched up.

Recognized Behavior Issues and Traits

Reported breed characteristics include: Outgoing, active, friendly, high trainability, and good with children. Heat tolerant, high grooming needs, good alarm barker, needs close human companionship, possesses high activity levels.

Normal Physiologic Variations

None Reported

Drug Sensitivities

None reported

Inherited Diseases

Hip Dysplasia: Polygenically inherited trait causing degenerative hip joint disease and arthritis. OFA reports 9.9% affected.[1]

Elbow Dysplasia: Polygenically inherited trait causing elbow arthritis. OFA reports 6.4% affected.[1]

Patella Luxation: Polygenically inherited laxity of patellar ligaments, causing luxation, lameness, and later degenerative joint disease. Treat surgically if causing clinical signs. OFA reports 2.8% affected.[1]

Disease Predispositions

Hypothyroidism: Inherited autoimmune thyroiditis. 22.6% positive for thyroid autoantibodies based on testing at Michigan State University. (Ave. for all breeds is 7.5%).[2,3]

Osteochondrodysplasia (OCD): Developmental anomaly causing premature growth plate closure and crooked or bowed front legs. Segregation analysis suggests that this may be a syndrome that could also include cataracts, hepatic abnormalities, and cardiac abnormalities. Unknown mode of inheritance with a heritability of 0.36. Reported at a frequency of 20% in the 2004 Havanese Health Survey.[4,5]

Portosystemic Shunt (PSS, Liver Shunt): Abnormal blood vessels connecting the systemic and portal blood flow. Can be intrahepatic or extrahepatic. Hepatic microvascular dysplasia may also be genetically related to this condition. Causes stunting, abnormal behavior, possible seizures, and can cause ammonium urate urinary calculi. Diagnose with paired fasted and feeding serum bile acid and/or ammonium levels, and abdominal ultrasound. Treatment of PSS includes partial ligation and/or medical and dietary control of symptoms. Molecular genetic studies show a complex inheritance with a single gene of major effect. Reported in 3.2% of Havanese presented to veterinary teaching hospitals. Reported at a frequency of 4% in the 2004 Havanese Health Survey.[4,6,7]

Cataracts: Posterior suture and punctate cataracts predominate in the breed. Unknown mode of inheritance. 11.57% of Havanese presented to veterinary teaching hospitals had cataracts. Identified in 2.61% of Havanese CERF examined by veterinary ophthalmologists between 2000-2005. Reported at a frequency of 5% in the 2004 Havanese Health Survey. CERF does not recommend breeding any Havanese with a cataract.[4,8,9]

Persistent Pupillary Membranes: Strands of fetal remnant connecting; iris to iris, cornea, lens, or involving sheets of tissue. The later three forms can impair vision, and dogs affected with these forms should not be bred. Identified in 7.34% of Havanese CERF examined by veterinary ophthalmologists between 2000-2005.[9]

Distichiasis: Abnormally placed eyelashes that irritate the cornea and conjunctiva. Can cause secondary corneal ulceration. Identified in 4.56% of Havanese CERF examined by veterinary ophthalmologists between 2000-2005.[9]

Vitreous Degeneration: A liquefaction of the vitreous gel which may predispose to retinal detachment and/or glaucoma. Identified in 1.69% of Havanese CERF examined by veterinary ophthalmologists between 2000-2005.[9]

Deafness: Congenital deafness can be unilateral of bilateral. Diagnosed by BAER testing. Unknown mode of inheritance. Reported at a frequency of 2% in the 2004 Havanese Health Survey.[1,4,10]

Oligodontia, progressive Retinal Atrophy, and **Retinal Dysplasia** are reported.[11]

Isolated Case Studies
None Reported

Genetic Tests
Tests of Genotype: Direct test for black/chocolate is available from VetGen.

Tests of Phenotype: CHIC Certification: Required testing includes hip radiographs, CERF eye examination, patella examination, and BAER test for deafness. (See CHIC website; www.caninehealthinfo.org).

Recommended tests include blood ammonia and bile acids test for PSS, elbow radiographs, thyroid profile including autoantibodies, and cardiac evaluation.

Miscellaneous
- **Breed name synonyms:** Havana Silk Dog (historical), Spanish Silk Dog (historical), Bichon Havanais.
- **Registries:** AKC, UKC, ANKC (Australian National Kennel Club), NKC (National Kennel Club)
- **AKC rank (year 2008):** 36 (4,435 dogs registered)
- **Internet resources: Havanese Club of America:** www.havanese.org
  Havanese Fanciers of Canada: www.havanesefanciers.com
  Havanese Club of Great Britain: www.havaneseclub.co.uk

References
1. OFA Website breed statistics: www.offa.org Last accessed July 1, 2010.
2. Nachreiner RF, Refsal KR, Graham PA, et. al.: Prevalence of serum thyroid hormone autoantibodies in dogs with clinical signs of hypothyroidism. *J Am Vet Med Assoc* 2002 Feb 15;220(4):466-71.
3. Nachreiner R & Refsal K: Personal communication, Diagnostic Center for Population and Animal Health, Michigan State University. April, 2007.
4. Havanese Club of America: 2004 Havanese Health Survey. 2004.
5. Starr AN, Famula TR, Markward NJ, et. al.: Hereditary evaluation of multiple developmental abnormalities in the Havanese dog breed. J Hered. 2007;98(5):510-7.
6. Tobias KM, Rohrbach BW: Association of breed with the diagnosis of congenital portosystemic shunts in dogs: 2,400 cases (1980-2002). *J Am Vet Med Assoc.* 2003 Dec 1;223(11):1636-9.
7. Center SA: Portosystemic Vascular Anomalies & Hepatic MVD: Evidence of Common Genetics in Small Dogs. Proceedings, 2008 ACVIM Forum. 2008.
8. Gelatt KN, Mackay EO: Prevalence of primary breed-related cataracts in the dog in North America. *Vet Ophthalmol.* 2005 Mar-Apr;8(2):101-11.
9. *Ocular Disorders Presumed to be Inherited in Purebred Dogs.* American College of Veterinary Ophthalmologists. ACVO, 2007.
10. Strain GM: Deafness prevalence and pigmentation and gender associations in dog breeds at risk. *Vet J.* 2004 Jan;167(1):23-32.
11. *The Genetic Connection: A Guide to Health Problems in Purebred Dogs.* L Ackerman. p. 222. AAHA Press, 1999.
12. *The Complete Dog Book, 20th Ed.* The American Kennel Club. Howell Book House, NY 2006. p. 470-473.

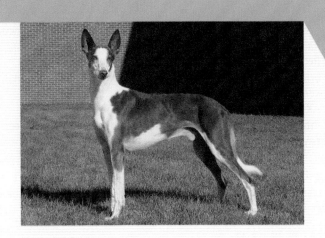

is well tucked up, and the thin, low-set tail reaches to the tarsus and may be curved, ring or saber shaped. The tail is carried high while in action. Limbs are straight and long, fine-boned, and the hare-type feet have thick pads and white nails. Characteristically, there is lots of interdigital hair. The gait is springy, fairly high, and appears effortless. This breed has the ability to jump high and wide, and is as fast as any sight hounds. The eyes are small, oblique and amber to caramel in color. The ears may rest folded when the dog is relaxed. Front dewclaws may be removed.

The Breed History

Like the Pharaoh hound, these dogs are ancient and originate in Egypt. First records date to about 3100 BC. Like the Pharaoh hound, the claim is that this dog is the source for the image of *Anubis*, the canine deity that watches over the souls of the departed. From Egypt, the Phoenicians took these dogs to the Mediterranean Isle of Ibiza, one of the Balearic Islands off of Spain by about 800 BC. The breed became extinct in Egypt. They were common also in mainland Spain. First American imports date to the year 1956. AKC registry first accepted this breed in 1979.

Breeding for Function

As Pharaoh's dogs, they were keen hunting partners and companions. They hunted by both sight and sound. Later, in the Isle of Ibiza, they were selected based on their rabbit hunting ability, and also for their ability to be sustained on a small amount of food. They were valued as watchdogs. Good sturdy constitution and physical health is highly valued, so breeding programs selected only the most vigorous specimens. Today, they are often shown in tracking, obedience and lure coursing and are valued as companion dogs.

Physical Characteristics

Height at Withers: female 22.5-26" (57-66 cm), male 23.5-27.5" (60-70 cm).

Weight: females 45 lb (20.5 kg), males 50 lb (22.5 kg).

Coat: Two types of coat exist—short and wirehaired. The latter may carry a prominent moustache, though the coat is still only 1.5-3" (3.5-7.5 cm) in length. White, red, or a mixture of the two is accepted. A red color varies from deep rich red to light yellow-red.

Longevity: 11-14 years

Points of Conformation: Very chiseled and lithe, these strong athletic dogs are noted for their large pricked up pointed ears and greyhound-type stature. Muscle mass is lean. The head is shaped like a long cone with a minimal stop, they possess a prominent occipital protuberance, and no facial wrinkles are present. Nose and lip margins are flesh colored and the nose is prominent. The long, slender neck is slightly arched, the topline is level with a gradual drop off to the tail at the croup. The thorax is moderately deep, breastbone prominent, and ribs only slightly sprung. The abdomen

Recognized Behavior Issues and Traits

Reported breed characteristics include: Active, enjoy human companionship, good with children and other dogs, stable temperament, loyal, high trainability, aloof with strangers, alarm barker, groom themselves like a cat, off leash in a fenced enclosure only; can jump up to 6' so fence should be sturdy and high. Good trainability, adaptable, high exercise needs, but low activity around the house. Low grooming needs, good in country or city settings.

Normal Physiologic Variations

Sight hounds have lower normal ranges for T4 and T3 concentrations compared to other breeds.[1]

Drug Sensitivities

Anesthesia: Sight hounds require particular attention during anesthesia. Their lean body conformation with high surface-area-to-volume ratio predisposes them to hypothermia during anesthesia. Impaired biotransformation of drugs by the liver results in prolonged recovery from barbiturate and thiobarbiturate intravenous anesthetics. Propofol, and ketamine/diazepam combination are recommended induction agents.[2]

Inherited Diseases

Hip Dysplasia: Polygenically inherited trait causing degenerative joint disease and hip arthritis. OFA reports 2.8% affected.[3]

Elbow Dysplasia: Polygenically inherited trait causing elbow arthritis. Too few Ibizan Hounds have been screened by OFA to determine an accurate frequency.[3]

Patella Luxation: Polygenically inherited laxity of patellar ligaments, causing luxation, lameness, and later degenerative joint disease. Treat surgically if causing clinical signs. Too few Ibizan Hounds have been screened by OFA to determine an accurate frequency.[3]

Axonal Dystrophy: A rare, fatal, autosomal recessive disorder, causing an uncoordinated, spastic gait. Affected dogs initially present between five and sixteen weeks of age with a lack of balance, spasticity, and weaving, often worse in the hind limbs. Some dogs have stressful episodes manifested by high fever, recumbency, stiffening of the limbs, and seizures. Variable progression of clinical signs necessitates euthanasia by 5 to 24 months of age. The disorder is caused by a dying off of neurons in the spinal cord and brain. No genetic test is available.

Disease Predispositions

Hypothyroidism: Inherited autoimmune thyroiditis. 6.3% positive for thyroid autoantibodies based on testing at Michigan State University. (Ave. for all breeds is 7.5%).[4,5]

Persistent Pupillary Membranes: Strands of fetal remnant connecting; iris to iris, cornea, lens, or involving sheets of tissue. The later three forms can impair vision, and dogs affected with these forms should not be bred. Identified in 6.09% of Ibizan Hounds CERF examined by veterinary ophthalmologists between 2000-2005.[6]

Cataracts: Nuclear intermediate and punctate cataracts predominate in the breed. Identified in 3.91% of Ibizan Hounds CERF examined by veterinary ophthalmologists between 2000-2005. CERF does not recommend breeding any Ibizan Hound with a cataract.[6]

Allergies: Inhalant or food allergy. Presents with pruritis (itching) and pyotraumatic dermatitis (hot spots). Reported as a problem in the breed on the IHCUS website.

Idiopathic Epilepsy (Inherited Seizures): Generalized or partial seizures. Control with anti-seizure medication. Reported as a problem in the breed on the IHCUS website. Unknown mode of inheritance.

Retinal Dysplasia: Focal retinal dysplasia/folds are recognized in the breed. Can casue retinal detachment and blindness. Reported in 1.30% of Ibizan Hounds CERF-examined by veterinary ophthalmologists between 2000-2005.[6]

Deafness: Congenital deafness can be unilateral of bilateral. Diagnosed by BAER testing. Reported to occur in the breed by Strain, and the IHCUS.[7]

Brachygnathism, Cardiomyopathy, Elongated Soft Palate, Oligodontia, Polydontia, and **Prognathism** are reported.[8]

Isolated Case Studies

Arteriovenous Fistula: A nine-year-old male Ibizan hound had a network of large tortuous pulsating blood vessels on the prepuce that enlarged gradually over a five month period.[9]

Genetic Tests

Tests of Genotype: none

Tests of Phenotype: CHIC Certification: Required testing includes hip radiographs, CERF eye examination, brainstem audio-evoked response (BAER) test for deafness, and thyroid profile including autoantibodies. (See CHIC website; www.caninehealthinfo.org).

Recommend elbow radiographs, patella evaluation, and cardiac evaluation.

Miscellaneous

- **Breed name synonyms:** Galgo Hound, Ibizan, Podenco Ibicenco, Ca Ebisenc, Balaeric Dog, Charnique (Fr.).
- **Registries:** AKC-P, UKC-P, CKC, KCGB (Kennel Club of Great Britain), ANKC (Australian National Kennel Club), NKC (National Kennel Club).
- **AKC rank (year 2008):** 134 (146 dogs registered)
- **Internet resources:** Ibizan Hound Club of the United States: www.ihcus.org

References

1. Kintzer PP & Peterson ME: Progress in the Diagnosis and Treatment of Canine Hypothyroidism. 2007. Proceedings, ACVIM 2007.
2. Court MH: Anesthesia of the sighthound. Clin Tech Small Anim Pract 1999 Feb;14(1):38-43.
3. OFA Website breed statistics: www.offa.org Last accessed July 1, 2010.
4. Nachreiner RF, Refsal KR, Graham PA, et. al.: Prevalence of serum thyroid hormone autoantibodies in dogs with clinical signs of hypothyroidism. *J Am Vet Med Assoc* 2002 Feb 15;220(4):466-71.
5 Nachreiner R & Refsal K: Personal communication, Diagnostic Center for Population and Animal Health, Michigan State University. April, 2007.
6. *Ocular Disorders Presumed to be Inherited in Purebred Dogs.* American College of Veterinary Ophthalmologists. ACVO, 2007.
7. Strain GM: Deafness prevalence and pigmentation and gender associations in dog breeds at risk. *The Veterinary Journal* 2004; 167(1):23-32.
8. *The Genetic Connection: A Guide to Health Problems in Purebred Dogs.* L Ackerman. p. 223. AAHA Press, 1999.
9. Trower ND, White RN, Lamb CR: Arteriovenous fistula involving the prepuce of a dog. *J Small Anim Pract.* 1997 Oct;38(10):455-8.
10. *The Complete Dog Book, 20th Ed.* The American Kennel Club. Howell Book House, NY 2006. p. 184-187.

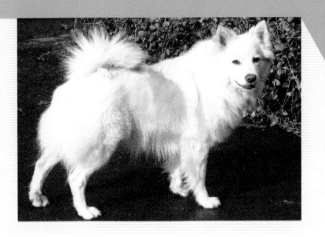

Icelandic Sheepdog

The Breed History
The Icelandic Sheepdog came to Iceland with the Vikings in AD 874-930 and was used to work sheep, cattle, and horses. The breed adapted its working style to Iceland's local terrain and farming techniques so well that it became indispensable to the Icelandic people. It is thought to be one of the oldest breeds of dogs in the world and happens to be Iceland's only native dog. A population genetic study of European Icelandic Sheepdogs shows low genetic diversity.[1] AKC recognition occurred in 2010.

Breeding for Function
The Icelandic Sheepdog was used to work sheep, cattle and horses.

Physical Characteristics
Height at withers: Dogs 18 inches (46 cm); Bitches 16.5 inches (42 cm).

Weight: 20-30 pounds (9-14 kg).

Coat: Double coat, thick and weatherproof. There are two types: short-haired and long-haired. Short-haired: The outer coat of medium length, fairly coarse, with a thick, soft undercoat. Long-haired: The outer coat is longer than the above, fairly coarse, with a thick, soft undercoat. In both lengths, the hair is shorter on the face, top of the head, ears and front of the legs; and longer on the neck, chest and back of the thighs. Several colors are permitted but a single color should always be predominant. The predominant colors are: various shades of tan, ranging from cream to reddish brown; chocolate brown, grey, and black. White always accompanies the predominant color. The most common white markings, which are often irregular, are a blaze or a part of the face, collar, chest, socks of varying lengths and tip of tail. On tan and grey dogs, a black mask, black tips to the outer hairs and even occasional black hairs often occur. Black (tri-color) dogs have a black coat, white markings as mentioned above and traditional markings in any of the various tan colors on the cheeks, over the eyes (eyebrows) and on the legs.

Longevity: Around 12 years.

Points of Conformation: The Icelandic Sheepdog is a Nordic herding Spitz, slightly under medium sized with prick ears and a curled tail. Seen from the side the dog is rectangular. The head is triangular when seen from above or the side, with a defined stop. Scissors bite. Eyes are medium size and almond shaped. Level back, muscular and strong. Forelegs are straight, parallel and strong, with single or double dewclaws. Hindlegs are also straight, with double dewclaws being more desirable. The gait displays agility and endurance with good driving action covering the ground effortlessly.

Recognized Behavior Issues and Traits
Playful, friendly and inquisitive, the Icelandic Sheepdog is a hardy and agile dog. The breed is extremely social, loving, and patient with children, making them an ideal family dog. Intelligent and eager to please, Icelandic Sheepdogs are easily trained. The breed sheds its undercoat twice a year and needs to be brushed when it does.

Normal Physiologic Variations
None reported

Drug Sensitivities
None reported

Inherited Diseases
Hip Dysplasia: Polygenically inherited trait causing degenerative joint disease and hip arthritis. OFA reports 13.3% affected, but too few Icelandic Sheepdogs have been evaluated for statistical confidence.[2]

Elbow Dysplasia: Polygenically inherited trait causing elbow arthritis. Too few Icelandic Sheepdogs have been screened by OFA to determine an accurate frequency.[2]

Patella Luxation: Polygenically inherited laxity of patellar ligaments, causing luxation, lameness, and later degenerative joint disease. Treat surgically if causing clinical signs. Too few Icelandic Sheepdogs have been screened by OFA to determine an accurate frequency.[2]

Disease Predispositions
Persistent Pupillary Membranes: Strands of fetal remnant connecting; iris to iris, cornea, lens, or involving sheets of tissue. The later three forms can impair vision, and dogs affected with these forms should not be bred. Identified in 5.02% of Icelandic Sheepdogs CERF examined by veterinary ophthalmologists between 2000-2005.[3]

Entropion: A rolling in of the eyelids that can cause corneal irritation and ulceration. Entropion is reported in 1.83% of Icelandic Sheepdogs CERF examined by veterinary ophthalmologists between 2000-2005.[3]

Cataracts: Cortical and capsular cataracts predominate in the breed. Reported in 1.37% of Icelandic Sheepdogs CERF examined by veterinary ophthalmologists between 2000-2005. Reported as a breed health issue on the ISAA website.[3]

Retinal Dysplasia: Retinal folds, geographic, and generalized retinal dysplasia with detachment are recognized in the breed. Can lead to blindness. Reported in 1.37% of Icelandic Sheepdogs CERF examined by veterinary ophthalmologists between 2000-2005.[3]

Hypothyroidism: Inherited autoimmune thyroiditis. Not enough samples have been submitted for thyroid auto-antibodies to Michigan State University to determine an accurate frequency. (Ave. for all breeds is 7.5%).[4,5]

Cryptorchidism: Unilateral or bilateral undescended testicles. This is a sex-limited disorder with an unknown mode of inheritance. Reported as a breed health issue on the ISAA website.

Distichiasis: Abnormally placed eyelashes that irritate the cornea and conjunctiva. Can cause secondary corneal ulceration. Reported as a breed health issue on the ISAA website.

Deafness: Congenital deafness can be unilateral or bilateral. Diagnosed by BAER testing. Reported as a breed health issue on the Canadian Icelandic Sheepdog Club website.

Isolated Case Studies
None Reported

Genetic Tests
Tests of Genotype: Direct tests for coat color are available from VetGen.

Tests of Phenotype: CHIC Certification: Required testing includes hip radiograph, CERF eye examination and a blood donation to the CHIC DNA repository. Optional testing includes elbow radiographs, patella evaluation, cardiac evaluation (ECHO by a cardiologist preferred), thyroid profile including autoantibodies, and MDR1 genetic test for multidrug sensitivity (See CHIC website; www.caninehealthinfo.org).

Miscellaneous
- **Breed name synonyms:** Iceland Sheepdog, Islandsk Farehond, Friaar Dog, Islenkur Fjárhundur, Icelandic Dog.
- **Registries:** AKC, CKC, FCI
- **AKC rank (none):** Recognized June, 2010. Entire stud book entered.
- **Internet resources: Icelandic Sheepdog Association of America:** www.icelanddogs.com
  Canadian Icelandic Sheepdog Club: http://canadianicelandicsheepdogclub.blogspot.com

References
1. Oliehoek PA, Bijma P & van der Meijden A: History and structure of the closed pedigreed population of Icelandic Sheepdogs. Genet Sel Evol. 2009 Aug 6;41:39.
2. OFA Website breed statistics: www.offa.org Last accessed July 1, 2010.
3. *Ocular Disorders Presumed to be Inherited in Purebred Dogs.* American College of Veterinary Ophthalmologists. ACVO, 2007.
4. Nachreiner R & Refsal K: Personal communication, Diagnostic Center for Population and Animal Health, Michigan State University. April, 2007.
5. Nachreiner RF, Refsal KR, Graham PA, et. al.: Prevalence of serum thyroid hormone autoantibodies in dogs with clinical signs of hypothyroidism. *J Am Vet Med Assoc* 2002 Feb 15;220(4):466-71.
6. AKC Breed Website: www.akc.org/breeds/icelandic_sheepdog Last accessed July 1, 2010.

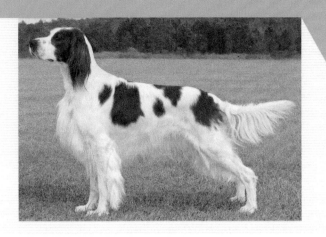

The Breed History

The Irish Red and White Setter was the predecessor of the solid red Irish Setter, and was established in the 17th century from other Setter, Pointer, and Spaniel breeds. By the end of the 19th century, the popularity of the solid red Irish Setter eclipsed the Irish Red and White, and they fell to near extinction. In 1920, Rev. Noble Huston collected breed members, and a breed association was formed in 1944. Mrs. Maureen Cuddy's efforts at establishing pedigrees allowed the breed to be admitted to the Irish Kennel Club in 1978. The breed is active in Field Trials and Shows. It attained full AKC recognition in 2009.

Breeding for Function

The Irish Red and White Setter is bred primarily for the field. The standard as set out hereunder must be interpreted chiefly from this point of view and all Judges at Bench Shows must be encouraged to judge the exhibits chiefly from the working standpoint. The appearance is strong and powerful, well balanced and proportioned without lumber; athletic rather than racy with an aristocratic, keen and intelligent attitude.

Physical Characteristics

Height at Withers: Dogs 24.5-26 inches (62-66 cm). Bitches 22.5-24 inches (57-61 cm). Field dogs tend to be smaller than show dogs.

Weight: 50-75 pounds (22.5 kg-34 kg).

Coat: The base color is white with solid red patches (clear islands of red color). Flecking but not roaning is permitted around the face and feet and up the foreleg as far as the elbow and up the hind leg as far as the hock. Feathering is present on the back of the fore and hind legs, on the outer ear flap, on the flank extending onto the chest and throat forming a fringe, and on the tail.

Longevity: 11-15 years.

Points of Conformation: The length of the body from point of shoulders to base of tail is not shorter than the height at the top of the withers. Bone is moderate in proportion to size. The eyes are round, and dark hazel or dark brown. The skull is broad in proportion to the body and domed without showing an occipital protuberance. The stop is distinct, but not exaggerated. The neck is

moderately long, very muscular, but not too thick. There is a level topline. The body is strong and muscular with a deep chest and well sprung ribs. The feet are close-knit with plenty of feathering between toes. The gait is long striding, very lively, graceful and efficient. The forelegs and hind legs move perpendicularly to the ground with no crossing or weaving.

Recognized Behavior Issues and Traits

The Irish Red and White Setter is a very friendly, dependable and easily trained gundog. The breed displays a kindly, friendly attitude, behind which should be discernible determination, courage and high spirit. His good and kind nature makes him a most acceptable companion and friend in the home and the field. The Irish Red and White Setter has a high activity requirement and needs a lot of exercise.

Normal Physiologic Variations
None Reported

Drug Sensitivities
None Reported

Inherited Diseases

Canine Leukocyte Adhesion Deficiency (CLAD): An autosomal recessive, fatal immunodeficiency disease found in Irish Red and White setters. Affected dogs present with severe recurrent infections, neutrophilia and low body weight. The mutation is the same as in Irish Setters, showing a common ancestral origin. One study in the US showed a 13% carrier frequency in the breed, and a study in the UK showed a 7.9% carrier frequency.[1,2,3]

Hip Dysplasia: Polygenically inherited trait causing degenerative joint disease and hip arthritis. OFA reports 4.5% affected.[4]

Elbow Dysplasia: Polygenically inherited trait causing elbow arthritis. Too few Irish Red and White Setters have been screened by OFA to determine an accurate frequency.[4]

Progressive Retinal Atrophy (PRA, RCD-1): Autosomal recessive, early onset rod, cone dysplasia form of PRA with an onset of 25 days of age, and progressing to blindness by one year old. The mutation is the same as in Irish Setters, showing a common ancestral origin. A genetic test is available. The frequency of carriers in the breed has not been established.[5,6,7]

von Willebrand's Disease Type 1 (vWD): Autosomal recessive genetic disorder causing a mild bleeding syndrome. A direct genetic test is available from the Animal Health Trust. Reported at a low frequency in the breed.

Patella Luxation: Polygenically inherited laxity of patellar ligaments, causing luxation, lameness, and later degenerative joint disease. Treat surgically if causing clinical signs. Too few Irish Red and White Setters have been screened by OFA to determine an accurate frequency.[4]

Disease Predispositions

Hypothyroidism: Inherited autoimmune thyroiditis. 12.5% positive for thyroid autoantibodies based on testing at Michigan State University. (Ave. for all breeds is 7.5%).[8,9]

Distichiasis: Abnormally placed eyelashes that irritate the cornea and conjunctiva. Can cause secondary corneal ulceration. Identified in 7.79% of Irish Red and White Setters CERF examined by veterinary ophthalmologists between 2000-2005.[10]

Persistent Pupillary Membranes: Strands of fetal remnant connecting; iris to iris, cornea, lens, or involving sheets of tissue. The later three forms can impair vision, and dogs affected with these forms should not be bred. Identified in 3.90% of Irish Red and White Setters CERF examined by veterinary ophthalmologists between 2000-2005.[10]

Gastric Dilatation-Volvulus (Bloat, GDV): Life-threatening twisting of the stomach within the abdomen. Requires immediate veterinary attention. Irish Red and White Setters are at increased risk versus other breeds. Dogs with the deepest thorax relative to width have the greatest risk for GDV.[11]

Cataracts: Anterior and posterior cortical cataracts predominate in the breed. Identified in 2.60% of Irish Red and White Setters CERF examined by veterinary ophthalmologists between 2000-2005.[10]

Chronic Superficial Keratitis (CSK)/Pannus: Corneal disease that can cause vision problems due to pigmentation. Treatment with topical ocular lubricants and anti-inflammatory medication. Identified in 2.60% of Irish Red and White Setters CERF examined by veterinary ophthalmologists between 2000-2005.[10]

Retinal Dysplasia: Focal retinal dysplasia and retinal folds are recognized in the breed. Identified in 2.60% of Irish Red and White Setters CERF examined by veterinary ophthalmologists between 2000-2005.[10]

Iris Cysts: Fluid filled sacs arising from the posterior surface of the iris, to which they may remain attached or break free and float into the anterior chamber. Usually occur in mature dogs. Can occasionally block the iridocorneal angle causing glaucoma. Identified in 1.30% of Irish Red and White Setters CERF examined by veterinary ophthalmologists between 2000-2005.[10]

Isolated Case Studies
None Reported

Genetic Tests

Tests of Genotype: Direct test for Canine Leukocyte Adhesion Deficiency is available from Optigen and the Animal Health Trust.

Direct test for Rcd-1 PRA is available from Optigen, and the Animal Health Trust.

Direct test for vWD is available from the Animal Health Trust.

Tests of Phenotype: CHIC certification: Required testing includes hip radiographs, CERF eye examination, thyroid profile including autoantibodies, and genetic tests for Rcd-1 PRA and Canine Leukocyte Adhesion Deficiency. (See CHIC Website: www.caninehealthinfo.org)

Recommend elbow radiographs, patella evaluation, and cardiac examination.

Miscellaneous

- **Breed name synonyms:** Red and White Irish Setter, Parti-Colored Setter.
- **Registries:** AKC, UKC, KCGB (Kennel Club of Great Britain), ANKC (Australian National Kennel Club), NKC (National Kennel Club), FCI.
- **AKC rank:** Became an AKC recognized breed Jan. 2009. Entire studbook registered.
- **Internet resources: Irish Red and White Setter Association:** www.irishredwhitesetterassociation.com
  Irish Red and White Setter Club of Great Britain: www.irishredandwhitesetterclub.com
  Irish Red and White Setter Club of Canada: www.irishredandwhitesetterclub.ca

References

1. Foureman P, Whiteley M, & Giger U: Canine leukocyte adhesion deficiency: presence of the Cys36Ser beta-2 integrin mutation in an affected US Irish Setter cross-breed dog and in US Irish Red and White Setters. J Vet Intern Med. 2002 Sep-Oct;16(5):518-23.

2. Kijas JM, Bauer TR Jr, Gafvert S, et. Al.: A missense mutation in the beta-2 integrin gene (ITGB2) causes canine leukocyte adhesion deficiency. Genomics. 1999 Oct 1;61(1):101-7.

3. Debenham SL, Millington A, Kijast J, et. al.: Canine leucocyte adhesion deficiency in Irish red and white setters. J Small Anim Pract. 2002 Feb;43(2):74-5.

4. OFA Website breed statistics: www.offa.org Last accessed July 1, 2010.

5. Schellenberg D, Yi Q, Glickman NW, et. al.: Influence of thoracic conformation and genetics on the risk of gastric dilatation-volvulus in Irish setters. J Am Anim Hosp Assoc. 1998 Jan-Feb;34(1):64-73.

8. Nachreiner RF, Refsal KR, Graham PA, et. al.: Prevalence of serum thyroid hormone autoantibodies in dogs with clinical signs of hypothyroidism. *J Am Vet Med Assoc* 2002 Feb 15;220(4):466-71.

9. Nachreiner R & Refsal K: Personal communication, Diagnostic Center for Population and Animal Health, Michigan State University. April, 2007.

10. *Ocular Disorders Presumed to be Inherited in Purebred Dogs.* American College of Veterinary Ophthalmologists. ACVO, 2007.

11. AKC Breed Website: www.akc.org/breeds/irish_red_white_setter/ Last accessed July 1, 2010.

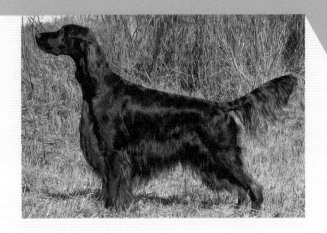

Irish Setter

moderate shedders and their grooming needs are average.

Normal Physiologic Variations
None reported

Drug Sensitivities
None reported

Inherited Diseases

Hip Dysplasia: Polygenically inherited trait causing degenerative joint disease and hip arthritis. OFA reports 12.1% affected. Reported at a frequency of 7.3% in the 2003 ISCA National Health Survey.[1,2]

Elbow Dysplasia: Polygenically inherited trait causing elbow arthritis. OFA reports 3.4% affected.[1]

Patella Luxation: Polygenically inherited laxity of patellar ligaments, causing luxation, lameness, and later degenerative joint disease. Treat surgically if causing clinical signs. Too few Irish Setters have been screened by OFA to determine an accurate frequency.[1]

Progressive Retinal Atrophy (PRA, RCD-1): Autosomal recessive, early onset rod, cone dysplasia form of PRA with an onset of 25 days of age, and progressing to blindness by one year old. A genetic test is available, revealing 7% carriers and 0.5% affected. A late-onset, **rcd-4 PRA** also occurs in the breed with a average age of onset of 10 years. A genetic test available.[3,4,5]

Canine Leukocyte Adhesion Deficiency (CLAD): An autosomal recessive, fatal immunodeficiency disease found in Irish setters. Affected dogs present with severe recurrent infections, neutrophilia and low body weight. A genetic test is available, showing 11% testing as carriers in Germany, and 7.6% testing as carriers in Australia. The frequency in the US population is not published.[6,7,8,9]

Hypochondroplastic Dwarfism: A rare, autosomal recessive form of dwarfism has been identified in the breed.[10]

Hereditary Quadriplegia and Amblyopia: A rare, congenital, autosomal recessive disorder causing inability to stand, tremor, amblyopia with nystagmus, and seizures has been identified in the breed.[11,12]

Disease Predispositions

Allergic Dermatitis: Inhalant or food allergy. Presents with pruritis and pyotraumatic dermatitis. Irish setters have a significantly increased risk for atopy versus other breeds. Reported at a frequency of 15.8% in the 2003 ISCA National Health Survey.[2,13]

Gastric Dilatation-Volvulus (Bloat, GDV): Life-threatening twisting of the stomach within the abdomen. Requires immediate veterinary attention. Irish setters with the deepest thorax relative to width had the greatest risk for GDV (8.45x odds ratio). A lifetime

The Breed History
In the 18th century in Ireland, this breed most probably originated from a mix of Pointer, Spaniel, English setter, and Gordon setter breeds. The early specimens of these scent dogs were red and white, but in the 19th century, they were progressively selected for the solid red color. Disney's "Big Red" helped to propel this breed's popularity. AKC registry began in 1878.

Breeding for Function
Bred to be a gun dog for both pointing and retrieving, they are now most widely seen in conformation shows, obedience trials, and as a household pet.

Physical Characteristics
Height at Withers: female 25" (63.5 cm), male 27" (69 cm)

Weight: females 60lb (27 kg), males 70 (32 kg).

Coat: The beautiful medium-length smooth, flat and glossy coat has a rich mahogany or chestnut red color. Small white markings are not faulted on feet or chest.

Longevity: 11-15 years.

Points of Conformation: A long, lean appearance with good bone, finely chiseled muzzle, dark to medium brown colored eyes, ears almost reaching the nose, well-defined stop and prominent occiput characterize these dogs. These dogs have prominent flews and the nose is pigmented black or brown. Their topline is gently inclined downward to the rear, and the tail should almost reach the tarsus, and is carried curving or straight nearly level with the back. They are very deep-chested.

Recognized Behavior Issues and Traits
These dogs progress slowly but steadily during development of their working skills, but excel at hunting tasks once fully trained. They are gentle, loyal, outgoing dogs, with a characteristically stable temperament. They are affectionate, have high energy levels and while some are reserved, others may be a bit high strung. They are not known to have well developed guarding instincts, instead they may seem to want to "clown around". They require high levels of exercise, and without adequate human contact, they may develop boredom vices such as barking, digging or chewing. They are

risk of 24.9% is reported, with 4.8% of all Irish Setters dying from the condition. Reported at a frequency of 12.8% in the 2003 ISCA National Health Survey.[2,14,15]

Hypothyroidism: Inherited autoimmune thyroiditis. 12.6% positive for thyroid autoantibodies based on testing at Michigan State University. (Ave. for all breeds is 7.5%) Reported at a frequency of 20.7% in the 2003 ISCA National Health Survey. Dorn reports a 1.87x odds ratio versus other breeds.[2,16,17,18]

Umbilical Hernias: Congenital opening of the abdominal wall at the umbilicus. Correct with surgery if large. Reported at a frequency of 10.3% in the 2003 ISCA National Health Survey.[2]

Distichiasis: Abnormally placed eyelashes that irritate the cornea and conjunctiva. Can cause secondary corneal ulceration. Identified in 5.83% of Irish setters CERF-examined by veterinary ophthalmologists between 2000-2005.[11]

Persistent Pupillary Membranes: Strands of fetal remnant connecting; iris to iris, cornea, lens, or involving sheets of tissue. The later three forms can impair vision, and dogs affected with these forms should not be bred. Identified in 5.56% of Irish Setters CERF examined by veterinary ophthalmologists between 2000-2005.[11]

Idiopathic Epilepsy: Inherited seizures can be generalized or partial seizures. Control with anticonvulsant medications. Reported at a frequency of 5.3% in the 2003 ISCA National Health Survey. Unknown mode of inheritance.[2]

Hypertrophic Osteodystrophy (HOD): Immune-mediated disorder causing fever, and painful, swollen joints and bones in young Irish Setters. Occurs mostly within 3-14 days post-vaccination. Age of onset is 8-16 weeks. Reported 14.3x odds ratio versus other breeds. Reported at a frequency of 5.0% in the 2003 ISCA National Health Survey. Unknown mode of inheritance.[2,19,20]

Urinary Incontinence: Spayed female Irish setters are over represented compared with other breeds for urinary incontinence. Reported at a frequency of 5.0% in the 2003 ISCA National Health Survey.[2,21,22]

Osteosarcoma: The Irish Setter is a breed with an increased frequency of malignant osteosarcoma, usually in the long bones of the limbs. Reported at a frequency of 4.6% in the 2003 ISCA National Health Survey.[2,23]

Cataracts: Anterior, posterior, and capsular intermediate and punctate cataracts predominate in the breed. Identified in 3.89% of Irish setters CERF-examined by veterinary ophthalmologists between 2000-2005. Reported at a frequency of 5.3% in the 2003 ISCA National Health Survey. CERF does not recommend breeding any Irish Setter with a cataract.[2,11]

Entropion: Rolling in of the eyelid. Can cause corneal irritation. Entropion is reported in 2.22% of Irish setters CERF-examined by veterinary ophthalmologists between 2000-2005. Reported at a frequency of 2.1% in the 2003 ISCA National Health Survey.[2,11]

Gluten (Wheat) Sensitive Enteropathy: Irish setters can demonstrate an inherited gluen sensitivity that produces poor weight gain or weight loss, with or without diarrhea. Pathologically

the intestinal crypts become blunted, with increased intestinal permeability. Reducing exposure to gluten (dietary cereal) will minimize clinical signs. The mode of inheritance has not been determined.[24,25]

Seborrheic Dermatitis: Skin disorder presenting with greasy skin and haircoat. Unknown mode of inheritance. Dorn reports a 2.51x odds ratio versus other breeds.[16]

Persistent Hyaloid Artery: Congenital defect resulting from abnormalities in the development and regression of the hyaloid artery. Identified in 1.11% of Irish Setters CERF examined by veterinary ophthalmologists between 2000-2005.[11]

IgA Deficiency: Inherited disorder seen in Irish setters causing recurrent bacterial pneumonia, diarrhea, poor weight gain, skin infections, allergies, and immune-mediated diseases.[26]

Laryngeal Paralysis: Irish setters are a breed at increased risk to develop geriatric laryngeal paralysis secondary to axonal degeneration of the recurrent laryngeal nerve. Clinical signs are exercise intolerance, inspiratory stridor, inspiratory dyspnea, gagging, coughing and dysphonia.[27]

Megaesophagus: Irish setters are identified as a breed at increased risk of developing acquired megaesophagus. Causes include peripheral neuropathy, laryngeal paralysis, acquired myasthenia gravis, esophagitis, and gastric dilatation. Hypothyroidism is not associated with megaesophagus. Clinical signs include regurgitation, excess salivation, and aspiration pneumonia.[28]

Degenerative Myelopathy (DM): Affected dogs show an insidious onset of upper motor neuron (UMN) paraparesis at an average age of 11.4 years. The disease eventually progresses to severe tetraparesis. Affected dogs have normal results on myelography, MRI, and CSF analysis. Necropsy confirms the condition. Unknown mode of inheritance. A direct genetic test for an autosomal recessive DM susceptibility gene is available. All affected dogs are homozygous for the gene, however, only a small percentage of homozygous dogs develop DM. Clinical DM is reported at a prevalence of 0.68% in the breed.[29]

Acral lick Dermatitis, Brachygnathism, Cervical Vertebral Instability, Color Dilution Alopecia, Cutaneous Asthenia, Ectropion, Factor VIII Deficiency, Lissencephaly, Lupoid Onychopathy, Narcolepsy, Optic Nerve Hypoplasia, Osteochondrodysplasia, Perianal Fistula, Prognathism, Retained Primary Teeth, Sebaceous Adenitis, Tricuspid Valve Dysplasia, Vascular Ring Anomaly, and **von Willebrand's Disease** are reported.[30]

Isolated Case Studies

Patent Ductus Arteriosis (PDA): A right to left shunting PDA was identified in a six-month-old, female Irish setter presented with a two-month history of progressive hindlimb weakness and collapse on exercise. Thoracic auscultation revealed a soft systolic murmur and a split second heart sound.[31]

Aortic Bulb/Valve Mineralization: Six of 20 affected dogs were Irish setters in one study. The mineralization was visible radiographically, but did not cause clinical signs.[32]

Globoid Cell Leukodystrophy (Krabbe disease): A rare, autosomal recessive lysosomal storage disease causing severe neurological symptoms including seizures, hypotonia, blindness, and death in young affected dogs was identified in a family of Irish setters. A genetic test was developed for this cohort.[33]

Genetic Tests

Tests of Genotype: Direct test for Canine Leukocyte Adhesion Deficiency is available from HealthGene, Optigen and the Animal Health Trust.

Direct test for Rcd-1 PRA is available from HealthGene, Optigen, VetGen, and the Animal Health Trust.

Direct test for Rcd-4 PRA is available from the Animal Health Trust.

Direct test for a DM susceptability gene is available from OFA.

Tests of Phenotype: CHIC Certification: Required testing includes hip radiographs, CERF eye examination or genetic test for PRA, and thyroid profile including autoantibodies. (See CHIC website; www.caninehealthinfo.org).

Recommend elbow radiographs, patella evaluation, and cardiac examination.

Miscellaneous

- **Breed name synonyms:** Irishman, Irish Red Setter (historical), Red Setter
- **Registries:** AKC, UKC, CKC, KCGB (Kennel Club of Great Britain), ANKC(Australian National Kennel Club), NKC (National Kennel Club)
- **AKC rank (year 2008):** 69 (1,291 dogs registered)
- **Internet resources: Irish Setter Club of America:** www.irishsetterclub.org
  Irish setter Club of Canada: www.irishsettercanada.org
  Irish Setter Association, England: www.isae.co.uk
  National Red Setter Field Trial Club: www.nrsftc.com

References

1. OFA Website breed statistics: www.offa.org Last accessed July 1, 2010.
2. Irish Setter Club of America: 2003 ISCA National Health Survey. 2004.
3. Djajadiningrat-Laanen SC, Boeve MH, Stades FC, van Oost BA: Familial non-rcd1 generalised retinal degeneration in Irish setters. *J Small Anim Pract.* 2003 Mar;44(3):113-6.
4. Suber ML, Pittler SJ, Qin N, Wright GC, Holcombe V, Lee RH, Craft CM, Lolley RN, Baehr W, Hurwitz RL: Irish setter dogs affected with rod/cone dysplasia contain a nonsense mutation in the rod cGMP phosphodiesterase beta-subunit gene. *Proc Natl Acad Sci U S A.* 1993 May 1;90(9):3968-72.
5. Aguirre GD, Baldwin V, Weeks KM, Acland GM, Ray K: Frequency of the codon 807 mutation in the cGMP phosphodiesterase beta-subunit gene in Irish setters and other dog breeds with hereditary retinal degeneration. *J Hered.* 1999 Jan-Feb;90(1):143-7.
6. Jobling AI, Ryan J, Augusteyn RC: The frequency of the canine leukocyte adhesion deficiency (CLAD) allele within the Irish Setter population of Australia. Aust Vet J. 2003 Dec;81(12):763-5.
7. Pfeiffer I, Brenig B: Frequency of the canine leucocyte adhesion deficiency (CLAD) mutation among Irish red setters in Germany. J Anim Breed Genet. 2005 Apr;122(2):140-2.
8. Kijas JM, Bauer TR Jr, Gafvert S, et. Al.: A missense mutation in the beta-2 integrin gene (ITGB2) causes canine leukocyte adhesion deficiency. Genomics. 1999 Oct 1;61(1):101-7.
9. Trowald-Wigh G, Hakansson L, Johannisson A, et. al.: Leucocyte adhesion protein deficiency in Irish setter dogs. Vet Immunol Immunopathol. 1992 May;32(3-4):261-80.
10. Hanssen I, Falck G, Grammeltvedt AT, Haug E, Isaksen CV: Hypochondroplastic dwarfism in the Irish setter. *J Small Anim Pract.* 1998 Jan;39(1):10-4.
11. *Ocular Disorders Presumed to be Inherited in Purebred Dogs.* American College of Veterinary Ophthalmologists. ACVO, 2007.
12. Palmer AC, Payne JE, Wallace ME: Hereditary quadriplegia and amblyopia in the Irish Setter. J Small Anim Pract. 1973 Jun;14(6):343-52.
13. Schick RO, Fadok VA: Responses of atopic dogs to regional allergens: 268 cases (1981-1984). J Am Vet Med Assoc. 1986 Dec 1;189(11):1493-6.
14. Ward MP, Patronek GJ, Glickman LT: Benefits of prophylactic gastropexy for dogs at risk of gastric dilatation-volvulus. *Prev Vet Med.* 2003 Sep 12;60(4):319-29.
15. Schellenberg D, Yi Q, Glickman NW, et. al.: Influence of thoracic conformation and genetics on the risk of gastric dilatation-volvulus in Irish setters. J Am Anim Hosp Assoc. 1998 Jan-Feb;34(1):64-73.
16. Dorn CR: Canine breed-specific risks of frequently diagnosed diseases at veterinary teaching hospitals. Monograph. AKC Canine Health Foundation. 2000.
17. Nachreiner RF, Refsal KR, Graham PA, et. al.: Prevalence of serum thyroid hormone autoantibodies in dogs with clinical signs of hypothyroidism. J Am Vet Med Assoc 2002 Feb 15;220(4):466-71.
18. Nachreiner R & Refsal K: Personal communication, Diagnostic Center for Population and Animal Health, Michigan State University. April, 2007.
19. McLaughlin R: Developmental Orthopedic Diseases in Dogs. 2003. Proceedings, Western Veterinary Conference 2003.
20. LaFond E, Breur GJ & Austin CC: Breed susceptibility for developmental orthopedic diseases in dogs. J Am Anim Hosp Assoc. 2002 Sep-Oct;38(5):467-77.
21. Holt PE, Thrusfield MV: Association in bitches between breed, size, neutering and docking, and acquired urinary incontinence due to incompetence of the urethral sphincter mechanism. Vet Rec. 1993 Aug 21;133(8):177-80.
22. Blendinger C, Blendinger K, Bostedt H: Urinary incontinence in spayed bitches. 1. Pathogenesis, incidence and disposition. Tierarztl Prax. 1995 Jun;23(3):291-9.
23. Misdorp W, Hart AA: Some prognostic and epidemiologic factors in canine osteosarcoma. J Natl Cancer Inst. 1979 Mar;62(3):537-45.
24. Polvi A, Garden OA, Houlston RS, Maki M, Batt RM, Partanen J: Genetic susceptibility to gluten sensitive enteropathy in Irish setter dogs is not linked to the major histocompatibility complex. *Tissue Antigens.* 1998 Dec;52(6):543-9.
25. Hall EJ, Batt RM: Dietary modulation of gluten sensitivity in a naturally occurring enteropathy of Irish setter dogs. Gut. 1992 Feb;33(2):198-205.
26. Norris CR, Gershwin LJ: Evaluation of systemic and secretory IgA concentrations and immunohistochemical stains for IgA-containing B cells in mucosal tissues of an Irish setter with selective IgA deficiency. *J Am Anim Hosp Assoc.* 2003 May-Jun;39(3):247-50.
27. Burbidge HM: A review of laryngeal paralysis in dogs. Br Vet J. 1995 Jan-Feb;151(1):71-82.
28. Gaynor AR, Shofer FS, Washabau RJ: Risk factors for acquired megaesophagus in dogs. J Am Vet Med Assoc. 1997 Dec 1;211(11):1406-12.
29. Coates JR & Wade C: Update on the Genetic Basis of Canine Degenerative Myelopathy. Proceedings, 2008 ACVIM Forum. 2008.
30. *The Genetic Connection: A Guide to Health Problems in Purebred Dogs.* L Ackerman. p. 223, AAHA Press, 1999.
31. Ferasin L, Rizzo F, Darke PG: Original investigation of right-to-left shunting patent ductus arteriosus in an Irish setter puppy. *Vet J.* 2007 Mar; 173(2): 443-8.
32. Douglass JP, Berry CR, Thrall DE, Malarkey DE, Spaulding KA: Radiographic features of aortic bulb/valve mineralization in 20 dogs. *Vet Radiol Ultrasound.* 2003 Jan-Feb;44(1):20-7.
33. McGraw RA, Carmichael KP: Molecular basis of globoid cell leukodystrophy in Irish setters. Vet J. 2006 Mar;171(2):370-2.
34. *The Complete Dog Book, 20th Ed.* The American Kennel Club. Howell Book House, NY 2006. p 72-75.

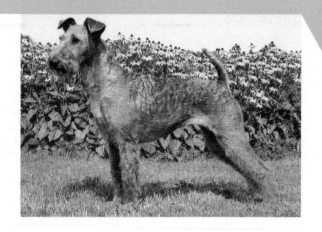

Irish Terrier

The Breed History
This is one of the oldest terrier breeds, possibly two centuries old. They may be related to Airedale Terrier, Wheaten Terrier and the Irish Wolfhound. The wire-haired Black and Tan Terrier may have been the primary breed ancestor. Early records originated in County Cork, Ireland. AKC recognition occurred in 1885.

Breeding for Function
They served as a small game hunter, for vermin control, dry and wet retrieving, guard dog, war dog (messenger, sentinel), police dog, and were sometimes even used for large game hunting. Today, they are primarily found in family pet roles. Speed and agility are retained.

Physical Characteristics
Height at Withers: 18" (45.5 cm)

Weight: female 25 lb (11 kg), male 27 lb (12 kg)

Coat: A rich red color, though it can be as light as wheaten (is the standard). Puppies are sometimes born with some black hair but as they mature, the normal red color takes over. The wiry dense hairs overlay a fine undercoat of soft, short, lighter hair. The coat is harshest over the topline. They require moderate grooming but bathing needs are minimal. The dog needs stripping once to twice yearly.

Longevity: 14-15 years

Points of Conformation: Though a terrier, the breed is more similar to the Irish wolfhound type in their overall lithe conformation than the typical stocky, short-legged terrier. The skull is long and narrow between the ears, they possess a minimal stop, and have a moderate beard and moustache which frame their large black nose. They have very bushy brows and the lips are black. Eyes are dark brown with an intense gaze, the ears are small and triangular in shape with moderate leather and the fold of the ear sits above skull level. The long neck is moderately muscled and not throaty. The thorax is deep and somewhat narrow. The topline is long and slightly arched only over the loin. The metatarsals and metacarpals are short, the tail is high set, and may be docked to three quarters of the length. Feet are compact, almost round, the nails dark and toes well arched. Limbs are long and straight boned, and not feathered. The gait is lively, animated and powerful.

Recognized Behavior Issues and Traits
Reported breed traits include: Loyal, high intelligence, high-spirited, fiery attitude, and always on guard. Adaptable, at home in city or rural environments, and enjoys children. Hardy; tolerates both warm and cold.

They are playful and affectionate with family members, including children, but aggressive with other dogs and animals. Their tendency to have contempt of danger was the genesis to their nickname of "Red Devil". They may dig, and are considered only moderately trainable due to stubbornness. Early obedience and socialization are important for these dogs. They have moderate exercise needs. If off leash, they require a fenced enclosure.

Normal Physiologic Variations
None reported

Drug Sensitivities
None reported.

Inherited Diseases
Digital Hyperkeratosis (Corny Feet): An autosomal recessive disease of abnormal hardening and proliferation of the footpads. Affected dogs develop abnormal footpads around 6 months of age, which then fissure and crack, predisposing them to secondary infection.[1]

Hip Dysplasia: Polygenically inherited trait causing degenerative joint disease and hip arthritis. Too few Irish Terriers have been screened to determine an accurate frequency.[2]

Patella Luxation: Polygenically inherited laxity of patellar ligaments, causing luxation, lameness, and later degenerative joint disease. Treat surgically if causing clinical signs. Too few Irish Terriers have been screened by OFA to determine an accurate frequency.[2]

Elbow Dysplasia: Polygenically inherited trait causing elbow arthritis. Too few Irish Terriers have been screened by OFA to determine an accurate frequency.[2]

Muscular Dystrophy/Myopathy: A rare, fatal, X-linked muscular dystrophy affecting primarily male Irish Terriers. This is a dystrophin deficient form of muscular dystrophy. There is no genetic test for female carriers.[3,4]

Disease Predispositions
Hypothyroidism: Inherited autoimmune thyroiditis. 6.1% positive for thyroid auto-antibodies based on testing at Michigan State University. (Ave. for all breeds is 7.5%).[5,6]

Cystinuria/Cystine Bladder Stones: Irish Terriers have an increased risk for developing cystine bladder stones. Caused by an error in cystine metabolism. Treat with surgical removal and life-long medical therapy. Unknown mode of inheritance in this breed.[7,8]

Progressive Retinal Atrophy (PRA): Progressive degeneration of the retina, eventually causing blindness. Typical age of onset is between 2 to 5 years. Presumed autosomal recessive inheritance. Too few Irish Terriers have been CERF eye examined to determine an accurate frequency in the breed.[9,10]

Distichiasis, Persistent Pupillary Membranes, and **Cataracts** are reported by CERF, but too few Irish Terriers have been CERF eye examined to determine an accurate frequency.[10]

Cryptorchidism, Degenerative Myelopathy, Microphthalmia, and **Uveodermatological Syndrome** are reported.[11]

Isolated Case Studies
None Reported

Genetic Tests
Tests of Genotype: none

Tests of Phenotype: Recommend patella evaluation, hip and elbow radiographs, CERF eye examination, thyroid profile including autoantibodies, and cardiac examination.

Miscellaneous
- **Breed name synonyms:** Irish Red Terrier
- **Registries:** AKC, UKC, CKC, KCGB (Kennel Club of Great Britain), ANKC (Australian National Kennel Club), NKC (National Kennel Club)
- **AKC rank (year 2008):** 130 (182 dogs registered)
- **Internet resources: Irish Terrier Club of America:** www.itca.info/ **U.K. Irish Terrier Association:** www.irishterrierassociation.co.uk **The Irish Terrier Association of Canada:** www.dogbiz.com/itac/index.html

References

1. Binder H, Arnold S, Schelling C, et. al.: Palmoplantar hyperkeratosis in Irish terriers: evidence of autosomal recessive inheritance. *J Small Anim Pract.* 2000 Feb;41(2):52-5.
2. OFA Website breed statistics: www.offa.org Last accessed July 1, 2010.
3. Schatzberg S, Olby N, Steingold S, et. al.: A polymerase chain reaction screening strategy for the promoter of the canine dystrophin gene. *Am J Vet Res.* 1999 Sep;60(9):1040-6.
4. Wentink GH, Meijer AE, van der Linde-Sipman JS, et. al.: Myopathy in an irish terrier with a metabolic defect of the isolated mitochondria. *Zentralbl Veterinarmed A.* 1974 Jan;21(1):62-74
5. Nachreiner RF, Refsal KR, Graham PA, et. al.: Prevalence of serum thyroid hormone autoantibodies in dogs with clinical signs of hypothyroidism. *J Am Vet Med Assoc* 2002 Feb 15;220(4):466-71.
6. Nachreiner R & Refsal K: Personal communication, Diagnostic Center for Population and Animal Health, Michigan State University. April, 2007.
7. Lewis LD, Morris ML Jr: Canine urolithiasis: diagnosis and treatment. *Mod Vet Pract.* 1984 May;65(5):375-8.
8. Allen LBA, Pratt A, Lulich J, et. al.: Canine Cystine Urolithiasis: Investigation of Cases Identified in the United Kingdom. Proceedings, 2008 British Small Animal Veterinary Congress. 2008.
9. Glaze MB: Fundus Interpretation Made Real. Proceedings, 2004 Northeast Veterinary Conference. 2004.
10. *Ocular Disorders Presumed to be Inherited in Purebred Dogs.* American College of Veterinary Ophthalmologists. ACVO, 2007.
11. *The Genetic Connection: A Guide to Health Problems in Purebred Dogs.* L Ackerman. p. 223. AAHA Press, 1999.
12. *The Complete Dog Book, 20th Ed.* The American Kennel Club. Howell Book House, NY 2006. p. 382-386.

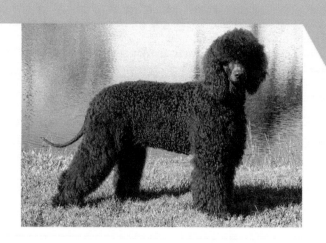

Irish Water Spaniel

The Breed History

The tallest of the spaniel breeds is also an ancient one, and original spaniel type fits the modern type of this breed. A member of the water spaniel group that includes the extinct Tweed water spaniel, these dogs are thought to have arisen from the South Country Water Spaniel and the North Country Water Spaniel. Written records begin in 1607. The first Irish Water Spaniels came to America around the year 1873. and became an AKC breed in 1884.

Breeding for Function

Their primary function was to perform as a high endurance waterfowl retriever. They were bred with a heavy oily coat to allow them to retrieve in cold waters. They were less commonly used for upland game hunting.

Physical Characteristics

Height at Withers: females 21-23" (53-58.5 cm), males 22-24" (56-61 cm).

Weight: females 45-58 lb (20.5-26 kg), males 55-65 lb (25-29.5 kg).

Coat: The tail, front of the neck and face are covered in very short hair. The main haircoat is a longer crisp, dense, oily, and tightly curly overcoat. The undercoat is short and dense. The standard coat color is liver. The liver haircoat has a purplish tinge referred to as *puce* liver.

Longevity: 12-14 years

Points of Conformation: The water-repelling curly coat, rat-tail, beard and sideburns and the loose curly topknot that reaches the eyes of this dog are distinctive breed characteristics. They possess a strong square conformation, and the wedge-shaped head is well chiseled. The skull is domed, stop is moderate, and occipital protuberance is prominent. The muzzle is long and square, the nose large and liver colored. Almond shaped eyes are medium sized and hazel in color. The very long pendulous ears are low set with extensive curly feathering at the tips. The neck is arched, long and muscular. The topline is level, though it may be slightly higher in the rear. The thorax is deep and the ribs are well sprung. The rib cage extends well back. Limbs are straight boned, feet large and spreading with webbed toes, and the low set tail is generally carried level. The ground-covering gait is long, low, smooth, and seems effortless.

Recognized Behavior Issues and Traits

Reported breed characteristics include: Loyal with family, some dogs are so reserved as to be aggressive with strangers, and intelligent. They have a strong willingness to please, high activity and exercise needs, and high trainability. Grooming needs consist of a weekly combing. They are a low to moderate shedder depending on the season. This breed is not always good with other pets. Early obedience training and socialization are recommended. This breed is considered a good watchdog, but has a low barking tendency otherwise. They are also considered an excellent swimmer.

Normal Physiologic Variations

Some Irish Water Spaniel females can have irregular heat cycles.

Drug Sensitivities

The Irish Water Spaniel breed club websites alert to possible reactions to potentiated sulfonamide antibiotics.

Inherited Diseases

Elbow Dysplasia: Polygenically inherited trait causing elbow arthritis. OFA reports 16.1% affected.[1]

Hip Dysplasia: Polygenically inherited trait causing degenerative joint disease and hip arthritis. OFA reports 12.0% affected.[1]

Patella Luxation: Polygenically inherited laxity of patellar ligaments, causing luxation, lameness, and later degenerative joint disease. Treat surgically if causing clinical signs. Too few Irish Water Spaniels have been screened by OFA to determine an accurate frequency.[1]

Disease Predispositions

Distichiasis: Abnormally placed eyelashes that irritate the cornea and conjunctiva. Can cause secondary corneal ulceration. Identified in 18.55% of Irish Water Spaniels CERF examined by veterinary ophthalmologists between 2000-2005.[2]

Follicular Dysplasia (Hair Loss): Hair loss may be somewhat cyclical, and typically affects the trunk and spares the head and distal extremities. Hair loss in IWS can be influenced by dietary factors and an abnormality of their sex hormone intermediates, especially an exaggerated response of 17-hydroxyprogesterone (17-OHP) in ACTH-response tests. Unknown mode of inheritance, although one study suggested a dominant mode of inheritance. Diagnosis by skin biopsy. Treatment with melatonin.[3,4,5]

Cataracts: Anterior and posterior cortex intermediate cataracts predominate in the breed. Age of onset averages 5 years of age. Unknown mode of inheritance. Identified in 5.43% of Irish Water Spaniels CERF examined by veterinary ophthalmologists between 2000-2005. CERF does not recommend breeding any Irish Water Spaniel with a cataract.[2]

Hypothyroidism: Inherited autoimmune thyroiditis. 2.5% positive for thyroid autoantibodies based on testing at Michigan State University. (Ave. for all breeds is 7.5%).[6,7]

Persistent Pupillary Membranes: Strands of fetal remnant connecting; iris to iris, cornea, lens, or involving sheets of tissue. The later three forms can impair vision, and dogs affected with these forms should not be bred. Identified in 2.26% of Irish Water Spaniels CERF examined by veterinary ophthalmologists between 2000-2005.[2]

Entropion: Rolling in of the eyelid. Can cause corneal irritation. Entropion is reported in 1.36% of Irish Water Spaniels CERF examined by veterinary ophthalmologists between 2000-2005.[2]

Inherited Epilepsy (Hereditary seizures): Generalized or partial seizures. Control with anticonvulsant medication. Reported as a problem in the breed on the IWSCA website. Unknown mode of inheritance.

Coat dilution Alopecia and **Progressive Retinal Atrophy** are reported.[8]

Isolated Case Studies

Epitheliotropic (T-cell) lymphoma: A 9-year-old Irish water spaniel with nodular areas of alopecia and erythematous skin lesions was diagnosed by biopsy with epitheliotropic lymphoma.[9]

Genetic Tests

Tests of Genotype: none

Tests of Phenotype: CHIC Certification: Hip and Elbow radiographs, CERF eye examination (after 2 years of age), and thyroid profile including autoantibodies. (See CHIC website; www.caninehealthinfo.org).

Recommend patella evaluation and cardiac examination.

Miscellaneous

- **Breed name synonyms:** IWS, Water Spaniel, Shannon Spaniel (historical), Rat-tail or Whip-tail Spaniels, Southern Irish Water Spaniel (all historical)
- **Registries:** AKC, CKC, ANKC (Australian National Kennel Club), NKC (National Kennel Club)
- **AKC rank (year 2008):** 144 (83 dogs registered)
- **Internet resources: Irish Water Spaniel Club of America:** http://iwsca.webs.com
  Irish Water Spaniel Association of Canada: www.iwsac.org
  UK Irish Water Spaniel Association: www.irishwaterspaniels.org.uk

References

1. OFA Website breed statistics: www.offa.org Last accessed July 1, 2010.
2. *Ocular Disorders Presumed to be Inherited in Purebred Dogs.* American College of Veterinary Ophthalmologists. ACVO, 2007.
3. Cerundolo R, Lloyd DH, Pidduck HG: Studies on the inheritance of hair loss in the Irish water spaniel. *Vet Rec.* 1999 Nov 6;145(19):542-4.
4. Cerundolo R, Lloyd DH, McNeil PE, et. al.: An Analysis of Factors Underlying Hypotrichosis and Alopecia in Irish Water Spaniels in the United Kingdom. *Vet Dermatol* 2000: 11[2]:107-122.
5. White SD: Update on Follicular Alopecias: "Pseudo-Endocrinopathies". Proceedings, 2005 ACVIM Forum. 2005.
6. Nachreiner RF, Refsal KR, Graham PA, et. al.: Prevalence of serum thyroid hormone autoantibodies in dogs with clinical signs of hypothyroidism. J Am Vet Med Assoc 2002 Feb 15;220(4):466-71.
7. Nachreiner R & Refsal K: Personal communication, Diagnostic Center for Population and Animal Health, Michigan State University. April, 2007.
8. *The Genetic Connection: A Guide to Health Problems in Purebred Dogs.* L Ackerman. p. 223. AAHA Press, 1999.
9. Bouchard H: Epitheliotropic lymphoma in a dog. *Can Vet J.* 2000 Aug;41(8):628-30.
10. *The Complete Dog Book, 20th Ed.* The American Kennel Club. Howell Book House, NY 2006. p. 102-105.

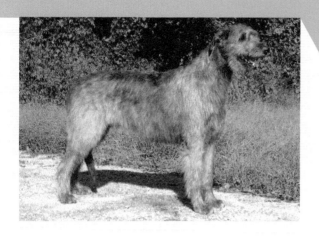

Irish Wolfhound

The Breed History

This breed is similar in type to the deerhound but is much larger; in fact it is the tallest breed of dog in the world. The first written records of this breed date to the year 391 in a document authored by a Roman, though evidence exists that they were in Ireland before that. At one point the breed almost became extinct but in 1862, remaining stock was gathered and restoration of the breed began. Infusion of Scottish Deerhound, Great Dane, and Borzoi bloodlines helped to widen the gene pool. The first breed standard was drawn up in 1885.

Breeding for Function

The Irish wolfhound was used for the hunt in pursuit of wolves and elk and was renowned for courage and an excellent gentle temperament. Bred for sight hunting and chase, these dogs were renowned athletes. They were not considered suitable for guarding, watchdog or other such work. The breed has become a valuable country companion, and also excels at coursing and obedience competitions. They are not built for draft.

Physical Characteristics

Height at Withers: female 30" (76 cm), male 32" (81 cm).

Weight: females 105 lb minimum (48 kg), males 120 lb minimum (54.5 kg). Some males have reached 180 lb and exceed 35"in height.

Coat: They possess a rough-coated hard, weather resistant haircoat with wire over eyes and under the mandible. A soft dense undercoat is present. Approved colors include red, brindle, black, fawn, gray, or white.

Longevity: 6-8 years

Points of Conformation: The Irish Wolfhound is often described as a heavy-set greyhound type. They possess moderate bone weight. They posses high head carriage, the head is long and the muzzle has a moderate point. Eyes and nose are dark, and the small ears are carried back. The neck is long, muscular and arched without a dewlap. The thorax is very deep and is wider at the front aspect. The ribs are well sprung. The long back transitions smoothly into arched loins and the tail is long and thickly coated, with a curved tip. The strong boned limbs are straight, feet are large and round, and the toes well knuckled. The gait is smooth, easy and elastic. Hips are broad, and the abdomen well tucked up.

Recognized Behavior Issues and Traits

Reported breed characteristics include: Requires a rural setting, preferably a property with a securely fenced perimeter so that the dog can freely exercise. They are very large in stature and may not fit in well in small rooms and homes. These dogs do settle down indoors, and are intelligent. They require close human companionship. Sensitive, they require a soft touch, and they require mental stimulation and physical activity; bored ones will become destructive. Early socialization and obedience training is important.

Though they do very well around children, puppies can easily weigh 75 lb and so care must be taken that rambunctious puppies do not inadvertently injure small children. Minimal grooming is needed (biweekly will suffice). They shed year-round, but tend not to blow the coat. Many chase cats and small dogs so ideally, they should be raised with them (even so, quick movements can trigger a chase reflex). Provide soft bedding or calluses and hygromas may form. Beard may need cleaning after a meal. Good trainability. Generally get along with other dogs.

Normal Physiologic Variations

Sight hounds have lower normal ranges for T4 and T3 concentrations compared to other breeds.[1]

Echocardiography: The predictive value of body weight for echocardiographic measurements was clinically not relevant. Sex had no influence on echocardiographic values.[2]

Echocardiographic Normal Values:[2]			
Parameter	Mean	Range	Mean ±2SD
LVIDs (mm)	35.4	25.4-41.5	29.8-41
LVIDd (mm)	53.2	42.7-65.5	45.2-61.2
FS (%)	34.0	25-48	25-43
FWs (mm)	14.9	9.7-21.3	10.6-19.2
FWd (mm)	9.8	6.6-13.8	6.6-13.0
IVSs (mm)	13.7	8.1-19.0	8.9-18.5
IVSd (mm)	9.3	5.2-13.5	5.7-12.9
LA (mm), M-mode	32.9	25.4-40.9	26.1-39.7
AO (mm), M-mode	33.1	23.1-39.7	27.7-38.7
EPSS (mm)	6.8	4.0-11.4	3.6-10.0
LA (mm), 2D	47.3	36.5-56.8	38.7-55.9
RA (mm), 2D	40.4	30.9-54.6	25.4-55.4
RVIDd (mm), 2D	29.1	17.9-37.6	21.4-36.8
ESVI (ml/m2)	29.0	15.3-40.6	17.2-40.8
Heart rate (bpm)	121	74-166	74-168
Age (yrs)	3.4	1-8.5	
Body weight (kg)	65.0	48-93	
N	262		

LVIDs, left ventricular end-systolic dimension; LVIDd, left ventricular end-diastolic dimension; FS, fractional shortening; FWs and FWd, left ventricular free wall thickness at end-systole and end-diastole; IVSs and IVSd, interventricular septum thickness at end-systole and end-diastole; LA, left atrial end-systolic dimension; AO, aortic root diameter at end-diastole; EPSS, E-point to septal separation; RA, right atrial end-systolic dimension; 2D, two-dimensional echocardiographic measurement; RVIDd, end-diastolic right ventricular internal dimension; ESVI, end-systolic volume index.

Blood Pressure: Irish wolfhounds have lower arterial blood pressure than other sight hounds. Arterial blood pressure measurements were obtained from 158 healthy Irish wolfhounds using the oscillometric technique. Mean systolic pressure was 116.0 mm Hg. Mean diastolic pressure was 69.2 mm Hg, and the average mean arterial pressure was 87.8 mm Hg. Blood pressure measurements were higher in older wolfhounds than in young dogs. There was no difference between systolic and mean arterial blood pressures in lateral recumbency compared to the standing position. However, diastolic pressure was slightly lower when standing. Calm dogs had lower pressure than anxious wolfhounds. There was a significant interaction between the effects of age, gender, and mood on systolic, diastolic, and mean arterial blood pressure values.[3]

A study in the UK reports 40.3% of Irish Wolfhound litters are delivered via **Cesarean section.**[4]

Drug Sensitivities

Anesthesia: Sight hounds require particular attention during anesthesia. Their lean body conformation with high surface-area-to-volume ratio predisposes them to hypothermia during anesthesia. Impaired biotransformation of drugs by the liver results in prolonged recovery from barbiturate and thiobarbiturate intravenous anesthetics. Propofol, and ketamine/diazepam combination are recommended induction agents.[5]

Inherited Diseases

Dilated Cardiomyopathy (DCM): Complexly inherited form of dilated cardiomyopathy with a 3:2 male/ female ratio. In one survey of 500 dogs, 24.2% had DCM, with 88% of those having an accompanying **Atrial Fibrillation** (AF). Another study reported a frequency of 12.1%. Right-sided congestive heart failure develops with pleural effusion and pulmonary edema. The mean age at which AF was first detected was 3.8 years in males and 4.9 years in females, and the mean time from the first detection of AF to CHF was 6.4 years in males and 2 years in females. Dorn reports a 3.43x odds ratio for cardiac disease versus other breeds.[6,7,8,9,10,11]

Elbow Dysplasia: Polygenically inherited trait causing elbow arthritis. OFA reports 12.1% affected. Reported 93.4x odds ratio for the fragmented coronoid process form of elbow dysplasia versus other breeds.[12,13]

Hip Dysplasia: Polygenically inherited trait causing degenerative joint disease and hip arthritis. OFA reports 5.3% affected.[12]

Patella Luxation: Polygenically inherited laxity of patellar ligaments, causing luxation, lameness, and later degenerative joint disease. Treat surgically if causing clinical signs. Too few Irish

Wolfhounds have been screened by OFA to determine an accurate frequency.[12]

Disease Predispositions

Epilepsy (Inherited Seizures): Partial or generalized seizures. Treat with anticonvulsant medications. Reported at a frequency of 18.3% in one study, with a heritability of 0.87. Suggested autosomal recessive inheritance with incomplete penetrance and a male prevalence.[14]

Iris Cysts: Fluid filled sacs arising from the posterior surface of the iris. They may remain affixed to the iris, or break free into the anterior chamber. Identified in 7.92% of Irish Wolfhounds CERF examined by veterinary ophthalmologists between 2000-2005.[15]

Cataracts: Anterior, posterior, intermediate and punctate cataracts occur in the breed. Age of onset 1-2 years with rapid progression, or 5-7 years with slow progression. Identified in 6.19% of Irish Wolfhounds CERF examined by veterinary ophthalmologists between 2000-2005. CERF does not recommend breeding any Irish Wolfhound with a cataract.[15]

Distichiasis: Abnormally placed eyelashes that irritate the cornea and conjunctiva. Can cause secondary corneal ulceration. Identified in 5.20% of Irish Wolfhounds CERF examined by veterinary ophthalmologists between 2000-2005.[15]

Osteosarcoma (Bone Cancer): Irish Wolfhounds are a breed with a predisposition to develop malignant osteosarcoma. It usually occurs in the extremities. Dorn reports a 27.50x odds ratio versus other breeds. Unknown mode of inheritance. One study showed an increased risk in castrated male Irish Wolfhounds.[6,16]

Optic Nerve Hypoplasia/Micropapilla: Congenital defect of optic nerve development affecting vision, or a small optic disc. Identified in 1.24% of Irish Wolfhounds CERF examined by veterinary ophthalmologists between 2000-2005.[15]

Gastric Dilatation-Volvulus (Bloat, GDV): Polygenically inherited, life-threatening twisting of the stomach within the abdomen. Requires immediate veterinary treatment. Dorn reports a 5.52x odds ratio versus other breeds.[6,17]

Corneal Dystrophy: Epithelial/stromal form of corneal opacities on the surface of the cornea. Unknown mode of inheritance. Identified in 2.48% of Irish Wolfhounds CERF-examined by veterinary ophthalmologists between 2000-2005.[15]

Hypothyroidism: Inherited autoimmune thyroiditis. 2.3% positive for thyroid auto-antibodies based on testing at Michigan State University. (Ave. for all breeds is 7.5%).[18,19]

Retinal Dysplasia: Retinal folds, geographic, and generalized retinal dysplasia with detachment are recognized in the breed. Reported in 2.23% of Irish Wolfhounds CERF examined by veterinary ophthalmologists between 2000-2005.[15]

Porto-Systemic Shunt (PSS, Liver Shunt): Congenital abnormality of abnormal blood vessels connecting the systemic and portal blood flow. Causes stunting, abnormal behavior and possible seizures. Tobias reports a 9.9 odds ratio versus other breeds. Post-prandial bile acids and blood ammonia tests are used for diagnosis, as fasting samples are often normal. Diagnosed in 2.1% of Irish Wolfhounds in the Netherlands. Appears to be complexly inherited without sex influence.[20,21,22,23]

Everted Cartilage of the Third Eyelid: A scroll-like curling of the cartilage of the third eyelid, usually everting the margin. Can be unilateral or bilateral, and cause ocular irritation. Identified in 1.24% of Irish Wolfhounds CERF-examined by veterinary ophthalmologists between 2000-2005.[15]

Osteochondritis Dissecans (OCD): Polygenically inherited cartilage defect of the humeral head or stifle. Causes joint pain and lameness in young growing dogs. Mild cases can resolve with rest, while more severe cases require surgery. There is a 2.24:1 male to female ratio. 75% of all cases are unilateral. Dorn reports a 3.65x odds ratio versus other breeds. Another study reports a 523.5x odds ratio for stifle OCD, and a 47.1x odds ratio for shoulder OCD versus other breeds. Shoulder OCD is reported at a frequency of 1.2% in the Irish Wolfhound.[6,13,24]

Progressive Retinal Atrophy (PRA): Inherited degeneration of the retinal leading to blindness. Onset is early with blindness developing in the young adult (2-3 years of age). Presumed autosomal recessive mode of inheritance. CERF does not recommend breeding any Irish Wolfhound with PRA.[15]

Rhinitis/Bronchopneumonia Syndrome: Affected Irish Wolfhounds present beginning at less than 1 year of age with transient to persistent mucoid or mucopurulent rhinorrhea, cough, and dyspnea. Affected dogs responded to antibiotics, but were chronically recurring. In one study, ciliary function tests were normal, but low circulating IgA levels were seen. Abnormal ciliary function is still being investigated. Occurs worldwide. Unknown mode of inheritance.[25,26]

Megaesophagus is also reported on the IWCA website.

Cervical Vertebral Instability, Entropion, Hypertrophic Osteodystrophy, and **von Willebrand's Disease** are reported.[27]

Isolated Case Studies

Fibrocartilaginous Embolism: Diagnosed in eight Irish Wolfhounds between eight and 13 weeks of age. Affected dogs have an acute onset of abnormal locomotion. Diagnosis by histopathologic identification of focal myelomalacia and Alcian blue-positive-nucleus-pulposus material in the spinal cord vasculature. Dogs with mild signs can improve and survive.[28]

Juvenile Nephropathy: Case report of one Irish Wolfhound presenting with severe polyuria and polydipsia, and progressing to chronic renal failure. Histopathology included immature glomeruli and/or tubules, and persistent mesenchyme.[29]

Spinal Nephroblastoma: A 1-year-old Irish wolfhound was presented with a history of slowly progressive left pelvic limb paresis. An intradural, extramedullary mass at the caudal aspect of T13 was diagnosed histologically as an extrarenal nephroblastoma.[30]

Genetic Tests

Tests of Genotype: None.

Tests of Phenotype: CHIC Certification: Elbow and hip radiographs, CERF eye examination, and cardiac evaluation. Optional testing includes serum bile acid test. (See CHIC website; www.caninehealthinfo.org).

Recommend thyroid profile including autoantibodies and patella evaluation.

Miscellaneous

- **Breed name synonyms:** Greyhound of Ireland, Wolfdog of Ireland, Irish dogs, Big dogs of Ireland, Great Hound of Ireland (all historical), wolfhound, IW, Cu Faoil.
- **Registries:** AKC, UKC, CKC, KCGB (Kennel Club of Great Britain), ANKC (Australian National Kennel Club), NKC (National Kennel Club).
- **AKC rank (year 2008):** 81 (863 dogs registered)
- **Internet resources: Irish Wolfhound Club of America:** www.iwclubofamerica.org
  Irish Wolfhound Club of Canada: www.irishwolfhoundclubofcanada.ca
  Irish Wolfhound Club (UK): www.irishwolfhoundclub.org.uk
  The Irish Wolfhound Foundation, Inc.: www.iwfoundation.org
  Irish Wolfhound Health Group: www.iwhealthgroup.co.uk

References

1. Kintzer PP & Peterson ME: Progress in the Diagnosis and Treatment of Canine Hypothyroidism. 2007. Proceedings, ACVIM 2007.
2. Vollmar AC: Echocardiographic measurements in the Irish wolfhound: reference values for the breed. *J Am Anim Hosp Assoc.* 1999 Jul-Aug;35(4):271-7.
3. Bright JM, Dentino M. Indirect arterial blood pressure measurement in nonsedated Irish wolfhounds: reference values for the breed. J Am Anim Hosp Assoc. 2002 Nov-Dec;38(6):521-6.
4. Evans KM & Adams VJ: Proportion of litters of purebred dogs born by caesarean section. J Small Anim Pract. 2010 Feb;51(2):113-8.
5. Court MH: Anesthesia of the sighthound. Clin Tech Small Anim Pract 1999 Feb;14(1):38-43.
6. Dorn CR: Canine breed-specific risks of frequently diagnosed diseases at veterinary teaching hospitals. Monograph. AKC Canine Health Foundation. 2000.
7. Broschk C, Distl O: Dilated cardiomyopathy (DCM) in dogs--pathological, clinical, diagnosis and genetic aspects. Dtsch Tierarztl Wochenschr. 2005 Oct;112(10):380-5.
8. Vollmar AC: The prevalence of cardiomyopathy in the Irish wolfhound: a clinical study of 500 dogs. *J Am Anim Hosp Assoc.* 2000 Mar-Apr;36(2):125-32.
9. Brownlie SE, Cobb MA: Observations on the development of congestive heart failure in Irish wolfhounds with dilated cardiomyopathy. *J Small Anim Pract.* 1999 Aug;40(8):371-7.
10. Vollmar A & Fox PR: Clinical, echocardiographic, and ECG findings in 232 sequentially examined Irish Wolfhounds. J Vet Intern Med. 2001 May-June;15(3):279.
11. Distl O, Vollmar AC, Broschk C, et. al.: Complex segregation analysis of dilated cardiomyopathy (DCM) in Irish wolfhounds. Heredity. 2007 Oct;99(4):460-5.
12. OFA Website breed statistics: www.offa.org Last accessed July 1, 2010.
13. LaFond E, Breur GJ & Austin CC: Breed susceptibility for developmental orthopedic diseases in dogs. J Am Anim Hosp Assoc. 2002 Sep-Oct;38(5):467-77.

14. Casal ML, Munuve RM, Janis MA, et. al.: Epilepsy in Irish Wolfhounds. J Vet Intern Med. 2006 Jan-Feb;20(1):131-5.

15. *Ocular Disorders Presumed to be Inherited in Purebred Dogs.* American College of Veterinary Ophthalmologists. ACVO, 2007.

16. Urfer SR, Gaillard C, & Steiger A: Lifespan and disease predispositions in the Irish Wolfhound: a review. Vet Q. 2007 Sep;29(3):102-11.

17. Glickman LT, Glickman NW, Schellenberg DB, et. al.: Incidence of and breed-related risk factors for gastric dilatation-volvulus in dogs. J Am Vet Med Assoc. 2000 Jan 1;216(1):40-5.

18. Nachreiner RF, Refsal KR, Graham PA, et. al.: Prevalence of serum thyroid hormone autoantibodies in dogs with clinical signs of hypothyroidism. *J Am Vet Med Assoc* 2002 Feb 15;220(4):466-71.

19. Nachreiner R & Refsal K: Personal communication, Diagnostic Center for Population and Animal Health, Michigan State University. April, 2007.

20. Kerr MG, van Doorn T: Mass screening of Irish wolfhound puppies for portosystemic shunts by the dynamic bile acid test. *Vet Rec.* 1999 Jun 19;144(25):693-6.

21. Meyer HP, Rothuizen J, Ubbink GJ, et. al.: Increasing incidence of hereditary intrahepatic portosystemic shunts in Irish wolfhounds in The Netherlands (1984 to 1992). *Vet Rec.* 1995 Jan 7;136(1):13-6.

22. Tobias KM, Rohrbach BW: Association of breed with the diagnosis of congenital portosystemic shunts in dogs: 2,400 cases (1980-2002). J Am Vet Med Assoc. 2003 Dec 1;223(11):1636-9.

23. van Steenbeek FG, Leegwater PA, van Sluijs FJ, et. al.: Evidence of inheritance of intrahepatic portosystemic shunts in Irish Wolfhounds. J Vet Intern Med. 2009 Jul-Aug;23(4):950-2.

24. Rudd RG, Whitehair JG, Margolis JH: Results of management of osteochondritis dissecans of the humeral head in dogs : 44 cases (1982 to 1987). J Am Anim Hosp Assoc 1990: 26[2]:173-178.

25. Leisewitz AL, Spencer JA, Jacobson LS, et. al.: Suspected primary immunodeficiency syndrome in three related Irish wolfhounds. *J Small Anim Pract.* 1997 May;38(5):209-12.

26. Clercx C, Reichler I, Peeters D, et. al.: Rhinitis/Bronchopneumonia syndrome in Irish Wolfhounds. *J Vet Intern Med.* 2003 Nov-Dec;17(6):843-9.

27. *The Genetic Connection: A Guide to Health Problems in Purebred Dogs.* L Ackerman. p. 224. AAHA Press, 1999.

28. Junker K, van den Ingh TS, Bossard MM, et. al.: Fibrocartilaginous embolism of the spinal cord (FCE) in juvenile Irish Wolfhounds. *Vet Q.* 2000 Jul;22(3):154-6.

29. Peeters D, Clercx C, Michiels L, et. al.: Juvenile nephropathy in a boxer, a rottweiler, a collie and an Irish wolfhound. *Aust Vet J.* 2000 Mar;78(3):162-5.

30. Vaughan-Scott T, Goldin J, Nesbit JW: Spinal nephroblastoma in an Irish wolfhound. *J S Afr Vet Assoc.* 1999 Mar;70(1):25-8.

31. *The Complete Dog Book, 20th Ed.* The American Kennel Club. Howell Book House, NY 2006. p. 188-191.

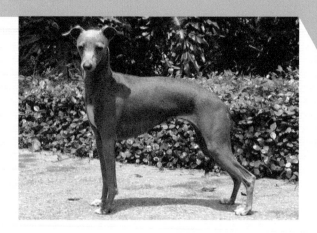

Italian Greyhound

The Breed History

The Italian Greyhound breed origins are not clear, though their place of origin is thought to be in Greece and Turkey, dating to the birth of Christ. In Italy in the 16th century, these dogs were portrayed in artwork of the Renaissance. The English Kennel club listed them in their first studbook, and in the AKC registry, they first appear in 1886, but were rare (less than 50 registrants) until the 1950s.

Breeding for Function

Historically, they were companion dogs and today they can be seen in obedience trials, agility, and in bench shows. They were possibly originally bred for small game hunting, deriving as they do from the sight hound group.

Physical Characteristics

Height at Withers: 13-15" (33-38 cm).

Weight: 5-15 lb (2.3-7 kg).

Coat: Any colors are acceptable except brindle or the black markings associated with black and tan color pattern. These are not accepted in the show ring. The fine, soft, shiny, smooth short haircoat lays flat.

Longevity: 13-14 years

Points of Conformation: The Italian Greyhound looks like a miniature Greyhound, though he is much finer in constitution. The action is much more animated and high stepping. The skull is long and narrow, the stop is slight, and the nose is darkly pigmented. The eyes are dark and medium-sized, ears are small, carried back and folded and the leather is fine; hair on pinnae is silky and short. The neck is long, arched and fine though well-muscled. The topline is curved starting at the loin. The tuck up in the abdomen is pronounced. The thorax is deep and chest is oval in cross section. The limbs are finely boned, long and straight; metacarpals and metatarsals are short. Dewclaws are usually removed. They possess a hare type foot with moderately arched toes. The tail tapers at the tip, though it is very fine along the full length, and is carried low, reaching the tarsus at rest.

Recognized Behavior Issues and Traits

Reported breed characteristics include: Very affectionate, slightly aloof with strangers, adapts well to rural or urban environment, needs regular exercise but quiet around the home. Playful, easy going, sensitive, intelligent, good with other pets and children (gentle ones); they are needy of human contact and do not do well if left alone. An Italian Greyhound demands lots of attention; some have a degree of stubbornness. Easily bored, has a short attention span. For their size, they have a loud bark. Not tolerant of extreme temperature, especially cold. Sweater coverage is needed in cold weather. Overall, not as easy to housetrain as some other breeds. Not an outdoor dog but adaptable to both rural and urban living. The Italian Greyhound is noted for high energy levels, particularly as puppies. In a pack, the dog may be assertive.

Normal Physiologic Variations

Sight hounds have lower normal ranges for T4 and T3 concentrations compared to other breeds.[1]

Drug Sensitivities

Anesthesia: Sight hounds require particular attention during anesthesia. Their lean body conformation with high surface-area-to-volume ratio predisposes them to hypothermia during anesthesia. Impaired biotransformation of drugs by the liver results in prolonged recovery from barbiturate and thiobarbiturate intravenous anesthetics. Propofol, and ketamine/diazepam combination are recommended induction agents.[2]

Inherited Diseases

Patella Luxation: Polygenically inherited laxity of patellar ligaments, causing luxation, lameness, and later degenerative joint disease. Treat surgically if causing clinical signs. OFA reports 3.1% affected.[3]

Elbow Dysplasia: Polygenically inherited trait causing elbow arthritis. Too few Italian Greyhounds have been screened by OFA to determine an accurate frequency.[3]

Hip Dysplasia and Legg-Calve Perthes Disease: Polygenically inherited traits causing degenerative hip joint disease and arthritis. Occuring at a very low frequency in Italian Greyhounds.[3]

Disease Predispositions

Vitreous Degeneration: A liquefaction of the vitreous gel which may predispose to **retinal detachment** or **glaucoma**. Identified in 22.11% of Italian Greyhounds CERF examined by veterinary ophthalmologists between 2000-2005.[4]

Dental Disease: Gingivitis (13.63%), Tooth Loss (9.67%), and **Retained Deciduous Teeth** (8.53%) are reported in the 1993 IGCA Health Survey.[5]

Cryptorchidism: Retained testicles. Can be bilateral or unilateral. Reported at a frequency of 11.26% in the 1993 IGCA Health Survey.[5]

Demodicosis: Demodectic mange dermatitis has an underlying immunodeficiency in its pathogenesis. Primarily seen as a focal disease in young Italian Greyhounds. Reported at a frequency of 10.42% in the 1993 IGCA Health Survey. Unknown mode of inheritance.[5]

Leg Fractures: Seen at an increased frequency due to reduced bone density in thin leg bones. Reported at a frequency of 9.81% in the 1993 IGCA Health Survey.[5]

Inherited Epilepsy: Generalized seizures. Control with anticonvulsant medication. Reported at a frequency of 6.55% in the 1993 IGCA Health Survey. Unknown mode of inheritance.[5]

Cataracts: Anterior or posterior intermediate and punctate cataracts occur in the breed. Onset 2-3 years of age. Identified in 5.86% of Italian Greyhounds CERF examined by veterinary ophthalmologists between 2000-2005. CERF does not recommend breeding any Italian Greyhound with a cataract.[4]

Hypothyroidism: Inherited autoimmune thyroiditis. 4.4% positive for thyroid auto-antibodies based on testing at Michigan State University. (Ave. for all breeds is 7.5%).[6,7]

Color Dilution Alopecia: Hair loss seen in some blue or dilute colored Italian Greyhounds. Reported at a frequency of 3.12% in the 1993 IGCA Health Survey. Unknown mode of inheritance.[5,8]

Deafness: Reported to occur in the breed. Congenital deafness can be unilateral or bilateral. Diagnosed by BAER testing.[9]

Progressive Retinal Atrophy (PRA): PRA is reported to occur in the breed. Causes retinal deterioration and progressive blindness. Identified in 1.89% of Italian Greyhounds CERF examined by veterinary ophthalmologists between 2000-2005. Assumed autosomal recessive inheritance.[4]

Primary Lens Luxation: Occurs at an increased frequency in the breed. Often progresses to secondary glaucoma and blindness. Reported relative risk of 8.44x versus other breeds.[10]

Persistent Pupillary Membranes: Strands of fetal remnant connecting; iris to iris, cornea, lens, or involving sheets of tissue. The later three forms can impair vision, and dogs affected with these forms should not be bred. Identified in 1.00% of Italian Greyhounds CERF examined by veterinary ophthalmologists between 2000-2005.[4]

Hemangiosarcoma and Hemangioma: Italian Greyhounds are at increased risk of developing visceral and nonvisceral hemangiosarcoma and hemangiomas.[11]

Brachygnathism, Corneal Dystrophy, Persistent Right Aortic Arch, Prognathism, and **von Willebrand's Disease** are reported.[12]

Isolated Case Studies
None Reported

Genetic Tests
Tests of Genotype: Direct genetic test for black, brown and fawn is available from HealthGene.

Tests of Phenotype: CHIC Certification: Required testing includes hip radiograph, CERF eye examination (at 36 months and then annually to age 10), thyroid profile including autoantibodies (at 3 years of age), and patella examination. (See CHIC website; www.caninehealthinfo.org).

Recommend elbow radiographs and cardiac examination.

Miscellaneous
- **Breed name synonyms:** Piccolo Levrieri Italiani.
- **Registries:** AKC, UKC, CKC, KCGB (Kennel Club of Great Britain), ANKC (Australian National Kennel Club), NKC (National Kennel Club).
- **AKC rank (year 2008):** 61 (1,450 dogs registered)
- **Internet resources: Italian Greyhound Club of America:** www.italiangreyhound.org
  The Italian Greyhound Club of Canada: www.igcc.ca
  The Italian Greyhound Club UK: www.theitaliangreyhoundclub.co.uk

References

1. Kintzer PP & Peterson ME: Progress in the Diagnosis and Treatment of Canine Hypothyroidism. 2007. Proceedings, ACVIM 2007.
2. Court MH: Anesthesia of the sighthound. Clin Tech Small Anim Pract 1999 Feb;14(1):38-43.
3. OFA Website breed statistics: www.offa.org Last accessed July 1, 2010.
4. *Ocular Disorders Presumed to be Inherited in Purebred Dogs.* American College of Veterinary Ophthalmologists. ACVO, 2007.
5. Italian Greyhound Club of America, Slater M: 1993 Survey on Health Problems in Italian Greyhounds. 1994.
6. Nachreiner RF, Refsal KR, Graham PA, et. al.: Prevalence of serum thyroid hormone autoantibodies in dogs with clinical signs of hypothyroidism. J Am Vet Med Assoc 2002 Feb 15;220(4):466-71.
7. Nachreiner R & Refsal K: Personal communication, Diagnostic Center for Population and Animal Health, Michigan State University. April, 2007.
8. Briggs OM et al. Color mutant alopecia in a blue Italian Greyhound. *J Amer Anim Hosp Assoc.* 1986; 22: 611-14.
9. Strain GM: Deafness prevalence and pigmentation and gender associations in dog breeds at risk. *Vet J.* 2004 Jan;167(1):23-32.
10. Sargan DR, Withers D, Pettitt L, et. al.: Mapping the mutation causing lens luxation in several terrier breeds. J Hered. 2007;98(5):534-8.
11. Schultheiss PC: A retrospective study of visceral and nonvisceral hemangiosarcoma and hemangiomas in domestic animals. *J Vet Diagn Invest.* 2004 Nov;16(6):522-6.
12. *The Genetic Connection: A Guide to Health Problems in Purebred Dogs.* L Ackerman. p. 222. AAHA Press, 1999.
13. *The Complete Dog Book, 20th Ed.* The American Kennel Club. Howell Book House, NY 2006. p. 474-476.

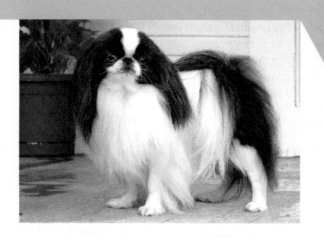

Japanese Chin

The Breed History
The chins were considered *above* regular dogs (inu) in status because of their ancient origins with aristocracy in China. Perhaps the Tibetan Spaniel was a breed ancestor. They were often given as gifts to visiting dignitaries. It is thought that they were given to the emperor of Japan perhaps in the 1700s, where they subsequently became very popular and were then subsequently named the Japanese Chin. In the 1800s some dogs were also given as gifts to Queen Victoria. The AKC first registered the Japanese Chin breed in 1977 using that name rather than the previously applied American designation: Japanese Spaniel (that had first entered the books in 1888). The CKC still retains Japanese Spaniel as the breed name. English breeders are thought to have introduced some Cavalier King Charles spaniel into the bloodlines.

Breeding for Function
Companionship has been the only function of the Japanese Chin.

Physical Characteristics
Height at Withers: 8-11" (20.5-28 cm)

Weight: 4-7 lb (2-3 kg), though some are up to 11 lb (5 kg)—the larger body size is not preferred.

Coat: The single layered soft, silky, thick (profuse) coat is straight. Most dogs are black and white, others are black and white with tan points; other markings may include white with red, lemon, sable and brindle. Markings on the face should be symmetrical—a blaze is preferred, and other markings have a preferred distribution laid out in the breed standard. Coat stands off, and ruff and trousers are present though the head has short hair cover.

Longevity: 12-14 years

Points of Conformation: They possess a high head carriage, square, solid and compact conformation. Movement is animated and straight, and they are described as having an "Oriental" expression. They have dark large eyes, the nose is matched to coat color, and the very heavily plumed tail is carried over the back and may be curved to either side. The muzzle is short, eyes are front facing and widely set, the stop is pronounced, head is broad, and the skull rounded. Note that a bit of white showing in the medial canthus and around the edge of the cornea is considered desirable

in the breed. The small ears are triangular and hang beside the head with copious feathering, and fine leather. The nose is upturned, nostrils wide and it sits between the eyes. The bite is only slightly off ideally. Neck is moderate in length, and muscling, topline is level, and thorax is moderately deep and round. They have a high set tail. The limbs are straight boned and dewclaw removal is optional. Feet are feathered and hare shaped.

Recognized Behavior Issues and Traits
Reported breed characteristics include: Sensitive, friendly, alert and active, tolerates temperature extremes well but should be kept as a housedog. The Chin is generally reserved with strangers, independent minded and even sometimes feisty. They are generally not considered for other than urban or suburban pet and are well suited to apartment life. They have low exercise and grooming needs. They are considered to be somewhat like a cat, being very clean and agile in climbing and jumping and in using their front feet for grasping.

Normal Physiologic Variations
None reported

Drug Sensitivities
None reported

Inherited Diseases
Patella Luxation: Polygenically inherited laxity of patellar ligaments, causing luxation, lameness, and later degenerative joint disease. Treat surgically if causing clinical signs. Reported 4.8x odds ratio versus other breeds. OFA reports 11.5% affected.[1,2]

Hip Dysplasia and Legg-Calve Perthes Disease: Polygenically inherited traits causing degenerative hip joint disease and arthritis. OFA reports 8.3% affected.[1]

Elbow Dysplasia: Polygenically inherited trait causing elbow arthritis. Too few Japanese Chin have been screened by OFA to determine an accurate frequency.[1]

GM2 Gangliosidosis: A rare, autosomal recessive glycogen storage disease causing neurological signs has been identified in young Japanese Chin. The biochemical and histopathologic diagnosis is GM2 gangliosidosis, with an increase in total beta-hexosaminidase activity measured in vitro. A genetic test is available.[9]

Disease Predispositions
Cataracts: Anterior, posterior, and equatorial cortex intermediate and punctate cataracts predominate in the breed. Reported in 4.89% of Japanese Chin presented to veterinary teaching hospitals. Identified in 12.27% of Japanese Chin CERF examined by veterinary ophthalmologists between 2000-2005. CERF does not recommend breeding any Japanese Chin with a cataract.[3,4]

Persistent Pupillary Membranes: Strands of fetal remnant connecting; iris to iris, cornea, lens, or involving sheets of tissue. The later three forms can impair vision, and dogs affected with these forms should not be bred. Identified in 11.19% of Japanese Chin CERF examined by veterinary ophthalmologists between 2000-2005.[3]

Hypothyroidism: Inherited autoimmune thyroiditis. 6.2% positive for thyroid auto-antibodies based on testing at Michigan State University. (Ave. for all breeds is 7.5%).[5,6]

Entropion: Rolling in of the eyelid. Can cause corneal irritation or ulceration. Entropion is reported in 5.42% of Japanese Chin CERF examined by veterinary ophthalmologists between 2000-2005.[3]

Distichiasis: Abnormally placed eyelashes that irritate the cornea and conjunctiva. Can cause secondary corneal ulceration. Identified in 5.05% of Japanese Chin CERF examined by veterinary ophthalmologists between 2000-2005.[3]

Persistent Hyaloid Artery: Congenital defect resulting from abnormalities in the development and regression of the hyaloid artery. Identified in 3.25% of Japanese Chin CERF examined by veterinary ophthalmologists between 2000-2005.[3]

Exposure Keratopathy Syndrome/Pigmentary Keratitis: Corneal reactivity and drying from ocular exposure secondary to shallow orbits, exophthalmos, and lagophthalmos. Identified in 2.53% of Japanese Chin CERF examined by veterinary ophthalmologists between 2000-2005.[3]

Persistent Hyperplastic Tunica Vasculosa Lentis and Primary Vitreous (PHTVL/PHPV): Congenital disorder presenting in the breed with variable lesions from spots on the posterior lens to posterior lenticonus, and posterior polar subcapsular cataracts. Identified in 2.53% of Japanese Chin CERF examined by veterinary ophthalmologists between 2000-2005.[3]

Lens Luxation/Subluxation: Can be primary, or secondary. Identified in 1.44% of Japanese Chin CERF examined by veterinary ophthalmologists between 2000-2005.[3]

Mitral Valve Disease (MVD): Japanese Chin dogs are prone to early age mitral regurgitation. This condition may eventually lead to congestive heart disease, cardiac arrhythmias and cardiac failure. Unknown mode of inheritance. (See JCCA website)

Atlantoaxial Subluxation: Subluxation of the atlantoaxial joint is seen at an increased frequency in the breed. It can occur subsequent to a variety of lesions of the dens or atlantoaxial ligaments. In each case, dorsal displacement of the axis results in compression of the cervical spinal cord. Unknown mode of inheritance.[7]

Epilepsy and **portosystemic (liver) shunts** are reported in the breed.

Cryptorchidism, Elbow Luxation, Hemivertebra, and **Progressive Retinal Atrophy** are reported.[8]

Isolated Case Studies
None reported

Genetic Tests
Tests of Genotype: Direct test for coat colors is available from HealthGene and VetGen.

Direct test for Gen2-gangliosidosis is available from the OFA.

Tests of Phenotype: CHIC Certification: Required testing includes CERF eye examination (minimum 3 years of age), patella examination (minimum 1 year), and cardiac evaluation (minimum 4 years by a cardiologist). (See CHIC website; www.caninehealthinfo.org).

Recommended tests include hip and elbow radiographs, and thyroid profile including autoantibodies.

Miscellaneous
- **Breed name synonyms:** Japanese Spaniel, Chin.
- **Registries:** AKC, UKC, CKC, KCGB (Kennel Club of Great Britain), ANKC (Australian National Kennel Club), NKC (National Kennel Club).
- **AKC rank (year 2008):** 74 (1,066 dogs registered)
- **Internet resources: Japanese Chin Club of America:** http://www.japanesechinonline.org/
  Japanese Chin Club UK: www.japanesechinclub.co.uk/
  Japanese Spaniel Club of Canada: www.japanesespanielclubofcanada.com

References
1. OFA Website breed statistics: www.offa.org Last accessed SJuly 1, 2010.
2. LaFond E, Breur GJ & Austin CC: Breed susceptibility for developmental orthopedic diseases in dogs. J Am Anim Hosp Assoc. 2002 Sep-Oct;38(5):467-77.
3. Ocular Disorders Presumed To Be Inherited In Purebred Dogs. American College Of Veterinary Ophthalmologists. ACVO,2007.
4. Gelatt KN, Mackay EO: Prevalence of primary breed-related cataracts in the dog in North America. Vet Ophthalmol. 2005 Mar-Apr;8(2):101-11.
5. Nachreiner RF, Refsal KR, Graham PA, et. al.: Prevalence of serum thyroid hormone autoantibodies in dogs with clinical signs of hypothyroidism. J Am Vet Med Assoc 2002 Feb 15;220(4):466-71.
6. Nachreiner R & Refsal K: Personal communication, Diagnostic Center for Population and Animal Health, Michigan State University. April, 2007.
7. Axlund TW: Canine Spinal Cord Disease: The Non-painful Diseases. Proceedings, 2004 Atlantic Coast Veterinary Conference. 2004.
8. *The Genetic Connection: A Guide to Health Problems in Purebred Dogs.* L Ackerman. p. 224. AAHA Press, 1999.
9. Cummings JF, Wood PA, Walkley SU, et. al.: GM2 gangliosidosis in a Japanese spaniel. Acta Neuropathol (Berl). 1985;67(3-4):247-53.
10. *The Complete Dog Book, 20th Ed.* The American Kennel Club. Howell Book House, NY 2006. p. 477-480.

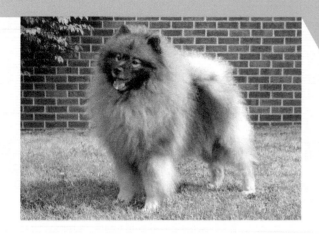

Keeshond

The Breed History
Originating in Holland about 300 years ago, Keeshonden (pl.) are the National Dog of their country. The name derives from the nickname of a politician, **"Kees"**. This Spitz-type dog is related to Northern breeds such as the Samoyed, Norwegian Elkhound and Finnish Spitz. The breed ancestors likely originally came to Holland from the North. Some also link this dog to the development of the Pomeranian. The first breed standard was drawn up in 1933. First AKC registration occurred in 1930. In Europe, they are considered the same breed as the **German Wolfspitz**.

Breeding for Function
The Keeshond has always served a companionship role. They were also used as a barge dog and a watchdog.

Physical Characteristics
Height at Withers: female 17" (43 cm), male 18" (45.5 cm)

Weight: 55-65 lb (25-29.5 kg)

Coat: The hair forms a lion's ruff and trousers particularly in the male, and breed specific markings around the eyes are termed *spectacles*. These markings include dark lines extending out from the eyes. The undercoat is dense and colored gray or cream. The ears are black or off-black, the tip of tail is black, and outer coat hairs are straight and harsh. Black, gray and cream are melded together in the coat, with the tips of the guard hairs colored black. The ruff and trousers are lighter than the main coat color, as are the feet. They go through a high shedding phase twice a year when they blow their coats otherwise they have moderate grooming needs.

Longevity: 12-14 years

Points of Conformation: These dogs are compact and squarely built, with moderately muscled and boned conformation and a profuse standoff coat, a fox face with high head carriage and a heavily plumed tail that rests closely over the back. The eyes are medium-brown in color, almond shaped and the palpebral margins are pigmented black. Ears are small and erect, high set, and the skull is wedge shaped with a definite stop. Lips are black and tight, neck is moderate in length, and the topline descends slightly towards the rear. The thorax is rounded, the abdomen has moderate tuck up, and limbs are straight boned. Feet are rounded and compact with black nails. The gait is strong, showing lots of drive.

Recognized Behavior Issues and Traits
Reported breed attributes include: Stable temperament, a good alert dog, playful, friendly with other dogs and especially good with children, though independent minded. They don't tend to nuisance bark. Their trainability is good. They don't tolerate hot humid weather very well. The do well in city or country settings.

Normal Physiologic Variations
Tendency to become overweight.

Drug Sensitivities
None reported

Inherited Diseases
Elbow Dysplasia: Polygenically inherited trait causing elbow arthritis. OFA reports 7.8% affected.[1]

Hip Dysplasia: Polygenically inherited trait causing degenerative joint disease and hip arthritis. OFA reports 6.3% affected.[1]

Patella Luxation: Polygenically inherited laxity of patellar ligaments, causing luxation, lameness, and later degenerative joint disease. Treat surgically if causing clinical signs. Reported 4.4x odds ratio versus other breeds. OFA reports 2.6% affected.[1,2]

Primary Hyperparathyroidism: Autosomal dominant disorder with age-dependant penetrance. Average age of onset is 11.2 years. Affected dogs present with hypercalcemia, inappetence, polyuria, polydipsia, and vomiting. Caused by a parathyroid gland adenoma. Progresses to hypercalcemic kidney failure. Reported at a frequency of 1.87% in the KCA Health Survey 2000. A linked-marker genetic test is available, reporting 4.1% affected.[1,3,4,5,6,7]

Cono-Truncal Septal Defect: A group of genetically and embryologically related cardiac malformations, including sub-clinical defects of the conal septum, conal ventricular septal defects, tetralogy of Fallot, and persistent truncus arteriosus. Three predisposing gene markers are identified, showing a polygenic mode of inheritance.[8,9]

Disease Predispositions
Hypothyroidism: Inherited autoimmune thyroiditis. 6.4% positive for thyroid auto-antibodies based on testing at Michigan State University. (Ave. for all breeds is 7.5%).[10,11]

Distichiasis: Abnormally placed eyelashes that irritate the cornea and conjunctiva. Can cause secondary corneal ulceration. Identified in 5.66% of Keeshonden CERF examined by veterinary ophthalmologists between 2000-2005.[12]

Cataracts: Posterior suture punctate cataracts predominate in the breed. Age of onset 1-3 years. Identified in 5.27% of Keeshonden CERF examined by veterinary ophthalmologists between 2000-2005. CERF does not recommend breeding any Keeshond with a cataract.[12]

Allergic Dermatitis (Atopy): Inhalant or food allergy. Presents with pruritis and pyotraumatic dermatitis (hot spots). Reported at a frequency of 3.19% in the KCA Health Survey 2000.[6]

Inherited Epilepsy: Generalized or partial seizures. Control with anticonvulsant medication. Age of onset 6 months to 3 years. Dorn reports a 9.36x odds ratio versus other breeds. One study suggests an autosomal recessive mode of inheritance. Seizures are reported at a frequency of 2.88% in the KCA Health Survey 2000.[6,13,14]

Alopecia-X (Coat Funk): Progressive, symmetrical, non-pruritic, truncal hair loss usually beginning in early adulthood. ACTH stimulation test, low-dose dexamethazone stimulation test, and thyroid panel results are normal. Elevated blood concentrations of 17-hydroxyprogesterone (17-OHP) are seen post ACTH stimulation. Partial hair regrowth is reported in Keeshonden treated with melatonin. Reported at a frequency of 2.41% in the KCA Health Survey 2000. Unknown mode of inheritance.[6,15,16]

Juvenile Diabetes Mellitus: Caused by a lack of insulin production by the pancreas. Controlled by insulin injections, diet, and glucose monitoring. Affected dogs also form glucose-related cataracts. Age of onset 2-6 months. Breeding studies suggest an autosomal recessive mode of inheritance. Reported at a frequency of 0.78% in the KCA Health Survey 2000.[6,17,18]

Bladder Stones: One study reports a 5.47x odds ratio of forming calcium oxalate stones versus other breeds. Dorn reports a 2.81x odds ratio versus other breeds. Composition of calculi not reported. Reported at a frequency of 0.31% in the KCA Health Survey 2000.[6,19,20]

Spontaneous Chronic Corneal Epithelial Defects (SCCED): Keeshonden are reported as a breed with an increased prevalence of spontaneous corneal epithelial defects. Research indicates a role of substance P.[21]

Central progressive Retinal Atrophy, Cutaneous Asthenia, Optic Nerve Hypoplasia, Oligodontia, and **von Willebrand's Disease** are reported.[22]

Isolated Case Studies

Renal Cortical Hypoplasia: Congenital kidney disease was reported in a litter of Keeshonds.[23]

Malignant Fibrous Histiocytoma: Identified in a retrobulbar location in a 12-year-old castrated male Keeshond dog.[24]

Genetic Tests

Tests of Genotype: Linked marker test is available for Primary Hyperparathyroidism from the Goldstein lab at Cornell (www.vet.cornell.edu/labs/goldstein/).

Tests of Phenotype: CHIC Certification: Hip and elbow radiographs, CERF eye examination, and patella evaluation. (See CHIC website; www.caninehealthinfo.org).

Recommend thyroid profile including autoantibodies and cardiac examination.

Miscellaneous

- **Breed name synonyms:** Keeshound, Wolfspitz (German), Chien Loup (Fr.), Lupini (Italy), Dutch Barge Dog (historical-England), Dutch Keeshond.
- **Registries:** AKC, UKC, CKC, KCGB (Kennel Club of Great Britain), ANKC (Australian National Kennel Club), NKC (National Kennel Club)
- **AKC rank (year 2008):** 95 (630 dogs registered)
- **Internet resources:** The Keeshond Club of America: www.keeshond.org
  The Keeshond Club UK: www.keeshondclub.org.uk
  The Keeshond Club of Canada: www.keeshondcanada.com

References

1. OFA Website breed statistics: www.offa.org Last accessed July 1, 2010.
2. LaFond E, Breur GJ & Austin CC: Breed susceptibility for developmental orthopedic diseases in dogs. J Am Anim Hosp Assoc. 2002 Sep-Oct;38(5):467-77.
3. Weir EC, Norrdin RW, Barthold SW, et. al.: Primary hyperparathyroidism in a dog: biochemical, bone histomorphometric, and pathologic findings. J Am Vet Med Assoc. 1986 Dec 1;189(11):1471-4.
4. Skelly B: Hyperparathyroidism in the keeshond dog. Vet Rec. 2004 May 22;154(21):672.
5. Gear RN, Neiger R, Skelly BJ, et. al.: Primary hyperparathyroidism in 29 dogs: diagnosis, treatment, outcome and associated renal failure. J Small Anim Pract. 2005 Jan;46(1):10-6.
6. Keeshond Club of America: KCA 2000 Health Survey.
7. Goldstein RE, Atwater DZ, Cazolli DM, et. al.: Inheritance, mode of inheritance, and candidate genes for primary hyperparathyroidism in Keeshonden. J Vet Intern Med. 2007 Jan-Feb;21(1):199-203.
8. Patterson DF, Pyle RL, Van Mierop L, et. al.: Hereditary defects the conotruncal septum in Keeshond dogs: pathologic and genetic studies. Am J Cardiol. 1974 Aug;34(2):187-205.
9. Werner P, Raducha MG, Prociuk U, et. al.: The keeshond defect in cardiac conotruncal development is oligogenic. Hum Genet. 2005 Apr;116(5):368-77
10. Nachreiner RF, Refsal KR, Graham PA, et. al.: Prevalence of serum thyroid hormone autoantibodies in dogs with clinical signs of hypothyroidism. J Am Vet Med Assoc 2002 Feb 15;220(4):466-71.
11. Nachreiner R & Refsal K: Personal communication, Diagnostic Center for Population and Animal Health, Michigan State University. April, 2007.
12. Ocular Disorders Presumed to be Inherited in Purebred Dogs. American College of Veterinary Ophthalmologists. ACVO, 2007.
13. Hall SJ, Wallace ME: Canine epilepsy: a genetic counselling programme for keeshonds. Vet Rec. 1996 Apr 13;138(15):358-60.
14. Wallace ME: Keeshonds: a genetic study of epilepsy and EEG readings. J Small Anim Pract. 1975 Jan;16(1):1-10.
15. Frank LA, Hnilica KA, Oliver JW: Adrenal steroid hormone concentrations in dogs with hair cycle arrest (Alopecia X) before and during treatment with melatonin and mitotane. Vet Dermatol. 2004 Oct;15(5):278-84.
16. Frank LA, Hnilica KA, Rohrbach BW, et. al.: Retrospective evaluation of sex hormones and steroid hormone intermediates in dogs with alopecia. Vet Dermatol. 2003 Apr;14(2):91-7.
17. Kramer JW, Klaassen JK, Baskin DG, et. al.: Inheritance of diabetes mellitus in Keeshond dogs. Am J Vet Res. 1988 Mar;49(3):428-31.
18. Kramer JW, Nottingham S, Robinette J, et. al.: Inherited, early onset,

insulin-requiring diabetes mellitus of Keeshond dogs. *Diabetes.* 1980 Jul;29(7):558-65.

19. Dorn CR: Canine breed-specific risks of frequently diagnosed diseases at veterinary teaching hospitals. Monograph. AKC Canine Health Foundation. 2000.

20. Lekcharoensuk C, Lulich JP, Osborne CA, et. al.: Patient and environmental factors associated with calcium oxalate urolithiasis in dogs. J Am Vet Med Assoc. 2000 Aug 15;217(4):515-9.

21. Murphy CJ, Marfurt CF, McDermott A, et. al.: Spontaneous chronic corneal epithelial defects (SCCED) in dogs: clinical features, innervation, and effect of topical SP, with or without IGF-1. *Invest Ophthalmol Vis Sci.* 2001 Sep;42(10):2252-61.

22. *The Genetic Connection: A Guide to Health Problems in Purebred Dogs.* L Ackerman. p. 224-5. AAHA Press, 1999.

23. Klopfer U, Neumann F, Trainin R: Renal cortical hypoplasia in a Keeshond litter. *Vet Med Small Anim Clin.* 1975 Sep;70(9):1081-3.

24. Lassaline ME, Gelatt KN, Brooks DE, et. al.: Orbitotomy for retrobulbar malignant fibrous histiocytoma in a dog. *Vet Ophthalmol.* 2005 Jan-Feb;8(1):1-6.

25. *The Complete Dog Book, 20th Ed.* The American Kennel Club. Howell Book House, NY 2006. p. 567-571.

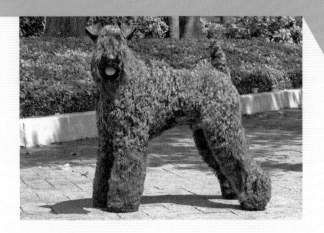

The Breed History

In counties Kerry, Tipperary, and elsewhere in Ireland the breed was selected as an all-round utility dog for the farm. It is reported that the Soft-coated Wheaten terrier, perhaps the Irish Wolfhound, and Bedlington and Welsh terriers contributed to breed development. Much of the breed development occurred in the 1800s. The breed standard was written in 1922. First exports to the USA occurred in 1918. The AKC first recognized the breed in 1924.

Breeding for Function

Some of the tasks the Kerry Blue excelled at included dry and wet retrieving, small game hunting, birddog, and sheep and cattle herding. Watchdog, companion, and police work round out his many modern accomplishments.

Physical Characteristics

Height at Withers: female 17.5-19" (44.5-48 cm), male 18-19.5" (45.5-49.5 cm)

Weight: 33-40 lb (15-18 kg)

Coat: The coat is dense and hairs are wavy and soft in texture. It takes about 1 1/2 years for the adult coat to mature. Puppies are often black and during early maturity, very dark gray and brownish hair may intermingle in the coat until they are gradually replaced by the correct final hair color of blue (this correct color varies from light gray-blue to deep slate gray). Extremities may keep a darker color. Black adults are not accepted.

Longevity: 14+ years

Points of Conformation: This breed is characterized by a sturdy conformation with lots of muscle and bone, and small dark eyes somewhat deep set, triangular ears that are small with moderately thick leather and folded forward. The ear fold is above the topline of the skull. The skull is flat with a very minimal stop. The nose is black. The neck is moderately long and strong, not throaty. The topline is short and level, and there is a slight abdominal tuck. The tail is high set, and carried high. The thorax is deep and somewhat narrow, metatarsals and metacarpals are short and sturdy. Feet are compact, small, and with deep strong footpads with black toenails. Rear dewclaws disqualify. Gait is smooth, true, elastic and ground covering with good rear drive.

Recognized Behavior Issues and Traits

Reported breed attributes include: They are considered to be good guard dogs. Kerry Blues get along with children well and tolerate play. They commonly exhibit inter-male aggression. They require an early introduction to and supervision with cats or other small pets. They have a low barking tendency, are diggers, and need regular exercise and stimulating games. Intelligent, but easily bored, they have an independent streak and can be stubborn. They need close human contact, and do not do well as kenneled dogs. The Kerry Blue does not tolerate hot weather well.

Normal Physiologic Variations

No undercoat, a no-shedding dog, though care of the coat should be done regularly to keep it tidy. Considered a high grooming needs dog. Reportedly no doggy odor even when wet.

Drug Sensitivities

None reported

Inherited Diseases

Hip Dysplasia and Legg–Calve Perthes Disease: Polygenically inherited traits causing degenerative hip joint disease and arthritis. OFA reports 5.9% affected.[1]

Elbow Dysplasia: Polygenically inherited trait causing elbow arthritis. OFA reports 5.0% affected.[1]

Patella Luxation: Polygenically inherited laxity of patellar ligaments, causing luxation, lameness, and later degenerative joint disease. Treat surgically if causing clinical signs. Too few Kerry Blue Terriers have been screened by OFA to determine an accurate frequency.[1]

von Willebrand's Disease Type 1 (vWD): Autosomal recessive genetic disorder causing a mild bleeding syndrome, usually after trauma or surgery. A genetic test is available.[2]

Progressive Neuronal Abiotrophy (PNA, Multiple System Degeneration): Fatal, autosomal recessive cerebellar disorder, with an onset between 9 and 16 weeks of age. Progresses to incapacity by 4-8 months of age. Histopathology shows progressive loss of cerebellar cortical Purkinje's cells, with bilateral symmetric degeneration of the olivary nuclei followed by degeneration of the substantia nigra and caudate nucleus. No genetic test is available.[3,4]

Factor XI Deficiency: Rare, autosomal recessive bleeding disorder causing a tendency for mild posttraumatic or postoperative bleeding. Clotting tests show a prolonged activated partial thromboplastin and activated clotting times. Treat with fresh-frozen plasma. A genetic test is available.[5]

Disease Predispositions

Sebaceous Cysts: Benign follicular skin cysts. Reported at a frequency of 22.7% in the KBTF Health Survey 2004. Unknown mode of inheritance.[6]

Spiculosis (Hard Hairs, Spikes): Hard keratinized hairs produced by abnormal hair follicles. Reported at a frequency of 6.7% in the KBTF Health Survey 2004. Unknown mode of inheritance.[6,7]

Cataracts: Anterior cortex punctate and posterior suture intermediate cataracts predominate in the breed. Reported at a frequency of 4.7% in the KBTF Health Survey 2004. Identified in 3.52% of Kerry Blue Terriers CERF examined by veterinary ophthalmologists between 2000-2005. CERF does not recommend breeding any Kerry Blue Terrier with a cataract.[6,8]

Keratoconjunctivitis Sicca (KCS, Dry Eye): Inadequate tear production causing drying of the cornea and conjunctiva. Reported at a frequency of 3.4% in the KBTF Health Survey 2004.[6]

Premolar Hypodontia: Multiple missing premolar syndromes are reported in the breed. The absence of the second premolars appears to be an autosomal recessive disorder, while missing fourth premolars appears to have a more complex, polygenic mode of inheritance. Studies show that Kerry Blue Terriers with missing teeth have smaller litter sizes (ave. 3.64 versus 5.72) suggesting a pleiotrophic effect. Missing teeth are reported at a frequency of 3.3% in the KBTF Health Survey 2004.[6,9,10,11]

Food Allergy (Food Hypersensitivity/Food Intolerance): Presents with pruritis and pyotraumatic dermatitis (hot spots). Average age of onset of 1.7 years. Reported at a frequency of 3.3% in the KBTF Health Survey 2004.[6]

Hypothyroidism: Inherited autoimmune thyroiditis. 2.6% positive for thyroid autoantibodies based on testing at Michigan State University. (Ave. for all breeds is 7.5%).[12,13]

Colitis/Chronic Large Bowel Diarrhea: Onset usually prior to 3 years of age. Reported at a frequency of 2.7% in the KBTF Health Survey 2004.[6]

Degenerative Myelopathy (DM): Affected dogs show an insidious onset of upper motor neuron (UMN) paraparesis at an average age of 11.4 years. The disease eventually progresses to severe tetraparesis with lower motor neuron signs. Affected dogs have normal results on myelography, MRI, and CSF analysis. Necropsy confirms the condition. Unknown mode of inheritance. A direct genetic test for an autosomal recessive DM susceptibility gene is available. All affected dogs are homozygous for the gene, however, only a small percentage of homozygous dogs develop DM. OFA reports DM susceptibility gene frequencies of 44% carrier, and 12% homozygous "at-risk". Clinical DM is reported at a frequency of 2.18% in the KBTC Health Survey 2004.[1,6,14,15]

Persistent Pupillary Membranes: Strands of fetal remnant connecting; iris to iris, cornea, lens, or involving sheets of tissue. The later three forms can impair vision, and dogs affected with these forms should not be bred. Identified in 1.76% of Kerry Blue Terriers CERF examined by veterinary ophthalmologists between 2000-2005.[8]

Distichiasis: Abnormally placed eyelashes that irritate the cornea and conjunctiva. Can cause secondary corneal ulceration. Identified in 1.32% of Kerry Blue Terriers CERF examined by veterinary ophthalmologists between 2000-2005.[8]

Vitreous Degeneration: A liquefaction of the vitreous gel which may predispose to retinal detachment and/or glaucoma. Identified in 1.32% of Kerry Blue Terriers CERF examined by veterinary ophthalmologists between 2000-2005.[8]

Craniomandibular Osteopathy, Dermoid Sinus, Entropion, Patent Ductus Arteriosus, Progressive Retinal Atrophy, and **XX Sex Reversal** are reported.[16]

Isolated Case Studies

Congenital Intestinal Atresia: Case report of a Kerry Blue Terrier with an undeveloped intestinal tract.[17]

Genetic Tests

Tests of Genotype: Direct gene test for vWD is available from VetGen.

Direct test for an autosomal recessive DM susceptibility gene is available from OFA.

Direct gene test for Factor XI deficiency is available from PennGen.

Tests of Phenotype: CHIC certification: Required testing includes hip radiographs and CERF eye examination. Optional testing includes direct tests for von Willebrands disease, Factor XI deficiency, and the susceptibility gene for DM. (See CHIC Website: www.caninehealthinfo.org)

Recommend thyroid profile including autoantibodies, elbow radiographs, patella evaluation, and cardiac examination.

Miscellaneous

- **Breed name synonyms:** Kerry Blue, Irish Blue Terrier
- **Registries:** AKC, UKC, CKC, KCGB (Kennel Club of Great Britain), ANKC (Australian National Kennel Club)
- **AKC rank (year 2008):** 120 (274 dogs registered)
- **Internet resources:** United States Kerry Blue Terrier Club: www.uskbtc.com
  The Kerry Blue Terrier Club of Canada: www.kbtcc.ca

References

1. OFA Website breed statistics: www.offa.org Last accessed July 1, 2010.
2. Wardrop KJ: Canine von Willebrand Disease. Proceedings, 2004 Western Veterinary Conference. 2004.
3. O'brien DP, Johnson GS, Schnabel RD, et. al.: Genetic mapping of canine multiple system degeneration and ectodermal dysplasia Loci. *J Hered.* 2005 Nov-Dec;96(7):727-34.
4. deLahunta A, Averill DR Jr: Hereditary cerebellar cortical and extrapyramidal nuclear abiotrophy in Kerry Blue Terriers. *J Am Vet Med Assoc.* 1976 Jun 15;168(12):1119-24.
5. Knowler C, Giger U, Dodds WJ, et. al.: Factor XI deficiency in Kerry Blue Terriers. *J Am Vet Med Assoc.* 1994 Dec 1;205(11):1557-61.
6. Kerry Blue Terrier Foundation, Sell E: Health Survey 2004. 2004.
7. McKeever PJ, Torres SMF, O'Brien TD: Spiculosis. J Am Anim Hosp Assoc 1992: 28[3]:257-262.
8. *Ocular Disorders Presumed to be Inherited in Purebred Dogs.* American College of Veterinary Ophthalmologists. ACVO, 2007.
9. Aksenovich TI, Zorkal'tsov IV, Aul'chenko IuS, et. al.: Inheritance of hypodontia in Kerry Blue Terrier dogs. *Genetika.* 2004 May;40(5):658-66.
10. Zorkaltseva IV, Akberdin IR, Kulikova AV, et. al.: Changes in litter size in Kerry blue terrier dogs with abnormal dentition. Genetika. 2006 Mar;42(3):427-9.

11. Aksenovich TI, Kulikova AV, Kniazev SP, et. al.: Polymorphism of dental formula and segregation of its variants in a pedigree of kerry blue terrier dogs. Genetika. 2006 Mar;42(3):414-20.

12. Nachreiner RF, Refsal KR, Graham PA, et. al.: Prevalence of serum thyroid hormone autoantibodies in dogs with clinical signs of hypothyroidism. J Am Vet Med Assoc 2002 Feb 15;220(4):466-71.

13. Nachreiner R & Refsal K: Personal communication, Diagnostic Center for Population and Animal Health, Michigan State University. April, 2007.

14. Shelton GD, Johnson GC, Johnson GS, et. al.: Peripheral Nerve Pathology in Canine Degenerative Myelopathy with Mutation in Superoxide Dismutase 1 Gene. Proceedings, 2009 ACVIM Forum. 2009.

15. Coates JR, Zeng R, Awano T, et. al.: An SOD1 Mutation Associated with Degenerative Myelopathy Occurs in Many Dog Breeds. Proceedings 2009 ACVIM Forum. 2009.

16. *The Genetic Connection: A Guide to Health Problems in Purebred Dogs.* L Ackerman. p. 225. AAHA Press, 1999.

17. Gough J: Congenital intestinal atresia in a Kerry blue terrier. *Can Vet J.* 1999 Nov;40(11):809.

18. *The Complete Dog Book, 20th Ed.* The American Kennel Club. Howell Book House, NY 2006. p. 387-390.

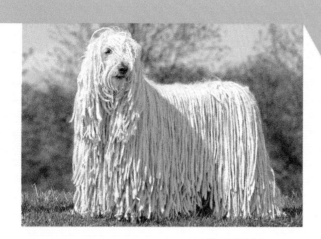

Komondor

Longevity: 12 years

Points of Conformation: The Komondor is large, with a large head and a distinctive coat of tightly coiled cords of hair. The thick haircoat covers all parts of the body. This well-muscled dog has a very heavy boned constitution. Eyes are dark brown in color, medium-sized and almond shaped. The palpebral margins are pigmented black or gray. Lip margins are black, and the nose is large and black, though a dark brown or gray nose is also accepted, stop is moderate. Ears are triangular, and fold to hang parallel to the face. Gingiva and palate tissues are usually also pigmented black. The neck is medium in length and arching with no throatiness. The topline is level, the thorax is deep and the abdomen moderately tucked up. The tail reaches the tarsus and is slightly curved and carried below the topline. Legs are straight boned and feet are large with toes well-knuckled up. Black nails are preferred. Rear dewclaws are removed in North America. The gait is long-strided and smooth; he covers lots of ground with a high level of agility.

Recognized Behavior Issues and Traits
Reported breed characteristics include: Devoted to their owners, reserved with strangers; don't tend to wander away from their home; excellent guard of home and family. They will follow their charges around the house in order to keep an eye on them. Early socialization and obedience training are important due to the well-developed guarding instinct. If not properly trained, may exhibit sudden aggression if a threat is perceived. Easily bored, and have strong talent for independent thinking so obedience training can be challenging. The Komondor has a high barking tendency; good alarm barker but calm when nothing threatens. Due to large body size and exercise needs, the Komondor is not a suitable apartment pet though he does have low activity levels and exercise needs as an adult.

Normal Physiologic Variations
The breed is considered slow to mature.

Drug Sensitivities
None Reported

Inherited Diseases
Hip Dysplasia: Polygenically inherited trait causing degenerative joint disease and hip arthritis. OFA reports 12.2% affected.[1]

Elbow Dysplasia: Polygenically inherited trait causing elbow arthritis. OFA reports 2.9% affected.[1]

Patella Luxation: Polygenically inherited laxity of patellar ligaments, causing luxation, lameness, and later degenerative joint disease. Treat surgically if causing clinical signs. Too few Komondorok have been screened by OFA to determine an accurate frequency.[1]

The Breed History
Komondorok (plural for Komondor) are ancient Hungarian working dogs. They are descended from the Aftscharka (some term them Owtcharka), a type of dogs originating in Russia. The Maygars that bred these dogs never allowed crossbreeding so the breed was closed for perhaps a millennium. This is not confirmed by written records, since none were kept, but by oral tradition and stories. First formal records date to the 16th century. The Komondorok almost became extinct during the Second World War. The Komondor is of a much larger and heavier build than the Hungarian Puli. The AKC recognized this rare breed in 1937.

Breeding for Function
Centuries of breeding led to a heavily coated dog that could tolerate low temperatures, important since they often lived outdoors. His function in the sheep and cattle herd was to be a protector (against wolves, bears and poachers), rather than acting as a herder. He was expected to be courageous, vigilant and self-reliant. Self-reliance was important because he was expected to act without herder commands. The white coat color may have helped him blend in with sheep herds so that predators would be surprised.

Physical Characteristics
Height at Withers: female 25.5" or taller (65 cm), male 27.5" or taller (70 cm).

Weight: females 80 lb or more (36.5 kg), males 100 lb or more (45.5 kg).

Coat: All-white, though a hint of buff or cream, especially in young dogs is seen. The corded double coat that reaches the ground takes at least 2 years to grow. Puppies appear to have a fluffy coat. Cording starts at close to 1 year of age. In the adult, there remains a wooly undercoat entwined in the cords. This gives the cords a soft "felt" feel.

No grooming is required but the ears need to be plucked and cleaned regularly, hair of the feet trimmed and cords need to be kept clean. As cords develop the fingers can be used to help divide hair into distinct quarter-sized cords, and the cords can be trimmed as needed. After bathing, the coat must be fully dried to prevent mildew in the cords.

Disease Predispositions

Cataracts: Anterior and equatorial cortex intermediate cataracts predominate in the breed, with an onset of 2-3 years. Juvenile cataracts are also reported to occur. Cataracts are identified in 7.14% of Komondorok CERF examined by veterinary ophthalmologists between 2000-2005. CERF does not recommend breeding any Komondor with a cataract.[2]

Hypothyroidism: Inherited autoimmune thyroiditis. 6.3% positive for thyroid auto-antibodies based on testing at Michigan State University. (Ave. for all breeds is 7.5%).[3,4]

Persistent Pupillary Membranes: Strands of fetal remnant connecting; iris to iris, cornea, lens, or involving sheets of tissue. The later three forms can impair vision, and dogs affected with these forms should not be bred. Identified in 2.38% of Komondorok CERF examined by veterinary ophthalmologists between 2000-2005.[2]

Gastric Dilation/Volvulus (Bloat): Life-threatening twisting of the stomach within the abdomen. Requires immediate veterinary attention. Unknown mode of inheritance.[5]

Entropion: Rolling in of the eyelid. Can cause corneal irritation. Entropion is reported in 1.19% of Komondorok CERF-examined by veterinary ophthalmologists between 2000-2005.[2]

Oligodontia, Prognathism, and **Retained Primary Teeth** are reported.[6]

Isolated Case Studies
None Reported

Genetic Tests

Tests of Genotype: None

Tests of Phenotype: Recommend hip and elbow radiographs, CERF eye examination, patella evaluation, thyroid profile including autoantibodies and cardiac examination.

Miscellaneous
- **Breed name synonyms:** Hungarian Sheepdog.
- **Registries:** AKC, UKC, CKC, KCGB (Kennel Club of Great Britain), ANKC (Australian National Kennel Club).
- **AKC rank (year 2008):** 151 (60 dogs registered)
- **Internet resources: The Komondor Club of America Inc.:** http://clubs.akc.org/kca/
  Komondor Club of Great Britain: www.komondor.co.uk/

References

1. OFA Website breed statistics: www.offa.org Last accessed July 1, 2010.
2. *Ocular Disorders Presumed to be Inherited in Purebred Dogs.* American College of Veterinary Ophthalmologists. ACVO, 2007.
3. Nachreiner RF, Refsal KR, Graham PA, et. al.: Prevalence of serum thyroid hormone autoantibodies in dogs with clinical signs of hypothyroidism. J Am Vet Med Assoc 2002 Feb 15;220(4):466-71.
4. Nachreiner R & Refsal K: Personal communication, Diagnostic Center for Population and Animal Health, Michigan State University. April, 2007.
5. Matushek KJ & Cockshutt JR: Mesenteric and gastric volvulus in a dog. J Am Vet Med Assoc. 1987 Aug 1;191(3):327-8.
6. *The Genetic Connection: A Guide to Health Problems in Purebred Dogs.* L Ackerman. p. 225. AAHA Press, 1999.
7. *The Complete Dog Book, 20th Ed.* The American Kennel Club. Howell Book House, NY 2006. p. 284-287.

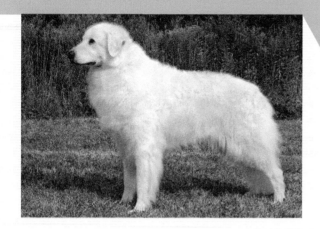

Kuvasz

The Breed History

The breed traces back perhaps five thousand years, and through much of this time, this dog was a favorite of the ruling class. The breed name derives from the Turkish word *kawasz*, which translates as "armed guard of nobility", or perhaps Arabic *kawwasz*, meaning archer. Breed ancestors were larger, and likely came from Tibet. The Komondor is likely related to this breed, and less well documented are possible ties to the Maremma Sheepdog and Akbash dog. Hungarian fanciers were responsible for much of the breed evolution and standardization. AKC recognition occured in 1931.

Breeding for Function

In early times, he was a valued guard dog. Later, once the nobility lost exclusive ownership, they were adapted for herding tasks as guards of the flock or herd. Now they are often kept for companionship.

Physical Characteristics

Height at Withers: female 26-28" (66-71 cm), male 28-30" (71-76.2 cm)

Weight: females 70-90 lb (32-41 kg), males 100-115 lb (45.5-52.5 kg).

Coat: The thick double coat is always white. The outer coat is coarse and straight to wavy, while the undercoat is fine and short. Coat length varies with the season. Skin is darkly pigmented.

Longevity: 8-12 years.

Points of Conformation: Strong build with medium bone, head is elongated, stop is defined, the muzzle is somewhat tapering, lips are pigmented black and fit close. The inside of the mouth is preferred black. The eyes are wide set and almond shaped, colored dark brown and the nictitans should not show. The nose is black and pointed. Ears are triangular with slight rounding at the tips, thick leathered, and folded. The neck is medium in length, well muscled and arched. For topline, the scapulae sit above the back, and the topline is straight until it slopes at the croup. Thorax is deep, while the fore-chest is prominent and ribs are well sprung. The abdomen is well tucked up. The tail reaches the tarsus, limbs are straight and dewclaws are left on in front, but removed behind, nails preferred dark. The feet are compact and round, though the rear feet may be longer. The gait is elastic and smooth, agile, low and long.

Recognized Behavior Issues and Traits

They are noted to be sensitive, devoted, protective, wary with strangers, courageous, intelligent, and possessing a gentle temperament when not guarding. They also go through seasonal shedding, are slow to mature, need early socialization and obedience training if adopted as a family dog with children and other pets, are independent minded, and some are aggressive. These dogs are not best for owners that have not handled dogs before. They also need regular exercise and games, and lots of human contact or they will develop boredom vices. They have average to high grooming needs.

Normal Physiologic Variations

None reported

Drug Sensitivities

None reported

Inherited Diseases

Hip Dysplasia: Polygenically inherited trait causing degenerative joint disease and hip arthritis. Reported 10.2x odds ratio versus other breeds. OFA reports 18.4% affected.[1,2]

Elbow Dysplasia: Polygenically inherited trait causing elbow arthritis. OFA reports 6.7% affected.[1]

Progressive Retinal Atrophy (PRA): Autosomal recessive progressive rod cone degeneration (prcd) form. Age of onset between 4-7 years, eventually causing blindness. CERF does not recommend breeding any Kuvaszok with PRA. A genetic test is available, showing a high frequency of carrier and affected dogs in the breed.[3]

Patella Luxation: Polygenically inherited laxity of patellar ligaments, causing luxation, lameness, and later degenerative joint disease. Treat surgically if causing clinical signs. OFA reports 0.8% affected.[1]

Disease Predispositions

Hypothyroidism: Inherited autoimmune thyroiditis. 15.1% positive for thyroid autoantibodies based on testing at Michigan State University. (Ave. for all breeds is 7.5%).[4,5]

Distichiasis: Abnormally placed eyelashes that irritate the cornea and conjunctiva. Can cause secondary corneal ulceration. Identified in 6.20% of Kuvaszok CERF examined by veterinary ophthalmologists between 2000-2005.[3]

Persistent Pupillary Membranes: Strands of fetal remnant connecting; iris to iris, cornea, lens, or involving sheets of tissue. The later three forms can impair vision, and dogs affected with these forms should not be bred. Identified in 4.65% of Kuvaszok CERF examined by veterinary ophthalmologists between 2000-2005.[3]

Humeral Osteochondritis Dissecans: Polygenically inherited cartilage defect of the humeral head. Causes shoulder joint pain and lameness in young growing dogs. Mild cases can resolve with rest, while more severe cases require surgery. There is a 2.24:1 male to female ratio. 75% of all cases are unilateral. Reported 29.1x odds ratio versus other breeds. Reported at a frequency of 2.96% in the Kuvasz.[2,6]

Corneal Dystrophy: The epithelial/stromal and endothelial forms occur in the breed, causing a bilateral, white to gray, non-inflammatory corneal opacity. Identified in 2.83% of Kuvaszok CERF examined by veterinary ophthalmologists between 2000-2005. CERF does not recommend breeding Kuvaszok with corneal dystrophy.[3]

Cataracts: Posterior cortical punctate cataracts predominate in the breed. Identified in 2.33% of Kuvaszok CERF examined by veterinary ophthalmologists between 2000-2005. CERF does not recommend breeding any Kuvaszok with a cataract.[3]

Hypertrophic Osteodystrophy (HOD): Puppies generally show swollen, painful ends of long bones and may have a fever as well as loss of appetite. If these puppies are not diagnosed early permanent damage may necessitate euthanasia. Research with Great Danes (the breed showing a relatively high incidence of H.O.D.) shows that a high energy, high protein diet or excess supplementation may predispose puppies to H.O.D. Treatment consists of putting the affected animal onto a high quality but more moderate diet as well as using analgesics to encourage the puppy to eat and stay mobile. The typical age of onset 12-20 weeks. Seen at a low frequency in the breed. (See KCA website)

Deafness: Congenital deafness occurs in the breed. Can be unilateral or bilateral. Diagnosed by BAER testing. Unknown mode of inheritance.[7]

Degenerative Myelopathy (DM): Affected dogs show an insidious onset of upper motor neuron (UMN) paraparesis at an average age of 11.4 years. The disease eventually progresses to severe tetraparesis with lower motor neuron signs. Affected dogs have normal results on myelography, MRI, and CSF analysis. Necropsy confirms the condition. Unknown mode of inheritance. A direct genetic test for an autosomal recessive DM susceptibility gene is available. All affected dogs are homozygous for the gene, however, only a small percentage of homozygous dogs develop DM. The gene is present at a frequency of 22% in the breed.[8,9]

Allergic Inhalant Dermatitis, Cruciate Ligament Rupture, Dermatomyositis, Gastric Dilatation-Volvulus, Prognathism, and **von Willebrand's Disease** are reported.[10]

Isolated Case Studies

Degenerative Encephalomyelopathy: Seven Kuvasz puppies from 2 same-parentage litters developed weakness and ataxia. Six necropsied dogs had lesions in caudate nucleus, cerebellar nuclei and folia, and spinal cord. Lesions seen were felt to be either familial or due to the effects of an amprolium-induced thiamine deficiency on the developing brains of these puppies.[11]

Genetic Tests

Tests of Genotype: Direct test for prcd-PRA is available from Optigen.

Direct test for an autosomal recessive DM susceptibility gene is available from OFA.

Tests of Phenotype: CHIC Certification: Required testing includes hip and elbow radiographs, and thyroid profile including autoantibodies. Optional recommended tests include patella examination, CERF eye examination, congenital cardiac evaluation, and genetic test for prcd PRA. (See CHIC website; www.caninehealthinfo.org).

Miscellaneous

- **Breed name synonyms:** Hungarian Kuvasz, Kuvaszok (pl)
- **Registries:** AKC, UKC, CKC, KCGB (Kennel Club of Great Britain), ANKC (Australian National Kennel Club), NKC (National Kennel Club)
- **AKC rank (year 2008):** 135 (145 dogs registered)
- **Internet resources: Kuvasz Club of America:** www.kuvasz.com **Kuvasz Club of Canada:** www.kuvaszclubofcanada.org **Kuvasz Fanciers of America Inc.:** http://hbalaw.com/KFA/index.htm

References

1. OFA Website breed statistics: www.offa.org Last accessed July 1, 2010.
2. LaFond E, Breur GJ & Austin CC: Breed susceptibility for developmental orthopedic diseases in dogs. J Am Anim Hosp Assoc. 2002 Sep-Oct;38(5):467-77.
3. Ocular Disorders Presumed to be Inherited in Purebred Dogs. American College of Veterinary Ophthalmologists. ACVO, 2007.
4. Nachreiner RF, Refsal KR, Graham PA, et. al.: Prevalence of serum thyroid hormone autoantibodies in dogs with clinical signs of hypothyroidism. J Am Vet Med Assoc 2002 Feb 15;220(4):466-71.
5. Nachreiner R & Refsal K: Personal communication, Diagnostic Center for Population and Animal Health, Michigan State University. April, 2007.
6. Rudd RG, Whitehair JG, Margolis JH: Results of management of osteochondritis dissecans of the humeral head in dogs : 44 cases [1982 to 1987]. J Am Anim Hosp Assoc 1990: 26[2]:173-178.
7. Strain GM: Deafness prevalence and pigmentation and gender associations in dog breeds at risk. Vet J. 2004 Jan;167(1):23-32.
8. Kathmann I, Cizinauskas S, Doherr MG, et. al.: Daily controlled physiotherapy increases survival time in dogs with suspected degenerative myelopathy. J Vet Intern Med. 2006 Jul-Aug;20(4):927-32.
9. Coates JR, Zeng R, Awano T, et. al.: An SOD1 Mutation Associated with Degenerative Myelopathy Occurs in Many Dog Breeds. Proceedings 2009 ACVIM Forum. 2009.
10. The Genetic Connection: A Guide to Health Problems in Purebred Dogs. L Ackerman. p. 225. AAHA Press, 1999.
11. Hazlett MJ, Smith-Maxie LL, de Lahunta A: A degenerative encephalomyelopathy in 7 Kuvasz puppies. Can Vet J. 2005 May;46(5):429-32.
12. The Complete Dog Book, 20th Ed. The American Kennel Club. Howell Book House, NY 2006. p. 288-292.

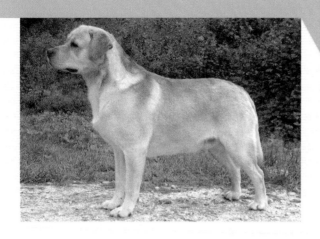

Labrador Retriever

The Breed History

This breed, the most popular breed in North America, took its name from the province of Labrador-Newfoundland in Canada, where this hardy breed was first reported in the early 1800s. They were exported to England not long after, and recognized by the English Kennel Club in 1903. AKC registrations began in 1917.

Breeding for Function

As their name implies, these solid, muscular dogs were bred to be gun dogs for retrieving waterfowl. They are much more versatile than that, and so have also become popular as assistance and therapy dogs, for companionship, obedience, agility, and as search and rescue and narcotics dogs. The field lines are leaner and taller than average.

Physical Characteristics

Height at Withers: female 21.5-23.5" (54.5-59.5cm), male 22.5-24.5" (57-62 cm)

Weight: females 55-70lb (25-32 kg) , males 65-80 lb (29.5-36.5 kg).

Coat: Their glossy water-resistant coat is flat, dense and short, and comes in three colors: black, chocolate and yellow. They have a soft wooly undercoat that provides insulation and water resistance.

Longevity: 11-13 years.

Points of Conformation: These are compact muscular dogs, a bit longer than tall that have a distinctive thick tail, referred to as "otter" type. These tails extend to the tarsus and taper from a thick origin, and are not feathered. The skull is broad and mesocephalic in type, with moderate stop and well-developed jaws and soft mouth for game handling. Eyes are medium-sized, dark, and express a gentle look, and the nose is wide and pigmented brown on chocolates, and black in black labs. The eyes are usually brown, but can be hazel in the chocolates. The ears are medium sized, leathered and pendulous in a triangular shape. The neck of medium length has moderate arch, and the topline is level. The chest is moderate in volume and depth and the abdomen is not tucked up. Limbs are straight and solid boned. Feet are compact and the toes are webbed and arched. The dewclaws may be removed. Their way of going is easy and straight, giving the impression of stamina and sturdy grace.

Recognized Behavior Issues and Traits

These dogs are famous for their placid, loving temperament. They enjoy play and need lots of human contact. Their loyalty and intelligence make them a treasured companion dog. Good with children and other pets, they are also easy to train but they need to be trained from an early age. They require both mental challenge and physical exercise for good health. If bored, they may resort to chewing. They are average shedders that need only routine grooming care. They gain weight easily.

Normal Physiologic Variations

None Reported

Drug Sensitivities

None Reported

Inherited Diseases

Hip Dysplasia: Polygenically inherited trait causing degenerative joint disease and hip arthritis. Reported at a frequency of 12.6% in one study. OFA reports 12.0% affected. Quantitative trait loci (QTL) have been identified in the breed that are linked to the development of hip dysplasia. Heritability estimated at 0.21 in the breed. Selection based on relatives (estimated breeding values) provide a greater response than selection based on phenotype alone.[1,2,3,4]

Elbow Dysplasia: Polygenically inherited trait causing elbow arthritis. Reported at a frequency of 17.8% with a male predilection in Labrador Retrievers in one study. OFA reports 11.0% affected. Reported 20.5x odds ratio for fragmented coronoid process, 8.5x odds ratio for ununited anconeal process forms of elbow dysplasia, and 109.4x odds ratio for elbow osteochondrosis versus other breeds.Heritability estimated at 0.12 in the breed. Dietary restriction slows the progression of elbow arthritis in affected dogs.[1,2,5,6,7]

Patella Luxation: Polygenically inherited laxity of patellar ligaments, causing luxation, lameness, and later degenerative joint disease. Treat surgically if causing clinical signs. Lateral patella luxation occurs in the Labrador Retriever, with a 3.3x relative risk versus other breeds. OFA reports 9.4% affected.[1,8]

Progressive Retinal Atrophy (prcd–PRA): Autosomal recessive progressive rod cone degeneration (prcd) form. Age of onset between 3-8 years of age, eventually causing blindness. Optigen reports 3% testing affected, and 20% testing carrier. A genetic test is available.[9,10,11,12]

Exercise Induced Collapse (EIC, Dynamin 1 Mutation): Average age of recognition is 12 months, especially in dogs being trained. An autosomal recessive disorder of muscle weakness, incoordination and life threatening collapse accompanied by hyperthermia after just five to fifteen minutes of intense exercise or excitement. After 10 to 30 minutes of rest, most dogs return to normal. Genetic testing shows 3% of Labrador Retrievers are affected, and over 30% carriers. A genetic test is available.[13,14,15]

Oculo-Skeletal Dysplasia/Retinal Dysplasia (RD/OSD): Autosomal recessive developmental disease causing ocular vitreous dysplasia, cataracts, retinal detachment, and dwarfism with valgus deformity of the carpi. Heterozygous carriers of the defective gene present with various forms of **retinal dysplasia** (folds, geographic, or detachment). Retinal dysplasia is identified in 2.31% of Labrador Retrievers CERF examined by veterinary ophthalmologists between 2000-2005. CERF does not recommend breeding any affected Labrador Retrievers. A genetic test is available.[2,9,16,17,18]

Centro-Nuclear Myopathy (CNM): Autosomal recessive disorder of muscle weakness. Onset of progressive weight loss and loss of tendon reflexes by 2 months of age, and an awkward gait, decreased exercise tolerance, and generalized muscle weakness between 2-5 months of age. Clinical signs stabilize in adult affected dogs. A genetic test is available.[19,20]

Tricuspid Valve (Right Atrioventricular) Dysplasia: Autosomal dominant disorder with incomplete penetrance. Congenital malformation of the tricuspid valve leaflets, chordae tendineae, and/or right ventricular papillary muscles. Mild cases have no clinical signs except tricuspid regurgitation on auscultation and echocardiography. Severely affected dogs show signs of ascites, pleural effusion, exercise intolerance, syncope, weight loss, arrythmia, and right sided heart failure. Labrador Retrievers have a 35x relative risk versus other breeds, with a heritability of 0.71. No genetic test is available.[21,22,23]

Cystinuria: Rare, autosomal recessive disease causing dysuria, stranguria, or obstruction due to cystine calculi, primarily in affected males. Caused by a defect in cystine metabolism. Affected females can have cystine crystals and calculi without clinical signs. A genetic test is available.[24,25]

Narcolepsy: Rare, autosomal recessive disorder causing sudden collapse and a sleep-like state elicited by excitement. Clinical episodes begin at four weeks of age, with maximal symptoms by 10-32 weeks of age. A genetic test is available.[26,27]

Disease Predispositions

Allergic Dermatitis: Inhalant or food allergies. Presents with pruritis and pyotraumatic dermatitis (hot spots). The breed has a significant frequency of allergies, with a computed heritability of 0.47.[28]

Hypothyroidism: Inherited autoimmune thyroiditis. 5.7% positive for thyroid autoantibodies based on testing at Michigan State University. (Ave. for all breeds is 7.5).[29,30]

Persistent Pupillary Membranes: Strands of fetal remnant connecting; iris to iris, cornea, lens, or involving sheets of tissue. The later three forms can impair vision, and dogs affected with these forms should not be bred. Identified in 3.41% of Labrador Retrievers CERF examined by veterinary ophthalmologists between 2000-2005.[9]

Epilepsy (Inherited Seizures): Can be generalized or partial seizures. Control with anticonvulsant medication. Occurs at a frequency of 3.1% in Danish Labrador Retrievers with 24% generalized, and 70% partial seizures. Proposed polygenic inheritance with a major recessive gene of influence.[31,32,33,34]

Cataracts: Polar subcapsular triangular cataracts predominate, usually developing between 6 and 18 months of age, with 75% of affected dogs developing cataracts by 5 years of age. Proposed autosomal recessive mode of inheritance. Identified in 2.64% of Labrador Retrievers CERF examined by veterinary ophthalmologists between 2000-2005. Identified in 8% of Labrador Retrievers in Holland, with offspring of affected dogs occuring at a much higher frequency. CERF does not recommend breeding any Labrador Retriever with a cataract.[9,35,36]

Cranial Cruciate Ligament (ACL) Rupture: Traumatic tearing of the ACL in the stifle, causing lameness and secondary arthritis. Treat with surgery. Reported at an increased incidence versus other breeds. In one study, 23% of large breed dogs with the diagnosis were Labrador Retrievers. Dorn reports a 2.17x odds ratio versus other breeds. There is no difference in tibial plateau angle between affected and unaffected Labrador Retrievers with ACL rupture.[37,38,39,40]

Osteochondritis Desicans (OCD): Inherited joint cartilage defect. Causes joint pain and lameness in young growing dogs. Mild cases can resolve with rest, while more severe cases require surgery. Reported 45.9x odds ratio for hock OCD, 27.6x odds ratio for stifle OCD and 13.1x odds ratio for shoulder OCD versus other breeds.[7]

Hypertrophic Osteodystrophy (HOD): Immune-mediated disorder causing fever, and painful, swollen joints and bones in young Labrador Retrievers. Occurs mostly within 3-14 days post-vaccination. Age of onset is 8-16 weeks. Reported 5.9x odds ratio versus other breeds.[7]

Chronic Hepatitis/Copper Associated Hepatitis: A breed-related hepatopathy occurs in Labrador Retrievers, characterized by vomiting, polyuria/polydipsia, icterus, and abdominal pain and distention. Liver enzymes are elevated, and histopathology shows chronic inflammation, fibrosis, and copper accumulation. Feeding low copper diets is helpful in controlling the disease. Incidence is 1.2% in the breed, with a median age at diagnosis of 9.3 years. Unknown mode of inheritance.[41,42,43,44]

Distichiasis: Abnormally placed eyelashes that irritate the cornea and conjunctiva. Can cause secondary corneal ulceration. Identified in 0.90% of Labrador Retrievers CERF examined by veterinary ophthalmologists between 2000-2005.[9]

Corneal Dystrophy: Non-inflammatory epithelial/stromal corneal opacity. Identified in 0.76% of Labrador Retrievers CERF examined by veterinary ophthalmologists between 2000-2005.[9]

Lymphoma/Lymphosarcoma: Malignant cancer of lymphoid tissue. Both B-cell and T-cell (mycosis fungoides) occur in the breed.[45]

Entropion: A rolling in of the eyelids, can cause corneal irritation and ulceration. Correct with surgery. Reported at an increased incidence versus other breeds. Identified in 0.44% of Labrador Retrievers CERF examined by veterinary ophthalmologists between 2000-2005.[9,46]

Acquired Laryngeal Paralysis: Late-onset disorder of laryngeal dysfunction secondary to axonal degeneration of the recurrent laryngeal nerve. Affected dogs show exercise intolerance, inspiratory stridor, inspiratory dyspnoea, gagging, coughing and dysphonia. There is a male:female ratio of 1.56:1 and the average age of presentation is 9.9 years. Labrador Retrievers are identified as the most frequently affected breed.[47,48]

Diabetes Mellitus (Sugar Diabetes): Treat with insulin injections. Age of onset between 5-12 years. Labrador Retrievers represent 17.4% of all diagnosed cases.[49]

Immune-Mediated Hemolytic Anemia (IMHA): Autoimmune destruction of red blood cells. Females are more frequently affected than males. Labrador Retrievers account for 8% of diagnosed cases. Unknown mode of inheritance.[50,51]

Nasal Parakeratosis: Inherited disorder of nasal hyperkeratotic lesions appearing between 6 and 12 months of age. Affected dogs have mild to severe lesions of dry and rough keratin affecting the dorsal aspect of the nasal planum. Fissures and erosions can develop in severe cases. Proposed autosomal recessive inheritance.[52,53]

Uveal Cysts: Labrador Retrievers have a higher frequency of uveal cysts than other breeds, with a mean age of cyst development of 9.1 years.[54]

Secondary Glaucoma: Glaucoma causes increased pressure within the eyeball and blindness due to damage to the retina. The breed is listed as predisposed to secondary glaucoma due to uveitis or lens luxation. Screen with tonometry.[55]

Limbal Melanoma: Benign eye mass, usually originating from the dorsal limbus. Labrador Retrievers have a 3.0x odds ratio of limbal melanomas versus other breeds.[56]

Lingual Squamous Cell Carcinoma (SCC): Labrador Retrievers have a 2.41x odds ratio versus other breeds of developing this tongue cancer. Females are overrepresented in one study.[57]

Atrioventricular (Heart) Block: Labrador Retrievers are found to be at increased risk of high-grade second- or third-degree atrioventricular block versus other breeds. Treatment is with a pacemaker.[58,59]

Histiocytic Sarcoma/Histiocytosis: Malignant cancer of CD11d+ macrophages, producing masses in the spleen, liver, lung, bone marrow, +/or eye. Mean age of diagnosis of 8.61 +/- 2.43 years, with a less than 6 month life expectancy. Labrador Retrievers are overrepresented in diagnoses versus other breeds.[60,61]

Ectopic Ureter: Congenital malformation where one or both ureters do not enter the body of the urinary bladder, often entering the bladder neck or urethra causing incontinence. Labrador Retrievers are at increased risk versus other breeds. Unknown inheritance.[62,63]

Digital Squamous Cell Carcinoma (SCC): Subungual (toe) squamous cell carcinoma occurs at increased frequency in black dogs. Treat with digital amputation. Labrador Retrievers account for 23.8% of all cases.[64]

Iridociliary Epithelial Tumors: These intraocular adenomas and adenocarcinomas occur more frequently in the Labrador Retriever. They rarely metastasize.[65]

Calcinosis Circumscripta: Calcinosis circumscripta is an uncommon syndrome of dystrophic, metastatic or iatrogenic mineralization of calcium salts in soft tissues. Lesions usually occur on the hind feet or tongue in 1-4 year old dogs. Nine percent of canine cases occur in Labrador Retrievers.[66]

Ossification of the Infraspinatus Tendon-Bursa: Disorder identified in 13 Labrador Retrievers with unilateral or bilateral forelimb lameness between 2 to 10 years of age. Diagnose via radiograph. Treat with rest, steroid injection, or surgery.[67]

Acral Lick Dermatitis, Central Axonopathy, Central PRA, Cervical Vertebral Instability, Cleft Lip/Palate, Degenerative Myelopathy, Ectropion, Factor VIII Deficiency, Fanconi Syndrome, Fibrinoid Leukodystrophy, Follicular Dysplasia, Gastric Dilatation w/Volvulus, Hypotrichosis, Juvenile Cellulitis, Lymphedema, Malignant Hyperthermia, Megaesophagus, Microphthalmia, Micropapilla, Mucinosis, Myelodysplasia, Myoclonus, Neuroaxonal Dystrophy, Optic Nerve Coloboma, Optic Nerve Hypoplasia, Panosteitis, Seasonal Flank Alopecia, Sebaceous Adenitis, Silica Urolithiasis, Spongiform Leukodystrophy, Supernumerary Teeth, Tetralogy of Fallot, Vitamin A Responsive Dermatosis, Vitiligo, and von Willebrand's Disease are reported.[68]

Isolated Case Studies

Hemophilia B (Factor IX deficiency): An affected male Labrador Retriever had clinically severe bleeding due to complete deletion of the Factor IX gene. A genetic test was developed for this X-linked recessive gene.[69]

Cerebellar Abiotrophy: Several cases of juvenile cerebellar degeneration have been diagnosed in Labrador Retrievers. Puppies between 9 and 17 weeks of age developed rapidly progressive hypermetria, ataxia, and intension tremors resulting in euthanasia.[70,71]

X-linked Muscular Dystrophy: A dystrophin deficient muscular dystrophy similar to human Duchenne's muscular dystrophy was identified in a 3.5 month-old, male Labrador retriever. The dog presented with difficulty swallowing, poor body condition and a protruding tongue.[72]

Mytubular Myopathy: Three to four-month-old, male, Labrador retrievers present with progressive weakness and muscle atrophy. Histology demonstrated central mitochondrial accumulations. A mutation in the MTM 1 gene causes this x-linked disease in the breed. Worldwide screening did not identify carriers outside of this affected kindred in Canada.[73,74]

Chondrodysplasia/Dwarfism: An apparently autosomal recessively inherited dwarfism without retinal lesions is identified in a kindred of Labrador Retrievers in the Netherlands. Candidate gene analysis was not successful in identifying a causative gene.[75]

Neuronal Ceroid-Lipofuscinosis (NCL): An 8-year-old, neutered male Labrador Retriever presented with an 11 month history of progressive partial seizure activity (facial and ear twitching), and a 2 week history of ataxia and dysphagia. Necropsy diagnosis confirmed NCL.[76]

Mucopolysaccharidosis Type II (MPSII): A 5-year-old male Labrador Retriever had progressive incoordination, visual impairment, exercise intolerance, coarse facial features, macrodactylia, unilateral corneal dystrophy, and generalized osteopenia. X-linked recessive MPSII was diagnosed.[77]

Sub-Follicular Panniculitis And Sebaceous Adenitis: A 6-year-old male black Labrador retriever presented with a 12 week course of nonpruritic multicentric, well-demarcated alopecia. Pathology revealed an inflammatory sebaceous adenitis and sub-follicular panniculitis. Alopecia was permanent in these areas.[78]

Genetic Tests

Tests of Genotype: Direct tests for prcd-PRA, and RD/OSD are available from Optigen.

Direct test for exercise induced collapse (EIC) is available from the University of Minnesota Veterinary Diagnostic Lab.

Direct test for centronuclear myopathy (CNM) is available from the Alfort Lab www.labradorcnm.com, and the Animal Health Trust.

Direct test for cystinuria is available from PennGen.

Direct test for Hemophilia B is available from HealthGene.

Direct test for Narcolepsy is available from Optigen and HealthGene.

Direct tests for black, chocolate (brown), yellow, and diluted coat colors and black and brown nose are available from HealthGene and VetGen.

Tests of Phenotype: CHIC Certification: Required testing includes hip and elbow radiographs, and CERF eye examination. Optional gene test for CNM (See CHIC website; www.caninehealthinfo.org).

Recommend thyroid profile including autoantibodies, patella evaluation, genetic test for EIC, and cardiac examination.

Miscellaneous

- **Breed name synonyms:** Lab, Labrador, Yellow Lab, Black Lab, Chocolate Lab, St. John's Retriever (historical)
- **Registries:** AKC, CKC, UKC, KCGB (Kennel Club of Great Britain), ANKC (Australian National Kennel Club), NKC (National Kennel Club)
- **AKC rank (year 2008):** 1 (100,736 dogs registered)
- **Internet resources: The Labrador Retriever Club, Inc.:** www.thelabradorclub.com
  Labrador Retriever Club of Canada: www.labradorretrieverclub.ca
  The Labrador Retriever Club of Great Britain: www.thelabradorretriverclub.com

References

1. OFA Website breed statistics: www.offa.org Last accessed July. 1, 2010.
2. Morgan JP, Wind A, Davidson AP, et. al.: Bone dysplasias in the labrador retriever: a radiographic study. J Am Anim Hosp Assoc. 1999 Jul-Aug;35(4):332-40.
3. Phavaphutanon J, Mateescu RG, Tsai KL, et. al.: Evaluation of quantitative trait loci for hip dysplasia in Labrador Retrievers. Am J Vet Res. 2009 Sep;70(9):1094-101.
4. Hou Y, Wang Y, Lust G, et. al.: Retrospective analysis for genetic improvement of hip joints of cohort labrador retrievers in the United States: 1970-2007. PLoS One. 2010 Feb 24;5(2):e9410.
5. Engler J, Hamann H & Distl O: Estimation of population genetic parameters for radiographical findings of elbow dsyplasia in the Labrador Retriever. Berl Munch Tierarztl Wochenschr. 2009 Sep-Oct;122(9-10):378-85.
6. Huck JL, Biery DN, Lawler DF, et. al.: A longitudinal study of the influence of lifetime food restriction on development of osteoarthritis in the canine elbow. Vet Surg. 2009 Feb;38(2):192-8.
7. LaFond E, Breur GJ & Austin CC: Breed susceptibility for developmental orthopedic diseases in dogs. J Am Anim Hosp Assoc. 2002 Sep-Oct;38(5):467-77.
8. Gibbons SE, Macias C, Tonzing MA, et. al.: Patellar luxation in 70 large breed dogs. J Small Anim Pract. 2006 Jan;47(1):3-9.
9. *Ocular Disorders Presumed to be Inherited in Purebred Dogs.* American College of Veterinary Ophthalmologists. ACVO, 2007.
10. Kommonen B, Kylmä T, Karhunen U, et. al.: Impaired retinal function in young labrador retriever dogs heterozygous for late onset rod-cone degeneration. Vision Res. 1997 Feb;37(3):365-70.
11. Morris Animal Foundation: Morris Animal Foundation Update: Genetic Tests Focus on Breed-Specific Vision Problems. Canine Pract 1999:24[4]:21.
12. Zangerl B, Goldstein O, Philp AR, et al.: Identical mutation in a novel retinal gene causes progressive rod–cone degeneration in dogs and retinitis pigmentosa in humans. Genomics 2006; 88:551–563.
13. Taylor SM, Shmon CL, Adams VJ, et. al.: Evaluations of labrador retrievers with exercise-induced collapse, including response to a standardized strenuous exercise protocol. J Am Anim Hosp Assoc. 2009 Jan-Feb;45(1):3-13.
14. Patterson EE, Minor KM, Tchernatynskaia AV, et. al.: A canine DNM1 mutation is highly associated with the syndrome of exercise-induced collapse. Nat Genet. 2008 Oct;40(10):1235-9.
15. Taylor SM, Shmon CL, Shelton GD, et. al.: Exercise-induced collapse of Labrador retrievers: survey results and preliminary investigation of heritability. J Am Anim Hosp Assoc. 2008 Nov-Dec;44(6):295-301.
16. Farnum CE, Jones K, Riis R, et. al.: Ocular-chondrodysplasia in labrador retriever dogs: a morphometric and electron microscopical analysis. Calcif Tissue Int. 1992 Jun;50(6):564-72.
17. Carrig CB, Sponenberg DP, Schmidt GM, et. al.: Inheritance of associated ocular and skeletal dysplasia in Labrador retrievers. J Am Vet Med Assoc. 1988 Nov 15;193(10):1269-72.
18. Goldstein O, Guyon R, Kukekova A, et. al.: COL9A2 and COL9A3 mutations in canine autosomal recessive oculoskeletal dysplasia. Mamm Genome. 2010 Aug;21(7-8):398-408.
19. Pelé M, Tiret L, Kessler JL, et. al.: SINE exonic insertion in the PTPLA gene leads to multiple splicing defects and segregates with the autosomal recessive centronuclear myopathy in dogs. Hum Mol Genet. 2005 Jun 1;14(11):1417-27.
20. Tiret L, Blot S, Kessler JL, et. al.: The cnm locus, a canine homologue of human autosomal forms of centronuclear myopathy, maps to chromosome 2. Hum Genet. 2003 Sep;113(4):297-306.
21. Chetboul V, Tran D, Carlos C, et. al.: Congenital malformations of the tricuspid valve in domestic carnivores: a retrospective study of 50 cases. Schweiz Arch Tierheilkd. 2004 Jun;146(6):265-75.
22. Famula TR, Siemens LM, Davidson AP, et. al.: Evaluation of the genetic basis of tricuspid valve dysplasia in Labrador Retrievers. Am J Vet Res. 2002 Jun;63(6):816-20.
23. Andelfinger G, Wright KN, Lee HS, et. al.: Canine tricuspid valve malformation, a model of human Ebstein anomaly, maps to dog chromosome 9. J Med Genet. 2003 May;40(5):320-4.

24. Crane CW & Turner AW: Amino acid patterns of urine and blood plasma in a cystinuric Labrador dog. Nature. 1956 Feb 4;177(4501):237-8.

25. Jones BR, Kirkman JH, Hogan J, et. al.: Analysis of uroliths from cats and dogs in New Zealand, 1993-96. N Z Vet J. 1998 Dec;46(6):233-6.

26. Foutz AS, Mitler MM, Cavalli-Sforza LL, et. al.: Genetic factors in canine narcolepsy. Sleep. 1979 Summer;1(4):413-21.

27. Hungs M, Fan J, Lin L, et. al.: Identification and functional analysis of mutations in the hypocretin (orexin) genes of narcoleptic canines. Genome Res. 2001 Apr;11(4):531-9.

28. Shaw SC, Wood JL, Freeman J, et. al.: Estimation of heritability of atopic dermatitis in Labrador and Golden Retrievers. Am J Vet Res. 2004 Jul;65(7):1014-20.

29. Nachreiner RF, Refsal KR, Graham PA, et. al.: Prevalence of serum thyroid hormone autoantibodies in dogs with clinical signs of hypothyroidism. *J Am Vet Med Assoc* 2002 Feb 15;220(4):466-71.

30. Nachreiner R & Refsal K: Personal communication, Diagnostic Center for Population and Animal Health, Michigan State University. April, 2007.

31. Jaggy A & Heynold Y: Idiopathic epilepsy in the dog. Schweiz Arch Tierheilkd. 1996;138(11):523-31.

32. Ellenberger C, Mevissen M, Doherr M, et. al.: Inhibitory and excitatory neurotransmitters in the cerebrospinal fluid of epileptic dogs. Am J Vet Res. 2004 Aug;65(8):1108-13.

33. Berendt M, Gredal H, Pedersen LG, et. al.: A cross-sectional study of epilepsy in Danish Labrador Retrievers: prevalence and selected risk factors. J Vet Intern Med. 2002 May-Jun;16(3):262-8.

34. Jaggy A, Faissler D, Gaillard C, et. al.: Genetic aspects of idiopathic epilepsy in Labrador retrievers. J Small Anim Pract. 1998 Jun;39(6):275-80.

35. Sidjanin DJ, McElwee J, Miller B, et. al.: Cloning of canine galactokinase (GALK1) and evaluation as a candidate gene for hereditary cataracts in Labrador retrievers. Anim Genet. 2005 Jun;36(3):265-6.

36. Kraijer-Huver IM, Gubbels EJ, Scholten J,, et. al.: Characterization and prevalence of cataracts in Labrador Retrievers in The Netherlands. Am J Vet Res. 2008 Oct;69(10):1336-40.

37. Dorn CR: Canine breed-specific risks of frequently diagnosed diseases at veterinary teaching hospitals. Monograph. AKC Canine Health Foundation. 2000.

38. Harasen G: Canine cranial cruciate ligament rupture in profile: 2002-2007. Can Vet J. 2008 Feb;49(2):193-4.

39. Duval JM, Budsberg SC, Flo GL, et. al.: Breed, sex, and body weight as risk factors for rupture of the cranial cruciate ligament in young dogs. J Am Vet Med Assoc. 1999 Sep 15;215(6):811-4.

40. Reif U & Probst CW: Comparison of tibial plateau angles in normal and cranial cruciate deficient stifles of Labrador retrievers. Vet Surg. 2003 Jul-Aug;32(4):385-9.

41. Shih JL, Keating JH, Freeman LM, et. al.: Chronic hepatitis in Labrador Retrievers: clinical presentation and prognostic factors. J Vet Intern Med. 2007 Jan-Feb;21(1):33-9.

42. Hoffmann G, van den Ingh TS, Bode P, et. al.: Copper-associated chronic hepatitis in Labrador Retrievers. J Vet Intern Med. 2006 Jul-Aug;20(4):856-61.

43. Smedley R, Mullaney T, Rumbeiha W, et. al.: Copper-associated hepatitis in Labrador Retrievers. Vet Pathol. 2009 May;46(3):484-90.

44. Hoffmann G, Jones PG, Biourge V, et. al.: Dietary management of hepatic copper accumulation in Labrador Retrievers. J Vet Intern Med. 2009 Sep-Oct;23(5):957-63

45. Wilkerson MJ, Dolce K, Koopman T, et. al.: Lineage differentiation of canine lymphoma/leukemias and aberrant expression of CD molecules. Vet Immunol Immunopathol. 2005 Jul 15;106(3-4):179-96.

46. Read RA & Broun HC: Entropion correction in dogs and cats using a combination Hotz-Celsus and lateral eyelid wedge resection: results in 311 eyes. Vet Ophthalmol. 2007 Jan-Feb;10(1):6-11.

47. Snelling SR & Edwards GA: A retrospective study of unilateral arytenoid lateralisation in the treatment of laryngeal paralysis in 100 dogs (1992-2000). Aust Vet J. 2003 Aug;81(8):464-8.

48. Burbidge HM: A review of laryngeal paralysis in dogs. Br Vet J. 1995 Jan-Feb;151(1):71-82.

49. Davison LJ, Herrtage ME, Catchpole B, et. al.: Study of 253 dogs in the United Kingdom with diabetes mellitus. Vet Rec. 2005 Apr 9;156(15):467-71.

50. Burgess K, Moore A, Rand W, et. al.: Treatment of immune-mediated hemolytic anemia in dogs with cyclophosphamide. J Vet Intern Med. 2000 Jul-Aug;14(4):456-62.

51. Stokol T, Blue JT & French TW: Idiopathic pure red cell aplasia and nonregenerative immune-mediated anemia in dogs: 43 cases (1988-1999). J Am Vet Med Assoc. 2000 May 1;216(9):1429-36.

52. Pagé N, Paradis M, Lapointe JM, et. al.: Hereditary nasal parakeratosis in Labrador Retrievers. Vet Dermatol. 2003 Apr;14(2):103-10.

53. Peters J, Scott DW, Erb HN, et. al.: Hereditary nasal parakeratosis in Labrador retrievers: 11 new cases and a retrospective study on the presence of accumulations of serum ('serum lakes') in the epidermis of parakeratotic dermatoses and inflamed nasal plana of dogs. Vet Dermatol. 2003 Aug;14(4):197-203.

54. Corcoran KA, Koch SA: Uveal cysts in dogs: 28 cases (1989-1991). J Am Vet Med Assoc. 1993 Aug 15;203(4):545-6.

55. Gelatt KN, MacKay EO: Secondary glaucomas in the dog in North America. *Vet Ophthalmol.* 2004 Jul-Aug;7(4):245-59.

56. Donaldson D, Sansom J, Scase T, et. al.: Canine limbal melanoma: 30 cases (1992-2004). Part 1. Signalment, clinical and histological features and pedigree analysis. Vet Ophthalmol. 2006 Mar-Apr;9(2):115-9.

57. Dennis MM, Ehrhart N, Duncan CG, et. al.: Frequency of and risk factors associated with lingual lesions in dogs: 1,196 cases (1995-2004).

58. Wess G, Thomas WP, Berger DM, et. al.: Applications, complications, and outcomes of transvenous pacemaker implantation in 105 dogs (1997-2002). J Vet Intern Med. 2006 Jul-Aug;20(4):877-84.

59. Schrope DP & Kelch WJ: Signalment, clinical signs, and prognostic indicators associated with high-grade second- or third-degree atrioventricular block in dogs: 124 cases (January 1, 1997-December 31, 1997). J Am Vet Med Assoc. 2006 Jun 1;228(11):1710-7.

60. Naranjo C, Dubielzig RR, & Friedrichs KR: Canine ocular histiocytic sarcoma. Vet Ophthalmol. 2007 May-Jun;10(3):179-85.

61. Moore PF, Affolter VK, Vernau W, et. al.: Canine hemophagocytic histiocytic sarcoma: a proliferative disorder of CD11d+ macrophages. Vet Pathol. 2006 Sep;43(5):632-45.

62. Lamb CR & Gregory SP: Ultrasonographic findings in 14 dogs with ectopic ureter. Vet Radiol Ultrasound. 1998 May-Jun;39(3):218-23.

63. Holt PE & Moore AH: Canine ureteral ectopia: an analysis of 175 cases and comparison of surgical treatments. Vet Rec. 1995 Apr 8;136(14):345-9.

64. O'Brien MG, Berg J & Engler SJ: Treatment by digital amputation of subungual squamous cell carcinoma in dogs: 21 cases (1987-1988) J Am Vet Med Assoc. 1992 Sep 1;201(5):759-61.

65. Dubielzig RR, Steinberg H, Garvin H, et. al.: Iridociliary epithelial tumors in 100 dogs and 17 cats: a morphological study. Vet Ophthalmol. 1998;1(4):223-231.

66. Tafti AK, Hanna P, Bourque AC: Calcinosis circumscripta in the dog: a retrospective pathological study. J Vet Med A Physiol Pathol Clin Med. 2005 Feb;52(1):13-7.

67. McKee WM, Macias C, May C, et. al.: Ossification of the infraspinatus tendon-bursa in 13 dogs. Vet Rec. 2007 Dec 22-29;161(25):846-52.

68. *The Genetic Connection: A Guide to Health Problems in Purebred Dogs.* L Ackerman. p 225-26, AAHA Press, 1999.

69. Brooks MB, Gu W & Ray K: Complete deletion of factor IX gene and inhibition of factor IX activity in a labrador retriever with hemophilia B. J Am Vet Med Assoc. 1997 Dec 1;211(11):1418-21.

70. Bildfell RJ, Mitchell SK & de Lahunta A: Cerebellar cortical degeneration in a Labrador retriever. Can Vet J. 1995 Sep;36(9):570-2.

71. Perille AL, Baer K, Joseph RJ, et. al.: Postnatal cerebellar cortical degeneration in Labrador Retriever puppies. Can Vet J. 1991 Oct;32(10):619-621.

72. Bergman RL, Inzana KD, Monroe WE, et. al.: Dystrophin-deficient muscular dystrophy in a Labrador retriever. J Am Anim Hosp Assoc. 2002 May-Jun;38(3):255-61.

73. Cosford KL, Taylor SM, Thompson L, et. al.: A possible new inherited myopathy in a young Labrador retriever. Can Vet J. 2008 Apr;49(4):393-7.

74. Shelton GD, Snead E, Böhm J, et. al.: A Missense Variant in the MTM1 Gene Associated with X-Linked Myotubular Myopathy in Labrador Retrievers. Proceedings, 2009 ACVIM Forum. 2009.

75. Smit JJ, Temwitchitr J, Brocks BA, et. al.: Evaluation of candidate genes as cause of chondrodysplasia in Labrador retrievers. Vet J. 2011 Feb;187(2):269-71.

76. Rossmeisl JH Jr, Duncan R, Fox J, et. al.: Neuronal ceroid-lipofuscinosis in a Labrador Retriever. J Vet Diagn Invest. 2003 Sep;15(5):457-60.

77. Wilkerson MJ, Lewis DC, Marks SL, et. al.: Clinical and morphologic features of mucopolysaccharidosis type II in a dog: naturally occurring model of Hunter syndrome. Vet Pathol. 1998 May;35(3):230-3.

78. Varjonen K, Rest J & Bond R: Alopecia in a black Labrador retriever associated with focal sub-follicular panniculitis and sebaceous adenitis. Vet Dermatol. 2010 Mar 30. [Epub ahead of print]

79. *The Complete Dog Book, 20th Ed.* The American Kennel Club. Howell Book House, NY 2006. p 52-57.

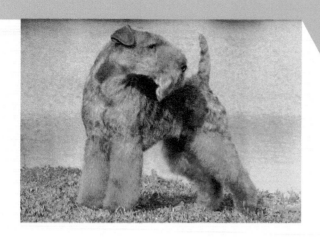

The Breed History

The breed derives its name from the **Lake** District of England where early development of the breed took place. This breed is considered one of the original terrier breeds. The Lakeland shares ancestors with the Bedlington, Patterdale, and Border Terriers. Perhaps the extinct Black and Tan Terrier was a progenitor. The first breed standard was drawn up in 1921. Registration in AKC occurred in 1934.

Breeding for Function

They were raised primarily for fox and otter hunting. They were renowned for going deep underground. These terriers were also used for vermin control and for guarding sheep flocks.

Physical Characteristics

Height at Withers: female 13-15" (33-38 cm), male 14-15" (35.5-38 cm)

Weight: males 17 lb (7.5 kg), females 15 lb (7 kg)

Coat: The double weather resistant coat is harsh and wiry, straight to slightly wavy in the outer coat layer, and the undercoat is dense and soft. The brows do not cover the eyes, and beard and moustache are trimmed for show. Blue, liver, wheaten, red, black, black and tan, blue and tan, and grizzled are accepted colors. Some dogs may have a dark saddle.

Longevity: 13-14 years

Points of Conformation: Lakelands possess sturdy square conformation, moderate muscling and bone, and their expression is alert. Smallish oval eyes are fairly wide set and colored to match the dog (hazel, brown, or dark brown), with dark palpebral margins. Ears are triangular, small and the leather is thick. They fold forward, with the fold above the topline of the skull. The skull is fairly flat and broad, muzzle is blocky, and there is a minimal stop. The nose is black, but may be liver on liver colored dogs. The lips are dark, neck is long and fine, not throaty, slightly arching, and there are prominent shoulders. Limbs are straight boned and metacarpals and metatarsals are short. Dewclaws are usually removed. The feet are compact, toes well arched, and the pads thick and darkly pigmented. The topline is level and the back is short, the thorax is deep and narrow with ribs well sprung, and the abdomen is moderately tucked up. The high set tail is carried up and curves

slightly forward at the tip. It is commonly docked. The gait is long, free and smooth.

Recognized Behavior Issues and Traits

Reported traits of this breed include: Courageous at the hunt, calm temperament, is an independent thinker, mischievous and playful. Lakelands make a good watchdog. These terriers will fight with other dogs, and should be socialized early to other pets in the household. Need close human companionship, plenty of exercise and mental stimulation to prevent boredom vices, including digging. Need to be in a fenced area if let off leash. Have moderate grooming needs.

Normal Physiologic Variations

None reported

Drug Sensitivities

None reported

Inherited Diseases

Hip Dysplasia: Polygenically inherited trait causing degenerative joint disease and hip arthritis. Too few Lakeland Terriers have been screened to determine an accurate frequency.[1]

Legg-Calvé-Perthes Disease: Polygenically inherited aseptic necrosis of the femoral head, resulting in degenerative joint disease. Can be unilateral or bilateral, with onset of degeneration usually between 6-9 months of age. Treat surgically if causing lameness/discomfort. Frequency and mode of inheritance in the breed has not been determined.

Patella Luxation: Polygenically inherited laxity of patellar ligaments, causing luxation, lameness, and later degenerative joint disease. Treat surgically if causing clinical signs. Too few Lakeland Terriers have been screened by OFA to determine an accurate frequency.[1]

Elbow Dysplasia: Polygenically inherited trait causing elbow arthritis. Too few Lakeland Terriers have been screened by OFA to determine an accurate frequency.[1]

Primary Lens Luxation (PLL): An autosomal recessive gene causes primary lens luxation. Homozygous affected dogs usually develop lens luxation between 4-8 years of age. Rarely, heterozygous carriers can develop lens luxation, but at a later age. Lens luxation can lead to secondary **glaucoma** and blindness. A genetic mutation has been identified, and a genetic test is available.

Disease Predispositions

Persistent Pupillary Membranes: Strands of fetal remnant connecting; iris to iris, cornea, lens, or involving sheets of tissue. The later three forms can impair vision, and dogs affected with these forms should not be bred. Identified in 9.38% of Lakeland Terriers CERF examined by veterinary ophthalmologists between 2000-2005.[2]

Hypothyroidism: Inherited autoimmune thyroiditis. 7.7% positive for thyroid auto-antibodies based on testing at Michigan State University. (Ave. for all breeds is 7.5%).[3,4]

Cataracts: Intermediate or punctate cataracts. Reported in 7.46% of Lakeland Terriers presented to veterinary teaching hospitals. CERF does not recommend breeding any Lakeland Terrier with a cataract.[5]

Glaucoma: Primary, narrow angle glaucoma occurs in the breed. Can cause secondary lens luxation. Screen with gonioscopy and tonometry. Frequency and mode of inheritance in the breed has not been determined.[2]

Other Eye Disorders: Distichiasis, Corneal Dystrophy, and other eye disorders are reported in the breed, but too few Lakeland Terriers have been CERF eye examined to determine an accurate frequency.[2]

Cryptorchidism, Microphthalmia, Prognathism, Progressive Retinal Atrophy, and **von Willebrand's Disease** are reported.[6]

Isolated Case Studies

Laryngeal Paralysis and Everted Laryngeal Saccules: The ultrasonographic appearance of laryngeal eversion due to bilateral laryngeal paralysis is described in a young Lakeland terrier.[7]

Osteochondroma: A Lakeland terrier puppy had progressive hind limb ataxia associated with pain in the thoracic spine. Plain radiographs revealed a lesion affecting the dorsal neural arch of the fourth thoracic vertebra and myelography revealed spinal cord compression. Surgical excision cured the dog's clinical signs. Histopathology revealed osteochondromatosis.[8]

Genetic Tests

Tests of Genotype: Direct test for PLL is available from OFA and the Animal Health Trust.

Tests of Phenotype: Recommend patella evaluation, hip and elbow radiographs, CERF eye examination, and thyroid profile including autoantibodies.

Miscellaneous

- **Breed name synonyms:** Lakeland, Patterdale Terrier (historical)
- **Registries:** AKC, UKC, CKC, KCGB (Kennel Club of Great Britain), ANKC (Australian National Kennel Club), NKC (National Kennel Club)
- **AKC rank (year 2008):** 131 (176 dogs registered)
- **Internet resources: The United States Lakeland Terrier Club:** www.uslakelandterrier.org
  Lakeland Terrier Club (UK): http://lakelandterrierclub.org.uk/

References

1. OFA Website breed statistics: www.offa.org Last accessed July 1, 2010.
2. *Ocular Disorders Presumed to be Inherited in Purebred Dogs.* American College of Veterinary Ophthalmologists. ACVO, 2007.
3. Nachreiner RF, Refsal KR, Graham PA, et. al.: Prevalence of serum thyroid hormone autoantibodies in dogs with clinical signs of hypothyroidism. J Am Vet Med Assoc 2002 Feb 15;220(4):466-71.
4. Nachreiner R & Refsal K: Personal communication, Diagnostic Center for Population and Animal Health, Michigan State University. April, 2007.
5. Gelatt KN, Mackay EO: Prevalence of primary breed-related cataracts in the dog in North America. Vet Ophthalmol. 2005 Mar-Apr;8(2):101-11.
6. *The Genetic Connection: A Guide to Health Problems in Purebred Dogs.* L Ackerman. p. 226. AAHA Press, 1999.
7. Rudorf H, Lane JG, Wotton PR: Everted laryngeal saccules: ultrasonographic findings in a young Lakeland terrier. *J Small Anim Pract.* 1999 Jul;40(7):338-9.
8. Ness MG: Osteochondroma causing progressive posterior paresis in a lakeland terrier puppy. *Vet Rec.* 1993 Jun 12;132(24):608-9.
9. *The Complete Dog Book, 20th Ed.* The American Kennel Club. Howell Book House, NY 2006. p. 391-395.

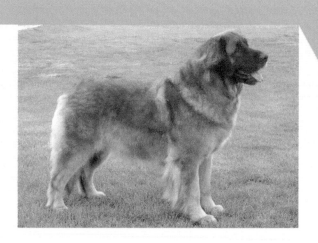

The Breed History

The Leonberger originated in the 1800s in Leonberg, Germany. The origins are from many breeds, including Landseer Newfoundland, St. Bernard, and Pyrenean Mountain Dog. The first breed clubs were established in 1889. Leonbergers almost became extinct after each World War, but were brought back by dedicated breeders. AKC recognition occurred in 2010.

Breeding for Function

Their original purpose was to be a family, farm and draft dog. Today's Leonberger excels as a multi-purpose working dog; the most important task being a reliable family companion.

Physical Characteristics

Height at withers: Males 28 to 31.5 inches (72-80 cm), Females 25.5 inches to 29.5 inches (65-74 cm),

Weight: Males 130-170 pounds (59-77 kg), Females 100-130 pounds (45-59 kg).

Coat: Leonbergers have a medium to long, water resistant, double coat on the body and short fine hair on the muzzle and front of limbs. Mature males carry a mane. Coat colors are lion–yellow, golden to red and red–brown, also sand colored (cream, pale yellow) and all combinations thereof, always with a black mask. A small, unobtrusive stripe or white patch on the chest and some white hairs on toes is tolerated.

Longevity: 8-9 years.

Points of Conformation: Proportion of height at withers to length of body is 9 to 10. Bone is medium to heavy and in proportion to size of body with sufficient muscle to support frame. Head is rectangular with parallel lines. Stop is moderate. Eyes are dark brown, medium size, oval to almond shaped. Ears are of medium size, triangular, fleshy, hanging flat and close to the head. Nose is large, black, with clearly outlined nostrils. Lips are tight, with no drooling. Teeth are scissors to level. Withers are set above a firm level back that flows with a gently sloping croup into the tail. Chest is broad, roomy, and deep, reaching at least to the level of the elbows. Fore and rear quarters are well muscled. Shoulders are well laid–back, 90 degrees to the foreleg. Hind end is well angulated. Legs are straight and powerful. Feet do not turn in or out, with

tight arched toes. Dewclaws are usually present in the front, and may be present in the back. The Leonberger has a ground–covering, even and balanced gait. The stride is powerful, easy, free and elastic, with good reach and strong drive giving the impression of effortless power. In motion, the Leonberger maintains a level topline. As the dog's speed increases, the legs tend to converge toward the centerline.

Recognized Behavior Issues and Traits

The gentle character and even temperament of the Leonberger is of utmost importance for fulfilling their role as a family companion. The Leonberger is self–assured and calm, with a steady, playful demeanor. He is willing to please and possesses a good capacity for learning. The Leonberger exhibits a marked friendliness towards children and is at ease in all situations, never showing fear, shyness or aggression. The Leonberger's profuse coat tends to shed a lot, requiring daily brushing. The breed needs moderate daily exercise.

Normal Physiologic Variations

None reported

Drug Sensitivities

None reported

Inherited Diseases

Hip Dysplasia: Polygenically inherited trait causing degenerative joint disease and hip arthritis. OFA reports 14.1% affected. In a Czech study, 22.4% were affected. Reported at a frequency of 17% (including PennHIP diagnoses) in the 2000 LCA Health Survey.[1,2,3]

Elbow Dysplasia: Polygenically inherited trait causing elbow arthritis. OFA reports 4.8% affected.[1]

Polyneuropathy/Inherited Motor And Sensory Neuropathy: It is believed that there are more than one causes of polyneuropathy in the Leonberger breed. Polyneuropathy is a disorder of axonal degeneration identified in the breed worldwide. Affected Leonbergers present with exercise intolerance, laryngeal paralysis, distal muscle atrophy and neuromuscular weakness. Affected dogs between 1–3 years of age have a more severe form of the disease compared to older affected dogs that present between 8–9 years of age. The ratio of affected males to affected females is approximately 2.5 to 1, and some research suggests that one form of the disease can be x-linked. An autosomal recessive mutation (LPN1) has been identified that accounts for approximately one-third of all cases of polyneuropathy in the breed. Dogs homozygous for this mutation will develop the severe form of the disease by 3 years of age. It is possible that dogs heterozygous (carrying one copy) for this mutation may develop the milder, later-age form of the disease. A direct genetic test for this mutation is available. The frequency of the disorder in the breed has not been determined. Genetic mutations for other forms of the disease have not been identified.[4,5,6]

Patella Luxation: Polygenically inherited laxity of patellar ligaments, causing luxation, lameness, and later degenerative joint disease. Treat surgically if causing clinical signs. Too few Leonbergers have been screened by OFA to determine an accurate frequency.[1]

Disease Predispositions

Persistent Pupillary Membranes: Strands of fetal remnant connecting; iris to iris, cornea, lens, or involving sheets of tissue. The later three forms can impair vision, and dogs affected with these forms should not be bred. Identified in 16.21% of Leonbergers CERF examined by veterinary ophthalmologists between 2000-2005.[7]

Osteoarthritis: Leonbergers have an increased incidence of arthritis. Reported at a frequency of 15% of all dogs over 5 years of age in the 2000 LCA Health Survey.[3]

Hypothyroidism: Inherited autoimmune thyroiditis 11.1% positive for thyroid auto-antibodies based on testing at Michigan State University. (Ave. for all breeds is 7.5%). Reported at a frequency of 5.5% (9.3% of all dogs over 5 years of age) in the 2000 LCA Health Survey.[3,8,9]

Panosteitis: A self-limiting disease of young, large breed dogs involving the diaphyseal and metaphyseal areas of the tubular long bones, characterized by medullary fibrosis and both endosteal and subperiosteal new bone deposition. Affected dogs show intermittent lameness. Treatment is with non-steroidal anti-inflammatory drugs and rest. Reported at a frequency of 11% in the 2000 LCA Health Survey.[3]

Cataracts: Nuclear, posterior nuclear, or posterior polar cataracts predominate in the breed. Identified in 5.94% of Leonbergers CERF examined by veterinary ophthalmologists between 2000-2005. In a UK study, 24.6% of Leonbergers had cataracts, with the posterior polar subcapsular form showing significant inheritance. Reported at a frequency of 2.7% (4.6% of all dogs over 5 years of age) in the 2000 LCA Health Survey. CERF does not recommend breeding any Leonberger with a cataract.[3,7,10]

Osteosarcoma: Malignant bone cancer, usually affecting the limbs. A Swedish study showed an increased risk in the breed, with a median age of onset of 7.2 years. Reported at a frequency of 3.2% (7.8% of all dogs over 5 years of age) in the 2000 LCA Health Survey.[3,11]

Umbilical Hernia: Congenital umbilical hernias are reported at a frequency of 5.4% in the 2000 LCA Health Survey.[3]

Entropion: Rolling in of eyelids, often causing corneal irritation or ulceration. Entropion is reported in 4.34% of Leonbergers CERF examined by veterinary ophthalmologists between 2000-2005. Reported at a frequency of 3.2% in the 2000 LCA Health Survey.[3,7]

Distichiasis: Abnormally placed eyelashes that irritate the cornea and conjunctiva. Can cause secondary corneal ulceration. Reported in 2.28% of Leonbergers CERF examined by veterinary ophthalmologists between 2000-2005.[7]

Cranial Cruciate Ligament Rupture (ACL): Traumatic tearing of the anterior cruciate ligament. Treatment is surgery. Reported at a

frequency of 2.2% (3% of all dogs over 5 years of age) in the 2000 LCA Health Survey. Unknown mode of inheritance.[3]

Ectropion: Rolling out of eyelids, often with a medial canthal pocket. Can cause secondary conjunctivitis. Can be secondary to **macroblepharon**; an abnormally large eyelid opening. Ectropion is reported in 1.60% and macroblepharon in 2.05% of Leonbergers CERF examined by veterinary ophthalmologists between 2000-2005.[7]

Dilated Cardiomyopathy: Leonbergers are a predisposed breed for this condition, resulting in heart failure. Undetermined mode of inheritance. Reported at a frequency of 0.75% (2.1% of all dogs over 5 years of age) in the 2000 LCA Health Survey.[3,13]

Hypoadrenocorticism (Addison's disease): Immune mediated destruction of the adrenal gland. Typical presentation of lethargy, poor appetite, vomiting, weakness, and dehydration can occur from 4 months to several years of age. Treatment with DOCA injections or oral fludrocortisone. Some affected Leonbergers were diagnosed with concurrent hypothyroidism, suggesting a polyglandular syndrome. Reported at a frequency of 1% (2% of all dogs over 5 years of age) in the 2000 LCA Health Survey.[3,12]

Third Eyelid Eversion/Cartilage Anomaly: Developmental anomaly of the cartilage of the nictitating membrane. Eversion causes conjunctival drying and inflammation. Identified in 1.14% of Leonbergers CERF examined by veterinary ophthalmologists between 2000-2005.[7]

Osteochondritis Dissecans (OCD): Abnormality of cartilage development causing lameness in the shoulder, elbow, hock or knee. Severe cases may require surgery. Reported at a frequency of 1% in the 2000 LCA Health Survey.[3]

Gastric Dilatation-Volvulus (bloat, GDV): Polygenically inherited, life-threatening twisting of the stomach within the abdomen. Requires immediate treatment. Reported as a breed health issue on the LCA website.

Perianal Fistula/Furunculosis: Inflammatory disorder creating perianal ulceration and fistulas. Treat with anti-inflammatory medications and tacrolimus. Reported as a breed health issue on the LCA website.

Isolated Case Studies

Leukoencephalomyelopathy: Two unrelated 2 year old Leonbergers (a male and a female) presenting with signs of progressive ataxia of all 4 limbs, proprioceptive deficits, and thoracic limb hypermetria. were found to have a slowly progressive demyelinating leukoencephalomyelopathy. This disorder must be differentiated from the polyneuropathies identified in the breed.[14]

Genetic Tests

Tests of Genotype: Direct test for an autosomal recessive polyneuropathy gene (LPN1) is available from the University of Minnesota Veterinary Diagnostic Lab and University of Bern, Switzerland.

Tests of Phenotype: CHIC Certification: Required testing includes hip and elbow radiographs, CERF eye examination, and thyroid profile including autoantibodies. Optional testing includes a cardiac evaluation for congenital disease, canine good citizen certification, DNA submission to the CHIC DNA repository and a genetic test for LPN1. (See CHIC website; www.caninehealthinfo.org).

Recommended testing: Patella evaluation

Miscellaneous
- **Breed name synonyms:** Leo
- **Registries:** AKC, UKC, CKC, FCI, KCGB (Kennel Club of Great Britain), ANKC (Australian National Kennel Club), NKC (National Kennel Club).
- **AKC rank (None):** AKC recognized in June, 2010. Entire stud book entered.
- **Internet resources: Leonberger Club of America:** www.leonbergerclubofamerica.com
  Leonberger Club of Great Britain: http://leonbergerclub.org.uk
  Leonberger Club of Canada: www.leonbergerclubofcanada.com/temp/index.htm
  LCA Health Committee website: www.leowatch.org

References

1. OFA Website breed statistics: www.offa.org Last accessed July 1, 2010.
2. Doskarova B, Kyllar M & Paral V: Morphometric assessment of the canine hip joint using the acetabular angle of retrotorsion. Vet Comp Orthop Traumatol. 2010, 23(5).
3. Zieher W & Leonberger Club of America Health Research and Education Committee: Summary of the 2000 Health Survey Findings. Leowatch Vol. 2; Spring, 2002.
4. Shelton GD, Podell M, Poncelet L, et. al.: Inherited polyneuropathy in Leonberger dogs: a mixed or intermediate form of Charcot-Marie-Tooth disease? Muscle Nerve. 2003 Apr;27(4):471-7.
5. Granger N: Canine inherited motor and sensory neuropathies: An updated classification in 22 breeds and comparison to Charcot-Marie-Tooth disease. Vet J. 2011 Jun;188(3):274-85.
6. Granger, N, Escriou, C, Thibaud, JL, et. al.: Polyneuropathy in Leonberger dogs: an emerging pan-Europea polyneuropathy. Proceedings 2007 BSAVA Congress. 2007:488–489.
7. *Ocular Disorders Presumed to be Inherited in Purebred Dogs.* American College of Veterinary Ophthalmologists. ACVO, 2007.
8. Nachreiner R & Refsal K: Personal communication, Diagnostic Center for Population and Animal Health, Michigan State University. April, 2007.
9. Nachreiner RF, Refsal KR, Graham PA, et. al.: Prevalence of serum thyroid hormone autoantibodies in dogs with clinical signs of hypothyroidism. *J Am Vet Med Assoc* 2002 Feb 15;220(4):466-71.
10. Heinrich CL, Lakhani KH, Featherstone HJ, et. al: Cataract in the UK Leonberger population. Vet Ophthalmol. 2006 Sep-Oct;9(5):350-6.
11. Egenvall A, Nødtvedt A & von Euler H: Bone tumors in a population of 400 000 insured Swedish dogs up to 10 y of age: incidence and survival. Can J Vet Res. 2007 Oct;71(4):292-9.
12. Smallwood LJ & Barsanti JA: Hypoadrenocorticism in a family of leonbergers. J Am Anim Hosp Assoc. 1995 Jul-Aug;31(4):301-5.
13. Haggstrom J: Dilated Cardiomyopathy in Dogs: Diagnosis and Treatment. Proceedings, 2008 World Small Animal Veterinary Association World Congress. 2008.
14. Oevermann A, Bley T, Konar M, et. al.: A novel leukoencephalomyelopathy of Leonberger dogs. J Vet Intern Med. 2008 Mar-Apr;22(2):467-71.
15. AKC Breed Website: www.akc.org/breeds/leonberger Last accessed July 1, 2010.

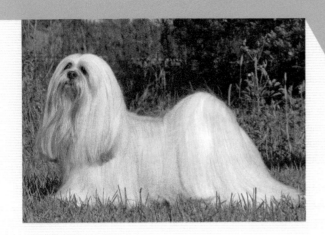

Lhasa Apso

The Breed History

This breed originated in the mountains of Tibet, in the city of Lhasa where the harsh environment and high elevations led to the selection of a very hardy dog type. They had been bred for their heavy insulating coat to cope with the extremes of climate. They were so prized in Tibet that they were considered good luck and over a few thousand years, were only found in monasteries or in the houses of nobles. They were also sent as gifts to China, where they contributed to the Shih Tzu and Pekingese breeds. They join the Tibetan Terrier and Tibetan Spaniel in the same group from this region. This breed was first accepted into the AKC registry in 1935. The first US imports came as gifts from the 13th Dalai Lama.

Breeding for Function

They served as guard and alarm dogs for dwellings and monasteries, and also for companionship.

Physical Characteristics

Height at Withers: female 10 " (25.4 cm), male 11" (28 cm)

Weight: females 13-15 lb (6-7 kg), males 13-18 lb (6-8 kg).

Coat: Many colors are accepted, but the haircoat density is significantly developed as protection against harsh conditions. The beard is often dark, and hairs are often mixed color throughout the coat, and have a straight medium texture. The colors most often seen are described as leonine (lion-like); honey, wheaten with dark on the extremities. Parti-color, white, black, and slate are less commonly seen.

Longevity: 14-15 years.

Points of Conformation: The dog is built longer than high, and the head, carried high, is well endowed with whiskers and beard hairs, the nose is black and the face profile is straight. Eyes should be dark brown in pigment, with keen bright expression, and the ears are pendulous and well covered with long hair. The skull is brachycephalic, and jaw is normally mildly prognathic. The tail should be carried well up, and sometimes a screw tip is noted at the terminus of the tail. The topline is straight with a slight slope, and the back is short. The feet are compact and hair-covered as well for warmth.

Recognized Behavior Issues and Traits

Reported breed characteristics include: They are dogs that generally train easily, though some are a bit independent. They will respond to gentle handling and are a trustworthy companion to their families and are loyal. They enjoy plenty of close human contact. They are wary of strangers and should be socialized when young to both other pets and people.Some are aggressive; especially males. They are good alarm barkers, and because of their historical function as a watchdog they will respond to intruders. They are active dogs, but require low exercise levels. High shedding, and high grooming requirements characterize Lhasas so some owners elect to have them clipped once or twice per annum. They do well in town or country settings.

Normal Physiologic Variations

None reported

Drug Sensitivities

None reported

Inherited Diseases

Patella Luxation: Polygenically inherited laxity of patellar ligaments, causing luxation, lameness, and later degenerative joint disease. Treat surgically if causing clinical signs. Reported 3.4x odds ratio versus other breeds. OFA reports 10.3% affected.[1,2]

Hip Dysplasia and Legg-Calve-Perthes Disease: Polygenically inherited traits causing degenerative hip joint disease and arthritis. Reported 6.7x odds ratio for Legg-Calve-Perthes versus other breeds. OFA reports 6.4% affected.[1,2]

Renal Dysplasia: Autosomal dominant disorder with incomplete penetrance causing renal failure. Affected dogs can succumb to renal failure from birth to two years of age. Mildly affected dogs can live with compensated renal insufficiency. Biopsy studies suggest that a large portion of the breed is affected, although only a small percentage dies from the condition. A direct genetic test for a susceptibility gene is available. (Affected dogs all have one copy of the gene, but most dogs with the gene will not develop kidney failure.)[3,4]

Progressive Retinal Atrophy (PRA): Autosomal recessive progressive degeneration of the retina leading to blindness. Age of onset in the breed 2-8 years of age. There is no test for carriers. Identified in 1.06% of Lhasa Apsos CERF examined by veterinary ophthalmologists between 2000-2005.[5,6]

Factor IX Deficiency (Hemophilia B): Rare X-linked inherited bleeding disorder identified in the breed. A genetic test is available.[7]

Elbow Dysplasia: Polygenically inherited trait causing elbow arthritis. Too few Lhasa Apsos have been screened by OFA to determine an accurate frequency.[1]

Disease Predispositions

Distichiasis: Abnormally placed eyelashes that irritate the cornea and conjunctiva. Can cause secondary corneal ulceration. Identified in 3.72% of Lhasa Apsos CERF examined by veterinary ophthalmologists between 2000-2005.[5]

Cataracts: Anterior or posterior cortex intermediate and punctate cataracts predominate in the breed. In one large study, 4.61% of Lhasa Apsos had cataracts. Identified in 3.27% of Lhasa Apsos CERF examined by veterinary ophthalmologists between 2000-2005. CERF does not recommend breeding any Lhasa Apso with a cataract.[5,8]

Brachycephalic Complex: The brachycephalic complex includes **Stenotic Nares, Elongated Soft Palate, Everted Laryngeal Saccules, Laryngeal Collapse,** and occasionally **Hypoplastic Trachea.** Can cause respiratory distress, apnea, and hypoxia.[9]

Hypothyroidism: Inherited autoimmune thyroiditis. 3.2% positive for thyroid auto-antibodies based on testing at Michigan State University. (Ave. for all breeds is 7.5%).[10,11]

Allergic Dermatitis: Inhalant or food allergy. Presents with pruritis and pyotraumatic dermatitis. Lhasa Apsos have a significantly increased risk for atopy versus other breeds. Dorn reports a 1.19x odds ratio versus other breeds.[12,13]

Exposure Keratopathy Syndrome/Pigmentary Keratopathy: Corneal reactivity and drying from ocular exposure secondary to shallow orbits, exophthalmos, and lagophthalmos. Identified in 2.66% of Lhasa Apsos CERF examined by veterinary ophthalmologists between 2000-2005.[5]

Corneal Dystrophy: Lhasa Apsos can have an epithelial/stromal form of corneal dystrophy. Identified in 2.13% of Lhasa Apsos CERF-examined by veterinary ophthalmologists between 2000-2005.[5]

Entropion: Rolling in of eyelids, often causing corneal irritation or ulceration. Reported in 1.60% of Lhasa Apsos CERF-examined by veterinary ophthalmologists between 2000-2005.[5]

Chronic Superficial Keratitis: This condition can cause conjunctivitis, corneal ulcerations, and vision problems due to corneal pigmentation. Age of onset 2-5 years. Treatment with topical ocular lubricants and anti-inflammatory medication. Identified in 1.60% of Lhasa Apsos CERF-examined by veterinary ophthalmologists between 2000-2005.[5]

Keratoconjunctivitis Sicca (KCS, Dry Eye): Ocular condition causing lack of tear production and secondary conjunctivitis, corneal ulcerations, and vision problems. Age of onset 2-5 years. CERF does not recommend breeding any Lhasa Apso with KCS.[5,14]

Prolapsed Gland of the Nictitans (Cherry Eye): This condition occurs secondary to inflammation of the gland. Reported at an increased frequency in the breed.[15]

Primary (Narrow Angle) Glaucoma: Ocular condition causing increased pressure within the eyeball, and secondary blindness due to damage to the retina. Diagnose with tonometry and gonioscopy. Diagnosed in 1.33% of Lhasa Apsos presented to veterinary teaching hospitals.[16]

Retinal Dysplasia: Geographic retinal dysplasia occurs in the breed. Can lead to blindness. Reported in 1.06% of Lhasa Apsos CERF-examined by veterinary ophthalmologists between 2000-2005.[5]

Persistent Pupillary Membranes: Strands of fetal remnant connecting; iris to iris, cornea, lens, or involving sheets of tissue. The later three forms can impair vision, and dogs affected with these forms should not be bred. Identified in 1.06% of Lhasa Apsos CERF-examined by veterinary ophthalmologists between 2000-2005.[5]

Urinary Calculi: The breed is found to be at an increased risk of developing **struvite** and **oxalate** calculi. One study reported an odds ratio of 10.95x for calcium oxalate stones versus other breeds.[17,18]

Intervertebral Disc Disease (IVDD): Lhasa Apsos have an increased risk of developing spinal cord disease due to prolapsed disk material. Clinical signs include back pain, scuffing of paws, spinal ataxia, limb weakness, and paralysis. Requires immediate veterinary attention.[19]

Sebaceous Adenitis: Disorder of immune mediated sebaceous gland destruction, presenting with hair loss, usually beginning with the dorsal midline and ears. Diagnosis by skin biopsy. Treat with isotretinoin. An autosomal recessive mode of inheritance is suspected.[20,21]

Portosystemic shunt (PSS, liver shunt): Congenital abnormal blood vessel connecting the portal and systemic circulation. Can be intrahepatic or extrahepatic. Causes stunting, abnormal behavior, possible seizures, and secondary ammonium urate urinary calculi. Treatment of PSS includes partial ligation and/or medical and dietary control of symptoms. Tobias reports a 5.4x odds ratio versus other breeds.[22]

Lissencephaly: A rare, inherited, congenital absence of cerebrocortical convolutions. Clinical signs include behavioral, abnormalities, blindness, and seizures that occur during the first year of life. Diagnosis with MRI.[23,24,25]

Demodicosis, Ectodermal Defect, Epilepsy, Hydrocephalus, Hypotrichosis, Juvenile Cellulitis, Oligodontia, Pancreatitis, Seasonal Flank Alopecia, Vertebral Stenosis, and **von Willebrand's Disease** are reported.[26]

Isolated Case Studies

Hydrocephalus, Syringomyelia, and Spinal Cord Angiodysgenesis: A Lhasa Apso pup with weakness and ataxia was diagnosed with this combination of disorders.[27]

Genetic Tests

Tests of Genotype: Direct test for a renal dysplasia susceptibility gene is available from Dogenes (www.dogenes.com).

Direct test for Factor XI deficiency is available from HealthGene.

Tests of Phenotype: Recommended tests are; CERF eye examination, hip and elbow radiographs, patella examination, thyroid profile including autoantibodies, genetic test for renal dysplasia susceptability, and cardiac examination.

Miscellaneous

- **Breed name synonyms:** Abso Seng Kye (Engl: Bark Lion Sentinel Dog), Lhasa, Tibetan Apso, Lion Dog
- **Registries:** AKC, CKC, UKC, KCGB (Kennel Club of Great Britain), ANKC (Australian National Kennel Club), NKC (National Kennel Club)
- **AKC rank (year 2008):** 56 (2,020 dogs registered)
- **Internet resources: American Lhasa Apso Club:** www.lhasaapso.org
  Lhasa Apso Canada: http://lhasa-apso-canada.com
  The Lhasa Apso Club (UK): www.lhasa-apso-club.org.uk

References

1. OFA Website breed statistics: www.offa.org Last accessed July 1, 2010.

2. LaFond E, Breur GJ & Austin CC: Breed susceptibility for developmental orthopedic diseases in dogs. J Am Anim Hosp Assoc. 2002 Sep-Oct;38(5):467-77.

3. Manderino DM, DeVries JG, Tamarkin J: Primary renal disease in a dog. Mod Vet Pract. 1984 Aug;65(8):633-5.

4. O'Brien TD, Osborne CA, Yano BL, et. al.: Clinicopathologic manifestations of progressive renal disease in Lhasa Apso and Shih Tzu dogs. J Am Vet Med Assoc. 1982 Mar 15;180(6):658-64.

5. Ocular Disorders Presumed to be Inherited in Purebred Dogs. American College of Veterinary Ophthalmologists. ACVO, 2007.

6. Bedford PGC: Retinopathies--Old and New. 2004. Proceedings, World Small Animal Veterinary Association World Congress, 2004.

7. Mauser AE, Whitlark J, Whitney KM, et. al.: A deletion mutation causes hemophilia B in Lhasa Apso dogs. Blood. 1996 Nov 1;88(9):3451-5.

8. Gelatt KN, Mackay EO: Prevalence of primary breed-related cataracts in the dog in North America. Vet Ophthalmol. 2005 Mar-Apr;8(2):101-11.

9. Koch DA, Arnold S, Hubler M, et. al.: Brachycephalic Syndrome in Dogs. Compend Contin Educ Pract Vet. January 2003;25(1):48-55.

10. Nachreiner RF, Refsal KR, Graham PA, et. al.: Prevalence of serum thyroid hormone autoantibodies in dogs with clinical signs of hypothyroidism. J Am Vet Med Assoc 2002 Feb 15;220(4):466-71.

11. Nachreiner R & Refsal K: Personal communication, Diagnostic Center for Population and Animal Health, Michigan State University. April, 2007.

12. Dorn CR: Canine breed-specific risks of frequently diagnosed diseases at veterinary teaching hospitals. Monograph. AKC Canine Health Foundation. 2000.

13. Schick RO, Fadok VA: Responses of atopic dogs to regional allergens: 268 cases (1981-1984). J Am Vet Med Assoc. 1986 Dec 1;189(11):1493-6.

14. Herrera D: Canine Keratoconjunctivitis Sicca. 2005. Proceedings, World Small Animal Veterinary Association World Congress, 2005.

15. Herrera D: Surgery of the Eyelids. 2005. Proceedings, World Small Animal Veterinary Association Congress, 2005.

16. Gelatt KN, MacKay EO: Prevalence of the breed-related glaucomas in pure-bred dogs in North America. Vet Ophthalmol. 2004 Mar-Apr;7(2):97-111.

17. Houston DM & Moore AE: Canine and feline urolithiasis: examination of over 50 000 urolith submissions to the Canadian veterinary urolith centre from 1998 to 2008. Can Vet J. 2009 Dec;50(12):1263-8.

18. Lekcharoensuk C, Lulich JP, Osborne CA, et. al.: Patient and environmental factors associated with calcium oxalate urolithiasis in dogs. J Am Vet Med Assoc. 2000 Aug 15;217(4):515-9.

19. LeCouteur RA: Spinal Cord Diseases of Small Breed Dogs. 2006. Proceedings, Western Veterinary Conference.

20. White S: Sebaceous Adenitis. 2001. Proceedings, World Small Animal Veterinary Association World Congress, 2001

21. Hernblad Tevell E, Bergvall K, & Egenvall A: Sebaceous adenitis in Swedish dogs, a retrospective study of 104 cases. Acta Vet Scand. 2008 May 25;50:11.

22. Tobias KM & Rohrbach BW: Association of breed with the diagnosis of congenital portosystemic shunts in dogs: 2,400 cases (1980-2002). J Am Vet Med Assoc. 2003 Dec 1;223(11):1636-9.

23. Zaki FA: Lissencephaly in Lhasa Apso dogs. J Am Vet Med Assoc. 1976 Dec 1;169(11):1165, 1168.

24. Greene CE, Vandevelde M, Braund K: Lissencephaly in two Lhasa Apso dogs. J Am Vet Med Assoc. 1976 Aug 15;169(4):405-10.

25. Saito M, Sharp NJ, Kortz GD, et. al.: Magnetic resonance imaging features of lissencephaly in 2 Lhasa Apsos. Vet Radiol Ultrasound. 2002 Jul-Aug;43(4):331-7.

26. The Genetic Connection: A Guide to Health Problems in Purebred Dogs. L Ackerman. p 227, AAHA Press, 1999.

27. Schmahl W, Kaiser E: Hydrocephalus, syringomyelia, and spinal cord angiodysgenesis in a Lhasa-apso dog. Vet Pathol. 1984 Mar;21(2):252-4.

28. The Complete Dog Book, 20th Ed. The American Kennel Club. Howell Book House, NY 2006. p. 572-574

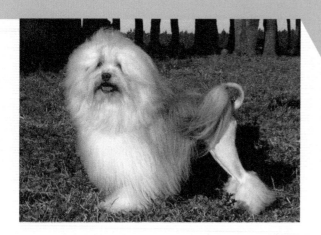

and other pets. Good alarm barkers. May dig or bark excessively if bored. Possessing good trainability. Fine for apartment or city living. Low to moderate exercise needs. The Lowchen has moderate to high grooming needs but a low shedding tendency.

Normal Physiologic Variations
None reported

Drug Sensitivities
None reported

Inherited Diseases

Patella Luxation: Polygenically inherited laxity of patellar ligaments, causing luxation, lameness, and later degenerative joint disease. Treat surgically if causing clinical signs. OFA reports 5.3% affected.[1]

Hip Dysplasia and Legg–Calve Perthes Disease: Polygenically inherited traits causing degenerative hip joint disease and arthritis. OFA reports 3.3% affected.[1]

Elbow Dysplasia: Polygenically inherited trait causing elbow arthritis. Too few Lowchen have been screened by OFA to determine an accurate frequency.[1]

Progressive Retinal Atrophy (PRA): PRA in the Lowchen causes progressive blindness, beginning with night blindness from 6 months to 2 years of age. Autosomal recessive mode of inheritance. There is no test for carriers.[2]

Disease Predispositions

Persistent Pupillary Membranes: Strands of fetal remnant connecting; iris to iris, cornea, lens, or involving sheets of tissue. The later three forms can impair vision, and dogs affected with these forms should not be bred. Identified in 8.14% of Lowchen CERF examined by veterinary ophthalmologists between 2000-2005.[2]

Distichiasis: Abnormally placed eyelashes that irritate the cornea and conjunctiva. Can cause secondary corneal ulceration. Identified in 4.46% of Lowchen CERF examined by veterinary ophthalmologists between 2000-2005.[2]

Cataracts: Anterior or posterior cortex intermediate cataracts predominate in the breed. Unknown mode of inheritance. Identified in 2.71% of Lowchen CERF examined by veterinary ophthalmologists between 2000-2005. CERF does not recommend breeding any Lowchen with a cataract.[2]

Vitreous Degeneration: A liquefaction of the vitreous gel which may predispose to retinal detachment and/or glaucoma. Reported in 1.74% of Lowchen dogs CERF examined by veterinary ophthalmologists between 2000-2005.[2]

The Breed History
Records show that this European breed has been in existence since the mid 15th century.[1] The Lowchen belongs to the Bichon breed class. The nickname of *"Little Lion Dog"* can be traced back to the breed specific clip that results in a lion-like short coat over the hindquarters and rear limbs down to the tarsus and the thick natural mane hair which is left on. In the period between the end of the Second World War and the 1960s, it was among the rarest of breeds in the world, but has recently resurged in popularity. The AKC admitted them to the non-sporting group in 1999.

Breeding for Function
This breed was primarily developed for companionship.

Physical Characteristics
Height at Withers: 12-14" (30.5-35.5 cm)

Weight: 8-18 lb (4-8 kg)

Coat: The long dense haircoat is straight to slightly wavy and fairly soft in texture. There are no coat color limitations.

Longevity: 13-14 years

Points of Conformation: The Lowchen has a square conformation, the skull is broad, the stop is moderate and muzzle is short and rounded. High head carriage during activity is characteristic. Deep-set eyes are wide-set, face forward and are darkly colored. The mildly pendulous ears have plenty of feathering, the nose is large and black or brown in pigmentation. The neck is moderate in length and muscling, is slightly arched, and the thorax is moderate in depth, ribs are well sprung, and the abdomen is slightly tucked up. The tail is carried over the back unless at rest and is high set. The limbs are straight boned, metacarpals and metatarsals are short, dewclaws may be removed; especially the rear ones. The feet are small, tight and compact, with the 3rd and 4th toe appearing longer than the 1st and 5th; with well-developed pads; hind feet are smaller than forefeet. The gait is a long, low stride.

Recognized Behavior Issues and Traits
Reported breed characteristics include: Lively, friendly, intelligent, strong-willed and may challenge other dogs or household members for dominance. Generally, they are considered good with children

Hypothyroidism: Inherited autoimmune thyroiditis. Too few Lowchen have been tested by Michigan State University for thyroid autoantibodies to determine an accurate frequency. (Ave. for all breeds is 7.5%).[3,4]

Deafness, Diabetes Mellitus, and Patent Ductus Arteriosus are reported in the breed.

Isolated Case Studies
None Reported

Genetic Test
Tests of Genotype: Direct tests for presence of black, brown and red colors, and black and brown nose are available from HealthGene.

Tests of Phenotype: Recommend CERF eye examination, hip and elbow radiographs, patella evaluation, thyroid profile including autoantibodies, and cardiac examination.

Miscellaneous
- **Breed name synonyms:** Little Lion Dog, Petit Chien Lion.
- **Registries:** AKC, UKC, CKC, KCGB (Kennel Club of Great Britain), ANKC (Australian National Kennel Club), NKC (National Kennel Club).
- **AKC rank (year 2008):** 137 (131 dogs registered)
- **Internet resources: The Lowchen Club of America:** www.thelowchenclubofamerica.org
  The Lowchen Club of Canada: www.lowchenclubofcanada.com
  The Lowchen Club (UK): www.thelowchenclubuk.com
  Lowchen World: http://lowchenworld.com

References
1. OFA Website breed statistics: www.offa.org Last accessed July 1, 2010.
2. *Ocular Disorders Presumed to be Inherited in Purebred Dogs.* American College of Veterinary Ophthalmologists. ACVO, 2007.
3. Nachreiner RF, Refsal KR, Graham PA, et. al.: Prevalence of serum thyroid hormone autoantibodies in dogs with clinical signs of hypothyroidism. J Am Vet Med Assoc 2002 Feb 15;220(4):466-71.
4. Nachreiner R & Refsal K: Personal communication, Diagnostic Center for Population and Animal Health, Michigan State University. April, 2007.
5. *The Complete Dog Book, 20th Ed.* The American Kennel Club. Howell Book House, NY 2006. p. 575-578.

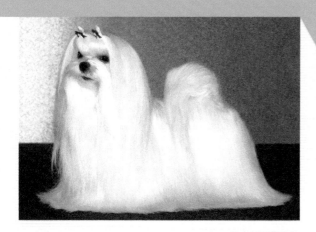

The Breed History

Records of this breed in art can be found on the Isle of Malta dated thousands of years ago. Roman, Greek and Egyptian records trace the breed back to very early times. The AKC registered this Bichon-type breed in 1888. They are somewhat spaniel in type though they were sometimes called Maltese Terriers historically.

Breeding for Function

In early history, the Maltese dogs may have served for vermin control. A companion dog exclusively for a very long time, Maltese dogs were particularly sought after by women of high social standing in the past.

Physical Characteristics

Height at Withers: 10" (25 cm).

Weight: 4-6 lb (2-3 kg).

Coat: The single haircoat hangs flat, is white, and the hairs are long, straight and silky. The coat often reaches the floor or longer at maturity and the topknot is usually tied up. The thick, luxurious coat needs regular grooming. Due to the long white coat, this is essentially an indoor dog and is suitable for apartment life.

Longevity: 14-15 years

Points of Conformation: This is a toy dog with naturally high head carriage, moderate stop, the skull slightly rounded, and the muzzle is tapered and of medium length; the nose is black. Eyes are moderately set apart, dark, large, and palpebral margins are black. Ears are well feathered and hanging from a low set position. Neck is moderately short, body is square in conformation, the topline level, thorax moderate in depth, and ribs are well sprung. The abdomen is only slightly tucked up. Limbs are fine and straight boned, feet are small and round in shape, pads thick and black. The tail is high set and sits over the back; is well plumed with hair. The gait is straight, energetic, quick and smoothly flowing.

Recognized Behavior Issues and Traits

The reported breed characteristics include: Gentle nature, playful, intelligent, affectionate, and loves children. Exercise needs are low. Activity levels are moderate. The Maltese is noted to be a vigorous alarm barker. Needs to have quiet, gentle children in the family or can be snappy. Some can be difficult to house train. The Maltese is considered a low shedding, low allergy dog.

Normal Physiologic Variations

Regular hygiene around the eyes is needed due to chronic epiphora.[1]

Some are picky eaters.

Drug Sensitivities

None reported

Inherited Diseases

Patella Luxation: Polygenically inherited laxity of patellar ligaments, causing luxation, lameness, and later degenerative joint disease. Treat surgically if causing clinical signs. Dorn reports a 1.92x odds ratio in Maltese versus other breeds. Another study reports a 6.5x odds ratio versus other breeds. OFA reports 5.0% affected.[2,3,4]

Hip Dysplasia and Legg-Calve-Perthes Disease: Polygenically inherited traits causing degenerative hip joint disease and arthritis. Reported at a high frequency, but too few Maltese have been screened by OFA to determine an accurate frequency.[2]

Elbow Dysplasia: Polygenically inherited trait causing elbow arthritis. Too few Maltese have been evaluated by the OFA to determine an accurate frequency in the breed.[2]

Disease Predispositions

Hypothyroidism: Inherited autoimmune thyroiditis. 16.5% positive for thyroid auto-antibodies based on testing at Michigan State University. (Ave. for all breeds is 7.5%).[5,6]

Cataracts: Anterior and posterior cortex intermediate cataracts predominate in the breed. Identified in 7.23% of Maltese CERF examined by veterinary ophthalmologists between 2000-2005. CERF does not recommend breeding any Maltese with a cataract.[7]

Persistent Pupillary Membranes: Strands of fetal remnant connecting; iris to iris, cornea, lens, or involving sheets of tissue. The later three forms can impair vision, and dogs affected with these forms should not be bred. Identified in 7.23% of Maltese CERF examined by veterinary ophthalmologists between 2000-2005.[7]

Retinal Dysplasia: Retinal folds and geographic dysplasia are recognized in the breed. Can lead to blindness. Reported in 2.41% of Maltese CERF-examined by veterinary ophthalmologists between 2000-2005.[7]

Hydrocephalus: The breed is one with an increased frequency of hydrocephalus. Diagnosis by radiography, MRI, or ultrasound (through an open fontanel). Dorn reports an 11.61x odds ratio in Maltese versus other breeds.[3,8]

Distichiasis: Abnormally placed eyelashes that irritate the cornea and conjunctiva. Can cause secondary corneal ulceration. Identified in 1.20% of Maltese CERF-examined by veterinary ophthalmologists between 2000-2005.[7]

Portosystemic Shunt (PSS, Liver Shunt): Abnormal blood vessels connecting the systemic and portal blood flow. Vessels can be intrahepatic or extrahepatic. Hepatic **microvascular dysplasia** is genetically related to PSS. Causes stunting, abnormal behavior and possible seizures. Diagnose with paired fasted and feeding serum bile acid and/or ammonium levels, and abdominal ultrasound. Treatment of PSS includes partial ligation and/or medical and dietary control of symptoms. 1.6% of Maltese presented to veterinary teaching hospitals had PSS, with an odds ratio of 32x versus other breeds. Undetermined mode of inheritance.[9,10]

Patent Ductus Arteriosus (PDA): Polygenically inherited congenital heart disorder, where a fetal vessel remains open after birth, causing a mixing of oxygenated and unoxygenated blood. Affected dogs are usually stunted, and have a loud heart murmur. Diagnosis with Doppler ultrasound. Treat with surgery. Dorn reports a 30.09x odds ratio in Maltese versus other breeds.[3]

Deafness: Congenital deafness can be unilateral of bilateral. Diagnosed by BAER testing.[11,12]

Autoimmune Hemolytic Anemia (AIHA): Autoimmune destruction of red blood cells. Clinical features include pale mucous membranes, weakness, lethargy and collapse. Treat with immunosuppressive drugs. Reported 2.8x odds ratio versus other breeds in an Australian Study.[13]

Protein Losing Enteropathy (PLE, Lymphangiectasia): Presents with diarrhea, weight loss, and/or abdominal effusion due to dilation of lymph vessels in the intestine. Inflammatory cell buildup blocks normal absorption of nutrients. Can occur at any age, but primarily affects middle-aged dogs. Maltese are a breed with a predilection for the condition. Treatment consists of chronic anti-inflammatory medication and dietary restriction. Some dogs with severe cases have a poor prognosis.[14]

Necrotizing Meningoencephalitis: An inherited disorder in Maltese dogs of progressive seizures with or without other neurologic signs, resulting in death. CSF reveals pleocytosis and elevated levels of protein. Pathology shows mild to moderate asymmetrical dilation of the lateral ventricles, and focal areas of necrosis and generalized non-suppurative inflammation. Homozygosity of DLA class II genes is associated with the disease in the breed. Unknown mode of inheritance.[15,16,17,18]

White Shaker Dog Syndrome: Affected dogs present between 6 months to 5 years of age, with diffuse, fine, whole body tremor, and can also show nystagmus, menace response abnormalities, proprioceptive deficits, and seizures. CSF usually is abnormal containing a mild lymphocytic pleocytosis. Protein concentration may be normal or mildly increased. Treat with tapering doses of corticosteroid. Unknown mode of inheritance.[19]

Gastrointestinal Mast Cell Tumor: The Maltese breed was over-represented in a study of mast cell tumors of the gastrointestinal tract.[20]

Testicular Tumors: A study in Taiwan suggests an increased frequency of testicular tumors in intact males in the breed. This occurred with and without concurrent cryptorchidism.[21]

Splenic Masses: In an Australian study, Maltese were overrepresented versus other breeds for masses in the spleen. Histopathological diagnoses included benign and malignant masses.[22]

Atresia Ani (Imperforate Anus): An increased incidence of this congenital condition is reported in the breed, with a frequency of 0.069%, and an odds ratio of 13.39x. Treatment is surgery.[23]

Brachygnathism, Cleft Lip/Plate, Mitral Valve Disease, Oligodontia, Prognathism, Retained Primary Teeth, Sebaceous Adentitis, Tracheal Collapse, and **Wry Mouth** are reported.[24]

Isolated Case Studies

Exocrine Pancreatic Insufficiency: A 1.8-year-old female Maltese dog was presented because of a history of chronic diarrhea, polyphagia, weight loss, and coprophagia. A definite diagnosis of exocrine pancreatic insufficiency was made based on low serum trypsin-like immunoreactivity activity. The clinical signs disappeared after porcine pancreatic powder supplementation.[25]

Malonic Aciduria: A family of Maltese dogs with malonic aciduria is reported. Affected dogs presented with episodes of seizures and stupor with hypoglycemia, acidosis, and ketonuria. Urinary organic acid assays showed elevated malonic acid without elevation of methylmalonic acid. Treatment with frequent feedings of a low-fat diet high in medium-chain triglycerides resulted in normalization of clinical signs and a resolution of the malonic aciduria.[26]

Gallbladder Aplasia: Two cases of gallbladder aplasia are found in the literature. Affected dogs present with persistent mild hepatopathy and intermittent vomiting of bile. Absence of the gallbladder with malformation of the quadrate lobe of the liver, with histological evidence of bile duct proliferation and portal fibrosis are found.[27,28]

Urinary Bladder Rhabdomyosarcoma: A two-year-old female Maltese presented with hematuria and pollakiuria. A urinary bladder tumor was diagnosed. Histopathology identified a rhabdomyosarcoma. The dog died of metastatic liver disease 2 months later.[29]

Glycogen Storage Disease Type Ia (GSD Ia): An autosomal recessive storage disease, GSD 1a causes affected puppies to exhibit tremors, weakness, and neurologic signs when hypoglycemic. They have postnatal growth retardation and progressive hepatomegaly. Present in research colonies from a natural mutation.[30,31]

Oculocutaneous Albinism: A 4-month-old female Maltese dog was evaluated for photophobia and complete absence of pigment resulting in white hair, pink muzzle, eyelids and foot-pads. Ophthalmoscopic examination revealed a yellow tapetal fundus but no pigment in the nontapetal fundus.[32]

Genetic Tests

Tests of Genotype: none

Tests of Phenotype: Recommend patella evaluation, hip and elbow radiographs, CERF eye examination, thyroid profile including autoantibodies, and cardiac examination.

Miscellaneous

- **Breed name synonyms:** Bichon Maltaise, Maltese Terrier (historical).
- **Registries:** AKC, UKC, CKC, KCGB (Kennel Club of Great Britain), ANKC (Australian National Kennel Club), NKC (National Kennel Club).
- **AKC rank (year 2008):** 20 (10,056 dogs registered)
- **Internet resources: American Maltese Association:** www.americanmaltese.org

References

1. Yi NY, Park SA, Jeong MB, et. al.: Medial canthoplasty for epiphora in dogs: a retrospective study of 23 cases. J Am Anim Hosp Assoc. 2006 Nov-Dec;42(6):435-9.
2. OFA Website breed statistics: www.offa.org Last accessed July 1, 2010.
3. Dorn CR: Canine breed-specific risks of frequently diagnosed diseases at veterinary teaching hospitals. Monograph. AKC Canine Health Foundation. 2000.
4. LaFond E, Breur GJ & Austin CC: Breed susceptibility for developmental orthopedic diseases in dogs. J Am Anim Hosp Assoc. 2002 Sep-Oct;38(5):467-77.
5. Nachreiner RF, Refsal KR, Graham PA, et. al.: Prevalence of serum thyroid hormone autoantibodies in dogs with clinical signs of hypothyroidism. J Am Vet Med Assoc 2002 Feb 15;220(4):466-71.
6. Nachreiner R & Refsal K: Personal communication, Diagnostic Center for Population and Animal Health, Michigan State University. April, 2007.
7. Ocular Disorders Presumed to be Inherited in Purebred Dogs. American College of Veterinary Ophthalmologists. ACVO, 2007.
8. Axlund TW: Managing the Hydrocephalic Patient: Medical and Surgical Options. Proceedings, 2004 Atlantic Coast Veterinary Conference. 2004.
9. Hunt GB: Effect of breed on anatomy of portosystemic shunts resulting from congenital diseases in dogs and cats: a review of 242 cases. Aust Vet J. 2004 Dec;82(12):746-9.
10. Tobias KM, Rohrbach BW: Association of breed with the diagnosis of congenital portosystemic shunts in dogs: 2,400 cases (1980-2002). J Am Vet Med Assoc. 2003 Dec 1;223(11):1636-9.
11. Coppens AG, Resibois A, Poncelet L: Bilateral deafness in a maltese terrier and a great pyrenean puppy: inner ear morphology. J Comp Pathol. 2000 Feb-Apr;122(2-3):223-8.
12. Strain GM: Deafness prevalence and pigmentation and gender associations in dog breeds at risk. The Veterinary Journal 2004; 167(1):23-32.
13. McAlees TJ: Immune-mediated haemolytic anaemia in 110 dogs in Victoria, Australia. Aust Vet J. 2010 Jan;88(1-2):25-8.
14. Marks S: Diagnosis and Management of Protein-Losing Enteropathies. Proceedings, 2009 Western Veterinary Conference. 2009.
15. Fearnside SM, Kessell AE, Powe JR: Cervical hyperaesthesia in a Maltese Terrier with necrotising meningoencephalitis. Aust Vet J. 2004 Sep;82(9):550-2.
16. Stalis IH, Chadwick B, Dayrell-Hart B, et. al.: Necrotizing meningoencephalitis of Maltese dogs. Vet Pathol. 1995 May;32(3):230-5.
17. Pedersen NC, Vernau K, Dickinson P, et. al.: DLA Association in Various Toy Breeds with Immune Mediated Encephalopathies. Proceedings, 2009 Tufts' Canine and Feline Breeding and Genetics Conference. 2009.
18. Maehara T, Shimada A, Morita T, et. al.: Distribution of the inflammatory lesions in the central nervous system of dogs affected with disseminated and ocular form of granulomatous meningoencephalomyelitis. J Vet Med Sci. 2009 Apr;71(4):509-12.
19. Bagley RS: Differential Diagnosis of Animals with Peripheral Nervous System Disease. Proceedings, 2002 Atlantic Coast Veterinary Conference. 2002.
20. Ozaki K, Yamagami T, Nomura K, et. al.: Mast cell tumors of the gastrointestinal tract in 39 dogs. Vet Pathol. 2002 Sep;39(5):557-64.
21. Liao AT, Chu PY, Yeh LS, et. al.: A 12-year retrospective study of canine testicular tumors. J Vet Med Sci. 2009 Jul;71(7):919-23.
22. Christensen N, Canfield P, Martin P, et. al.: Cytopathological and histopathological diagnosis of canine splenic disorders. Aust Vet J. 2009 May;87(5):175-81.
23. Vianna ML, Tobias KM: Atresia ani in the dog: a retrospective study. J Am Anim Hosp Assoc. 2005 Sep-Oct;41(5):317-22.
24. The Genetic Connection: A Guide to Health Problems in Purebred Dogs. L Ackerman. p. 227. AAHA Press, 1999.
25. Kim JW, Jung DI, Kang BT, et. al.: Canine exocrine pancreatic insufficiency treated with porcine pancreatic extract. J Vet Sci. 2005 Sep;6(3):263-6.
26. O'Brien DP, Barshop BA, Faunt KK, et. al.: Malonic aciduria in Maltese dogs: normal methylmalonic acid concentrations and malonyl-CoA decarboxylase activity in fibroblasts. J Inherit Metab Dis. 1999 Dec;22(8):883-90.
27. Liptak JM, Swinney GR, Rothwell TL, et. al.: Aplasia of the gallbladder in a dog. J Small Anim Pract. 2000 Apr;41(4):175-7.
28. Austin B, Tillson DM, & Kuhnt LA: Gallbladder agenesis in a Maltese dog. J Am Anim Hosp Assoc. 2006 Jul-Aug;42(4):308-11.
29. Takiguchi M, Watanabe T, Okada H, et. al.: Rhabdomyosarcoma (botryoid sarcoma) of the urinary bladder in a Maltese. J Small Anim Pract. 2002 Jun;43(6):269-71.
30. Kishnani PS, Faulkner E, VanCamp S, et. al.: Canine model and genomic structural organization of glycogen storage disease type Ia (GSD Ia). Vet Pathol. 2001 Jan;38(1):83-91.
31. Brix AE, Howerth EW, McConkie-Rosell A, et. al.: Glycogen storage disease type Ia in two littermate Maltese puppies. Vet Pathol. 1995 Sep;32(5):460-5.
32. Park SA, Yi NY, Kim MS, et. al.: A Case of oculocutaneous albinism in a Maltese. J Vet Sci. 2005 Dec;6(4):361-2.
33. The Complete Dog Book, 20th Ed. The American Kennel Club. Howell Book House, NY 2006. p. 481-483.

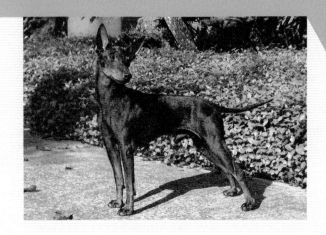

The Breed History

Originating in the British Isles, the original Black and Tan progenitor terrier for this breed was a heavier set dog with a coarser coat. In Manchester England, history records that a fancier who wanted a dog for both hare coursing and rat killing bred a whippet and a crossbred ratter terrier. Other breed ancestors potentially include Greyhound, Italian Greyhound and Dachshunds. AKC recognition occurred in 1886 (Toy) and 1887 (Standard). Until 1959, the two sizes of Manchester were two separate breeds. The toy was developed from the standard.

Breeding for Function

Vermin control was the primary purpose for these dogs. As a ratter in the field and in pub pit rat killing contests they excelled. They were courageous enthusiastic hunting companions. The toy variety was a lady's pet. Both varieties are now valued show and companion dogs.

Physical Characteristics

Height at Withers: Standard 15-16 inches (39-40 cm).

Weight of Standard: 12-22 lb (5.5-10 kg)

Height at Withers: Toy 10-12 inches (25-30 cm).

Weight of Toy: 7 up to 12 lb (3-5.5 kg).

Coat: The sleek short hair coat is black with mahogany markings; distinct, not smudgy borders—well defined pattern.

Longevity: 14-15 years.

Points of Conformation: These dogs have a long muzzle, flat wedge-shaped skull, slight stop, and their bone structure is sleek and athletic. Ears are naturally pricked up, and the dogs are a bit longer than high. Almond-shaped slanting close-set dark eyes, and a strong jaw ending in a black nose characterizes the face. Ears vary only slightly with Standard ears being erect, cropped, or button. Toys must have naturally erect ears only. The neck is slim, slightly arched and moderately long, the topline has a slight arch, chest is narrow but deep, abdomen is mildly tucked, and a slightly curved tail tapers to finish just short of the tarsal joint.

Recognized Behavior Issues and Traits

Reported breed characteristics include that they are: Agile, loyal, intelligent, they respond well to obedience training. They maintain a well-developed chase instinct, so should not be left off-leash unless in an enclosure. They are excellent watchdogs, and enjoy close contact with humans. They require minimal grooming and are low to moderate shedders. They should be socialized early to other pets and people.

Normal Physiologic Variations

None reported

Drug Sensitivities

None reported

Inherited Diseases

von Willebrand's Disease Type 1 (vWD): Autosomal recessive genetic disorder causing a mild bleeding syndrome. A direct genetic test is available from VetGen that reports 4% affected, and 37% carrier in the breed. Reported at a frequency of 2.72% in the Manchester Terrier Health and Genetics Survey.[1]

Hip Dysplasia and Legg-Calve Perthes Disease: Polygenically inherited traits causing degenerative hip joint disease and arthritis. Too few Manchester Terriers have been screened by OFA to determine an accurate frequency. Breeding studies in Manchester Terriers show a high heritability for Legg-Calve Perthes Disease. Reported at a frequency of 1.46% in the Manchester Terrier Health and Genetics Survey.[1,2,3]

Patella Luxation: Polygenically inherited laxity of patellar ligaments, causing luxation, lameness, and later degenerative joint disease. Treat surgically if causing clinical signs. Too few Manchester Terriers have been screened by OFA to determine an accurate frequency. Reported at a frequency of 1.17% in the Manchester Terrier Health and Genetics Survey.[1,2]

Elbow Dysplasia: Polygenically inherited trait causing elbow arthritis. Too few Manchester Terriers have been screened by OFA to determine an accurate frequency.[2]

Disease Predispositions

Missing Teeth: Reported at a frequency of 18.37% in the Manchester Terrier Health and Genetics Survey. Unknown mode of inheritance.[1]

Hypothyroidism: Inherited autoimmune thyroiditis. 8.9% positive for thyroid auto-antibodies based on testing at Michigan State University. (Ave. for all breeds is 7.5%).[4,5]

Anal Gland Disease: Anal sacculitis and anal gland infection. Dorn reports a 2.92x odds ratio in Manchester Terriers versus other breeds. Reported at a frequency of 3.40% in the Manchester Terrier Health and Genetics Survey.[1,6]

Cryptorchidism: Can be bilateral or unilateral. Reported at a frequency of 3.21% in the Manchester Terrier Health and Genetics Survey.[1]

Demodicosis: Demodectic mange dermatitis has an underlying immunodeficiency in its pathogenesis. Reported at a frequency of 2.53% in the Manchester Terrier Health and Genetics Survey. Unknown mode of inheritance.[1]

Seasonal Flank Alopecia: Bilateral, symmetrical hair loss affecting the flank, dorsum and tail. Dorn reports a 10.55x odds ratio in Manchester Terriers versus other breeds. Reported at a frequency of 1.85% in the Manchester Terrier Health and Genetics Survey.[1,6]

Umbilical Hernia: Congenital opening in the body wall from where the umbilical cord was attached. Correct surgically if large. Reported at a frequency of 1.75% in the Manchester Terrier Health and Genetics Survey. Unknown mode of inheritance.[1]

Deafness: Congenital sensorineural deafness can be unilateral of bilateral. Diagnosed by BAER testing. Reported at a frequency of 1.46% in the Manchester Terrier Health and Genetics Survey. Unknown mode of inheritance.[1]

Cataracts: Too few Manchester Terriers have been CERF eye examined to determine an accurate frequency in the breed. Reported in 3.81% of Manchester Terriers presented to veterinary teaching hospitals. Reported at a frequency of 1.36% in the Manchester Terrier Health and Genetics Survey.[1,7,8]

Diabetes Mellitus: Sugar diabetes. Caused by a lack of insulin production by the pancreas. Controlled by insulin injections, diet, and glucose monitoring. Dorn reports a 8.81x odds ratio in Manchester Terriers versus other breeds.[6]

Juvenile Cardiomyopathy: Several Manchester Terriers under the age of one year have died in heart failure with a post-mortum diagnosis of juvenile cardiomyopathy. Research at Prince Edward Island and the University of Pennsylvania is looking into the cause of this disorder.

Other Ocular Disorders: Too few Manchester Terriers have been CERF examined to determine an accurate breed frequency of ocular disorders.[7]

Cleft Lip/Palate, Cutaneous Asthenia, Hydrocephalus, Lens Luxation, Oligodontia, Progressive Retinal Atrophy, and **Retained Primary Teeth** are reported.[9]

Isolated Case Studies

X-linked Myotubular Myopathy: Three male Manchester Terriers presented at 2 months of age due to weakness and failure to thrive. Other males in the dam's previous litter showed similar symptoms. Muscle biopsy revealed a myotubular myopathy, and genetic analysis found a mutation in the MTM1 gene on the X-chromosome.[10]

Genetic Tests

Tests of Genotype: Direct test for vWD is available from VetGen.

Tests of Phenotype: CHIC Certification: Required testing includes hip radiographs, thyroid profile including autoantibodies, and genetic test for VWD. (See CHIC website: www.caninehealthinfo.org).

Recommend patella evaluation, elbow radiographs, CERF eye examination, and cardiac examination.

Miscellaneous

- **Breed name synonyms:** Toy Manchester Terrier, Black and Tan Terrier (historical), Toy Black and Tan Terrier (historical), English Toy Terrier, Gentleman's Terrier (historical)
- **Registries:** AKC, CKC, UKC, KCGB (Kennel Club of Great Britain), ANKC (Australian National Kennel Club), NKC (National Kennel Club)
- **AKC rank (year 2008):** 107 (404 dogs registered)
- **Internet resources: American Manchester Terrier Club:** http://clubs.akc.org/mtca
  Canadian Manchester Terrier Club: www.canadamt.com
  British Manchester Terrier Club: www.british-manchester-terrier-club.co.uk

References

1. American & Canadian Manchester Terrier Clubs: Manchester Terrier Health and Genetics Survey. 2002.
2. OFA Website breed statistics: www.offa.org Last accessed July 1, 2010.
3. Vasseur PB, Foley P, Stevenson S, et. al.: Mode of inheritance of Perthes' disease in Manchester terriers. *Clin Orthop Relat Res.* 1989 Jul;(244):281-92.
4. Nachreiner RF, Refsal KR, Graham PA, et. al.: Prevalence of serum thyroid hormone autoantibodies in dogs with clinical signs of hypothyroidism. *J Am Vet Med Assoc* 2002 Feb 15;220(4):466-71.
5. Nachreiner R & Refsal K: Personal communication, Diagnostic Center for Population and Animal Health, Michigan State University. April, 2007.
6. Dorn CR: Canine breed-specific risks of frequently diagnosed diseases at veterinary teaching hospitals. Monograph. AKC Canine Health Foundation. 2000.
7. *Ocular Disorders Presumed to be Inherited in Purebred Dogs.* American College of Veterinary Ophthalmologists. ACVO, 2007.
8. Gelatt KN, Mackay EO: Prevalence of primary breed-related cataracts in the dog in North America. Vet Ophthalmol. 2005 Mar-Apr;8(2):101-11.
9. *The Genetic Connection: A Guide to Health Problems in Purebred Dogs.* L Ackerman. p.228, AAHA Press, 1999.
10. Robinson FL, Misizin AP, O'Brien DP, et. al.: Myotubular Myopathy in a Family of Manchester Terrier Dogs. Proceedings, 2008 ACVIM Forum. 2008.
11. *The Complete Dog Book, 20th Ed.* The American Kennel Club. Howell Book House, NY 2006. p.396-400.

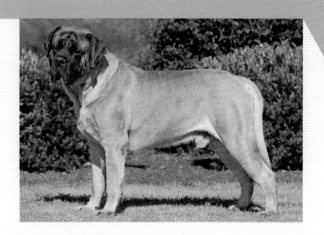

Mastiff

Points of Conformation: A massive well muscled and heavily boned dog with an equally massive square head, the Mastiff is a picture of brute strength. Medium-sized eyes are dark brown in color and no nictitans should be showing. Ears are v-shaped with rounded tips and possess fairly fine leather. They lie close to the cheeks at rest. A prominent furrow up the center of the forehead is present. The stop is moderate. The muzzle is short, blunt and deep, and forehead wrinkles appear when alerted. The nose is always dark, and the lips somewhat pendulous. The neck is muscular and medium in length, with little loose skin. The topline is straight, until gently curving down over the croup, and the thorax is deep and wide. There is a moderate abdominal tuck up. The tail reaches to the tarsus or a bit longer. The Tail tapers and is straight to slightly curved. The limbs are straight boned and wide set, feet are large and toes well knuckled up. The gait is best described as smooth and ground covering.

The Breed History

This popular and widespread breed was known in England for a few centuries as a pit fighter and watchdog. In ancient times they likely originated in Southwest Asia, moving through Tibet to the west of the continent. Phoenicians were thought to have brought Molosser and Alaunt type dogs westward to Britain by 2000 years BC. Other breeds deriving from the ancient Molosser type dogs include Tibetan Mastiff, Bullmastiff, Neopolitan Mastiff, Dogue de Bordeaux and Fila Brasileiro. First written accounts of this breed in England date to 55 BC when Caesar made note of them during his invasions. Many were sent back to Italy, and became fighting dogs in the Roman Empire. AKC recognition occurred in 1885.

The term *Mastiff* is actually a generic term for gigantic defense dogs but over the Centuries types emerged, of which the English Mastiff, now simply termed Mastiff is one. At the times of the World Wars of the twentieth century, they became almost extinct in England, but because of breeders sending dogs back from North America, the breed was revived.

Breeding for Function

Pit fighting, police and military work, war cart dog and watchdog duties are the best-known historical duties. Importantly, the peasant class kept these dogs to help with guarding, vermin and wolf control. Many were kept by butchers who were able to afford the high cost of feeding them because they fed the Mastiff dogs their meat scraps. The other function that the breed was prized for was as group hunting dogs for lion and deer. Power, courage and agility are characteristics thoroughly bred into the Mastiff.

Physical Characteristics

Height at Withers: female 27.5" (70 cm), male 30" minimum (76 cm).

Weight: 170-190 lb (79-86 kg).

Coat: The double coat consists of very dense short undercoat and an outer coat consisting of straight, coarse and moderately short hairs. Brindle, apricot and fawn are accepted colors, and in brindle the background should be fawn or apricot. There is generally a black mask and ear coloration irrespective of coat coloration.

Longevity: Approximately 8-9 years.

Recognized Behavior Issues and Traits

Reported breed characteristics include: Courageous but docile to handle represents the ideal breed temperament. A dignified manner is also selected for. They are loyal, and well-developed guarding instincts are the standard. They are wary of strangers and vigorous in defense of perceived threats. Early socialization and obedience are essential. These dogs have high human companionship needs and need lots of room due to the large body size. High exercise levels need to be allowed for. This dog, though calm with family is not recommended for toddlers due to massive size. They tend to drool significantly. Grooming needs are low.

Normal Physiologic Variations

None reported

According to a study in the UK 64.6% of Mastiff litters were born via cerserean section.[1]

Drug Sensitivities

None reported

Inherited Diseases

Hip Dysplasia: Polygenically inherited trait causing degenerative joint disease and hip arthritis. OFA reports 19.4% affected.[2]

Elbow Dysplasia: Polygenically inherited trait causing elbow arthritis. OFA reports 14.7% affected. Reported 48.4x odds ratio for fragmented coronoid process, and 20.2x odds ratio for ununited anconeal process forms of elbow dysplasia versus other breeds.[2,3]

Multifocal Retinopathy/Retinal Dysplasia: Autosomal recessive retinal pigment epithelial dysplasia causing localized multifocal retinal detachments. Age of onset from 11 to 13 weeks of age. Can lead to blindness. Reported in 7.63% of Mastiffs CERF examined by veterinary ophthalmologists between 2000-2005. A genetic test is available.[4]

Dominant Progressive Retinal Atrophy (PRA): An autosomal dominant PRA exists in the breed, with an onset of 6 months to 3-1/2 years of age. Causes blindness. Optigen reports 1% of Mastiffs are affected based on the available genetic test.[4,5]

Patella Luxation: Polygenically inherited laxity of patellar ligaments, causing luxation, lameness, and later degenerative joint disease. Treat surgically if causing clinical signs. OFA reports 0.3% affected.[2]

Disease Predispositions

Allergic Dermatitis (Atopy): Inhalant or food allergy. Presents with pruritis and pyotraumatic dermatitis (hot spots). Reported at a frequency of 10.2% in the Mastiff Health Survey.[6]

Hypothyroidism: Inherited autoimmune thyroiditis. 8.7% positive for thyroid auto-antibodies based on testing at Michigan State University. (Ave. for all breeds is 7.5%).[7,8]

Persistent Pupillary Membranes: Strands of fetal remnant connecting; iris to iris, cornea, lens, or involving sheets of tissue. In the Mastiff, the strands most often bridge from the iris to the cornea and may potentially cause vision impairment. Identified in 7.63% of Mastiffs CERF examined by veterinary ophthalmologists between 2000-2005. CERF does not recommend breeding a Mastiff with any form of PPM.[4]

Cranial Cruciate Ligament Rupture (ACL): Traumatic tearing of the anterior cruciate ligament. The breed is found to be one with an increased incidence. Treatment is surgery. Reported at a frequency of 7.5% in the Mastiff Health Survey.[6,9]

Ectropion: Rolling out of eyelids, often with a medial canthal pocket. Can also cause conjunctivitis. Ectropion is reported in 6.26% of Mastiffs CERF examined by veterinary ophthalmologists between 2000-2005.[4]

Cystine Urolithiasis/Cystinuria: Cystine uroliths are a sequela to cystinuria, an inherited renal tubular defect in reabsorption of cystine and some other amino acids. The mode of inheritance in the breed is not determined. Diagnosis with nitroprusside urine test. PennGen testing shows 9.9% of males and 0.2% of females tested are affected.[10,11]

Entropion: Rolling in of eyelids, often causing corneal irritation or ulceration. Entropion is reported in 4.18% of Mastiffs CERF examined by veterinary ophthalmologists between 2000-2005.[4]

Macroblepharon: Abnormally large eyelid opening; may lead to secondary conditions associated with corneal exposure. Reported in 4.11% of Mastiffs CERF examined by veterinary ophthalmologists between 2000-2005.[4]

Gastric Dilation/Volvulus (GDV, Bloat): Life-threatening twisting of the stomach within the abdomen. Requires immediate veterinary attention. Cause of 16.3% of deaths in Mastiffs in one survey. Reported at a frequency of 4.0% in the Mastiff Health Survey.[6,12]

Osteosarcoma (OSA): Malignant bone cancer, most often seen in the humerus or femur. Reported at a frequency of 3.8% in the OFA on-line Mastiff Health Survey.[2]

Cataracts: Anterior cortex punctate cataracts predominate in the breed. Identified in 2.82% of Mastiffs CERF examined by veterinary ophthalmologists between 2000-2005.[4]

Idiopathic Epilepsy: Inherited seizures. Control with anti-seizure medication. Onset of seizures from 6 months to 5 years of age. Reported at a frequency of 1.4% in the Mastiff Health Survey.[6]

Osteochondritis Dissecans (OCD): Polygenically inherited cartilage defect. Causes joint pain and lameness in young growing dogs. Mild cases can resolve with rest, while more severe cases require surgery. Reported 1006.8xx odds ratio for stifle OCD, and 11.9x odds ratio for shoulder OCD versus other breeds. Shoulder OCD is reported at a frequency of 1.30% in the Mastiff.[3,13]

Corneal Dystrophy: Endothelial form occurs in the breed due to edema from the loss of the inner lining of the cornea. Results in keratitis and decreased vision. Identified in 1.02% of Mastiffs CERF examined by veterinary ophthalmologists between 2000-2005.[4]

Panosteitis: Self-limiting disease of young, large breed dogs involving the diaphyseal and metaphyseal areas of the tubular long bones. Affected dogs show intermittent lameness. Reported 3.5x odds ratio versus other breeds.[3]

Cervical Malformation/Malarticulation (Wobblers disease): A congenital anatomical disorder that causes compression of the cervical spinal cord. Clinical signs include limb weakness, proprioceptive deficits, and paralysis. A breed predisposition is found in the Mastiff. Unknown mode of inheritance.[14,15]

Pulmonic Stenosis (PS) and Dysplasia of the Atrioventricular Valves (DAV): Two congenital heart disorders identified in the breed. Screen with auscultation and echocardiography. Unknown mode of inheritance.[16]

Microphthalmia, Prognathism, and **Subaortic Stenosis** are reported.[17]

Isolated Case Studies

Sacral Osteochondrosis: Several case reports of this condition are in the literature. In one, a Mastiff dog showed chronic signs of pain in its pelvic limbs. Radiography revealed a triangular mineralized opacity at the craniodorsal aspect of the sacrum consistent with sacral osteochondrosis. A T2-weighted spin-echo MRI revealed dorsal and lateral compression of the cauda equina. The osteochondral fragment was removed via a dorsal laminectomy, and the clinical signs resolved.[18,19]

Extradural Synovial Cyst Myelopathy: Three male Mastiffs presented with progressive ataxia and tetraparesis. Degenerative arthritis of the articular facet joints was noted on survey spinal radiographs. Myelography disclosed lateral axial compression of the cervical spinal cord medial to the articular facets. Extradural compressive cystic structures adjacent to articular facets were identified on magnetic resonance imaging (1 dog). Dorsal laminectomies cured all 3 dogs. The cysts were identified as synovial cysts.[20]

Mesenchymal Chondrosarcoma: A young adult female Mastiff dog developed a large retroperitoneal mass, pleural effusion, and multiple pulmonary and pleural nodules. All masses were diagnosed as mesenchymal subtype chondrosarcomas, using histological and immunohistochemical criteria.[21]

Genetic Tests

Tests of Genotype: Direct tests for PRA and Multifocal Retinopathy are available from Optigen.

Tests of Phenotype: CHIC Certification: Required testing includes hip and elbow radiographs, CERF eye examination (minimum of 2 years) and congenital cardiac evaluation. Optional tests include thyroid profile including autoantibodies, and nitroprusside urine test for cystinuria from PennGen. (See CHIC website; www.caninehealthinfo.org).

Recommend patella evaluation.

Miscellaneous

- **Breed name synonyms:** Old English Mastiff, English Mastiff, Alan/Alaunts (historical terms in Italian-French).
- **Registries:** AKC, UKC, CKC, KCGB (Kennel Club of Great Britain), ANKC (Australian National Kennel Club), NKC (National Kennel Club)
- **AKC rank (year 2008):** 28 (6,657 dogs registered)
- **Internet resources: Mastiff Club of America Inc.:**
  http://mastiff.org/
  Canadian Mastiff Club: www.mastiffcanada.org
  Old English Mastiff Club (UK): www.mastiffclub.com

References

1. Evans KM & Adams VJ: Proportion of litters of purebred dogs born by caesarean section. J Small Anim Pract. 2010 Feb;51(2):113-8.
2. OFA Website breed statistics: www.offa.org Last accessed July 1, 2010 .
3. LaFond E, Breur GJ & Austin CC: Breed susceptibility for developmental orthopedic diseases in dogs. J Am Anim Hosp Assoc. 2002 Sep-Oct;38(5):467-77.
4. *Ocular Disorders Presumed to be Inherited in Purebred Dogs.* American College of Veterinary Ophthalmologists. ACVO, 2007.
5. Kijas JW, Miller BJ, Pearce-Kelling SE, et. al.: Canine models of ocular disease: outcross breedings define a dominant disorder present in the English mastiff and bull mastiff dog breeds. *J Hered.* 2003 Jan-Feb;94(1):27-30.
6. Mastiff Club of America: Mastiff Health Survey; preliminary statistics – first 570. 2005.
7. Nachreiner RF, Refsal KR, Graham PA, et. al.: Prevalence of serum thyroid hormone autoantibodies in dogs with clinical signs of hypothyroidism. *J Am Vet Med Assoc* 2002 Feb 15;220(4):466-71.
8. Nachreiner R & Refsal K: Personal communication, Diagnostic Center for Population and Animal Health, Michigan State University. April, 2007.
9. Duval JM, Budsberg SC, Flo GL, et. al.: Breed, sex, and body weight as risk factors for rupture of the cranial cruciate ligament in young dogs. *J Am Vet Med Assoc.* 1999 Sep 15;215(6):811-4.
10. Osborne CA, Sanderson SL, Lulich JP, et. al: Canine cystine urolithiasis. Cause, detection, treatment, and prevention. *Vet Clin North Am Small Anim Pract.* 1999 Jan;29(1):193-211, xiii.
11. Case LC, Ling GV, Franti CE, et. al.: Cystine-containing urinary calculi in dogs: 102 cases (1981-1989). J Am Vet Med Assoc. 1992 Jul 1;201(1):129-33.
12. Evans KM & Adams VJ: Mortality and morbidity due to gastric dilatation-volvulus syndrome in pedigree dogs in the UK. J Small Anim Pract. 2010 Jul;51(7):376-81.
13. Rudd RG, Whitehair JG, Margolis JH: Results of management of osteochondritis dissecans of the humeral head in dogs : 44 cases [1982 to 1987]. *J Am Anim Hosp Assoc* 1990: 26[2]:173-178.
14. Berry WL: Common Cervical Myelopathies. Proceedings, 2004 Western Veterinary Conference. 2004.
15. Lyman R: Surgical Treatment of Caudal Cervical Spondylomyeopathy: A Discussion of the Controversy III. Proceedings, 2004 ACVIM Forum. 2004.
16. Fernández del Palacio MJ: Congenital Heart Diseases: Part I. Proceedings, 2002 WSAVA Congress. 2002.
17. *The Genetic Connection: A Guide to Health Problems in Purebred Dogs.* L Ackerman. p. 228. AAHA Press, 1999.
18. Glyde M, Doyle R, McAllister H, et. al.: Magnetic resonance imaging in the diagnosis and surgical management of sacral osteochondrosis in a mastiff dog. *Vet Rec.* 2004 Jul 17;155(3):83-6.
19. Snaps FR, Heimann M, Saunders J, et. al.: Osteochondrosis of the sacral bone in a mastiff dog. *Vet Rec.* 1998 Oct 24;143(17):476-7.
20. Levitski RE, Chauvet AE, Lipsitz D: Cervical myelopathy associated with extradural synovial cysts in 4 dogs. *J Vet Intern Med.* 1999 May-Jun;13(3):181-6.
21. Munday JS, Prahl A: Retroperitoneal extraskeletal mesenchymal chondrosarcoma in a dog. *J Vet Diagn Invest.* 2002 Nov;14(6):498-500.
22. *The Complete Dog Book, 20th Ed.* The American Kennel Club. Howell Book House, NY 2006. p. 293-297.

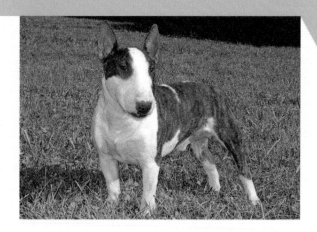

Miniature Bull Terrier

an early introduction to children (and small pets or other dogs) in the household. Needs human companionship, has low grooming needs and is a low shedder. Good in town or country but has high energy levels so adequate exercise and mental gymnastics are recommended to prevent boredom vices.

The Breed History
The Bull-and-Terrier (white English terrier X Bulldog) was the progenitor of the miniature version of the bull terrier. Additional crosses with the Spanish terrier and the Black and Tan may have also contributed to the final type. Some records show Dalmation crosses also occurred. The goal was to produce the miniature version of the bull terrier. AKC accepted this breed in 1991.

Breeding for Function
These downsized bull terriers were not specifically bred for fighting as were their larger counterparts, but they have inherited the feisty courageous personality from their forbearers. This makes them a formidable watchdog.

Physical Characteristics
Height at Withers: 10-14" (24.5-35.5 cm)

Weight: 24-33 lb (11-15 kg)

Coat: They possess a short hard glossy flat haircoat either white or colored, with or without markings.

Longevity: 12-13 years

Points of Conformation: A sturdy square constitution characterizes the breed. The skull is full, the forehead flat and egg-shaped as in the bull terrier. The small triangular shaped obliquely set eyes are dark in color and deep set, resulting in a piercing look. High set ears are close set, small and pricked when alert, and the leather is moderate. The nose is black. The neck is long, arched and muscular, not throaty. The back is short with a moderate arch over the loin. The chest is very broad, and the thorax is deep with the broadness and depth extending well back in the rib cage. They have a moderate abdominal tuck, and the tapering fine curved tail is set low and carried high. Limbs have straight heavy bone and moderate musculature. The small compact feet have well knuckled up toes.

Recognized Behavior Issues and Traits
Reported breed attributes include: Though fiery if faced with opponents, in the home they are expected to be tractable. Courageous, playful, devoted, tenacious, generally friendly but need

Normal Physiologic Variations
According to a study in the UK, 52.4% of Miniature Bull Terrier litters are delivered via cesarean section.[1]

Drug Sensitivities
None reported

Inherited Diseases
Primary Lens Luxation: An autosomal recessive lens luxation occurs in the breed due to abnormalities of the suspensory apparatus of the lens (zonule). Often progresses to secondary glaucoma. Relative risk of 48.44x versus other breeds. Identified in 3.88% of Miniature Bull Terriers CERF examined by veterinary ophthalmologists between 2000-2005. Reported at a frequency of 6.33%, and glaucoma at a frequency of 3.80% in the 2002-2004 MBTCA Breed Health Survey. Homozygous affected dogs usually develop lens luxation between 4-8 years of age. Rarely, heterozygous carriers can develop lens luxation, but at a later age. A genetic test is available from OFA, showing 52% carrier, and 13% affected.[2,3,4,5,6]

Hip Dysplasia: Polygenically inherited trait causing degenerative joint disease and hip arthritis. Too few Miniature Bull Terriers have been screened by OFA to determine an accurate frequency.[2]

Patella Luxation: Polygenically inherited laxity of patellar ligaments, causing luxation, lameness, and later degenerative joint disease. Treat surgically if causing clinical signs. Too few Miniature Bull Terriers have been screened by OFA to determine an accurate frequency.[2]

Elbow Dysplasia: Polygenically inherited trait causing elbow arthritis. Too few Miniature Bull Terriers have been screened by OFA to determine an accurate frequency.[2]

Hereditary Nephritis: Autosomal dominant disorder causing renal failure at variable ages in affected dogs due to abnormal kidney basement membrane protein and structure. No genetic test is available.[7]

Disease Predispositions
Persistent Pupillary Membranes: Strands of fetal remnant connecting; iris to iris, cornea, lens, or involving sheets of tissue. The later three forms can impair vision, and dogs affected with these forms should not be bred. Identified in 11.34% of Miniature Bull Terriers CERF examined by veterinary ophthalmologists between 2000-2005.[3]

Hypothyroidism: Inherited autoimmune thyroiditis. 4.5% positive for thyroid auto-antibodies based on testing at Michigan State University. (Ave. for all breeds is 7.5%).[8,9]

Deafness: Congenital deafness can be unilateral or bilateral. Diagnosed by BAER testing. Reported at a frequency of 3.80% in the 2002-2004 MBTCA Breed Health Survey. Unknown mode of inheritance.[5]

Corneal Dystrophy: Endothelial form occurs in the breed due to the edema from the loss of the inner lining of the cornea. Results in keratitis and decreased vision. Identified in 1.49% of Miniature Bull Terriers CERF examined by veterinary ophthalmologists between 2000-2005.[3]

Vitreous Degeneration: Liquefaction of the vitreous gel which may predispose to retinal detachment. Identified in 1.49% of Miniature Bull Terriers CERF examined by veterinary ophthalmologists between 2000-2005.[3]

Cataracts: Anterior cortex and capsular punctate cataracts predominate in the breed. Identified in 1.19% of Miniature Bull Terriers CERF examined by veterinary ophthalmologists between 2000-2005. CERF does not recommend breeding any Miniature Bull Terrier with a cataract.[3]

Left Ventricular Outflow Tract Obstruction (LVOTO): Reported as a problem in the breed. Screen by echocardiography. The MBTCA recommends only breeding dogs with LVOT rates of less than 2.2 m/sec with no multiple minor or any major structural defects present.

Compulsive Tail Chasing and Spinning: Disorder of persistent spinning observed in the breed. Possibly a behavioral compulsion, as 75% of affected dogs respond to clomipramine administration. However a neurological partial seizure disorder cannot be ruled out, as some dogs have abnormal electroencephalograms and respond to anticonvulsants.[10,11]

Isolated Case Studies

None reported

Genetic Tests

Tests of Genotype: Direct genetic test for Lens Luxation is available from OFA and AHT.

Tests of Phenotype: CHIC Certification: Required testing includes cardiac evaluation with echocardiogram, CERF eye examination, BAER test for deafness, and kidney disease screening with urine protein:creatinine ratio. (See CHIC website; www.caninehealthinfo.org).

Recommended tests include hip and elbow radiographs, patella examination, and thyroid profile including autoantibodies.

Miscellaneous

- **Breed name synonyms:** Mini Bull
- **Registries:** AKC, UKC, CKC, KCGB (Kennel Club of Great Britain), ANKC (Australian National Kennel Club), NKC (National Kennel Club)
- **AKC rank (year 2008):** 124 (236 dogs registered)

- **Internet resources: Miniature Bull Terrier Club of America:** www.minibull.org
  Miniature Bull Terrier Club UK: www.miniaturebullterrierclub.co.uk
  Miniature Bull Terrier Club of Canada: www.minibullyclub.com

References

1. Evans KM & Adams VJ: Proportion of litters of purebred dogs born by caesarean section. J Small Anim Pract. 2010 Feb;51(2):113-8.
2. OFA Website breed statistics: www.offa.org Last accessed July 1, 2010.
3. *Ocular Disorders Presumed to be Inherited in Purebred Dogs.* American College of Veterinary Ophthalmologists. ACVO, 2007.
4. Curtis R, Barnett KC, Startup FG: Primary lens luxation in the miniature bull terrier. *Vet Rec.* 1983 Apr 2;112(14):328-30.
5. Miniature Bull Terrier Club of America: 2002-2004 Health Survey Report. 2004.
6. Sargan DR, Withers D, Pettitt L, et. al.: Mapping the mutation causing lens luxation in several terrier breeds. J Hered. 2007;98(5):534-8.
7. Hood JC, Craig AJ: Hereditary nephritis in a miniature bull terrier. *Vet Rec.* 1994 Aug 6;135(6):138-40.
8. Nachreiner RF, Refsal KR, Graham PA, et. al.: Prevalence of serum thyroid hormone autoantibodies in dogs with clinical signs of hypothyroidism. J Am Vet Med Assoc 2002 Feb 15;220(4):466-71.
9. Nachreiner R & Refsal K: Personal communication, Diagnostic Center for Population and Animal Health, Michigan State University. April, 2007.
10. Moon-Fanelli AA, Dodman NH: Description and development of compulsive tail chasing in terriers and response to clomipramine treatment. *J Am Vet Med Assoc.* 1998 Apr 15;212(8):1252-7.
11. Dodman NH, Knowles KE, Shuster L, et. al.: Behavioral changes associated with suspected complex partial seizures in bull terriers. *J Am Vet Med Assoc.* 1996 Mar 1;208(5):688-091.
12. *The Complete Dog Book, 20th Ed.* The American Kennel Club. Howell Book House, NY 2006. p. 401-403.

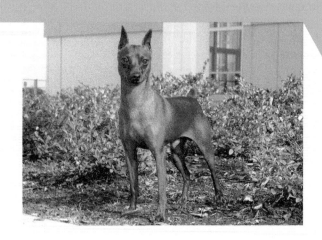

Miniature Pinscher

The Breed History

The Miniature Pinscher is not bred down in size from Doberman Pinscher stock, in fact, the MinPin is a much older breed (predates the Doberman by about 200 years). In the 1800s, writings suggest Italian Greyhound and Dachshund were contributors to breed development. Records date back perhaps 2000 years and the German Pinscher may in fact be the original larger breed ancestor. The origins of the breed are in Scandinavia and particularly, later in Germany. Pinscher means *biter* or *terrier*. The AKC registry admitted the breed in 1929.

Breeding for Function

Historically, they served as valuable rodent control dogs. Watchdog and companionship are two other roles that they play.

Physical Characteristics

Height at Withers: 10-12.5" (25.5-32 cm).

Weight: 8-10 lb (4-4.5 kg).

Coat: The glossy, short flat-lying coat has a hard, smooth hair texture. Red, stag red (red and black hairs), chocolate with rust, black with tan (red) are the accepted coat colors.

Longevity: 13-14 years

Points of Conformation: Small, compact and almost square in conformation, the MinPin has oval large dark eyes; palpebral margins are black or self in chocolates. The head is flat, they have a tapering narrow muzzle, the stop is slight, nose is black or self in chocolates, and lips are close and dry. The ears are prick and large, the neck is moderate in length and muscling, slightly arched, and not throaty. The topline is level to mildly sloping down to the rear, and the thorax deep with well sprung ribs. The abdomen is moderately tucked up. Limbs are straight boned and dewclaws are usually removed. Feet are compact, with well knuckled up toes, and nails are thick. The tail is high set, carried high and may be docked to a short length. The gait is described as "hackney-like" due to the very high stepping, quick action similar to the hackney horse.

Recognized Behavior Issues and Traits

Reported breed characteristics include: Low grooming needs, loyal and affectionate, good watchdog, high spirited, alert, can be snappy, brave against dogs much larger, curious, extremely high activity levels, good with sensible, quiet gentle children, moderately good trainability, good escape artists, and should not be off leash unless in a fenced enclosure. They are known to have a moderate barking tendency.

Normal Physiologic Variations

Dilute coat color is due to the homozygous recessive expression of a mutation in the melanophilin gene (MLPH). This can predispose to color dilution alopecia.[1]

Drug Sensitivities

None reported

Inherited Diseases

Legg–Calve Perthes Disease and Hip Dysplasia: Polygenically inherited traits causing degenerative hip joint disease and arthritis. Legg-Calves Perthes disease is considered a significant problem in the breed, however too few Miniature Pinschers have been screened by OFA to determine an accurate frequency. Reported 71.5x odds ratio for Legg-Calve-Perthes versus other breeds.[2,3]

Patella Luxation: Polygenically inherited laxity of patellar ligaments, causing luxation, lameness, and later degenerative joint disease. Treat surgically if causing clinical signs. Dorn reports an 4.87x odds ratio for the disorder versus other breeds. Another study reports a 14.4x odds ratio versus other breeds. OFA reports 3.2% affected.[2,3,4,5]

Mucopolysaccharidosis VI (MPS VI): Autosomal recessive disorder causing skeletal deformities, including defects in the sternum, vertebrae and particularly the hip joints. To varying degrees they may also experience corneal cloudiness and facial dysmorphia. A genetic test is available.[6,7,8]

Elbow Dysplasia: Polygenically inherited trait causing elbow arthritis. Too few Miniature Pinschers have been screened by OFA to determine an accurate frequency.[2]

Disease Predispositions

Corneal Dystrophy: Epithelial/stromal form causes opacities on the surface of the cornea. Average age of onset is 1-2 years. Unknown mode of inheritance. Identified in 5.80% of Miniature Pinschers CERF examined by veterinary ophthalmologists between 2000-2005.[9]

Cataracts: Anterior or posterior intermediate and punctate cataracts occur in the breed. Onset 1.5-3 years of age. Reported in 4.58% of Miniature Pinschers presented to veterinary teaching hospitals. Identified in 1.79% of Miniature Pinschers CERF examined by veterinary ophthalmologists between 2000-2005. CERF does not recommend breeding any Miniature Pinscher with a cataract.[9,10]

Vitreous Degeneration: Liquefaction of the vitreous gel which may predispose to **retinal detachment** or **glaucoma**. Identified in 4.46% of Miniature Pinschers CERF examined by veterinary ophthalmologists between 2000-2005.[9]

Hypothyroidism: Inherited autoimmune thyroiditis. 3.6% positive for thyroid auto-antibodies based on testing at Michigan State University. (Ave. for all breeds is 7.5%).[11,12]

Persistent Pupillary Membranes: Strands of fetal remnant connecting; iris to iris, cornea, lens, or involving sheets of tissue. The later three forms can impair vision, and dogs affected with these forms should not be bred. Identified in 3.57% of Miniature Pinschers CERF examined by veterinary ophthalmologists between 2000-2005.[9]

Color-Dilution Alopecia: Condition seen in some blue or fawn (dilute) colored Miniature Pinschers. Starts as a gradual onset of dry, dull and poor hair coat quality. Progresses to poor hair regrowth, follicular papules and comedomes. Hair loss and comedome formation are usually most severe on the trunk. Dorn reports an 8.54x odds ratio for developing alopecia versus other breeds.[1,4,13]

Optic Nerve Hypoplasia/Micropapilla: Congenital defect of optic nerve development affecting vision, or a small optic disc. Identified in 1.34% of Miniature Pinschers CERF examined by veterinary ophthalmologists between 2000-2005.[9]

Inherited Epilepsy: Grand-mal seizures. Control with anticonvulsant medication. Dorn reports a 5.39x odds ratio versus other breeds. Unknown mode of inheritance.[4]

Demodicosis: Demodectic mange dermatitis has an underlying immunodeficiency in its pathogenesis. Dorn reports a 1.95x odds ratio versus other breeds. Unknown mode of inheritance.[4]

Immune-Mediated Hemolytic Anemia: Auto-immune disorder where the body produces antibodies against its own red blood cells. Treat with immunosuppressive drugs. There is generally a female preponderance with this disorder. Miniature Pinschers have an increased risk versus other breeds.[14]

Cystinuria/Cystine Bladder Stones: Miniature Pinschers have an increased risk for developing cystine bladder stones, due to an error in cystine metabolism. Treat with surgical removal and life-long medical therapy. Unknown mode of inheritance in this breed.[15]

Portosystemic shunt (PSS, liver shunt): Congenital abnormal blood vessel connecting the portal and systemic circulation. More frequently intrahepatic in this breed versus extrahepatic. Causes stunting, abnormal behavior, possible seizures, and secondary ammonium urate urinary calculi in the breed. Treatment of PSS includes partial ligation and/or medical and dietary control of symptoms. Tobias reports a 7.0x odds ratio versus other breeds.[16]

Progressive Retinal Atrophy (PRA): Degeneration of the retina leading to blindness. Unknown mode of inheritance. Identified in 0.45% of Miniature Pinschers CERF examined by veterinary ophthalmologists between 2000-2005. CERF does not recommend breeding any Miniature Pinscher with PRA.[9]

Diabetes Mellitus: Sugar diabetes. Control with insulin injection, diet, and glucose monitoring. Reported at an increased prevalence in the breed. Unknown mode of inheritance.[17]

Deafness, Ebow Luxation, Keratoconjunctivitis Sicca, and **Sebaceous Adenitis** are reported.[18]

Isolated Case Studies

Sry-Negative XX True Hermaphrodite (XX Sex Reversal): A phenotypically male Miniature Pinscher was examined. The chromosomal sex was female (XX), and there was an absence of "male" causing Sry. XX Sex-reversal is familial in other breeds.[19]

Genetic Tests

Tests of Genotype: Direct test for MPS VI is available from PennGen.

Direct test for black and chocolate coat color is available from VetGen.

Tests of Phenotype: Recommend patella examination, CERF eye examination, hip and elbow radiographs, thyroid profile including autoantibodies, and cardiac evaluation.

Miscellaneous

- **Breed name synonyms:** MinPin, Zwergpinscher, Reh Pinscher, King of Toys (nickname).
- **Registries:** AKC, UKC, CKC, KCGB (Kennel Club of Great Britain), ANKC (Australian National Kennel Club), NKC (National Kennel Club).
- **AKC rank (year 2008):** 32 (5,848 dogs registered)
- **Internet resources: Miniature Pinscher Club of America:** www.minpin.org
  The Canadian Miniature Pinscher Club: www.cdn-miniaturepinscherclub.com
  Miniature Pinscher Club of Great Britain: www.miniaturepinscherclub.co.uk

References

1. Drögemüller C, Philipp U, Haase B, et. al.: A noncoding melanophilin gene (MLPH) SNP at the splice donor of exon 1 represents a candidate causal mutation for coat color dilution in dogs. J Hered. 2007;98(5):468-73.
2. OFA Website breed statistics: www.offa.org Last accessed July 1, 2010.
3. LaFond E, Breur GJ & Austin CC: Breed susceptibility for developmental orthopedic diseases in dogs. J Am Anim Hosp Assoc. 2002 Sep-Oct;38(5):467-77.
4. Dorn CR: Canine breed-specific risks of frequently diagnosed diseases at veterinary teaching hospitals. Monograph. AKC Canine Health Foundation. 2000.
5. Stark D: Luxating patella in miniature pinschers. *Vet Rec.* 1991 Sep 14;129(11):251.
6. Neer TM, Dial SM, Pechman R, et. al.: Clinical vignette. Mucopolysaccharidosis VI in a miniature pinscher. *J Vet Intern Med.* 1995 Nov-Dec;9(6):429-33.
7. Wang P, Seng A, Huff A, et. al.: Mucopolysaccharidosis in Dogs and Cats: Clinical Signs to DNA Tests. Proceedings, 2005 Tufts' Canine and Feline Breeding and Genetics Conference. 2005.
8. Foureman P, Berman L, Stieger K, et. al.: Mucopolysaccharidosis Type VI in Miniature Pinschers: Screening For the Mutation. Proceedings, 2004 ACVIM Forum. 2004.
9. *Ocular Disorders Presumed to be Inherited in Purebred Dogs.* American College of Veterinary Ophthalmologists. ACVO, 2007.
10. Gelatt KN, Mackay EO: Prevalence of primary breed-related cataracts in the dog in North America. Vet Ophthalmol. 2005 Mar-Apr;8(2):101-11.
11. Nachreiner RF, Refsal KR, Graham PA, et. al.: Prevalence of serum thyroid hormone autoantibodies in dogs with clinical signs of hypothyroidism. J Am Vet Med Assoc 2002 Feb 15;220(4):466-71.
12. Nachreiner R & Refsal K: Personal communication, Diagnostic Center for Population and Animal Health, Michigan State University. April, 2007.
13. Kim JH, Kang KI, Sohn HJ, et. al.: Color-dilution alopecia in dogs. *J Vet Sci.* 2005 Sep;6(3):259-61.

14. Miller SA, Hohenhaus AE, Hale AS: Case-control study of blood type, breed, sex, and bacteremia in dogs with immune-mediated hemolytic anemia. *J Am Vet Med Assoc.* 2004 Jan 15;224(2):232-5.

15. Case LC, Ling GV, Franti CE, et. al.: Cystine-containing urinary calculi in dogs: 102 cases (1981-1989). *J Am Vet Med Assoc.* 1992 Jul 1;201(1):129-33.

16. Tobias KM, Rohrbach BW: Association of breed with the diagnosis of congenital portosystemic shunts in dogs: 2,400 cases (1980-2002). J Am Vet Med Assoc. 2003 Dec 1;223(11):1636-9.

17. Scott-Moncrieff JC: Canine and Feline Diabetes Mellitus I. Proceedings, 2009 Western Veterinary Conference. 2009.

18. *The Genetic Connection: A Guide to Health Problems in Purebred Dogs.* L Ackerman. p. 228. AAHA Press, 1999.

19. Nowacka J, Nizanski W, Klimowicz M, et. al.: Lack of the SOX9 Gene Polymorphism in Sex Reversal Dogs (78,XX; SRY negative). *J Hered.* 2005 Nov-Dec;96(7):797-802.

20. *The Complete Dog Book, 20th Ed.* The American Kennel Club. Howell Book House, NY 2006. p. 488-490.

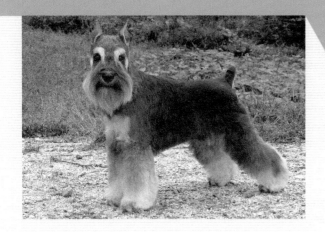

Miniature Schnauzer

The Breed History

In artwork of the 15th century, a dog with features consistent with the Miniature Schnauzer is pictured. By 1900, the breed was well established and was being shown. The origin of this dog is thought to be a mixture of Standard Schnauzer, with perhaps Poodle, Miniature pinscher, and Affenpinscher. They were brought to America around the year 1925. The name derives from the German word for nose (schnauzer). The AKC recognized this breed in 1933.

Breeding for Function

These dogs were widely used on the farm to control vermin such as rats, but the temperament of this breed varies from the classic terrier. Currently, they serve primarily as companion animals.

Physical Characteristics

Height at Withers: 12-14" (30.5-35.5 cm).

Weight: 14-16 lb (6.5-7.5 kg).

Coat: The double wiry, thick coat is commonly seen in salt and pepper (black and white intermixed in bands on some hairs to produce a grey appearance). Silver and black, and solid black are also seen. A small white patch is sometimes found on the black-coated dogs. Coat color may fade with age. The undercoat varies widely in color and can be beige, black, or gray.

Longevity: 14 years

Points of Conformation: This alert expressive terrier-type dog is similar in appearance to the Standard Schnauzer. Miniature Schnauzers are stocky in build, and the head is rectangular, and the flat forehead is free of wrinkles. The stop is slight, and oval ears are small, triangular, high-set, and lie close to the head. Some ears are cropped to have pointed tips, and to rest pricked up; if not cropped they fold forward. The eyes, overlain with bushy brows are dark brown, deep-set and small. Body skin is pigmented. Whiskers on the chin are left long to accentuate the face. The black nose is prominent with wide nostrils. The neck is well muscled and arched, and no throatiness is evident. The topline is straight but descends slightly as it goes toward the rear, the thorax is deep and ribs well sprung. No tuck up of abdomen is evident. The tail is carried up, and often docked short. Limbs are straight boned and feet are round, with well-arched toes and possessing thick, black pads. The gait is quick and agile.

Recognized Behavior Issues and Traits

Reported breed characteristics include: Grooming requirements are moderate, and they are low shedding dogs, though the coat must be stripped at least every 6 months; ideally they should not be clipped to maintain the outer coat. Daily grooming, with emphasis on limbs and whiskers should be done. Whiskers need a wash clean after meals. The Miniature Schnauzer dogs are obedient and friendly and like close human companionship. They are of high intelligence, possess high trainability, are active, affectionate, and are good with children. They do well in both city and country, and do well with other dogs; considered less scrappy than the other terriers. They possess a well-developed guarding instinct. Easy to train, but like to alarm bark; some lines have nervous temperaments. When off leash, should be in a fenced enclosure.

Normal Physiologic Variations

Idiopathic Hyperlipoproteinemia: Miniature Schnauzers have a non-pathological condition of hypertriglyceridemia, characterized by increased very low density lipoproteins with or without accompanying chylomicronemia. Both the prevalence and severity of hypertriglyceridemia increase with age. Dogs with high serum triglyceride concentrations can also have associated high serum alkaline phosphatase (AlkP) and alanine aminotransferase (ALT)levels.[1,2,3]

Hereditary Stomatocytosis (HSt): Miniature Schnauzers can have an autosomal recessive HSt, characterized by a normal hematocrit with macrocytic and hypochromic erythrocytes. The cause is erythrocyte overhydration due to a defect in cation exchange.[4]

Drug Sensitivities

Miniature Schnauzers are overrepresented for adverse reactions to **potentiated sulfonamides**. Clinical signs included hypersensitivity, thrombocytopenia and hepatopathy, and infrequently can include neutropenia, keratoconjunctivitis sicca, hemolytic anemia, arthropathy, uveitis, skin and mucocutaneous lesions, proteinuria, facial palsy, suspected meningitis, hypothyroidism, pancreatitis, facial edema, and pneumonitis.[5]

Inherited and Congenital Diseases

Myotonia Congenita: Autosomal recessive disorder causing hypertrophic skeletal muscles, difficulty in rising after a period of rest, a stiff and stilted gait when walking, and a bunnyhop-type movement when running. In addition, there are increased respiratory sounds, difficulty when swallowing, ptyalism, dental abnormalities, and superior prognathism. Worldwide genetic testing in the breed shows 20.4% carriers and 1.1% affected. A genetic test is available.[6,7]

Hip Dysplasia and Legg-Calve Perthes Disease: Polygenically inherited traits causing degenerative hip joint disease and arthritis. Too few Miniature Schnauzers have been screened by OFA to determine an accurate frequency.[8]

Patella Luxation: Polygenically inherited laxity of patellar ligaments, causing luxation, lameness, and later degenerative joint disease. Treat surgically if causing clinical signs. Too few Miniature Schnauzers have been screened by OFA to determine an accurate frequency.[8]

Type-A Progressive Retinal Atrophy (PRA)/Photoreceptor Dysplasia (PD): Partially dominant form of PRA identified in Miniature Schnauzers causing progressive blindness with age of onset around three years of age. Dogs homozygous for the mutated gene are always affected. Heterozygous dogs can be clinically normal or affected. A genetic test for Type-A PRA is available. There are other forms of PRA in the breed that are not caused by Type-A PRA, and that do not have a genetic test. CERF does not recommend breeding any Miniature Schnauzer with PRA.[9,10]

Retinal Dysplasia: Autosomal recessive congenital disorder of the retina causing regional retinal dysplasia and associated retinal detachment leading to blindness. The disorder is also associated with a mild unilateral or bilateral **persistent hyperplastic primary vitreous** (PHPV). CERF does not recommend breeding any Miniature Schnauzer with retinal dysplasia. There is no genetic test for carriers.[10,11]

Elbow Dysplasia: Polygenically inherited trait causing elbow arthritis. Too few Miniature Schnauzers have been screened by OFA to determine an accurate frequency.[8]

Congenital Cataracts and Microphthalmia: A simple autosomal recessive disorder of congenital cataract and microphthalmia occurs in the breed caused by a mutation in the MISRII receptor gene. The opacity is primarily in the lens nucleus and posterior cortex. There is no test for carriers.[12,13]

Persistent MÜllerian Duct Syndrome: Autosomal recessive intersex disorder in the breed caused by a mutation in the MISRII gene. Genetically normal males have a normal male karyotype (78, XY), bilateral testes, and a complete Mullerian duct system (oviducts, uterus, cervix and cranial vagina). A genetic test is available.[14,15,16]

Mucopolysaccharidosis VI (MPS VI): PennGen reports MPS VI identified in the Miniature Schnauzer. This is an autosomal recessive disorder causing skeletal deformities, including defects in the sternum, vertebrae and particularly the hip joints. To varying degrees they may also experience corneal cloudiness and facial dysmorphia. A genetic test is available.

Disease Predispositions

Urolithiasis: The breed has a high incidence of bladder stones compared to other breeds. Reported in 5.9% of Miniature Schnauzers examined at veterinary school hospitals. Of bladder stone submissions from Miniature Schnauzers in a Canadian study, 61.2% were **Calcium Oxalate**, 23.1% were **Struvite**, and 1.7% were **Urate**. Mean age of recognition of bladder stones in the breed is 4.9 years. Dorn reports a 7.77x odds ratio versus other breeds.[17,18,19,20]

Cataracts: Anterior or posterior intermediate and punctate cataracts occur in the breed. Unknown mode of inheritance. 4.98% of Miniature Schnauzers presented to veterinary teaching hospitals had cataracts. The breed has a 3.7x odds ratio for developing cataracts versus other breeds mean age of onset of 5.4 years. Identified in 1.54% of Miniature Schnauzers CERF examined by veterinary ophthalmologists between 2000-2005. CERF does not recommend breeding any Miniature Schnauzer with a cataract.[10,21,22,23]

Hyperadrenocorticism (Cushing's disease): Caused by a functional adrenal or pituitary tumor. Clinical signs may include increased thirst and urination, symmetrical truncal alopecia, and abdominal distention. Dorn reports a 3.77x odds ratio versus other breeds. Reported in 4.3% of Miniature Schnauzers examined at veterinary school hospitals.[17,20]

Diabetes Mellitus: Sugar diabetes. Control with insulin injection, diet, and glucose monitoring. Reported in 4.0% of Miniature Schnauzers examined at veterinary school hospitals. Odds ratios versus other breeds range from 10.01x (Dorn) to 9.87x (Hess). Genetic predisposition is linked to mutations in the CTLA4 promotior. Unknown mode of inheritance.[14,17,20,24,25]

Chronic Mitral Valve Disease/Mitral Prolapse: Systolic heart murmurs caused by chronic mitral valve disease. Can progress to congestive heart failure. Screen with auscultation. Reported in 3.9% of Miniature Schnauzers examined at veterinary school hospitals. Unknown mode of inheritance.[20]

Pancreatitis: Inflammation of the pancreas causing vomiting and peritonitis. Can be life threatening if severe. Hypertriglyceridemia in the breed is not a risk factor for pancreatitis. Reported in 3.5% of Miniature Schnauzers examined at veterinary school hospitals. Dorn reports a 55.06x odds ratio versus other breeds. Breed prevalence may be related to mutations in the SPINK 1 gene.[17,20,26,27]

Persistent Pupillary Membranes: Strands of fetal remnant connecting; iris to iris, cornea, lens, or involving sheets of tissue. The later three forms can impair vision, and dogs affected with these forms should not be bred. Identified in 2.78% of Miniature Schnauzers CERF examined by veterinary ophthalmologists between 2000-2005.[10]

Distichiasis: Abnormally placed eyelashes that irritate the cornea and conjunctiva. Can cause secondary corneal ulceration. Identified in 1.93% of Miniature Schnauzers CERF examined by veterinary ophthalmologists between 2000-2005.[10]

Schnauzer Comedome Syndrome: The breed is prone to developing follicular dermatitis with comedones (blackheads); hair follicles filled with keratin and sebum.[28]

Sick Sinus Syndrome: Arrhythmia characterized by sinus bradycardia and sinoatrial arrest due to abnormal firing of the sinoatrial node. Clinical signs include lethargy and syncopy. Occurs at an increased frequency in older Miniature Schnauzers. Treatment is with a pacemaker. Reported in 1.9% of Miniature Schnauzers examined at veterinary school hospitals.[20,29]

Hypothyroidism: Inherited autoimmune thyroiditis. 1.3% positive for thyroid auto-antibodies based on testing at Michigan State University. (Ave. for all breeds is 7.5%.)[30,31]

Portosystemic Shunt (PSS, Liver Shunt): Undetermined mode of inheritance. Vessels can be intrahepatic or extrahepatic. Causes stunting, with abnormal behavior and possible seizures. Diagnose with paired fasted and feeding serum bile acid and/or ammonium levels, and abdominal ultrasound. In one study, 23% of Miniature Schnauzers with PSS were not diagnosed until they were over 7 years of age (due to hepatic encephalopathy). Treatment of PSS includes partial ligation and/or medical and dietary control of symptoms. Reported in 1.3% of Miniature Schnauzers examined at veterinary school hospitals with an odds ratio of 19.8x versus other breeds.[20,32,33,34]

Immune-Mediated Hemolytic Anemia (IMHA): Auto-immune disorder where the body produces antibodies against its own red blood cells. Treat with immunosuppressive drugs. There is generally a female preponderance with this disorder. Occurs with an increased frequency in the breed versus other breeds. Reported in 1.0% of Miniature Schnauzers examined at veterinary school hospitals.[20,35]

Atherosclerosis: Miniature Schnauzers have a higher prevalence versus other breeds. Most common clinical signs are lethargy, anorexia, weakness, dyspnea, collapse, and vomiting. Hypercholesterolemia, lipidemia, and hypothyroidism were common in affected dogs. Myocardial fibrosis, infarction, and thickened arteries with narrow lumens are found on necropsy.[36]

Pulmonic Valve Stenosis: Miniature Schnauzers are a breed at increased risk (3.5x odds ratio) for this congenital heart anomaly. Clinical signs can include exercise intolerance, stunting, dyspnea, syncope and ascites, leading to heart failure. Screen with auscultation and echocardiography.[37]

Fibrocartilaginous Embolic Myelopathy (FCEM): Acute release of fibrocartilage into the spinal cord. Causes spinal weakness or paralysis. Seen at an increased frequency in Miniature Schnauzers versus other breeds.[38]

Sudden Acute Retinal Degeneration (SARDS): Degenerative retinal disease causing acute blindness. Age of onset from 1.5 to 15 years, with an average of 8.4 years. In one study, 10% of affected dogs were Miniature Schnauzers. Diagnose with ERG.[39,40]

Neuronal Ceroid-Lipofuscinosis (NCL): Miniature Schnauzers have a fatal form of NCL that causes rapidly progressive blindness and mental deterioration from 2-4 years of age. An autosomal recessive mode of inheritance is suspected. There is no test for carriers.[41,42]

Juvenile Renal Disease: Disorder of progressive renal failure in young Miniature Schnauzers. Affected dogs are polyuric and polydipsic, uremic, and anemic. Unknown mode of inheritance.[43]

Achalasia, Megaesophagus: A neonatal condition of esophageal dysfunction is identified in the breed. Clinical signs are regurgitation, poor weight gain, and secondary aspiration pneumonia. The condition spontaneously resolves by 4-6 months in most affected dogs. Breeding studies suggest a polygenic mode of inheritance.[44]

Superficial Suppurative Necrolytic Dermatitis (SSND): Rare, cutaneous and systemic reaction consisting of erythematous papules and plaques that progress to necrosis and ulcers. Systemic signs consist of fever, depression and leucocytosis. Most cases of SSND improve in 1 to 2 weeks with symptomatic treatment, but

some cases may culminate with death. Thought to be caused by a severe contact dermatitis to elements in shampoo.[45,46,47]

Aquired Aurotrichia, Allergic Inhalant Dermatitis, Anterior Crossbite, Base narrow Canines, Brachygnathism, Cleft Lip/Palate, Cryptorchidism, Cutaneous Asthenia, Deafness, Factor VII Deficiency, Fanconi Syndrome, Glaucoma, IgA Deficiency, Keratoconjunctivitis Sicca, Muscular Dystrophy, OCD Stifle, Optic Nerve Hypoplasia, Prognathism, Seasonal Flank Alopecia, von Willebrand's Disease, and **Wry Mouth** are reported.[48]

Isolated Case Studies

***Mycobacterium Avium* Infection (Tuberculosis):** Several Miniature Schnauzers worldwide have been diagnosed with M. Avium TB. The primary clinical sign is lymph node enlargement. All affected dogs die of the infection. A genetic predisposition/immune defect is suggested.[49]

Intraocular Xanthogranuloma (Foam Cell Tumor): Three Miniature Schnauzers whose eyes were enucleated secondary to diabetes mellitus, chronic bilateral uveitis, and glaucoma were diagnosed with this solid intraocular mass of foam cells and birefringent crystals.[50]

Cerebellar Abiotrophy: Rapidly progressive signs of cerebellar ataxia began at three months of age. The puppy was euthanized at six weeks. Diagnosis was confirmed with pathology.[51]

Cerebellar Vermis Hypoplasia: A 3 month old male Miniature Schnauzer with non-progressive ataxia, dysmetria, intention tremors, and loss of balance was found to have cerebellar vermis hypoplasia.[52]

Microglossia: Three of five two-day-old Miniature Schnauzer puppies were diagnosed as having "bird-tongue", a microglossia that prevents normal nursing. A multi-system defect was suspected, though no primary neuromuscular abnormality could be determined.[53]

Sperm Knobbed Acrosome Defect (KAD): Four closely related Miniature Schnauzer dogs had between 8 and 44% sperm with KAD. No reduction in fertility was found.[54]

Demyelinating Polyneuropathy: A kindred of Miniature Schnauzers was identified with a demyelinating polyneuropathy characterized by varying degrees of megaesophagus, laryngeal paralysis, and/or mild proprioceptive defecits. Pathology includes demyelination with focally folded myelin sheaths. Most affected dogs stabilized if aspiration pneumonia was controlled. An autosomal recessive mode of inheritance was suspected.[55]

Genetic Tests

Tests of Genotype: Direct test for PRA-Type A is available from Optigen.

Direct test for Myotonia Congenita is available from PennGen and HealthGene.

Direct test for Persistent Mullerian Duct Syndrome is available from the Meyers-Wallen lab: 607-256-5683, vnm1@cornell.edu.

Direct test for MPS is available from PennGen.

Direct test for black color and mask is available from HealthGene and VetGen.

Tests of Phenotype: CHIC Certification: CERF eye examination, and cardiac evaluation. Optional testing includes the genetic test for myotonia congenita. (See CHIC website; www.caninehealthinfo.org).

Recommend patella evaluation, hip and elbow radiographs, and thyroid profile including autoantibodies.

Miscellaneous

- **Breed name synonyms:** Zwergschauzer.
- **Registries:** AKC, UKC, CKC, KCGB (Kennel Club of Great Britain), ANKC (Australian National Kennel Club), NKC (National Kennel Club).
- **AKC rank (year 2008):** 11 (17,040 dogs registered)
- **Internet resources:** The American Miniature Schnauzer Club Inc.: http://amsc.us
  Miniature Schnauzer Club of Canada: www.mscc.ca
  The Miniature Schnauzer Club (UK):
  http://the-miniature-schnauzer-club.co.uk
  Schnauzer Club of Great Britain: www.schnauzerclub.co.uk

References

1. Whitney MS, Boon GD, Rebar AH, et. al.: Ultracentrifugal and electrophoretic characteristics of the plasma lipoproteins of miniature schnauzer dogs with idiopathic hyperlipoproteinemia. J Vet Intern Med. 1993 Jul-Aug;7(4):253-60.
2. Xenoulis PG, Suchodolski JS, Levinski MD, et. al.: Investigation of hypertriglyceridemia in healthy Miniature Schnauzers. J Vet Intern Med. 2007 Nov-Dec;21(6):1224-30.
3. Xenoulis PG, Suchodolski JS, Levinski MD, et. al.: Serum liver enzyme activities in healthy Miniature Schnauzers with and without hypertriglyceridemia. J Am Vet Med Assoc. 2008 Jan 1;232(1):63-7.
4. Di Terlizzi R: Erythrocyte Membrane Disorders in Domestic Animals. Proceedings, 2008 ACVIM Forum. 2008.
5. Trepanier LA, Danhof R, Toll J, et. al.: Clinical findings in 40 dogs with hypersensitivity associated with administration of potentiated sulfonamides. J Vet Intern Med. 2003 Sep-Oct;17(5):647-52.
6. Bhalerao DP, Rajpurohit Y, Vite CH, et. al.: Detection of a genetic mutation for myotonia congenita among Miniature Schnauzers and identification of a common carrier ancestor. Am J Vet Res. 2002 Oct;63(10):1443-7.
7. Vite CH, Melniczek J, Patterson D, et. al.: Congenital myotonic myopathy in the miniature schnauzer: an autosomal recessive trait. J Hered. 1999 Sep-Oct;90(5):578-80.
8. OFA Website breed statistics: www.offa.org Last accessed July 1, 2010.
9. Zhang Q, Acland GM, Parshall CJ, et. al.: Characterization of canine photoreceptor phosducin cDNA and identification of a sequence variant in dogs with photoreceptor dysplasia. Gene. 1998 Jul 30;215(2):231-9.
10. Ocular Disorders Presumed to be Inherited in Purebred Dogs. American College of Veterinary Ophthalmologists. ACVO, 2007.
11. Grahn BH, Storey ES, McMillan C: Inherited retinal dysplasia and persistent hyperplastic primary vitreous in Miniature Schnauzer dogs. Vet Ophthalmol. 2004 May-Jun;7(3):151-8.
12. Gelatt KN, Samuelson DA, Bauer JE, et. al.: Inheritance of congenital cataracts and microphthalmia in the Miniature Schnauzer. Am J Vet Res. 1983 Jun;44(6):1130-2.
13. Shastry BS, Reddy VN: Studies on congenital hereditary cataract and microphthalmia of the miniature schnauzer dog. Biochem Biophys Res Commun. 1994 Sep 30;203(3):1663-7.

14. Meyers-Wallen VN: Genetics of sexual differentiation and anomalies in dogs and cats. J Reprod Fertil Suppl. 1993;47:441-52.
15. Pujar S & Meyers-Wallen VN: A molecular diagnostic test for persistent Müllerian duct syndrome in miniature schnauzer dogs. Sex Dev. 2009;3(6):326-8.
16. Wu X, Wan S, Pujar S, et. al.: A single base pair mutation encoding a premature stop codon in the MIS type II receptor is responsible for canine persistent Müllerian duct syndrome. J Androl. 2009 Jan-Feb;30(1):46-56.
17. Dorn CR: Canine breed-specific risks of frequently diagnosed diseases at veterinary teaching hospitals. Monograph. AKC Canine Health Foundation. 2000.
18. Houston DM & Moore AE: Canine and feline urolithiasis: examination of over 50 000 urolith submissions to the Canadian veterinary urolith centre from 1998 to 2008. Can Vet J. 2009 Dec;50(12):1263-8.
19. Klausner JS, Osborne CA, Clinton CW, et. al.: Mineral composition of urinary calculi from miniature schnauzer dogs. J Am Vet Med Assoc. 1981 May 15;178(10):1082-3.
20. Veterinary Medical Database, Purdue University: Search of diagnoses for Miniature Schnauzers. July 18, 2000.
21. Gelatt KN, Mackay EO: Prevalence of primary breed-related cataracts in the dog in North America. Vet Ophthalmol. 2005 Mar-Apr;8(2):101-11.
22. Adkins EA, Hendrix DV: Outcomes of dogs presented for cataract evaluation: a retrospective study. J Am Anim Hosp Assoc. 2005 Jul-Aug;41(4):235-40.
23. Park SA, Yi NY, Jeong MB, Kim WT, et. al.: Clinical manifestations of cataracts in small breed dogs. Vet Ophthalmol. 2009 Jul-Aug;12(4):205-10.
24. Hess RS, Kass PH, Ward CR: Breed distribution of dogs with diabetes mellitus admitted to a tertiary care facility. J Am Vet Med Assoc. 2000 May 1;216(9):1414-7.
25. Short AD, Saleh NM, Catchpole B, et. al.: CTLA4 promoter polymorphisms are associated with canine diabetes mellitus. Tissue Antigens. 2010 Mar;75(3):242-52.
26. Xenoulis PG, Suchodolski JS, Ruaux CG, et. al.: Association between serum triglyceride and canine pancreatic lipase immunoreactivity concentrations in miniature schnauzers. J Am Anim Hosp Assoc. 2010 Jul-Aug;46(4):229-34.
27. Bishop MA, Xenoulis PG, Levinski MD, et. al.: Identification of variants of the SPINK1 gene and their association with pancreatitis in Miniature Schnauzers. Am J Vet Res. 2010 May;71(5):527-33.
28. Campbell, KL: Diagnosis and management of keratinization disorders in dogs. 1997 Proceedings, 15th Annual ACVIM Veterinary Medical Forum. 1997.
29. Kraus MS: Syncope in Small Breed Dogs. 2003 Proceedings ACVIM Forum. 2003.
30. Nachreiner RF, Refsal KR, Graham PA, et. al.: Prevalence of serum thyroid hormone autoantibodies in dogs with clinical signs of hypothyroidism. J Am Vet Med Assoc 2002 Feb 15;220(4):466-71.
31. Nachreiner R & Refsal K: Personal communication, Diagnostic Center for Population and Animal Health, Michigan State University. April, 2007.
32. Hunt GB: Effect of breed on anatomy of portosystemic shunts resulting from congenital diseases in dogs and cats: a review of 242 cases. Aust Vet J. 2004 Dec;82(12):746-9.
33. Tobias KM, Rohrbach BW: Association of breed with the diagnosis of congenital portosystemic shunts in dogs: 2,400 cases (1980-2002). J Am Vet Med Assoc. 2003 Dec 1;223(11):1636-9.
34. Mertens M, Fossum TW, Willard MD, et. al.: Diagnosis of congenital portosystemic shunt in miniature schnauzers 7 years of age or older (1997-2006). J Am Anim Hosp Assoc. 2010 Jul-Aug;46(4):235-40.
35. Weinkle TK, Center SA, Randolph JF, et. al.: Evaluation of prognostic factors, survival rates, and treatment protocols for immune-mediated hemolytic anemia in dogs: 151 cases (1993-2002). J Am Vet Med Assoc. 2005 Jun 1;226(11):1869-80.
36. Liu SK, Tilley LP, Tappe JP, et. al.: Clinical and pathologic findings in dogs with atherosclerosis: 21 cases (1970-1983). J Am Vet Med Assoc. 1986 Jul 15;189(2):227-32.

37. Buchanan JW: Causes and prevalence of cardiovascular diseases. In Kirk RW, Bonagura JD, eds: Current veterinary therapy XI, Philadelphia, 1992, WB Saunders.

38. Hawthorne JC, Wallace LJ, Fenner WR, et. al.: Fibrocartilaginous embolic myelopathy in miniature schnauzers. J Am Anim Hosp Assoc. 2001 Jul-Aug;37(4):374-83.

39. van der Woerdt A, Nasisse MP, Davidson MG. Sudden acquired retinal degeneration in the dog. Progress in Veterinary and Comparative Ophthalmology 1991; 1: 11–18.

40. Montgomery KW, van der Woerdt A, & Cottrill NB: Acute blindness in dogs: sudden acquired retinal degeneration syndrome versus neurological disease (140 cases, 2000-2006). Vet Ophthalmol. 2008 Sep-Oct;11(5):314-20.

41. Palmer DN, Tyynela J, van Mil HC, et. al.: Accumulation of sphingolipid activator proteins (SAPs) A and D in granular osmiophilic deposits in miniature Schnauzer dogs with ceroid-lipofuscinosis. J Inherit Metab Dis. 1997 Mar;20(1):74-84.

42. Jolly RD, Sutton RH, Smith RI, e. al.: Ceroid-lipofuscinosis in miniature Schnauzer dogs. Aust Vet J. 1997 Jan;75(1):67.

43. Morton LD, Sanecki RK, Gordon DE, et. al.: Juvenile renal disease in miniature schnauzer dogs. Vet Pathol. 1990 Nov;27(6):455-8.

44. Cox VS, Wallace LJ, Anderson VE, et. al.: Hereditary esophageal dysfunction in the Miniature Schnauzer dog. Am J Vet Res. 1980 Mar;41(3):326-30.

45. Rosenkrantz WS, Griffin CE & Walder E: Superficial suppurative necrolytic dermatitis in miniature schnauzers: retrospective analysis. Proceedings, 7th AAVD/ACVD Meeting. 1991: 99.

46. Gross TL, Ihrke PJ, Walder EJ, et. al.: Sterile pustular erythroderma of miniature schnauzers. In: Skin Diseases of the Dog and Cat. Oxford: Blackwell Science, 2005: 20–3.

47. Murayama N, Midorikawa K & Nagata M: A case of superficial suppurative necrolytic dermatitis of miniature schnauzers with identification of a causative agent using patch testing. Vet Dermatol. 2008 Dec;19(6):395-9.

48. The Genetic Connection: A Guide to Health Problems in Purebred Dogs. L Ackerman. p. 237. AAHA Press, 1999.

49. Eggers JS, Parker GA, Braaf HA, et. al.: Disseminated Mycobacterium avium infection in three miniature schnauzer litter mates. J Vet Diagn Invest. 1997 Oct;9(4):424-7.

50. Zarfoss MK & Dubielzig RR: Solid intraocular xanthogranuloma in three Miniature Schnauzer dogs. Vet Ophthalmol. 2007 Sep-Oct;10(5):304-7.

51. Berry ML, Blas-Machado U: Cerebellar abiotrophy in a miniature schnauzer. Can Vet J. 2003 Aug;44(8):657-9.

52. Choi H, Kang S, Jeong S, et. al.: Imaging diagnosis-cerebellar vermis hypoplasia in a Miniature Schnauzer. Vet Radiol Ultrasound. 2007 Mar-Apr;48(2):129-31.

53. Wiggs RB, Lobprise HB, de Lahunta A: Microglossia in three littermate puppies. J Vet Dent. 1994 Dec;11(4):129-33.

54. Santos NR, Krekeler N, Schramme-Jossen A, et. al.: The knobbed acrosome defect in four closely related dogs. Theriogenology. 2006 Oct;66(6-7):1626-8.

55. Vanhaesebrouck AE, Couturier J, Cauzinille L, et. al.: Demyelinating polyneuropathy with focally folded myelin sheaths in a family of Miniature Schnauzer dogs. J Neurol Sci. 2008 Dec 15;275(1-2):100-5.

56. The Complete Dog Book, 20th Ed. The American Kennel Club. Howell Book House, NY 2006. p. 404-408.

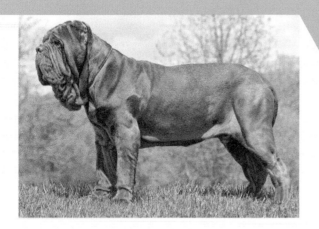

Neopolitan Mastiff

The Breed History

This is an ancient breed with reports dating back 5000 years, but only recognized as a distinct breed since the 1940s. Very early origins trace back to the war dogs (Macedonian, Sumerian, Assyrian) in the middle east and Asia. Alexander the Great was reported to have crossed war dogs with short-haired Indian dogs, giving rise to the Molossus. The Romans crossed these Molossus dogs with English Mastiffs when they invaded, increasing their size. In southern Italy in the Neapolitan region, these crossbreds were further selected for guarding and inbred over the years. Breed characteristics that define the Neapolitan Mastiff include extensive loose skin, enormous body and head, and a smooth lumbering gait. First reported imports to the USA occurred in the 1970s, and now estimates are that 6000 dogs are in the country, especially along the eastern seaboard. AKC recognition occurred in 2004.

Breeding for Function

These dogs fulfilled many roles including guard dog, war dog, hunting dog, and draft dog.

Physical Characteristics

Height at Withers: female 24-29" (61-74 cm), male 26-31" (66-79 cm)

Weight: bitches: 110 lb (50 kg), dogs 150 lb (68 kg)

Coat: Smooth, short (1") and dense, the hairs are straight. Lacks furnishings anywhere. Colors include black, tawny, mahogany, grey (also termed blue). Sometimes brindling may occur, but must be tan. Any white markings must meet the breed standard—if outside defined areas, these are a disqualification. Blue color is most desired as he blends into the shadows during guarding.

Longevity: 8-10 years

Points of Conformation: Massive! Heavy boned. If not, the dog is eliminated. The head is substantially larger than a typical dog and the skull top is broad, flat and parallel to the muzzle profile. The stop is very well defined, muzzle is square. The head has specified folds that must be present. Bite is scissors or slightly undershot. A little longer than tall, the first thing that strikes you is the masses of folded and wrinkled loose skin over the dog, with an extensive dewlap merging with massive flews. The eyes are expressive, deep

set, with large overhanging dorsal palpebral, and lower palpebral sags, showing the third eyelid. Eye color and rim synchronize with coat color, and usually are brown to amber. Ears may be cropped to a triangular shape. The neck is short and well muscled. The thorax is deep and ribs are well sprung. The topline is level. The abdomen is not tucked up. Front dewclaws are not to be removed but rear ones are. Feet are large, round and the front feet are slightly turned out. Tail is tapered, and docked to 1/3 of the length to the tarsus. Carriage is horizontal to slightly elevated when working. The gait is slow, steady and a rolling swaying attitude is normal, especially if pace rather than trot. The head is carried just above the topline level usually, and front feet may paddle a bit. There is a low shedding tendency except during seasonal coat turnover.

Recognized Behavior Issues and Traits

Breed attributes ascribed include: Loyal—even devoted, gentle, well tempered, calm yet wary of strangers, fearsome when provoked. Not recommended for young children due to extreme large size and weight. They are droolers. Tolerate cool weather better than hot. Need enough room to move around. They are not well suited to small apartments. Low to moderate need for exercise.

Normal Breed Variations

Late maturing—about 3 years of age

Tend to need cesarian section and occasionally cannot breed without artificial insemination. In a UK study, 36.4% of litters were delivered via **Cesarian section**.[1]

Drug Sensitivities

None reported

Inherited Diseases

Hip Dysplasia: Polygenically inherited trait causing degenerative joint disease and hip arthritis. Reported at a frequency of 60% in a Polish study. OFA reports 47.7% affected.[2,3]

Elbow Dysplasia: Polygenically inherited trait causing elbow arthritis. OFA reports 37.5% affected.[2]

Patella Luxation: Polygenically inherited laxity of patellar ligaments, causing luxation, lameness, and later degenerative joint disease. Treat surgically if causing clinical signs. Too few Neapolitan Mastiffs have been screened by OFA to determine an accurate frequency.[2]

Disease Predispositions

Hypothyroidism: Inherited autoimmune thyroiditis. 7.9% positive for thyroid auto-antibodies based on testing at Michigan State University. (Ave. for all breeds is 7.5%).[4,5]

Prolapsed Gland of the Nictitans (Cherry Eye): The breed is reported to have a high frequency of this condition secondary to inflammation of the gland. Some surgeons report frequent relapses after tacking surgery due to a defect in the cartilage, and removal should be considered.[6,7]

Gastric Dilatation–Volvulus (bloat, GDV): Polygenically inherited, life-threatening twisting of the stomach within the abdomen. Requires immediate treatment. Reported cause of death of 28.6% of Neapolitan Mastiffs in one study.[8]

Cranial Cruciate Ligament (ACL) Rupture: Traumatic tearing of the ACL in the stifle, causing lameness and secondary arthritis. Treat with surgery. Reported at an increased incidence versus other breeds.[9]

Entropion: Rolling in of eyelids, often causing corneal irritation or ulceration. Reported to be common in the breed, but too few Neapolitan Mastiffs have been CERF eye examined to determine an accurate frequency.[6,7,10]

Ectropion: Rolling out of eyelids, often with a medial canthal pocket. Can also cause conjunctivitis. Reported to be common in the breed, but too few Neapolitan Mastiffs have been CERF eye examined to determine an accurate frequency.[6,7,10]

Cataracts: Inherited cataracts occur in the breed, but too few Neapolitan Mastiffs have been CERF eye examined to determine an accurate frequency. CERF does not recommend breeding any Neapolitan Mastiff with a cataract.[10]

Distichiasis: Abnormally placed eyelashes that irritate the cornea and conjunctiva. Can cause secondary corneal ulceration. Too few Neapolitan Mastiffs have been CERF eye examined to determine an accurate frequency.[10]

Cardiomyopathy, Allergies, Demodecosis, Leishmaniasis, and **Cryptorchidism** are reported problems in the breed.

Patent Ductus Arteriosis and **Progressive Retinal Atrophy** are reported.[11]

Isolated Case Studies

Teratoid Medulloepithelioma: A 4-year-old Neapolitan mastiff presented with acute glaucoma of the left eye and progressive neurologic signs. A tumor of the left eye was identified. On necropsy, the ocular tumor originated from the ciliary body, metastases with the same morphology were present in the brain and in one kidney. The diagnosis was malignant teratoid medulloepithelioma.[12]

Myocardial Myxosarcoma: A two years and eight months old male Neapolitan mastiff presented with a history of chronic diarrhea and weight loss. No primary gastrointestinal or metabolic cause for the diarrhea could be identified. Echocardiography revealed a large, multilocular, cyst-like structure within the pericardium compressing the heart. The mass was surgically excised from the left ventricular myocardium, and identified as a low-grade malignant myxosarcoma. The dog made a full recovery, but returned with diarrhea, weight loss, tumor recurrence and local metastasis 11 months later.[13]

Undifferentiated Sarcoma: A six-month-old Neapolitan mastiff presented for a rapidly growing cervical mass. Necropsy revealed undifferentiated sarcoma with metastases to the mediastinum, pleura, lungs, liver, kidneys, omentum, mesentery, and multiple lymph nodes.[14]

Genetic Tests

Tests of Genotype: none

Tests of Phenotype: Recommend hip and elbow radiographs, CERF eye examination, cardiac evaluation, patella evaluation, and thyroid profile including autoantibodies.

Miscellaneous
- **Breed name synonyms:** Mastino Napoletano, Italian Mastiff, Mastino
- **Registries:** AKC, UKC, CKC, KCGB (Kennel Club of Great Britain), ANKC (Australian National Kennel Club), NKC (National Kennel Club), FCI.
- **AKC rank (year 2008):** 112 (357 dogs registered)
- **Breed resources: United States Neapolitan Mastiff Club:** www.neapolitan.org
  The Neapolitan Mastiff Club UK: www.uknmc.org.uk
  The Mastino Health Foundation: www.mastinohealth.org

References

1. Evans KM & Adams VJ: Proportion of litters of purebred dogs born by caesarean section. J Small Anim Pract. 2010 Feb;51(2):113-8.
2. OFA Website breed statistics: www.offa.org Last accessed July 1, 2010.
3. Aleksiewicz R, Budziska Z, Nowicki M, et. al.: Canine hip dysplasia of selected breeds--results obtained by two Polish clinics based on radiological examination conducted in 1997-2006. Pol J Vet Sci. 2008;11(2):139-42
4. Nachreiner RF, Refsal KR, Graham PA, et. al.: Prevalence of serum thyroid hormone autoantibodies in dogs with clinical signs of hypothyroidism. J Am Vet Med Assoc 2002 Feb 15;220(4):466-71.
5. Nachreiner R & Refsal K: Personal communication, Diagnostic Center for Population and Animal Health, Michigan State University. April, 2007.
6. Herrera D: Surgery of the Eyelids. Proceedings, 2005 World Small Animal Veterinary Association Congress. 2005.
7. Guandalini A: Ocular Disorders Presumed to be Inherited in Four Italian Breeds: Italian Spitz, Neapolitan Mastiff, Cane Corso and Pastore Maremmano-Abruzzese. Proceedings, 2005 World Small Animal Veterinary Association Congress. 2005.
8. Evans KM & Adams VJ: Mortality and morbidity due to gastric dilatation-volvulus syndrome in pedigree dogs in the UK. J Small Anim Pract. 2010 Jul;51(7):376-81.
9. Duval JM, Budsberg SC, Flo GL, et. al.: Breed, sex, and body weight as risk factors for rupture of the cranial cruciate ligament in young dogs. J Am Vet Med Assoc. 1999 Sep 15;215(6):811-4.
10. Ocular Disorders Presumed to be Inherited in Purebred Dogs. American College of Veterinary Ophthalmologists. ACVO, 2007.
11. The Genetic Connection: A Guide to Health Problems in Purebred Dogs. L Ackerman. p. 228. AAHA Press, 1999.
12. Aleksandersen M, Bjerkas E, Heiene R, et. al.: Malignant teratoid medulloepithelioma with brain and kidney involvement in a dog. Vet Ophthalmol. 2004 Nov-Dec;7(6):407-11.
13. Foale RD, White RA, Harley R, et. al.: Left ventricular myxosarcoma in a dog. J Small Anim Pract. 2003 Nov;44(11):503-7.
14. Sanders NA, Kerlin RL, Dambach DM: Aggressive, undifferentiated sarcoma with widespread metastasis in a six-month-old Neapolitan mastiff. J Am Anim Hosp Assoc. 1996 Mar-Apr;32(2):97-101.
15. The Complete Dog Book, 20th Ed. The American Kennel Club. Howell Book House, NY 2006. p. 298-302.

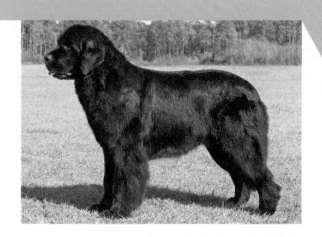

Newfoundland

the breed is heavily boned and muscled and possesses a gait that is smooth and covers a lot of ground with apparent ease. The skull is broad, the head is massive and the occipital protuberance is well developed. Eyes are generally dark brown in color, though some lighter colored dogs have lighter eye pigmentation. A gentle expression is emphasized. Palpebral rims are dark and the deep-set eyes are small and wide-set. Triangular ears sit close to the head and have rounded tips. A deep square muzzle and moderate stop characterize the profile. The neck is muscular and thick. The topline is level, thorax is deep and ribs well sprung. The tail is strong and distally it reaches the tarsus. Limbs are straight and heavily boned, feet are large and webbed with compact knuckled up toes. Front dewclaw removal is optional, but they are taken off in the rear.

The Breed History

Named after the Canadian province of Newfoundland, these hardy dogs were descended from European breeds such as Great Pyrenees and others brought over with early settlers. Others place the origins of the breed in North America back to the time when the Vikings explored Newfoundland and brought their bear dogs with them, about 1000 AD. This may explain the presence of this type of dog skeletons in Indian burial sites dating to the 5th century AD. First written records in Newfoundland date to 1732. The breed actually underwent most modern development in Europe, where breeders imported the Newfoundland dogs back. AKC recognition occurred in 1886.

Breeding for Function

Newfies were selected for their natural instinct to retrieve those in need from water. The breed characteristics reflect adaptation to the harsh climate of Newfoundland. Thick coats, webbed feet for moving over snow and marsh and swimming, and stamina characterize the breed. They excelled at both water and dry land work, especially helpful for pulling nets and boats for fishermen, and were noted for their courage and loyalty in search and rescue type work. Because of their size and strength, they were also favored as draft dogs, pulling carts on farms and carrying heavy packs. The characteristics that are placed first in priority for breeding are a docile, sweet temperament and well-developed life saving instinct. These are considered a hallmark of the breed.

Physical Characteristics

Height at Withers: female 26" (66 cm), male 28" (71 cm).

Weight: females 100-120 lb (45.5-54.5 kg), males 130-150 lb (59-68 kg).

Coat: White, gray, black and brown are recognized. A landseer coloring is white background with black markings, controlled by an autosomal recessive MIFT gene.[1] The dense, double coat is oily and thus waterproof. Outer hairs are coarse and may be straight to wavy, and are moderately long. The undercoat is soft and dense. The face and muzzle are covered by a much shorter haircoat. Limbs are feathered.

Longevity: 8-10 years

Points of Conformation: Large, strong, muscular, and thick coated,

Recognized Behavior Issues and Traits

Reported breed characteristics include: Very loyal, very intelligent, are able to work on their own but at the same time be obedient to commands. Possessing a gentle disposition and at the same time, having good guarding instincts for home and family. Newfoundland dogs are devoted to, and good with children. They possess a drooling tendency. Need daily brushing and shed year-round. Tolerates temperature extremes well, especially the cold. Moderate exercise requirements. Not an alarm barker.

Normal Physiologic Variations

Irregularities in bone remodeling in the distal radius and ulna can be observed between 6-24 months of age in growing Newfoundland dogs. These changes resolve and are not associated with clinical disease.[2,3]

Echocardiographic Normal Values:[4]	
Parameter	90% Confidence Interval
AO (cm)	2.6-3.3
AOexc (cm)	0.5-1.3
LA (cm)	2.4-3.3
LA/AO	0.8-1.25
LVd (cm)	4.4-6.0
LVs (cm)	2.9-4.4
%FS	22-37
%EF	44-66
LVET (sec)	0.14-0.20
Vcf (cir/sec)	1.1-2.5
EPSS (cm)	0.3-1.4
VSd (cm)	0.7-1.5
VSs (cm)	1.1-2.0
VS%Δ	0-45
VSexc (cm)	0.4-1.0
LVWd (cm)	0.8-1.3
LVWs (cm)	1.1-1.6
LVW%Δ	11-40
LVWexc (cm)	0.8-1.7
HR	70-120
Kg	47-70
N	27

AO, aorta; LA, left atrium; LV, left ventricle; FS, fractional shortening; EF, ejection fraction; LVET, left ventricular ejection time; Vcf, velocity of circumferential; EPSS, E-point to septal separation; VS, ventricular septum; VS%Δ, change in VS thickness between diastole and systole; LVW, left ventricular wall; HR, heart rate; N, number of animals.

Drug Sensitivities

None reported

Inherited Diseases

Hip Dysplasia: Polygenically inherited trait causing degenerative joint disease and hip arthritis. Dorn reports a 2.46x odds ratio versus other breeds. Another study reports a 7.7x odds ratio versus other breeds. OFA reports 25.2% affected.[5,6,7]

Elbow Dysplasia: Polygenically inherited trait causing elbow arthritis. OFA reports 24.2% affected. Reported 10.9x odds ratio for fragmented coronoid process, and 13.8x odds ratio for ununited anconeal process forms of elbow dysplasia versus other breeds.[5,7]

Cystinuria: Autosomal recessive disease of cystine metabolism causing dysuria, stranguria, or obstruction due to cystine calculi, primarily in affected males. Affected females can have cystine crystals and calculi without clinical signs. PennGen testing finds 2.3% affected, and 28% carrier. A genetic test is available.[8,9,10]

Dilated Cardiomyopathy (DCM): An autosomal dominant disease with late onset and reduced penetrance in this breed. Affected dogs have reduced shortening fraction (FS) in the presence of clinical and radiographic signs of left-sided or biventricular heart failure. Atrial fibrillation is the most common arrhythmia. Studies show 1.3-2.5% of Newfoundland dogs are affected. Some affected Newfoundlands have low plasma taurine levels, and improve on taurine supplementation, suggesting an abnormality in taurine metabolism.[11,12,13]

Patella Luxation: Polygenically inherited laxity of patellar ligaments, causing luxation, lameness, and later degenerative joint disease. Treat surgically if causing clinical signs. OFA reports 0.5% affected.[5]

Disease Predispositions

Allergic Dermatitis: Inhalant or food allergy. Presents with pruritis and pyotraumatic dermatitis. Padgett reports a frequency of 12.6% in the breed.[14]

Entropion: Rolling in of eyelids, often causing corneal irritation or ulceration. Reported in 8.04% of Newfoundlands CERF-examined by veterinary ophthalmologists between 2000-2005.[15]

Ectropion: Rolling out of eyelids, often with a medial canthal pocket. Can cause secondary conjunctivitis. Can be secondary to macroblepharon; an abnormally large eyelid opening. Ectropion is reported in 7.21% of Newfoundlands CERF-examined by veterinary ophthalmologists between 2000-2005.[15]

Hypothyroidism: Inherited autoimmune thyroiditis. 4.0% positive for thyroid auto-antibodies based on testing at Michigan State University. (Ave. for all breeds is 7.5%)[16,17]

Cataracts: Anterior or posterior intermediate and punctate cataracts occur in the breed. Identified in 3.90% of Newfoundlands CERF-examined by veterinary ophthalmologists between 2000-2005.[15]

Gastric Dilatation-Volvulus (Bloat, GDV): Polygenically inherited, life-threatening twisting of the stomach within the abdomen. Requires immediate veterinary attention. Reported at a frequency of 3.4% in the breed.[18]

Cranial Cruciate Ligament (ACL) Rupture: Traumatic tearing of the ACL in the stifle, causing lameness and secondary arthritis. Treat with surgery. Dorn reports a 1.38x odds ratio versus other breeds. One study found a heritability of 0.27 in the breed. A genome scan identified 4 chromosomal locations associated with the disorder, indicating a complex mode of inheritance.[6,19,20,21]

Osteochondritis Dessicans (OCD): Defect in cartilage maturation in young dogs, causing joint lesions and lameness. Treatment with rest, or surgery in severe cases. Severe cases can result in later arthritis and degenerative joint disease. Padgett reports a frequency of 2.0% in the breed. Odds ratios for elbow OCD is 261x, and shoulder OCD 18.7x versus other breeds.[7,14]

Retinal Dysplasia: Retinal folds, geographic, and generalized retinal dysplasia with detachment are recognized in the breed. Reported in 1.77% of Newfoundlands CERF examined by veterinary ophthalmologists between 2000-2005.[15]

Iris Cysts: Fluid filled sacs originating from the iris. They can remain attached or break free and float in the anterior chamber. Usually seen in mature dogs. Reported in 1.06% of Newfoundlands CERF examined by veterinary ophthalmologists between 2000-2005.[15]

Persistent Pupillary Membranes: Strands of fetal remnant connecting; iris to iris, cornea, lens, or involving sheets of tissue. The later three forms can impair vision, and dogs affected with these forms should not be bred. Identified in 1.06% of Newfoundlands CERF examined by veterinary ophthalmologists between 2000-2005.[15]

Third Eyelid Eversion/Cartilage Anomaly: Developmental anomaly of the cartilage of the nictitating membrane. Eversion causes conjunctival drying and inflammation. Identified in 1.06% of Newfoundlands CERF examined by veterinary ophthalmologists between 2000-2005.[15]

Subaortic Stenosis (SAS): Congenital narrowing of the aortic outflow tract from the heart, causing a murmur, endocarditis, left heart failure, or sudden death. Diagnosis is by doppler ultrasound. Newfoundland dogs have a 88.0x odds ratio for the disorder versus other breeds. Padgett reports a frequency of 0.8% affected. Unknown mode of inheritance.[14,22,23]

Osteosarcoma (OSA): Malignant bone cancer, most often seen in the humerus or femur. Occurs at an increased frequency in the breed.[24]

Laryngeal Paralysis: Newfoundlands are a breed at increased risk to develop geriatric laryngeal paralysis secondary to axonal degeneration of the recurrent laryngeal nerve. Clinical signs are exercise intolerance, inspiratory stridor, inspiratory dyspnea, gagging, coughing and dysphonia.[25]

Pemphigus Foliaceus: An increased risk of developing immune mediated pemphigus foliaceus was noted in the breed. Typical lesions include dorsal muzzle and head symmetric scaling, crusting, and alopecia with peripheral collarettes, characteristic footpad lesions, with erythematous swelling at the pad margins, cracking, and villous hypertrophy. Average age of onset is 50 months. Treatment with corticosteroid and cytotoxic medications. Unknown mode of inheritance.[26]

Glaucoma: Primary, narrow angle glaucoma (goniodysgenesis) occurs in the breed. Can cause secondary lens luxation. Screen with gonioscopy and tonometry. Frequency and mode of inheritance in the breed has not been determined. CERF does not recommend breeding Newfoundlands with goniodysgenesis.[15]

Ectopic Ureters: Newfoundland dogs are an over-represented breed for ectopic ureters that do not enter the bladder normally. Clinical signs are urinary incontinence and dribbling. The anomaly can be unilateral or bilateral. Unknown mode of inheritance.[27]

Myasthenia Gravis: Acquired myasthenia gravis is identified in multiple relatives of different breeding lines, suggesting an inherited disorder. This is an autoimmune disease characterized by exercise induced muscle weakness and/or megaesophagus.[28]

Inflammatory Myopathy: Newfoundland dogs are a breed with increased incidence of inflammatory muscle disease. Many affected dogs have high circulating autoantibodies to sarcolemma antigens.[29]

Osteochondritis Dissecans of the Stifle, Prognathism, Tricuspid Valve Dysplasia, and **Ventricular Septal Defect** are reported.[30]

Isolated Case Studies

Primary Ciliary Dyskinesia: Three Newfoundland dogs with histories of chronic rhinitis and bronchopneumonia from an early age were diagnosed with the disorder. Pedigree analysis indicated an autosomal recessive mode of inheritance.[31]

Glomerulosclerosis with Proteinuria: Three littermates were euthanized due to progressive kidney disease characterized by growth retardation, anorexia, proteinuria, hypoalbuminemia, and uremia. Histopathology revealed glomerulosclerosis and glomerulofibrosis.[32]

Genetic Tests

Tests of Genotype: Direct test for cystinuria is available from HealthGene, Optigen, PennGen, and VetGen.

Direct tests for black, gray and brown coat colors, and black and brown nose are available from HealthGene and VetGen.

Tests of Phenotype: CHIC Certification: Required tests are; hip and elbow radiographs, cardiac examination by a cardiologist, and genetic test for cystinuria. (See CHIC website: www.caninehealthinfo.org) Recommended tests include CERF eye examination, patella evaluation, and thyroid profile including autoantibodies.

Miscellaneous

- **Breed name synonyms:** Newfie, Landseer.
- **Registries:** AKC, UKC, CKC, KCGB (Kennel Club of Great Britain), ANKC (Australian National Kennel Club), NKC (National Kennel Club).
- **AKC rank (year 2008):** 46 (2,938 dogs registered)
- **Internet resources:** Newfoundland Dog Club of America Inc.: www.newfdogclub.org
  Newfoundland Dog Club of Canada: www.newfoundlanddogclub.ca
  The Newfoundland Club UK: www.thenewfoundlandclub.co.uk/

References

1. Rothschild MF, Van Cleave PS, Glenn KL, et. al.: Association of MITF with white spotting in Beagle crosses and Newfoundland dogs. Anim Genet. 2006 Dec;37(6):606-7.
2. Trangerud C, Sande RD, Rorvik AM, et. al.: A new type of radiographic bone remodeling in the distal radial and ulnar metaphysis in 54 Newfoundland dogs. *Vet Radiol Ultrasound.* 2005 Mar-Apr;46(2):108-13.
3. Trangerud C, Grøndalen J, & Ytrehus B: Bone dysplasia in the radial and ulnar metaphysis of a Newfoundland dog. Vet Pathol. 2008 Mar;45(2):197-200.
4. Koch J, Pedersen HD, Jensen AL, et al: M-mode echocardiographic diagnosis of dilated cardiomyopathy in giant breed dogs. *J Vet Med A.* 1996; 43:297-304.
5. OFA Website breed statistics: www.offa.org Last accessed July 1, 2010.
6. Dorn CR: Canine breed-specific risks of frequently diagnosed diseases at veterinary teaching hospitals. Monograph. AKC Canine Health Foundation. 2000.
7. LaFond E, Breur GJ, Austin CC: Breed susceptibility for developmental orthopedic diseases in dogs. *J Am Anim Hosp Assoc.* 2002 Sep-Oct;38(5):467-77.
8. Henthorn PS, Liu J, Gidalevich T, et. al.: Canine cystinuria: polymorphism in the canine SLC3A1 gene and identification of a nonsense mutation in cystinuric Newfoundland dogs. *Hum Genet.* 2000 Oct;107(4):295-303.
9. Casal ML, Giger U, Bovee KC, et. al.: Inheritance of cystinuria and renal defect in Newfoundlands. *J Am Vet Med Assoc.* 1995 Dec 15;207(12):1585-9.
10. Giger U, Rajpurohit Y, Liu J: Prevalence of type i cystinuria in Newfoundland dogs. *J Vet Internal Med.* 2000;14:353.
11. Backus RC, Ko KS, Fascetti AJ, et. al.: Low plasma taurine concentration in Newfoundland dogs is associated with low plasma methionine and cyst(e)ine concentrations and low taurine synthesis. *J Nutr.* 2006 Oct;136(10):2525-33.
12. Tidholm A, Jonsson L: Dilated cardiomyopathy in the Newfoundland: a study of 37 cases (1983-1994). *J Am Anim Hosp Assoc.* 1996 Nov-Dec;32(6):465-70.
13. Wiersma AC, Stabej P, Leegwater PA, et. al.: Evaluation of 15 candidate genes for dilated cardiomyopathy in the Newfoundland dog. J Hered. 2008 Jan-Feb;99(1):73-80.
14. Control of Canine Genetic Diseases. Padgett GA. pp. 166-167. Howell Book House, NY. 1998.
15. *Ocular Disorders Presumed to be Inherited in Purebred Dogs.* American College of Veterinary Ophthalmologists. ACVO, 2007.
16. Nachreiner RF, Refsal KR, Graham PA, et. al.: Prevalence of serum thyroid hormone autoantibodies in dogs with clinical signs of hypothyroidism. J Am Vet Med Assoc 2002 Feb 15;220(4):466-71.
17. Nachreiner R & Refsal K: Personal communication, Diagnostic Center for Population and Animal Health, Michigan State University. April, 2007.
18. Glickman LT, Glickman NW, Schellenberg DB, et. al.: Incidence of and breed-related risk factors for gastric dilatation-volvulus in dogs. *J Am Vet Med Assoc.* 2000 Jan 1;216(1):40-5.
19. Duval JM, Budsberg SC, Flo GL, et. al.: Breed, sex, and body weight as risk factors for rupture of the cranial cruciate ligament in young dogs. *J Am*

Vet Med Assoc. 1999 Sep 15;215(6):811-4.

20. Wilke VL, Conzemius MG, Kinghorn BP, et. al.: Inheritance of rupture of the cranial cruciate ligament in Newfoundlands. *J Am Vet Med Assoc.* 2006 Jan 1;228(1):61-4.

21. Wilke VL, Zhang S, Evans RB, et. al.: Identification of chromosomal regions associated with cranial cruciate ligament rupture in a population of Newfoundlands. Am J Vet Res. 2009 Aug;70(8):1013-7

22. Kienle RD, Thomas WP, Pion PD: The natural clinical history of canine congenital subaortic stenosis. *J Vet Intern Med.* 1994 Nov-Dec;8(6):423-31.

23. Pyle RL, Patterson DF, Chacko S: The genetics and pathology of discrete subaortic stenosis in the Newfoundland dog. *Am Heart J.* 1976 Sep;92(3):324-34.

24. Dawe J: Osteosarcoma in a 6-year-old Newfoundland dog: limb-sparing surgery and cisplatin chemotherapy. Can Vet J. 2007 Nov;48(11):1169-71.

25. Burbidge HM: A review of laryngeal paralysis in dogs. Br Vet J. 1995 Jan-Feb;151(1):71-82.

26. Ihrke PJ, Stannard AA, Ardans AA, et. al.: Pemphigus foliaceus in dogs: a review of 37 cases. *J Am Vet Med Assoc.* 1985 Jan 1;186(1):59-66.

27. Westropp JL & Chew DJ: Urinary Incontinence in Dogs: Overview and Management. Proceedings 2005 ACVIM Forum. 2005.

28. Lipsitz D, Berry JL, Shelton GD: Inherited predisposition to myasthenia gravis in Newfoundlands. *J Am Vet Med Assoc.* 1999 Oct 1;215(7):956-8, 946.

29. Hankel S, Shelton GD, Engvall E: Sarcolemma-specific autoantibodies in canine inflammatory myopathy. *Vet Immunol Immunopathol.* 2006 Sep 15;113(1-2):1-10.

30. *The Genetic Connection: A Guide to Health Problems in Purebred Dogs.* L Ackerman. p. 228-29. AAHA Press, 1999.

31. Watson PJ, Herrtage ME, Peacock MA, et. al.: Primary ciliary dyskinesia in Newfoundland dogs. *Vet Rec.* 1999 Jun 26;144(26):718-25.

32. Koeman JP, Biewenga WJ, Gruys E: Proteinuria associated with glomerulosclerosis and glomerular collagen formation in three Newfoundland dog littermates. *Vet Pathol.* 1994 Mar;31(2):188-93.

33. *The Complete Dog Book, 20th Ed.* The American Kennel Club. Howell Book House, NY 2006. p. 303-307.

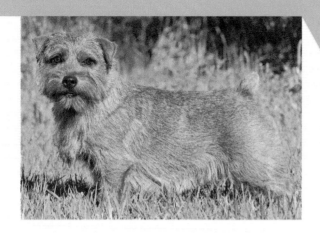

Norfolk Terrier

The Breed History

The Norwich and Norfolk terriers share a common background, originating in the Eastern Counties of Britain. Yorkshire and other terriers were used in breed development. First brought to the U.S. in 1914, they were classified as one breed until the mid 1960s in England at which time they were split into two breeds based on ear carriage. The AKC split them into two breeds in 1979. The Norfolk has folded ears, the Norwich has prick ears.

Breeding for Function

These dogs were valued as ratters and used for fox hunting—including going to ground (fox bolter). They hunted singly or in packs. Today, they are commonly kept for companionship. They enjoy playing games such as agility and earthdog trials.

Physical Characteristics

Height at Withers: 9-11" (23-28 cm)

Weight: 11-12 lb (5-5.5 kg)

Coat: The weather resistant coat is wiry and straight and about 1.5-2" (3.75-5 cm) in length, lies close, and the undercoat is short and dense. Coat colors include red, grizzle, black and tan and wheaten. They may have dark points. White markings are undesirable. The male has a longer thick ruff. Regular brushing is important and stripping is usually performed twice a year. They are moderate shedding dogs.

Longevity: 12-15 years

Points of Conformation: The skull is wide and roundish, the muzzle wedge-shaped, the face fox-like and the stop is well defined. Eyes are small and oval in shape, dark, and the palpebral margins are black. The ears, which are the distinguishing feature of the breed fold forward and are small and triangular, with slightly rounded tips. They possess a compact conformation, are longer than tall, and fairly heavily boned. The neck is medium in length and well muscled, the topline level, and thorax rounded with well-sprung ribs. The tail is high set and usually docked. They have short fairly straight limbs, with short metacarpals and metatarsals. The feet are compact, round and nails are black. The gait is low and smooth.

Recognized Behavior Issues and Traits

Reported breed characteristics include: Enjoys the company of people, possesses a stable temperament, fearless, a good guard dog, good in both rural and urban environments. He is a loyal dog with a charming personality, independently minded, moderately trainable; one should start obedience training early. Introduce to children, cats and other pets early. This terrier will view small pets as prey. Generally, they are very good with children. A Norfolk must be exercised in a fenced enclosure if off the leash.

They have moderate exercise requirements. Norfolk terriers need close human contact and have a moderate barking tendency. Norfolks may bark or dig if bored. They are easy to housetrain. They are high-energy dogs around the home.

Normal Physiologic Variations

None reported

Drug Sensitivities

None reported

Inherited Diseases

Hip Dysplasia: Polygenically inherited trait causing degenerative joint disease and hip arthritis. OFA reports 33.1% affected.[1]

Patella Luxation: Polygenically inherited laxity of patellar ligaments, causing luxation, lameness, and later degenerative joint disease. Treat surgically if causing clinical signs. OFA reports 6.4% affected.[1]

Elbow Dysplasia: Polygenically inherited trait causing elbow arthritis. Too few Norfolk Terriers have been screened by OFA to determine an accurate frequency.[1]

Epidermolytic Hyperkeratosis (Ichthyosis): An autosomal recessive cornification defect in Norfolk Terriers causing hyperpigmented skin with scaling following mild trauma. The lesions are generalized but most prominent in the glabrous skin of the axillary and inguinal regions. A genetic test is available.[2,3]

Disease Predispositions

Mitral Valve Disease (MVD): Norfolk Terriers are prone to early age mitral regurgitation. This condition may eventually lead to congestive heart disease, cardiac arrhythmias (irregular heart beats) and cardiac failure. Unknown mode of inheritance.

Persistent Pupillary Membranes: Strands of fetal remnant connecting; iris to iris, cornea, lens, or involving sheets of tissue. The later three forms can impair vision, and dogs affected with these forms should not be bred. Identified in 17.57% of Norfolk Terriers CERF examined by veterinary ophthalmologists between 2000-2005.[4]

Cataracts: Posterior cortex punctate cataracts predominate in the breed. Identified in 3.38% of Norfolk Terriers CERF examined by veterinary ophthalmologists between 2000-2005. CERF does not recommend breeding any Norfolk Terrier with a cataract.[4]

Optic Nerve Coloboma: A congenital cavity in the optic nerve which, if large, may cause blindness or vision impairment. Identified in 3.04% of Norfolk Terriers CERF examined by veterinary ophthalmologists between 2000-2005. CERF does not recommend breeding any affected Norfolk Terrier.[4]

Optic Nerve Hypoplasia: A congenital defect of the optic nerve causing blindness. Reported in 2.70% of Norfolk Terriers CERF-examined by veterinary ophthalmologists between 2000-2005.[4]

Hypothyroidism: Inherited autoimmune thyroiditis. 1.1% positive for thyroid auto-antibodies based on testing at Michigan State University. (Ave. for all breeds is 7.5%).[5,6]

Retinal Dysplasia: Retinal folds are recognized in the breed. Can lead to retinal detachment and blindness. Reported in 1.01% of Norfolk Terriers CERF-examined by veterinary ophthalmologists between 2000-2005.[4]

Portosystemic shunt (PSS, liver shunt): Congenital abnormal blood vessel connecting the portal and systemic circulation. More frequently intrahepatic in this breed versus extrahepatic. Causes stunting, abnormal behavior, possible seizures, and secondary ammonium urate urinary calculi in the breed. Treatment of PSS includes partial ligation and/or medical and dietary control of symptoms. Reported to occur at an increased frequency in the breed.[7]

Glaucoma: Primary, narrow angle glaucoma occurs in the breed. Can cause secondary lens luxation. Screen with gonioscopy and tonometry. Frequency and mode of inheritance in the breed has not been determined.[8]

Progressive Retinal Atrophy (PRA): Inherited retinal degeneration leading to complete blindness. Onset between 2 and 3 years of age with initial loss of night vision. Undetermined mode of inheritance.[4]

Allergic Inhalant Dermatitis, Brachygnathism, Inguinal Hernia, Micropapilla, and **Prognathism** are reported.[9]

Isolated Case Studies
None Reported

Genetic Tests
Tests of Genotype: Direct test for Ichthyosis is available from the Venta Lab at Michigan State University (517-355-6463 x1552).

Tests of Phenotype: CHIC Certification: Cardiac evaluation by a cardiologist with color doppler echocardiogram, CERF eye examination, and patella evaluation. Optional tests include hip evaluation, and genetic test for Ichthyosis. (See CHIC website; www.caninehealthinfo.org).

Recommend elbow radiographs, and thyroid profile including autoantibodies.

Miscellaneous
- **Breed name synonyms:** Jones Terrier (historical), Norfolk.
- **Registries:** AKC, UKC, CKC, KCGB (Kennel Club of Great Britain), ANKC (Australian National Kennel Club).
- **AKC rank (year 2008):** 115 (314 dogs registered)
- **Internet resources: The Norfolk Terrier Club:** www.norfolkterrierclub.org
  American Norfolk Terrier Association: http://www.norfolkterrier.org/
  Norfolk Terrier Club of Great Britain: www.norfolkterrierclub.co.uk/
  Norfolk Terrier Club of Canada: www.norfolkterrierclubofcanada.ca

References
1. OFA Website breed statistics: www.offa.org Last accessed July 1, 2010.
2. Barnhart KF, Credille KM, Ambrus A, et. al.: A heritable keratinization defect of the superficial epidermis in norfolk terriers. *J Comp Pathol.* 2004 May;130(4):246-54.
3. Credille KM, Barnhart KF, Minor JS, et. al.: Mild recessive epidermolytic hyperkeratosis associated with a novel keratin 10 donor splice-site mutation in a family of Norfolk terrier dogs. *Br J Dermatol.* 2005 Jul;153(1):51-8.
4. *Ocular Disorders Presumed to be Inherited in Purebred Dogs.* American College of Veterinary Ophthalmologists. ACVO, 2007.
5. Nachreiner RF, Refsal KR, Graham PA, et. al.: Prevalence of serum thyroid hormone autoantibodies in dogs with clinical signs of hypothyroidism. J Am Vet Med Assoc 2002 Feb 15;220(4):466-71.
6. Nachreiner R & Refsal K: Personal communication, Diagnostic Center for Population and Animal Health, Michigan State University. April, 2007.
7. Center S: Portosystemic Vascular Anomalies & Hepatic MVD: Evidence of Common Genetics in Small Dogs. Proceedings, 2008 ACVIM Forum. 2008.
8. Ketring KL: Schirmer Testing & Tonometry Are "Good Medicine". Proceedings, 2005 Western Veterinary Conference. 2005.
9. *The Genetic Connection: A Guide to Health Problems in Purebred Dogs.* L Ackerman. p. 229 AAHA Press, 1999.
10. *The Complete Dog Book, 20th Ed.* The American Kennel Club. Howell Book House, NY 2006. p. 409-411 .

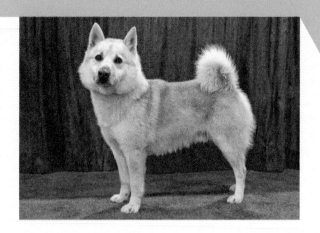

Norwegian Buhund

The Breed History

In the ancient Gokstad excavation in Norway, where a Viking grave from about the year 900 was opened, skeletons from six dogs of various sizes were found. They would be the representatives of modern-day Buhunds. These dogs travelled with Vikings on their many journeys, by sea and by land. The first Buhund show was held at Jaeren in the 1920's. The Norsk Buhundklubb was established in 1939. AKC recognition occurred in 2009.

Breeding for Function

Nurtured in the rainy western coastlands of Norway, they herded sheep and guarded farms. Besides working ability, Buhunds are trained to aid the hearing handicapped, perform some types of police work, and score well in obedience and agility trials. In olden times they hunted bear and wolf. Today they work with livestock and guard home and family.

Physical Characteristics

Height at Withers: female 16-17.5 inches (41-45 cm), male 17 to 18.5 inches (43-47 cm).

Weight: females 26.5-35.5 pounds (12-16 kg), males 31-40 pounds (14-18 kg).

Coat: Outer coat is thick and hard, but rather smooth lying. The under coat is soft and dense. The coat on the head and front of the legs is comparatively short. The coat on the neck, chest and back of the thighs is longer. Acceptable coat colors are: Wheaton (pale cream to bright orange) with or without a black mask, or black without too much bronzing. As little white as possible is permissible around the neck, face, chest, toes, or tail tip.

Longevity: 13-15 years.

Points of Conformation: The Buhund is square in profile. The skull is wedge-shaped, almost flat, and parallel with the bridge of the nose. The lips should be black and tightly closed. The teeth should meet in a scissors bite. The eyes are oval shaped, color as dark as possible, with black eye rims. The ears are medium sized, prick ears with pointed tips. The nose is black. The back is level; croup with as little slope as possible. The tail is set high, tightly curled and carried over the center line of the back. The feet are oval in shape with tightly closed toes. The action is free and effortless. The topline remains level while moving. Sound movement is essential for working ability.

Recognized Behavior Issues and Traits

Self confident, alert, lively, and very affectionate with people. The Buhund is considered by many researchers to be the easiest of the Spitz breeds to train due to their innate desire to please plus a quick learning aptitude. As it is extremely intelligent by nature, consistent training is needed from early puppyhood. Their Spitz independence is an asset if they have to be left alone for awhile. The Buhund has a lot of energy, strength and stamina. This is an active dog who needs ample amounts of exercise.

Normal Physiologic Variations

None Reported

Drug Sensitivities

None Reported

Inherited Diseases

Hip Dysplasia: Polygenically inherited trait causing degenerative joint disease and hip arthritis. OFA reports 10.7% affected.[1]

Pulverulent Nuclear Cataract: Autosomal dominant pulverulent nuclear cataracts with high penetrance occur in the breed. They start as small dots at 6-1/2 weeks, and extending throughout the fetal nucleus by 4 to 5-1/2 years of age. Identified in 9.66% of Norwegian Buhunds CERF examined by veterinary ophthalmologists between 2000-2005.[2,3]

Elbow Dysplasia: Polygenically inherited trait causing elbow arthritis. Too few Norwegian Buhunds have been screened by OFA to determine an accurate frequency.[1]

Patella Luxation: Polygenically inherited laxity of patellar ligaments, causing luxation, lameness, and later degenerative joint disease. Treat surgically if causing clinical signs. Too few Norwegian Buhunds have been screened by OFA to determine an accurate frequency.[1]

Disease Predispositions

Cataracts: Besides the dominant nuclear cataracts, posterior cortical cataracts predominate in the breed. Identified in 11.93% of Norwegian Buhunds CERF examined by veterinary ophthalmologists between 2000-2005. CERF does not recommend breeding any Norwegian Buhund with a cataract.[2]

Hypothyroidism: Inherited autoimmune thyroiditis. Too few Norwegian Buhunds have been test for thyroid autoantibodies at Michigan State University to determine an accurate frequency for the breed. (Ave. for all breeds is 7.5%).[4,5]

Isolated Case Studies

None Reported

Genetic Tests

Tests of Genotype: None

Tests of Phenotype: CHIC Certification: Required testing includes hip radiographs, CERF eye examination (after 24 months), and blood sample in the CHIC DNA Repository. (See CHIC website; www.caninehealthinfo.org).

Recommend patella evaluation, elbow radiographs, thyroid profile including autoantibodies, and cardiac examination.

Miscellaneous

- **Breed name synonyms:** Norwegian Sheepdog, Norsk Buhund, Nordiske Sitz-hunde.
- **Registries:** AKC, UKC, KCGB (Kennel Club of Great Britain), ANKC (Australian National Kennel Club), NKC (National Kennel Club), FCI.
- **AKC rank:** (None) Became an AKC recognized breed Jan. 2009. Entire studbook registered.
- **Internet resources: Norwegian Buhund Club of America:** www.buhund.org
  Norwegian Buhund Club (UK): www.norwegian-buhund.org.uk

References

1. OFA Website breed statistics: www.offa.org Last accessed July 1, 2010.
2. *Ocular Disorders Presumed to be Inherited in Purebred Dogs.* American College of Veterinary Ophthalmologists. ACVO, 2007.
3. Bjerkås E & Haaland MB: Pulverulent nuclear cataract in the Norwegian buhund. J Small Anim Pract. 1995 Nov;36(11):471-4.
4. Nachreiner RF, Refsal KR, Graham PA, et. al.: Prevalence of serum thyroid hormone autoantibodies in dogs with clinical signs of hypothyroidism. *J Am Vet Med Assoc* 2002 Feb 15;220(4):466-71.
5. Nachreiner R & Refsal K: Personal communication, Diagnostic Center for Population and Animal Health, Michigan State University. April, 2007.
6. AKC Breed Website: www.akc.org/breeds/norwegian_buhund/ Last accessed July 1, 2010.

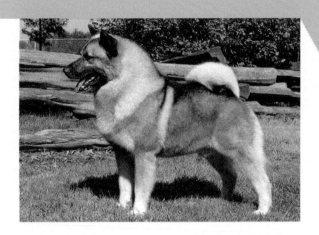

The Breed History

Six thousand years ago is the estimated timeline given for the origins of this ancient breed, also termed the "Dog of the Vikings". Archeological records show skeletal remains that match the breed in size and constitution dating from between 4000-5000 BC alongside stone weapon remnants. The first breed standard was drawn up in 1877. This is one of the Scandinavian elkhounds (Swedish Elkhound, Norwegian Buhund are others) included in the Spitz dog family. AKC recognition occurred in 1913.

Breeding for Function

Working as a chicken and duck herder, a guard dog, hunter for moose, elk, lynx, raccoon, fox and bear and as a sled dog, this was truly a versatile dog. Courageous enough to defend against bear and wolf, but gentle enough to be a companion. Stamina is a hallmark of the breed rather than extreme speed. Their short-coupled stature allows them the agility to hold quarry at bay; avoiding harm while sounding a strong voice for the hunter.

Physical Characteristics

Height at Withers: female 19.5" (49.5 cm), male 20.5" (cm)

Weight: females 48 lb (22 kg), males 55 lb (25 kg)

Coat: They have a distinctive double gray coat. Hairs are straight, and the coat lies smoothly. The overcoat hairs are black-tipped. The undercoat is wooly and dense and silvery shaded as is the underside and legs of the dog. There is a black tip on the tail; ears and muzzle are also black. They undergo twice-yearly shedding and have moderate grooming needs and no doggy odor.

Longevity: 12-13 years

Points of Conformation: These dogs possess heavy bone and well-developed musculature and a compact conformation. The wedge-shaped head is broad and ears are held pricked up. The high-set tail is carried curled over the back. Eyes are medium-sized, oval, and dark brown in color. The stop is clearly defined, skull is broad, and the muzzle tapers. The neck is muscular, of medium length and slightly arched, without throatiness. The thorax is large and deep, and the ribs well sprung. The topline gradually slopes down to the rear. The legs are straight boned, dewclaws are usually left on, and paws are small with a compact oval shape. The gait is smooth and ground covering.

Norwegian Elkhound

Recognized Behavior Issues and Traits

Reported breed attributes include: Intelligent, reliable, enjoys close human companionship, loyal, friendly, good alarm barker and watchdog, and will capably protect home and family. These dogs are eager to please. They have very high exercise needs. Noted to be sensitive, independent and headstrong, this type of dog needs mental stimulation to prevent boredom vices. Though needing human companionship, they are aloof with strangers. They are good with older, mature children, and may see small pets as prey. If off leash, they must be in a fenced enclosure because they are prone to roaming.

Normal Physiologic Variations

Tendency to become obese without dietary restriction.

Drug Sensitivities

None reported

Inherited Diseases

Hip Dysplasia: Polygenically inherited trait causing degenerative joint disease and hip arthritis. OFA reports 19.5% affected. Reported at a frequency of 23% in the NEAA Health Survey 2007 Summary.[1,2]

Patella Luxation: Polygenically inherited laxity of patellar ligaments, causing luxation, lameness, and later degenerative joint disease. Treat surgically if causing clinical signs. Too few Norwegian Elkhounds have been screened by OFA to determine an accurate frequency.[1]

Elbow Dysplasia: Polygenically inherited trait causing elbow arthritis. Too few Norwegian Elkhounds have been screened by OFA to determine an accurate frequency.[1]

Early Retinal Degeneration (ERD): An autosomal recessive early onset form of progressive retinal atropy. Affected dogs are nightblind by 6 weeks of age, and become totally blind between 12- and 18 months. No genetic test is available. CERF does not recommend breeding affected dogs.[3,4]

Rod Dysplasia (RD): An autosomal recessive form of PRA manifested by night blindness by 6 months of age, and total blindness at 3-5 years. No genetic test is available. CERF does not recommend breeding affected dogs.[4,5]

Chondrodysplasia: Autosomal recessive dwarfism in the Norwegian Elkhound occurrs due to a generalized disturbance in endochondral ossification. Radiographic changes included flaring and increased width of the distal metaphyses of the radius and ulna, delayed ossification of the cuboid bones of the carpus, and reduction in length of the vertebral bodies. A direct genetic test is available.[6]

Sry Negative XX Sex-Reversal: Autosomal recessive disorder of sexual differentiation. Affected dogs can appear to be female with enlarged clitori, or male with bilateral aspermatogenic testes. All have a 78 XX karyotype. Gonads can be ovotestes, but lack Sry, the testis-determining gene. No genetic test is available.[7]

Disease Predispositions

Sebaceous Cysts: Benign accumulation of sebum within plugged hair follicles. Reported at a frequency of 20.8% in the NEAA Health Survey 2007 Summary.[2]

Allergies: Inhalant or food allergy. Presents with pruritis (itching) and pyotraumatic dermatitis (hot spots). Reported at a frequency of 5.2% in the NEAA Health Survey 2007 Summary.[2]

Cataracts: Posterior and equatorial cortex intermediate cataracts predominate in the breed. Age of onset 1-3 years. Identified in 3.87% of Norwegian Elkhounds CERF examined by veterinary ophthalmologists between 2000-2005. Reported at a frequency of 12.3% in the NEAA Health Survey 2007 Summary. CERF does not recommend breeding any Norwegian Elkhound with a cataract.[2,4]

Hypothyroidism: Inherited autoimmune thyroiditis. 3.1% positive for thyroid auto-antibodies based on testing at Michigan State University. (Ave. for all breeds is 7.5%). Reported at a frequency of 2.4% in the NEAA Health Survey 2007 Summary.[2,8,9]

Primary (Narrow Angle) Glaucoma: Ocular condition causing increased pressure within the eyeball, and secondary blindness due to damage to the retina. The breed can have primary goniodysgenesis with pectinate ligament dysplasia and/or trabecular meshwork dysplasia. Many affected dogs have cystic degeneration of the iridociliary epithelial and/or peripheral retina. Age of onset of 4-7 years. Classified as an open-angle, closed-cleft glaucoma. Diagnose with tonometry and gonioscopy. Dorn reports a 3.48x odds ratio for glaucoma versus other breeds. Incidence in the Norwegian Elkhound is estimated at 1.98%.[10,11,12]

Persistent Pupillary Membranes: Strands of fetal remnant connecting; iris to iris, cornea, lens, or involving sheets of tissue. The later three forms can impair vision, and dogs affected with these forms should not be bred. Identified in 1.83% of Norwegian Elkhounds CERF examined by veterinary ophthalmologists between 2000-2005.[4]

Idiopathic Epilepsy: Inherited seizures. Control with anticonvulsant medication. Seizures are reported at a frequency of 1.8% in the NEAA Health Survey 2007 Summary.[2]

Distichiasis: Abnormally placed eyelashes that irritate the cornea and conjunctiva. Can cause secondary corneal ulceration. Identified in 1.63% of Norwegian Elkhounds CERF examined by veterinary ophthalmologists between 2000-2005.[4]

Mast Cell Tumor (MCT): Skin tumors that produce histamine, causing inflammation and ulceration. They can reoccur locally or with distant metastasis. Reported at a frequency of 1.6% in the NEAA Health Survey 2007 Summary.[2]

Irritable Bowel Syndrome: Causes chronic bouts of diarrhea. Control with diet and/or medications. Reported at a frequency of 1.4% in the NEAA Health Survey 2007 Summary.[2]

Juvenile Renal Disease: A kidney basement membrane disorder causing an impaired ability to concentrate urine, and progressive azotemia. Periglomerular and interstitial fibrosis are the earliest renal lesions. Results of glomerular counts, kidney size, and dissection of the nephron indicated that nephron numbers and size are adequate early in the disease, but that numbers decrease as the disease progresses. Dorn reports a 9.41x odds ratio for kidney disease versus other breeds. Unknown mode of inheritance.[10,13,14,15,16]

Renal Glucosuria/Fanconi Syndrome: Causes glucosuria, hyposthenuria, metabolic acidosis, hyperchloremia, and reduction in glomerular filtration rate. May be part of Norwegian Elkhound juvenile renal disease, or a separate inherited disorder. In a study of Norwegian Elkhounds at dog show in Norway, 27.3% had glucosuria. Dorn reports a 9.41x odds ratio for kidney disease versus other breeds. Unknown mode of inheritance. Diagnose by finding glucosuria with normal blood glucose levels, and urine amino acids. A phenotypic test is available.[10,15,16,17]

Diabetes Mellitus: Sugar diabetes caused by a lack of insulin production by the pancreas. Controlled by insulin injections, diet, and glucose monitoring. Reported at an increased frequency versus other breeds, with a female predominance. Unknown mode of inheritance.[18]

Intracutaneous Cornifying Epithelioma: Benign skin tumors consisting of keratin-filled crypts in the dermis and subcutis that open to the skin surface. Most of these tumors occur on the back, neck, sides of the thorax, and the shoulders. Usually occur prior to 5 years of age, with a male predominance. Etretinate treatment is successful in 50% of affected dogs.[19,20]

Brachygnathism, Ciliary Dyskenesia, Entropion, Oligodontia, Osteochondrodysplasia, Osteogenesis Imperfecta, and **Prognathism** are reported.[21]

Isolated Case Studies
None Reported

Genetic Tests
Tests of Genotype: Direct test for chondrodysplasia is available from Genoscoper: www.genoscoper.com.

Tests of Phenotype: CHIC Certification: Required testing includes hip radiograph, CERF eye examination (minimum 5 years of age), thyroid profile including autoantibodies (minimum 5 years of age), and kidney disease screening with urine protein:creatinine ratio (minimum of 5 years of age). Optional recommended tests include elbow radiographs, patella examination, and urine amino acid test for Fanconi syndrome from PennGen. (See CHIC website; www.caninehealthinfo.org).

Recommend cardiac examination.

Urine amino acid test for Fanconi syndrome is available from PennGen.

Miscellaneous

- **Breed name synonyms:** Elkhound, Norsk Elghund, Grahund, Gray Norwegian Elkhound, Norsk Elghund (Gra).
- **Registries:** AKC, UKC, CKC, ANKC (Australian National Kennel Club), NKC (National Kennel Club)
- **AKC rank (year 2008):** 100 (544 dogs registered)
- **Internet resources: Norwegian Elkhound Association of America:** www.neaa.net
  Norwegian Elkhound Club of Canada: www.elkhounds.net/necc/
  Norwegian Elkhound Club of Great Britain: www.necgb.co.uk/

References

1. OFA Website breed statistics: www.offa.org Last accessed July 1, 2010.

2. Norwegian Elkhound Association of America: NEAA Health Survey 2007 Summary. Sept. 18, 2007.

3. Acland GM, Aguirre GD: Retinal degenerations in the dog: IV. Early retinal degeneration (erd) in Norwegian elkhounds. *Exp Eye Res.* 1987 Apr;44(4):491-521.

4. *Ocular Disorders Presumed to be Inherited in Purebred Dogs.* American College of Veterinary Ophthalmologists. ACVO, 2007.

5. Aguirre GD, Rubin LF: Progressive retinal atrophy (rod dysplasia in the Norwegian Elkhound. J Am Vet Med Assoc. 1971 Jan 15;158(2):208-18.

6. Bingel SA, Sande RD: Chondrodysplasia in the Norwegian Elkhound. *Am J Pathol.* 1982 May;107(2):219-29.

7. Melniczek JR, Dambach D, Prociuk U, et. al.: Sry-negative XX sex reversal in a family of Norwegian Elkhounds. *J Vet Intern Med.* 1999 Nov-Dec;13(6):564-9.

8. Nachreiner R & Refsal K: Personal communication, Diagnostic Center for Population and Animal Health, Michigan State University, April, 2007.

9. Nachreiner RF, Refsal KR, Graham PA, et. al.: Prevalence of serum thyroid hormone autoantibodies in dogs with clinical signs of hypothyroidism. *J Am Vet Med Assoc* 2002 Feb 15;220(4):466-71.

10. Dorn CR: Canine breed-specific risks of frequently diagnosed diseases at veterinary teaching hospitals. Monograph. AKC Canine Health Foundation. 2000.

11. Oshima Y, Bjerkas E, Peiffer RL Jr: Ocular histopathologic observations in Norwegian Elkhounds with primary open-angle, closed-cleft glaucoma. *Vet Ophthalmol.* 2004 May-Jun;7(3):185-8.

12. Gelatt KN, MacKay EO: Prevalence of the breed-related glaucomas in pure-bred dogs in North America. *Vet Ophthalmol.* 2004 Mar-Apr;7(2):97-111.

13. Wiersma AC, Millon LV, van Dongen AM, et. al.: Evaluation of Canine COL4A3 and COL4A4 as Candidates for Familial Renal Disease in the Norwegian Elkhound. *J Hered.* 2005 Nov-Dec;96(7):739-44.

14. Finco DR, Kurtz HJ, Low DG, et. al.: Familial renal disease in Norwegian Elkhound dogs. *J Am Vet Med Assoc.* 1970 Mar 15;156(6):747-60.

15. Finco DR: Familial renal disease in Norwegian Elkhound dogs: physiologic and biochemical examinations. *Am J Vet Res.* 1976 Jan;37(1):87-91.

16. Finco DR, Duncan JD, Crowell WA, et. al.: Familial renal disease in Norwegian Elkhound dogs: morphologic examinations. *Am J Vet Res.* 1977 Jul;38(7):941-7.

17. Heiene R, Bjørndal H, & Indrebø A: Glucosuria in Norwegian elkhounds and other breeds during dog shows. Vet Rec. 2010 Apr 10;166(15):459-62.

18. Fall T, Hamlin HH, Hedhammar A, et. al.: Diabetes mellitus in a population of 180,000 insured dogs: incidence, survival, and breed distribution. J Vet Intern Med. 2007 Nov-Dec;21(6):1209-16.

19. Stannard AA, Pulley LT: Intracutaneous cornifying epithelioma (keratoacanthoma) in the dog: a retrospective study of 25 cases. *J Am Vet Med Assoc.* 1975 Sep 1;167(5):385-8.

20. White SD, Rosychuk RA, Scott KV, et. al.: Use of isotretinoin and etretinate for the treatment of benign cutaneous neoplasia and cutaneous lymphoma in dogs. *J Am Vet Med Assoc.* 1993 Feb 1;202(3):387-91.

21. *The Genetic Connection: A Guide to Health Problems in Purebred Dogs.* L Ackerman. p. 229. AAHA Press, 1999.

22. *The Complete Dog Book, 20th Ed.* The American KennelClub. Howell Book House, NY 2006. p. 192-195.

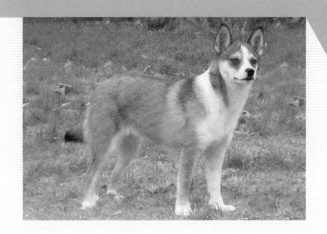

Norwegian Lundehund

Points of Conformation: The Lundehund should be athletic and agile. The head is wedge-shaped, tapering gradually to the end of the muzzle. Nose and lips are black. Scissors bite is preferred, but level and reverse scissors bite are permitted. Missing premolars on both sides of the upper and lower jaws are common and allowed. Eyes are almond-shaped, light yellow-brown to brown with a brown ring around the pupil. Eye rims are dark and complete. Ears are medium-size, triangular, and carried erect. Level back, short loin and slightly sloping croup. The tail is high-set. When moving, the tail may be carried trailing or in a graceful arch over the back. When at rest, the tail hangs with a slight curve. Moderate angulation with very elastic shoulders so that the front legs can extend out to the side. The legs are straight with slightly outward-turned feet. The forefeet are oval with at least six fully developed toes, five of which should reach the ground. Eight pads on each foot. The additional toes consist of one three jointed toe, like a thumb, and one two-jointed toe along with corresponding tendons and muscles that give the foot a strong appearance. Strong muscular upper and lower thighs. Hind feet are oval, slightly outward turned with a minimum of six toes, of which four support the dog's weight. There are seven pads with the center pad elongated. When viewed from behind, the rear legs are close but parallel. An elastic gait with a unique rotary front movement.

The Breed History

The name Lundehund is a combination of the Norwegian words "lunde," the Puffin bird, and "hund," meaning dog. Originally, they were bred to hunt and retrieve the Puffin, a meat and feather crop for the Norwegian farmer of past centuries living along the fjords and on the islands off the west coast. Written references to the breed date back to the fifteenth century. When the Puffin bird became a protected species in the 1800's, the dogs were no longer useful to the farmers and breed numbers were allowed to dwindle. The breed was saved from near extinction after World War II through the friendship of two concerned Norwegians, but even today there are a thousand dogs worldwide. AKC recognition occurred in 2011.

Breeding for Function

Their unique foot structure (at least six toes on each foot and elongated rear foot pads) and unusual flexibility enabled them to climb the steep, rocky cliffs and navigate the small burrows and crevices where Puffins nest. They have an elastic neck that allows the head to bend backward to touch the spine, letting the dog turn around in narrow puffin bird caves; and shoulders flexible enough to allow the front legs to extend flat to the side in order to hug the cliffs. This shoulder structure produces a peculiar rotary movement. Finally, the ears close and fold forward or backward to protect from debris.

Physical Characteristics

Height at withers: Males 13-15 inches (33-38 cm); Females 12-14 inches (30.5-35.5 cm).

Weight: 13-20 pounds (6-9 kg)

Coat: Double coat with a harsh outer coat and a dense, soft undercoat. The coat is short on the head and front of the legs, longer and thicker around the neck and back of thighs. It is dense on the tail with little feathering. Color is fallow to reddish brown to tan with black hair tips and white markings or white with red or dark markings. More black hair tips with maturity.

Longevity: Around 12 years.

Recognized Behavior Issues and Traits

A Lundehund is alert, very energetic, loyal and protective. He can be wary of strangers but never aggressive toward people. He is playful, curious, and intelligent. May be difficult to house train. Has a tendancy to barking. Can be stubborn.

Normal Physiologic Variations

At least six toes on each foot and elongated rear foot pads.

Drug Sensitivities

None reported

Inherited Diseases

Patella Luxation: Polygenically inherited laxity of patellar ligaments, causing luxation, lameness, and later degenerative joint disease. Treat surgically if causing clinical signs. Reported 7.7% affected, however too few Norwegian Lundehunds have been screened by OFA to determine an accurate frequency.[1]

Hip Dysplasia: Polygenically inherited trait causing degenerative joint disease and hip arthritis. Too few Norwegian Lundehunds have been screened by OFA to determine an accurate frequency.[1]

Elbow Dysplasia: Polygenically inherited trait causing elbow arthritis. Too few Norwegian Lundehunds have been screened by OFA to determine an accurate frequency.[1]

Disease Predispositions

Gastroenteropathy (Lundehund Syndrome): The collective term for a group of gastrointestinal disorders that include **chronic atrophic gastritis, intestinal lymphangiectasia, and lymphoplasmacytic enteritis.** Secondary disease includes **bacterial overgrowth in the small intestine, and protein-losing enteropathy (PLE)** which causes abnormal protein loss in the intestines. Clinical signs are intermittent diarrhea, vomiting, weight loss, lethargy, ascites, and subcutaneous edema of the hind legs. Laboratory changes include hypoalbuminemia (with or without hypoglobulinemia), hypocalcemia, a decrease in the serum cobalamin concentration, and an increase or decrease in the serum folate concentration; reflecting microbial synthesis or malabsorption respectively. Pathology includes chronic atrophic gastritis, segmental distention of lymphatics, atrophy, fusion and balloon-like swelling of villi with occasional rupture of lacteals. Undetermined mode of inheritance. Studies suggest that the majority of the breed is affected to some extent. Treatment is symptomatic.[2,3,4,5]

Hypothyroidism: Inherited autoimmune thyroiditis. Not enough samples have been submitted for thyroid auto-antibodies to Michigan State University to determine an accurate frequency. (Ave. for all breeds is 7.5%).[6,7]

Inherited Ocular Disorders: Too few Norwegian Lundehunds have been CERF examined by veterinary ophthalmologists to determine an accurate frequency of inherited ocular disorders.[8]

Gastric Carcinoma: Norwegian Lundehunds with chronic atrophic gastritis and hypergastrinemia are predisposed to the development of gastric carcinoma.[4,9]

Isolated Case Studies
None Reported

Genetic Tests

Tests of Genotype: None

Tests of Phenotype: Tests of Phenotype: **CHIC Certification:** CERF eye examination (after 24 months of age), patella evaluation, and a blood donation to the CHIC DNA repository. (See CHIC website; www.caninehealthinfo.org).

Recommend hip and elbow radiographs, thyroid profile including autoantibodies, and cardiac examination.

Miscellaneous

- **Breed name synonyms:** Lundehund, Norwegian Puffin Dog, Norsk Lundehund, Lundies
- **Registries:** AKC, UKC, CKC, FCI, NKC (National Kennel Club)
- **AKC rank (none):** AKC recognized in January, 2011. Entire stud book entered.
- **Internet resources: Norwegian Lundehund Association of America:** www.nlaainc.com
  Norwegian Lundehund Club Of America: www.lundehund.com
  American Norwegian Lundehund Club:
  www.americannorwegianlundehundclub.com

References

1. OFA Website breed statistics: www.offa.org Last accessed July 1, 2010.
2. Berghoff N, Ruaux CG, Steiner JM, et. al.: Gastroenteropathy in Norwegian Lundehunds. Compend Contin Educ Vet. 2007 Aug;29(8):456-65, 468-70; quiz 470-1.
3. Landsverk T & Gamlem H: Intestinal lymphangiectasia in the Lundehund. Scanning electron microscopy of intestinal mucosa. Acta Pathol Microbiol Immunol Scand A. 1984 Sep;92(5):353-62.
4. Kolbjørnsen O, Press CM & Landsverk T: Gastropathies in the Lundehund. I. Gastritis and gastric neoplasia associated with intestinal lymphangiectasia. APMIS. 1994 Sep;102(9):647-61.
5. Flesjå K & Yri T: Protein-losing enteropathy in the Lundehund. J Small Anim Pract. 1977 Jan;18(1):11-23.
6. Nachreiner R & Refsal K: Personal communication, Diagnostic Center for Population and Animal Health, Michigan State University. April, 2007.
7. Nachreiner RF, Refsal KR, Graham PA, et. al.: Prevalence of serum thyroid hormone autoantibodies in dogs with clinical signs of hypothyroidism. J Am Vet Med Assoc 2002 Feb 15;220(4):466-71.
8. Ocular Disorders Presumed to be Inherited in Purebred Dogs. American College of Veterinary Ophthalmologists. ACVO, 2007.
9. Qvigstad G, Kolbjørnsen Ø, Skancke E, et. al.: Gastric neuroendocrine carcinoma associated with atrophic gastritis in the norwegian lundehund. J Comp Pathol. 2008 Nov;139(4):194-201.
10. AKC Breed Website: www.akc.org/breeds/norwegian_lundehund Last accessed July 1, 2010.

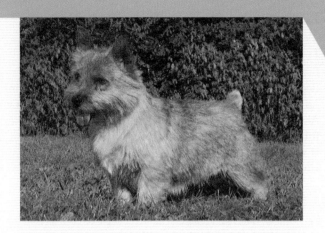

with a charming personality, independently minded, and moderately trainable so it is important to start obedience training early. Introduce to children, cats and other pets early. This terrier will view small pets as prey. Generally, they are very good with children. A Norwich must be exercised in a fenced enclosure if off the leash.

They are moderate shedding dogs. They enjoy playing and they have moderate exercise requirements. Norwich terriers like close human contact and have a moderate barking tendency. These dogs may bark or dig if bored. They are easy to housetrain.

The Breed History

The Norwich and Norfolk terriers share a common background, originating in the Eastern Counties of Britain. Yorkshire and Irish terriers were used during breed development. They were classified as one breed until the mid 1960s in England, when they were split into two breeds based on ear carriage. The AKC split them into two breeds also in 1979. The Norfolk has folded ears, the Norwich prick ears.

Breeding for Function

They were valued as ratters, and were used in fox hunting, including going to ground (fox bolter). They were hunted singly or in packs. Today, they are valued as companion dogs and excel at earthdog and agility.

Physical Characteristics

Height at Withers: 9-10" (24.5-25.5 cm)

Weight: 11-12 lb (5-5.5 kg)

Coat: The weather resistant coat is wiry and straight and about 1.5-2" (3.75-5 cm) in length, lies close, and the undercoat is short and dense. Coat colors in red, grizzle, black and tan and wheaten are accepted. The Norwich may have dark points. Regular brushing is important and stripping is usually performed twice a year.

Longevity: 12-15 years

Points of Conformation: The skull is wide and somewhat rounded, the muzzle wedge shaped, the face fox-like, and the stop is well defined. Eyes are small and oval in shape, dark, and the palpebral margins black. The ears, which are the distinguishing feature of the breed are small, pricked and triangular in shape, with slightly rounded tips. They possess a compact conformation, are longer than tall, and fairly heavily boned. The neck is medium in length and well muscled, the topline level, and thorax rounded with well-sprung ribs. The tail is high set and usually docked. They have short, fairly straight limbs, with short metacarpals and metatarsals. The feet are compact, round and nails are black. The gait is low and smooth.

Recognized Behavior Issues and Traits

Reported breed characteristics include: Enjoys the company of people, possesses a stable temperament, fearless, a good guard dog, good in both rural and urban environments. The Norwich is loyal

Normal Physiologic Variations

In a UK study, 36.6% of litters were born via **Cesarian section**.[1]

Drug Sensitivities

None reported

Inherited Diseases

Hip Dysplasia: Polygenically inherited trait causing degenerative joint disease and hip arthritis. OFA reports 13.1% affected.[2]

Patella Luxation: Polygenically inherited laxity of patellar ligaments, causing luxation, lameness, and later degenerative joint disease. Treat surgically if causing clinical signs. OFA reports 3.6% affected. Reported at a frequency of 4.5% in the 2003 Norwich Terrier General Health Survey.[2,3]

Elbow Dysplasia: Polygenically inherited trait causing elbow arthritis. Too few Norwich Terriers have been screened by OFA to determine an accurate frequency.[2]

Disease Predispositions

Missing Teeth: Reported at a frequency of 20.9% in the 2003 Norwich Terrier General Health Survey. Unknown mode of inheritance.[3]

Cataracts: Posterior and equatorial cortex intermediate cataracts predominate in the breed. Reported at a frequency of 10.5% in the 2003 Norwich Terrier General Health Survey. Identified in 2.26% of Norwich Terriers CERF examined by veterinary ophthalmologists between 2000-2005. CERF does not recommend breeding any Norwich Terrier with a cataract.[3,4]

Idiopathic Epilepsy: Inherited seizures can be generalized or partial seizures. The breed has an epileptic condition called **Epileptoid Cramping Syndrome**, which presents as paroxysmal episodes of hypertonicity affecting the pelvic limbs and lumbar muscles. Control with anticonvulsant medication. Reported at a frequency of 9.9% in the 2003 Norwich Terrier General Health Survey.[3]

Elongated Soft Palate: Can cause dyspnea, and is part of the **Brachycephalic Complex**. Surgery is indicated in severe cases. Reported at a frequency of 6.1% in the 2003 Norwich Terrier General Health Survey.[3]

Allergic Dermatitis (Atopy): Inhalant or food allergy. Presents with pruritis and pyotraumatic dermatitis (hot spots). Reported at a frequency of 6.0% in the 2003 Norwich Terrier General Health Survey.[3]

Persistent Pupillary Membranes: Strands of fetal remnant connecting; iris to iris, cornea, lens, or involving sheets of tissue. The later three forms can impair vision, and dogs affected with these forms should not be bred. Identified in 5.71% of Norwich Terriers CERF examined by veterinary ophthalmologists between 2000-2005.[4]

Deafness: Congenital sensorineural deafness can be unilateral of bilateral. Diagnosed by BAER testing. Reported at a frequency of 3.6% in the 2003 Norwich Terrier General Health Survey. Unknown mode of inheritance.[3]

Collapsing Trachea: Caused by diminished integrity of the cartilage rings in the trachea. Can produce increased coughing, stridor, and respiratory distress. Reported at a frequency of 2.1% in the 2003 Norwich Terrier General Health Survey. Unknown mode of inheritance.[3]

Glaucoma: Primary, narrow angle glaucoma occurs in the breed. Can cause secondary lens luxation and blindness due to retinal degeneration. Screen with gonioscopy and tonometry. Frequency and mode of inheritance in the breed has not been determined.[5]

Hypothyroidism: Inherited autoimmune thyroiditis. 2.8% positive for thyroid auto-antibodies based on testing at Michigan State University. (Ave. for all breeds is 7.5%). Reported at a frequency of 2.8% in the 2003 Norwich Terrier General Health Survey.[3,6,7]

Portosystemic shunt (PSS, liver shunt): Congenital abnormal blood vessel connecting the portal and systemic circulation. More frequently intrahepatic in this breed versus extrahepatic. Causes stunting, abnormal behavior, possible seizures, and secondary ammonium urate urinary calculi in the breed. Treatment of PSS includes partial ligation and/or medical and dietary control of symptoms. Reported to occur at an increased frequency in the breed.[8]

Corneal Dystrophy: Epithelial/stromal form causes opacities on the surface of the cornea. Unknown mode of inheritance. Identified in 0.93% of Norwich Terriers CERF examined by veterinary ophthalmologists between 2000-2005.[3]

Brachygnathism and **Prognathism** are reported.[9]

Isolated Case Studies
None reported

Genetic Tests
Tests of Genotype: none

Tests of Phenotype: CHIC Certification: CERF eye examination, hip radiographs, and patella evaluation. (See CHIC website; www.caninehealthinfo.org).

Recommend elbow radiographs, thyroid profile including autoantibodies, and cardiac examination.

Miscellaneous
- **Breed name synonyms:** Norwich, Jones Terrier.
- **Registries:** AKC, UKC, CKC, KCGB (Kennel Club of Great Britain), ANKC (Australian National Kennel Club), NKC (National Kennel Club).
- **AKC rank (year 2008):** 97 (616 dogs registered)
- **Internet resources:** The Norwich Terrier Club of America: www.norwichterrierclub.org
  Norwich Terrier Club (UK): www.norwichterrierclub.co.uk/

References
1. Evans KM & Adams VJ: Proportion of litters of purebred dogs born by caesarean section. J Small Anim Pract. 2010 Feb;51(2):113-8.
2. OFA Website breed statistics: www.offa.org Last accessed July 1, 2010.
3. Slater M, The Norwich and Norfolk Terrier Club: 2003 Norwich Terrier General Health Survey. 2003.
4. *Ocular Disorders Presumed to be Inherited in Purebred Dogs.* American College of Veterinary Ophthalmologists. ACVO, 2007.
5. Ketring KL: Schirmer Testing & Tonometry Are "Good Medicine". Proceedings, 2005 Western Veterinary Conference. 2005.
6. Nachreiner RF, Refsal KR, Graham PA, et. al.: Prevalence of serum thyroid hormone autoantibodies in dogs with clinical signs of hypothyroidism. J Am Vet Med Assoc 2002 Feb 15;220(4):466-71.
7. Nachreiner R & Refsal K: Personal communication, Diagnostic Center for Population and Animal Health, Michigan State University. April, 2007.
8. Center S: Portosystemic Vascular Anomalies & Hepatic MVD: Evidence of Common Genetics in Small Dogs. Proceedings, 2008 ACVIM Forum. 2008.
9. *The Genetic Connection: A Guide to Health Problems in Purebred Dogs.* L Ackerman. p. 229 AAHA Press, 1999.
10. *The Complete Dog Book, 20th Ed.* The American Kennel Club. Howell Book House, NY 2006. p. 412-413.

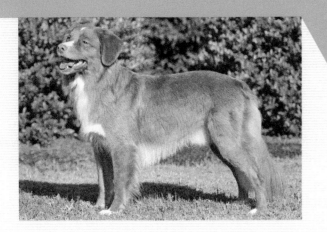

Nova Scotia Duck Tolling Retriever

The Breed History

In the southern tip of Nova Scotia in Yarmouth in the early part of the 19th century, the Toller was developed to toll or decoy (lure) the waterfowl and then retrieve them. The dogs will play at the water's edge in response to thrown balls and sticks, and this activity engages the attention of the ducks. They will then come into range for the gunner and once the job is done, the dog swims out to bring in the bird. Breed origins are sketchy, but the Europeans may have brought with them the red decoy dog which was crossed with the local retriever and spaniel types. The first registry to accept this breed, affectionately called "the little red dog" was the Canadian Kennel Club (1945). The AKC first accepted the dog into the Miscellaneous Class in 2001 and accepted it into the Sporting group in 2003. This is the official dog of the province of origin, Nova Scotia.

Breeding for Function

Strictly bred for hunter function, these dogs have continued to be encouraged to prove in field tests (Working Certificates WC, WCI, WCX) to ensure that their original suitability for the tolling and retrieving is maintained. They are gradually gaining in popularity as a companion animal. While working, they usually keep their feathered tail in motion.

Physical Characteristics

Height at Withers: female 17-20" (43-51 cm), male 18-21" (45.5-53 cm)

Weight: 35-45 lb (16-20 kg)

Coat: The medium length water resistant coat is double. Overall, the coat is straight, though slightly wavy over the back. The undercoat is short, soft and dense. Moderate feathering of legs, tail, underside of body and pantaloons is present, while muzzle hair is short. Colors are red shades, with a range from golden red to copper red. Specific markings are set out in the standard—usually at least one white marking is present. In winter, a heavy coat may curl under the neck. The hairs growing alongside the back of the ears may become fluffy and kinky and long. The ear hairs are gently plucked a few at a time to maintain the outline of the leather. The paws may also become excessively shaggy. To maintain a groomed look, these fuzz feet can be carefully trimmed of excess hair. Weekly brushing is recommended.

Longevity: 12-14 years

Points of Conformation:

A sturdy well balanced conformation is the hallmark of this medium-sized powerful working dog. Smallest of all of the retriever type dogs, utility has dictated all aspects of conformation. They possess a broad slightly wedge-shaped and rounded skull, a strong profile with moderate stop, the muzzle tapers and lips are tight, and the broad nose matches the coat color or is black. Cheeks are flat. Ears are high and wide set and well back on the skull. Ears are medium in size and length, triangular, and held slightly erect. Eyes are wide set and almond shaped. Eye and eyelid margin color should match the coat or be darker. Rims can also be black. The neck is strong and medium in thickness and length, without throatiness. Deep-chested, back is short and straight, abdomen has moderate tuck. The tail is richly feathered, broader at its base, reaching to the tarsus and is carried above the back while active, and held following the curve of the croup when resting. Medium in bone, these dogs should be slightly longer than high. Feet are medium-sized, webbed, oval and well knuckled up in the toes. Pads are thick, and the front dewclaws can be removed. Rear dewclaws disqualify. Moves with a springy gait, with straight alignment.

Recognized Behavior Issues and Traits

Breed attributes ascribed include: Agile, keen to work, quick to learn, loves to please. Very intense attitude is typical while working. Highly intelligent, good with children, affectionate, some puppies may be reserved but shyness is a fault. Outgoing in the field. Training—can be easily distracted and bored—need to keep sessions short and fun.

Normal Physiologic Variations

Sometimes the ears are taped to maintain proper folding if they become wonky (folded, rosebud). This frequently occurs when the pup is around 3-4 months of age, and the taping is left on for about 1 month. Sometimes a second one month application is required. The abnormal folding of the ear may be an inherited trait.

Drug Sensitivities

None reported in the literature

Inherited Diseases

Progressive Retinal Atrophy (prcd–PRA): Autosomal recessive progressive rod cone degeneration (prcd) form. Age of onset between 3-8 years of age, eventually causing blindness. A genetic test from Optigen reports 7% affected, and 45% carrier in Nova Scotia Duck Tolling Retrievers.[1,2]

Hip Dysplasia: Polygenically inherited trait causing degenerative joint disease and hip arthritis. OFA reports 6.5% affected.[3]

Collie Eye Anomaly/Choroidal Hypoplasia (CEA/CH): Autosomal recessive disorder of eye development that can lead to retinal detachment and blindness. CERF does not recommend breeding affected dogs. A genetic test is available from Opigen, which reports 2% affected, 16% carrier in the breed.[1,4]

Elbow Dysplasia: Polygenically inherited trait causing elbow arthritis. OFA reports 2.7% affected.[3]

Patella Luxation: Polygenically inherited laxity of patellar ligaments, causing luxation, lameness, and later degenerative joint disease. Treat surgically if causing clinical signs. OFA reports 1.9% affected.[3]

Hypoadrenocorticism (Addison's Disease): Immune mediated destruction of the adrenal gland. Inherited form is present at a reported incidence of 1.4%. Typical presentation of lethargy, poor appetite, vomiting, weakness, and dehydration can occur from 4 months to several years of age, with a median age of onset of 2.6 years in the breed. Controlled by a major autosomal recessive gene, with a heritability of 0.98. Reported at a frequency of 1.02% in the 2002 NSDTR Health Survey. Associated with DLA class II genes conferring increased risk for the disease. Treatment with DOCA injections or oral fludrocortisone.[5,6,7,8]

Systemic Lupus Erythematosus (SLE)-Related Disease: An inherited SLE-related disease occurs in the breed that includes both both antinuclear antibody (ANA)-positive **Immune-Mediated Rheumatic Disease (IMRD)** and **Steroid-Responsive Meningitis-Arteritis (SRMA)**. Affected dogs with IMRD present with persistent lameness, stiffness mainly after resting, and palpable pain from several joints of the extremities. Dogs with SRMA present with fever and neck pain. Both presentations respond to steroid treatment. Seen at a prevalence of 2.5% in a Norwegian population of Nova Scotia Duck Tolling Retrievers. Complexly inherited and associated with multiple gene loci conferring increased risk for the disease complex.[9,10,11,12,13]

Disease Predispositions

Hypothyroidism: 17.6% positive for thyroid auto-antibodies based on testing at Michigan State University. (Ave. for all breeds is 7.5%).[14,15]

Cryptorchidism: Unilateral or bilateral undescended testicles occurred in 14.08% of males in the 2002 NSDTR Health Survey. This is a sex-limited disorder with an unknown mode of inheritance.[6]

Distichiasis: Abnormally placed eyelashes that irritate the cornea and conjunctiva. Can cause secondary corneal ulceration. Identified in 11.74% of Nova Scotia Duck Tolling Retrievers CERF examined by veterinary ophthalmologists between 2000-2005.[1]

Deafness: Congenital sensorineural deafness can be unilateral of bilateral. Diagnosed by BAER testing. Reported at a frequency of 4.66% in the 2002 NSDTR Health Survey. Unknown mode of inheritance.[6,16]

Persistent Pupillary Membranes: Strands of fetal remnant connecting; iris to iris, cornea, lens, or involving sheets of tissue. The later three forms can impair vision, and dogs affected with these forms should not be bred. Identified in 4.47% of Nova Scotia Duck Tolling Retrievers CERF examined by veterinary ophthalmologists between 2000-2005.[1]

Umbilical Hernia: Congenital defect of abdominal wall closure at the umbilicus. Close surgically if large. Reported at a frequency of 4.41% in the 2002 NSDTR Health Survey. Unknown mode of inheritance.[6]

Corneal Dystrophy: Causes opacities on the surface of the cornea. Unknown mode of inheritance. Identified in 2.16% of Nova Scotia Duck Tolling Retrievers CERF examined by veterinary ophthalmologists between 2000-2005. CERF does not recommend breeding any Nova Scotia Duck Tolling Retriever with the condition.[1]

Cataracts: Anterior cortex, punctate, and capsular cataracts predominate in the breed. Identified in 1.68% of Nova Scotia Duck Tolling Retrievers CERF examined by veterinary ophthalmologists between 2000-2005. CERF does not recommend breeding any Nova Scotia Duck Tolling Retrievers with a cataract.[1]

Idiopathic Epilepsy (Inherited Seizures): Control with anticonvulsant medication. Reported at a low frequency in the 2002 NSDTR Health Survey. Unknown mode of inheritance.[6,17]

Pulmonic Stenosis: Clinical signs can include exercise intolerance, stunting, dyspnea, syncope and ascites, leading to heart failure. Diagnosis by auscultation for a heart murmur, and echocardiography. Reported at a low frequency in the 2002 NSDTR Health Survey. Unknown mode of inheritance.[6]

Skeletal Dysplasia: This disorder causes asynchronous growth of the radius and ulna, leading to bowing of the radius and valgus deformity of the front limbs. It is being researched at UC-Davis: http://faculty.vetmed.ucdavis.edu/faculty/dlbannasch/lab/projects/sd.htm

Isolated Case Studies
None reported

Genetic Tests
Tests of Genotype: Direct tests for prcd-PRA and CEA/CH are available from Optigen.

Tests of Phenotype: CHIC Certification: Required testing includes hip radiographs, CERF eye examination, and direct test for prcd-PRA. (See CHIC website; www.caninehealthinfo.org).

Direct tests for coat color are available from VetGen.

Recommend elbow radiographs, thyroid profile including autoantibodies, BAER testing for deafness, cardiac evaluation, and patella evaluation.

Miscellaneous
- **Breed name synonyms:** Historical SYN: Yarmouth Toller, Little River Duck Dog. Toller.
- **Registries:** AKC, CKC, UKC, KCGB (Kennel Club of Great Britain), ANKC (Australian National Kennel Club), NKC (National Kennel Club)
- **AKC rank (year 2008):** 102 (474 dogs registered)
- **Breed resources: Nova Scotia Duck Tolling Retriever Club (USA):** www.nsdtrc-usa.org/
  Nova Scotia Duck Tolling Retriever Club of Canada: www.toller.ca
  Nova Scotia Duck Tolling Retriever Club of UK: www.toller-club.co.uk/
  Toller Health Coalition (& health database): www.toller.ca/tollerhealth/index.html

References

1. *Ocular Disorders Presumed to be Inherited in Purebred Dogs.* American College of Veterinary Ophthalmologists. ACVO, 2007.

2. Morris Animal Foundation: Morris Animal Foundation Update: Genetic Tests Focus on Breed-Specific Vision Problems. Canine Pract 1999:24[4]:21.

3. OFA Website breed statistics: www.offa.org Last accessed July 1, 2010.

4. Parker HG, Kukekova AV, Akey DT, et. al.: Breed relationships facilitate fine-mapping studies: a 7.8-kb deletion cosegregates with Collie eye anomaly across multiple dog breeds. Genome Res. 2007 Nov;17(11):1562-71.

5. Burton S, DeLay J, Holmes A, et. al.: Hypoadrenocorticism in young related Nova Scotia duck tolling retrievers. Can Vet J. 1997 Apr;38(4):231-4.

6. Toller Health Coalition: 2002 Nova Scotia Duck Tolling Retriever Health Survey. 2002.

7. Hughes AM, Nelson RW, Famula TR, et. al.: Clinical features and heritability of hypoadrenocorticism in Nova Scotia Duck Tolling Retrievers: 25 cases (1994-2006).

8. Hughes AM, Jokinen P, Bannasch DL, et. al.: Association of a dog leukocyte antigen class II haplotype with hypoadrenocorticism in Nova Scotia Duck Tolling Retrievers. Tissue Antigens. 2010 Jun;75(6):684-90.

9. Wilbe M, Jokinen P, Truvé K, et. al.: Genome-wide association mapping identifies multiple loci for a canine SLE-related disease complex. Nat Genet. 2010 Mar;42(3):250-4.

10. Wilbe M, Jokinen P, Hermanrud C, et. al.: MHC class II polymorphism is associated with a canine SLE-related disease complex. Immunogenetics. 2009 Aug;61(8):557-64.

11. Hansson-Hamlin H & Lilliehöök I: A possible systemic rheumatic disorder in the Nova Scotia duck tolling retriever. Acta Vet Scand. 2009 Mar 30;51:16.

12. Anfinsen KP, Berendt M, Liste FJ, et. al.: A retrospective epidemiological study of clinical signs and familial predisposition associated with aseptic meningitis in the Norwegian population of Nova Scotia duck tolling retrievers born 1994-2003. Can J Vet Res. 2008 Jul;72(4):350-5.

13. Redman J: Steroid-responsive meningitis-arteritis in the Nova Scotia duck tolling retriever. Vet Rec. 2002 Dec 7;151(23):712.

14. Nachreiner RF, Refsal KR, Graham PA, et. al.: Prevalence of serum thyroid hormone autoantibodies in dogs with clinical signs of hypothyroidism. J Am Vet Med Assoc 2002 Feb 15;220(4):466-71.

15. Nachreiner R & Refsal K: Personal communication, Diagnostic Center for Population and Animal Health, Michigan State University. April, 2007.

16. Strain GM: Deafness prevalence and pigmentation and gender associations in dog breeds at risk. Vet J. 2004 Jan;167(1):23-32.

17. Parent J: The Diagnostic and Therapeutic Approach to Recurrent Seizures in the Dog. Proceedings World Small Animal Veterinary Association Congress, 2004.

18. *The Complete Dog Book, 20th Ed.* The American Kennel Club. Howell Book House, NY 2006. p. 58-62.

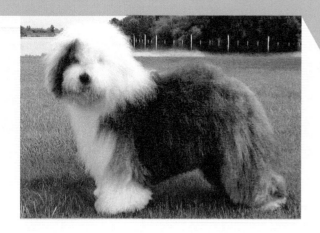

Old English Sheepdog

gait is long and elastic and they tend to do a rolling pace, or amble much like a bear's way of going.

Recognized Behavior Issues and Traits

These are loyal intelligent dogs. They need fairly intensive grooming including a schedule of a thorough brush-through every 2 to 3 days. Their shedding varies with the seasons, but they're considered heavy shedders. This breed is often shaved down to a short coat for purposes of practical care. They tend to possess a stable temperament, but some can be aggressive. They have been known to try to herd children in the family. They are quite independent so their training should start early. Their bark is a very loud one, with a distinct bell-overtone. They benefit from early socialization to other dogs, particularly male, and to children. They need lots of exercise, human contact and activities that provide mental stimulation.

Normal Physiologic Variations

None reported

Drug Sensitivities

MDR1 Mutation (Ivermectin/Drug Toxicity): Autosomal recessive disorder in the MDR1 gene allows high CNS drug levels of ivermectin, doramectin, loperamide, vincristine, moxidectin, and other drugs. Causes neurological signs, including tremors, seizures, and coma. A genetic test is now available for the mutated gene. Testing at various labs shows 2.5 to 7.3% of Old English Sheepdogs are carriers. The carrier frequency in Germany was found to be 12.5%.[1,2,3,4]

Inherited Disease

Hip Dysplasia: Polygenically inherited trait causing degenerative joint disease and hip arthritis. OFA reports 18.7% affected. Dorn reports a 2.03x odds ratio versus other breeds. Another study reports a 5.2x odds ratio versus other breeds.[5,6,7]

Elbow Dysplasia: Polygenically inherited trait causing elbow arthritis. OFA reports 3.9% affected.[5]

Patella Luxation: Polygenically inherited laxity of patellar ligaments, causing luxation, lameness, and later degenerative joint disease. Treat surgically if causing clinical signs. Too few Old English Sheepdogs have been screened by OFA to determine an accurate frequency.[5]

Cerebellar Abiotrophy (Cerebellar Ataxia, CA): Rare, simple autosomal recessive disorder causing muscular incoordination with an onset between six months and three years of age. Clinical signs are mild in most affected dogs and do not progress to recumbency.[8]

Primary Ciliary Dyskinesia: A rare, autosomal recessive ciliary dyskinesia is identified in Old English Sheepdogs. Affected dogs present with chronic, recurrent rhinitis and bronchopneumonia, male subfertility and situs-inversus in half of the cases. A genetic test is not available.[9,10]

The Breed History

This breed originates in England and many believe that the Bearded Collie is an important ancestor. Other breeds listed in various accounts include Briard, Russian Owtchar, Bergamasco and others. About 150 years ago, the first breed representations appeared in works of art. The first AKC registration occurred in 1905. These dogs have gained popular recognition via many television, film and cartoon appearances.

Breeding for Function

These were drover's dogs, or dogs used to drive cattle and sheep. They tolerated cold, damp and hot environmental conditions well. Their coats were considered such good insulators that the shepherds would shear their dogs along with the sheep, and the dog hair was used to make clothing.

They are also excellent companion animals and are sometimes also used as sled dogs. The tradition of tail docking them was started during their early working days in order to designate them as working dogs, and thus their owners would be granted tax-exempt status for the dog.

Physical Characteristics

Height at Withers: female 21" (53 cm) and up, male 22" (56 cm) and up.

Weight: females 60 lb (27 kg), males 65 lb (29.5 kg).

Coat: Their heavy coat is pigmented blue, blue-gray, blue merle, or gray with or without white markings.

Longevity: 10-12 years

Points of Conformation: The shaggy profuse coat and square athletic build characterize this breed. The eyes are brown or blue or sometimes one of each. They have a large black nose and medium ears falling against the head, a well-defined stop and strong jaw and muzzle. The topline is slightly arched, and lower at the withers than loin; the latter being a distinct breed characteristic. They are deep-chested but not too wide, and a body wider at the rump than shoulders are also distinguishing breed features. The tail is docked very short to the body when not born bobbed. Good solid bone and straight limbs with small, arched round feet are characteristic. The

Disease Predispositions

Hypothyroidism: Inherited autoimmune thyroiditis. 21.9% positive for thyroid auto-antibodies based on testing at Michigan State University. (Ave. for all breeds is 7.5%.)[11,12]

Persistent Pupillary Membranes: Strands of fetal remnant connecting; iris to iris, cornea, lens, or involving sheets of tissue. The later three forms can impair vision, and dogs affected with these forms should not be bred. Identified in 8.30% of Old English Shepdogs CERF-examined by veterinary ophthalmologists between 2000-2005.[13]

Cryptorchidism (Retained Testicles): Can be bilateral or unilateral. Reported at a frequency of 6.38% in the 2003-2004 OESCA Health Survey.[14]

Allergic Dermatitis: Inhalant or food allergy. Presents with pruritis and pyotraumatic dermatitis (hot spots). Food allergy is reported at a frequency of 4.05%, and inhalant allergies at 2.38% in the 2009 OESCA Health Survey.[15]

Cataracts: Anterior cortex punctate cataracts predominate in the breed. Reported in 2.61% of Old English Sheepdogs presented to veterinary teaching hospitals. Identified in 3.08% of Old English Sheepdogs CERF-examined by veterinary ophthalmologists between 2000-2005. Juvenile cataracts are reported at a frequency of 1.81% in the 2003-2004 OESCA Health Survey. CERF does not recommend breeding any Old English Sheepdog with a cataract.[13,14,16]

Lymphoma/Lymphosarcoma: Malignant cancer of lymphocytes. Can be of B-cell or T-cell origin. Treatment is with chemotherapy. Reported at a frequency of 2.76% in the 2009 OESCA Health Survey.[15]

Retinal Dysplasia: Retinal folds, geographic, and generalized retinal dysplasia with detachment are recognized in the breed. Can progress to blindness. Reported in 2.05% of Old English Sheepdogs CERF examined by veterinary ophthalmologists between 2000-2005.[13]

Gastric Dilatation-Volvulus (Bloat, GDV): Life-threatening twisting of the stomach within the abdomen. Requires immediate veterinary attention. GDV is the cause of death of 7.7% of Old English Sheepdogs in the British Kennel Club Old English Sheepdog Health Survey. Reported at a frequency of 1.93% in the 2003-2004 OESCA Health Survey.[14,17]

Deafness: Congenital deafness can be unilateral or bilateral. Diagnose by BAER testing. Bilateral deafness is reported at a frequency of 1.28% and unilateral deafness at 0.70% in the 2009 OESCA Health Survey.[15,18]

Osteosarcoma (OSA): Malignant bone cancer, most often seen in the humerus or femur. Reported at a frequency of 1.73% in the 2009 OESCA Health Survey.[15]

Portosystemic Shunt (PSS, Liver Shunt): Congenital abnormal blood vessel connecting the portal and systemic circulation. More frequently intrahepatic in this breed versus extrahepatic. Causes stunting, abnormal behavior, possible seizures, and secondary ammonium urate urinary calculi in the breed. Treatment of PSS includes partial ligation and/or medical and dietary control of symptoms. Tobias reports a 5.2x odds ratio versus other breeds.[19]

Autoimmune Hemolytic Anemia (AIHA): Auto-immune disorder where the body produces antibodies against its own red blood cells. Old English Sheepdogs account for one-third of all cases of AIHA in one study. Clinical features included pale mucous membranes, weakness, lethargy and collapse. The intravascular hemolytic form of the disease is characterized by bilirubinemia. Treatment with prednisone is successful in most cases. Reported at a frequency of 1.46% in the 2009 OESCA Health Survey.[15,20]

Sebaceous Adenitis: Disorder of immune mediated sebaceous gland destruction, presenting with hair loss, usually beginning with the dorsal midline and ears. Diagnosis by skin biopsy. Treat with isotretinoin. An autosomal recessive mode of inheritance is suspected. Reported at a frequency of 1.19% in the 2009 OESCA Health Survey.[15,25]

Distichiasis: Abnormally placed eyelashes that irritate the cornea and conjunctiva. Can cause secondary corneal ulceration. Identified in 1.11% of Old English Sheepdogs CERF examined by veterinary ophthalmologists between 2000-2005.[13]

Immune-Mediated Thrombocytopenia (ITP): Auto-immune disorder where the body produces antibodies against its own platelets. Most common presentation is in middle aged females. Old English Sheepdogs have a breed predilection for ITP. Reported at a frequency of 0.97% in the 2009 OESCA Health Survey.[15,21]

Osteochondritis Dissecans (OCD): Abnormality of cartilage development causing lameness in the shoulder, elbow, hock or knee. Severe cases may require surgery. Reported 7.1x odds ratio for shoulder OCD versus other breeds. Dorn reports a 5.10x odds ratio versus other breeds.[6,7]

Demodicosis (Generalized): Demodectic mange dermatitis has an underlying immunodeficiency in its pathogenesis. Dorn reports a 2.67x odds ratio versus other breeds.[6]

Silica Bladder Stones: Old English Sheepdogs are found to be at increased risk of developing silica-containing urinary calculi.[22]

Perineal Hernia: Old English Sheepdogs are predisposed to developing perineal hernias. Treat with surgery.[23,24]

Uveodermatologic (VKH-like) Syndrome: An autoimmune disease manifested by progressive uveitis and depigmenting dermatitis that closely resembles the human Vogt-Koyanagi-Harada syndrome. Affected Old English Sheepdogs often have heterochromia irides. Onset 1-1/2 to 4 years of age. CERF does not recommend breeding any affected dogs.[13,26]

Degenerative Myelopathy (DM): Affected dogs show an insidious onset of upper motor neuron (UMN) paraparesis at an average age of 11.4 years. The disease eventually progresses to severe tetraparesis. Affected dogs have normal results on myelography, MRI, and CSF analysis. Necropsy confirms the condition. Unknown mode of inheritance. A direct genetic test for an autosomal recessive DM susceptibility gene is available. All affected dogs are homozygous for the gene, however, only a small percentage of homozygous dogs develop DM. Reported as a clinical disease in the breed with a prevalence of 0.38%.[27]

Microphthalmia with Multiple Ocular Abnormalities: Affected litters have congenital non-progressive microphthalmia, cataracts and retinal abnormalities including retinal detachment. Unknown mode of inheritance. Affected dogs should not be bred.[13,28]

Anasarca, Atrial Septal Defect, Brachygnathism, Cardiomyopathy, Cervical Vertebral Instability, Diabetes Mellitus, Entropion, Factor IX Deficiency, Hypoadrenocorticism, Lymphedema, Micropapilla, Optic Nerve Hypoplasia, Prognathism, Progressive Retinal Atrophy, Tricuspid Valve Dysplasia, and **von Willebrand's Disease** are reported.[29]

Isolated Case Studies

Juvenile Renal Failure: Chronic renal failure was diagnosed in three young Old English Sheepdogs. Clinical signs included ill-thrift, polydipsia, polyuria, and behavioral changes. Clinical pathology included azotemia, anemia, hyperphosphatemia, and isosthenuria.[30]

Lactic Acidosis and Myopathy: Two littermates presented with exercise-induced weakness, lactic acidosis, increased muscle enzyme activity, an increased lactate/pyruvate ratio, and increased venous PO2. The authors suggested the possibility of defective mitochondrial oxygen utilization.[31]

Muscular Dystrophy: An 11 month old male Old English Sheepdog in the UK was diagnosed with dystrophin deficient muscular dystrophy.[32]

Giant Hypertrophic Gastritis: An 11-year-old, male Old English sheepdog with weight loss and vomiting had a mass-like stomach, anemia, hypoproteinemia, and hypoalbuminemia. The significantly thickened gastric wall had multilobulated folds protruding into the gastric lumen, with pronounced gastric glandular hyperplasia. The condition was poorly responsive to medications.[33]

Genetic Tests

Tests of Genotype: Direct test for Mdr1 drug sensitivity is available from Washington State University-VCPL.

Direct test for a DM susceptibility gene is available from OFA.

Tests of Phenotype: CHIC Certification: Required tests are: CERF eye examination (yearly until 5, then every other year), thyroid profile including autoantibodies (yearly until 5, then every other year), and hip radiograph. Optional recommended tests are; Cardiac certification by a cardiologist, BAER test for deafness and genetic test for MDR1. (See CHIC website: www.caninehealthinfo.org)

Recommend elbow radiographs and patella evaluation.

Miscellaneous

- **Breed name synonyms:** Bob, Bobtail, Sheepdog
- **Registries:** AKC, CKC, UKC, KCGB (Kennel Club of Great Britain), ANKC (Australian National Kennel Club), NKC (National Kennel Club)
- **AKC rank (year 2008):** 75 (1,024 registered)

- **Internet resources:** Old English Sheepdog Club of America: www.oldenglishsheepdogclubofamerica.org
  Greater London Old English Sheepdog Club: www.gloesc.co.uk
  Old English Sheepdog and Owners Club of Canada: www.oesocc.com

References

1. Neff MW, Robertson KR, Wong AK, et. al.: Breed distribution and history of canine mdr1-1Delta, a pharmacogenetic mutation that marks the emergence of breeds from the collie lineage. Proc Natl Acad Sci U S A. 2004 Aug 10;101(32):11725-30.
2. Geyer J, Döring B, Godoy JR, et. al.: Frequency of the nt230 (del4) MDR1 mutation in Collies and related dog breeds in Germany. J Vet Pharmacol Ther. 2005 Dec;28(6):545-51.
3. Mealey KL & Meurs KM: Breed distribution of the ABCB1-1Delta (multidrug sensitivity) polymorphism among dogs undergoing ABCB1 genotyping. J Am Vet Med Assoc. 2008 Sep 15;233(6):921-4.
4. Gramer I, Leidolf R, Döring B, et. al.: Breed distribution of the nt230(del4) MDR1 mutation in dogs. Vet J. 2011 Jul;189(1):67-71.
5. OFA Website breed statistics: www.offa.org Last accessed July 1, 2010.
6. Dorn CR: Canine breed-specific risks of frequently diagnosed diseases at veterinary teaching hospitals. Monograph. AKC Canine Health Foundation. 2000.
7. LaFond E, Breur GJ & Austin CC: Breed susceptibility for developmental orthopedic diseases in dogs. J Am Anim Hosp Assoc. 2002 Sep-Oct;38(5):467-77.
8. Steinberg HS, Van Winkle T, Bell JS, et. al.: Cerebellar degeneration in Old English Sheepdogs. J Am Vet Med Assoc. 2000 Oct 15;217(8):1162-5.
9. Merveille AC, Battaille G, Davis E, et. al.: Detection of a New Mutation Responsible For Primary Ciliary Dyskinesia in a Pedigree of Old English Sheepdogs. Proceedings, 19th ECVIM-CA Congress. 2009.
10. Billen F, Binst D, Geyskens V, et. al.: Primary Ciliary Dyskinesia in a Family of Old English Sheepdogs. Proceedings, 17th ECVIM-CA Congress. 2007.
11. Nachreiner RF, Refsal KR, Graham PA, et. al.: Prevalence of serum thyroid hormone autoantibodies in dogs with clinical signs of hypothyroidism. J Am Vet Med Assoc 2002 Feb 15;220(4):466-71.
12. Nachreiner R & Refsal K: Personal communication, Diagnostic Center for Population and Animal Health, Michigan State University. April, 2007.
13. *Ocular Disorders Presumed to be Inherited in Purebred Dogs.* American College of Veterinary Ophthalmologists. ACVO, 2007.
14. Old English Sheepdog Club of America. 2003-2004 OESCA General Health Survey. 2004.
15. Old English Sheepdog Club Of America Health and Research Committee. 2009 Breed Health Survey Report. 2009.
16. Gelatt KN, Mackay EO: Prevalence of primary breed-related cataracts in the dog in North America. Vet Ophthalmol. 2005 Mar-Apr;8(2):101-11.
17. The Kennel Club/British Small Animal Veterinary Association Scientific Committee: Summary results of the Purebred Dog Health Survey for Old English Sheepdogs. 2006.
18. Strain GM: Deafness prevalence and pigmentation and gender associations in dog breeds at risk. Vet J. 2004 Jan;167(1):23-32.
19. Tobias KM, Rohrbach BW: Association of breed with the diagnosis of congenital portosystemic shunts in dogs: 2,400 cases (1980-2002). J Am Vet Med Assoc. 2003 Dec 1;223(11):1636-9.
20. Mills JN, Day MJ, Shaw SE, et. al.: Autoimmune haemolytic anaemia in dogs. Aust Vet J. 1985 Apr;62(4):121-3.
21. Mackin A: Immune-Mediated Thrombocytopenia: Pathophysiology And Diagnosis. 2002 ACVIM Forum. 2002.
22. Aldrich J, Ling GV, Ruby AL, et. al.: Silica-containing urinary calculi in dogs (1981-1993). J Vet Intern Med. 1997 Sep-Oct;11(5):288-95.
23. Sjollema BE, van Sluijs FJ: Perineal hernia in the dog: developments in its surgical treatment and retrospective study in 197 patients. Tijdschr Diergeneeskd. 1991 Feb 1;116(3):142-7.

24. Elkins AD: Perineal Hernias: Medical & Surgical Management. Proceedings 2004 Western Veterinary Conference. 2004.

25. White S: Sebaceous Adenitis. 2001. Proceedings, World Small Animal Veterinary Association World Congress, 2001.

26. Sigle KJ, McLellan GJ, Haynes JS, et. al.: Unilateral uveitis in a dog with uveodermatologic syndrome. J Am Vet Med Assoc. 2006 Feb 15;228(4):543-8.

27. Coates JR & Wade C: Update on the Genetic Basis of Canine Degenerative Myelopathy. Proceedings, 2008 ACVIM Forum. 2008.

28. Barrie K, et al: Posterior lenticonus, microphthalmia, cataracts and retinal folds in Old English Sheepdogs. J Am Anim Hosp Assoc 15:715, 1979.

29. *The Genetic Connection: A Guide to Health Problems in Purebred Dogs.* L Ackerman. p 230, AAHA Press, 1999.

30. Jones BR, Jones JM, Chen W, et. al.: Chronic renal failure in young Old English Sheepdogs. N Z Vet J. 1990 Sep;38(3):118-21.

31. Breitschwerdt EB, Kornegay JN, Wheeler SJ, et. al.: Episodic weakness associated with exertional lactic acidosis and myopathy in Old English sheepdog littermates. J Am Vet Med Assoc. 1992 Sep 1;201(5):731-6.

32. Wieczorek LA, Garosi LS, & Shelton GD: Dystrophin-deficient muscular dystrophy in an old English sheepdog. Vet Rec. 2006 Feb 25;158(8):270-3.

33. Rallis TS, Patsikas MN, Mylonakis ME, et. al.: Giant hypertrophic gastritis (Menetrier's-like disease) in an Old English sheepdog. J Am Anim Hosp Assoc. 2007 Mar-Apr;43(2):122-7.

34. *The Complete Dog Book, 20th Ed.* The American Kennel Club. Howell Book House, NY 2006. p 671-674.

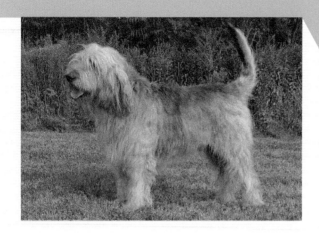

The Breed History

Dating to early in the 1300s, the first tentative records of a dog meeting this description originate in Britain. Described as a mix of hound and terrier, these dogs likely arose from Bloodhound, Welsh terrier and other southern hound mixes, though some evidence points to the inclusion of Vendéé hound of France or French Griffon. Otterhounds are one of the Airedale terrier's ancestors. First imports to the USA occurred around 1900. AKC first recognized the breed in 1907. This is a rare breed.

Breeding for Function

As the name implies, hunting otter was the purpose for which these dogs were developed. They are versatile enough for land or water and excel at scent tracking. The webbed feet of this breed help to ensure good swimming ability.

Physical Characteristics

Height at Withers: females 24" (61 cm), males 27" (68.5 cm)

Weight: female 75-85 lb (34-38.5 kg), male 100-115 lb (45.5-52 kg)

Coat: The rough-coated double oily coat makes him almost waterproof. It sits close, not flat, and the hairs are hard, crisp and broken in texture. The outer coat is 1.5-2" (3.75-5 cm) long though hairs are longer over the back (up to 6" or 15 cm). The undercoat is dense, short and wooly. Blue and white is the favored coat color, but they also commonly appear as black and tan grizzle and many other combinations.

Longevity: 12-13 years

Points of Conformation: These large dogs are noted for their excellent nose and are of sturdy constitution, being both well muscled and boned. The large narrow head is well covered with hair, the stop is not obvious, and the dark eyes are deeply set with minimal nictitans exposure. Long, pendulous ears fold in hound fashion and are low set and close hanging. There is a square muzzle, the flews are deep and the darkly pigmented nose is large. The neck is muscular, and the topline level. The thorax is deep, ribs are well sprung, and chest depth extends well back. The high set tail is tapering, feathered and held up but not over the back when alert; the tail is arched and reaches the tarsus. Limbs are straight boned, fore and rear dewclaws may be removed, the feet are large

and broad, and toes webbed. The Otterhound gait is long, low and smooth and appears effortless. The walk is loose and shuffling.

Recognized Behavior Issues and Traits

Reported breed characteristics include: Devoted, energetic (boisterous), playful, friendly but possessing an independent streak. They are vocal dogs, with a well-developed voice and are good watch dogs, not guard dogs. They should only be left off leash in a fenced enclosure. Good with children and other pets if raised with them. Some consider them a bit too active for seniors and infants and they are not recommended for apartment living. They have moderate grooming needs. They may need some hygiene around mealtime since food can be trapped in the beard, ear hair and moustache. Moderate exercise and early obedience training are recommended.

Normal Physiologic Variations

Slow maturing

Drug Sensitivities

None reported

Inherited Diseases

Hip Dysplasia: Polygenically inherited trait causing degenerative joint disease and hip arthritis. OFA reports 52.3% affected. Reported at a frequency of 31.9% in the 2003 OHCA Health Survey.[1,2]

Elbow Dysplasia: Polygenically inherited trait causing elbow arthritis. OFA reports a high incidence, but very few Otterhounds have been screened to determine an accurate frequency.[1]

Glanzmann's Thrombasthenia (GT): This autosomal recessive defect causes frequent epistaxis, and gingival bleeding during teething in young dogs. Caused by a defect in intrinsic platelet function involving glycoprotein complex IIb-IIIa. Affected dogs have normal platelet numbers, and normal coagulation panels. A genetic test is available.[3,4]

Patella Luxation: Polygenically inherited laxity of patellar ligaments, causing luxation, lameness, and later degenerative joint disease. Treat surgically if causing clinical signs. Too few Otterhounds have been screened by OFA to determine an accurate frequency.[1]

Disease Predispositions

Sebaceous Cysts: Benign accumulation of sebum within plugged hair follicles. OHCA 2003 health survey reports 46.2% of Otterhounds develop sebaceous cysts.[2]

Allergic Dermatitis (Atopy): Inhalant or food allergy. Presents with pruritis and pyotraumatic dermatitis (hot spots). Reported at a frequency of 15.1% in the 2003 OHCA Health Survey.[2]

Hypothyroidism: Inherited autoimmune thyroiditis. 2.3% positive for thyroid autoantibodies based on testing at Michigan State University. (Ave. for all breeds is 7.5%). Reported at a frequency of 11.8% in the 2003 OHCA Health Survey.[2,5,6]

Idiopathic Epilepsy: Inherited seizures can be generalized or partial seizures. Control with anticonvulsant medication. Reported at a frequency of 10.0% in the 2003 OHCA Health Survey.[2]

Gastric Dilation/Volvulus (GDV, Bloat): Life-threatening twisting of the stomach within the abdomen. Requires immediate veterinary attention. Reported breed prevalence of 9.0%, and cause of death of 7.4% of Otterhounds in a UK study.[7]

Cataracts: Reported at a frequency of 5.04% in the 2003 OHCA Health Survey.[2]

Ocular Disorders: Not enough Otterhounds have had CERF eye examinations to determine accurate frequencies for ocular disorders.[8]

Brachygnathism, Factor II Deficiency, and **Prognathism** are reported.[9]

Isolated Case Studies

Malignant Lymphoma of the Myocardium: Identified in a male Otterhound and two sibling offspring.[10]

Genetic Tests

Tests of Genotype: Direct test for Glannzmann's thrombasthenia (GT) is available from the Boudreaux Lab: http://www.vetmed.auburn.edu/faculty/pathobiology-faculty/boudreaux (334-844-2692).

Tests of Phenotype: CHIC Certification: Required testing includes hip radiographs, DNA(blood sample) in OFA/CHIC repository, and genetic test for GT. (See CHIC website; www.caninehealthinfo.org).

Recommend elbow radiographs, CERF eye examination, patella evaluation, thyroid profile including autoantibodies, and cardiac examination.

Miscellaneous

- **Breed name synonyms:** none
- **Registries:** AKC, UKC, CKC, KCGB (Kennel Club of Great Britain), ANKC (Australian National Kennel Club), NKC (National Kennel Club).
- **AKC rank (year 2008):** 154 (36 dogs registered)
- **Internet resources: The Otterhound Club of America:**
  http://clubs.akc.org/ohca/
  The Otterhound Club (UK): www.otterhoundclub.co.uk

References

1. OFA Website breed statistics: www.offa.org Last accessed July 1, 2010.
2. Otterhound Club of America: 2003 Otterhound Health Survey. 2003.
3. Boudreaux MK, Lipscomb DL: Clinical, biochemical, and molecular aspects of Glanzmann's thrombasthenia in humans and dogs. *Vet Pathol.* 2001 May;38(3):249-60.
4. Boudreaux MK, Catalfamo JL: Molecular and genetic basis for thrombasthenic thrombopathia in otterhounds. *Am J Vet Res.* 2001 Nov;62(11):1797-804.
5. Nachreiner RF, Refsal KR, Graham PA, et. al.: Prevalence of serum thyroid hormone autoantibodies in dogs with clinical signs of hypothyroidism. J Am Vet Med Assoc 2002 Feb 15;220(4):466-71.
6. Nachreiner R & Refsal K: Personal communication, Diagnostic Center for Population and Animal Health, Michigan State University. April, 2007.
7. Evans KM & Adams VJ: Mortality and morbidity due to gastric dilatation-volvulus syndrome in pedigree dogs in the UK. J Small Anim Pract. 2010 Jul;51(7):376-81
8. *Ocular Disorders Presumed to be Inherited in Purebred Dogs.* American College of Veterinary Ophthalmologists. ACVO, 2007
9. *The Genetic Connection: A Guide to Health Problems in Purebred Dogs.* L Ackerman. p. 230 AAHA Press, 1999.
10. Teske E, de Vos JP, Egberink HF, et. al.: Clustering in canine malignant lymphoma. Vet Q. 1994 Jul;16(2):134-6.
11. *The Complete Dog Book, 20th Ed.* The American Kennel Club. Howell Book House, NY 2006. p. 196-199.

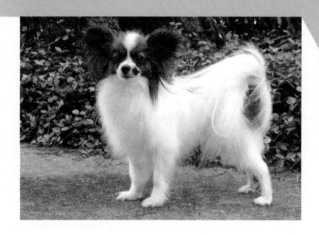

Papillon

The Breed History

Dwarf or toy spaniels of Italy and Spain were the likely breed progenitors. The origins of the word *Spaniel* derive from the presumed origin country, Spain. Since the 16th century the Papillon (French for butterfly) has been depicted in paintings. The early breed characteristic of the drooping ears was gradually replaced by the popular modern day "butterfly ears" (erect, feathered and obliquely set). Both types of ears are still found, even within a single litter. The drop eared variety is termed **Phalene**. Much of the Continental Toy Spaniel (syn. Phalene) breed development occurred in France and Belgium. The AKC accepted the breed in 1935.

Breeding for Function

Though not bred specifically as ratters, they characteristically perform this function well. Primarily companion dogs, they are also more recently being adapted for work as therapy dogs.

Physical Characteristics

Height at Withers: 8-11" (20-28 cm)

Weight: 9-10 lb (4-4.5 kg), though weights down to 3 lb (1.5 kg) are not uncommon.

Coat: White is the dominant color in the coat and patches may include any color, but these patches must conform to a specific distribution on the head. The coat is single, flat, profuse, long, straight and silky in texture.

Longevity: 13-15 years.

Points of Conformation: Fine boned, and almost square in conformation, the skull is medium in width, slightly rounded, stop is well defined, muzzle is thin and tapering, black nose is small, and lips are also black. Eyes are dark, round, medium in size, and palpebral margins are black. Ears are large with rounded tips. Those with erect ears must have them stay up, and in the Phalene strain dogs, ears must be consistently folded. The topline is level, neck is medium in length, thorax is moderate in depth and the ribs are well sprung. The abdomen is moderately tucked up, limbs slender and straight, and dewclaws may be removed (fronts), and in America only, the rear dewclaws are removed. The long tail is high set and sits over the body, with prominent plume. Toes are fine, and feet are hare-like. Action is described as light, quick and dainty.

Recognized Behavior Issues and Traits

Descriptions of the breed traits include: Good in rural or urban environments, tolerate temperature extremes well, friendly and likes to be a lapdog, playful.

Likes other dogs and children, intelligent, trainable, requires daily brushing, low barking tendency, active in the home, some may be possessive of owner. Low exercise needs, low odor, moderate shedder. Needs gentle handling by children to prevent injury. Noted for their steady stable temperament.

Normal Physiologic Variations

None reported

Drug Sensitivities

None reported

Inherited Diseases

Patella Luxation: Polygenically inherited laxity of patellar ligaments, causing luxation, lameness, and later degenerative joint disease. Treat surgically if causing clinical signs. Reported 8.4x odds ratio versus other breeds. OFA reports 3.9% affected. Reported at a frequency of 18% in the 2002 PCA Health Survey.[1,2,3]

von Willebrand's Disease (vWD) Type 1: Autosomal recessive genetic disorder causing a mild bleeding syndrome in this breed. Reported at a high frequency in the 2002 PCA Health Survey. A genetic test is available, showing a high gene frequency in the breed.[2]

Progressive Retinal Atrophy (PRA): More than one non-prcd autosomal recessive forms of PRA exist in the breed, with an onset of 7-8 years of age. A reliable age for diagnosis using electroretinogram is considered to be 1.5 years. PRA is reported at a frequency of 2% in the 2002 PCA Health Survey. Identified in 0.84% of Papillons CERF examined by veterinary ophthalmologists between 2000-2005. A direct genetic test for one form of PRA in the breed is available.[2,4,5,6]

Hip Dysplasia and Legg-Calve-Perthes Disease: Polygenically inherited traits causing degenerative joint disease and hip arthritis. Too few Papillons have been screened by OFA to determine an accurate frequency.[1]

Elbow Dysplasia: Polygenically inherited trait causing elbow arthritis. Too few Papillions have been screened by OFA to determine an accurate frequency.[1]

Disease Predispositions

Cryptorchidism (Retained Testicles): Can be unilateral or bilateral. Reported at a frequency of 14% in the 2002 PCA Health Survey.[2]

Idiopathic Epilepsy: Inherited seizures can be generalized or partial seizures. First seizure usually occurs between 1-2 years of age. Must differentiate from seizures due to portosystemic shunts, hydrocephalus, and other causes. Control with anticonvulsant medication. Reported at a high frequency in the 2002 PCA Health Survey.[2]

Hypothyroidism: Inherited autoimmune thyroiditis. 4.5% positive for thyroid auto-antibodies based on testing at Michigan State University. (Ave. for all breeds is 7.5%).[7,8]

Portosystemic Shunt (PSS, Liver Shunt): Abnormal blood vessels connecting the systemic and portal blood flow. Vessels can be intrahepatic or extrahepatic. Causes stunting, abnormal behavior, possible seizures, and secondary ammonium urate urinary calculi. Test with fasted and post-feeding bile acids and blood ammonia, and abdominal ultrasound. Reported at a frequency of 3% in the 2002 PCA Health Survey. Undetermined mode of inheritance.[2]

Vitreous Degeneration: A liquefaction of the vitreous gel which may predispose to retinal detachment resulting in blindness. Identified in 2.93% of Papillons CERF examined by veterinary ophthalmologists between 2000-2005.[6]

Persistent Pupillary Membranes: Strands of fetal remnant connecting; iris to iris, cornea, lens, or involving sheets of tissue. The later three forms can impair vision, and dogs affected with these forms should not be bred. Identified in 2.70% of Papillons CERF examined by veterinary ophthalmologists between 2000-2005.[6]

Cataracts: Anterior cortex intermediate and punctate cataracts predominate in the breed. Age of onset 1.5-3 years. Identified in 2.17% of Papillons CERF examined by veterinary ophthalmologists between 2000-2005. CERF does not recommend breeding any Papillon with a cataract.[6]

Distichiasis: Abnormally placed eyelashes that irritate the cornea and conjunctiva. Can cause secondary corneal ulceration. Identified in 1.67% of Papillons CERF examined by veterinary ophthalmologists between 2000-2005.[6]

Deafness: Congenital deafness can be unilateral or bilateral. Diagnosed by BAER testing. Reported to occur in the breed by Strain, possibly associated with the piebald gene. Reported at a frequency of 1% in the 2002 PCA Health Survey.[2,9]

Birth Defects: Open Fontanels, Hydrocephalus, and **Cleft Palate** are reported as birth defects in the breed, according to the 2002 PCA Health Survey.[2]

Neuroaxonal Dystrophy: Affected dogs present with pelvic limb ataxia, hypermetria and depressed postural reflexes affecting all four limbs. Affected dogs show clinical signs by 14 weeks of age, with deterioration to euthanasia by 5 months of age. Pathological examination revealed changes include widespread changes in the dorsolateral white matter of the spinal cord, characterized by axonal swellings typical of neuroaxonal dystrophy.[10,11,12,13]

Black Hair Follicular Dysplasia, Inguinal Hernia, and **Retained Primary Teeth** are reported.[14]

Isolated Case Studies

Cerebellar Cortical Abiotrophy (CCA): Reported in a 6 month old male Papillon with broad-based stance, pelvic limb ataia, truncal ataxia, head tremor, intension tremor, and loss of menace response. Pathology showed loss of Purkinji cells and thinning of the granular cell layer of the cerebellum, but also had other CNS changes more consistent with **Neuroaxonal Dystrophy.**[11,13]

Genetic Tests

Tests of Genotype: Direct test for vWD is available from VetGen.

Direct tests for coat color are available from VetGen.

Direct test for one form of PRA is available from Genoscoper: www.genoscoper.com.

Tests of Phenotype: CHIC Certification: Required testing includes CERF eye examination, patella evaluation, and congenital cardiac screening. (See CHIC website; www.caninehealthinfo.org).

Recommend hip and elbow radiographs, and thyroid profile including autoantibodies.

Miscellaneous
- **Breed name synonyms:** Pap, Continental Toy Spaniel, Phalene, Epagneul Nain Continental, Dwarf Spaniel (historical)
- **Registries:** AKC, UKC, CKC, KCGB (Kennel Club of Great Britain), ANKC (Australian National Kennel Club), NKC (National Kennel Club)
- **AKC rank (year 2008):** 37 (4,396 dogs registered)
- **Internet resources: Papillon Club of America:** www.papillonclub.org
  Papillon Canada: www.papilloncanada.org
  Papillon (Butterfly Dog) Club UK: www.papillonclub.co.uk/

References

1. OFA Website breed statistics: www.offa.org Last accessed July 1, 2010.
2. Papillon Club of America: 2002 PCA Health Survey. 2002.
3. LaFond E, Breur GJ & Austin CC: Breed susceptibility for developmental orthopedic diseases in dogs. J Am Anim Hosp Assoc. 2002 Sep-Oct;38(5):467-77.
4. Narfstrom K, Wrigstad A: Clinical, electrophysiological and morphological changes in a case of hereditary retinal degeneration in the Papillon dog. *Vet Ophthalmol.* 1999;2(1):67-74.
5. Narfstrom K, Ekesten B: Electroretinographic evaluation of Papillons with and without hereditary retinal degeneration. Am J Vet Res. 1998 Feb;59(2):221-6.
6. *Ocular Disorders Presumed to be Inherited in Purebred Dogs.* American College of Veterinary Ophthalmologists. ACVO, 2007.
7. Nachreiner RF, Refsal KR, Graham PA, et. al.: Prevalence of serum thyroid hormone autoantibodies in dogs with clinical signs of hypothyroidism. *J Am Vet Med Assoc* 2002 Feb 15;220(4):466-71.
8. Nachreiner R & Refsal K: Personal communication, Diagnostic Center for Population and Animal Health, Michigan State University. April, 2007.
9. Strain GM: Deafness prevalence and pigmentation and gender associations in dog breeds at risk. *The Veterinary Journal* 2004; 167(1):23-32.
10. Franklin RJ, Jeffery ND, Ramsey IK: Neuroaxonal dystrophy in a litter of papillon pups. J Small Anim Pract. 1995 Oct;36(10):441-4.
11. Nibe K, Kita C, Morozumi M, et. al.: Clinicopathological features of canine neuroaxonal dystrophy and cerebellar cortical abiotrophy in Papillon and Papillon-related dogs. J Vet Med Sci. 2007 Oct;69(10):1047-52.
12. Diaz JV, Duque C, & Geisel R: Neuroaxonal dystrophy in dogs: case report in 2 litters of Papillon puppies. J Vet Intern Med. 2007 May-Jun;21(3):531-4.
13. Nibe K, Nakayama H, Uchida K, et. al.: Immunohistochemical features of dystrophic axons in Papillon dogs with neuroaxonal dystrophy. Vet Pathol. 2009 May;46(3):474-83.
14. *The Genetic Connection: A Guide to Health Problems in Purebred Dogs.* L Ackerman. p. 230. AAHA Press, 1999.
15. *The Complete Dog Book, 20th Ed.* The American Kennel Club. Howell Book House, NY 2006. p. 491-494.

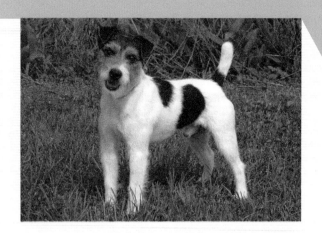

Parson Russell Terrier

The Breed History

The breed was cultivated for over 200 years in the south of England. The breed progenitors are thought to be the extinct Black-and-Tan terrier and the Old English White Terrier. The first Jack Russell terrier dogs were brought to America around 1930. Breed nomenclature is quite confusing. *Parson Jack Russell Terrier* was often used as a synonym for this breed, but in England and in the UKC standard, the Parson Jack Russell Terrier breed is different. Differences in the Parson terrier standard include inclusion of three coat types, longer legs and shorter body, and being larger in stature. In those constituencies, the Jack Russell Terrier breed name is limited to terriers standing less than twelve inches.

Parson John Russell was considered to be the original breeder of this general type of terriers. The Jack Russell terrier breed is popular with the horsy set, and further gained popularity following feature roles in television series as the Eddie and Wishbone characters.

Breeding for Function

Fox hunting and ratting was the original purpose for which the breed determination, fearlessness and agility were bred into them. They were baying terriers, and were not developed to kill the quarry, just bolt them out.

Physical Characteristics

Height at Withers: AKC ideal size is for the male, 14" (35.5 cm), and female 13" (33 cm)

Weight: 9 lb (4 kg) up to 13-17 lb (6-7.5 kg)

Coat: Two coat types in the AKC standard:
Smooth: Double coated with a hard outer flat layer and a dense undercoat.
Broken: Also double coated, but the outer coat stands flat and is broken, with some curling and waving of the hairs.

White or predominantly white with tan or black, and also tri-color are accepted colors. Brindle is disqualifying but grizzled is acceptable. Markings are preferred on extremities such as the face, ears and tail tip.

Longevity: 13-15 years

Points of Conformation:
Jack Russell Terriers are medium-boned and well muscled with almost square conformation. They possess a keen expression and lively attitude. The eyes are moderate in size, dark in color and almond-shaped. They have small triangular ears with moderately thick leathers, pointed tips, and ears are folded forward with the fold at the level of the top of the skull or slightly higher. The head is also characterized by a flat skull, well-defined stop and black nose. The moderately long and arched neck is free of throatiness. The topline is level, abdomen is moderately tucked up, and the thorax is moderate in depth and narrow. The tail is high set and thick and normally docked to provide a handhold length at maturity (4" or 10 cm), Limbs are straight boned, feet are compact with tough pads, and the gait is powerful with long strides.

Recognized Behavior Issues and Traits

Reported breed attributes include: High activity, sometmes hyperactive in fact, happy, but can be snappy or aggressive with moving targets and other dogs. May see small pets as prey even after being socialized to them. Also described as intelligent, bouncy, springy, lively (exuberant), friendly with family and strangers, though some are aloof with strangers. They have low grooming needs. Considered good in town or country but not for condo or apartment life. They have a moderate shedding tendency. They are diggers, and have high exercise needs. Fences need to be high and secure since they can climb over and dig under fences quite effectively. They like close human companionship, and activities that provide mental stimulation to help prevent boredom vices. They have a high barking tendency, and are good alarm barkers. Their assertive nature means that early socialization to children and other pets, and obedience training are important. Not recommended for homes with children under 6 years of age since they do not always tolerate young children well.

Normal Physiologic Variations
None reported

Drug Sensitivities
None reported

Inherited Diseases

Primary Lens Luxation (PLL) and Secondary Glaucoma: An autosomal recessive gene causes partial or complete displacement of the lens from its normal anatomic site behind the pupil. Relative risk of 9.03x versus other breeds. Parson Russell terriers have a 7.1x odds ratio for secondary glaucoma with blindness due to lens luxation versus other breeds. Homozygous affected dogs usually develop lens luxation between 4-8 years of age. Rarely, heterozygous carriers can develop lens luxation, but at a later age. A genetic mutation has been identified, and a genetic test is available. OFA testing shows 23% carrier, and 1% affected for Parson Russell Terriers, and 36% carrier and 3% affected for Jack Russell Terriers.[1,2,3,4,5,6]

Deafness: Polygenically inherited congenital deafness can be unilateral or bilateral. Diagnosed by BAER testing. Strain reports 16.1% testing unilaterally or bilaterally deaf based on BAER testing. Heritability is between 0.22-0.31. There is a pigmentation association with deafness in this breed, as mostly white dogs are more likely to be deaf.[7,8]

Hip Dysplasia and Legg-Calve Perthes Disease: Polygenically inherited traits causing degenerative hip joint disease and arthritis. OFA reports 4.0% affected with hip dysplasia, and 3.0% affected with Legg-Calve-Perthes disease.[1]

Elbow Dysplasia: Polygenically inherited trait causing elbow arthritis. OFA reports 2.7% affected.[1]

Cataracts: Polygenically inherited in this breed. Posterior cortex intermediate cataracts predominate in the breed. Heritability estimate of 0.73. Identified in 3.78% of Parson Russell terriers CERF-examined by veterinary ophthalmologists between 2000-2005. CERF does not recommend breeding any Parson Russell Terrier with a cataract.[2,3]

Patella Luxation: Polygenically inherited laxity of patellar ligaments, causing luxation, lameness, and later degenerative joint disease. Treat surgically if causing clinical signs. OFA reports 0.8% affected.[1]

Hereditary Ataxia (Axonopathy, Neuroaxonal Dystrophy): An inherited axonopathy in the breed produces a gait disturbance between 2-9 months of age with symmetric generalized ataxia and hypermetric and spastic movements. Seizures and respiratory distress can also occur. Pathological lesions occur throughout the central nervous system. The disorder appears to have a polygenic mode of inheritance.[9,10]

Hyperuricosuria (HUU)/Urate Bladder Stones: An autosomal recessive mutation in the SLC2A9 gene causes urate urolithiasis and can predispose male dogs to urinary obstruction. Estimated at a carrier frequency of 7.75% in the breed. A genetic test is available.[36]

Myasthenia Gravis: An autosomal recessive, congenital form of myasthenia gravis occurs in Parson Russell terriers. Clinical signs are evident from six to eight weeks of age, and include exercise induced weakness without megaesophagus. Raised antibody levels to acetylcholine receptor do not occur, although the amount of receptor in the end-plates is decreased.[11,12]

Severe Combined Immunodeficiency (SCID): Autosomal recessive disorder, where affected dogs cannot generate antigen-specific immune responses. Parson Russell terrier puppies with SCID succumb to infections at a few months of age. A commercial genetic test is not available.[13,14]

Nonepidermolytic Ichthyosis: A rare, autosomal recessive disease in Jack Russell Terriers presenting with congenital, non-alopecic or pruritic, thick, adherent, scales. As adults, the scales persist and secondary infections with coccoid bacteria and yeasts are common. Pathology reveals orthokeratotic hyperkeratosis that extends into follicular infundibula. The disease is caused by an insertion of a LINE-1 into the TGM1 gene. A genetic test is not available.[15,16]

Disease Predispositions

Hypothyroidism: 4.1% positive for thyroid auto-antibodies based on testing at Michigan State University. (Ave. for all breeds is 7.5%).[17,18]

Persistent Pupillary Membranes: Strands of fetal remnant connecting; iris to iris, cornea, lens, or involving sheets of tissue. The later three forms can impair vision, and dogs affected with these forms should not be bred. Identified in 3.47% of Parson Russell terriers CERF-examined by veterinary ophthalmologists between 2000-2005.[2]

Secondary Glaucoma: Increased intraocular pressure can cause retinal deterioration and blindness. Can occur after cataract formation, lens luxation, or uveitis. Screen with tonometry. One report found an odds ratio of 7.1x for secondary glaucoma in Jack Russell Terriers.[19]

Autoimmune Hemolytic Anemia (AIHA): Auto-immune destruction of red blood cells. Parson Russell terriers have a 2.8x risk of developing AIHA versus other breeds. Females are more frequently affected than males. Clinical features included pale mucous membranes, weakness, lethargy and collapse. Treatment with prednisone is successful in most cases.[20]

Distichiasis: Abnormally placed eyelashes that irritate the cornea and conjunctiva. Can cause secondary corneal ulceration. Identified in 2.42% of Parson Russell terriers CERF-examined by veterinary ophthalmologists between 2000-2005.[2]

Primary (Narrow Angle) Glaucoma: Ocular condition causing increased pressure within the eyeball, and secondary blindness due to damage to the retina. Diagnose with tonometry and gonioscopy. Diagnosed in 1.37% of Parson Russell Terriers presented to veterinary teaching hospitals.[5]

Pulmonic Stenosis: Clinical signs can include exercise intolerance, stunting, dyspnea, syncope and ascites, leading to heart failure. Diagnosis by auscultation for a heart murmur, and echocardiography. Parson Russell Terriers are overrepresented versus other breeds.[21]

Portosystemic Shunt (PSS, Liver Shunt): Abnormal blood vessels connecting the systemic and portal blood flow. Vessels can be intrahepatic or extrahepatic. Causes stunting, abnormal behavior, possible seizures, and secondary ammonium urate urinary calculi. Diagnose with paired fasting and post-feeding bile acids and blood ammonia, and abdominal ultrasound. Tobias reports a 8.5x odds ratio versus other breeds. Undetermined mode of inheritance.[22,23]

Malassezia Pachydermatis infection: Yeast skin infection. Affected dogs present with pruritus, alopecia and lichenification. Parson Russell terriers are significantly overrepresented versus other breeds. Can also be secondary to ichthiosis in the breed.[24]

Episodic Myokymia and Neuromyotonia: Jack Russell Terriers affected with Hereditary Ataxia can develop episodes of generalized muscle stiffness and delayed muscle relaxation resulting in collapse into lateral recumbency. Episodes can be preceded by intense facial rubbing, and can be associated with severe hyperthermia. An underlying neuronal ion channel dysfunction is suspected.[25,26]

Black Hair Follicular Dysplasia, Brachygnathism, Compulsive Tail Chasing, Epilepsy, Oligodontia, Prognathism, and Progressive Retinal Atrophy, are reported.[27]

Isolated Case Studies

Sry-Negative XX Sex Reversal (Hermaphrodism): Identified in a Parson Russell terrier. An autosomal recessive disorder, where outwardly male dogs are chromosomal females (XX), and there is an absence of male causing SRY.[28]

Colonic Duplication: Identified in a 4-month-old male Parson Russell terrier because of stranguria and tenesmus.[29]

Factor X Deficiency: Deficiency in Factor X (Stuart-Prower factor) was identified in a 7-month-old spayed female Parson Russell terrier following recurrent bleeding episodes. Low Factor X was also identified in the father and paternal grandmother. Factor X deficiency may be an autosomal dominant trait with variable expression.[30]

Mitochondrial Myopathy: A stunted, thin four month old Parson Russell terrier with a stilted gait and progressive exercise intolerance was examined. The dog had raised lactate levels before and after feeding and a raised lactate/pyruvate ratio after feeding, indicating a metabolic abnormality. Ultrastructural examination of the muscle confirmed the presence of subsarcolemmal accumulations of mitochondria.[31]

Mitochondrial Encephalomyopathy: A 10-month-old female Parson Jack Russell terrier was euthanized because of therapy-resistant ataxia, hypermetria, and deafness that had first been observed at 10 weeks of age. Pathological findings included severe, bilateral, symmetrical neuronal degeneration and mineralization of the brain, and hepatocytes and cardiac myocytes with increased numbers of enlarged or misshapen mitochondria.[32]

Acute Necrotising Pulmonary Vasculitis: Identified in a 5 month-old female Jack Russell terrier with acute lethargy, coughing, and respiratory distress. Tests revealed severe pulmonary hypertension, cor pulmonale and right-sided heart failure. Pathology revealed acute necrotising pulmonary arteritis without any cardiac abnormalities or immune complex disease.[33]

Myotonia Congenita: A 4-month-old male Jack Russell terrier was evaluated for non-painful muscle spasms and exercise induced hindquarter bunny-hopping and collapse. He had non-painful hypertrophic muscles, and was found to have a mutation in the chloride ion channel gene for MC.[34]

Genetic Tests

Tests of Genotype: Direct test for lens luxation is available from OFA and AHT.

Direct test for HUU is available from the UC-Davis VGL and the Animal Health Trust.

Tests of Phenotype: CHIC Certification: Required testing includes CERF eye examination, patella examination, and BAER test for deafness. (See CHIC website; www.caninehealthinfo.org).

Recommended tests include hip and elbow radiographs, thyroid profile including autoantibodies, and cardiac examination.

Miscellaneous

- **Breed name synonyms:** Jack Russell, JRT, Jack, Parson Jack Russell Terrier, English Jack Russell Terrier
- **Registries:** AKC, UKC (Parson Russell Terrier), KCGB (Kennel Club of Great Britain) (also as Jack Parson Russell Terrier), ANKC (Australian National Kennel Club), NKC (National Kennel Club)
- **AKC rank (year 2008):** 84 (802 dogs registered)
- **Internet resources: Parson Russell Terrier Association of America:** www.prtaa.org
  The Parson Russell Terrier Club (UK):
  www.parsonrussellterrierclub.co.uk
  Association of Parson Russell Terrier Fanciers (Canada):
  http://aprtf.webs.com
  English Jack Russell Terrier Club Alliance Inc.: www.ejrtca.com (under 12" height dog registry)
  Jack Russell Terrier Club of America: www.therealjackrussell.com
  Jack Russell Terrier Club of Canada: www.jrtca.com

References

1. OFA Website breed statistics: www.offa.org Last accessed July 1, 2010.
2. *Ocular Disorders Presumed to be Inherited in Purebred Dogs.* American College of Veterinary Ophthalmologists. ACVO, 2007.
3. Oberbauer AM, Hollingsworth SR, Belanger JM, et. al.: Inheritance of cataracts and primary lens luxation in Jack Russell Terriers. Am J Vet Res. 2008 Feb;69(2):222-7.
4. Johnsen DA, Maggs DJ, Kass PH: Evaluation of risk factors for development of secondary glaucoma in dogs: 156 cases (1999-2004). J Am Vet Med Assoc. 2006 Oct 15;229(8):1270-4.
5. Gelatt KN, MacKay EO: Prevalence of the breed-related glaucomas in pure-bred dogs in North America. Vet Ophthalmol. 2004 Mar-Apr;7(2):97-111.
6. Sargan DR, Withers D, Pettitt L, et. al.: Mapping the mutation causing lens luxation in several terrier breeds. J Hered. 2007;98(5):534-8.
7. Strain GM: Deafness prevalence and pigmentation and gender associations in dog breeds at risk. *Vet J.* 2004 Jan;167(1):23-32.
8. Famula TR, Cargill EJ, & Strain GM: Heritability and complex segregation analysis of deafness in Jack Russell Terriers. BMC Vet Res. 2007 Nov 13;3:31.
9. Wessmann A, Goedde T, Fischer A, et. al.: Hereditary ataxia in the Jack Russell Terrier--clinical and genetic investigations. J Vet Intern Med. 2004 Jul-Aug;18(4):515-21.
10. Sacre BJ, Cummings JF, De Lahunta A: Neuroaxonal dystrophy in a Jack Russell terrier pup resembling human infantile neuroaxonal dystrophy. Cornell Vet. 1993 Apr;83(2):133-42.
11. Wallace ME, Palmer AC: Recessive mode of inheritance in myasthenia gravis in the Jack Russell terrier. Vet Rec. 1984 Apr 7;114(14):350.
12. Palmer AC, Goodyear JV: Congenital myasthenia in the Jack Russell terrier. Vet Rec. 1978 Nov 4;103(19):433-4.
13. Perryman LE: Molecular pathology of severe combined immunodeficiency in mice, horses, and dogs. *Vet Pathol.* 2004 Mar;41(2):95-100.
14. Bell TG, Butler KL, Stickle JE, et. al.: Autosomal recessive severe combined immunodeficiency of Jack Russell terriers. J Vet Diagn Invest 2002; 14:194-204.
15. Credille KM, Minor JS, Barnhart KF, et. al.: Transglutaminase 1-deficient recessive lamellar ichthyosis associated with a LINE-1 insertion in Jack Russell terrier dogs. Br J Dermatol. 2009 Aug;161(2):265-72.
16. Lewis DT, Ford MJ, & Kwochka KW: Characterization and management of a Jack Russell terrier with congenital ichthyosis. Vet Dermatol 1998; 9:111-18.
17. Nachreiner RF, Refsal KR, Graham PA, et. al.: Prevalence of

serum thyroid hormone autoantibodies in dogs with clinical signs of hypothyroidism. J Am Vet Med Assoc 2002 Feb 15;220(4):466-71.

18. Nachreiner R & Refsal K: Personal communication, Diagnostic Center for Population and Animal Health, Michigan State University. April, 2007.

19. Johnsen DA, Maggs DJ, Kass PH: Evaluation of risk factors for development of secondary glaucoma in dogs: 156 cases (1999-2004). J Am Vet Med Assoc. 2006 Oct 15;229(8):1270-4.

20. Miller SA, Hohenhaus AE, Hale AS: Case-control study of blood type, breed, sex, and bacteremia in dogs with immune-mediated hemolytic anemia. J Am Vet Med Assoc. 2004 Jan 15;224(2):232-5.

21. Baumgartner C, Glaus TM: Congenital cardiac diseases in dogs: a retrospective analysis. Schweiz Arch Tierheilkd. 2003 Nov;145(11):527-33, 535-6.

22. Hunt GB: Effect of breed on anatomy of portosystemic shunts resulting from congenital diseases in dogs and cats: a review of 242 cases. Aust Vet J. 2004 Dec;82(12):746-9.

23. Tobias KM, Rohrbach BW: Association of breed with the diagnosis of congenital portosystemic shunts in dogs: 2,400 cases (1980-2002). J Am Vet Med Assoc. 2003 Dec 1;223(11):1636-9.

24. Carlotti DN: Malassezia Dermatitis in the Dog. Proceedings 2005 World Small Animal Veterinary Association World Congress. 2005.

25. Van Ham L, Bhatti S, Polis I, et. al.: "Continuous muscle fibre activity" in six dogs with episodic myokymia, stiffness and collapse. Vet Rec. 2004 Dec 11;155(24):769-74.

26. Vanhaesebrouck AE, Van Soens I, Poncelet L, et. al.: Clinical and electrophysiological characterization of myokymia and neuromyotonia in jack russell terriers. J Vet Intern Med. 2010 Jul-Aug;24(4):882-9.

27. *The Genetic Connection: A Guide to Health Problems in Purebred Dogs.* L Ackerman. p. 224. AAHA Press, 1999.

28. Kuiper H, Bunck C, Gunzel-Apel AR, et. al.: SRY-negative XX sex reversal in a Jack Russell Terrier: a case report. Vet J. 2005 Jan;169(1):116-7.

29. Arthur EG, Fox DB, Essman SC, et. al.: Surgical treatment of noncommunicating duplication of the colon in a dog. J Am Vet Med Assoc. 2003 Jul 15;223(2):210-4, 196.

30. Cook AK, Werner LL, O'Neill SL, et. al.: Factor X deficiency in a Jack Russell terrier. Vet Clin Pathol. 1993;22(3):68-71.

31. Olby NJ, Chan KK, Targett MP, et. al.: Suspected mitochondrial myopathy in a Jack Russell terrier. J Small Anim Pract. 1997 May;38(5):213-6.

32. Gruber AD, Wessmann A, Vandevelde M, et. al.: Mitochondriopathy with regional encephalic mineralization in a Jack Russell Terrier. Vet Pathol. 2002 Nov;39(6):732-6.

33. Russell NJ, Irwin PJ, Hopper BJ, et. al.: Acute necrotising pulmonary vasculitis and pulmonary hypertension in a juvenile dog. J Small Anim Pract. 2008 Jul;49(7):349-55.

34. Lobetti RG: Myotonia congenita in a Jack Russell terrier. J S Afr Vet Assoc. 2009 Jun;80(2):106-7.

35. *The Complete Dog Book, 20th Ed.* The American Kennel Club. Howell Book House, NY 2006. p. 415-418.

36. Karmi N, Brown EA, Hughes SS, et. al.: Estimated frequency of the canine hyperuricosuria mutation in different dog breeds. J Vet Intern Med. 2010 Nov-Dec;24(6):1337-42.

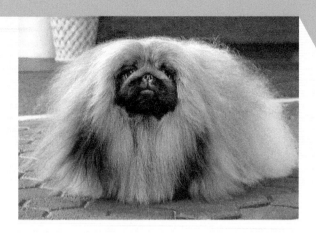

The Breed History

The Pekingese is an ancient Chinese dog breed that was so highly esteemed that they became a symbol of good fortune, and artistic representations of them, (Foo Dog idols) became family heirlooms. In Buddhism, the lion is a symbol of Buddha, and this may be the origin of the special position the dog held since in legend, these dogs were thought to originate from union of monkey and lion. A favorite of the Imperial families, a theft of one of these dogs was punishable by death. Earliest records indicate the breed was distinctive by the 8th century. First specimens arrived in Britain in the year1860; one was given to Queen Victoria. The AKC first registered the breed in 1906.

Breeding for Function

These dogs have always been kept purely for companionship.

Physical Characteristics

Height at Withers: 6-9" (15-23 cm)

Weight: < 14 lb (6 kg).

Coat: Profuse long coat is straight, stands off, and texture of the hairs is coarse. All colors are allowed. The undercoat is dense and soft.

Longevity: 12-13 years.

Points of Conformation: The overall conformation is stocky and compact; slightly longer than tall. The nickname *lion dog* derives from the fact that the dog is much heavier in the fore than behind, and with a full mane somewhat resembles a little lion in profile. They are not dainty. The head is wider than deep with a broad flat top, jaw is wide at the base, skull is brachycephalic, with correct standard placing the brow in the same plane as the chin and nose. The nose is pigmented black and—sitting up between the prominent eyes. The eyes are very dark and wide set, and palpebral margins are black. A prominent v-shaped wrinkle extends cheek to cheek over the nose, and the stop is deep and well defined. The muzzle is broad and short, and the hair is pigmented black. The jaw is slightly undershot. Ears are folded, heavily feathered, and hang to frame the face on each side. They possess a short thick neck, moderate thorax depth, moderate but distinct abdominal tuck up, the topline is level; the high-set tail is also profusely feathered and carried over the back, hanging to the side. Forelimbs are short and slightly bowed in

Pekingese

the radius. Feet are outturned, large, flat and well feathered. Gait is rolling in front and not fast moving.

Recognized Behavior Issues and Traits

Breed characteristics reported include: Regal carriage, bold and courageous, good alarm barker. Stubborn and independent minded (this is a significant characteristic that is encouraged with a resulting personality peculiar to the breed). Calm, good-tempered and affectionate, with condescending air (others term this noble bearing or dignified), and loyal.

Socialized early, they are generally good with other pets and children but are aloof with strangers. Some can be aggressive. They have low exercise needs, tolerate heat poorly, and have a snoring tendency.

Daily brushing is needed, and they have a high shedding tendency; need lots of human contact. Care around eyes and anus is needed due to the facial fold and in the latter case, hair.

Normal Physiologic Variations

In a UK study, 43.8% of litters were delivered via **Cesarean section.**[1]

Drug Sensitivities

None reported

Inherited Diseases

Patella Luxation: Polygenically inherited laxity of patellar ligaments, causing luxation, lameness, and later degenerative joint disease. Treat surgically if causing clinical signs. Reported at an increased frequency in the breed, but too few Pekingese have been screened by OFA to determine an accurate frequency.[2]

Hip Dysplasia and Legg-Calve Perthes Disease: Polygenically inherited trait causing degenerative hip joint disease and arthritis. Reported at a high frequency by the OFA, but too few Pekingese have been screened to determine an accurate frequency.[2]

Elbow Dysplasia: Polygenically inherited trait causing elbow arthritis. Too few Pekingese have been screened by OFA to determine an accurate frequency.[2]

Disease Predispositions

Intervertebral Disc Disease (IVDD): Pekingese dogs have an increased risk of developing spinal cord disease due to prolapsed disk material. Requires immediate treatment to prevent permanent paralysis. Reported at a frequency of 4.5% in the breed. Dorn reports a 2.50x odds ratio versus other breeds.[3,4,5]

Brachycephalic Airway Syndrome: The brachycephalic syndrome causes breathing difficulties, especially in hot weather. It includes **Stenotic Nares, Elongated Soft Palate, Everted Laryngeal Saccules, Laryngeal Collapse,** and occasionally **Hypoplastic Trachea.**[6]

Chronic Valvular Heart Disease: Heart failure due to valvular insufficiency, usually involving the mitral valve. Treat with heart medications. Pekingese have a 3.4x odds ratio for chronic valvular disease versus other breeds.[7]

Cataracts: A partial or complete opacity of the lens and/or its capsule. CERF reports a high frequency, but too few Pekenese have been examined to determine an accurate frequency. Reported in 2.14% of Pekingese presented to veterinary teaching hospitals. CERF does not recommend breeding any Pekingese with a cataract.[8,9]

Keratoconjunctivitis Sicca (KCS, Dry Eye): Ocular condition causing lack of tear production and secondary conjunctivitis, corneal ulcerations, and vision problems. Age of onset 2-5 years. CERF reports a high frequency, but too few Pekenese have been examined to determine an accurate frequency. CERF does not recommend breeding any Pekingese with KCS.[8]

Anal Gland Disease: Anal sacculitis and anal gland infection. Dorn reports a 3.03x odds ratio versus other breeds.[3]

Chronic Superficial Keratitis (Pannus), Ectopic Cilia, Entropion, Exposure Keratopathy Syndrome, Lens Luxation, Macroblepharon, and **Progressive Retinal Atrophy** are all reported in multiple Pekingese by CERF examination. Too few Pekingese have been CERF examined to determine an accurate frequency in the breed. Dorn reports a 2.55x odds ratio for eye disease versus other breeds.[3,8]

Hypothyroidism: Inherited autoimmune thyroiditis. 2.0% positive for thyroid autoantibodies based on testing at Michigan State University. (Ave. for all breeds is 7.5%).[10,11]

Distichiasis: Abnormally placed eyelashes that irritate the cornea and conjunctiva. Can cause secondary corneal ulceration. Dorn reports a 2.02x odds ratio versus other breeds. CERF reports a high frequency, but too few Pekenese have been examined to determine an accurate frequency.[3,8]

Primary (Narrow Angle) Glaucoma: Ocular condition causing increased pressure within the eyeball, and secondary blindness due to damage to the retina. Diagnose with tonometry and gonioscopy. Diagnosed in 1.22% of Pekingese presented to veterinary teaching hospitals.[12]

Cystic Calculi: Pekingese are found to have a predisposition to forming bladder stones. Mineral composition is not reported. Staphylococcus intermedius was isolated from 67.9% of female Pekingese with uroliths.[13,14,15]

Portosystemic shunt (PSS, liver shunt): Congenital abnormal blood vessel connecting the portal and systemic circulation. Can be intrahepatic or extrahepatic. Causes stunting, abnormal behavior, possible seizures, and secondary ammonium urate urinary calculi. Treatment of PSS includes partial ligation and/or medical and dietary control of symptoms. Tobias reports a 7.1x odds ratio versus other breeds.[16]

Perineal Hernia: Pekingese have a predisposition to developing perineal hernias. Treatment is surgery.[17,18]

Sertoli Cell Testicular Tumor: Pekingese males have a greater risk of developing sertoli cell tumors than other breeds.[19]

Atlantoaxial Subluxation: Pekingese have an increased risk for atlantoaxial subluxation due to a congenital abnormality of the dens or atlantoaxial ligaments. Dorsal displacement of the axis results in compression of the cervical spinal cord. Treatment is surgery. Unknown mode of inheritance.[20]

Necrotizing Meningoencephalitis: Affected dogs have clinical signs of recurrent seizures and progressive abnormal gait and behavior, which do not respond to treatment. At necropsy, histopathological features of the inflammatory lesions are consistent with necrotizing meningoencephalitis and resembled those described as Pug dog encephalitis.[21,22,23]

Cleft Lip/Palate, Cryptorchidism, Fold Dermatitis, Hydrocephalus, Microphthalmia, Prognathism, Pseudo-Hermaphrodism, Renal Dysplasia, and **Wry Mouth** are reported.[24]

Isolated Case Studies

Multiple Congenital Urinary System Abnormalities: An eight-month-old Pekingese bitch with urinary incontinence was found to have three congenital anomalies of the urinary tract: left renal agenesis, bilateral ectopic ureters with a left cranial blind-ending ureter, and urinary bladder hypoplasia.[25]

Ureterocele: Report of a 5-year-old female Pekingese with a ureterocele, ipsilateral hydroureter, and bilateral renal dysfunction.[26]

Osteochondritis Dissecans of the Femoral Head: An 8-month-old male Pekingese with a 1-month history of right hind limb lameness and crepitus in the right coxofemoral joint treated by femoral head ostectomy. Gross and microscopic examination of the femoral head resulted in a diagnosis of osteochondritis dissecans.[27]

Cervical Syringohydromyelia: An 11-year-old male Pekingese presented with a right-sided head tilt, ataxia, scoliosis, and proprioceptive deficits. MRI of the head and neck revealed a mass in the brainstem, cerebellar herniation, and syringohydromyelia. The dog responded to corticosteroids and radiation therapy of the mass.[28]

Genetic Tests

Tests of Genotype: Direct tests for coat color are available from VetGen.

Tests of Phenotype: Recommend hip and elbow radiographs, patella examination, CERF eye examination, thyroid profile including autoantibodies, and cardiac examination.

Miscellaneous

- **Breed name synonyms:** Peke, Pekinese, Peking Palasthund. In Chinese, fond historical nicknames include Lion Dog, Sun Dog (those with red-gold coats) and Sleeve Dog (small breed specimens that were carried in the sleeves)
- **Registries:** AKC, UKC, CKC, KCGB (Kennel Club of Great Britain), ANKC (Australian National Kennel Club), NKC (National Kennel Club)
- **AKC rank (year 2008):** 55 (2,056 dogs registered)
- **Internet resources: Pekingese Club of America Inc.:** www.thepekingeseclubofamerica.com
  The Pekingese Club (UK): www.thepekingeseclub.co.uk

References

1. Evans KM & Adams VJ: Proportion of litters of purebred dogs born by caesarean section. J Small Anim Pract. 2010 Feb;51(2):113-8.

2. OFA Website breed statistics: www.offa.org Last accessed July 1, 2010.

3. Dorn CR: Canine breed-specific risks of frequently diagnosed diseases at veterinary teaching hospitals. Monograph. AKC Canine Health Foundation. 2000.

4. Nakama S, Taura Y, Tabaru H, et. al.: A retrospective study of ventral fenestration for disk diseases in dogs. J Vet Med Sci. 1993 Oct;55(5):781-4.

5. Jerram RM, Dewey CW: Acute Thoracolumbar Disk Extrusion in Dogs - Part I. Compend Contin Educ Pract Vet 1999: 21[10]:922-930.

6. Monnet M: Brachycephalic Airway Syndrome. Proceedings, 2004 World Small Animal Veterinary Association Congress. 2004.

7. Petric AD, Hozjan E & Blejec A: Chronic Valvular Disease. Proceedings, 17th ECVIM-CA Congress. 2007.

8. Ocular Disorders Presumed to be Inherited in Purebred Dogs. American College of Veterinary Ophthalmologists. ACVO, 2007.

9. Gelatt KN, Mackay EO: Prevalence of primary breed-related cataracts in the dog in North America. Vet Ophthalmol. 2005 Mar-Apr;8(2):101-11.

10. Nachreiner RF, Refsal KR, Graham PA, et. al.: Prevalence of serum thyroid hormone autoantibodies in dogs with clinical signs of hypothyroidism. J Am Vet Med Assoc 2002 Feb 15;220(4):466-71.

11. Nachreiner R & Refsal K: Personal communication, Diagnostic Center for Population and Animal Health, Michigan State University. April, 2007.

12. Gelatt KN, MacKay EO: Prevalence of the breed-related glaucomas in pure-bred dogs in North America. Vet Ophthalmol. 2004 Mar-Apr;7(2):97-111.

13. Bovee KC, McGuire T: Qualitative and quantitative analysis of uroliths in dogs: definitive determination of chemical type. J Am Vet Med Assoc. 1984 Nov 1;185(9):983-7.

14. Ling GV, Franti CE, Johnson DL, et. al.: Urolithiasis in dogs. IV: Survey of interrelations among breed, mineral composition, and anatomic location of calculi, and presence of urinary tract infection. Am J Vet Res. 1998 May;59(5):650-60.

15. Weichselbaum RC, Feeney DA, Jessen CR, et. al.: Evaluation of the morphologic characteristics and prevalence of canine urocystoliths from a regional urolith center. Am J Vet Res. 1998 Apr;59(4):379-87.

16. Tobias KM, Rohrbach BW: Association of breed with the diagnosis of congenital portosystemic shunts in dogs: 2,400 cases (1980-2002). J Am Vet Med Assoc. 2003 Dec 1;223(11):1636-9.

17. Hosgood G, Hedlund CS, Pechman RD, et. al.: Perineal herniorrhaphy: perioperative data from 100 dogs. J Am Anim Hosp Assoc. 1995 Jul-Aug;31(4):331-42.

18. Robertson JJ: Perineal hernia repair in dogs. Mod Vet Pract. 1984 May;65(5):365-8.

19. Weaver AD: Survey with follow-up of 67 dogs with testicular sertoli cell tumours. Vet Rec. 1983 Jul 30;113(5):105-7.

20. McCarthy RJ, Lewis DD, Hosgood G: Atlantoaxial Subluxation in Dogs. Compendium Contin Educ Pract Vet 1995: 17(2):215-226.

21. Cantile C, Chianini F, Arispici M, et. al.: Necrotizing meningoencephalitis associated with cortical hippocampal hamartia in a Pekingese dog. Vet Pathol. 2001 Jan;38(1):119-22.

22. Sorjonen DC: Clinical and histopathological features of granulomatous meningoencephalomyelitis in dogs. J Am Anim Hosp Assoc 1990: 26[2]:141-147.

23. Pedersen NC, Vernau K, Dickinson P, et. al.: DLA Association in Various Toy Breeds with Immune Mediated Encephalopathies. Proceedings, 2009 Tufts' Canine and Feline Breeding and Genetics Conference. 2009.

24. The Genetic Connection: A Guide to Health Problems in Purebred Dogs. L Ackerman. p. 230-31. AAHA Press, 1999.

25. Agut A, Fernandez del Palacio MJ, Laredo FG, et. al.: Unilateral renal agenesis associated with additional congenital abnormalities of the urinary tract in a Pekingese bitch. J Small Anim Pract. 2002 Jan;43(1):32-5.

26. Stiffler KS, Stevenson MA, Mahaffey MB, et. al.: Intravesical ureterocele with concurrent renal dysfunction in a dog: a case report and proposed classification system. J Am Anim Hosp Assoc. 2002 Jan-Feb;38(1):33-9.

27. Johnson AL, Pijanowski GJ, Stein LE: Osteochondritis dissecans of the femoral head of a Pekingese. J Am Vet Med Assoc. 1985 Sep 15;187(6):623-5.

28. da Costa RC, Parent JM, Poma R, et. al.: Cervical syringohydromyelia secondary to a brainstem tumor in a dog. J Am Vet Med Assoc. 2004 Oct 1;225(7):1061-4, 1048.

29. The Complete Dog Book, 20th Ed. The American Kennel Club. Howell Book House, NY 2006. p. 495-498.

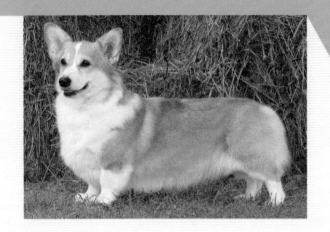

Pembroke Welsh Corgi

Forelegs are bowed due to the chondrodystrophic type of the breed. Feet are well arched, and the dewclaws are generally removed all around. They move with a long low stride.

Recognized Behavior Issues and Traits

This is considered an ideal small housedog because of their friendly intelligence. They are also reported to be loud vigilant alarm barkers. Breed standards are firm that the dog should not be shy or vicious. They may try to herd their humans by nipping at heels, but can be trained away from this behavior. They are devoted, and are a bit more active on average than the Cardigan Corgis, though perhaps gentler on average. The coat just needs routine grooming and they are considered moderate shedders. At the very least, a few brisk walks daily are needed, and they should only be turned out into fenced enclosures. Obedience training is strongly recommended, along with early training and socialization. They need close human contact, and if left alone for long periods, they may chew or bark.

Normal Physiologic Variations

Echocardiographic Normal Values:[1]	
Parameter	Median Range
Weight (kg)	15 (8-19)
Heart rate (bpm)	120 (80-160)
LVPWD (mm)	8 (6-10)
LVPWS (mm)	12 (8-13)
LVD (mm)	32 (28-40)
LVS (mm)	19 (12-23)
FS (%)	44 (33-57)
EPSS (mm)	2 (0-5)
RVd (mm)	10 (6-14)
IVSd (mm)	8 (6-9)
IVSs (mm)	12 (10-14)
AOD (mm)	18 (15-22)
LAS (mm)	21 (12-24)
N	20

LVPWD, LV posterior wall dimension at end-diastole; LVPWS, LV posterior wall thickness at end-systole; LVD, LV chamber dimension at end-diastole; LVS, LV chamber dimension at end-systole; FS, percent fractional shortening; EPSS, E-point septal separation; RVD, RV chamber dimension at end-diastole; IVSd, interventricular septal thickness at end-diastole; IVSs, interventricular septal thickness at end-systole; AOD, aortic root at end-diastole; LAS, left atrium at end-systole; N, number of animals.

Natural Bob-Tail: Pembroke Welsh Corgis exist due to the heterozygous dominant expression of the *T* gene. Most genetic studies find that homozygous dominant individuals are pre-natally lethal. However, one study found that homozygous dominant Pembroke Welsh Corgis were born tailless, with anorectal atresia and multiple spinal defects. Due to this finding, natural bob-tail

The Breed History

Though often considered an offshoot of the Cardigan Welsh Corgi family, the Pembroke Corgis may trace further back, to about the year 1107. Various breeds are thought to have contributed to the corgi type including Shipperke, Finnish Spitz, Keeshond, Swedish Vallhunds, and Samoyed. Cross breeding with Cardigans occurred, and only in the last 75 years have the registries bred separately. The Pembroke lines matured in Pembrokeshire, Wales. Corgi is thought to mean dog in Celtic, or in Welsh, dwarf dog. This breed was brought to the public's attention as the chosen pets of Queen Elizabeth. AKC first recognized Pembrokes in 1934.

Breeding for Function

Bred originally as cattle driving dogs, they are also excellent watchdogs, and are successful at obedience trials. Their talents also include tracking and agility. They are valued for their loyal companionship.

Physical Characteristics

Height at Withers: female 10-12" (25.4-30.5 cm), male 10-12" (25.4-30.5 cm)

Weight: females under 28 lb (12.5 kg), males under 30 lb (13.5 kg).

Coat: A short to medium length, it is composed of an undercoat and coarser outer coat. The dog is shown basically untrimmed. White is acceptable in markings of chest, leg, neck and small amounts only on face. Body colors are black and tan, red, fawn, and sable. Predominantly white coats, or coats with a bluish/smoky cast are serious faults. Some dogs are tri-colored.

Longevity: 12-15 years.

Points of Conformation: The Pembroke is finer boned and smaller than the Cardigan, but still gives the impression of strength. Pembrokes have pointed erect ears and are short-tailed, while the Cardigan's ears are less pointed and they have a long tail. A low-set dog, Pembrokes are well known for their agility and stamina. They are longer than high, topline is level, neck is long, and the head is large with moderate stop and fox-like proportions with a keen expression. The eyes are oval, oblique and brown, and the nose is black. Ribs are deep and well sprung. Tails are usually docked short, though puppies are sometimes born with naturally short tails.

Pembroke Welsh Corgis should not be bred together, and should only be bred to normal-tailed dogs. This will produce 50% bob-tail and 50% normal-tail offspring.[2,3,4]

Fluffy Coat Length: An autosomal recessive condition causing a long, fluffy coat exists in the Pembroke Welsh Corgi. Dogs with this coat type are not eligible for competition. A genetic test is available.

In a UK study, 35.7% of litters were born via **Cesarean section**.[5]

Drug Sensitivities
None reported

Inherited Diseases
Hip Dysplasia: Polygenically inherited trait causing degenerative joint disease and hip arthritis. OFA reports 18.4% affected.[6]

von Willebrand's Disease Type 1 (vWD): Autosomal recessive genetic disorder causing a mild bleeding syndrome. A direct genetic test is available from VetGen, reporting 6% affected, and 37% carrier in the breed.

Elbow Dysplasia: Polygenically inherited trait causing elbow arthritis. OFA reports 3.0% affected.[6]

Patella Luxation: Polygenically inherited laxity of patellar ligaments, causing luxation, lameness, and later degenerative joint disease. Treat surgically if causing clinical signs. Too few Pembroke Welsh Corgis have been screened by OFA to determine an accurate frequency.[6]

Disease Predispositions
Persistent Pupillary Membranes: Strands of fetal remnant connecting; iris to iris, cornea, lens, or involving sheets of tissue. The later three forms can impair vision, and dogs affected with these forms should not be bred. Identified in 19.19% of Pembroke Welsh Corgis CERF examined by veterinary ophthalmologists between 2000-2005. Dorn reports a 9.01x increased odds ratio versus other breeds.[7,8]

Retinal Dysplasia: Retinal folds, geographic, and generalized retinal dysplasia with detachment are recognized in the breed. Reported in 4.92% of Pembroke Welsh Corgis CERF examined by veterinary ophthalmologists between 2000-2005. Suspected autosomal recessive inheritance. CERF does not recommend breeding any Pembroke Welsh Corgi with retinal dysplasia.[8]

Cataracts: Anterior, posterior, and nuclear cortex intermediate cataracts predominate in the breed. Identified in 3.15% of Pembroke Welsh Corgis CERF examined by veterinary ophthalmologists between 2000-2005. CERF does not recommend breeding any Pembroke Welsh Corgi with a cataract.[8]

Hypothyroidism: Inherited autoimmune thyroiditis. 2.1% positive for thyroid auto-antibodies based on testing at Michigan State University. (Ave. for all breeds is 7.5%).[9,10]

Distichiasis: Abnormally placed eyelashes that irritate the cornea and conjunctiva. Can cause secondary corneal ulceration. Identified in 1.49% of Pembroke Welsh Corgis CERF examined by veterinary ophthalmologists between 2000-2005.[8]

Intervertebral Disc Disease (IVDD): Serious neurological condition where disk degeneration and rupture into spinal nerves and the spinal cord causes pain and possible paralysis. Requires immediate veterinary attention. Occurs at an increased frequency in the breed.

Degenerative Myelopathy (DM): Affected dogs show an insidious onset of upper motor neuron (UMN) paraparesis at an average age of 11.4 years. The disease eventually progresses to severe tetraparesis. Affected dogs have normal results on myelography, MRI, and CSF analysis. Necropsy confirms the condition. Reported at a frequency of 0.58% in Pembroke Welsh Corgis. Unknown mode of inheritance. A direct genetic test for an autosomal recessive DM susceptibility gene is available. All affected dogs are homozygous for the gene, however, only a small percentage of homozygous dogs develop DM. OFA testing shows 39% carrier and 52% homozygous "at risk" for the DM susceptability gene.[11,12,13,14]

Bladder Stones: The breed has a predisposition to develop bladder stones. Stone composition is not identified. Dorn reports a 4.20x increased odds ratio versus other breeds.[7,15,16]

Cystinuria/Cystine Bladder Stones: Caused by a metabolic abnormality in cystine metabolism. Welsh Corgis have an increased risk for developing cystine bladder stones. Treat with surgical removal and life-long medical therapy. Unknown mode of inheritance in this breed.[17]

Perineal Hernia: An Australian study identified the Corgi breed as most commonly affected with perineal hernias. The mean age of affected dogs was 9.4 years. Treatment is herniorrhaphy surgery.[18]

Patent Ductus Arteriosus (PDA): Polygenically inherited congenital heart disorder, where a fetal vessel remains open after birth, causing a mixing of oxygenated and unoxygenated blood. Affected dogs are usually stunted, and have a loud heart murmur. Diagnosis with Doppler ultrasound. Treat with surgery. Some Pembroke Welsh Corgis have been reported with concurrent pulmonary hypertension or plexogenic pulmonary arteriopathy.[19,20,21]

Steroid Responsive Meningitis/Arteritis: Affected dogs present with apathy, fever, delayed proprioception, ataxia, and/or increased head and cervical pain. Histopathology shows necrotizing vasculitis in the CNS, with perivascular granulomatous inflammation. Treat with steroids. Unknown mode of inheritance.[22]

Brachygnathism, Corneal Dystrophy, Cryptorchidism, Cutaneous Asthenia, Dermatomyositis, Epilepsy, Methemoglobin Reductase Deficiency, Narcolepsy, Prognathism, and **Progressive Retinal Atrophy** are reported.[23]

Isolated Case Studies
Telangiectasia: Multiple vascular lesions involving kidneys and various other organs consisting of cavernous, blood-filled spaces lined by endothelial cells with various amounts of mural collagen. Described in eight Pembroke Welsh Corgi dogs. The most common clinical sign associated with this condition is hematuria.[24]

Juvenile Nephropathy: Two related Pembroke Welsh corgi puppies presented at three and five months of age, respectively, for lethargy, diarrhoea, poor body condition, polyuria and proteinuria. Based upon the clinical presentation, urinalysis and serum biochemistry, chronic renal failure was diagnosed. Renal histopathology was consistent with juvenile nephropathy.[25]

Tongue Atrophy due to Polymyositis: A three-year-old female Pembroke Welsh Corgi exhibited symptomatic tongue atrophy, dysphagia and excessive salivation following a bout of masticatory polymyositis. The dog died of aspiration pneumonia 2 years later.[26]

Genetic Tests

Tests of Genotype: Direct tests for vWD and coat colors are available from VetGen.

Direct test for an autosomal recessive DM susceptibility gene is available from the OFA.

Direct test for the fluffy coat gene is available from the Animal Health Trust, DDC Veterinary and VetGen.

Tests of Phenotype: CHIC Certification: Required testing includes hip radiographs, and CERF eye examination. (See CHIC website; www.caninehealthinfo.org).

Recommended testing includes patella examination, elbow radiographs, thyroid profile including autoantibodies, genetic test for vWD, and cardiac examination.

Miscellaneous

- **Breed name synonyms:** Pembroke, Corgi
- **Registries:** AKC, CKC, UKC, KCGB (Kennel Club of Great Britain), ANKC (Australian National Kennel Club), NKC (National Kennel Club)
- **AKC rank (year 2008):** 24 (8,102 dogs registered)
- **Internet resources: Pembroke Welsh Corgi Club of America:** www.pembrokecorgi.org
  Pembroke Welsh Corgi Association (Canada): www.pembrokewelshcorgis.ca
  The Welsh Corgi League (UK): www.pembrokewelshcorgileague.co.uk

References

1. Morrison SA, Moise NS, Scarlett J, et. al.: Effect of breed and body weight on echocardiographic values in four breeds of dogs of differing somatotype. J Vet Intern Med. 1992 Jul-Aug;6(4):220-4.
2. Indrebø A, Langeland M, Juul HM, et. al.: A study of inherited short tail and taillessness in Pembroke Welsh corgi. J Small Anim Pract. 2008 May;49(5):220-4.
3. Haworth K, Putt W, Cattanach B, et. al.: Canine homolog of the T-box transcription factor T; failure of the protein to bind to its DNA target leads to a short-tail phenotype. Mamm Genome. 2001 Mar;12(3):212-8.
4. Hytönen MK, Grall A, Hédan B, et. al.: Ancestral T-box mutation is present in many, but not all, short-tailed dog breeds. J Hered. 2009 Mar-Apr;100(2):236-40.
5. Evans KM & Adams VJ: Proportion of litters of purebred dogs born by caesarean section. J Small Anim Pract. 2010 Feb;51(2):113-8.
6. OFA Website breed statistics: www.offa.org Last accessed July 1, 2010.
7. Dorn CR: Canine breed-specific risks of frequently diagnosed diseases at veterinary teaching hospitals. Monograph. AKC Canine Health Foundation. 2000.
8. Ocular Disorders Presumed to be Inherited in Purebred Dogs. American College of Veterinary Ophthalmologists. ACVO, 2007
9. Nachreiner RF, Refsal KR, Graham PA, et. al.: Prevalence of serum thyroid hormone autoantibodies in dogs with clinical signs of hypothyroidism. J Am Vet Med Assoc 2002 Feb 15;220(4):466-71.
10. Nachreiner R & Refsal K: Personal communication, Diagnostic Center for Population and Animal Health, Michigan State University. April, 2007.
11. Coates JR: Degenerative Myelopathy of Pembroke Welsh Corgi Dogs. Proceedings, 2005 ACVIM Forum. 2005.
12. Coates JR, March PA, Oglesbee M, et. al.: Clinical characterization of a familial degenerative myelopathy in Pembroke Welsh Corgi dogs. J Vet Intern Med. 2007 Nov-Dec;21(6):1323-31.
13. March PA, Coates JR, Abyad RJ, et. al.: Degenerative myelopathy in 18 Pembroke Welsh Corgi dogs. Vet Pathol. 2009 Mar;46(2):241-50.
14. Awano T, Johnson GS, Wade CM, et. al.: Genome-wide association analysis reveals a SOD1 mutation in canine degenerative myelopathy that resembles amyotrophic lateral sclerosis. Proc Natl Acad Sci U S A. 2009 Feb 24;106(8):2794-9.
15. Weichselbaum RC, Feeney DA, Jessen CR, et al,: Evaluation of the morphologic characteristics and prevalence of canine urocystoliths from a regional urolith center. Am J Vet Res. 1998 April; 59(4):379-87.
16. Bovee KC, McGuire T: Qualitative and quantitative analysis of uroliths in dogs: definitive determination of chemical type. J Am Vet Med Assoc. 1984 Nov 1;185(9):983-7.
17. Case LC, Ling GV, Franti CE, et. al.: Cystine-containing urinary calculi in dogs: 102 cases (1981-1989). J Am Vet Med Assoc. 1992 Jul 1;201(1):129-33.
18. Bellenger CR: Perineal hernia in dogs. Aust Vet J. 1980 Sep;56(9):434-8.
19. Kolm US, Amberger CN, Boujon CE, et. al.: Plexogenic pulmonary arteriopathy in a Pembroke Welsh corgi. J Small Anim Pract. 2004 Sep;45(9):461-6.
20. Tanaka R, Hoshi K, Nagashima Y, et. al.: Detachable coils for occlusion of patent ductus arteriosus in 2 dogs. Vet Surg. 2001 Nov-Dec;30(6):580-4.
21. Oswald GP, Orton EC: Patent ductus arteriosus and pulmonary hypertension in related Pembroke Welsh corgis. J Am Vet Med Assoc. 1993 Mar 1;202(5):761-4.
22. Cherubini GB: Steroid-responsive meningitis-arteritis in the Pembroke Welsh corgi. Vet Rec. 2008 Mar 29;162(13):424.
23. The Genetic Connection: A Guide to Health Problems in Purebred Dogs. L Ackerman. p.243, AAHA Press, 1999.
24. Moore FM, Thornton GW: Telangiectasia of Pembroke Welsh Corgi dogs. Vet Pathol. 1983 Mar;20(2):203-8.
25. McKay LW, Seguin MA, Ritchey JW, et. al.: Juvenile nephropathy in two related Pembroke Welsh corgi puppies. J Small Anim Pract. 2004 Nov;45(11):568-71.
26. Ito D, Okada M, Jeffery ND, et. al.: Symptomatic tongue atrophy due to atypical polymyositis in a Pembroke Welsh Corgi. J Vet Med Sci. 2009 Aug;71(8):1063-7.
27. The Complete Dog Book, 20th Ed. The American Kennel Club. Howell Book House, NY 2006. p.675-679.

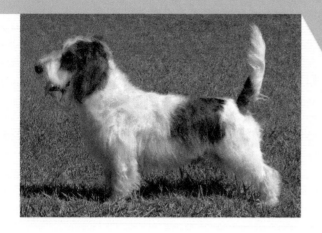

The Breed History

An ancient hound originating in France, old records there from the 16th century indicate early development of the Griffon Vendéen. Note that the Grand Griffon Vendéen breed also originates from this common ancestor. Basset means low to the ground, and petite is French for small. The term Griffon refers to the wiry coat, and the Vendéen portion of the name refers to the section of France (Vendée) where this breed is known to have originated. The first breed standard of 1909 differentiated between Petit and Grand varieties in the breed, and the definitive breed standard version was drawn up in the 1950s. It was not until 1975 that interbreeding between Grand and Petit was discontinued. The AKC first admitted the breed in 1990.

Breeding for Function

This is an exceptional scent hound, hardy, with good stamina, bold, and especially bred for rabbit and hare. Well suited for heavy underbrush and rough rocky terrain. They possess a loud voice. Today they are found in obedience, tracking and agility, and bench shows or as a companion.

Physical Characteristics

Height at Withers: 13-15 " (33-38 cm)

Weight: females 31-40 lb (14-18 kg).

Coat: Overall, he has a tousled rough appearance with a long beard and well-defined brows, a large moustache, and an outer coat that is harsh and long. The undercoat is short and dense, but not soft or wooly. Colors include white with lemon, orange, tricolor, grizzle or black markings.

Longevity: 12-14 years.

Points of Conformation: Compact, but longer than tall, strong in muscle and bone, alert and lively, large eyes are dark and the expression is friendly. The low set ears fold and are narrow with rounded tips. The domed skull has a prominent occipital protuberance, the stop is well defined, muzzle is square, and nose is very large, and black, though in light dogs a lighter nose is tolerated. The neck is long, with no throatiness, the topline is level with a slight arch over the loin, and the thorax is moderately deep and rounded. The well-feathered curved high set tail is held

erect, and tapers towards the tip. The limbs may be straight but commonly are somewhat bowed, which is acceptable. Dewclaws may be removed. Forefeet may be slightly turned out and are longer than wide. The gait is smooth and ground covering.

Recognized Behavior Issues and Traits

Breed characteristics reported in the literature include: Willing to please, loyal, affectionate, extroverted, active, not possessing high heat tolerance, and may argue with other dogs, though they generally get along well with other pets. Needs lots of human contact, like being in packs, independent thinkers, have a moderate to high barking tendency, and need mental stimulation to prevent boredom vices. Off leash exercise should be in fenced enclosures only. They are good with children. They require moderate to high levels of exercise. They have low grooming needs.

Normal Physiologic Variations

None reported

Drug Sensitivities

None reported

Inherited Diseases

Hip Dysplasia: Polygenically inherited trait causing degenerative joint disease and hip arthritis. OFA reports 11.2% affected.[1]

Patella Luxation: Polygenically inherited laxity of patellar ligaments, causing luxation, lameness, and later degenerative joint disease. Treat surgically if causing clinical signs. OFA reports 7.7% affected.[1]

Elbow Dysplasia: Polygenically inherited trait causing elbow arthritis. OFA reports 4.0% affected.[1]

Disease Predispositions

Persistent Pupillary Membranes: Strands of fetal remnant connecting; iris to iris, cornea, lens, or involving sheets of tissue. The later three forms can impair vision, and dogs affected with these forms should not be bred. Identified in 23.76% of Petit Basset Griffon Vendéen CERF examined by veterinary ophthalmologists between 2000-2005.[2]

Hypothyroidism: Inherited autoimmune thyroiditis. 9.4% positive for thyroid autoantibodies based on testing at Michigan State University. (Ave. for all breeds is 7.5%).[3,4]

Retinal Dysplasia: Retinal folds, geographic, and generalized retinal dysplasia with detachment are recognized in the breed. Can progress to blindness. Reported in 3.87% of Petit Basset Griffon Vendéen CERF examined by veterinary ophthalmologists between 2000-2005.[2]

Sterile Meningitis/Neck Pain Syndrome: An episodic condition in affected dogs usually between 2-4 years of age where the neck is held extended and low, with pain. Possibly related to necrotizing vasculitis identified in Beagle pain syndrome. Episodes respond to corticosteroids. Reported at a frequency of 3.75% in the 2000 PBGV Health Survey.[5]

Idiopathic Epilepsy: Inherited seizures can be generalized or partial seizures. Control with anticonvulsant medication. Reported at a frequency of 3.28% in the 2000 PBGV Health Survey.[5]

Allergic Dermatitis (Atopy): Inhalant or food allergy. Presents with pruritis and pyotraumatic dermatitis (hot spots). Reported at a frequency of 3.12% in the 2000 PBGV Health Survey.[5]

Cataracts: Anterior, posterior, intermediate and punctate cataracts occur in the breed. Reported at a frequency of 3.28% in the 2000 PBGV Health Survey. Identified in 3.04% of PBGV CERF examined by veterinary ophthalmologists between 2000-2005. CERF does not recommend breeding any PBGV with a cataract.[2,5]

Lens Luxation: Partial or complete displacement of the lens from its normal anatomic site behind the pupil. Can cause Secondary Glaucoma. CERF does not recommend breeding any PBGV with lens luxation or glaucoma.[2,6]

Corneal Dystrophy is reported.[7]

Isolated Case Studies

Systemic Hypertension and Severe Arteriosclerosis: A 12-year-old sexually intact male Vendee Griffon Basset was presented for acute pulmonary edema. Severe systemic systolic arterial hypertension (SAH) was diagnosed (290 mmHg). Three months later, the dog underwent euthanasia because of an acute episode of distal aortic thromboembolism. Necropsy revealed severe aortic and iliac arteriosclerosis. SAH related to arteriosclerosis is an uncommon finding in dogs.[8]

Genetic Tests

Tests of Genotype: none

Tests of Phenotype: CHIC Certification: Hip radiographs and CERF eye examination. (See CHIC website; www.caninehealthinfo.org)

Recommend patella evaluation, elbow radiographs, thyroid profile including autoantibodies, and cardiac examination

Miscellaneous

- **Breed name synonyms:** PBGV, Small Vendeen Basset, Little Griffon Vendeen Basset, Roughies or Griffs (England nicknames), Petites or Griffs (nickname in Denmark) and in America, Petites. (pl. Petits Bassets Griffons Vendeens)
- **Registries:** AKC, UKC, CKC, KCGB (Kennel Club of Great Britain), ANKC (Australian National Kennel Club)
- **AKC rank (year 2008):** 119 (275 dogs registered)
- **Internet resources: Petit Basset Griffon Vendéen Club of America:** www.pbgv.org
  Petit Basset Griffon Vendeen Fanciers of Canada: www.angelfire.com/bc2/PBGVFC/ClubInfo.html
  Basset Griffon Vendee Club (UK): www.bgvclub.co.uk

References

1. OFA Website breed statistics: www.offa.org Last accessed July 1, 2010.
2. *Ocular Disorders Presumed to be Inherited in Purebred Dogs.* American College of Veterinary Ophthalmologists. ACVO, 2007.
3. Nachreiner RF, Refsal KR, Graham PA, et. al.: Prevalence of serum thyroid hormone autoantibodies in dogs with clinical signs of hypothyroidism. *J Am Vet Med Assoc* 2002 Feb 15;220(4):466-71.
4. Nachreiner R & Refsal K: Personal communication, Diagnostic Center for Population and Animal Health, Michigan State University. April, 2007.
5. Petit Basset Griffon Vendéen Club of America: 2000 PBGV Health Survey. 2000.
6. Chaudidu G., Clerc B, et. al.: Primary Lens Luxation in the Petite Bassett Griffon Vendeen in France. ECVO Proceedings 2002.
7. *The Genetic Connection: A Guide to Health Problems in Purebred Dogs.* L Ackerman. p. 231. AAHA Press, 1999.
8. Nicolle AP, Carlos Sampedrano C, Fontaine JJ, et. al.: Longitudinal left ventricular myocardial dysfunction assessed by 2D colour tissue Doppler imaging in a dog with systemic hypertension and severe arteriosclerosis. *J Vet Med A Physiol Pathol Clin Med.* 2005 Mar;52(2):83-7.
9. *The Complete Dog Book, 20th Ed.* The American Kennel Club. Howell Book House, NY 2006. p. 200-204.

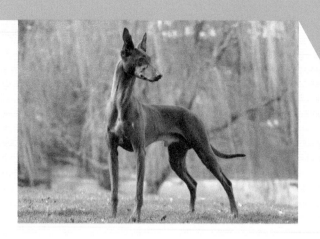

Pharaoh Hound

is minimal. The neck is long and muscular, with a small degree of arching and no throatiness. The topline is level, except for a slight slope down the croup. The tail is tapering and whip-like at the terminus, reaching below the tarsus while at rest. The thorax is deep, ribs are well sprung, and there is moderate tucking up of the abdomen. Limbs are straight boned, and the feet are medium in size with well knuckled up toes and strong large pads. Dewclaws fore and hind may be removed. The gait is long striding and smooth, and appears both powerful and effortless. When compared with the Ibizan hound, the Pharaoh hounds are smaller, have less extreme conformation and less white marking.

The Breed History

This breed is among the most ancient and mimics the depictions of the Egyptian god, Anubis, the guide for the souls of the departed. First records date back to around 3000 BC. Skeletal remains that match Pharaoh hound body structure date back to about 5000 BC. Paintings and many Egyptian hieroglyphs depict this dog. So highly prized were these dogs that some were mummified along with the nobility. Some of these dogs were exported to the Isle of Malta, where they were carefully bred for over 2000 years. This rare breed is the National Dog of Malta. It was not until 1983 that the AKC registered the breed.

Breeding for Function

The historical record shows that this dog was used for hunting and as a companion. In Malta, they were used specifically for hunting rabbit. Their need for low food intake, agility, power, speed and grace are traits that were valued and selected for. They can hunt using scent and sight, plus sound. They have been successful in obedience and coursing competitions.

Physical Characteristics

Height at Withers: female 21-24" (53-61 cm), male 23-25" (58.5-63.5 cm)

Weight: 45-55 lb (20-25 kg)

Coat: Short glossy hairs lie flat and the hairs are hard in texture. The coat is a rich red rust, tan or chestnut with limited white markings. A white star on the chest (The Star) and a white tail tip are especially acceptable.

Longevity: 12-14 years

Points of Conformation: These dogs are medium-sized with a high head carriage. All of the body structures are lithe and finely chiseled. There is an unusual breed trait called blushing. When very excited, because the blood vessels are so superficial, their dilation results in an increased rosy red flush affecting the ears and nose. Another breed characteristic is the strong amber pigment of the eyes. Palpebral margins, lip margins, and nose are all flesh colored. Eyes are moderately deep and close set, and ears are medium-large in size, set high and carried pricked high; leather is fine, and the pinnae are very broad at the base. The skull is long and the stop

Recognized Behavior Issues and Traits

Reported breed characteristics include: Intelligent, easily trained, friendly, and love children. They remain playful even as adults. They need close human contact. Pharaoh hounds have low grooming needs and don't get doggy odor even after becoming wet. They are active dogs and without adequate exercise they become obese easily. Not considered an apartment dog. They should be off leash in a fenced enclosure only. They are not considered watch or guard dogs, though they are aloof with strangers generally.

Normal Physiologic Variations

Sight hounds have lower normal ranges for T4 and T3 concentrations compared to other breeds.[1]

Drug Sensitivities

Anesthesia: Sight hounds require particular attention during anesthesia. Their lean body conformation with high surface-area-to-volume ratio predisposes them to hypothermia during anesthesia. Impaired biotransformation of drugs by the liver results in prolonged recovery from barbiturate and thiobarbiturate intravenous anesthetics. Propofol, and ketamine/diazepam combination are recommended induction agents.[2]

Inherited Disease

Hip Dysplasia: Polygenically inherited trait causing degenerative joint disease and hip arthritis. OFA reports 2.4% affected.[3]

Elbow Dysplasia: Polygenically inherited trait causing elbow arthritis. OFA reports 1.5% affected.[3]

Patella Luxation: Polygenically inherited laxity of patellar ligaments, causing luxation, lameness, and later degenerative joint disease. Treat surgically if causing clinical signs. Reported in the breed, but too few Pharaoh Hounds have been screened by OFA to determine an accurate frequency.[3]

Disease Predispositions

Hypothyroidism: Inherited autoimmune thyroiditis. Reported as a problem in the breed, but too few Pharaoh Hounds have been screened for thyroid autoantibodies by Michigan State University to determine an accurate frequency. (Ave. for all breeds is 7.5%).[4,5]

Cataracts: Anterior or posterior intermediate and punctate cataracts occur in the breed. Reported in the breed, but too few Pharaoh Hounds have been CERF eye examined to determine an accurate frequency. CERF does not recommend breeding any Pharaoh Hound with a cataract.[6]

Retinal Dysplasia: Retinal folds are recognized in the breed, but too few Pharaoh Hounds have been CERF eye examined to determine an accurate frequency.[6]

Distichiasis: Abnormally placed eyelashes that irritate the cornea and conjunctiva. Can cause secondary corneal ulceration. Reported in the breed, but too few Pharaoh Hounds have been CERF eye examined to determine an accurate frequency.[6]

Persistent Pupillary Membranes: Strands of fetal remnant connecting; iris to iris, cornea, lens, or involving sheets of tissue. The later three forms can impair vision, and dogs affected with these forms should not be bred. Reported in the breed, but too few Pharaoh Hounds have been CERF eye examined to determine an accurate frequency.[6]

The Pharaoh Hound is a rare breed, and there is little documented in the literature on health issues. **Allergies, Demodicosis, Epilepsy,** and **Gastric Dilitation-Volvulus** are reported to occur in the breed.

Shoulder Luxation is reported.[7]

Isolated Case Studies

Severe Zinc Responsive Dermatosis: Three of five puppies in a litter of 3-month-old Pharaoh Hounds presented with severe generalized erythematous-crusted papules, pruritus, footpad exfoliation, inappetence, lethargy, and retarded growth. Histologically, there was marked epidermal hyperplasia with a disorganized appearance of the epidermis and massive parakeratotic hyperkeratosis. Low serum zinc levels were documented, and the pups responded to intravenous, but not oral zinc supplementation. The affected dogs received IV zinc supplementation every three weeks to control their symptoms, but all expired over a course of 3 years.[8]

Genetic Tests

Tests of Genotype: None

Tests of Phenotype: CHIC Certification: Hip radiographs, thyroid profile including autoantibodies, CERF eye examination, and patella evaluation. (See CHIC website; www.caninehealthinfo.org).

Recommend elbow radiographs and cardiac examination.

Miscellaneous

- **Breed name synonyms:** Kelb-tal Fenek (means rabbit dog), Pharoah Hound, Pharaoh.
- **Registries:** AKC, UKC, CKC, KCGB (Kennel Club of Great Britain)-P, ANKC (Australian National Kennel Club), NKC (National Kennel Club).
- **AKC rank (year 2008):** 148 (72 dogs registered)
- **Internet resources: Pharaoh Hound Club of America:** www.ph-club.org
  The Pharaoh Hound Club (UK): www.pharaohhoundclub.co.uk

References

1. Kintzer PP & Peterson ME: Progress in the Diagnosis and Treatment of Canine Hypothyroidism. 2007. Proceedings, ACVIM 2007.
2. Court MH: Anesthesia of the sighthound. Clin Tech Small Anim Pract 1999 Feb;14(1):38-43.
3. OFA Website breed statistics: www.offa.org Last accessed July 1, 2010.
4. Nachreiner RF, Refsal KR, Graham PA, et. al.: Prevalence of serum thyroid hormone autoantibodies in dogs with clinical signs of hypothyroidism. J Am Vet Med Assoc 2002 Feb 15;220(4):466-71.
5. Nachreiner R & Refsal K: Personal communication, Diagnostic Center for Population and Animal Health, Michigan State University. April, 2007.
6. *Ocular Disorders Presumed to be Inherited in Purebred Dogs.* American College of Veterinary Ophthalmologists. ACVO, 2007.
7. *The Genetic Connection: A Guide to Health Problems in Purebred Dogs.* L Ackerman. p. 231-02. AAHA Press, 1999.
8. Campbell GA & Crow D: Severe zinc responsive dermatosis in a litter of Pharaoh Hounds. J Vet Diagn Invest. 2010 Jul;22(4):663-6.
9. *The Complete Dog Book, 20th Ed.* The American Kennel Club. Howell Book House, NY 2006. p. 205-208.

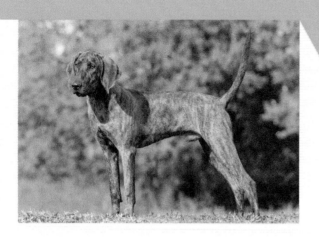

deep with well sprung ribs. The topline is higher at the withers than the hip, merging into slightly arched loins and a well tucked up abdomen. They possess fine, medium length straight boned limbs, with compact feet, toes well knuckled up. Nails are usually dark, but if white feet markings are present, there may be white nails and in brindles, reddish brown is permissible. A very long, medium weight curving tail tapers, and is normally held high in a saber like carriage. There can be a slight brush. Their gait is long, low, rhythmic, smooth and appearing tireless.

The Breed History

This breed was developed by the Plott family in the southeastern region of America during the late 1700s, and refined over seven family generations. The breed originated from imported German Hanoverian Hounds. One documented outcross to the American Blevins black saddle hound is recorded. AKC recognized this breed in 2006.

Breeding for Function

Originally developed for bear, mountain lion and boar hunting, the Plott hound became a valued coonhound because of their treeing instinct and ability to track a cold scent. Noted for their stamina and courage during the hunt, they are slow to tire and use a distinctive loud ringing high-pitched voice during the hunt. They can tolerate extreme terrain and weather. They can also do water work. Still primarily kept for hunting in the southeastern United States; coyotes and wildcats are also common quarry.

Physical Characteristics

Height at Withers: female 20-25" (51-58 cm), male 20-23" (51-58 cm).

Weight: females 40-55 lb (18-25 kg), males 50-65 lb (23-30 kg).

Coat: A short to medium length dense haircoat set close to the skin surface is standard. Sometimes these dogs are double coated. Some have a black saddle. The most common color pattern of brindle may be any shade (including yellow, brown, chocolate, red, black, gray, Maltese, blue or tan); some brindles have a black saddle. Other accepted colors include solid black, black with brindle trim, and buckskin (rarely). A small amount of white on the chest and feet is permissible; in older dogs a graying effect is also accepted.

Longevity: 11-14 years

Points of Conformation: The Plott is a muscular athletic medium-sized dog. Points include a moderately flat skull with a moderate stop, high head carriage, and prominent hazel to brown eyes with alert expression. The large pendulous high-set ears are semi-erect when working. They have a medium length neck and it is free of dewlap or throatiness. Palpebral margins, flews, nose, and lips are black. The muzzle is almost square, moderate in length and flews are present but not pendulous. The thorax is moderately

Recognized Behavior Issues and Traits

Reported breed characteristics include: Active, intelligent, bold, eager to please, vocal and responsive, alert. They are fearless on the hunt, and some variation in temperament occurs between strains. Plotts are generally good with children if socialized at an early age. They have very high exercise needs, and are generally suited to a hunting lifestyle only. They tend to drool, have low grooming needs, and have a moderate shedding tendency.

Normal Physiologic Variations

None reported

Drug Sensitivities

None reported

Inherited Diseases

Hip Dysplasia: Polygenically inherited trait causing degenerative joint disease and hip arthritis. Too few Plott Hounds have been screened to determine an accurate frequency.[1]

Patella Luxation: Polygenically inherited laxity of patellar ligaments, causing luxation, lameness, and later degenerative joint disease. Treat surgically if causing clinical signs. Too few Plott Hounds have been screened by OFA to determine an accurate frequency.[1]

Elbow Dysplasia: Polygenically inherited trait causing elbow arthritis. Too few Plott Hounds have been screened by OFA to determine an accurate frequency.[1]

Mucopolysaccharidosis I (MPS-I): A rare autosomal recessive disease discovered in three Plott Hound littermates was found to be associated with a profound and specific deficiency of alpha-L-iduronidase (mucopolysaccharide alpha-L-iduronohydrolase) in fibroblasts and leukocytes. Clinical signs of neurological, skeletal, and corneal abnormalities appear around 6-9 months of age. A direct test for MPS is available from PennGen.[2]

Disease Predispositions

Hypothyroidism: Inherited autoimmune thyroiditis. 6.3% positive for thyroid autoantibodies based on testing at Michigan State University. (Ave. for all breeds is 7.5%).[3,4]

Ocular Disorders: Too few Plott Hounds have been CERF examined to determine accurate frequencies for inherited ocular disorders.[5]

The Plott Hound is a rare breed, and there is little documented in the literature on health issues. **Gastric Dilatation-Volvulus** has been reported in the breed.

Isolated Case Studies
None reported

Genetic Tests
Tests of Genotype: Direct test for MPS is available from PennGen.

Tests of Phenotype: Recommend hip and elbow radiographs, CERF eye examination, patella evaluation, thyroid profile including autoantibodies, and cardiac examination.

Miscellaneous
- **Breed name synonyms:** Plotts.
- **Registries:** AKC, UKC, CKC, NKC (National Kennel Club).
- **AKC rank (year 2008):** 127 (220 dogs registered)
- **Internet resources: The Plott Hound:**
  http://www.akc.org/breeds/plott/index.cfm
  Plott Dogs: www.plottdogs.com

References
1. OFA Website breed statistics: www.offa.org Last accessed July 1, 2010.
2. Spellacy E, Shull RM, Constantopoulos G, et. al.: A canine model of human alpha-L-iduronidase deficiency. *Proc Natl Acad Sci U S A.* 1983 Oct;80(19):6091-5.
3. Nachreiner RF, Refsal KR, Graham PA, et. al.: Prevalence of serum thyroid hormone autoantibodies in dogs with clinical signs of hypothyroidism. *J Am Vet Med Assoc* 2002 Feb 15;220(4):466-71.
4. Nachreiner R & Refsal K: Personal communication, Diagnostic Center for Population and Animal Health, Michigan State University. April, 2007.
5. *Ocular Disorders Presumed to be Inherited in Purebred Dogs.* American College of Veterinary Ophthalmologists. ACVO, 2007.
6. *The Complete Dog Book, 20th Ed.* The American Kennel Club. Howell Book House, NY 2006. p. 700-702.

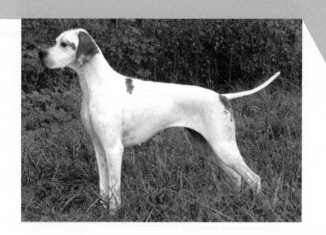

Pointer
(SYN: English Pointer)

long, slightly arched and well muscled. Limbs are straight boned and long bones are oval in cross section. The thorax is deep, ribs well sprung, and topline slightly descending towards the rear with a slight arch though loin and croup. The abdomen is moderately tucked up. The tapering tail reaches no longer than the tarsus and is carried slightly above the topline when active. Feet are compact and oval, have well knuckled up toes. Dewclaws on forelimbs may be removed.

The Breed History

The Pointer, often termed English Pointer is likely the original pointer-type dog. The Pointer was primarily developed in Britain though dogs of this general type existed earlier on the Continent, especially in Portugal and Spain regions (e.g., Italian and Spanish Pointer). First records in England date to the mid 1600s and ancestral bloodlines are thought to include Greyhound, Foxhound and Bloodhound mixed with the primitive setting spaniel dogs. Spanish, French and German pointer bloodlines were also admixed. Subsequently, Setter lines were also crossed with Pointers. AKC recognition occurred in 1884.

Breeding for Function

An on-foot hunt birddog (then subsequently a gundog) was the primary function for which this breed was developed and refined. The Pointer was also used to track and set hares for Greyhounds. During breed development a strong pointing instinct was highly prioritized. Popular uses today include companion, field trials, and obedience.

Physical Characteristics

Height at Withers: female 23-26" (58.5-66 cm), male 25-28" (63.5-71 cm).

Weight: females 45-65 lb (20.5-29.5 kg), males 55-75 lb (25-34 kg).

Coat: The dense, flat laying short glossy hard coat is most commonly liver and white, though other acceptable colors include solid liver, black, black and white, and orange, orange and white or lemon, lemon and white.

Longevity: 13-14 years

Points of Conformation: A lithe, compact, athletic build with an alert expression, high head carriage, and a powerful elastic graceful gait characterizes these dogs. They have a well-chiseled face, a prominent stop, a fairly flat skull with a prominent occipital protuberance, and slight furrow running between the eyes on the midline. The muzzle is deep and long, with a slight dishing, eyes are round, dark and moderately sized. The ears are pendulous with a moderately pointed tip, velvety hair cover and moderate leather thickness. The nose pigmentation matches the coat color and ranges from black through brown to flesh tone. The neck is

Recognized Behavior Issues and Traits

Reported breed characteristics include: Adaptable, does well in kennel, farm or home environments. Not considered an ideal apartment pet. He has lower needs for human companionship than many of the other gundogs but if housed inside with the family, becomes closely attached. Good with children, good alarm barker, early obedience training and socialization is very important. A very high energy and activity dog, he needs plenty of exercise or may become destructive. Possessing an independent will, high endurance, strong pointing instinct, intelligent, even temperament, low grooming needs, low shedding tendency, needs to be kept in during very cold weather.

Normal Physiologic Variations

Echocardiographic Normal Values:[1]	
Parameter	Mean ± SD
AO (mm)	24.1 ± 1.7
LA (mm)	22.6 ± 2.0
LA/AO	0.94 ± 0.07
LVd (mm)	39.2 ± 2.4
LVs (mm)	25.3 ± 2.4
%FS	35.5 ± 4.0
VSd (mm)	6.9 ± 1.1
VSs (mm)	10.6 ± 1.0
LVWd (mm)	7.1 ± 0.7
LVWs (mm)	11.5 ± 1.3
Kg	19.2 ± 2.8
N	16
HR	107 ± 17
Drugs	No

AO, aorta; LA, left atrium; LV, left ventricle; FS, fractional shortening; VS, ventricular septum; VS%Δ, change in VS thickness between diastole and systole; LVW, left ventricular wall; HR, heart rate; N, number of animals.

In a UK study, 26% of litters were delivered via **Cesarean section**.[2]

Drug Sensitivities

None reported

Inherited Diseases

Hip Dysplasia: Polygenically inherited trait causing degenerative joint disease and hip arthritis. OFA reports 8.0% affected.[3]

Elbow Dysplasia: Polygenically inherited trait causing elbow arthritis. OFA reports 3.1% affected.[3]

Patella Luxation: Polygenically inherited laxity of patellar ligaments, causing luxation, lameness, and later degenerative joint disease. Treat surgically if causing clinical signs. Too few Pointers have been screened by OFA to determine an accurate frequency.[3]

Hereditary Sensory Neuropathy: Rare, autosomal recessive disorder causing loss of sensation in the toes. Multiple feet can be involved, and affected dogs severely mutilate their paws.[4]

Spinal Muscle Atrophy: Rare, autosomal recessive disorder causing weakness and incoordination from 4-6 months of age. Progresses over a few months to paralysis of all muscles except the head and tail.[5]

X-Linked Cerebellar Ataxia: Rare, x-linked recessive disorder causing muscular incoordination, but not muscle weakness. Affected dogs slowly progress to constant falling.[6]

Deafness: Autosomal recessive deafness is identified in an inbred research strain of Pointers. It is not known whether this form of deafness exists in the general population. Congenital deafness can be unilateral of bilateral. Diagnosed by BAER testing.[7,8]

Disease Predispositions

Hypothyroidism: Inherited autoimmune thyroiditis. 13.1% positive for thyroid auto-antibodies based on testing at Michigan State University. (Ave. for all breeds is 7.5%).[9,10]

Demodicosis: Dorn reports an 8.52x odds ratio of developing demodectic mange versus other breeds. This disorder has an underlying immunodeficiency in its pathogenesis.[11]

Cataracts: Anterior cortex punctate cataracts predominate in the breed. Identified in 2.14% of Pointers CERF examined by veterinary ophthalmologists between 2000-2005. CERF does not recommend breeding any Pointer with a cataract.[12]

Retinal Dysplasia: Focal, folds and geographic retinal dysplasia occur in the breed. Can lead to blindness. Reported in 1.43% of Pointers CERF-examined by veterinary ophthalmologists between 2000-2005. CERF does not recommend breeding Pointers with any form of retinal dysplasia.[12]

Corneal Dystrophy: Pointers can have an epithelial/stromal form of corneal dystrophy. Identified in 1.43% of Pointers CERF-examined by veterinary ophthalmologists between 2000-2005.[12]

Abnormal/Lack of Semen, Allergies, Bloat (Gastric Dilitation-Volvulus), Cancer, Dwarfism, Ectropion/Entropion, Overbite/Underbite, Seizure Disorders, Skin Disease, and **Umbilical Hernias** are reported in the 2002 APC Health and Research Survey.[13]

Black Hair Follicular Dysplasia, Central PRA, Cleft Lip/Palate, Hypoadrenocorticism, Juvenile Cellulitis, Malignant Hyperthermia, Pannus, Prognathism, Progressive Retinal Atrophy, and **Subaortic Stenosis** are reported.[14]

Isolated Case Studies

Ciliary Dyskinesia: Electron microscopy was used to diagnose primary ciliary dyskinesia in a litter of English pointer dogs. Affected dogs present with chronic cough and nasal infection.[15]

Hemangioblastoma: A 6-year-old male Pointer dog was presented with a 4-week history of progressive hind-limb stiffness. Magnetic resonance imaging demonstrated a focal intramedullary lesion at the first thoracic vertebra. Necropsy revealed an intramedullary hemangioblastoma.[16]

Myoblastoma: A granular cell tumor (GCT; myoblastoma) was diagnosed on the tongue of a 12-year-old English Pointer with clinical signs of mild oral dysphagia. Surgical removal was cruative.[17]

Nervous Pointer Dogs: A family of pathologically "nervous Pointers" was inbred and established for psychiatric research in the late 1970s. Affected dogs "freeze" when nervous. This disorder is not reported in the general population.[18]

Genetic Tests

Tests of Genotype: Direct test for black, liver, lemon, and orange coat color genes available from VetGen and HealthGene.

Tests of Phenotype: CHIC Certification: Required testing includes hip radiographs, thyroid profile including autoantibodies, and CERF eye examination. Optional recommended testing includes congenital cardiac examination by a specialist, and BAER hearing test. (See CHIC website; www.caninehealthinfo.org).

Recommend elbow radiographs and patella evaluation.

Miscellaneous

- **Breed name synonyms:** English Pointer
- **Registries:** AKC, UKC as English Pointer, CKC, KCGB (Kennel Club of Great Britain), ANKC (Australian National Kennel Club), NKC (National Kennel Club) under English Pointer.
- **AKC rank (year 2008):** 111 (369 dogs registered)
- **Internet resources: American Pointer Club Inc.:** www.americanpointerclub.org
  The Pointer Club (UK): www.thepointerclub.co.uk/
  Pointer Club of Canada: www.pawsandeffects.com/PCC/PCC/PCC.html

References

1. Sisson D, Schaeffer D: Changes in linear dimensions of the heart, relative to body weight as measured by M-mode echocardiography in growing dogs. *Am J Vet Res.* 1991; 52:1591-1596.
2. Evans KM & Adams VJ: Proportion of litters of purebred dogs born by caesarean section. J Small Anim Pract. 2010 Feb;51(2):113-8.
3. OFA Website breed statistics: www.offa.org Last accessed July 1, 2010.
4. Cummings JF, de Lahunta A, Braund KG, et. al.: Hereditary sensory neuropathy. Nociceptive loss and acral mutilation in pointer dogs: canine

hereditary sensory neuropathy. *Am J Pathol.* 1983 Jul;112(1):136-8.

5. Sillevis Smitt PA, de Jong JM: Animal models of amyotrophic lateral sclerosis and the spinal muscular atrophies. *J Neurol Sci.* 1989 Jul;91(3):231-58.

6. O'Brien DP, Shibuya H, Zhou T: X-Linked Cerebellar Ataxia in English Pointer Dogs: Phenotype and Linkage Data. Proceedings, 1997 AKC Canine Health Foundation Canine Health Conference. 1997.

7. Coppens AG, Gilbert-Gregory S, Steinberg SA, et. al.: Inner ear histopathology in "nervous Pointer dogs" with severe hearing loss. *Hear Res.* 2005 Feb;200(1-2):51-62.

8. Steinberg SA, Klein E, Killens RL, et. al.: Inherited deafness among nervous pointer dogs. *J Hered.* 1994 Jan-Feb;85(1):56-9.

9. Nachreiner RF, Refsal KR, Graham PA, et. al.: Prevalence of serum thyroid hormone autoantibodies in dogs with clinical signs of hypothyroidism. J Am Vet Med Assoc 2002 Feb 15;220(4):466-71.

10. Nachreiner R & Refsal K: Personal communication, Diagnostic Center for Population and Animal Health, Michigan State University. April, 2007.

11. Dorn CR: Canine breed-specific risks of frequently diagnosed diseases at veterinary teaching hospitals. Monograph. AKC Canine Health Foundation. 2000.

12. *Ocular Disorders Presumed to be Inherited in Purebred Dogs.* American College of Veterinary Ophthalmologists. ACVO, 2007.

13. American Pointer Club: 2002 APC Health & Research Survey. 2002.

14. *The Genetic Connection: A Guide to Health Problems in Purebred Dogs.* L Ackerman. p. 231 AAHA Press, 1999.

15. Morrison WB, Wilsman NJ, Fox LE, et. al.: Primary ciliary dyskinesia in the dog. J Vet Intern Med. 1987 Apr-Jun;1(2):67-74.

16. Cantile C, Baroni M, Tartarelli CL, et. al.: Intramedullary hemangioblastoma in a dog. *Vet Pathol.* 2003 Jan;40(1):91-4.

17. Rallis TS, Tontis DK, Soubasis NH, et. al.: Immunohistochemical study of a granular cell tumor on the tongue of a dog. *Vet Clin Pathol.* 2001;30(2):62-66.

18. Reese WG, Newton JE, Angel C, et. al.: Induced immobility in nervous and normal Pointer dogs. *J Nerv Ment Dis.* 1982 Oct;170(10):605-13.

19. *The Complete Dog Book, 20th Ed.* The American Kennel Club. Howell Book House, NY 2006. p. 20-23.

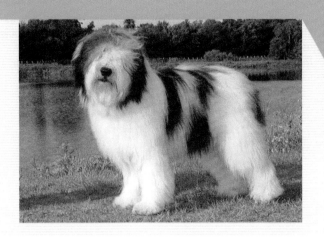

The Breed History

The Polski Owczarek Nizinny or PON was accepted into the AKC registry in 2001. The breed may have derived from the Hungarian group of herding dogs; some perhaps of the corded coat type. In Poland, first records of the breed trace to about the year 1500. During the Second World War, the breed came close to extinction. After the war, one breeder had six bitches and two dogs which were used to recover the breed. This is still a rare breed.

Breeding for Function

Though a sheepdog primarily developed for herding, this dog was originally used for hunting, and also was widely valued for companionship.

Physical Characteristics

Height at Withers: 16-20" (40.5-51 cm).

Weight: 30-35 lb (13.5-16 kg).

Coat: The double coat is accepted in any color. The coarse profuse outer coat is shaggy and long, and the inner coat short, dense and wooly. Colors may include white with black, or gray or sandy patches, gray and white, or chocolate. A fading factor (dominant inheritance) results in puppy coats fading as they mature; this does not affect white puppies.

Longevity: 13-15 years

Points of Conformation: In general appearance, they are often considered to be a small version of the Bearded Collie, a breed that the PON may have acted as an ancestor for. Their overall conformation is slightly longer than tall, cobby and heavily boned. The skull is heavy and broad and slightly domed. The hair normally covers the brown or hazel oval shaped eyes. The head appears to be larger than it really is because of profuse hair, especially in the brows, moustache and beard. The muzzle is long. The nose is large and dark brown or black. Ears are moderate in size, hanging down and well covered in hair. The neck is short and strong. These dogs possess a broad level topline, and the legs are well haired. The thorax is deep with moderately sprung ribs and the abdomen is moderately tucked up. Limbs are straight boned and the feet are oval, compact, and the forefeet are larger than the rear feet. Puppies may be born tailless; if a tail is present, it is usually docked

to 2 vertebrae in length. The tail is low set. The gait is long and low striding with an ambling appearance. These dogs may tend to toe in somewhat.

Recognized Behavior Issues and Traits

Reported breed characteristics include: Moderate grooming needs, friendly, high intelligence and trainability, likes to please, adaptable to city or country living. Aloof with strangers, he makes a good watchdog. The PON needs human companionship and regular exercise. He is considered to have an excellent memory. Early obedience training is strongly recommended as some of these dogs tend to be dominant in personality.

Normal Physiologic Variations

None reported

Drug Sensitivities

None reported

Inherited Diseases

Hip Dysplasia: Polygenically inherited trait causing degenerative joint disease and hip arthritis. OFA reports 15.8% affected.[1]

Elbow Dysplasia: Polygenically inherited trait causing elbow arthritis. Too few Polish Lowland Sheepdogs have been screened by OFA to determine an accurate frequency.[1]

Patella Luxation: Polygenically inherited laxity of patellar ligaments, causing luxation, lameness, and later degenerative joint disease. Treat surgically if causing clinical signs. Too few Polish Lowland Sheepdogs have been screened by OFA to determine an accurate frequency.[1]

Disease Predispositions

Hypothyroidism: Inherited autoimmune thyroiditis. 28.4% positive for thyroid autoantibodies based on testing at Michigan State University. (Ave. for all breeds is 7.5%).[2,3]

Persistent Pupillary Membranes: Strands of fetal remnant connecting; iris to iris, cornea, lens, or involving sheets of tissue. The later three forms can impair vision, and dogs affected with these forms should not be bred. Identified in 6.50% of Polish Lowland Sheepdogs CERF examined by veterinary ophthalmologists between 2000-2005.[4]

Corneal Dystrophy: Epithelial/stromal form causes a bilateral non-inflammatory corneal opacity (white to gray). Identified in 3.11% of Polish Lowland Sheepdogs CERF-examined by veterinary ophthalmologists between 2000-2005.[4]

Cataracts: Anterior cortex punctate cataracts predominate in the breed. Identified in 2.26% of Polish Lowland Sheepdogs CERF examined by veterinary ophthalmologists between 2000-2005.

CERF does not recommend breeding any Polish Lowland Sheepdog with a cataract.[4]

Neuronal Ceroid Lipofuscinosis (NCL, CL): A slowly progressive disorder, beginning with retinal degeneration and nyctalopia from 6 months to 4-5 years of age. Affected dogs then progress to cerebellar ataxia and dementia. Stored material in nerve and retinal cells consisting of sphingolipid activation proteins. Suspected autosomal recessive mode of inheritance.[5,6,7]

Central Progressive Retinal Atrophy (CPRA): A progressive photoreceptor degeneration secondary to an underlying abnormal metabolism of Vitamin E. Progression is slow and some animals may never lose vision. Undetermined mode of inheritance. CERF does not recommend breeding any Polish Lowland Sheepdog with CPRA.[4]

Entropion and **Patent Ductus Arteriosus** are reported.[8]

Isolated Case Studies

Intracranial Medulloblastoma: A caudal fossa, cerebellar medullobastoma was identified in a Polish Lowland Sheepdog by MRI. The tumor arose laterally and extended to the surface of the cerebellar hemisphere.[9]

Genetic Tests

Tests of Genotype: None

Tests of Phenotype: Recommend hip and elbow radiographs, CERF eye examination, patella evaluation, thyroid profile including autoantibodies, and cardiac examination.

Miscellaneous

- **Breed name synonyms:** Polski Owczarek Nizinny, Valee Sheepdog, Nizinny, PON.
- **Registries:** AKC, UKC (as Polski Owczarek Nizinny), KCGB (Kennel Club of Great Britain), ANKC (Australian National Kennel Club).
- **AKC rank (year 2008):** 145 (78 dogs registered)
- **Internet resources: The American Polish Lowland Sheepdog Club:** www.aponc.org
  Canadian Polish Lowland Sheepdog Club: www.cponc.com
  Polish Lowland Sheepdog Club (UK): www.plsc.org.uk

References

1. OFA Website breed statistics: www.offa.org Last accessed July 1, 2010.
2. Nachreiner RF, Refsal KR, Graham PA, et. al.: Prevalence of serum thyroid hormone autoantibodies in dogs with clinical signs of hypothyroidism. J Am Vet Med Assoc 2002 Feb 15;220(4):466-71.
3. Nachreiner R & Refsal K: Personal communication, Diagnostic Center for Population and Animal Health, Michigan State University. April, 2007.
4. *Ocular Disorders Presumed to be Inherited in Purebred Dogs.* American College of Veterinary Ophthalmologists. ACVO, 2007.
5. Wrigstad A, Nilsson SE, Dubielzig R, et. al.: Neuronal ceroid lipofuscinosis in the Polish Owczarek Nizinny (PON) dog. A retinal study. *Doc Ophthalmol.* 1995;91(1):33-47.
6. Narfstrom K, Wrigstad A: Clinical, electrophysiological, and morphological findings in a case of neuronal ceroid lipofuscinosis in the Polish Owczarek Nizinny (PON) dog. *Vet Q.* 1995 Apr;17 Suppl 1:S46.
7. Narfström K, Wrigstad A, Ekesten B, et. al.: Neuronal ceroid lipofuscinosis: clinical and morphologic findings in nine affected Polish Owczarek Nizinny (PON) dogs. Vet Ophthalmol. 2007 Mar-Apr;10(2):111-20.
8. *The Genetic Connection: A Guide to Health Problems in Purebred Dogs.* L Ackerman. p. 231. AAHA Press, 1999.
9. McConnell JF, Platt S, Smith KC: Magnetic resonance imaging findings of an intracranial medulloblastoma in a Polish Lowland Sheepdog. *Vet Radiol Ultrasound.* 2004 Jan-Feb;45(1):17-22.
10. *The Complete Dog Book, 20th Ed.* The American Kennel Club. Howell Book House, NY 2006. p. 680-683

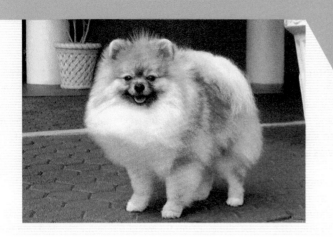

The Breed History

Pomeranians are a Spitz-type breed that originated from sled dogs in Iceland and Lapland. They were bred down from much larger dogs in Pomerania and Germany. They are similar in type to the modern Klein German Spitz. Queen Victoria brought them into the limelight in Britain.

Breeding for Function

Bred for companionship after downsizing, though early in breed development they were used for sheep herding.

Physical Characteristics

Height at Withers: 8-11" (20-28 cm)

Weight: 3-7 lb (1.5-3 kg).

Coat: Double coated, with a profuse fluffy glossy outer coat consisting of long harsh hairs, and a soft dense undercoat. Feathering includes a frill over neck and chest, and limb and tail feathering. All colors and patterns are allowed, though the red-orange coat is most popular. It takes a few years for the coat to reach full density and length.

Longevity: 15 years.

Points of Conformation: Sturdy, compact conformation, high head carriage, profusely plumed tail sits flat over the short back, expression is described as fox-like, wide set eyes are large and dark, almond shaped and set low on the skull. The top of the skull is mildly domed, and the muzzle short and fine. Ears are high and pricked, the stop well defined, nose and eyelid margins are black (or self in some colors such as blue and brown). The short neck is well muscled and the back is short. The topline is level, thorax fairly deep with well sprung ribs, limbs are straight and short, feet are compact and straight. Dewclaws are often removed. The gait is smooth, quick and active.

Recognized Behavior Issues and Traits

Traits ascribed to the breed include: Gentle temperament, very active and outgoing, alert, curious, and intelligent. Good alarm barker/watchdog. Moderate exercise requirements, good with children, some are finicky eaters, and regular grooming is needed,

Pomeranian

particularly during the shedding season. They enjoy learning games, tricks and obedience training.

Normal Physiologic Variations
None reported

Drug Sensitivities
None reported

Inherited Diseases

Patella Luxation: Polygenically inherited laxity of patellar ligaments, causing luxation, lameness, and later degenerative joint disease. Treat surgically if causing clinical signs. Dorn reports a 10.15x odds ratio in Pomeranians versus other breeds. Another study reports an 18.6x odds ratio versus other breeds. OFA reports 42.6% affected.[1,2,3]

Hip Dysplasia and Legg-Calve Perthes Disease: Polygenically inherited traits causing degenerative hip joint disease and arthritis. Too few Pomeranians have been screened by OFA to determine an accurate incidence.[1]

Elbow Dysplasia: Polygenically inherited trait causing elbow arthritis. Reported 3.7x odds ratio for ununited anconeal process form of elbow dysplasia versus other breeds. Too few Pomeranians have been screened by OFA to determine an accurate incidence.[1,3]

Patent Ductus Arteriosus (PDA): Polygenically inherited congenital heart disorder, where a fetal vessel remains open after birth, causing a mixing of oxygenated and unoxygenated blood. Affected dogs are usually stunted, and have a loud heart murmur. Diagnosis with Doppler ultrasound. Treat with surgery. Dorn reports a 10.15x odds ratio in Pomeranians versus other breeds.[2,4]

Hyperuricosuria (HUU)/Urate Bladder Stones: An autosomal recessive mutation in the SLC2A9 gene causes urate urolithiasis and can predispose male dogs to urinary obstruction. Estimated at a carrier frequency of 1.12% in the breed. A genetic test is available.[24]

Disease Predispositions

Tracheal Collapse: Caused by diminished integrity of the cartilage rings in the trachea. Can produce increased coughing, stridor, and respiratory distress, especially when excited. Usually occurs in middle-aged to older dogs. Usually poorly responsive to surgery. Many cases can be controlled medically. Dorn reports a 11.61x odds ratio for tracheal collapse versus other breeds.[2,5]

Distichiasis: Abnormally placed eyelashes that irritate the cornea and conjunctiva. Can cause secondary corneal ulceration. Identified in 5.52% of Pomeranians CERF examined by veterinary ophthalmologists between 2000-2005.[6]

Persistent Pupillary Membranes: Strands of fetal remnant connecting; iris to iris, cornea, lens, or involving sheets of tissue. The later three forms can impair vision, and dogs affected with these forms should not be bred. Identified in 3.31% of Pomeranians CERF examined by veterinary ophthalmologists between 2000-2005.[6]

Cataracts: Anterior and posterior cortex punctate and intermediate cataracts predominate in the breed. Identified in 2.76% of Pomeranians CERF examined by veterinary ophthalmologists between 2000-2005. CERF does not recommend breeding any Pomeranian with a cataract.[6]

Hypothyroidism: Inherited autoimmune thyroiditis. 2.5% positive for thyroid autoantibodies based on testing at Michigan State University. (Ave. for all breeds is 7.5%).[7,8]

Alopecia-X (Black Skin Disease, BSD, Coat Funk, Severe Hair Loss, SHL): Progressive, symmetrical, non-pruritic, truncal hair loss usually beginning in early adulthood. ACTH stimulation test, low-dose dexamethazone suppression test, and thyroid panel results are normal. Urinary corticoid:creatinine ratio may be normal to elevated. Elevated blood concentrations of 17-hydroxypro-gesterone (17-OHP) have been seen post ACTH stimulation. Oral trilostane reverses the condition in some cases. The disorder appears familial, with a male predilection.[9,10,11]

Chronic Valvular Heart Disease: Heart failure due to valvular insufficiency, usually involving the mitral valve. Treat with heart medications. Pomeranians have a high odds ratio for chronic valvular disease versus other breeds.[12]

Vitreous Degeneration: A liquefaction of the vitreous gel which may predispose to retinal detachment resulting in blindness. Identified in 1.66% of Pomeranians CERF examined by veterinary ophthalmologists between 2000-2005.[6]

Progressive Retinal Atrophy (PRA): Inherited degeneration of the retina resulting in blindness. Unknown mode of inheritance in this breed. Generalized or suspicious PRA was identified in 1.66% of Pomeranians CERF examined by veterinary ophthalmologists between 2000-2005.[6]

Hydrocephalus: Congenital increased volume of cerebrospinal fluid (CSF), with a concurrent dilation of the ventricular system and reduction of brain tissue. Can have an associated open fontanel. Can cause behavior changes, visual defects, impaired motor function, or seizures.[13]

Necrotizing Meningoencephalitis: Affected dogs have clinical signs of recurrent seizures and progressive abnormal gait and behavior, which do not respond to treatment. At necropsy, histopathological features of the inflammatory lesions are consistent with necrotizing meningoencephalitis and resembled those described as Pug dog encephalitis.[14,15]

Atlantoaxial Subluxation: Subluxation of the atlantoaxial joint is seen at an increased frequency in the breed. It can occur subsequent to a variety of lesions of the dens or atlantoaxial ligaments. In each case, dorsal displacement of the axis results in compression of the cervical spinal cord, resulting in ataxia or paresis.[16,17]

Cryptorchidism, Cyclic Hematopoeisis, Deafness, Entropion, **Globoid Cell Leukodystrophy, Intervertebral Disk Disease, Oligodontia, Prognathism,** and **Sebaceous Adenitis** are reported.[18]

Isolated Case Studies

Vitamin D-Resistant Rickets: A female Pomeranian was followed from 2 to 8.5 months of age with low Vitamin D levels, progressive hypocalcemia, secondary hyperparathyroidism, hypomineralization and fracture of bones, rickets, and alopecia that was not responsive to Vitamin D supplementation. An autosomal recessive mutation was identified in the vitamin D receptor gene.[19]

Congenital Methemoglobinemia: A six-month-old Pomeranian was referred for evaluation of cyanosis, occurring since it was acquired at six weeks of age. Blood assays diagnosed methemoglo-binemia due to deficiency of methemoglobin reductase enzyme.[20]

Occipital Dysplasia: Congenital malformation of the foramen magnum was diagnosed in a 4-year-old Pomeranian dog, causing caudal displacement of the cerebellum and hydrocephalus.[21]

Hydrocephalus and Secondary Syringomyelia: A 7-year-old spayed female Pomeranian with a 6-month history of progressive paraparesis was determined to have syringomyelia secondary to hydrocephalus. Magnetic resonance imaging clearly revealed severe syringomyelia in the cervical portion of the spinal cord, which was directly connected to the marked dilated fourth ventricle. Laminectomy provided partial amelioration of clinical signs, without further deterioration.[22]

Genetic Tests

Tests of Genotype: Direct tests for black, brown and red (cream and orange) coat colors, and black and brown nose are available from HealthGene and VetGen.

Direct test for HUU is available from the UC-Davis VGL and the Animal Health Trust

Tests of Phenotype: CHIC Certification: Required testing includes CERF eye examination, congenital cardiac examination (with re-evaluation between 3 and 5 years of age), and patella evaluation. Optional recommended testing includes hip radiographs and thyroid profile including autoantibodies. (See CHIC website; www.caninehealthinfo.org).

Recommend elbow radiographs.

Miscellaneous

- **Breed name synonyms:** Pom, LouLou, Zwergspitz, Dwarf Spitz
- **Registries:** AKC, UKC, CKC, KCGB (Kennel Club of Great Britain), ANKC (Australian National Kennel Club), NKC (National Kennel Club)
- **AKC rank (year 2008):** 13 (13,215 dogs registered)
- **Internet resources: American Pomeranian Club Inc.:** http://americanpomeranianclub.org
  The Pomeranian Club of Canada: www.pcoc.net
  The Pomeranian Club (UK): www.thepomeranianclub.co.uk

References

1. OFA Website breed statistics: www.offa.org Last accessed July 1, 2010.
2. Dorn CR: Canine breed-specific risks of frequently diagnosed diseases at

veterinary teaching hospitals. Monograph. AKC Canine Health Foundation. 2000.

3. LaFond E, Breur GJ & Austin CC: Breed susceptibility for developmental orthopedic diseases in dogs. J Am Anim Hosp Assoc. 2002 Sep-Oct;38(5):467-77.

4. Ackerman N, Burk R, Hahn AW, et. al.: Patent ductus arteriosus in the dog: a retrospective study of radiographic, epidemiologic, and clinical findings. Am J Vet Res. 1978 Nov;39(11):1805-10.

5. Buback JL, Boothe HW, Hobson HP: Surgical treatment of tracheal collapse in dogs: 90 cases (1983-1993). J Am Vet Med Assoc. 1996 Feb 1;208(3):380-4.

6. *Ocular Disorders Presumed to be Inherited in Purebred Dogs.* American College of Veterinary Ophthalmologists. ACVO, 2007.

7. Nachreiner RF, Refsal KR, Graham PA, et. al.: Prevalence of serum thyroid hormone autoantibodies in dogs with clinical signs of hypothyroidism. J Am Vet Med Assoc 2002 Feb 15;220(4):466-71.

8. Nachreiner R & Refsal K: Personal communication, Diagnostic Center for Population and Animal Health, Michigan State University. April, 2007.

9. Cerundolo R, Lloyd DH, Persechino A, et. al: Treatment of canine Alopecia X with trilostane. Vet Dermatol. 2004 Oct;15(5):285-93.

10. Schmeitzel LP, Lothrop CD Jr: Hormonal abnormalities in Pomeranians with normal coat and in Pomeranians with growth hormone-responsive dermatosis. J Am Vet Med Assoc. 1990 Nov 15;197(10):1333-41.

11. Cerundolo R, Lloyd DH, Vaessen MM, et. al.: Alopecia in pomeranians and miniature poodles in association with high urinary corticoid:creatinine ratios and resistance to glucocorticoid feedback. Vet Rec. 2007 Mar 24;160(12):393-7.

12. Petric AD, Hozjan E & Blejec A: Chronic Valvular Disease. Proceedings, 17th ECVIM-CA Congress. 2007.

13. Axlund TW: Managing the Hydrocephalic Patient: Medical and Surgical Options. Proceedings, 2004 Atlantic Coast Veterinary Conference. 2004.

14. Pedersen NC, Vernau K, Dickinson P, et. al.: DLA Association in Various Toy Breeds with Immune Mediated Encephalopathies. Proceedings, 2009 Tufts' Canine and Feline Breeding and Genetics Conference. 2009.

15. Matsuki N, Takahashi M, Yaegashi M, et. al.: Serial examinations of anti-GFAP autoantibodies in cerebrospinal fluids in canine necrotizing meningoencephalitis. J Vet Med Sci. 2009 Jan;71(1):99-100.

16. McCarthy RJ, Lewis DD, Hosgood G: Atlantoaxial Subluxation in Dogs. Compend Contin Educ Pract Vet 1995: 17[2]:215-226.

17. Denny HR, Gibbs C, Waterman A: Atlanto-axial subluxation in the dog : A review of thirty cases and an evaluation of treatment by lag screw fixation. J Small Anim Pract 1988: 29[1]:37-47.

18. The Genetic Connection: A Guide to Health Problems in Purebred Dogs. L Ackerman. p. 231-32. AAHA Press, 1999.

19. LeVine DN, Zhou Y, Ghiloni RJ, et. al.: Hereditary 1,25-dihydroxyvitamin D-resistant rickets in a Pomeranian dog caused by a novel mutation in the vitamin D receptor gene. J Vet Intern Med. 2009 Nov-Dec;23(6):1278-83.

20. Fine DM, Eyster GE, Anderson LK, et. al.: Cyanosis and congenital methemoglobinemia in a puppy. J Am Anim Hosp Assoc. 1999 Jan-Feb;35(1):33-5.

21. van Herpen H, Voorhout G: Occipital dysplasia in a Pomeranian dog. Tijdschr Diergeneeskd. 1993 May 15;118(10):327-8.

22. Itoh T, Nishimura R, Matsunaga S, et. al.: Syringomyelia and hydrocephalus in a dog. J Am Vet Med Assoc. 1996 Sep 1;209(5):934-6.

23. The Complete Dog Book, 20th Ed. The American Kennel Club. Howell Book House, NY 2006. p. 499-502.

24. Karmi N, Brown EA, Hughes SS, et. al.: Estimated frequency of the canine hyperuricosuria mutation in different dog breeds. J Vet Intern Med. 2010 Nov-Dec;24(6):1337-42.

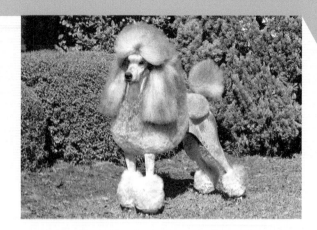

Poodle

The Breed History

"Poodle" likely derives from *Pudel*, a German term describing one who plays and splashes in water or puddles. The exact lines of genetic origin are obscured, but ancient breeds such as the Irish water spaniel, Rough haired water dog and others contribute to the type, and perhaps the first of the smaller types of poodles originated by crosses with terrier type for use in truffle hunting. German history records poodle type dogs in the 15th century. The toy version of poodle first widely entered the history record in the 18th century. Very early records in the Mediterranean place poodle type dogs in the first century. Though often referred to as the French poodle, the breed is not though to have originated there. AKC recognition occurred in 1887.

Breeding for Function

Originally these dogs were bred as gundogs for waterfowl hunting, as a water retriever. The origins of the fancy coat clips trace back to early times when the hunters clipped the bulk of the dog coat so that they would dry quickly, and to minimize the weight of the wet hair for ease of swimming, but they left fur over bony prominences to help insulate joints from the cold. In France, the dog was also used extensively as a circus dog. Toy, miniature, and standard poodles are all popular as companion dogs, and the smaller types were bred down in size from the standard; it was the larger standard poodle that was originally used for hunting. Guide dogs, therapy dogs, police work and obedience and agility competitions round out some of their modern functions.

Physical Characteristics

All three types share the same breed standard, only the size and weight varies between the three.

Toy

Height at Withers: female up to 10" (25.4 cm), male up to 10" (25.4 cm)
Weight: females 6-9 lb (2.5-4 kg), males 6-9 lb (2.5-4 kg).

Miniature

Height at Withers: female 10-15" (25.5-38 cm), male 10-15" (25.5-38 cm)
Miniature Weight: females 15-17 lb (7-8 kg), males 15-17 lb (7-8 kg).

Standard

Height at Withers: female 15 " (38 cm) or more, male 15" (38 cm) or more.
Standard Weight: females 45-60 lb (20-27 kg), males 45-70 lb (20-32 kg).

Coat: All solid colors accepted (e.g., apricot, black, gray, silver, blue, café-au-lait, cream) and the coat is dense, wiry and curly. If left unclipped, it tends to form ringlets (cording) and waves. There are specific clips used in show, and their coat is a distinguishing breed feature.

Longevity: 12-15 years. The smaller types may reach 15-17 years on average.

Points of Conformation: A long face, with medium-sized and leathered triangular ears lying flat, and wide, almond-shaped dark brown eyes, a slight stop, and fairly narrow muzzle typify the poodle head. They possess a level topline, feet are compact and webbed, and they have straight limbs with the dewclaws generally removed. Tails are usually docked to one half length, and they are proportioned to be as high as they are long. Their gait is lively and elastic, and they move straight.

Recognized Behavior Issues and Traits

Extreme intelligence, sociability, and excellent trainability are well known poodle traits. Very lively, they do tend to bark, and need to be socialized to other pets and people or else they can potentially be nippy. They need close human companionship and tend to be aloof with strangers. They are good alarm barkers.The poodles require regular clip and grooming (every 6-8 weeks), and are low shedding and low allergy dogs. They tend to need more frequent dental care. They do well in town or country and need moderate levels of exercise. They are high activity around the house, though the standard poodles are often less active indoors.

Normal Physiologic Variations

Echocardiographic Normal Values for Miniature Poodles:[1]	
Parameter	Median (Range)
Weight (kg)	3 (1.4-9)
Heart rate (bpm)	150 (100-200)
LVPWD (mm)	5 (4-6)
LVPWS (mm)	8 (6-10)
LVD (mm)	20 (16-28)
LVS (mm)	10 (8-16)
FS (%)	47 (35-57)
EPSS (mm)	0 (0-2)
RVd (mm)	4 (2-9)
IVSd (mm)	5 (4-6)
IVSs (mm)	8 (6-10)
AOD (mm)	10 (8-13)
LAS (mm)	12 (8-18)
N	20

LVPWD, LV posterior wall dimension at end-diastole; LVPWS, LV posterior wall thickness at end-systole; LVD, LV chamber dimension at end-diastole; LVS, LV chamber dimension at end-systole; FS, percent fractional shortening; EPSS, E-point septal separation; RVD, RV chamber dimension at end-diastole; IVSd, interventricular septal thickness at end-diastole; IVSs, interventricular septal thickness at end-systole; AOD, aortic root at end-diastole; LAS, left atrium at end-systole; N, number of animals.

Drug Sensitivities
None Reported

Inherited Diseases
Hip Dysplasia: Polygenically inherited trait causing degenerative joint disease and hip arthritis. OFA reports 12.3% affected.[2]

Patella Luxation: Polygenically inherited laxity of patellar ligaments, causing luxation, lameness, and later degenerative joint disease. Treat surgically if causing clinical signs. Reported 9.7x odds ratio in Toy Poodles, 4.1x odds ratio in Miniature Poodles, and 3.2x odds ratio in Standard Poodles versus other breeds. OFA reports 4.4% affected.[2,3]

Progressive Retinal Atrophy (PRA): Autosomal recessive progressive rod cone degeneration (prcd) form seen in Minature and Toy Poodles. Age of onset between 3-8 years of age, eventually causing blindness. Optigen reports 3% testing affected, and 28% testing carrier in Miniature Poodles, and 5% testing affected, and 29% testing carrier in Toy Poodles. Dorn reports a 9.71x odds ratio versus other breeds. A genetic test is available.[4,5,6,7,8]

Elbow Dysplasia: Polygenically inherited trait causing elbow arthritis. OFA reports 2.8% affected.[2]

Legg-Perthes Disease: Polygenically inherited aseptic necrosis of the femoral head seen in Toy and Miniature Poodles. Causes degenerative joint disease and hip arthritis. Usually presents unilaterally. Reported 22.4x odds ratio in Toy Poodles, and 12.1x odds ratio in Miniature Poodles for Legg-Calve-Perthes versus other breeds. OFA reports 1.0% affected.[2,3,9]

von Willebrand's Disease Type 1 (vWD): Autosomal recessive genetic disorder causing a mild bleeding syndrome. A direct genetic test is available from VetGen, reporting 1% affected, and 9% carrier in the breed.[10]

Hypoadrenocorticism (Addison's disease): Controlled by a major autosomal recessive gene, but not a simple recessive disorder. Immune mediated destruction of the adrenal gland seen in Standard Poodles. Typical presentation of lethargy, poor appetite, vomiting, weakness, and dehydration occuring from 4 months to several years of age. Can also present with painful muscle cramping. Treatment with DOCA injections or oral fludrocortisone. Heritabililty of 0.75 in the breed. No genetic test is available.[11,12,13,14]

Neonatal Encephalopathy: Rare, autosomal recessive disorder causing poor growth, ataxia, whole body tremor, and tonic-clonic seizures between 1-5 weeks of age. A genetic test is available.[15]

Mucopolysaccharidosis VI (MPS VI): PennGen reports MPS VI identified in the Miniature and Toy Poodle. This is an autosomal recessive disorder causing skeletal deformities, including defects in the sternum, vertebrae and particularly the hip joints. To varying degrees they may also experience corneal cloudiness and facial dysmorphia. A genetic test is available.

Disease Predispositions
Gastric Dilation/Volvulus (GDV, Bloat): Life-threatening twisting of the stomach within the abdomen. Requires immediate veterinary attention. There is a 25.3% lifetime risk of developing GDV in Standard Poodles, with 6.3% of all Standard Poodles dying from the condition.[16,17,18]

Epiphora: Ocular tear drainage with hair staining is reportedly a common occurrence in Toy Poodles. Can occur secondary to medial canthal trichiasis and/or entropion. Treat by keeping hair clipped short, and daily cleaning. Medial canthoplasty is curative in severe cases.[19]

Distichiasis: Abnormally placed eyelashes that irritate the cornea and conjunctiva. Can cause secondary corneal ulceration. Identified in 11.72% of Toy Poodles, 9.08% of Miniature Poodles, and 1.04% of Standard Poodles CERF examined by veterinary ophthalmologists between 2000-2005.[5]

Cataracts: Cortical and nuclear cataracts predominate in the breed. Reported at a frequency of 10.79% in Miniature Poodles, 10.21% in Toy Poodles, and 7.00% in Standard Poodles. Reported at a frequency of 13.8% in Toy Poodles in Brazil. Dorn reports a 3.10x odds ratio in Standard Poodles versus other breeds. One study showed a 6.1x odds ratio for Toy Poodles, and a 4.3x odds ratio for Miniature Poodles versus other breeds. Mean age at onset of 9.6 years in Miniature and Toy Pooodles. Identified in 3.95% of Toy Poodles, 3.63% of Standard Poodles, and 2.82% of Miniature Poodles CERF examined by veterinary ophthalmologists between 2000-2005. CERF does not recommend breeding any Poodle with a cataract.[4,5,20,21,22,23]

Periodontal Disease: Miniature and Toy Poodles are found to be predisposed to periodontal disease and tooth loss.[24]

Persistent Pupillary Membranes: Strands of fetal remnant connecting; iris to iris, cornea, lens, or involving sheets of tissue. The later three forms can impair vision, and dogs affected with these forms should not be bred. Identified in 5.54% of Miniature Poodles, 4.12% of Toy Poodles, and 2.08% of Standard Poodles CERF examined by veterinary ophthalmologists between 2000-2005.[5]

Bronchiectasis: Clinical signs of chronic cough with excessive airway mucous. Diagnosis with radiographs. Reported at a frequency of 5.2% and an odds ratio of 2.99x in the Miniature Poodle, and a frequency of 2.4% and an odds ratio of 1.83x in the Toy Poodle versus other breeds. Treatment is with bronchodilators and possibly corticosteroids.[25]

Hypothyroidism: Inherited autoimmune thyroiditis. 4.2% positive for thyroid autoantibodies based on testing at Michigan State University. (Ave. for all breeds is 7.5).[26,27]

Otitis Externa (Chronic Ear Infection): Bacterial, yeast, or mixed infections. Miniature Poodles are one of the breeds with the highest incidence. In one study, 39.29% of dogs with Malassezia (yeast) ear infection were Poodles.[28,29]

Tracheal Collapse: Seen in Toy and Miniature Poodles. Causes persistent "honking" cough, especially when excited. Dorn reports a 5.92x odds ratio for tracheal collapse versus other breeds. Usually occurs in middle-aged to older dogs. Usually poorly responsive to surgery. Many cases can be controlled medically.[4,30]

Mitral Valve Disease (MVD): Elderly Miniature and Toy Poodles are prone to mitral valvular regurgitation, at an average age of 9.8 years. Can lead to **congestive heart disease**, cardiac arrhythmias (irregular heartbeats) and cardiac failure. Treat with heart drugs.[31]

Cryptorchidism (Retained Testicles): Can be unilateral or bilateral. Reported at an increased frequency in all three varieties of Poodle; with a significant risk in Toy Poodles, moderate risk in Miniature Poodles, and increased risk in Standard Poodles versus other breeds.[32]

Atrial Septal Defect (ASD): Limited echocardiographic screening of Standard Poodles show approximately 5% affected with an ostium secundum atrial septal defect. Some families have up to 40% of dogs affected. If small, an ASD may not produce clinical disease. Medium to large ASD have hemodynamically significant left to right shunting resulting in right atrial and ventricular enlargement and clinical signs of heart failure. Screen with Doppler echocardiography. Undetermined mode of inheritance.[33,34]

Sebaceous Adenitis: Disorder of immune mediated sebaceous gland destruction, presenting with hair loss, hyperkeratosis and seborrhoea, usually beginning with the dorsal midline and ears. Diagnosis by skin biopsy. Treat with isotretinoin. An autosomal recessive mode of inheritance is suspected. Poodles are reported at a frequency of 0.9% in Sweden. OFA reports 2.8% affected.[2,35,36]

Idiopathic Epilepsy: Inherited Seizures can be generalized or partial seizures. In a study of one family, 93% had focal-onset seizures with a median age of onset of 3.7 years, an equal sex ratio, and a possible simple autosomal mode of inheritance. In Standard Poodles, 17.1% start as generalized seizures, and 68.3% begin as partial seizures (with the rest mixed) at a mean age of 2.8 years. 81% of affected Standard Poodles progress to generalized seizures. Control with anticonvulsant medications.[37,38]

Diabetes Mellitus: Caused by a lack of insulin production by the pancreas. Controlled by insulin injections, diet, and glucose monitoring. Miniature Poodles have an odds ratio of 4.01x, and Toy Poodles have an odds ratio of 3.27x versus other breeds.[39]

Hyperadrenocorticism (Cushing's disease): Hyperfunction of the adrenal gland caused by a pituitary or adrenal tumor. Clinical signs may include increased thirst and urination, symmetrical truncal alopecia, and abdominal distention. Reported at an increased frequency in Poodles, representing 38.14% of all cases. Dorn reports a 2.72x odds ratio versus other breeds.[4,40,41]

Secondary Glaucoma: Increased intraocular pressure and blindness can occur after cataract formation, lens luxation (predominantly Miniature Poodles), hyphema (predominantly Toy Poodles), or uveitis (predominantly Standard Poodles). One report found an odds ratio of 4.7x for secondary glaucoma in Poodles.[42,43]

Vitreous Degeneration: A liquefaction of the vitreous gel which may predispose to retinal detachment and/or glaucoma. Identified in 1.85% of Toy Poodles CERF examined by veterinary ophthalmologists between 2000-2005.[5]

Primary (Narrow Angle) Glaucoma: Ocular condition causing increased pressure within the eyeball, and secondary blindness due to damage to the retina. Diagnose with tonometry and gonioscopy. Diagnosed in 1.68% of Miniature Poodles, 1.20% of Toy Poodles, and 0.73% of Standard Poodles presented to veterinary teaching hospitals. CERF does not recommend breeding any Poodle with glaucoma.[5,44]

Patent Ductus Arteriosus (PDA): Polygenically inherited congenital heart disorder; affected dogs are usually stunted, and have a loud heart murmur. Diagnosis is via Doppler ultrasound. Treatment is surgical. Miniature and Toy Poodles have an increased incidence versus other breeds.[45]

Calcium Oxalate Urolithiasis: Miniature and Toy Poodles have a predisposition to develop calcium oxalate bladder stones, with a 3.85x odds ratio versus other breeds.[46]

Lens Induced Uveitis: Occurs secondary to cataract formation. 35% of all cases are in Toy and Miniature Poodles, with a mean age of 9.0 years. One-third of cases are bilateral. Can progress to glaucoma.[47]

Juvenile Renal Disease: Young Standard Poodles can develop a progressive renal dysfunction. Typically presents with increased drinking and urination, weight loss or unthriftiness, consistently dilute urine, and elevated kidney blood tests. Late in the disease, affected dogs can leak urinary protein, have non-regenerative anemia, and fibrous osteodystrophy. Onset from weeks of age to over a year in age. Some dogs remain with mild signs, while others rapidly progress to kidney failure. Unknown mode of inheritance. Diagnosis by kidney biopsy or pathology.[48]

Mammary Gland Osteosarcoma: Female Miniature Poodles have predisposition to develop this malignant cancer, with an odds ratio of 2.7x versus other breeds.[49]

Alopecia-X/ Hyperadrenocorticism Associated with Sex Steroid Excess (Black Skin Disease, BSD, Coat Funk, Severe Hair Loss, SHL): Miniature Poodles are overrepresented. Progressive, symmetrical, non-pruritic, truncal hair loss usually beginning in early adulthood. ACTH stimulation test, low-dose dexamethazone suppression test, and thyroid panel results are normal. Alkaline phosphatase and ALT are elevated. Urinary corticoid:creatinine ratio may be normal to elevated. Elevated blood concentrations of 17-hydroxyprogesterone (17-OHP) have been seen post ACTH stimulation. Oral trilostane reverses the condition in some cases. The disorder appears familial, with a male predilection.[50,51,52]

Dilated Cardiomyopathy: Can present with ventricular arrhythmias, leading to cardiac dilation and heart failure. Increased incidence reported in Standard Poodles. There is a two to one ratio of affected males to females.[53]

Perineal Hernia: Miniature Poodles have a predisposition to developing perineal hernias. Treatment is surgery.[54]

Optic Nerve Hypoplasia/Micropapilla: Failure of development of the optic nerve. Identified in 0.90% of Miniature Poodles CERF examined by veterinary ophthalmologists between 2000-2005. CERF does not recommend breeding any Poodle with the condition.[5]

Digital Squamous Cell Carcinoma (SCC): Subungual squamous cell carcinoma occurs at increased frequency in black dogs. Treat with digital amputation. Standard Poodles account for 14.3% of all cases.[55]

Shoulder Instability: In a one study, the most frequent breed was Standard Poodles, representing 13% of all cases. Clinical signs included pain and muscle atrophy. Surgerical stabilization provided the best outcome.[56]

Lingual Squamous Cell Carcinoma (SCC): Poodles have a 4.61x odds ratio versus other breeds of developing this cancer. Females are overrepresented in one study.[57]

Degenerative Myelopathy (DM): Identified as a rare disorder in Standard Poodles, though Miniature Poodles have also been pathologically diagnosed. Affected dogs show an insidious onset of upper motor neuron (UMN) paraparesis at an average age of 11.4 years. The disease eventually progresses to severe tetraparesis. Affected dogs have normal results on myelography, MRI, and CSF analysis. Necropsy confirms the condition. Unknown mode of inheritance. A direct genetic test for an autosomal recessive DM susceptibility gene is available from OFA showing 17% carrier and 1% homozygous genes "at risk" in Poodles. All affected dogs are homozygous for the gene, however, only a small percentage of homozygous dogs develop DM.[2,58]

Atresia Ani (Imperforate Anus): An increased incidence of this congenital condition is reported in Miniature and Toy Poodles, with a frequency of 0.02%, and an odds ratio of 4.28x. Treatment is surgery.[59]

Polymicrogyria: Affected Standard Poodles present between 7 weeks and 4 months of age with clinical signs that can include blindness, behavior changes, hypermetric gait, complex partial motor seizures, delayed proprioceptive hopping, and resting nystagmus. (1/5), and decreased pupillary light response. Some dogs also demonstrated progressive aggression toward the owner. EEG readings were abnormal. Imaging, and gross and histological examination revealed polymicrogyria that variously involved the occipital, temporal, or entire cerebral lobes of the brain. Undetermined mode of inheritance.[60,61]

Allergic Inhalant Dermatitis, Anterior Crossbite, Base-Narrow Canines, Brachygnathism, Cerebellar Abiotrophy, Ceroid Lipofuscinosis, Corneal Dystrophy, Cystinuria, Deafness, Entropion, Factor VIII Deficiency, Factor XII Deficiency, Fibrinoid Leukodystrophy, Globoid Cell Leukodystrophy, Growth Hormone Responsive Dermatosis, Hemeralopia, Hydrocephalus, Ichthyosis, Intervertebral Disc Disease, Keratoconjunctivits Sicca, Lafora Body Disease, Leukodystrophy Lymphedemamacrocytosis/ Dyshematopoiesis, Methemaglobin Reductase Deficiency, Microphthalmia, Osteogenesis Imperfecta, Narcolepsy,
Nodular Panniculitis, Oligodontia, Pancreatitis, Prognathism, Prolapsed Nictitans, Proliferative Episcleritis, Prekallikrein Deficiency, Pseudohermaphrodism, Retinal Dysplasia, Shoulder Osteochondritis Dessicans, Sphingomyelinosis, Tetralogy of Fallot, Vertebral Stenosis, and **Wry Mouth** are reported.[62]

Isolated Case Studies

Chronic Hepatitis: Three related Standard Poodles with chronic liver disease were pathologically diagnosed with lobular dissecting hepatitis.[63]

Nonspherocytic Hemolytic Anemia: A family of Miniature Poodles developed nonspherocytic hemolytic anemia, marked reticulocytosis, hepatosplenomegaly, hemosiderosis of reticuloendothelial organs, bone marrow myelofibrosis, and osteosclerosis by 1 year of age. The disease was fatal by 3 years of age. A pathogenesis was not determined.[64]

Congenital Ectodermal Defect: X-linked recessive disorder reported in male Miniature Poodle siblings. Affected dogs are born without hair (hypotrichosis), have a reduced number or absence of sweat glands, and missing or malformed teeth.[65,66]

Amelogenesis Imperfecta/Familial Enamel Defect: A multi-generational family of Standard Poodles in Sweden was identified with discolored teeth due to enamel malformation. Defective enamel mineralization was documented histologically.[67]

Junctional Epidermolysis Bullosa: A newborn Toy Poodle developed vesicles and bullae on the pads of the feet, oral mucous membranes, and skin if the ventral abdomen. The lesions progressed rapidly, and the pup was euthanized on day 2.[68]

Genetic Tests

Tests of Genotype: Direct test for pcrd-PRA is available from Optigen.

Direct test for von Willebrand's disease (vWD) is available from VetGen

Direct test for neonatal encephalopathy is available from the OFA.

A direct test for an autosomal recessive DM susceptibility gene is available from the OFA.

Direct test for MPS is available from PennGen.

Direct tests for black, brown, cream, white, red, and apricot coat colors, and black and brown nose are available from HealthGene and VetGen.

Tests of Phenotype: Miniature Poodles: CHIC Certification: Required testing includes hip radiographs, CERF eye examination, direct test for prcd-PRA, and patella evaluation. (See CHIC website; www.caninehealthinfo.org).

Recommend thyroid profile including autoantibodies, elbow radiographs, and cardiac evaluation.

Standard Poodles: CHIC Certification: Required testing includes hip radiographs, CERF eye examination, and one of the following: thyroid profile including autoantibodies, biopsy for sebaceous adenitis, or cardiac evaluation including echocardiogram. (See CHIC website; www.caninehealthinfo.org).

Recommend elbow radiographs and patella evaluation.

Toy Poodles: CHIC Certification: Required testing includes CERF eye examination, patella evaluation, and direct test for prcd-PRA. (See CHIC website; www.caninehealthinfo.org).

Recommend hip and elbow radiographs, thyroid profile including autoantibodies, and cardiac evaluation.

Miscellaneous

- **Breed name synonyms:** Pudel, Toy Poodle, Caniche, Chien Canne, Standard Poodle. Barbone, French duck dog, French Poodle, Toy Poodle, Miniature Poodle.
- **Registries:** AKC, UKC, CKC, KCGB (Kennel Club of Great Britain), ANKC(Australian National Kennel Club), NKC (National Kennel Club)
- **AKC rank (year 2008):** 9 (21,545 dogs registered)
- **Internet resources: The Poodle Club of America:**
  www.poodleclubofamerica.org
  Poodle Club of Canada: www.poodleclubcanada.com
  The Standard Poodle Club (UK): http://standardpoodleclub.com
  The Miniature Poodle Club (UK):
  www.miniaturepoodleclub.org.uk

References

1. Morrison SA, Moise NS, Scarlett JM, et al: Effect of breed and body weight on echocardiographic values of four breeds of dogs of differing weight and somatotype. *J Vet Intern Med.* 1992; 6:220.
2. OFA Website breed statistics: www.offa.org Last accessed July 1, 2010.
3. LaFond E, Breur GJ & Austin CC: Breed susceptibility for developmental orthopedic diseases in dogs. J Am Anim Hosp Assoc. 2002 Sep-Oct;38(5):467-77.
4. Dorn CR: Canine breed-specific risks of frequently diagnosed diseases at veterinary teaching hospitals. Monograph. AKC Canine Health Foundation. 2000.
5. *Ocular Disorders Presumed to be Inherited in Purebred Dogs.* American College of Veterinary Ophthalmologists. ACVO, 2007.
6. Morris Animal Foundation: Morris Animal Foundation Update: Genetic Tests Focus on Breed-Specific Vision Problems. Canine Pract 1999:24[4]:21.
7. Acland GM, Halloran-Blanton S, Boughman JA, et. al.: Segregation distortion in inheritance of progressive rod cone degeneration (prcd) in miniature poodle dogs. Am J Med Genet. 1990 Mar;35(3):354-9.
8. Zangerl B, Goldstein O, Philp AR, et. al.: Identical mutation in a novel retinal gene causes progressive rod-cone degeneration in dogs and retinitis pigmentosa in humans. Genomics. 2006 Nov;88(5):551-63.
9. Pidduck H & Webbon PM: The genetic control of Perthes' disease in toy poodles--a working hypothesis. J Small Anim Pract. 1978 Dec;19(12):729-33.
10. Dodd WJ: Bleeding Disorders in Animals. Proceedings, 2005 World Small Animal Veterinary Association World Congress. 2005.
11. Famula TR, Belanger JM, Oberbauer AM, et. al.: Heritability and complex segregation analysis of hypoadrenocorticism in the standard poodle. J Small Anim Pract. 2003 Jan;44(1):8-12.
12. Saito M, Olby NJ, Obledo L, et. al.: Muscle cramps in two standard poodles with hypoadrenocorticism. J Am Anim Hosp Assoc. 2002 Sep-Oct;38(5):437-43.
13. Peterson ME, Kintzer PP, Kass PH: Pretreatment clinical and laboratory findings in dogs with hypoadrenocorticism: 225 cases (1979-1993). J Am Vet Med Assoc. 1996 Jan 1;208(1):85-91.
14. Shaker E, Hurvitz AI & Peterson ME: Hypoadrenocorticism in a family of Standard poodles. J Am Vet Med Assoc. 1988 Apr 15;192(8):1091-2.
15. Chen X, Johnson GS, Schnabel RD, et. al.: A neonatal encephalopathy with seizures in standard poodle dogs with a missense mutation in the canine ortholog of ATF2. Neurogenetics. 2008 Feb;9(1):41-9.
16. Ward MP, Patronek GJ, Glickman LT: Benefits of prophylactic gastropexy for dogs at risk of gastric dilatation-volvulus. Prev Vet Med. 2003 Sep 12;60(4):319-29.
17. Glickman LT, Glickman NW, Schellenberg DB, et. al.: Incidence of and breed-related risk factors for gastric dilatation-volvulus in dogs. J Am Vet Med Assoc. 2000 Jan 1;216(1):40-5.
18. Brockman DJ, Washabau RJ, Drobatz KJ, et. al.: Canine gastric dilatation/volvulus syndrome in a veterinary critical care unit: 295 cases (1986-1992). J Am Vet Med Assoc. 1995 Aug 15;207(4):460-4.
19. Yi NY, Park SA, Jeong MB, et. al.: Medial canthoplasty for epiphora in dogs: a retrospective study of 23 cases. J Am Anim Hosp Assoc. 2006 Nov-Dec;42(6):435-9.
20. Adkins EA, Hendrix DV: Outcomes of dogs presented for cataract evaluation: a retrospective study. J Am Anim Hosp Assoc. 2005 Jul-Aug;41(4):235-40.
21. Gelatt KN, Mackay EO: Prevalence of primary breed-related cataracts in the dog in North America. Vet Ophthalmol. 2005 Mar-Apr;8(2):101-11.
22. Baumworcel N, Soares AM, Helms G, et. al.: Three hundred and three dogs with cataracts seen in Rio de Janeiro, Brazil. Vet Ophthalmol. 2009 Sep-Oct;12(5):299-301.
23. Park SA, Yi NY, Jeong MB, et. al.: Clinical manifestations of cataracts in small breed dogs. Vet Ophthalmol. 2009 Jul-Aug;12(4):205-10.
24. Hoffmann T & Gaengler P: Epidemiology of periodontal disease in poodles. J Small Anim Pract. 1996 Jul;37(7):309-16.
25. Hawkins EC, Basseches J, Berry CR, et. al.: Demographic, clinical, and radiographic features of bronchiectasis in dogs: 316 cases (1988-2000). J Am Vet Med Assoc. 2003 Dec 1;223(11):1628-35.
26. Nachreiner RF, Refsal KR, Graham PA, et. al.: Prevalence of serum thyroid hormone autoantibodies in dogs with clinical signs of hypothyroidism. *J Am Vet Med Assoc* 2002 Feb 15;220(4):466-71.
27. Nachreiner R & Refsal K: Personal communication, Diagnostic Center for Population and Animal Health, Michigan State University. April, 2007.
28. Girão MD, Prado MR, Brilhante RS, et. al.: Malassezia pachydermatis isolated from normal and diseased external ear canals in dogs: a comparative analysis. Vet J. 2006 Nov;172(3):544-8.
29. Baba E & Fukata T: Incidence of otitis externa in dogs and cats in Japan. Vet Rec. 1981 May 2;108(18):393-5.
30. Buback JL, Boothe HW, Hobson HP: Surgical treatment of tracheal collapse in dogs: 90 cases (1983-1993). J Am Vet Med Assoc. 1996 Feb 1;208(3):380-4.
31. Serfass P, Chetboul V,Sampedrano CC, et. al.: Retrospective Study of 942 Small-Sized Dogs: Prevalence of Left Apical Systolic Heart Murmur and Left-Sided Heart Failure, Critical Effects of Breed and Sex. J Vet Cardiol. May 2006;8(1):11-18.
32. Hayes HM Jr, Wilson GP, Pendergrass TW, et. al.: Canine cryptorchism and subsequent testicular neoplasia: case-control study with epidemiologic update. Teratology. 1985 Aug;32(1):51-6.
33. Gordon SG, Nelson DA, Achen SE, et. al.: Open heart closure of an atrial septal defect by use of an atrial septal occluder in a dog. J Am Vet Med Assoc. 2010 Feb 15;236(4):434-9.
34. Gordon SG & Meurs K: ASD in Standard Poodles: An Update. Proceedings, 2008 ACVIM Forum. 2008.
35. Hernblad Tevell E, Bergvall K & Egenvall A: Sebaceous adenitis in Swedish dogs, a retrospective study of 104 cases. Acta Vet Scand. 2008 May 25;50:11.
36. White SD, Rosychuk RA, Scott KV, et. al.: Sebaceous adenitis in dogs and results of treatment with isotretinoin and etretinate: 30 cases (1990-1994).

J Am Vet Med Assoc. 1995 Jul 15;207(2):197-200.

37. Licht BG, Lin S, Luo Y, et. al.: Clinical characteristics and mode of inheritance of familial focal seizures in Standard Poodles. J Am Vet Med Assoc. 2007 Nov 15;231(10):1520-8.

38. Licht BG, Licht MH, Harper KM, et. al.: Clinical presentations of naturally occurring canine seizures: similarities to human seizures. Epilepsy Behav. 2002 Oct;3(5):460-470.

39. Hess RS, Kass PH, Ward CR: Breed distribution of dogs with diabetes mellitus admitted to a tertiary care facility. J Am Vet Med Assoc. 2000 May 1;216(9):1414-7.

40. Nothelfer HB & Weinhold K: Formal pathogenesis, average age and breed distribution in the comparison of 61 Lysodren-treated and 36 untreated cases of canine hyperadrenocorticism which were dissected in the years 1975 to 1991 at the Institute for Veterinary Pathology of the Free University of Berlin. Berl Munch Tierarztl Wochenschr. 1992 Sep 1;105(9):305-11.

41. Ling GV, Stabenfeldt GH, Comer KM, et. al.: Canine hyperadrenocorticism: pretreatment clinical and laboratory evaluation of 117 cases. J Am Vet Med Assoc. 1979 Jun 1;174(11):1211-5.

42. Johnsen DA, Maggs DJ, Kass PH: Evaluation of risk factors for development of secondary glaucoma in dogs: 156 cases (1999-2004). J Am Vet Med Assoc. 2006 Oct 15;229(8):1270-4.

43. Gelatt KN, MacKay EO: Secondary glaucomas in the dog in North. Vet Ophthalmol. 2004 Jul-Aug;7(4):245-59.

44. Gelatt KN, MacKay EO: Prevalence of the breed-related glaucomas in pure-bred dogs in North America. Vet Ophthalmol. 2004 Mar-Apr; 7(2):97-111.

45. Ackerman N, Burk R, Hahn AW, et. al.: Patent ductus arteriosus in the dog: a retrospective study of radiographic, epidemiologic, and clinical findings. Am J Vet Res. 1978 Nov;39(11):1805-10.

46. Lekcharoensuk C, Lulich JP, Osborne CA, et. al.: Patient and environmental factors associated with calcium oxalate urolithiasis in dogs. J Am Vet Med Assoc. 2000 Aug 15;217(4):515-9.

47. van der Woerdt A, Nasisse MP & Davidson MG: Lens-induced uveitis in dogs: 151 cases (1985-1990). J Am Vet Med Assoc. 1992 Sep 15;201(6):921-6.

48. DiBartola SP, Chew DJ & Boyce JT: Juvenile renal disease in related Standard Poodles. J Am Vet Med Assoc. 1983 Sep 15;183(6):693-6.

49. Langenbach A, Anderson MA, Dambach DM, et. al.: Extraskeletal osteosarcomas in dogs: a retrospective study of 169 cases (1986-1996). J Am Anim Hosp Assoc. 1998 Mar-Apr;34(2):113-20.

50. Greco DS: Hyperadrenocorticism associated with sex steroid excess. Clin Tech Small Anim Pract. 2007 Feb;22(1):12-7.

51. Cerundolo R, Lloyd DH, Persechino A, et. al: Treatment of canine Alopecia X with trilostane. Vet Dermatol. 2004 Oct;15(5):285-93

52. Cerundolo R, Lloyd DH, Vaessen MM, et. al.: Alopecia in pomeranians and miniature poodles in association with high urinary corticoid:creatinine ratios and resistance to glucocorticoid feedback. Vet Rec. 2007 Mar 24;160(12):393-7.

53. Tidholm A, Jonsson L : A retrospective study of canine dilated cardiomyopathy (189 cases). J Am Anim Hosp Assoc. 1997 Nov-Dec;33(6):544-50.

54. Hosgood G, Hedlund CS, Pechman RD, et. al.: Perineal herniorrhaphy: perioperative data from 100 dogs. J Am Anim Hosp Assoc. 1995 Jul-Aug;31(4):331-42.

55. O'Brien MG, Berg J & Engler SJ: Treatment by digital amputation of subungual squamous cell carcinoma in dogs: 21 cases (1987-1988) J Am Vet Med Assoc. 1992 Sep 1;201(5):759-61.

56. Pucheu B & Duhautois B: Surgical treatment of shoulder instability. A retrospective study on 76 cases (1993-2007). Vet Comp Orthop Traumatol. 2008;21(4):368-74.

57. Dennis MM, Ehrhart N, Duncan CG, et. al.: Frequency of and risk factors associated with lingual lesions in dogs: 1,196 cases (1995-2004).

58. Matthews NS & de Lahunta A: Degenerative myelopathy in an adult miniature poodle. J Am Vet Med Assoc. 1985 Jun 1;186(11):1213-5.

59. Vianna ML, Tobias KM: Atresia ani in the dog: a retrospective study. J Am Anim Hosp Assoc. 2005 Sep-Oct;41(5):317-22.

60. Jurney C, Haddad J, Crawford N, et. al.: Polymicrogyria in standard poodles. J Vet Intern Med. 2009 Jul-Aug;23(4):871-4.

61. Van Winkle TJ, Fyfe JC, Dayrell-Hart B, et. al.: Blindness due to polymicrogyria and asymmetrical dilation of the lateral ventricles in Standard Poodles. Prog Vet Neurol 1994;5:66-71.

62. The Genetic Connection: A Guide to Health Problems in Purebred Dogs. L Ackerman. p 232-233, AAHA Press, 1999.

63. Jensen AL & Nielsen OL: Chronic hepatitis in three young standard poodles. Zentralbl Veterinarmed A. 1991 Apr;38(3):194-7.

64. Randolph JF, Center SA, Kallfelz FA, et. al.: Familial nonspherocytic hemolytic anemia in poodles. Am J Vet Res. 1986 Mar;47(3):687-95.

65. Selmanowitz VJ, Kramer KM & Orentreich N: Congenital ectodermal defect in miniature poodles. J Hered. 1970 Sep-Oct;61(5):196-9.

66. Selmanowitz VJ, Kramer KM, Orentreich N, et. al.: Congenital ectodermal dysplasia in male miniature poodle siblings. Arch Dermatol. 1970 May;101(5):613-5.

67. Mannerfelt T & Lindgren I: Enamel defects in standard poodle dogs in Sweden. J Vet Dent. 2009 Winter;26(4):213-5.

68. Dunstan RW, Sills RC, Wilkinson JE, et. al.: A disease resembling junctional epidermolysis bullosa in a toy poodle. Am J Dermatopathol. 1988 Oct;10(5):442-7.

69. *The Complete Dog Book, 20th Ed.* The American Kennel Club. Howell Book House, NY 2006. p 503-506 TOY, p 579-587 MINIATURE, STANDARD.

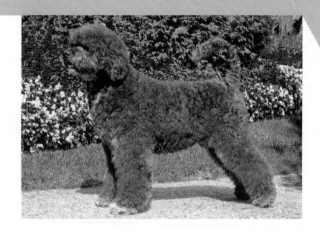

Portuguese Water Dog

or brown. The neck is short and strongly muscled, head carriage is high, and the throat is clean. Thorax is deep, the ribs are well sprung and moderate tuck up of abdomen is evident. The well-plumed tail extends to just above or just to the tarsus. When alert, the tail is held over the croup in a ring. Limbs are well muscled and straight boned. Dewclaws may be removed on the forelimbs. There are no rear dewclaws. Feet are flat and round in shape and are well covered in hair. The energetic gait is short-strided and quick.

The Breed History

The breed name in Portuguese means dog (cão) of the water (de agua). These dogs were a fisherman's working dogs, at home on the trawlers and in the water. Early breed origins may trace back to Asia. It is thought that breed progenitors entered Portugal (Iberia) around the 8th century via the Goths. Irish Water Spaniel dogs are thought to have derived from Portuguese Water Dog stock, and Poodles may share a common progenitor with the Portuguese Water dog. First breed specimens were exported to the USA in 1958. The AKC first accepted this breed into the stud book in 1983.

Breeding for Function

As Portuguese fishing dogs, the ideal dog was selected for stamina, excellent swimming ability and a weatherproof coat; along with a tractable nature. These dogs were fish herders, retrievers of equipment and a messenger dog between boats, and from boat-to-shore.

Physical Characteristics

Height at Withers: female 17-21" (43-53 cm), male 20-23" (51-58.5 cm).

Weight: female 35-50 lb (16-22.5 kg), male 40-60 lb (18-27 kg).

Coat: If clipped, a lion clip or retriever clip is done. The coat is single, dense, waterproof, and two distinct coat varieties exist. One type is a curly coat, the other a wavy haircoat. Accepted colors include black, white, black and white, brown, brown and white. Those with black and/or white in the coat have a bluish tinge to the skin.

Longevity: 12-14 years

Points of Conformation: A medium sized dog of strong constitution, well muscled and boned and slightly longer than high, the Portuguese Water Dogs are characterized by a domed wide skull, their coat, and the thick strong tail which is very useful for swimming since it acts like a rudder. Feet are also webbed. Roundish eyes are wide set, and are black or brown in color. Palpebral margins are black or brown. Ears are folded with the tips resting against the head, and the ear leather is fine. The occipital protuberance and the stop are both prominent. The muzzle is long and blocky. The nose is black or brown and possesses large open nostrils. The mucous membranes under the tongue and gingiva are black ticked, black,

Recognized Behavior Issues and Traits

Reported breed characteristics include: Intelligent, spirited in work but a calm demeanor, very hardy, excellent stamina. For some, this breed can be a low allergy choice and has a non-shedding coat. The Portuguese water dog is a good watchdog and very loyal. This breed of dog needs close human companionship. Some individuals have an independent streak. They have high exercise needs; preferably some swimming as well as running. Good with children and other pets. Generally, these dogs are aloof with strangers. Grooming is needed at least a few times per week at a minimum; is considered a high grooming needs dog.

Normal Physiologic Variations

Improper Coat: An autosomal recessive condition. An improperly coated wavy PWD will tend to look like a Flat Coated Retriever or Border Collie and a curly PWD like an American Water Spaniel or Curly Coated Retriever. Improperly coated dogs can also have some undercoat and shed. Caused by a mutation in the RSPO2 gene. Reported at a frequency of 0.68% in the 2005 PWD Health Survey. A genetic test is available.[1,2]

Drug Sensitivities

None Reported

Inherited Diseases

Hip Dysplasia: Polygenically inherited trait causing degenerative joint disease and hip arthritis. OFA reports 13.0% affected. Molecular genetic research suggests left and right hip status may be controlled by different genes. Reported at a frequency of 6.9% in the 2005 PWD Health Survey.[1,3,4]

Progressive Retinal Atrophy (PRCD-PRA): Autosomal recessive progressive rod cone degeneration (prcd) form. Age of onset between 3-8 years of age, eventually causing blindness. Optigen testing reports 4% affected, and 35% carriers in Portuguese Water Dogs. Reported at a frequency of 1.1% affected in the 2005 PWD Health Survey. A genetic test is available.[1,5,6]

GM1-Gangliosidosis (Storage Disease): Fatal autosomal recessive disorder causing rapidly progressive ataxia, intention tremors, wide-based stance, dysmetria, and weakness beginning around 3 to 5 months of age. 2% of the breed tests as carriers. A genetic test is available.[7,8]

Elbow Dysplasia: Polygenically inherited trait causing elbow arthritis. OFA reports 1.7% affected.[3]

Hypoadrenocorticism (Addison's Disease): Immune mediated destruction of the adrenal gland. Typical presentation of lethargy, poor appetite, vomiting, weakness, and dehydration can occur from 4 months to several years of age. Treatment with DOCA injections or oral fludrocortisone. Heritabililty of 0.49. Reported incidence of 1.5% affected. Controlled by a major autosomal recessive gene, but not a simple recessive disorder. No genetic test is available. Reported at a frequency of 1.7% in the 2005 PWD Health Survey.[1,9,10,11]

Juvenile Dilated Cardiomyopathy (JDCM): Fatal autosomal recessive disorder causing sudden death between 2-32 weeks of age from congestive heart failure. Echocardiograms are normal until 3-7 days prior to death. Occurring at a low frequency in the breed. A direct genetic test is available, showing a 12% carrier frequency worldwide.[12,13,14,15,16]

Patella Luxation: Polygenically inherited laxity of patellar ligaments, causing luxation, lameness, and later degenerative joint disease. Treat surgically if causing clinical signs. Reported at a high frequency by OFA, but too few Portuguese Water Dogs have been screened to determine an accurate frequency.[3]

Disease Predispositions

Sebaceous Cysts: Benign subcutaneous cysts of sebaceous material. Reported at a frequency of 10.0% in the 2005 PWD Health Survey.[1]

Cryptorchidism: Undescended testicles can be unilateral or bilateral. This is a sex-limited disorder with an unknown mode of inheritance. Reported in 10.0% of litters in the 2005 PWD Health Survey.[1]

Aggression and Behavior: Based on the 2005 PWD Health Survey, 7.4% show dog to dog aggression, and 3.4% show aggression towards people. 7.1% show noise phobia, and 5.7% show shyness.[1]

Allergies: Presents with pruritis and pyotraumatic dermatitis (hot spots). Based on the 2005 PWD Health Survey, 6.2% show food allergy and 3.4% show inhalant allergies.[1]

Persistent Pupillary Membranes: Strands of fetal remnant connecting; iris to iris, cornea, lens, or involving sheets of tissue. The later three forms can impair vision, and dogs affected with these forms should not be bred. Identified in 5.52% of Portuguese Water Dogs CERF examined by veterinary ophthalmologists between 2000-2005. Reported at a frequency of 1.6% in the 2005 PWD Health Survey.[1,5]

Otitis Externa (Chronic Ear Infections): Can be bacterial or yeast infection. Reported at a frequency of 5.4% in the 2005 PWD Health Survey.[1]

Hypothyroidism: Inherited autoimmune thyroiditis. 4.8% positive for thyroid autoantibodies based on testing at Michigan State University. (Ave. for all breeds is 7.5%). Reported at a frequency of 4.3% in the 2005 PWD Health Survey.[1,17,18]

Undershot Jaw (Overbite): Reported at a frequency of 3.7% in the 2005 PWD Health Survey.[1]

Malignant Cancer: Based on the 2005 PWD Health Survey, 3.1% were diagnosed with hemangiosarcoma, 1.6% with lymphosarcoma, 1.4% with mammary gland cancer (some of which may be benign), and 1.1% with mast cell cancer.[1]

Distichiasis: Abnormally placed eyelashes that irritate the cornea and conjunctiva. Can cause secondary corneal ulceration. Identified in 3.04% of Portuguese Water Dogs CERF examined by veterinary ophthalmologists between 2000-2005. Reported at a frequency of 1.2% in the 2005 PWD Health Survey.[1,5]

Cataracts: Anterior cortex punctate cataracts predominate in the breed. Identified in 2.87% of Portuguese Water Dogs CERF examined by veterinary ophthalmologists between 2000-2005. Reported at a frequency of 5.9% in the 2005 PWD Health Survey. CERF does not recommend breeding any Portuguese Water Dog with a cataract.[1,5]

Umbilical Hernia: Congential body wall defect at the umbilicus. Correct surgically if large. Reported in 2.7% of litters in the 2005 PWD Health Survey.[1]

Cleft Palate: Congenital disorder of incomplete closure of the maxillary processes to form the roof of the mouth. Reported in 2.3% of litters in the 2005 PWD Health Survey.[1]

Inflammatory Bowel Disease (IBD): Inflammatory condition of the gastrointestinal tract causing chronic vomiting, diarrhea, and/or weight loss. A low frequency of Portuguese Dogs suffers from IBD. Affected dogs can usually be controlled with diet and/or medications. Reported at a frequency of 2.1% in the 2005 PWD Health Survey.[1]

Bladder Stones: Based on the 2005 PWD Health Survey, 2.1% developed bladder stones. The composition of the stones was not indicated.[1]

Seizures/Epilepsy: Generalized or partial seizures. Based on the 2005 PWD Health Survey, 1.7% are reported with seizures or epilepsy.[1]

Keratoconjunctivitis Sicca (KCS, Dry Eye): Ocular condition causing lack of tear production and secondary conjunctivitis, corneal ulcerations, and vision problems. Reported at a frequency of 1.2% in the 2005 PWD Health Survey.[1]

Follicular Dysplasia (Hair Loss): Inherited, non-inflammatory, truncal, symmetrical, cyclic hair loss. Only occurs in curly dogs from two curly parents. Unknown mode of inheritance. Reported at a frequency of 0.62% in the 2005 PWD Health Survey.[1,19]

Coat Dilution Alopecia and **Microphthalmia** are reported.[20]

Isolated Case Studies

Juvenile Renal Disease: Cases of death due to renal failure in young Portuguese Water Dogs have been reported over the years. Some have had pathological findings of renal dysplasia.

Gastrinoma and Somatostatinoma: Case study of a ten year old Portuguese Water Dog with multiple endocrine tumors consisting of a pancreatic islet cell somatostatinoma, and a gastrinoma in the mesenteric lymph nodes and liver.[21]

Genetic Tests

Tests of Genotype: Direct test for JDCM is available from PennGen.

Direct tests for prcd-PRA and improper coat are available from Optigen.

Direct test for GM1-Gangliosidosis available from New York University Neurogenetics Laboratory: http://www.pwdca.org/health/tests/instructions/GM1TestInstructions.html.

Test for black and brown colors, and black or brown nose is available from HealthGene and VetGen.

Tests of Phenotype: CHIC Certification: Hip radiographs, CERF eye examination (annually until age 10), and direct genetic tests for GM-1 and prcd-PRA. Optional tests include congenital cardiac evaluation by a cardiologist, elbow radiographs, thyroid profile including autoantibodies, skin biopsy for sebaceous adenitis, patella evaluation, and genetic test for JDCM. (See CHIC website; www.caninehealthinfo.org).

Miscellaneous

- **Breed name synonyms:** Portie, Cão de Agua, Cão de Agua de Pelo Ondulado (longhaired variety), Cão de Agua de Pelo Encaradolado (curly-coated variety).
- **Registries:** AKC, UKC, CKC, KCGB (Kennel Club of Great Britain), ANKC (Australian National Kennel Club).
- **AKC rank (year 2008):** 64 (1,427 dogs registered)
- **Internet resources: Portuguese Water Dog Club of America:** www.pwdca.org
  Portuguese Water Dog Club of Canada: www.pwdcc.org
  Portuguese Water Dog Club of Great Britain: www.portuguesewaterdogs.org.uk
  Portuguese Water Dog Health Foundation: www.pwdfoundation.org

References

1. Slater M: The 2005 Portuguese Water Dog Health Survey. July 1, 2010.
2. Parker HG, Chase K, Cadieu E, et. al.: An insertion in the RSPO2 gene correlates with improper coat in the Portuguese water dog. J Hered. 2010 Sep-Oct;101(5):612-7.
3. OFA Website breed statistics: www.offa.org Last accessed July 1, 2010.
4. Chase K, Lawler DF, Adler FR, et. al.: Bilaterally asymmetric effects of quantitative trait loci (QTLs): QTLs that affect laxity in the right versus left coxofemoral (hip) joints of the dog (Canis familiaris). Am J Med Genet A. 2004 Jan 30;124(3):239-47.
5. Ocular Disorders Presumed to be Inherited in Purebred Dogs. American College of Veterinary Ophthalmologists. ACVO, 2007.
6. Zangerl B, Goldstein O, Philp AR, et. al.: Identical mutation in a novel retinal gene causes progressive rod-cone degeneration in dogs and retinitis pigmentosa in humans. Genomics. 2006 Nov;88(5):551-63.
7. Shell LG, Potthoff AI, Carithers R, et. al.: Neuronal-visceral GM1 gangliosidosis in Portuguese water dogs. J Vet Intern Med. 1989 Jan-Mar;3(1):1-7.
8. Wang ZH, Zeng B, Shibuya H, et. al.: Isolation and characterization of the normal canine beta-galactosidase gene and its mutation in a dog model of GM1-gangliosidosis. J Inherit Metab Dis. 2000 Sep;23(6):593-606.
9. Peterson ME, Kintzer PP, Kass PH: Pretreatment clinical and laboratory findings in dogs with hypoadrenocorticism: 225 cases (1979-1993). J Am Vet Med Assoc. 1996 Jan 1;208(1):85-91.
10. Chase K, Sargan D, Miller K, et. al.: Understanding the genetics of autoimmune disease: two loci that regulate late onset Addison's disease in Portuguese Water Dogs. Int J Immunogenet. 2006 Jun;33(3):179-84.
11. Oberbauer AM, Bell JS, Belanger JM, et. al.: Genetic evaluation of Addison's disease in the Portuguese Water Dog. BMC Vet Res. 2006 May 2;2:15.
12. Alroy J, Rush JE, Freeman L, et. al.: Inherited infantile dilated cardiomyopathy in dogs: genetic, clinical, biochemical, and morphologic findings. Am J Med Genet. 2000 Nov 6;95(1):57-66.
13. Sleeper MM, Henthorn PS, Vijayasarathy C, et. al.: Dilated cardiomyopathy in juvenile Portuguese Water Dogs. J Vet Intern Med. 2002 Jan-Feb;16(1):52-62.
14. Alroy J, Rush JE, Sarkar S: Infantile dilated cardiomyopathy in Portuguese water dogs: correlation of the autosomal recessive trait with low plasma taurine at infancy. Amino Acids. 2005 Feb;28(1):51-6.
15. Werner P, Raducha MG, Prociuk U, et. al.: A novel locus for dilated cardiomyopathy maps to canine chromosome 8. Genomics. 2008 Jun;91(6):517-21.
16. Dambach DM, Lannon A, Sleeper MM, et. al.: Familial dilated cardiomyopathy of young Portuguese water dogs. J Vet Intern Med. 1999 Jan-Feb;13(1):65-71.
17. Nachreiner RF, Refsal KR, Graham PA, et. al.: Prevalence of serum thyroid hormone autoantibodies in dogs with clinical signs of hypothyroidism. J Am Vet Med Assoc 2002 Feb 15;220(4):466-71.
18. Nachreiner R & Refsal K: Personal communication, Diagnostic Center for Population and Animal Health, Michigan State University. April, 2007.
19. Miller Jr WH, & Scott DW: Follicular Dysplasia of the Portuguese Water Dog. Vet Dermatol. 1995:6[2]:67-74.
20. The Genetic Connection: A Guide to Health Problems in Purebred Dogs. L Ackerman. p. 233-234 AAHA Press, 1999.
21. Hoenerhoff M, Kiupel M: Concurrent gastrinoma and somatostatinoma in a 10-year-old Portuguese water dog. J Comp Pathol. 2004 May;130(4):313-8.
22. The Complete Dog Book, 20th Ed. The American Kennel Club. Howell Book House, NY 2006. p. 308-313.

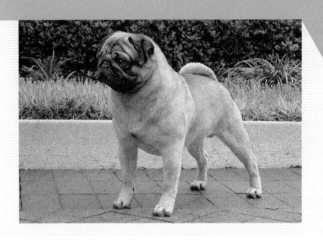

The Breed History

Records of this breed go back as far as 400 BC. The breed ancestors may have been Tibetan Mastiffs and later, Pomeranian stock brought over from China. Originally exported to Holland, it is possible that the breed name derives from the word applied to pet monkeys, *"pug"*. They were considered to have similar facial expressions as Marmosets. Another possible source for the name is the term *"pugnus"*, which is Latin for fist, presumably reflecting their very round head. These dogs became popular with English royalty. First registry for Pugs with AKC registry occurred in 1885.

Breeding for Function

Bred solely for companionship.

Physical Characteristics

Height at Withers: 10-11" (25-28 cm)

Weight: 14-18 lb (6.5-8 kg).

Coat: The fine short double glossy coat lies flat and breed colors include fawn and apricot, black, and silver. Markings follow a set pattern and are black or dark including ears, muzzle and sometimes a line is present down the back.

Longevity: 13-15 years.

Points of Conformation: Their cobby, stout, and compact square constitution gives them a lot of apparent substance for their size. Though they are classed as a toy, their heavy build makes them look larger. The head is massive and round, the high set ears are soft, the leather is thin and ears either in a rose or button type. Muzzle is very short and square and the bite is mildly undershot. Top of the head has prominent forehead wrinkles, eyes are dark, shallow set, and very large. Neck is short and strong, topline level, the thorax is barrel shaped, tail is high set and ideally, doubly curled to rest tightly over the hip joint. Legs are straight, moderate in length, and feet are moderately sized and oval in shape, toenails are black and dewclaws are generally removed. Their gait is strong, free, and hindquarters typically have some roll.

Recognized Behavior Issues and Traits

These dogs have been described as being: Loving of children and family, good alarm barkers, playful, "pugnacious", independently minded, stable, liking lots of human companionship.

Considered good for rural or urban environments, they have low grooming needs and may snore. They enjoy children and other pets, tend to obesity, have low exercise needs but some activity is needed to help them keep a proper body weight. They don't tolerate hot weather. They have low grooming needs; just a quick daily brush will do, and hygiene is needed around facial folds especially at eyes.

Normal Physiologic Variations

A UK study showed 27.4% of litters were born via **Cesarean section**.[1]

Drug Sensitivities

None reported

Inherited Diseases

Hip Dysplasia and Legg-Perthes Disease: Polygenically inherited traits causing degenerative joint disease and hip arthritis. Reported 65.6x odds ratio for Legg-Calve-Perthes versus other breeds. OFA reports 64.1% affected.[2,3]

Elbow Dysplasia: Polygenically inherited trait causing elbow arthritis. Reported 3.3x odds ratio versus other breeds. OFA reports 61.4% affected.[2,3]

Patella Luxation: Polygenically inherited laxity of patellar ligaments, causing luxation, lameness, and later degenerative joint disease. Treat surgically if causing clinical signs. OFA reports 7.3% affected.[2]

Disease Predispositions

Brachycephalic Complex: Can cause dyspnea, and collapse. Includes **Elongated Soft Palate, Stenotic Nares, Hypoplastic Trachea,** and **Everted Laryngeal Saccules**. Clinical signs are associated with bronchial collapse. Nasopharyngeal turbinates may also play a role. Surgery is indicated in severe cases. Identified in 26.0% of Pugs in an Australian study. Dorn reports a 13.3x odds ratio in Pugs versus other breeds.[4,5,6,7,8]

Entropion: A rolling in of the eyelids that can cause corneal irritation and ulceration. Dorn reports a 2.94x odds ratio in Pugs versus other breeds. Entropion is reported in 21.00% of Pugs CERF examined by veterinary ophthalmologists between 2000-2005.[4,9]

Exposure Keratopathy Syndrome/Pigmentary Keratitis: Corneal reactivity and drying from ocular exposure secondary to shallow orbits, exophthalmos, and lagophthalmos. Identified in 16.55% of Pugs CERF examined by veterinary ophthalmologists between 2000-2005.[9]

Persistent Pupillary Membranes: Strands of fetal remnant connecting; iris to iris, cornea, lens, or involving sheets of tissue. The later three forms can impair vision, and dogs affected with these forms should not be bred. Identified in 9.87% of Pugs CERF examined by veterinary ophthalmologists between 2000-2005.[9]

Distichiasis: Abnormally placed eyelashes that irritate the cornea and conjunctiva. Can cause secondary corneal ulceration. Identified in 8.62% of Pugs CERF examined by veterinary ophthalmologists between 2000-2005.[9]

Hypothyroidism: Inherited autoimmune thyroiditis. 5.6% positive for thyroid autoantibodies based on testing at Michigan State University. (Ave. for all breeds is 7.5%).[10,11]

Allergic Dermatitis (Atopy): Inhalant or food allergy. Presents with pruritis and pyotraumatic dermatitis (hot spots). Pugs have a significantly increased risk for atopy versus other breeds.[12]

Chronic Superficial Keratitis (Pannus): Chronic corneal inflammatory process that can cause vision problems due to corneal pigmentation. Treatment with topical ocular lubricants and anti-inflammatory medication. Identified in 3.20% of Pugs CERF examined by veterinary ophthalmologists between 2000-2005. CERF does not recommend breeding any Pug with the condition.[9]

Macroblepharon: Abnormally large eyelid opening; may lead to secondary conditions associated with corneal exposure. Identified in 3.06% of Pugs CERF examined by veterinary ophthalmologists between 2000-2005.[9]

Mast Cell Tumor (MCT): Histamine producing skin tumors that produce inflammation and ulceration. Can metastasize or reoccur locally following surgical removal. Pugs have a 4 to 8 times greater risk for developing cutaneous mast cell tumors than other breeds.[13]

Cataracts: Anterior, posterior, intermediate and punctate cataracts occur in the breed. Unknown mode of inheritance. Reported in 2.28% of Pugs presented to veterinary teaching hospitals. Identified in 1.53% of Pugs CERF examined by veterinary ophthalmologists between 2000-2005. CERF does not recommend breeding any Pug with a cataract.[9,14]

Portosystemic Shunt (PSS, Liver Shunt): Abnormal blood vessels connecting the systemic and portal blood flow. Vessels can be intrahepatic, extrahepatic or microvascular dysplasia. Causes stunting, abnormal behavior and possible seizures. Diagnose with paired fasted and feeding serum bile acid and/or ammonium levels, and abdominal ultrasound. Treatment of PSS includes partial ligation and/or medical and dietary control of symptoms. The Pug is a breed at increased risk of having PSS, with an incidence of 1.3% and an odds ratio of 26.2x versus other breeds. Undetermined mode of inheritance.[15]

Pug Dog Encephalitis (PDE): A sporadic, necrotizing meningoencephalitis affecting adolescent and mature pug dogs. Acute and chronic forms occur, with a median age of 19 months, and mean survival of 23 days. Presents with clinical signs of depression, ataxia, or generalized seizures. Anticonvulsants are helpful to control seizures. MRI along with clinical history can be diagnostic. Undetermined mode of inheritance, with a high heritability. Estimated frequency of 1.25% in the breed. Associated with a specific DLA Type II haplotype, especially in the heterozygous state (12.75x Odds Ratio; 75% of affected Pugs have this haplotype) A genetic test for the susceptibility haplotype is available.[16,17,18,19]

Bladder Stones: The Pug is a breed predisposed to develop bladder stones. Stone composition is not identified.[20,21]

Diabetes Mellitus: Sugar diabetes caused by a lack of insulin production by the pancreas. Controlled by insulin injections, diet, and glucose monitoring. Identified as a breed at increased risk of developing diabetes, with an odds ratio of 3.87x versus other breeds.[22]

Hemivertebra and Butterfly Vertebra: Malformed veterbra can cause scoliosis, pain or spinal cord compression if severe. Can produce **Spina Bifida** or **Sacrocaudal Dysgenesis**. Associated with selection for the screw tail. Seen at an increased frequency in the breed. Undetermined mode of inheritance.[23,24]

Pigmented Plaques: Pugs are predisposed to the development of deeply pigmented, slightly elevated hyperkeratotic noncancerous plaques on the abdomen and limbs. A novel papilloma virus (CPV4) has been isolated from these plaques.[25]

Lung Lobe Torsion: Pugs have a predisposition for spontaneous lung lobe torsion. Median age of 1.5 years, with a male prevalence. Histories included increased weakness, increased respiratory effort, tachypnea, acute collapse, lethargy, anorexia, and cyanosis. Surgical correction is curative, though one reported case had another lobe torsion 2 years later.[26,27,28,29]

Hydrops Fetalis: A previously unreported syndrome of transient mid-gestational hydrops fetalis identified by ultrasound was diagnosed in 16 litters of 16 different Pugs. There was 7.4% fetal resorption, 8.4% abortion, 8.0% stillbirths, 15% neonatal mortality, and 9.6% congenital abnormalities. Pugs were significantly (22.8 times) more likely to be affected than other breeds.[30]

Degenerative Myelopathy (DM): Affected dogs show an insidious onset of upper motor neuron (UMN) paraparesis. The disease eventually progresses to severe tetraparesis. Affected dogs have normal results on myelography, MRI, and CSF analysis. Necropsy confirms the condition. Unknown mode of inheritance. A direct genetic test for an autosomal recessive DM susceptibility gene is available. All affected dogs are homozygous for the gene, however only a small percentage of homozygous dogs develop DM. OFA reports DM susceptibility gene frequencies of 29% carrier, and 2% homozygous "at-risk".[2]

Brachygnathism, Cleft Palate, Cryptorchidism, Demodicosis, Fold Dermatitis, Lentigo, Oligodontia, and Progressive Retinal Atrophy are reported.[31]

Isolated Case Studies

Second Degree Heart Block: A colony of Pugs was established with intermittent sinus pauses and paroxysmal second degree heart block. Pathological findings included stenosis of the midportion of the His bundle, which appears to be a heritable trait in these purebred Pug dogs.[32]

Pigmented Cutaneous Papillomatosis (Pigmented Epidermal Nevus): Three cases of pigmented cutaneous papillomatosis (previously described also as CPEN) in pug dogs were investigated histopathologically, immunohistochemically and electron microscopically. PCR amplification targeted for the L1 gene of papillomavirus cloned from a case of CPEN yielded an expected fragment of 194-bp in the two CPEN cases examined but not in a case of canine oral papilloma.[33]

XX–Sex Reversal: A case of a male appearing Pug with Sry-negative XX-sex reversal was identified in Italy. The dog had a prepuce and an enlarged clitoris. A uterus was present. The gonads had seminiferous tubules lined by Sertoli cells.[34]

Double–Chambered Right Ventricle: A 32-month-old spayed female Pug was identified with a ventricular septal defect and double chambered right ventricle by echocardiography and pathological examinations. An anomalous muscle bundle crossed the right ventricular outflow tract, dividing the right ventricle into 2 chambers. There were no clinical abnormalities found.[35]

Genetic Tests

Tests of Genotype: A direct susceptibility test for PDE is available frm UC-Davis VGL.

A direct test for a DM susceptibility gene is available from OFA.

Direct test for black and fawn coat color is available from HealthGene and VetGen.

Tests of Phenotype: CHIC Certification: Hip radiographs, patella evaluation, CERF eye examination (every 3 years), and genetic test for PDE. (See CHIC website; www.caninehealthinfo.com).

Recommend elbow radiographs, thyroid profile including autoantibodies, and cardiac examination.

Miscellaneous

- **Breed name synonyms:** Mops (Germany), Mopshond (Dutch for Grumbler), Carlin (France), Dutch Pug, Lo-Sze (Chinese word for ancient pug)
- **Registries:** AKC, UKC, CKC, KCGB (Kennel Club of Great Britain), ANKC (Australian National Kennel Club), NKC (National Kennel Club)
- **AKC rank (year 2008):** 15 (12,202 dogs registered)
- **Internet resources: Pug Dog Club of America:** www.pugs.org
  Pug Club of Canada: www.pugcanada.com
  The Pug Dog Club (UK): www.pugdogclub.org.uk

References

1. Evans KM & Adams VJ: Proportion of litters of purebred dogs born by caesarean section. J Small Anim Pract. 2010 Feb;51(2):113-8.
2. OFA Website breed statistics: www.offa.org Last accessed July 1, 2010.
3. LaFond E, Breur GJ & Austin CC: Breed susceptibility for developmental orthopedic diseases in dogs. J Am Anim Hosp Assoc. 2002 Sep-Oct;38(5):467-77.
4. Dorn CR: Canine breed-specific risks of frequently diagnosed diseases at veterinary teaching hospitals. Monograph. AKC Canine Health Foundation. 2000.
5. Riecks TW, Birchard SJ, & Stephens JA: Surgical correction of brachycephalic syndrome in dogs: 62 cases (1991-2004). J Am Vet Med Assoc. 2007 May 1;230(9):1324-8.
6. Torrez CV & Hunt GB: Results of surgical correction of abnormalities associated with brachycephalic airway obstruction syndrome in dogs in Australia. J Small Anim Pract. 2006 Mar;47(3):150-4.
7. De Lorenzi D, Bertoncello D, Drigo M, et. al.: Bronchial abnormalities found in a consecutive series of 40 brachycephalic dogs. J Am Vet Med Assoc. 2009 Oct 1;235(7):835-40.
8. Ginn JA, Kumar MS, McKiernan BC, et. al.: Nasopharyngeal turbinates in brachycephalic dogs and cats. J Am Anim Hosp Assoc. 2008 Sep-Oct;44(5):243-9.
9. *Ocular Disorders Presumed to be Inherited in Purebred Dogs.* American College of Veterinary Ophthalmologists. ACVO, 2007.
10. Nachreiner RF, Refsal KR, Graham PA, et. al.: Prevalence of serum thyroid hormone autoantibodies in dogs with clinical signs of hypothyroidism. J Am Vet Med Assoc 2002 Feb 15;220(4):466-71.
11. Nachreiner R & Refsal K: Personal communication, Diagnostic Center for Population and Animal Health, Michigan State University. April, 2007.
12. Griffies JD: Atopic Disease–Clinical Presentation. Proceedings, 2002 Western Veterinary Conference. 2002.
13. Moore AS: Cutaneous Mast Cell Tumors in Dogs. Proceedings, 2005 World Small Animal Veterinary Association Congress. 2005.
14. Gelatt KN, Mackay EO: Prevalence of primary breed-related cataracts in the dog in North America. Vet Ophthalmol. 2005 Mar-Apr;8(2):101-11.
15. Tobias KM, Rohrbach BW: Association of breed with the diagnosis of congenital portosystemic shunts in dogs: 2,400 cases (1980-2002). J Am Vet Med Assoc. 2003 Dec 1;223(11):1636-9.
16. Levine JM, Fosgate GT, Porter B, et. al.: Epidemiology of necrotizing meningoencephalitis in pug dogs. J Vet Intern Med. 2008 Jul-Aug;22(4):961-8.
17. Greer KA, Wong AK, Liu H, et. al.: Necrotizing meningoencephalitis of Pug Dogs associates with dog leukocyte antigen class II and resembles acute variant forms of multiple sclerosis. Tissue Antigens. 2010 Aug 1;76(2):110-8.
18. Young BD, Levine JM, Fosgate GT, et. al.: Magnetic resonance imaging characteristics of necrotizing meningoencephalitis in Pug dogs. J Vet Intern Med. 2009 May-Jun;23(3):527-35.
19. Greer KA, Schatzberg SJ, Porter BF, et. al.: Heritability and transmission analysis of necrotizing meningoencephalitis in the Pug. Res Vet Sci. 2009 Jun;86(3):438-42.
20. Bovee KC, McGuire T: Qualitative and quantitative analysis of uroliths in dogs: definitive determination of chemical type. J Am Vet Med Assoc. 1984 Nov 1;185(9):983-7.
21. Brown NO, Parks JL, Greene RW: Canine urolithiasis: retrospective analysis of 438 cases. J Am Vet Med Assoc. 1977 Feb 15;170(4):414-8.
22. Hess RS, Kass PH, Ward CR: Breed distribution of dogs with diabetes mellitus admitted to a tertiary care facility. J Am Vet Med Assoc. 2000 May 1;216(9):1414-7.
23. Knipe, M: Spinal Cord Diseases of Small Breed Dogs. Proceedings, 2010 UC-Davis Veterinary Neurology Symposium. 2010.
24. Done SH, Drew RA, Robins GM, et. al: Hemivertebra in the dog: clinical and pathological observations. Vet Rec. 1975 Apr 5;96(14):313-7.
25. Tobler K, Lange C, Carlotti DN, et. al.: Detection of a novel papillomavirus in pigmented plaques of four pugs. Vet Dermatol. 2008 Feb;19(1):21-5.
26. Spranklin DB, Gulikers KP, Lanz OI: Recurrence of spontaneous lung lobe torsion in a pug. J Am Anim Hosp Assoc. 2003 Sep-Oct;39(5):446-51.
27. Teunissen GH, Wolverkamp WT, Goedegebuure SA: Necrosis of a pulmonary lobe in a dog. Tijdschr Diergeneeskd. 1976 Oct 15;101(20):1129-33.
28. Rooney MB, Lanz O, Monnet E: Spontaneous lung lobe torsion in two pugs. J Am Anim Hosp Assoc. 2001 Mar-Apr;37(2):128-30.
29. Murphy KA & Brisson BA: Evaluation of lung lobe torsion in Pugs: 7 cases (1991-2004). J Am Vet Med Assoc. 2006 Jan 1;228(1):86-90.
30. Hopper BJ, Richardson JL, Lester NV: Spontaneous antenatal resolution of canine hydrops fetalis diagnosed by ultrasound. J Small Anim Pract. 2004 Jan;45(1):2-8.
31. *The Genetic Connection: A Guide to Health Problems in Purebred Dogs.* L Ackerman. p. 234. AAHA Press, 1999.
32. James TN, Robertson BT, Waldo AL, et. al.: De subitaneis mortibus. XV. Hereditary stenosis of the His bundle in Pug dogs. Circulation. 1975 Dec;52(6):1152-60.
33. Narama I, Kobayashi Y, Yamagami T, et. al.: Pigmented cutaneous papillomatosis (pigmented epidermal nevus) in three pug dogs; histopathology, electron microscopy and analysis of viral DNA by the polymerase chain reaction. J Comp Pathol. 2005 Feb-Apr;132(2-3):132-8.
34. Rota A, Cucuzza AS, Iussich S, et al.: The case of an Sry-negative XX male Pug with an inguinal gonad. Reprod Domest Anim. 2010 Aug;45(4):743-5.
35. Koie H, Kurotobi EN, Sakai T: Double-chambered right ventricle in a dog. J Vet Med Sci. 2000 Jun;62(6):651-3.
36. *The Complete Dog Book, 20th Ed.* The American Kennel Club. Howell Book House, NY 2006. P 507-509.
37. Awano T, Johnson GS, Wade CM, et. al.: Genome-wide association analysis reveals a SOD1 mutation in canine degenerative myelopathy that resembles amyotrophic lateral sclerosis. Proc Natl Acad Sci U S A. 2009 Feb 24;106(8):2794-9.

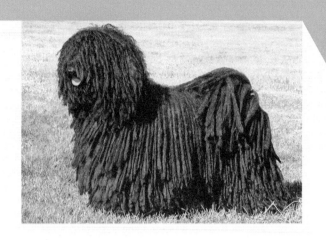

The Breed History

This ancient Hungarian breed is termed Puli in the singular and Pulik in plural. The Magyar people bred these shepherding dogs for at least a millennium. It is likely that the Tibetan terrier was the main source of foundation genes. In the 16th century, European invaders brought other sheepdogs with them and these were crossed with the Pulik, resulting in a dog termed Pumi, though the terms Pumi and Puli were used interchangeably. The breed was rescued from obscurity in the early 1900s. In 1915 the first breed standard was drawn up and in the shows, various size categories were recognized. First AKC registration occurred in 1936. This dog may be an ancestor of the Poodle.

Breeding for Function

These dogs were used exclusively for daytime sheep herding. Today, they are a popular companion dog, used for watchdog and police work purposes, and enjoy water retrieving.

Physical Characteristics

Height at Withers: female 16" (40.5 cm), male 17" (43 cm).

Weight: 30-40 lb (13.5-18 kg).

Coat: An off-black, which is tinged with bronze or grey is the standard breed color, though especially in Hungary, white and gray are seen. A small white spot on the chest is allowed. Body skin is darkly pigmented. The undercoat is wooly, short and soft. It naturally intermingles with the long outer coat. As the puppy matures, the tangle evolves into the cords that characterize the adult coat. Cording normally begins around the time of sexual maturity. This adult coat development process can take 4 or 5 years to complete. Cords may reach the ground if untrimmed. The dog may be shown corded or groomed.

Longevity: 11-14 years

Points of Conformation: The profuse corded coat is the trademark feature of this breed. The compact, square, medium build is hard to assess through the profuse coat. The head is medium in size, large, and the almond shaped eyes are dark brown with dark palpebral margins. Cords normally hang over the eyes in mature dogs. Ears are medium sized, triangular, high set, and hang down beside the head. The stop is average, skull is slightly domed, and the nose is black and large. The muzzle tapers moderately. Flews are tight. The neck is medium in length and muscling, not throaty, the topline is level, and the thorax is deep with well-sprung ribs. The abdomen is moderately tucked up. The tail is carried up over the back and limbs are straight boned. The feet have thick pads and well-arched toes, are round and compact. Dewclaws may be removed. They have a very elastic stride, and are very agile and fast on their feet as would be expected of a sheep herding dog.

Recognized Behavior Issues and Traits

Reported breed characteristics include: Excellent watchdogs, they are intelligent and friendly in temperament. Pulik are easy to obedience train and are playful. Good for country or city living. As cords form, they should be separated down to the skin to prevent matting. Though they do not tend to get a doggy odor, after bathing it is important to fully dry the dog to prevent mildew in the cords. The cords do not shed.

Normal Physiologic Variations

None reported

Drug Sensitivities

None reported

Inherited Diseases

Hip Dysplasia: Polygenically inherited trait causing degenerative joint disease and hip arthritis. OFA reports 10.1% affected.[1]

Elbow Dysplasia: Polygenically inherited trait causing elbow arthritis. OFA reports 5.9% affected.[1]

Patella Luxation: Polygenically inherited laxity of patellar ligaments, causing luxation, lameness, and later degenerative joint disease. Treat surgically if causing clinical signs. OFA reports 5.2% affected.[1]

Disease Predispositions

Persistent Pupillary Membranes: Strands of fetal remnant connecting; iris to iris, cornea, lens, or involving sheets of tissue. The later three forms can impair vision, and dogs affected with these forms should not be bred. Identified in 26.88% of Pulik CERF examined by veterinary ophthalmologists between 2000-2005.[2]

Retinal Dysplasia: Retinal folds, geographic, and generalized retinal dysplasia with detachment are recognized in the breed. Can progress to blindness. Reported in 7.50% of Pulik CERF examined by veterinary ophthalmologists between 2000-2005.[2]

Cataracts: Anterior cortex punctate cataracts predominate in the breed. Unknown mode of inheritance. Identified in 3.44% of Pulik CERF examined by veterinary ophthalmologists between 2000-2005. CERF does not recommend breeding any Puli with a cataract.[2]

Hypothyroidism: Inherited autoimmune thyroiditis. 2.9% positive for thyroid autoantibodies based on testing at Michigan State University. (Ave. for all breeds is 7.5%).[3,4]

Corneal Dystrophy: Epithelial/stromal form causes opacities on the surface of the cornea. Unknown mode of inheritance. Identified in 1.25% of Pulik CERF examined by veterinary ophthalmologists between 2000-2005.[2]

Diabetes Mellitus: Sugar diabetes caused by a lack of insulin production by the pancreas. Control with insulin injections, diet, and glucose monitoring. Identified as a breed at increased risk of developing diabetes.[5]

Deafness: Congenital deafness can be unilateral or bilateral. Diagnosed by BAER testing. Reported as a breed at risk by Strain.[6]

Micropapilla, Oligodontia, and **Progressive Retinal Atrophy** are reported.[7]

Isolated Case Studies
None Reported

Genetic Tests
Tests of Genotype: none

Tests of Phenotype: CHIC Certification: Required testing includes hip radiographs, CERF eye examination, and patella evaluation. Recommended tests include BAER hearing test, elbow radiographs, and congenital cardiac disease evaluation by a cardiologist or specialist. (See CHIC website; www.caninehealthinfo.org).

Recommend thyroid profile including autoantibodies.

Miscellaneous
- **Breed name synonyms:** Hungarian Puli, Hungarian Water Dog.
- **Registries:** AKC, UKC, CKC, KCGB (Kennel Club of Great Britain), ANKC (Australian National Kennel Club), NKC (National Kennel Club).
- **AKC rank (year 2008):** 142 (102 dogs registered)
- **Internet resources: The Puli Club of America:** www.puliclub.org
  Puli Canada: www.pulicanada.ca
  Hungarian Puli Club of Great Britain:
  www.hungarianpuliclubofgb.co.uk

References
1. OFA Website breed statistics: www.offa.org Last accessed July 1, 2010.
2. *Ocular Disorders Presumed to be Inherited in Purebred Dogs.* American College of Veterinary Ophthalmologists. ACVO, 2007.
3. Nachreiner RF, Refsal KR, Graham PA, et. al.: Prevalence of serum thyroid hormone autoantibodies in dogs with clinical signs of hypothyroidism. J Am Vet Med Assoc 2002 Feb 15;220(4):466-71.
4. Nachreiner R & Refsal K: Personal communication, Diagnostic Center for Population and Animal Health, Michigan State University. April, 2007.
5. Hannah SS: Genetic Considerations in Companion Animal Nutrition. Proceedings, 2003 Tufts' Canine and Feline Breeding and Genetics Conference. 2003.
6. Strain GM: Deafness prevalence and pigmentation and gender associations in dog breeds at risk. *Vet J.* 2004 Jan;167(1):23-32.
7. *The Genetic Connection: A Guide to Health Problems in Purebred Dogs.* L Ackerman. p. 234. AAHA Press, 1999.
8. *The Complete Dog Book, 20th Ed.* The American Kennel Club. Howell Book House, NY 2006. p. 684-687.

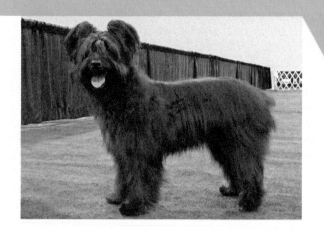

Pyrenean Shepherd

The Breed History

Evidence of sheepdogs in the Pyrenean mountains dates back to 6000 BC. Pyrenean Sheepdogs were used solely for herding and companionship, and not for protection; that role was left to the Great Pyrenees. It is believed that when the Virgin Mary appeared to the young shepherdess Bernadette Soubirous in the grotto at Lourdes in 1858, her little Pyrenean Shepherd was by her side. They are often referred to as "the dog that saw God." Pyrenean Shepherds distinguished themselves in the Pyrenees during World War II as couriers, and search and rescue dogs. The smooth-faced variety was used to establish the Australian Shepherd breed. The majority of Pyrenean Shepherd breeding stock was imported to the US in the 1970s and 1980s. AKC recognition occurred in 2009.

Breeding for Function

Pyrenean shepherds are breed to maintain a high degree of herding instinct and soundness. Their small size allows them to be quicker and more sure-footed on windy mountain crags. They should be selected to maintain breed type and working ability.

Physical Characteristics

Height at Withers: Rough-Faced: females 15-18" (38-46 cm), males: 15-1/2-18-1/2" (39-47 cm). Smooth-Faced: females 15-1/2-20-1/2" (39-52 cm), males 151/4-21" (39-53 cm).

Weight: 15-32 lbs (7-15 kg). To be kept lean, muscular, and never fat.

Coat: Rough-Faced: The Rough-Faced dog's coat can be of long or demi-long hair. Demi-long dogs have culottes on the rump, while the long-haired dogs are more heavily furnished with woollier hair that may cord. Smooth-Faced: The muzzle is covered with short, fine hairs. The hair becomes longer on the sides of the head, blending into a modest ruff. The hair on the body is fine and soft, attaining a maximum length of no more than 3 inches for the ruff and culottes, 2 inches along the back. Various shades of fawn from tan to copper, with or without a mixture of black hairs; grey, ranging from charcoal to silver to pearl grey; merles of diverse tones; brindle; black; black with white markings not exceeding 30% of the body surface. A little white is acceptable on the chest, head, and feet.

Longevity: 9-12 years.

Points of Conformation:

The dog in good working condition is lightly boned and sinewy. In rough faced dogs the body is clearly long in proportion to the height of the dog, whereas Smooth-Faced dogs appear much more square. The head is triangular in shape, and small in proportion to the size of the dog. The eyes are almond-shaped and dark brown in color, except in merles where blue or partially blue eyes are acceptable. Eye rims must be black. Ears can be cropped and erect, or natural and semi-prick. The head is a triangular wedge shape, with no stop. The nose is black. The back is level. The tail can be docked, natural bob, or long. The feet are oval, with double, single, or no rear dewclaws. The gait is flowing, with the feet barely leaving the ground.

Recognized Behavior Issues and Traits

The Pyrenean Shepdog is a high energy, intelligent, and mischievous dog that is always on alert, suspicious, ready for action. An ardent herder of all kinds of livestock. The Pyr Shep is naturally distrustful of strangers, but when well-socialized from a young age, he or she has a very lively, cheerful disposition. He is very affectionate with the members of his immediate family. He has the tendency to become passionately attached to his owner to the complete exclusion of all others and is astonishingly sensitive to his owner's moods. As a companion, he is very active and enthusiastic and insists upon being involved in the day's activities whatever they may be.

Normal Physiologic Variations

Merle Coat Color: Caused by a dominant mutation in the SILV gene. Breeding two merle dogs together should be avoided, as homozygous dogs can be born with multiple defects, including blindness, deafness, and heart anomalies.[1,2]

Drug Sensitivities

None Reported

Inherited Diseases

Hip Dysplasia: Polygenically inherited trait causing degenerative joint disease and hip arthritis. OFA reports 20.0% affected. Reported at a frequency of 11.8% in France.[3,4]

Elbow Dysplasia: Polygenically inherited trait causing elbow arthritis. Too few Pyrenean Shepherds have been screened by OFA to determine an accurate frequency.[3]

Patella Luxation: Polygenically inherited laxity of patellar ligaments, causing luxation, lameness, and later degenerative joint disease. Treat surgically if causing clinical signs. Reported as a breed problem on the Pyrenean Shepherd Club of America website. Too few Pyrenean Shepherds have been screened by OFA to determine an accurate frequency.[3]

Disease Predispositions

Cataracts: Anterior cortex punctate cataracts predominate in the breed. Reported in 7.14% of Pyrenean Shepherds CERF examined by veterinary ophthalmologists between 2000-2005. CERF does not recommend breeding any Pyrenean Shepherd with a cataract.[5]

Choroidal Hypoplasia: Inadequate development of the choroid present at birth and non-progressive. This condition is more commonly identified in the Collie breed where it is a manifestation of "Collie Eye Anomaly". CERF does not recommend breeding any Pyrenean Shepherd affected with the disorder. No genetic test is available in the breed. Identified in 5.36% of Pyrenean Shepherds CERF examined by veterinary ophthalmologists between 2000-2005.[5]

Persistent Pupillary Membranes: Strands of fetal remnant connecting; iris to iris, cornea, lens, or involving sheets of tissue. The later three forms can impair vision, and dogs affected with these forms should not be bred. Identified in 3.57% of Pyrenean Shepherds CERF examined by veterinary ophthalmologists between 2000-2005.[5]

Idiopathic Epilepsy (Inherited Seizures): Control with anti-seizure medication. Reported as a breed problem on the Pyrenean Shepherd Club of America website.

Hypothyroidism: Inherited autoimmune thyroiditis. Too few Pyrenean Shepherds have been test for thyroid autoantibodies at Michigan State University to determine an accurate frequency for the breed. (Ave. for all breeds is 7.5%).[6,7]

Progressive Retinal Atrophy (PRA): Progressive degeneration of the retina, eventually causing blindness. Reported as a breed problem on the Pyrenean Shepherd Club of America website. No genetic test is available.

Primary Lens Luxation: Partial (subluxation) or complete displacement of the lens from the normal anatomic site behind the pupil. Can progress to **secondary glaucoma** and blindness. Reported as a breed at risk by CERF; who does not recommend breeding any affected Pyrenean Shepherd.[5]

Patent Ductus Arteriosus (PDA): Inherited congenital heart disorder; affected dogs are usually stunted, and have a loud heart murmur. Diagnosis is via Doppler ultrasound. Treatment is surgical. Reported as a breed problem on the Pyrenean Shepherd Club of America website.[8]

Isolated Case Studies
None Reported

Genetic Tests
Tests of Genotype: None

Tests of Phenotype: CHIC certification: Required testing includes hip radiographs, CERF eye examination, patella evaluation, and DNA donation to the CHIC DNA repository. Optional testing includes cardiac evaluation. (See CHIC website; www.caninehealthinfo.org).

Recommend thyroid profile including autoantibodies and elbow radiographs.

Miscellaneous
- **Breed name synonyms:** Berger Des Pyrenees, Petit Berger, Labrit
- **Registries:** AKC, Canadian Kennel Club, UKC, KCGB (Kennel Club of Great Britain), FCI.
- **AKC rank:** (None) Became an AKC recognized breed Jan. 2009. Entire studbook registered.
- **Internet resources: Pyrenean Shepherd Club of America:** www.pyrshep.com
  The Pyrenean Sheepdog Club of Great Britain: www.pyreneansheepdog.co.uk/

References
1. Clark LA, Wahl JM, Rees CA, et. al.: Retrotransposon insertion in SILV is responsible for merle patterning of the domestic dog. Proc Natl Acad Sci U S A. 2006 Jan 31;103(5):1376-81.
2. Hedan B, Corre S, Hitte C, et al.: Coat colour in dogs: identification of the merle locus in the Australian shepherd breed. BMC Vet Res. 2006 Feb 27;2:9.
3. OFA Website breed statistics: www.offa.org Last accessed July 1, 2010.
4. Genevois JP, Remy D, Viguier E, et. al.: Prevalence of hip dysplasia according to official radiographic screening, among 31 breeds of dogs in France. Vet Comp Orthop Traumatol. 2008;21(1):21-4.
5. *Ocular Disorders Presumed to be Inherited in Purebred Dogs.* American College of Veterinary Ophthalmologists. ACVO, 2007.
6. Nachreiner RF, Refsal KR, Graham PA, et. al.: Prevalence of serum thyroid hormone autoantibodies in dogs with clinical signs of hypothyroidism. *J Am Vet Med Assoc* 2002 Feb 15;220(4):466-71.
7. Nachreiner R & Refsal K: Personal communication, Diagnostic Center for Population and Animal Health, Michigan State University. April, 2007.
8. Jacquet J, Nicolle AP, Chetboul V, et. al.: Echocardiographic and Doppler characteristics of postoperative ductal aneurysm in a dog. Vet Radiol Ultrasound. 2005 Nov-Dec;46(6):518-20.
9. AKC Breed Website: www.akc.org/breeds/pyrenean_shepherd/ Last accessed July 1, 2010.

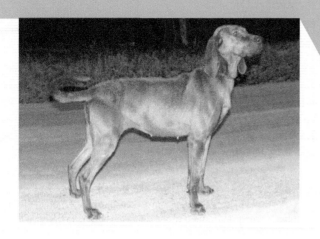

Redbone Coonhound

brush and saber-like. The gait should have good reach and drive.

Recognized Behavior Issues and Traits
The breed is even-tempered and trainable in the home, and wants to please its owner. They tend to be excellent with children. The Redbone should be well socialized at an early age and taught simple obedience like walking on a leash. They may not do well with cats, as they have a strong treeing instinct. They should be kept in a well fenced yard. They do best with a firm, but calm and consistent owner.

Normal Physiologic Variations
None reported

Drug Sensitivities
None reported

Inherited Diseases
Hip Dysplasia: Polygenically inherited trait causing degenerative joint disease and hip arthritis. OFA reports 36.4% affected, but too few Redbone Coonhounds have been evaluated for statistical confidence.[1]

Elbow Dysplasia: Polygenically inherited trait causing elbow arthritis. Too few Redbone Coonhounds have been screened by OFA to determine an accurate frequency.[1]

Patella Luxation: Polygenically inherited laxity of patellar ligaments, causing luxation, lameness, and later degenerative joint disease. Treat surgically if causing clinical signs. Too few Redbone Coonhounds have been screened by OFA to determine an accurate frequency.[1]

Disease Predispositions
Hypothyroidism: Inherited autoimmune thyroiditis. Not enough samples have been submitted for thyroid auto-antibodies to Michigan State University to determine an accurate frequency. (Ave. for all breeds is 7.5%).[2,3]

Coonhound Paralysis (polyradiculoneuritis): Disorder of acute paralysis due to transient demyelination, similar to Guillain-Barré syndrome. Caused by exposure to raccoon saliva in genetically susceptible dogs. Affected dogs can recover, but must be supported during remyelinization.[4,5]

Inherited Ocular Disorders: Too few Redbone Coonhounds have been CERF examined by veterinary ophthalmologists to determine an accurate frequency of inherited ocular disorders.[6]

Ectropion, Entropion, and **Progressive Retinal Atrophy** are reported.[7]

Isolated Case Studies
None Reported

The Breed History
Dating back to red foxhounds brought to the United States by Scottish immigrants in the late 1700s and red foxhounds imported from Ireland before the Civil War. By the late 18th century, some coon hunters began breeding for hotter-nosed, faster dogs that were swifter at locating and faster at treeing raccoons. They used the hot, swift Irish hounds in their breeding programs and the Redbone Coonhound evolved into a recognized, respected breed well before 1900. While other coonhound breeders selected only for function, Redbone breeders, for a period of several years, concentrated on breeding a nearly solid-colored, flashy, red dog, bred also for looks. As soon as the eye-catching color bred true, these serious hunters once again selected for performance. Today both attributes are well established in the breed. AKC recognition occurred in 2009.

Breeding for Function
The Redbone has been bred for the purpose of treeing raccoon and small game, and is acclaimed for its speed and agility from lowlands to steep, rocky hills. An excellent swimmer with a pleasant, if not constant voice.

Physical Characteristics
Height at withers: Males - 22 to 27 inches (56-69 cm). Females - 21 to 26 inches (53-66 cm).

Weight: 50-70 pounds (23-32 kg).

Coat: Short, smooth, coarse enough to provide protection. Solid red preferred. Dark muzzle and small amount of white on brisket and feet permissible.

Longevity: 11-12 years.

Points of Conformation: Should be equal in height from highest point of the shoulder blade to the ground as long measured from sternum to the buttocks. Slightly taller at shoulder than at hips. Pleading. Eyes - Dark brown to hazel in color, dark preferred. Set well apart. No drooping eyelids. Eyes round in shape. Ears are set moderately low, and fine in texture. The muzzle is square, and nostrils wide. Nose is black. Deep broad chest with ribs well sprung. Shoulder angulation should have a perfect 90-degree angle or close. Legs are straight and well boned. Tail is medium length, very slight

Genetic Tests

Tests of Genotype: None

Tests of Phenotype: Recommend hip and elbow radiographs, CERF eye examination, thyroid profile including autoantibodies, cardiac examination, and patella evaluation.

Miscellaneous

- **Breed name synonyms:** Redbone
- **Registries:** AKC, UKC, CKC, NKC (National Kennel Club)
- **AKC rank:** (none) AKC recognized in Dec. 2009. Entire stud book entered.
- **Internet resources: Redbone Coonhound Association of America:** www.redbonecaa.com

References

1. OFA Website breed statistics: www.offa.org Last accessed July 1, 2010.

2. Nachreiner R & Refsal K: Personal communication, Diagnostic Center for Population and Animal Health, Michigan State University. April, 2007.

3. Nachreiner RF, Refsal KR, Graham PA, et. al.: Prevalence of serum thyroid hormone autoantibodies in dogs with clinical signs of hypothyroidism. *J Am Vet Med Assoc* 2002 Feb 15;220(4):466-71.

4. Cummings JF, Haas DC: Coonhound paralysis. An acute idiopathic polyradiculoneuritis in dogs resembling the Landry-Guillain-Barre syndrome. *J Neurol Sci.* 1966 Jan-Feb;4(1):51-81.

5. Holmes DF, Schultz RD, Cummings JF, et. al.: Experimental coonhound paralysis: animal model of Guillain-Barre syndrome. *Neurology.* 1979 Aug;29(8):1186-7.

6. *Ocular Disorders Presumed to be Inherited in Purebred Dogs.* American College of Veterinary Ophthalmologists. ACVO, 2007.

7. *The Genetic Connection: A Guide to Health Problems in Purebred Dogs.* L Ackerman. p. 234. AAHA Press, 1999.

8. *The Complete Dog Book, 20th Ed.* The American Kennel Club. Howell Book House, NY 2006. p. 703-705.

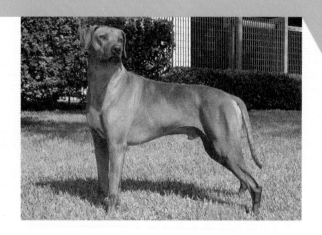

The Breed History

In South Africa, native Hottentot tribe dogs were crossed with imported European breeds such as Danes, Mastiffs and others. The native dogs had the unique breed signature "ridge" which is a patch of hair growing in reverse to the normal direction of hair on the topline. They were imported to the USA in the mid 1900s, and first AKC registration occurred in 1955.

Breeding for Function

The harsh environment of arid temperature extremes and rough bush required a dog that was hardy and could both hunt and protect. This loyal dog was used for lion hunting in Rhodesia starting in the late 1800s, and the standard breed arose from this Zimbabwe breeder group in 1922. These dogs have also been used for other large game such as bear and bobcat, and are now shown in obedience and conformation and are popular for hunting, watchdog, and companionship.

Physical Characteristics

Height at Withers: female 24-26" (61-66 cm), male 25-27" (63.5-68.5 cm)

Weight: females 70 lb (32 kg), males 85 lb (38.5 kg).

Coat: The sleek short coat is wheaten; a range of shades is permissible, with only very small white patches on chest or toes allowed.

Longevity: 10-12 years.

Points of Conformation: A lean, muscular athletic dog with excellent endurance, this breed is slightly longer than they are tall. The stop is defined, and eyes are round. Ears are wide at the base, tapering to a point and nose is black, brown or liver. Chest is deeper than wide, and the topline is slightly arched. Limbs are straight and strong but not coarse, and dewclaws may be removed. The signature characteristic, the ridge, should be symmetrical and start at the level of the shoulder, then taper as it reaches the wing of the ileum level. Exactly two whorls should be present and are placed opposite each other at the anterior end of the ridge.

Rhodesian Ridgeback

Recognized Behavior Issues and Traits

This dog is protective, gentle and loyal. He is easily trained, even-tempered and enjoys a family with children. They are known to be wary with strangers, and only rarely bark. Gentle obedience training should be combined with socialization to people and other pets when the dog is young. They need regular exercise and stimulation to prevent boredom. Average shedders, they require minimal grooming. They are not ideal city dogs, unless they get vigorous exercise.

Normal Physiologic Variations

Ridgelessness: The distinct dorsal ridge is inherited as an autosomal dominant trait. Ridgelessness is reported at a frequency of 10.6% in the RRCUS Health Survey 2001 Update. It is reported at a frequency of 5.6% in a study of Swedish Rhodesian Ridgebacks. The gene has been identified, but a commercial genetic test is not available.[1,2,3,4]

Drug Sensitivities

None reported

Inherited Diseases

Elbow Dysplasia: Polygenically inherited trait causing elbow arthritis. OFA reports 6.4% affected.[5]

Hip Dysplasia: Polygenically inherited trait causing degenerative joint disease and hip arthritis. OFA reports 5.1% affected.[5]

Patella Luxation: Polygenically inherited laxity of patellar ligaments, causing luxation, lameness, and later degenerative joint disease. Treat surgically if causing clinical signs. OFA reports 1.3% affected.[5]

Deafness: Rhodesian Ridgebacks have a rare, autosomal recessive form of deafness that develops after 8 weeks of age, and causes bilateral deafness by 1 year of age. Diagnosed by BAER testing. The gene has been identified, but a commercial genetic test is not available.[6,7]

Hemophilia B: An X-linked severe form of hemophilia B occurs in the breed due to a mutation in the Factor IX gene. Most affected Rhodesian Ridgebacks are male, with non-clinical carrier mothers. The frequency of the mutation in the breed is not known, but is thought to be low. A commercial genetic test is not available.[8]

Disease Predispositions

Hypothyroidism: Inherited autoimmune thyroiditis. 16.8% positive for thyroid autoantibodies based on testing at Michigan State University. (Ave. for all breeds is 7.5%).[9,10]

Dermoid Sinus (DS): A dermoid sinus is a congenital, dorsal midline tube extending from the skin to the dorsal spinous ligament or dura matter. They usually occur in the neck area, but can be located anywhere over the spine. The sinus is lined with epithelial cells, and may contain hair follicles, sebaceous glands and sweat glands. A DS can be palpated as a cord running between the skin and the spine, and most form a small external opening which can be readily seen once the hair has been shaved. A dog can have multiple DS. Dermoid sinuses become infected over time, which can spread into the CNS. All affected dogs should have the DS removed surgically, which often requires a partial dorsal laminectomy. The frequency in the Swedish Rhodesian ridgeback population is estimated to be between 8 and 10 per cent. DS is reported at a frequency of 4.8% in the RRCUS Health Survey 2001 Update. Undetermined mode of inheritance, but highly correlated to the presence of the dominantly inherited dorsal ridge. It is suggested that dogs homozygous for the dominant ridge gene may be more susceptible than heterozygous dogs. Difficulty in determining heredity pattern may be caused by undetected DS.[1,2,3,4,11,12,13,14]

Persistent Pupillary Membranes: Strands of fetal remnant connecting; iris to iris, cornea, lens, or involving sheets of tissue. The later three forms can impair vision, and dogs affected with these forms should not be bred. Identified in 5.26% of Rhodesian Ridgebacks CERF examined by veterinary ophthalmologists between 2000-2005.[15]

Allergic Dermatitis (Atopy): Inhalant or food allergy. Presents with pruritis and pyotraumatic dermatitis (hot spots). Reported at a frequency of 4.6% in the RRCUS Health Survey 2001 Update.[1]

Mast Cell Tumor (MCT): Skin tumors that produce histamine and cause inflammation and ulceration. Can reoccur locally or with distant metastasis. Reported at a frequency of 4.1% in the RRCUS Health Survey 2001 Update.[1]

Cataracts: Posterior cortex intermediate and punctate cataracts predominate in the breed. Age of onset 3 years. Identified in 3.41% of Rhodesian Ridgebacks CERF examined by veterinary ophthalmologists between 2000-2005. CERF does not recommend breeding any Rhodesian Ridgeback with a cataract.[15]

Distichiasis: Abnormally placed eyelashes that irritate the cornea and conjunctiva. Can cause secondary corneal ulceration. Identified in 2.73% of Rhodesian Ridgebacks CERF examined by veterinary ophthalmologists between 2000-2005.[15]

Soft Tissue Sarcoma: The Rhodesian Ridgeback is a breed at increased risk for developing soft tissue sarcomas, with 5.7% of all STS cases in one study occurring in Rhodesian Ridgebacks. Aggressive surgical management is associated with a low incidence of local recurrence.[16]

Secondary Glaucoma: Rhodesian Ridgebacks are listed as having a 4.1x risk for developing secondary glaucoma versus other breeds. Causes of secondary glaucoma include **anterior uveitis, lens luxation,** and **cataract**.[17]

Degenerative Myelopathy (DM): Affected dogs show an insidious onset of upper motor neuron (UMN) paraparesis at an average age of 11.4 years. The disease eventually progresses to severe tetraparesis. Affected dogs have normal results on myelography, MRI, and CSF analysis. Necropsy confirms the condition. Reported at a frequency of 0.74% in Rhodesian Ridgebacks. Unknown mode of inheritance. A direct genetic test for an autosomal recessive DM susceptibility gene is available, showing 41% carrier and 7% homozygous gene "at risk". All affected dogs are homozygous for the gene, however, only a small percentage of homozygous dogs develop DM.[18,19]

Cervical Vertebral Instability, Entropion, and **Hemivertebra** are reported.[20]

Isolated Case Studies

Renal Dysplasia: A six-month-old Rhodesian ridgeback dog was presented in chronic renal failure, with facial swelling due to fibrous osteodystrophy. Post mortem examination revealed renal dysplasia.[21]

Cerebellar Degeneration and Coat Color Dilution: Rhodesian Ridgebacks from two related litters presented with growth retardation, diluted coat color, and ataxia that progressed to lateral recumbency with tremors. Histopathology showed cerebellar Purkinje cell degeneration, and uneven distribution of macromelanosomes within hair shafts. Pedigree analysis suggested an autosomal recessive mode of inheritance.[22]

Acute Nonlymphocytic Leukemia: Diagnosed in a 1-year-old Rhodesian Ridgeback. Clinical signs of disease included weight loss, anorexia, lethargy, lymphadenopathy, splenomegaly, and hepatomegaly.[23]

Myotonic Dystrophy: A mature female Rhodesian Ridgeback had a progressive degenerative myopathy, associated with myotonia, dysphagia, and marked muscle wasting. Clinical findings revealed percussion dimpling, creatine kinase elevation, and a paroxysmal atrial tachycardia.[24]

Renal Adenocarcinoma: Concurrent renal adenocarcinoma and polycythemia were diagnosed in a 19-month-old, female Rhodesian ridgeback. Clinical signs included brick-red mucous membranes, lethargy, a periodic systolic heart murmur, and engorged retinal vessels. A large retroperitoneal mass and pulmonary metastatic nodules were found. Polycythemia was the result of excessive erythropoietin production.[25]

Osteochondrosarcoma of the Hard Palate: A 14-year-old castrated male Rhodesian Ridgeback was presented with a history of sneezing and epistaxis. A multilobular osteochondrosarcoma of the hard palate with pulmonary metastases was diagnosed.[26]

Spinal Meningioma: A 5-month-old male Rhodesian Ridgeback was diagnosed with a meningothelial meningioma with focal mineralization that extended from the cervical to the lumbosacral spine. There was a concurrent hydrocephalus.[27]

Genetic Tests

Tests of Genotype: Direct test for an autosomal recessive DM susceptibility gene is available from the OFA.

The genes for ridgelessness, deafness, and hemophilin B have been identified, however, commercial tests have not yet been developed.

Tests of Phenotype: CHIC certification: Required testing includes hip and elbow radiographs, CERF eye examination (annually to age 9), and thyroid profile including autoantibodies (at age 2, 3, 4, 5, 6 and 8). Optional recommended tests include cardiac evaluation, and BAER testing for deafness (minimum age of 12 months). (See CHIC website; www.caninehealthinfo.org).

Recommend patella evaluation.

Miscellaneous

- **Breed name synonyms:** African Lion Hound, Ridgeback
- **Registries:** AKC, CKC, UKC, KCGB (Kennel Club of Great Britain), ANKC (Australian National Kennel Club), NKC (National Kennel Club)
- **AKC rank (year 2008):** 50 (2,199 dogs registered)
- **Internet resources: Rhodesian Ridgeback Club of the United States:** www.rrcus.org
  RRCUS Health Website: www.rhodesianridgebackhealth.org
  Rhodesian Ridgeback Club of Canada: www.rrclubofcanada.org
  Rhodesian Ridgeback Club of Great Britain:
  www.rhodesianridgebacks.org

References

1. Pethick BJ, Brown DS: Rhodesian Ridgeback Club of the United States, Inc. 1996 National Health Survey Update. April 2001.
2. Hillbertz NH, Andersson G: Autosomal dominant mutation causing the dorsal ridge predisposes for dermoid sinus in Rhodesian ridgeback dogs. J Small Anim Pract. 2006 Apr;47(4):184-8.
3. Salmon Hillbertz NH, Isaksson M, Karlsson EK, et. al.: Duplication of FGF3, FGF4, FGF19 and ORAOV1 causes hair ridge and predisposition to dermoid sinus in Ridgeback dogs. Nat Genet. 2007 Nov;39(11):1318-20.
4. Karlsson EK, Baranowska I, Wade CM, et. al.: Efficient mapping of mendelian traits in dogs through genome-wide association. Nat Genet. 2007 Nov;39(11):1321-8.
5. OFA Website breed statistics: www.offa.org Last accessed July 1, 2010.
6. Strain GM: Deafness prevalence and pigmentation and gender associations in dog breeds at risk. Vet J. 2004 Jan;167(1):23-32.
7. Neff M: Personal communication. UC-Davis Veterinrary Genetics Laboratory. May, 2007.
8. Mischke R, Kühnlein P, Kehl A, et. al.: G244E in the canine factor IX gene leads to severe haemophilia B in Rhodesian Ridgebacks. Vet J. 2011 Jan;187(1):113-8.
9. Sist MD, Refsal KR, & Nachreiner RF: A Laboratory Survey of Autoimmune Thyroiditis and Hypothyroidism in Selected Sight Hound Breeds. Proceedings, 2009 Tufts' Canine and Feline Breeding and Genetics Conference. 2009.
10. Nachreiner RF, Refsal KR, Graham PA, et. al.: Prevalence of serum thyroid hormone autoantibodies in dogs with clinical signs of hypothyroidism. J Am Vet Med Assoc 2002 Feb 15;220(4):466-71.
11. Hillbertz NH: Inheritance of dermoid sinus in the Rhodesian ridgeback. J Small Anim Pract. 2005 Feb;46(2):71-4.
12. Kasa F, Kasa G, Kussinger S: Dermoid sinus in a Rhodesian ridgeback. Case report. Tierarztl Prax. 1992 Dec;20(6):628-31.
13. Antin IP: Dermoid sinus in a Rhodesian Ridgeback dog. J Am Vet Med Assoc. 1970 Oct 1;157(7):961-2.
14. Mann GE, Stratton J: Dermoid sinus in the Rhodesian Ridgeback. J Small Anim Pract. 1966 Oct;7(10):631-42.
15. *Ocular Disorders Presumed to be Inherited in Purebred Dogs.* American College of Veterinary Ophthalmologists. ACVO, 2007.
16. Baker-Gabb M, Hunt GB, France MP: Soft tissue sarcomas and mast cell tumours in dogs; clinical behaviour and response to surgery. Aust Vet J. 2003 Dec;81(12):732-8.
17. Johnsen DA, Maggs DJ, Kass PH: Evaluation of risk factors for development of secondary glaucoma in dogs: 156 cases (1999-2004). J Am Vet Med Assoc. 2006 Oct 15;229(8):1270-4.
18. Coates JR: Degenerative Myelopathy of Pembroke Welsh Corgi Dogs. Proceedings, 2005 ACVIM Forum. 2005.
19. Awano T, Johnson GS, Wade CM, et. al.: Genome-wide association analysis reveals a SOD1 mutation in canine degenerative myelopathy that resembles amyotrophic lateral sclerosis. Proc Natl Acad Sci U S A. 2009 Feb 24;106(8):2794-9.
20. *The Genetic Connection: A Guide to Health Problems in Purebred Dogs.* L Ackerman. p.234, AAHA Press, 1999.
21. Lobetti RG, Pearson J, Jimenez M: Renal dysplasia in a Rhodesian ridgeback dog. J Small Anim Pract. 1996 Nov;37(11):552-5.
22. Chieffo C, Stalis IH, Van Winkle TJ, et. al.: Cerebellar Purkinje's cell degeneration and coat color dilution in a family of Rhodesian Ridgeback dogs. J Vet Intern Med. 1994 Mar-Apr;8(2):112-6.
23. Hamlin RH, Duncan RC: Acute nonlymphocytic leukemia in a dog. J Am Vet Med Assoc. 1990 Jan 1;196(1):110-2.
24. Simpson ST, Braund KG: Myotonic dystrophy-like disease in a dog. J Am Vet Med Assoc. 1985 Mar 1;186(5):495-8.
25. Crow SE, Allen DP, Murphy CJ, et. al.: Concurrent renal adenocarcinoma and polycythemia in a dog. J Am Anim Hosp Assoc. 1995 Jan-Feb;31(1):29-33.
26. Banks TA, Straw RC: Multilobular osteochondrosarcoma of the hard palate in a dog. Aust Vet J. 2004 Jul;82(7):409-12.
27. Yeomans SM: SHORT PAPER - extensive spinal meningioma in a young dog. J Comp Pathol. 2000 May;122(4):303-6.
28. *The Complete Dog Book, 20th Ed.* The American Kennel Club. Howell Book House, NY 2006. p. 209-213.

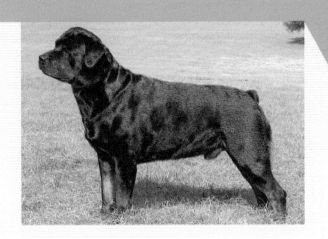

The Breed History

This Mastiff-type breed is thought to originate from the large drover dogs of Rome. The name of the breed derives from the German *"das Rote Wil"*, a name meaning *"the red tile"*, a reference to a building tile used in Roman structures which in addition to the Rottweiler dogs, were left behind in Germany. In the town named Rottweil, the breed thrived until cattle droving was outlawed. In the late 1800s there were few dogs left to represent the breed. Early in the 1900s breed resurgence was correlated with their new use as a police dog. The first stud book was put together in 1924. The first AKC studbook entry occurred in 1931.

Breeding for Function

These willing, dependable herding and guarding dogs were used by the Roman armies during their extensive war campaigns. Endurance, sure-footedness, strength and willingness to work characterized these dogs. Today, they are valued as companion dogs and police dogs.

Physical Characteristics

Height at Withers: female 22-25" (56-63.5 cm), male 24-27" (61-68.5 cm).

Weight: females 80-100 lb (36.5-45.5 kg), males 95-135 lb (43-61.5 kg).

Coat: There is only one coat color for the breed; black with rust marking. The inner coat is found on neck and the thighs, the outer coat lies down close to the skin and is hard and glossy. It is a dense coat, of medium to short length, with straight hairs.

Longevity: 12 years

Points of Conformation: Robust, compact constitution and black coloration with standard well-demarcated tan (rust to mahogany) markings characterize this breed. Males are distinctly more massive than females. This breed also has a characteristic long, swinging trot. The skull is very broad and somewhat arched between the ears, the head is large with heavy broad jaws, and the stop well defined. The eyes are dark brown, medium-sized, moderately deep set, and almond shaped. Ears are triangular, pendant and moderately sized so that the tips lie against the masseter muscle. The black nose is large and the lips are black. The neck is moderately short in length,

well muscled and slightly arched without throatiness. The topline is level. The thorax is deep and broad, and the ribs well sprung. Slight tuck up in the abdomen is standard. In North America, the tail is normally closely docked. The tail is carried slightly above horizontal while moving. Limbs are straight and heavily boned. Feet are compact, and round with well-arched toes. Dewclaws may be removed. Nails are black and the pads are thick and tough.

Recognized Behavior Issues and Traits

Reported breed traits include: Intensely developed guarding instinct, protective of family and home, high intelligence with aloof, self-assured attitude, calm, though some lines have tendencies to aggressiveness or shyness. Regular grooming needs and moderate tendency to shed characterize this breed. Moderate exercise needs. Good for country or city. Moderate barking tendency, and a low digging tendency unless bored. They possess a mild tendency to drool. Slow to mature. Early and thorough socialization and obedience training is essential. High trainability is notable. Males are more likely to exhibit dominance or inter-male aggression. Need mental stimulation and close human contact to prevent boredom vices.

Recommended for an experienced dog owner. Tolerance towards children is variable. Some do not recommend the breed for homes with toddlers or for the elderly or infirm. One reason is that the breed tends to "bump", a behavior left over from the drover days, when the dog would use a body check to move livestock. A full-grown dog can knock even an adult down. Tend to obesity. If let off leash, should be in a securely fenced enclosure (6' recommended). Tolerates cold weather but not heat.

Normal Physiologic Variations

None reported

Drug Sensitivities

None reported

Inherited Diseases

Elbow Dysplasia: Polygenically inherited trait causing elbow arthritis. Fragmented coronoid process is a common finding in the breed. Reported 36.1x odds ratio for fragmented coronoid process, 27.4x odds ratio for ununited anconeal process forms of elbow dysplasia, and 174x odds ratio for elbow osteochondrosis versus other breeds. OFA reports 40.3% affected. Elbow dysplasia has an estimated heritability of 0.34-0.39 in the breed.[1,2,3,4,5]

Hip Dysplasia: Polygenically inherited trait causing degenerative joint disease and hip arthritis. OFA reports 20.3% affected. Dorn reports a 1.94x odds ratio versus other breeds. Another study reports a 6.5x odds ratio versus other breeds. Hip dysplasia has an estimated heritability of 0.38 in the breed.[1,3,5,6]

Patella Luxation: Polygenically inherited laxity of patellar ligaments, causing luxation, lameness, and later degenerative joint disease. Treat surgically if causing clinical signs. OFA reports 1.2% affected.[1]

Disease Predispositions

Osteoarthritis: Rottweilers have an increased incidence of arthritis. Dorn reports a 3.82x odds ratio versus other breeds. Reported at a frequency of 20.0% in the Rottweiler Health Foundation Health Survey.[6,7]

Aggression: Towards other dogs reported at a frequency of 10.4%, and towards people at 3.6% in the Rottweiler Health Foundation Health Survey.[7]

Cranial Cruciate Ligament (ACL) Rupture: Traumatic tearing of the ACL in the stifle, causing lameness and secondary arthritis. Treat with surgery. Dorn reports a 2.19x odds ratio versus other breeds. Affected dogs have a significantly greater tibial plateau angle (TPA). TPA measurements may be helpful to screen prospective breeding dogs. Reported at a frequency of 9.1% in the Rottweiler Health Foundation Health Survey.[6,7,8]

Cataracts: Posterior polar cataracts predominate in the breed. Identified in 8.22% of Rottweilers CERF-examined by veterinary ophthalmologists between 2000-2005. Possible autosomal dominant inheritance, with incomplete penetrance. Reported at a frequency of 6.6% in the Rottweiler Health Foundation Health Survey. CERF does not recommend breeding any Rottweiler with a cataract.[7,9,10]

Hypothyroidism: Inherited autoimmune thyroiditis. 7.7% positive for thyroid autoantibodies based on testing at Michigan State University. (Ave. for all breeds is 7.5%). Reported at a frequency of 7.2% in the Rottweiler Health Foundation Health Survey.[7,11,12]

Osteosarcoma (OSA): Malignant bone cancer. Rottweilers are a breed with a predisposition for developing osteosarcoma versus other breeds. Mean age of appendicular OSA in the breed is 8.3 years, with preference for the forelimbs, and a breed frequency of 5.3%. Affected Rottweilers tend to have an increased immunohistochemical expression of p53 protein, and breed specific tumor chromosomal changes. Reported at a frequency of 7.3% in the Rottweiler Health Foundation Health Survey.[7,13,14,15,16]

Panosteitis: Self-limiting disorder of intermittent lameness involving the diaphyseal and metaphyseal areas of the tubular long bones in young dogs prior to skeletal maturation. Reported at a frequency of 5.0% in the Rottweiler Health Foundation Health Survey.[7]

Allergic Dermatitis: Inhalant or food allergy. Presents with pruritis and pyotraumatic dermatitis. Food allergy reported at a frequency of 5.0%, and inhalant at 3.2% in the Rottweiler Health Foundation Health Survey.[7]

Sebaceous Cysts: Benign skin cysts filled with sebum. Reported at a frequency of 4.7% in the Rottweiler Health Foundation Health Survey.[7]

Osteochondritis Dessicans/Osteochondrosis (OCD): Rottweilers have an increased incidence of hock OCD due to cartilage lesions in the lateral trochlear ridge of the talus, as well as shoulder and stifle OCD. Treatment with rest, or surgery in severe cases. Dorn reports a 3.35x odds ratio versus other breeds. Reported 206.2x odds ratio for hock OCD, 66.3x odds ratio for stifle OCD and 22.8x odds ratio for shoulder OCD versus other breeds. Reported at a frequency of 3.6% in the Rottweiler Health Foundation Health Survey.[3,6,7,17]

Subaortic Stenosis (SAS): Congenital narrowing of the aortic outflow tract from the heart, causing a murmur, endocarditis, left heart failure, or sudden death. Diagnosis is by doppler ultrasound. Rottweilers have a 19.3x odds ratio for the disorder versus other breeds.[18]

Multicentric Lymphoma (Lymphosarcoma): Malignant cancer of lymphocytes, expecially B-cells in the breed. Studies show an increased prevalence in the breed, with a 6.01x odds ratio versus other breeds. Treatment is with chemotherapy. Reported at a frequency of 3.3% in the Rottweiler Health Foundation Health Survey.[7,19,20,21]

Gastric Dilation/Volvulus (GDV, Bloat): Polygenically inherited, life-threatening twisting of the stomach within the abdomen. Requires immediate veterinary attention. There is a 3.9% lifetime risk of developing GDV in Rottweilers. Risk of death from GDV after prophylactic gastropexy decreased 2.2x fold. Reported at a frequency of 2.6% in the Rottweiler Health Foundation Health Survey.[7,22,23]

Umbilical Hernia: Congenital opening in the body wall from where the umbilical cord was attached. Correct surgically if large. Reported at a frequency of 2.3% in the Rottweiler Health Foundation Health Survey.[7]

Inflammatory Bowel Disease (IBD)/Protein-Losing Enteropathy (PLE): Immune mediated inflammatory disease of the intestines resulting in malabsorbtion. Rottweilers can present with a severe form of protein-losing enteropathy due to lymphoplasmacellular enteritis, with lymphangiectasia and eosinophil infiltration. Affected dogs present with chronic diarrhea, anorexia and weight loss, and a 1 year survival rate of 47% despite treatment with immunosuppressive drugs. IBD is reported at a frequency of 2.1% in the Rottweiler Health Foundation Survey.[7,24,25]

Idiopathic Epilepsy: Inherited seizures can be generalized or partial seizures. Control with anticonvulsant medication. Reported at a frequency of 2.0% in the Rottweiler Health Foundation Health Survey.[7]

Demodicosis, Generalized: Overgrowth of demodex mites in hair follicles due to an underlying immunodeficiency. Causes hair loss and inflammation. Reported at a frequency of 1.9% in the Rottweiler Health Foundation Health Survey.[7]

Persistent Pupillary Membranes: Strands of fetal remnant connecting; iris to iris, cornea, lens, or involving sheets of tissue. The later three forms can impair vision, and dogs affected with these forms should not be bred. Identified in 1.42% of Rottweilers CERF examined by veterinary ophthalmologists between 2000-2005.[9]

Cryptorchidism: Retained testicles. Can be unilateral or bilateral. Reported at a frequency of 1.3% in the Rottweiler Health Foundation Health Survey.[7]

Intervertebral Disc Disease (IVDD): Expulsion of disc material into the spinal cord causing pain, and spinal weakness or paralysis. Requires immediate veterinary attention. Reported at a frequency of 1.3% in the Rottweiler Health Foundation Health Survey.[7]

Retinal Dysplasia: Retinal folds, geographic, and generalized retinal dysplasia with detachment are recognized in the breed. Can progress to blindness. Reported in 1.05% of Rottweilers CERF-examined by veterinary ophthalmologists between 2000-2005.[9]

Corneal Dystrophy: Rottweilers can have an epithelial/stromal form of corneal dystrophy. Identified in 0.98% of Rottweilers CERF examined by veterinary ophthalmologists between 2000-2005.[9]

Entropion: A rolling in of the eyelids that can cause corneal irritation and ulceration. Reported in 0.73% of Rottweilers CERF-examined by veterinary ophthalmologists between 2000-2005. Dorn reports a 1.53x odds ratio versus other breeds.[6,9]

Progressive Retinal Atrophy (PRA): Inherited degeneration of the retina resulting in blindness. CERF does not recommend breeding any Rottweiler with PRA. Undetermined mode of inheritance in the breed.[9]

Susceptibility to Parvovirus Infection: Rottweilers have a 6.0x odds ratio for parvovirus enteritis versus other breeds. This is assumed to be due to an inherited immune impairment.[26]

Hypereosinophilia: Rottweilers are a breed found with higher frequencies of hypereosinophilia. Causes include pulmonary infiltrates with eosinophils, gastrointestinal disease, meningoencephalitis, and idiopathic hypereosinophilic syndrome (IHES).[27,28,29,30,31]

Metacarpal Sesamoid Disease: Young Rottweilers have a propensity for lameness due to forelimb sesamoid inflammation. Lameness resolves with rest. Many Rottweilers have subclinical sesamoid disease based on X-rays.[32]

Histiocytic Sarcomas: Rottweilers are a breed at increased risk for developing disseminated histiocytic sarcomas of the eye, synovium, subcutis, extremities, spleen, lung, brain, nasal cavity, and bone marrow. Histiocytic sarcoma should be considered as a differential diagnosis when a soft tissue mass is associated with a bone lesion on radiographs or myelography in Rottweilers over 5 years of age, or with aggressive periarticular, vertebral, or proximal humeral bone lesions.[33,34,35]

Cervical Spondylomyelopathy/Vertebral Instability (Wobbler Syndrome): Presents with UMN spasticity and ataxia. Imaging studies suggest that the primary lesion is foramenal stenosis and intervertebral instability at C6-7. MRI is superior to myelography in determining site, severity, and nature of the spinal cord compression. Seen an an increased frequency versus other breeds. Undetermined mode of inheritance.[36]

Hypoadrenocorticism (Addison's Disease): Immune-mediated destruction of the adrenal glands. Cited as a breed at significantly higher risk. Treat with life-long medication. Unknown mode of inheritance.[37]

Juvenile Nephropathy: Young affected Rottweilers present with severe polyuria and polydipsia, and progress to chronic renal failure. Histopathology included immature glomeruli and/or tubules, and persistent mesenchyme. A type IV collagen defect is suspected. Undetermined mode of inheritance.[38,39,40]

Calcinosis Circumscripta: Calcinosis circumscripta is an uncommon syndrome of dystrophic, metastatic or iatrogenic mineralization of calcium salts in soft tissues. Lesions usually occur on the hind feet or tongue in 1-4 year old dogs. Thirteen percent of canine cases occur in Rottweilers.[41]

Bronchiectasis: Rottweilers in Brazil have been reported with severe diffuse bronchiectasis with a history of chronic cough, respiratory distress, and progressive weight loss. Radiographic signs include lung lob consolidation, mild pleural effusion, and bilateral, diffuse saccular bronchiectasis.[42]

Neuronal Vacuolation and Spinocerebellar Degeneration: Rare, inherited disorder of Rottweilers presenting with generalized weakness, ataxia, and laryngeal paralysis starting at six weeks of age, and progressing to severe placing deficits, knuckling, severe ataxia, and quadraparesis by eight months of age. Pathology includes intracytoplasmic neuronal vacuolation in the cerebellar roof nuclei and extrapyramidal system, and symmetrical spinal cord axonal degeneration. Undetermined mode of inheritence.[43,44,45]

Neuroaxonal Dystrophy: Rare, inherited disorder of Rottweilers presenting with progressive four limb ataxia and head tremors of several months to years duration. There is no weakness associated with this disorder. Pathology shows neuroaxonal dystrophy, and immunoreactivity shows disruption of axonal transport. Undetermined mode of inheritence.[46,47]

Spinal Subarachnoid Cysts/Pseudocysts: Studies show Rottweilers under 12 months of age can have a predisposition to form cystic lesions in the subarachnoid space that can compress the spinal cord causing weakness and ataxia. Diagnosis with CT or MRI. Treatment is with surgery.[48,49]

Leucoencephalomyelopathy: Rare, inherited disorder of Rottweilers presenting with progressive ataxia and paresis from 1.5 to 3.5 years of age. In most dogs the forelimbs were affected prior to the hind limbs. Pathology reveals demyelinating lesions in the cervical spinal cord and brain stem. Undetermined mode of inheritence.[50]

Juvenile Distal Myopathy/Muscular Dystrophy: Rare disorder observed in multiple Rottweilers with decreased activity, plantigrade and palmigrade stance and splayed forepaw digits. Electromyography reveals a primary myopathy. Pathology revealed myofiber atrophy of the distal muscles.[51]

Distal Sensorimotor Polyneuropathy: Rare, slowly progressive paraparesis that progresses to tetraparesis, spinal hyporeflexia and hypotonia, and appendicular muscle atrophy in 1.5 to 4 year old Rottweilers. Histopathology suggests a dying-back distal sensorimotor polyneuropathy.[52]

Brachygnathism, Ciliary Dyskenesis, Deafness, Hemivertebra, Hypertrophic Osteodystrophy, Incomplete Ossification of the Humeral Condyle, Leukodystrophy, Lymphedema, Microphthalmia, Oligodontia, Prognathism, Seasonal Flank Alopecia, Spinal Muscular Atrophy, Ulcerative Keratitis, Vasculitis, Vitiligo, von Willebrand's Disease, and **Wry Mouth** are reported.[53]

Isolated Case Studies

Aortic Bulb/Valve Mineralization: Seven of 20 affected dogs were Rottweilers in one study. The mineralization is visible radiographically, but does not cause clinical signs.[54]

Narcolepsy: Case report of a one year old female Rottweiler with narcolepsy and cataplexy responsive to imipramine.[55]

Congenital Holoprosencephaly/Otocephaly: A stillborn Rottweiler puppy was born with severe craniofacial malformations including absence of the eyes, upper and lower jaws, mouth, teeth and tongue. Repeat breedings of the parents produced similarly affected pups.[56]

Genetic Tests

Tests of Genotype: None

Tests of Phenotype: CHIC Certification: Required testing includes hip and elbow radiographs, CERF eye examination, and cardiac evaluation. (See CHIC website; www.caninehealthinfo.org).

Recommended thyroid profile including autoantibodies, and patella evaluation.

Miscellaneous

- **Breed name synonyms:** Rottweiler Metzgerhund (means butcher dog) Rottie, Rottwieler.
- **Registries:** AKC, UKC, CKC, KCGB (Kennel Club of Great Britain), ANKC (Australian National Kennel Club), NKC (National Kennel Club).
- **AKC rank (year 2008):** 14 (13,059 dogs registered)
- **Internet resources: American Rottweiler Club (AKC parent club):** www.amrottclub.org
  Rottweiler Club of Canada: www.rottclub.ca
  The Rottweiler Club (UK): www.therottweilerclub.co.uk
  United States Rottweiler Club: www.usrconline.org
  Rottweiler Health Foundation: www.rottweilerhealth.org

References

1. OFA Website breed statistics: www.offa.org Last accessed July 1, 2010.
2. Meyer-Lindenberg A, Langhann A, Fehr M, et. al.: Prevalence of fragmented medial coronoid process of the ulna in lame adult dogs. Vet Rec. 2002 Aug 24;151(8):230-4.
3. LaFond E, Breur GJ & Austin CC: Breed susceptibility for developmental orthopedic diseases in dogs. J Am Anim Hosp Assoc. 2002 Sep-Oct;38(5):467-77.
4. Heine A, Hamann H, Tellhelm B, et. al.: Estimation of population genetic parameters and breeding values for elbow dysplasia in Rottweilers. Berl Munch Tierarztl Wochenschr. 2009 Mar-Apr;122(3-4):100-7.
5. Malm S, Fikse WF, Danell B, et. al.: Genetic variation and genetic trends in hip and elbow dysplasia in Swedish Rottweiler and Bernese Mountain Dog. J Anim Breed Genet. 2008 Dec;125(6):403-12.
6. Dorn CR: Canine breed-specific risks of frequently diagnosed diseases at veterinary teaching hospitals. Monograph. AKC Canine Health Foundation. 2000.
7. Rottweiler Health Foundation, Slater MR: Rottweiler Health Foundation Health Survey. 2001.
8. Morris E, Lipowitz AJ: Comparison of tibial plateau angles in dogs with and without cranial cruciate ligament injuries. J Am Vet Med Assoc. 2001 Feb 1;218(3):363-6.
9. *Ocular Disorders Presumed to be Inherited in Purebred Dogs.* American College of Veterinary Ophthalmologists. ACVO, 2007.
10. Bjerkas E, Bergsjo T: Hereditary cataract in the Rottweiler dog. Progress in Veterinary and Comparative Ophthalmol 1991;1:7.
11. Nachreiner RF, Refsal KR, Graham PA, et. al.: Prevalence of serum thyroid hormone autoantibodies in dogs with clinical signs of hypothyroidism. *J Am Vet Med Assoc* 2002 Feb 15;220(4):466-71.
12. Nachreiner R & Refsal K: Personal communication, Diagnostic Center for Population and Animal Health, Michigan State University. April, 2007.
13. Misdorp W, Hart AA: Some prognostic and epidemiologic factors in canine osteosarcoma. J Natl Cancer Inst. 1979 Mar;62(3):537-45.
14. Loukopoulos P, Thornton JR, Robinson WF: Clinical and pathologic relevance of p53 index in canine osseous tumors. Vet Pathol. 2003 May;40(3):237-48.
15. Rosenberger JA, Pablo NV, Crawford PC, et. al.: Prevalence of and intrinsic risk factors for appendicular osteosarcoma in dogs: 179 cases (1996-2005). J Am Vet Med Assoc. 2007 Oct 1;231(7):1076-80.
16. Thomas R, Wang HJ, Tsai PC, et. al.: Influence of genetic background on tumor karyotypes: evidence for breed-associated cytogenetic aberrations in canine appendicular osteosarcoma. Chromosome Res. 2009;17(3):365-77.
17. Wisner ER, Berry CR, Morgan JP, et. al.: Osteochondrosis of the lateral trochlear ridge of the talus in seven Rottweiler dogs. Vet Surg. 1990 Nov-Dec;19(6):435-9.
18. Kienle RD, Thomas WP, Pion PD: The natural clinical history of canine congenital subaortic stenosis. J Vet Intern Med. 1994 Nov-Dec;8(6):423-31.
19. Jagielski D, Lechowski R, Hoffmann-Jagielska M, et. al.: A retrospective study of the incidence and prognostic factors of multicentric lymphoma in dogs (1998-2000). J Vet Med A Physiol Pathol Clin Med. 2002 Oct;49(8):419-24.
20. Pastor M, Chalvet-Monfray K, Marchal T, et. al.: Genetic and environmental risk indicators in canine non-Hodgkin's lymphomas: breed associations and geographic distribution of 608 cases diagnosed throughout France over 1 year. J Vet Intern Med. 2009 Mar-Apr;23(2):301-10.
21. Lobetti RG: Lymphoma in 3 related Rottweilers from a single household. J S Afr Vet Assoc. 2009 Jun;80(2):103-5.
22. Glickman LT, Glickman NW, Schellenberg DB, et. al.: Incidence of and breed-related risk factors for gastric dilatation-volvulus in dogs. J Am Vet Med Assoc. 2000 Jan 1;216(1):40-5.
23. Ward MP, Patronek GJ, Glickman LT: Benefits of prophylactic gastropexy for dogs at risk of gastric dilatation-volvulus. Prev Vet Med. 2003 Sep 12;60(4):319-29.
24. Dijkstra M, Kraus JS, Bosje JT, et. al.: Protein-losing enteropathy in Rottweilers. Tijdschr Diergeneeskd. 2010 May 15;135(10):406-12.
25. Lecoindre P, Chevallier M & Guerret S: Protein-losing enteropathy of non neoplastic origin in the dog: a retrospective study of 34 cases. Schweiz Arch Tierheilkd. 2010 Mar;152(3):141-6.
26. Glickman LT, Domanski LM, Patronek GJ, et. al.: Breed-related risk factors for canine parvovirus enteritis. J Am Vet Med Assoc. 1985 Sep 15;187(6):589-94.
27. Lilliehook I, Tvedten H: Investigation of hypereosinophilia and potential treatments. Vet Clin North Am Small Anim Pract. 2003 Nov;33(6):1359-78, viii.
28. Sykes JE, Weiss DJ, Buoen LC, et. al.: Idiopathic hypereosinophilic

syndrome in 3 Rottweilers. J Vet Intern Med. 2001 Mar-Apr;15(2):162-6.

29. Olivier AK, Parkes JD, Flaherty HA, et. al.: Idiopathic eosinophilic meningoencephalomyelitis in a Rottweiler dog. J Vet Diagn Invest. 2010 Jul;22(4):646-8.

30. Lyles SE, Panciera DL, Saunders GK, et. al.: Idiopathic eosinophilic masses of the gastrointestinal tract in dogs. J Vet Intern Med. 2009 Jul-Aug;23(4):818-23.

31. James FE & Mansfield CS: Clinical remission of idiopathic hypereosino-philic syndrome in a Rottweiler. Aust Vet J. 2009 Aug;87(8):330-3.

32. Read RA, Black AP, Armstrong SJ, et. al.: Incidence and clinical significance of sesamoid disease in rottweilers. Vet Rec. 1992 Jun 13;130(24):533-5.

33. Affolter VK, Moore PF: Localized and disseminated histiocytic sarcoma of dendritic cell origin in dogs. Vet Pathol. 2002 Jan;39(1):74-83.

34. Schultz RM, Puchalski SM, Kent M, et. al.: Skeletal lesions of histiocytic sarcoma in nineteen dogs. Vet Radiol Ultrasound. 2007 Nov-Dec;48(6):539-43.

35. Naranjo C, Dubielzig RR, & Friedrichs KR: Canine ocular histiocytic sarcoma. Vet Ophthalmol. 2007 May-Jun;10(3):179-85.

36. Casimiro da Costa R: Cervical Spondylomyelopathy: Recent Advances. Proceedings, World Small Animal Veterinary Association World Congress. 2009.

37. Peterson ME, Kintzer PP, Kass PH: Pretreatment clinical and laboratory findings in dogs with hypoadrenocorticism: 225 cases (1979-1993). J Am Vet Med Assoc. 1996 Jan 1;208(1):85-91.

38. Peeters D, Clercx C, Michiels L, et. al.: Juvenile nephropathy in a boxer, a rottweiler, a collie and an Irish wolfhound. Aust Vet J. 2000 Mar;78(3):162-5.

39. Cook SM, Dean DF, Golden DL, et. al.: Renal failure attributable to atrophic glomerulopathy in four related rottweilers. J Am Vet Med Assoc. 1993 Jan 1;202(1):107-9.

40. Wakamatsu N, Surdyk K, Carmichael KP, et. al.: Histologic and ultrastructural studies of juvenile onset renal disease in four Rottweiler dogs. Vet Pathol. 2007 Jan;44(1):96-100.

41. Tafti AK, Hanna P, Bourque AC: Calcinosis circumscripta in the dog: a retrospective pathological study. J Vet Med A Physiol Pathol Clin Med. 2005 Feb;52(1):13-7.

42. Duarte R: Severe Bronchiectasis in Rottweilers: An Unnamed Disease. Proceedings, 2009 World Small Animal Veterinary Association World Congress. 2009.

43. Salvadori C, Tartarelli CL, Baroni M, et. al.: Peripheral nerve pathology in two rottweilers with neuronal vacuolation and spinocerebellar degeneration. Vet Pathol. 2005 Nov;42(6):852-5.

44. Kortz GD, Meier WA, Higgins RJ, et. al.: Neuronal vacuolation and spinocerebellar degeneration in young Rottweiler dogs. Vet Pathol. 1997 Jul;34(4):296-302.

45. Mahony OM, Knowles KE, Braund KG, et. al.: Laryngeal paralysis-polyneuropathy complex in young Rottweilers. J Vet Intern Med. 1998 Sep-Oct;12(5):330-7.

46. Siso S, Ferrer I, Pumarola M: Juvenile neuroaxonal dystrophy in a Rottweiler: accumulation of synaptic proteins in dystrophic axons. Acta Neuropathol (Berl). 2001 Nov;102(5):501-4.

47. Chrisman CL, Cork LC, Gamble DA: Neuroaxonal dystrophy of Rottweiler dogs. J Am Vet Med Assoc. 1984 Feb 15;184(4):464-7.

48. Gnirs K, Ruel Y, Blot S, et. al.: Spinal subarachnoid cysts in 13 dogs. Vet Radiol Ultrasound. 2003 Jul-Aug;44(4):402-8.

49. Jurina K, Grevel V: Spinal arachnoid pseudocysts in 10 rottweilers. J Small Anim Pract. 2004 Jan;45(1):9-15.

50. Wouda W, van Nes JJ: Progressive ataxia due to central demyelination in Rottweiler dogs. Vet Q. 1986 Apr;8(2):89-97.

51. Hanson SM, Smith MO, Walker TL, et. al.: Juvenile-onset distal myopathy in Rottweiler dogs. J Vet Intern Med. 1998 Mar-Apr;12(2):103-8.

52. Braund KG, Toivio-Kinnucan M, Vallat JM, et. al.: Distal sensorimotor polyneuropathy in mature Rottweiler dogs. Vet Pathol. 1994 May;31(3):316-26.

53. The Genetic Connection: A Guide to Health Problems in Purebred Dogs. L Ackerman. p. 235. AAHA Press, 1999.

54. Douglass JP, Berry CR, Thrall DE, Malarkey DE, Spaulding KA: Radiographic features of aortic bulb/valve mineralization in 20 dogs. Vet Radiol Ultrasound. 2003 Jan-Feb;44(1):20-7.

55. Hendricks JC, Hughes C: Treatment of cataplexy in a dog with narcolepsy. J Am Vet Med Assoc. 1989 Mar 15;194(6):791-2.

56. Martínez JS, Velázquez IR, Reyes H, et. al.: Congenital holoprosen-cephaly with severe otocephaly in a rottweiler puppy. Vet Rec. 2006 Apr 15;158(15):518-9.

57. The Complete Dog Book, 20th Ed. The American Kennel Club. Howell Book House, NY 2006. p. 314-318.

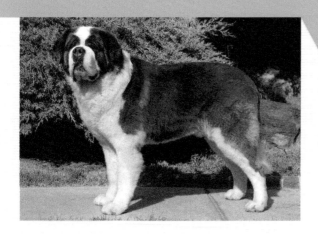

The Breed History

The St. Bernard dogs are thought to have originated from crosses of Asian Molosser dogs (Canis molossus) that were introduced to Switzerland by the Romans with local dogs. Augustine Monks bred these dogs primarily in the main pass between Switzerland and Italy; later named the Great St. Bernard Pass. Documentation of their use as rescue dogs in the Alps dates to the late 1600s. In 1830, outcrossing to Newfoundland dogs was done to increase breed vigor because of extensive inbreeding. This resulted in the first of the longhair subtype of the breed which turned out not to be desirable as the long hair trapped snow and ice. The breed was formally named in 1880. The original breed standard was developed in 1884 but some differences persisted in type between Swiss and English dogs. AKC recognition occurred in 1885. The English wrote a separate standard in 1887. The St. Bernard Club of America follows the original Swiss standard.

Breeding for Function

St. Bernard's were primarily used for draft, clearing trails in snow, guarding, and for herding. In the Swiss Alps, they became invaluable to the Monks, particularly at the Hospice St. Bernard de Menthon in the St. Bernard pass. Their live-saving role helped travelers safely traverse the treacherous mountain passes, and they provided search and rescue. They used their excellent tracking skills to find those lost in avalanches for example. No records were kept on how many lives were saved, but estimates run in the thousands.

Physical Characteristics

Height at Withers: ideal height for female 25.5" (65 cm), male 27.5" (70 cm).

Weight: 110-200 lb (50-91 kg).

Coat: The coat is very dense, and the hairs lie smoothly down; hairs are strong but not coarse, short, and the tail hair is longer near the body than at the tip. Colors include red with white markings, white with red markings, and brindle with white. Red may be a browny-yellow without fault. There is a specified pattern of markings. Dark mask and ears are favored. There is a longhaired and shorthaired variety. The autosomal recessive longhaired variety is actually a medium length coat. Hair is slightly wavy, though face and ears have a short straight coat.

Saint Bernard

Longevity: 8-9 years

Points of Conformation: A powerful figure, this breed is noted for the imposing stature and massive head with an intelligent expression. The wide skull is characterized by strong cheek bones, marked stop, and a furrow runs over the midline of the skull, including the muzzle, wrinkles are present over the forehead, and the muzzle is square, with well-developed flews on both upper and lower lips. Usually the palate is pigmented black. The nose and lips are also black. Ears are high set and triangular in shape, floppy, with a broad base. The front margin of the pinna sits against the head. Eyes are dark brown ,medium-sized and moderately deep set. The lower lids normally form a triangle and rest in an everted position. The neck is strong, of medium length and the dewlap is well developed. The thorax is of moderate depth and ribs are well sprung. The topline is level, though it gently curves down to the tail in the croup. The tail is heavy and long, straight to slightly curved. Limbs are straight, heavily boned and muscled. Dewclaws are undesirable and may be removed. Feet are large and broad, with good knuckling up of the toes.

Recognized Behavior Issues and Traits

Reported breed characteristics include: Docile, placid temperament, strong on a leash, not suitable for apartment living due to size. Slow to mature physically. Most are excellent with children and eager to please, but need to have early obedience training due to their size. Some can be aggressive. Low shedding tendency except during spring and fall when they blow the coat. They possess a moderate drooling tendency. Not a watchdog, but they will alarm bark. Will defend a family member if directly threatened. Good with other dogs, especially lacking inter-male aggression due to their history of work in male dog rescue teams.

Normal Physiologic Variations

In a UK study, 41.2% of litters were born via **Cesarean section.**[1]

Drug Sensitivities

None reported

Inherited Diseases

Hip Dysplasia: Polygenically inherited trait causing degenerative joint disease and hip arthritis. Reported 7.2x odds ratio versus other breeds. OFA reports 46.7% affected.[2,3]

Elbow Dysplasia: Polygenically inherited trait causing elbow arthritis. OFA reports 16.2% affected. Reported 53.4x odds ratio for fragmented coronoid process, and 14.2x odds ratio for ununited anconeal process forms of elbow dysplasia versus other breeds.[2,3]

Patella Luxation: Polygenically inherited laxity of patellar ligaments, causing luxation, lameness, and later degenerative joint disease. Treat surgically if causing clinical signs. Too few Saint Bernard's have been screened by OFA to determine an accurate frequency.[2]

Disease Predispositions

Ectropion: Rolling out of eyelids, often with a medial canthal pocket. Can cause secondary conjunctivitis. Can be secondary to macroblepharon; an abnormally large eyelid opening. Ectropion is reported in 28.33% and macroblepharon in 15.00% of Saint Bernards CERF examined by veterinary ophthalmologists between 2000-2005. Dorn reports a 4.64x odds ratio in Saint Bernard's versus other breeds.[4,5]

Entropion: Rolling in of eyelids, often causing corneal irritation or ulceration. Dorn reports a 4.64x odds ratio in Saint Bernards versus other breeds. Entropion is reported in 11.67% of Saint Bernards CERF examined by veterinary ophthalmologists between 2000-2005.[4,5]

Cataracts: Intermediate cataracts predominate in the breed. Identified in 11.67% of Saint Bernards CERF examined by veterinary ophthalmologists between 2000-2005. CERF does not recommend breeding any Saint Bernard with a cataract.[5]

Persistent Pupillary Membranes: Strands of fetal remnant connecting; iris to iris, cornea, lens, or involving sheets of tissue. The later three forms can impair vision, and dogs affected with these forms should not be bred. Identified in 8.33% of Saint Bernards CERF examined by veterinary ophthalmologists between 2000-2005.[5]

Hypothyroidism: Inherited autoimmune thyroiditis. 7.2% positive for thyroid autoantibodies based on testing at Michigan State University. (Ave. for all breeds is 7.5%).[6,7]

Gastric Dilatation-Volvulus (Bloat, GDV): Polygenically inherited, life-threatening twisting of the stomach within the abdomen. Requires immediate veterinary attention. Dorn reports a 2.91x odds ratio of developing GDV versus other breeds. Glickman reports a 4.2x odds ratio.[4,8]

Humeral Osteochondritis Dissecans (OCD): Polygenically inherited cartilage defect of the humeral head. Causes shoulder joint pain and lameness in young growing dogs. Mild cases can resolve with rest, while more severe cases require surgery. There is a 2.24:1 male to female ratio. 75% of all cases are unilateral. Reported 12.2x odds ratio versus other breeds. Dorn reports a 3.19x odds ratio of developing OCD versus other breeds.[3,4]

Cranial Cruciate Ligament (ACL) Rupture: Traumatic tearing of the ACL in the stifle, causing lameness and secondary arthritis. Treat with surgery. Reported at an increased incidence versus other breeds.[9]

Osteosarcoma (Bone Cancer): The Saint Bernard is a breed predisposed to develop malignant osteosarcoma, usually in the long bones of the limbs. A swiss study showed 4.0% of the breed affected by age 6, and 8.2% by age 10, with a median age of onset of 7.3 years.[10,11,12]

Distichiasis: Abnormally placed eyelashes that irritate the cornea and conjunctiva. Can cause secondary corneal ulceration. Reported in 3.33% of Saint Bernards CERF examined by veterinary ophthalmologists between 2000-2005.[5]

Dilated Cardiomyopathy: Saint Bernards are a predisposed breed for this condition, resulting in heart failure. Prevalence of 2.6%. Average age of clinical signs is 5.3 years. Unknown mode of inheritance.[13]

Corneal Dystrophy: Saint Bernards can have an epithelial/stromal form of corneal dystrophy. Reported in 1.67% of Saint Bernards CERF examined by veterinary ophthalmologists between 2000-2005.[5]

Idiopathic Epilepsy (inherited seizures): Seizures can be partial or generalized. Control with anti-seizure medication. Seen at an increased frequency in the breed.[14]

Primary Hypoparathyroidism: Identified in several Saint Bernards. Clinical signs included anorexia, behavioral changes, muscle tremors, seizures, panting, and cataracts. Serum calcium was low, phosphorus elevated, and the immunoreactive parathyroid hormone level low in all dogs. Most dogs responded to synthetic vitamin D and oral calcium. Unknown etiology.[15,16]

Multiple Ocular Defects: Rare disorder seen in Saint Bernard puppies. Characterized by microphthalmia, aphakia, acoria, peripheral anterior synechia, and retinal dysplasia. CERF does not recommend breeding any Saint Bernard with the condition.[5,17]

Cutaneous Asthenia, Deafness, Dermoid Sinus, Factor IX Deficiency, Hypofibrinogenemia, Malignant Hyperthermia, Narcolepsy, Panosteitis, and **Sebaceous Adenitis** are reported.[18]

Isolated Case Studies

Liver Lobe Torsion: A 5-month-old, male Saint Bernard was presented for acute collapse and abdominal discomfort. Exploratory surgery revealed torsion of both the left lateral and middle liver lobes. Early diagnosis and prompt surgical intervention is required.[19]

Occipito-Atlanto-Axial Malformation: A male Saint Bernard dog became suddenly tetraplegic at 8 weeks, was recumbent, had generalized muscle atrophy, but was alert and responsive. Pain was elicited on manipulation of the head-neck junction and the cervical vertebrae. Radiographs revealed malformation of the occipital bones, atlas, and axis, unilateral atlanto-occipital fusion, and atlanto-axial subluxation.[20]

Hepatic Arteriovenous Fistula: Two Saint Bernard pups, 7 and 5 months old respectively, were examined because of anorexia, vomiting, and ascites. Exploratory laparotomy disclosed arteriovenous fistula of the right medial lobe of the liver in one dog, and in the right medial and quadrate lobes of the other one. Surgical removal of the affected lobes resulted in cessation of presenting signs. Both dogs remained healthy but had poor weight gain and vomited occasionally.[21]

Nasal Philtrum Arteritis: Related Saint Bernard's developed solitary, well-circumscribed, linear ulcers on the nasal philtrum, with repeated episodes of arterial bleeding. Onset 3-6 years. Histopathological findings included lymphoplasmacytic dermatitis, proliferating spindle cells of either myofibroblast or smooth muscle origin, and deep dermal arteries and arterioles subjacent to the ulcer. The lesions respond to steroidal treatment.[22]

Genetic Tests

Tests of Genotype: none

Tests of Phenotype: Recommended testing includes hip and elbow radiographs, CERF eye examination, patella evaluation, thyroid profile including autoantibodies, and cardiac examination.

Miscellaneous

- **Breed name synonyms:** St. Bernhardshund, St.Bernard, Alpine Mastiff, Talhund (historical - means Valley Dog), Bauerhund (historical-means Farm Dog), Hospice Dog (historical) Monastery Dog (historical), Barryhund (historical-in Switzerland, means Barry dog), Sacred Dog (historical-English), Alpenhund (historical-German).
- **Registries:** AKC, UKC, CKC, KCGB (Kennel Club of Great Britain), ANKC (Australian National Kennel Club), NKC (National Kennel Club).
- **AKC rank (year 2008):** 45 (3,007 dogs registered)
- **Internet resources: The Saint Bernard Club of America:** www.saintbernardclub.org
  English Saint Bernard Club: www.englishstbernardclub.co.uk

References

1. Evans KM & Adams VJ: Proportion of litters of purebred dogs born by caesarean section. J Small Anim Pract. 2010 Feb;51(2):113-8.

2. OFA Website breed statistics: www.offa.org Last accessed July 1, 2010.

3. LaFond E, Breur GJ & Austin CC: Breed susceptibility for developmental orthopedic diseases in dogs. J Am Anim Hosp Assoc. 2002 Sep-Oct;38(5):467-77.

4. Dorn CR: Canine breed-specific risks of frequently diagnosed diseases at veterinary teaching hospitals. Monograph. AKC Canine Health Foundation. 2000.

5. *Ocular Disorders Presumed to be Inherited in Purebred Dogs.* American College of Veterinary Ophthalmologists. ACVO, 2007.

6. Nachreiner RF, Refsal KR, Graham PA, et. al.: Prevalence of serum thyroid hormone autoantibodies in dogs with clinical signs of hypothyroidism. J Am Vet Med Assoc 2002 Feb 15;220(4):466-71.

7. Nachreiner R & Refsal K: Personal communication, Diagnostic Center for Population and Animal Health, Michigan State University. April, 2007.

8. Glickman LT, Glickman NW, Perez CM, et. al.: Analysis of risk factors for gastric dilatation and dilatation-volvulus in dogs. J Am Vet Med Assoc. 1994 May 1;204(9):1465-71.

9. Duval JM, Budsberg SC, Flo GL, et. al.: Breed, sex, and body weight as risk factors for rupture of the cranial cruciate ligament in young dogs. J Am Vet Med Assoc. 1999 Sep 15;215(6):811-4.

10. Bech-Nielsen S, Haskins ME, Reif JS, et. al.: Frequency of osteosarcoma among first-degree relatives of St. Bernard dogs. J Natl Cancer Inst. 1978 Feb;60(2):349-53.

11. Taylor GN, Lloyd RD, Mays CW, et. al.: Relationship of natural incidence and radiosensitivity for bone cancer in dogs. Health Phys. 1997 Oct;73(4):679-83.

12. Egenvall A, Nødtvedt A & von Euler H: Bone tumors in a population of 400 000 insured Swedish dogs up to 10 y of age: incidence and survival. Can J Vet Res. 2007 Oct;71(4):292-9.

13. Bishop L: Ultrastructural investigations of cardiomyopathy in the dog. J Comp Pathol. 1986 Nov;96(6):685-98.

14. Patterson EN: Clinical Characteristics and Inheritance of Idiopathic Epilepsy. Proceedings, 2007 Tufts' Canine and Feline Breeding and Genetics Conference. 2007.

15. Jones BR, Alley MR: Primary idiopathic hypoparathyroidism in St. Bernard dogs. N Z Vet J. 1985 Jun;33(6):94-7.

16. Russell NJ, Bond KA, Robertson ID, et. al.: Primary hypoparathyroidism in dogs: a retrospective study of 17 cases. Aust Vet J. 2006 Aug;84(8):285-90.

17. Martin CL, Leipold HW: Aphakia and multiple ocular defects in Saint Bernard puppies. Vet Med Small Anim Clin. 1974 Apr;69(4):448-53.

18. *The Genetic Connection: A Guide to Health Problems in Purebred Dogs.* L Ackerman. p. 235-36. AAHA Press, 1999.

19. von Pfeil DJ, Jutkowitz LA, & Hauptman J: Left lateral and left middle liver lobe torsion in a Saint Bernard puppy. J Am Anim Hosp Assoc. 2006 Sept-Oct; 42(5):381-5.

20. Watson AG, de Lahunta A, Evans HE: Morphology and embryological interpretation of a congenital occipito-atlanto-axial malformation in a dog. Teratology. 1988 Nov;38(5):451-9.

21. Easley JC, Carpenter JL: Hepatic arteriovenous fistula in two Saint Bernard pups. J Am Vet Med Assoc. 1975 Jan 15;166(2):167-71.

22. Torres SM, Brien TO, Scott DW: Dermal arteritis of the nasal philtrum in a Giant Schnauzer and three Saint Bernard dogs. Vet Dermatol. 2002 Oct;13(5):275-81.

23. *The Complete Dog Book, 20th Ed.* The American Kennel Club. Howell Book House, NY 2006. p. 319-324.

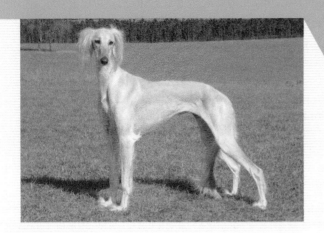

Saluki

The Breed History

This breed is thought to be one of the most ancient breeds of domesticated dogs. Excavations of ancient settlements (6500 BC, Sumerian empire), and Egyptian tomb carvings of 2100 BC reflect the presence of a distinctly "Saluki type" dog. They were highly esteemed and mummified remains of this type of dog have been found, attesting to their important status in Egyptian society. Muslim religion classed dogs as unclean, and termed them kelb but the Saluki on the other hand, was termed the "noble one" or *El Hor*, and accorded sacred status.

Originating in the region that includes Egypt, Arabia, Syria and Persia, and accompanying the Bedouin tribes, the first specimens were brought to England in the year 1840. The smooth (non-feathered) variety of Saluki is very much like the Sloughi dog. The latter was thought to have originated from the town of Saloug in Yemen. The Saluki likely originated in the town of Saluk, Yemen. The AKC recognized this breed in 1927.

Breeding for Function

Because of the harsh climate in which these dogs were kept, they became hardy and tolerated temperature extremes. They were also particularly sure-footed in rough going. Their speed, agility and endurance allowed them to hunt all day over difficult terrain. Arabs used these dogs to hunt gazelle, though they were also capable hunters of foxes, wild boar, and hares. In Europe and England the sport of saluki racing (which required clearing hurdles) was undertaken. They are found nowadays mostly in companionship and lure coursing or open field coursing roles.

Physical Characteristics

Height at Withers: female 22-26" (56-66 cm), male 23-28" (58.5-71 cm)

Weight: females 31-40 lb (14-18 kg), males 40-55 lb (18-25 kg).

Coat: Their coat is fine and silky, shorter over the body and well-developed feathers are present. Colors include white, cream, golden, red, fawn, grizzle and tan, black-and-tan, and tri-color. A smooth variety of this breed has the same body coat but without the feathers.

Longevity: 12 years

Points of Conformation: Long, with a very lean athletic build, exceptionally smooth and graceful bounding movements characterize Saluki dogs. Their ability to accelerate very quickly to speed allows them to be effective in gazelle hunts. The skull is long and narrow, the stop is not very pronounced, and the nose is either black or liver colored. The eyes are large, oval and colored dark brown to hazel. The ears are long, pendulous and fine-leathered with very long feathers. The neck is long and muscular, the thorax is somewhat narrow but very deep. The legs are straight and long. Tarsi are placed low on the hind limb. Feet are moderately arched, with good feathering between the toes. The inner digits can be longer than the outer digits. The tail is long, tapering, feathered on the underside, and carried in a curve. The back is broad with a slightly arched loin. They normally have prominent hip bones and the caudal rib cage is also clearly evident when they are in fit condition.

Recognized Behavior Issues and Traits

Reported breed characteristics include: Very athletic, and require lots of exercise and activity, friendly, clean, and they enjoy a soft bed inside the home. Saluki dogs are intelligent. Training should be started early, and socialization should be emphasized to counteract any nervous or shy/high strung tendencies. Introduce them to children, small dogs and household cats early. They thrive on close human companionship. They are sensitive, and obedience training is strongly recommended. Free exercise should only occur in a high fenced enclosure. They are somewhat independent minded. Though they do not like fetch type activities, they love to chase, so care should be taken to keep small animals such as cats out of their reach. Destructive behavior can occur if they become bored. Their coat has average care needs and they are average shedders. They will alarm bark, but are not considered defense dogs. Some recommend a snood, or ear hood to help prevent soiling of hair at mealtime.

Normal Physiologic Variations

Thyroid Hormone Levels: Sighthounds have lower normal ranges for T4 and T3 concentrations compared to other breeds. Median (reference limits) serum concentrations in Salukis are:[1,2]
Total T(4): 13.0 nmol/L (2.8 to 40.0 nmol/L)
Free T(4): 12.0 pmol/L (2.0 to 30.3 pmol/L)
Total T(3): 1.0 nmol/L (0.4 to 2.1 nmol/L)
Free T(3): 4.0 pmol/L (1.6 to 7.7 pmol/L)
TSH: 0.18 ng/mL (0 to 0.86 ng/mL)

Drug Sensitivities

Anesthesia: Sight hounds require particular attention during anesthesia. Their lean body conformation with high surface-area-to-volume ratio predisposes them to hypothermia during anesthesia. Impaired biotransformation of drugs by the liver results in prolonged recovery from barbiturate and thiobarbiturate intravenous anesthetics. Propofol, and ketamine/diazepam combination are recommended induction agents.[3]

Inherited Diseases

Hip Dysplasia: Polygenically inherited trait causing degenerative joint disease and hip arthritis. OFA reports 1.6% affected.[4]

Elbow Dysplasia: Polygenically inherited trait causing elbow arthritis. Too few Salukis have been screened by OFA to determine an accurate frequency.[4]

Patella Luxation: Polygenically inherited laxity of patellar ligaments, causing luxation, lameness, and later degenerative joint disease. Treat surgically if causing clinical signs. Too few Salukis have been screened by OFA to determine an accurate frequency.[4]

Disease Predispositions

Mitral Valve Disease (MVD): Salukis are reported with a high incidence of mitral regurgitation and thickening of the mitral valve. This condition can lead to congestive heart disease, cardiac arrhythmias (irregular heart beats) and cardiac failure. Unknown mode of inheritance. Reported as a breed problem in the 2000 SHR Inc. Saluki Health Survey.[5]

Hypothyroidism: Inherited autoimmune thyroiditis. 12.8% positive for thyroid autoantibodies based on testing at Michigan State University. (Ave. for all breeds is 7.5%).[2,6,7]

Persistent Pupillary Membranes: Strands of fetal remnant connecting; iris to iris, cornea, lens, or involving sheets of tissue. The later three forms can impair vision, and dogs affected with these forms should not be bred. Identified in 6.41% of Salukis CERF examined by veterinary ophthalmologists between 2000-2005.[8]

Cataracts: Nuclear intermediate and punctate cataracts predominate in the breed. Identified in 3.91% of Salukis CERF examined by veterinary ophthalmologists between 2000-2005. CERF does not recommend breeding any Saluki with a cataract.[8]

Vitreous Degeneration: A liquefaction of the vitreous gel which may predispose to retinal detachment resulting in blindness. Identified in 2.56% of Salukis CERF examined by veterinary ophthalmologists between 2000-2005.[8]

Cardiac Hemangiosarcoma/Sudden Death: In a necropsy study of Salukis with sudden death, 31% had cardiac hemangiosarcoma. The Saluki is found to have a 1% incidence of this type of cancer, with a 7.75x odds ratio of developing it versus other breeds. Almost one-third of all cases of cardiac hemangiosarcoma in dogs occur in Salukis. Unknown mode of inheritance. Reported as a breed problem in the 2000 SHR Inc. Saluki Health Survey.[5,9]

Immune-Mediated Hemolytic Anemia (IMHA): Autoimmune destruction of red blood cells. Treat with immunosuppressive drugs. Unknown mode of inheritance. Reported as a breed problem in the 2000 SHR Inc. Saluki Health Survey.[5]

Black Hair Follicular Dysplasia: Reported in Salukis in the UK. Loss of black hairs beginning around 4 weeks of age. Total loss of all black hair by 6-9 months of age. Melatonin may be effective. Unknown mode of inheritance.[10]

Ceroid Lipofuscinosis: Rare, fatal degenerative neurological disease. Onset 1-2 years. Unknown mode of inheritance.[11]

Brachygnathism, Color Dilution Alopecia, and **Prognathism,** are reported.[12]

Isolated Case Studies

Motor Neuron Abiotrophy: A nine-week-old saluki puppy presented for progressive, generalized weakness and bilateral forelimb deformities. Histopathology revealed a diffuse, symmetrical, degenerative motor neuronopathy of the ventral horn of the spinal cord.[13]

Multiple Cardiac Anomalies: A family of Salukis was identified where all affected dogs had patent ductus arteriosus or ductus diverticulum, and some members additionally had tricuspid valve insufficiency, pulmonic stenosis, or mitral valve insufficiency. Pedigree evaluation suggested a genetic cause.[14]

Intersex: A litter of five salukis was presented in which all of the individuals were intersexes or hermaphrodites. The external genitalia resembled a combination of penile sheath and vulva, and scrotal sacs. Internal anatomy consisted of two gonads in a position expected for ovaries, oviducts, uterus and cord-like structures lateral to the uterus which extended from gonad to inside of the scrotal sacs. Histologically, the gonads appeared to be ovaries which contained many dysgenic follicles.[15]

Genetic Tests

Tests of Genotype: Genetic tests for coat color and length are available from VetGen and HealthGene.

Tests of Phenotype: Recommended testing includes hip and elbow radiographs, CERF eye examination, cardiac evaluation, patella examination, and thyroid profile including autoantibodies.

Miscellaneous

- **Breed name synonyms:** Persian Greyhound (historical), Gazelle Hound, Arabian Hound, Saluqi, El Hor (Arabic for *"the noble one"*).
- **Registries:** AKC, UKC, CKC, KCGB (Kennel Club of Great Britain), ANKC (Australian National Kennel Club), NKC (National Kennel Club).
- **AKC rank (year 2008):** 118 (280 dogs registered)
- **Internet resources: Saluki Club of America:** www.salukiclub.org
  Saluki Club of Canada: www.salukicanada.com
  Saluki or Gazelle Hound Club of the U.K.: www.salukiclub.co.uk
  Saluki Health Research: www.salukihealthresearch.com

References

1. Kintzer PP & Peterson ME: Progress in the Diagnosis and Treatment of Canine Hypothyroidism. 2007. Proceedings, ACVIM 2007.
2. Shiel RE, Sist M, Nachreiner RF, et. al.: Assessment of criteria used by veterinary practitioners to diagnose hypothyroidism in sighthounds and investigation of serum thyroid hormone concentrations in healthy Salukis. J Am Vet Med Assoc. 2010 Feb 1;236(3):302-8.
3. Court MH: Anesthesia of the sighthound. Clin Tech Small Anim Pract 1999 Feb;14(1):38-43.
4. OFA Website breed statistics: www.offa.org Last accessed July 1, 2010.
5. Sist MD & Saluki Health Research, Inc.: Saluki Health Research, Inc. 2000 Saluki Health Survey. 2001.
6. Nachreiner RF, Refsal KR, Graham PA, et. al.: Prevalence of serum thyroid

hormone autoantibodies in dogs with clinical signs of hypothyroidism. J Am Vet Med Assoc 2002 Feb 15;220(4):466-71.

7. Sist MD, Refsal KR & Nachreiner RF: A Laboratory Survey of Autoimmune Thyroiditis and Hypothyroidism in Selected Sight Hound Breeds. Proceedings, 2009 Tufts' Canine and Feline Breeding and Genetics Conference. 2009.

8. *Ocular Disorders Presumed to be Inherited in Purebred Dogs.* American College of Veterinary Ophthalmologists. ACVO, 2007.

9. Ware WA, Hopper DL: Cardiac Tumors in Dogs: 1982–1995. J Vet Intern Med 1999;13:95–103.

10. Lewis CJ: Black hair follicular dysplasia in UK bred salukis. Vet Rec. 1995 Sep 16;137(12):294-5.

11. Appleby EC, Longstaffe JA, Bell FR: Ceroid-lipofuscinosis in two Saluki dogs. J Comp Pathol. 1982 Jul;92(3):375-80.

12. *The Genetic Connection: A Guide to Health Problems in Purebred Dogs.* L Ackerman. p. 236. AAHA Press, 1999.

13. Kent M, Knowles K, Glass E, et. al.: Motor neuron abiotrophy in a saluki. J Am Anim Hosp Assoc. 1999 Sep-Oct;35(5):436-9.

14. Ogburn PN, Peterson M, Jeraj K: Multiple cardiac anomalies in a family of Saluki dogs. J Am Vet Med Assoc. 1981 Jul 1;179(1):57-63.

15. Hinsch GW: Intersexes in the dog. Teratology. 1979 Dec;20(3):463-8.

16. *The Complete Dog Book, 20th Ed.* The American Kennel Club. Howell Book House, NY 2006. p. 214-217.

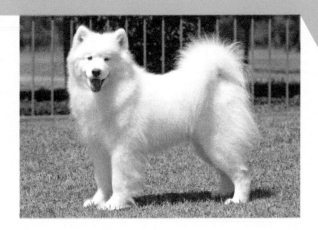

The Breed History

In ancient times, the early ancestral dogs of the Samoyed breed likely moved with migrating tribes from Iran through Mongolia to the Northwestern Siberian tundra. There they helped the Samoyede people in many ways, and were welcomed as family members into their nomadic dwellings. They were first brought to England in the late nineteenth century. The first dog was registered with AKC in 1906.

Breeding for Function

These dogs provided herding and guarding for the reindeer herds, and also were valued as close companions. They excelled as sled dogs in many of the early Arctic and Antarctic expeditions.

Physical Characteristics

Height at Withers: female 19-21" (48-53 cm), male 21-23.5" (53-60 cm).

Weight: 50-65 lb (23-29.5 kg).

Coat: The double coat is profuse, heavy and very resistant to the elements. Males have a particularly well-developed lion's type ruff. The undercoat is soft, short and wooly while outer hairs are straight, stand out from the body and are glistening silvery-white. Some dogs have a creamy or biscuit color.

Longevity: 12 years

Points of Conformation: The head is wedge-shaped, broad and the muzzle is moderate in all aspects, with some tapering. The nose is usually black (also liver and brown) and large. A well-defined stop is present, and the black rimmed lips are characteristically slightly upturned resulting in what breeders term the "Samoyed smile". Ears have thick leather and stand erect, and are short and triangular, though rounded at the tips. Eyes and palpebral rims are darkly pigmented. Blue eyes disqualify. Almond shaped and deep set, widely spaced, the eyes slant up laterally. Strong in bone and musculature, the thorax is deep and ribs are well sprung. The topline is highest at withers and straight. They possess a moderate abdominal tuck up. The muscular neck is fairly short. Limbs are moderate in length and straight boned. The feet are large (hare-foot) with arched toes and thick pads, with thick hair between the toes. Some feathering on the feet is often present. The

tail reaches the tarsus when held down, is profusely covered with hair, and when moving or alert, should be over the back and to one side. The proper gait is a trot, not a pace, and strides are quick and agile; springiness and speed are valued.

Recognized Behavior Issues and Traits

Reported breed characteristics include: Loyal guardian of home and family, not argumentative with other dogs generally, require lots of exercise, playful, curious, high grooming needs, tend to pull on leash; need early obedience training, gentle and intelligent but with an independent streak. Good with children. Need close human companionship, tolerate weather extremes well, particularly the cold. If not mentally or physically active and challenged, or given adequate time with family, they may become destructive. They have a high pitched bark.

Normal Physiologic Variations

None Reported

Drug Sensitivities

Samoyeds are overrepresented in the population of dogs with adverse reactions to **potentiated sulfonamides**. Clinical signs included hypersensitivity, thrombocytopenia and hepatopathy, and infrequently can include neutropenia, keratoconjunctivitis sicca, hemolytic anemia, arthropathy, uveitis, skin and mucocutaneous lesions, proteinuria, facial palsy, suspected meningitis, hypothyroidism, pancreatitis, facial edema, and pneumonitis.[1]

Inherited Diseases

Hip Dysplasia: Polygenically inherited trait causing degenerative joint disease and hip arthritis. OFA reports 11.1% affected. Dorn reports a 1.32x odds ratio versus other breeds. Reported at a frequency of 24% in the 1999 SCA Health Survey.[2,3,4]

Patella Luxation: Polygenically inherited laxity of patellar ligaments, causing luxation, lameness, and later degenerative joint disease. Treat surgically if causing clinical signs. Reported at a high frequency by the OFA, but too few Samoyeds have been screened to determine an accurate frequency.[2]

Elbow Dysplasia: Polygenically inherited trait causing elbow arthritis. OFA reports 2.3% affected.[2]

X-linked Progressive Retinal Atrophy (XLPRA): X-linked recessive degeneration of the retina. Causes blindness between 3-6 years of age. Reported in 0.21% of Samoyeds CERF examined by veterinary ophthalmologists between 1991-1999. A genetic test is available through Optigen, that reports 1% of Samoyeds test as affected, and 2% test as carriers. CERF does not recommend breeding any Samoyed with PRA. Reported at a frequency of 2.4% in the 1999 SCA Health Survey.[4,5,6,7]

Oculo-Skeletal Dysplasia (OSD): Autosomal recessive developmental disease causing ocular vitreous dysplasia, cataracts, retinal detachment, and dwarfism with valgus deformity of the carpi. Heterozygous carriers of the defective gene present with various forms of retinal dysplasia. CERF does not recommend breeding any affected Samoyeds. A genetic test for RD/OSD is available.[5,8,9,10]

Retinal Dysplasia (RD): Retinal dysplasia can be due to the incompletely dominant expression of the heterozygous form of the gene for oculo-skeletal dysplasia, though not all Samoyeds with retinal dysplasia are due to this testable gene. Focal retinal dysplasia and retinal folds can progress to retinal detachment. Reported in 2.24% of Samoyeds CERF examined by veterinary ophthalmologists between 2000-2005. CERF does not recommend breeding any Samoyed with retinal dysplasia. A genetic test for RD/OSD is available.[9,10,11]

Hereditary Nephritis (glomerulopathy): X-linked dominant inherited kidney disease. Affected males develop kidney disease from 3-5 months of age, and succumb to kidney failure by 15 months of age. Affected females have a less severe form of kidney disease that does not progress to failure. This disorder may no longer be present in the Samoyed breeding/pet population.[12,13]

Disease Predispositions

Hypothyroidism: Inherited autoimmune thyroiditis. 9.0% positive for thyroid autoantibodies based on testing at Michigan State University. (Ave. for all breeds is 7.5%). Reported at a frequency of 8% in the 1999 SCA Health Survey.[4,14,15]

Distichiasis: Abnormally placed eyelashes that irritate the cornea and conjunctiva. Can cause secondary corneal ulceration. Dorn reports a 1.19x odds ratio versus other breeds. Identified in 4.69% of Samoyeds CERF examined by veterinary ophthalmologists between 2000-2005.[3,5]

Diabetes Mellitus (Sugar Diabetes): Samoyeds have an inherited form of DM with an average age of onset of 7 years (range 4-10 years). Caused by immune-mediatd destruction of insulin producing beta cells of the pancreas. Research shows relationship to certain major histocompatability (MHC) genes, and mutations in the CTLAY promotor gene. Control by insulin injections, diet, and glucose monitoring. Odds ratios versus other breeds reported as 7.58x (Dorn), 11.83x (Hess), to 21.7x (Catchpole). Unknown mode of inheritance. Reported at a frequency of 4% in the 1999 SCA Health Survey.[3,4,16,17,18,19,20]

Corneal Dystrophy: The breed can form epithelial corneal opacities that do not lead to corneal edema. Identified in 2.51% of Samoyeds CERF examined by veterinary ophthalmologists between 2000-2005.[5]

Cataracts: Anterior or posterior punctate cataracts predominate in the breed. Juvenile cataracts are also seen, with an onset of 6 months to 2 years of age. Cataracts are identified in 2.40% of Samoyeds CERF examined by veterinary ophthalmologists between 2000-2005. Reported at a frequency of 7% in the 1999 SCA Health Survey. CERF does not recommend breeding any Samoyed with a cataract.[4,5]

Gastric Dilation/Volvulus (GDV, Bloat): Life-threatening twisting of the stomach within the abdomen. Requires immediate veterinary attention. Samoyeds are at increased risk. Reported at a frequency of 4.2% in the 1999 SCA Health Survey.[4,21]

Persistent Pupillary Membranes: Strands of fetal remnant connecting; iris to iris, cornea, lens, or involving sheets of tissue. The later three forms can impair vision, and dogs affected with these forms should not be bred. Identified in 2.29% of Samoyeds CERF examined by veterinary ophthalmologists between 2000-2005.[5]

Pulmonic Valve Stenosis: Samoyeds are a breed at increased risk (5.4x odds ratio) for this congenital heart anomaly. Clinical signs can include exercise intolerance, stunting, dyspnea, syncope and ascites, leading to heart failure. Screen with auscultation and echocardiography.[22]

Primary (Narrow Angle) Glaucoma: Ocular condition causing increased pressure within the eyeball, and secondary blindness due to damage to the retina. Diagnose with tonometry and gonioscopy. Reported at a frequency of 1.59% in the breed, with a female preponderance. Dorn reports a 1.76x odds ratio versus other breeds. CERF does not recommend breeding any Samoyed with glaucoma.[3,5,23,24]

Uveodermatologic (VKH-Like) Syndrome: This is an autoimmune disease manifested by progressive uveitis and depigmenting dermatitis that closely resembles the human Vogt - Koyanagi - Harada syndrome. The disease presents between 1-1/2 to 4 years of age, and can progress to blindness. Treatment is with steroids. CERF does not recommend breeding any affected Samoyeds.[5,25]

Alopecia-X (Black Skin Disease, BSD, Coat Funk): Progressive, symmetrical, non-pruritic, truncal hair loss usually beginning in early adulthood. ACTH, LDDS, and thyroid panel results are normal. Oral trilostane reverses the condition in some cases. The disorder appears familial.[26]

Sebaceous Adenitis: Disorder of immune mediated sebaceous gland destruction, presenting with hair loss, usually beginning with the dorsal midline and ears. Diagnosis by skin biopsy. Treat with isotretinoin. An autosomal recessive mode of inheritance is suspected.[27]

Lingual Squamous Cell Carcinoma (SCC): Samoyeds have a 24.63x odds ratio versus other breeds of developing this tongue cancer. Females are overrepresented in one study.[28]

Atrial Septal Defect, Cerebellar Abiotrophy, Deafness, Factor VIII Deficiency, Growth Hormone Responsive Dermatosis, Mcrophthalmia, Muscular Dystrophy, Myasthenia Gravis, Osteochondritis Dessicans-Stifle, Oligodontia, Pelger-Huet Anomaly, Shaker Syndrome, Spina Bifida, Spongiform Leukodystrophy, Subaortic Stenosis, Ulcerative Keratitis, Ventricular Septal Defect, von Willebrand's Disease, and **Zinc Responsive Dermatosis** are reported.[29]

Isolated Case Studies

Tremors and Hypomyelination: Reported in several related litters of Samoyed pups. Clinical signs of tremors and an inability to stand occurred from 3-5 weeks of age. There was a lack of myelin in the central nervous system due to abnormal oligodendrocyte function.[30]

Genetic Tests

Tests of Genotype: Direct tests for XLPRA and RD/OSD are available from Optigen.

Tests of Phenotype: CHIC Certification: Required tests are; cardiac exam, CERF eye examination (minimum of 1 year of age), hip dysplasia radiograph, and DNA test for XLPRA. (See CHIC website: www.caninehealthinfo.org)

Recommended tests are; elbow radiographs, thyroid profile including autoantibodies, and patella evaluation.

Miscellaneous

- **Breed name synonyms:** Samoyedskaya, Sammies (nickname).
- **Registries:** AKC, UKC, CKC, KCGB (Kennel Club of Great Britain), ANKC (Australian National Kennel Club), NKC (National Kennel Club).
- **AKC rank (year 2008):** 73 (1,077 dogs registered)
- **Internet resources: The Samoyed Club of America:** www.samoyedclubofamerica.org
Samoyed Association of Canada: www.samoyed.ca
The British Samoyed Club: www.british-samoyed-club.co.uk
Samoyed Club of America Research Foundation: www.samoyedhealthfoundation.org

References

1. Trepanier LA, Danhof R, Toll J, et. al.: Clinical findings in 40 dogs with hypersensitivity associated with administration of potentiated sulfonamides. J Vet Intern Med. 2003 Sep-Oct;17(5):647-52.

2. OFA Website breed statistics: www.offa.org Last accessed July 1, 2010.

3. Dorn CR: Canine breed-specific risks of frequently diagnosed diseases at veterinary teaching hospitals. Monograph. AKC Canine Health Foundation. 2000.

4. Richardson D & Samoyed Club of America: 1999 Samoyed Club of America Health Survey. June, 2001.

5. Ocular Disorders Presumed to be Inherited in Purebred Dogs. American College of Veterinary Ophthalmologists. ACVO, 2007

6. Acland GM, Blanton SH, Hershfield B, et. al.: XLPRA: a canine retinal degeneration inherited as an X-linked trait. Am J Med Genet. 1994 Aug 1;52(1):27-33.

7. Zangerl B, Johnson JL, Acland GM, et. al.: Independent origin and restricted distribution of RPGR deletions causing XLPRA. J Hered. 2007;98(5):526-30.

8. Pellegrini B, Acland GM, Ray J: Cloning and characterization of opticin cDNA: evaluation as a candidate for canine oculo-skeletal dysplasia. Gene. 2002 Jan 9;282(1-2):121-31.

9. Meyers VN, Jezyk PF, Aguirre GD, et. al.: Short-limbed dwarfism and ocular defects in the Samoyed dog. J Am Vet Med Assoc. 1983 Nov 1;183(9):975-9.

10. Goldstein O, Guyon R, Kukekova A, et. al.: COL9A2 and COL9A3 mutations in canine autosomal recessive oculoskeletal dysplasia. Mamm Genome. 2010 Aug;21(7-8):398-408.

11. Acland GM, Aguirre, GD: Retinal dysplasia in the Samoyed dog is the heterozygous phenotype of the gene (drds) for short limbed dwarfism and ocular defects. Transactions of the American College Veterinary Ophthalmology 1991;22:44.

12. Jansen B, Tryphonas L, Wong J, et. al.: Mode of inheritance of Samoyed hereditary glomerulopathy: an animal model for hereditary nephritis in humans. J Lab Clin Med. 1986 Jun;107(6):551-5

13. Baumal R, Thorner P, Valli VE, et. al.: Renal disease in carrier female dogs with X-linked hereditary nephritis. Implications for female patients with this disease. Am J Pathol. 1991 Oct;139(4):751-64.

14. Nachreiner RF, Refsal KR, Graham PA, et. al.: Prevalence of serum thyroid hormone autoantibodies in dogs with clinical signs of hypothyroidism. J Am Vet Med Assoc 2002 Feb 15;220(4):466-71.

15. Nachreiner R & Refsal K: Personal communication, Diagnostic Center for Population and Animal Health, Michigan State University. April, 2007.

16. Kimmel SE, Ward CR, Henthorn PS, et. al.: Familial insulin-dependent diabetes mellitus in Samoyed dogs. J Am Anim Hosp Assoc. 2002 May-Jun;38(3):235-8.

17. Hess RS, Kass PH, Ward CR: Breed distribution of dogs with diabetes mellitus admitted to a tertiary care facility. J Am Vet Med Assoc. 2000 May 1;216(9):1414-7.

18. Catchpole B, Kennedy LJ, Davison LJ, et. al.: Canine diabetes mellitus: from phenotype to genotype. J Small Anim Pract. 2008 Jan;49(1):4-10.

19. Fall T, Hamlin HH, Hedhammar A, et. al.: Diabetes mellitus in a population of 180,000 insured dogs: incidence, survival, and breed distribution. J Vet Intern Med. 2007 Nov-Dec;21(6):1209-16.

20. Short AD, Saleh NM, Catchpole B, et. al.: CTLA4 promoter polymorphisms are associated with canine diabetes mellitus. Tissue Antigens. 2010 Mar;75(3):242-52.

21. Glickman LT, Glickman NW, Schellenberg DB, et. al.: Incidence of and breed-related risk factors for gastric dilatation-volvulus in dogs. J Am Vet Med Assoc. 2000 Jan 1;216(1):40-5.

22. Buchanan JW: Causes and prevalence of cardiovascular diseases. In Kirk RW, Bonagura JD, eds: Current veterinary therapy XI, Philadelphia, 1992, WB Saunders.

23. Gelatt KN, MacKay EO: Prevalence of the breed-related glaucomas in pure-bred dogs in North America. Vet Ophthalmol. 2004 Mar-Apr;7(2):97-111.

24. Ekesten B, Torrang I: Heritability of the depth of the opening of the ciliary cleft in Samoyeds. Am J Vet Res. 1995 Sep;56(9):1138-43.

25. Glaze MB: Canine and Feline Uveitis. Proceedings, 2004 Northeast Veterinary Conference. 2004.

26. Cerundolo R, Lloyd D: "Alopecia X" in chows, pomeranians and samoyeds. Vet Rec. 1998 Aug 8;143(6):176.

27. White S: Sebaceous Adenitis. 2001. Proceedings, World Small Animal Veterinary Association World Congress, 2001

28. Dennis MM, Ehrhart N, Duncan CG, et. al.: Frequency of and risk factors associated with lingual lesions in dogs: 1,196 cases (1995-2004).

29. The Genetic Connection: A Guide to Health Problems in Purebred Dogs. L Ackerman. p. 236. AAHA Press, 1999.

30. Cummings JF, Summers BA, de Lahunta A, et. al.: Tremors in Samoyed pups with oligodendrocyte deficiencies and hypomyelination. Acta Neuropathol (Berl). 1986;71(3-4):267-77.

31. The Complete Dog Book, 20th Ed. The American Kennel Club. Howell Book House, NY 2006. p. 325-329.

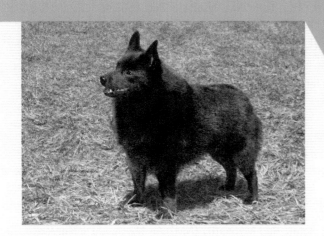

The Breed History

The Schipperke originates in Belgium, and is derived from Belgian Sheepdogs rather than Pomeranian or Spitz stock as some report, though it is possible some outcrosses occurred. These are close relatives to the Groenendael. Records of the breed extend back into the 1600s, though until 1888 they were known as Spits. About the same time, the first breed specimens arrived in America. AKC recognition occurred in1904. The word Schipperke derives from the Flemish word for "Little Captain, or Little Bargeman". Pronunciation of the breed name varies significantly; regional pronunciations include: Skip-er-kay, Skip-er-key, Ship-er-kee, Sheep-er-kay, and Sheep-er-ker.

Breeding for Function

Originally derived from Belgian sheep herding dogs, the Schipperke dogs were selected for small size and for watchdog qualities. They were also considered excellent for vermin control. They were popular with boat captains and tradesmen. Later in America, they were reported as being hunting dogs in the Midwest, successfully used for rabbits, raccoons and opossums.

Physical Characteristics

Height at Withers: female 10-12" (25.5-30.5 cm), male 11-13" (28-33 cm).

Weight: 7-16 lb (3-7.5 kg).

Coat: The thick black outer coat is straight and stands off, with a prominent ruff, jabot, coulotte and cape. These distinct coat features must be well developed in order to meet the breed standard. The undercoat is short, dense and may be lighter than the black outer coat.

Longevity: 13-16 years

Points of Conformation: Compact square, cobby, heavy set conformation, a profuse dense black coat, taillessness and foxy appearance all characterize this breed. They are also noted for their sharp, peppy personalities. Ears are high set, triangular, small and pricked. The eyes are oval, brown and close set, the face and head are fox-like in structure and the stop is defined. Nose is black and small. The neck is short and muscular and head carriage is high. The topline is level to slightly sloping towards the rear, but the coat

Schipperke

makes the dog appear higher in the withers than it really is. Thorax is broad and the ribs are well sprung. Though some are born tailless, those born with tails are usually docked to within 1" of the body wall. Dewclaws are usually removed on forelegs and are removed from the hind limbs. Limbs are straight boned, feet are compact and small. Nails are black. The gait is smooth, low and fast.

Recognized Behavior Issues and Traits

Reported breed characteristics include: Good with children but a plucky guardian of family and home (or boat). Known for his curiosity, high intelligence, stubborn streak and aloofness with strangers, the Schipperke has low grooming needs, and dogs typically shed twice a year. This type of dog needs close human companionship. These dogs are also known for their high activity levels, and they need mental stimulation or they will develop boredom vices such as chewing, barking or digging. They should be off leash only in a fenced enclosure. Schipperkes may see small pets as prey and should be socialized early to other pets, especially dogs, and to the children of the household. They have a high barking tendency and may snap if irritated.

Normal Physiologic Variations

In a UK study 27.7% of litters were born via **Cesarean section.**[1]

Drug Sensitivities

None reported

Inherited Diseases

Hip Dysplasia and Legg–Calve-Perthes: Polygenically inherited traits causing degenerative hip joint disease and arthritis. OFA reports 5.5% affected with hip dysplasia, and 2.0% affected with Legg-Calve-Perthes disease.[2,3]

Patella Luxation: Polygenically inherited laxity of patellar ligaments, causing luxation, lameness, and later degenerative joint disease. Treat surgically if causing clinical signs. OFA reports 5.0% affected.[2]

Elbow Dysplasia: Polygenically inherited trait causing elbow arthritis. OFA reports 1.8% affected.[2]

Mucopolysaccharidosis IIIB (MPS IIIb): Autosomal recessive metabolic storage disease causing cerebellar ataxia, mildly dystrophic corneas and small peripheral foci of retinal degeneration. Onset between 2-4 years of age. The disease is progressive and there is no effective treatment. A genetic test is available.[4,5]

Disease Predispositions

Hypothyroidism: Inherited autoimmune thyroiditis. 10.0% positive for thyroid autoantibodies based on testing at Michigan State University. (Ave. for all breeds is 7.5%).[6,7]

Persistent Pupillary Membranes: Strands of fetal remnant connecting; iris to iris, cornea, lens, or involving sheets of tissue. The later three forms can impair vision, and dogs affected with these forms should not be bred. Identified in 5.06% of Schipperkes CERF examined by veterinary ophthalmologists between 2000-2005.[8]

Collapsing Trachea: Caused by diminished integrity of the cartilage rings in the trachea. Can produce increased coughing, stridor, and respiratory distress. Dorn reports a 5.21x odds ratio versus other breeds.[9]

Cataracts: Anterior cortex punctate cataracts predominate in the breed. Identified in 4.49% of Schipperkes CERF examined by veterinary ophthalmologists between 2000-2005. CERF does not recommend breeding any Schipperke with a cataract.[8]

Distichiasis: Abnormally placed eyelashes that irritate the cornea and conjunctiva. Can cause secondary corneal ulceration. Identified in 3.37% of Schipperkes CERF examined by veterinary ophthalmologists between 2000-2005.[8]

Demodicosis: Dorn reports a 1.93x odds ratio of developing demodectic mange versus other breeds. This disorder has an underlying immunodeficiency in its pathogenesis.[9]

Vitreous Degeneration: A liquefaction of the vitreous gel which may predispose to retinal detachment resulting in blindness. Identified in 1.40% of Schipperkes CERF examined by veterinary ophthalmologists between 2000-2005.[8]

Retinal Dysplasia: Retinal folds, geographic, and detachment are recognized in the breed. Can progress to blindness. Identified in 1.12% of Schipperkes CERF examined by veterinary ophthalmologists between 2000-2005.[8]

Idiopathic Epilepsy: Inherited seizures can be generalized or partial seizures. Control with anticonvulsant medication. Reported as a problem in the breed on the SCA website. 1.98% of Schipperkes presenting for the first time to veterinary school hospitals are diagnosed with idiopathic epilepsy.[10]

Pemphigus Foliaceus: There is a significantly higher risk of developing pemphigus foliaceus versus other breeds. Typical lesions include dorsal muzzle and head symmetric scaling, crusting, and alopecia with peripheral collarettes, characteristic footpad lesions, with erythematous swelling at the pad margins, cracking, and villous hypertrophy. Average age of onset is 4.2 years. Treatment with corticosteroid and cytotoxic medications. One-year survival rate of 53%. Unknown mode of inheritance.[11]

Diabetes Mellitus: Sugar diabetes is caused by a lack of insulin production by the pancreas. Controlled by insulin injections, diet, and glucose monitoring. The Schipperke is reported as a breed predisposed to developing DM between 4-14 years of age.[12]

Progressive Retinal Atrophy (PRA): Inherited degeneration of the retina, causing blindness. Form, age of onset, and mode of inheritance are not defined. CERF does not recommend breeding any Schipperke with PRA.[8]

Black Hair Follicular Dysplasia: Rare condition causing loss of black hairs beginning around 4 weeks of age. Total loss of all black hair by 6-9 months of age. No treatment. Unknown mode of inheritance.[13]

Color Dilution Alopecia, Pancreatitis, and **Prognathism** are reported.[14]

Isolated Case Studies

Spinal Arachnoid Cyst: Two Schipperkes were diagnosed with dorsal midline spinal arachnoid cysts localized either at the second to third caudal vertebrae or between the eighth and tenth thoracic vertebrae. Surgical removal was curative.[15]

Nemaline Rod Myopathy (NM): An 11 year old Schipperke presented with exercise intolerance. Findings included abnormal electromyography, and the presence of nemaline rods in fresh, frozen, and glutaraldehyde-fixed biopsies from proximal appendicular limb muscles.[16]

Congenital Pulmonary Emphysema: A 4-month-old, intact female Schipperke was presented for evaluation and treatment of subcutaneous (SC) emphysema. Radiographs revealed pneumomediastinum and SC emphysema. Exploratory thoracotomy revealed an emphysematous right middle lung lobe. Lobectomy of the right middle lung lobe resolved both the pneumomediastinum and SC emphysema.[17]

Genetic Tests

Tests of Genotype: Direct test for MPS IIIB is available from PennGen.

Direct test for black, chocolate/brown, and fawn/cream coat colors are available from VetGen.

Tests of Phenotype: CHIC Certification: Required testing includes thyroid profile including autoantibodies, patella evaluation, and CERF eye examination. Optional recommended tests include genetic test for MPS IIIB, congenital cardiac disease evaluation, and hip radiographs. See CHIC website; www.caninehealthinfo.org).

Recommend elbow radiographs.

Miscellaneous

- **Breed name synonyms:** Skip, Little Skipper, Spits (historical)
- **Registries:** AKC, UKC, CKC, KCGB (Kennel Club of Great Britain), ANKC (Australian National Kennel Club), NKC (National Kennel Club)
- **AKC rank (year 2008):** 91 (639 dogs registered)
- **Internet resources:** The Schipperke Club of America Inc.: www.schipperkeclub-usa.org
  Schipperke Club of Canada: www.schipperkecanada.net
  The Schipperke Club (UK): www.schipperkeclub.co.uk
  Schipperke Health Foundation: www.schipperkefoundation.org

References

1. Evans KM & Adams VJ: Proportion of litters of purebred dogs born by caesarean section. J Small Anim Pract. 2010 Feb;51(2):113-8.
2. OFA Website breed statistics: www.offa.org Last accessed July 1, 2010.
3. Gibson KL, Lewis DD, Pechman RD: Use of external coaptation for the

treatment of avascular necrosis of the femoral head in a dog. *J Am Vet Med Assoc.* 1990 Oct 1;197(7):868-70.

4. Knowles K, Alroy J, Castagnaro M, et. al.: Adult-onset lysosomal storage disease in a Schipperke dog: clinical, morphological and biochemical studies. *Acta Neuropathol (Berl).* 1993;86(3):306-12.

5. Ellinwood NM, Wang P, Skeen T, et. al.: A model of mucopolysaccharidosis IIIB (Sanfilippo syndrome type IIIB): N-acetyl-alpha-D-glucosaminidase deficiency in Schipperke dogs. *J Inherit Metab Dis.* 2003;26(5):489-504.

6. Nachreiner RF, Refsal KR, Graham PA, et. al.: Prevalence of serum thyroid hormone autoantibodies in dogs with clinical signs of hypothyroidism. J Am Vet Med Assoc 2002 Feb 15;220(4):466-71.

7. Nachreiner R & Refsal K: Personal communication, Diagnostic Center for Population and Animal Health, Michigan State University. April, 2007.

8. *Ocular Disorders Presumed to be Inherited in Purebred Dogs.* American College of Veterinary Ophthalmologists. ACVO, 2007.

9. Dorn CR: Canine breed-specific risks of frequently diagnosed diseases at veterinary teaching hospitals. Monograph. AKC Canine Health Foundation. 2000.

10. Patterson EN: Clinical Characteristics and Inheritance of Idiopathic Epilepsy. Proceedings, 2007 Tufts' Canine and Feline Breeding and Genetics Conference. 2007.

11. Ihrke PJ, Stannard AA, Ardans AA, et. al.: Pemphigus foliaceus in dogs: a review of 37 cases. *J Am Vet Med Assoc.* 1985 Jan 1;186(1):59-66.

12. Kimmel SE, Ward CR, Henthorn PS, et al. Familial insulin-dependent diabetes mellitus in samoyed dogs. *J Am Anim Hosp Assoc* 2002;38:235-238

13. Carlotti DN: Non-Hormonal Alopecia. Proceedings, World Small Animal Veterinary Association Congress, 2005.

14. *The Genetic Connection: A Guide to Health Problems in Purebred Dogs.* L Ackerman. p. 236 AAHA Press, 1999.

15. Frykman OF: Spinal arachnoid cyst in four dogs: diagnosis, surgical treatment and follow-up results. *J Small Anim Pract.* 1999 Nov;40(11):544-9.

16. Delauche AJ, Cuddon PA, Podell M, et. al.: Nemaline rods in canine myopathies: 4 case reports and literature review. *J Vet Intern Med.* 1998 Nov-Dec;12(6):424-30.

17. Stephens JA, Parnell NK, Clarke K, et. al.: Subcutaneous emphysema, pneumomediastinum, and pulmonary emphysema in a young schipperke. *J Am Anim Hosp Assoc.* 2002 Mar-Apr;38(2):121-4.

18. *The Complete Dog Book, 20th Ed.* The American Kennel Club. Howell Book House, NY 2006. p. 588-592.

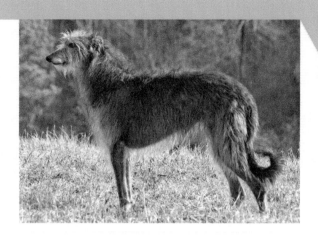

and straight boned with a lithe build, and feet are compact with well-arched toes, with little hair. The topline is arched through the loin, and drops off to the tail, which is long and tapering, reaching about 1/2 way down the metatarsals, and is gently curved. The gait is strong, long and low and appears effortless.

The Breed History

In the 16th century, early breed records first appeared in the British Isles. It is possible that the Irish Wolfhound was the main source of the genes of the Deerhound breed, and that they were crossed with Greyhounds to produce a finer body type. Deerhounds were highly esteemed at certain points in history such that only the aristocracy and Clan Chieftains could keep them. By severely limiting ownership, breed numbers dwindled to the brink of extinction and inbreeding further weakened the Scottish Deerhound, but later fanciers rejuvenated the bloodlines and though still a rare breed, they are once again thriving. AKC recognition occurred in 1886.

Breeding for Function

Bred for coursing or hunting deer alone or in pairs, this breed excels at scent tracking. In North America they were also used for hunting coyotes and wolves. They were also bred to be companions.

Physical Characteristics

Height at Withers: female 28" (71 cm) minimum, male 30-32" (76-81 cm).

Weight: females 75-95lb (34-43 kg), males 85-110 lb (38.5-50 kg).

Coat: The most common color is the dark gray-blue coat, but other shades of grays, brindles, faun and sandy red are accepted. White is not accepted, but the presence of a small white toe mark and white chest are tolerated. The haircoat consists of shaggy, crisp, hard hairs, though the haircoat has a softer texture on the ears and ventral abdomen. Averages about 4" (10 cm) in length.

Longevity: 8-11 years

Points of Conformation: The general conformation is similar to a very large Greyhound, with a wiry coat. They are smaller than Irish Wolfhounds and more refined in bone and in the head. The head gradually tapers through its length to a tapered muzzle, the skull is flat, and the nose black (though in blue fawn coated dogs, it may be blue). A black muzzle is preferred, ears are also black or dark in color, and prominent brows, with moderate whiskers and beard are present. The medium-sized ears are soft and folded, and high set. Eyes are dark brown or hazel in color, with black palpebral margins. The neck is long and well muscled. The thorax is deep and fairly narrow, and the abdomen is well tucked up. The limbs are long

Recognized Behavior Issues and Traits

Reported breed characteristics include: A very alert attitude, requires close human companionship, loyal and possessing high trainability; quiet in the home, and exhibit low energy unless outside on the run. It is best to start obedience training early; tend to be a "one-man" or one family dog. Scottish Deerhounds are sensitive and generally good with other dogs. Overall, they are good-natured and therefore not suitable as a watchdog. Because of the strong chase instinct, it is important that they are off leash in a fenced enclosure only. Deerhounds may exhibit chase reflex with small pets. They will show courageous response when necessary. They have low grooming needs except for the twice annual undercoat stripping. They have a low shedding tendency.

Normal Physiologic Variations

Sight hounds have lower normal ranges for T4 and T3 concentrations compared to other breeds.[1]

Echocardiographic and Electrocardiographic Values: The Deerhounds have relatively large hearts. Left ventricular echocardiographic measurements were similar to those obtained from Irish Wolfhounds. Normal end systolic volume index (ESVI) in the Deerhound was relatively high. It is concluded that an index greater than 70 ml/m^2 body surface area could be considered as abnormal. It is suggested that, due to the greater heart size/body weight ratio, as compared with other breeds of dogs, ECG analysis of Deerhounds produces a greater R-wave amplitude and a prolonged QRS duration than would be regarded normal in common large-breed dogs. In healthy Deerhounds, the mean R-wave amplitude was 3.8 +/- 1.5 mV for lead 2 and the mean QRS duration was 0.061 +/- 0.012 s.[2]

In a UK study, 28.1% of litters were born via **Cesarean section**.[3]

Drug Sensitivities

Anesthesia: Sight hounds require particular attention during anesthesia. Their lean body conformation with high surface-area-to-volume ratio predisposes them to hypothermia during anesthesia. Impaired biotransformation of drugs by the liver results in prolonged recovery from barbiturate and thiobarbiturate intravenous anesthetics. Propofol, and ketamine/diazepam combination are recommended induction agents.[4]

Inherited Disease

Factor VII Deficiency: Autosomal recessive disorder causing mild bleeding. Affected dogs may exhibit an increased bleeding tendency following trauma or surgery or rarely appear to develop spontaneous bleeding. Carriers are detected worldwide. A genetic test is available.[5]

Hip Dysplasia: Polygenically inherited trait causing degenerative hip joint disease and arthritis. Too few Scottish Deerhounds have been screened by OFA to determine an accurate incidence.[6]

Elbow Dysplasia: Polygenically inherited trait causing elbow arthritis. Too few Scottish Deerhounds have been screened by OFA to determine an accurate incidence.[6]

Patella Luxation: Polygenically inherited laxity of patellar ligaments, causing luxation, lameness, and later degenerative joint disease. Treat surgically if causing clinical signs. Too few Scottish Deerhounds have been screened by OFA to determine an accurate frequency.[6]

Disease Predispositions

Anal Gland Infection: A problem of young hounds, with an average age of onset of just over 2 years old. Males are affected about twice as often as bitches. Reported at a frequency of 11% in the 2000 SDCA Health Survey.[7]

Osteosarcoma: Malignant bone cancer, usually involving the long bones of the extremities. The average age of onset is 8 yrs of age. There is a female preponderance in the breed. Research estimate of 15% affected frequency. Heritability of 0.67. Appears to be influenced by a major autosomal dominant gene on chromosome 34. Reported at a frequency of 5% in the 2000 SDCA Health Survey.[7,8,9,10]

Gastric Dilation/Volvulus (GDV, Bloat): Polygenically inherited, life-threatening twisting of the stomach within the abdomen. Requires immediate veterinary attention. Reported at a frequency of 10% in the 2000 SDCA Health Survey.[7]

Inhalant Allergies (Atopy): Presents with pruritis and pyotraumatic dermatitis (hot spots). Reported at a frequency of 6% in the 2000 SDCA Health Survey.[7]

Dilated Cardiomyopathy (DCM)/Atrial Fibrillation: A high percentage of affected dogs initially present with atrial fibrillation, and progress to biventricular dilated cardiomyopathy. Clinical signs include sudden death, passing out, exercise intolerance, pulmonary edema, or ascites. Average age of onset of heart failure is 6-1/2 years of age. Not all dogs with atrial fibrillation will develop DCM, but these dogs should be carefully followed for the development of DCM and perhaps should be held out of breeding programs. DCM occurs in male Scottish Deerhounds 4x the frequency in females. DCM is reported at a frequency of 5-8%, heart failure at 5% and arrhythmia at 4% in the 2000 SDCA Health Survey. The mode of inheritance is not determined.[7,11]

Hypothyroidism: Inherited autoimmune thyroiditis. 4.5% positive for thyroid autoantibodies based on testing at Michigan State University. (Ave. for all breeds is 7.5%). Reported at a frequency of 4% in the 2000 SDCA Health Survey.[7,12,13]

Portosystemic Shunt (PSS, Liver Shunt): Abnormal blood vessels connecting the systemic and portal blood flow can be intrahepatic or extrahepatic. Causes stunting, abnormal behavior, and possible seizures. Diagnosis with paired fasted and feeding serum bile acid and/or ammonium levels, and abdominal ultrasound. Treatment of PSS includes partial ligation and/or medical and dietary control of symptoms. Unknown mode of inheritance.[14]

Cervical Vertebral Arthrosis (Deerhound Neck): Unilateral or bilateral arthrosis of the cervical facet joints between C2 and C3 was detected in nine Scottish Deerhounds, causing severe pain during lateral flexion. Lesions were evident radiographically. Myelography did not reveal abnormalities of the spinal cord or canal. Long-lasting relief was gained through intra-articular administration of corticosteroids.[15]

Cystinuria: Cystine bladder stones form in affected dogs at 3-4 years of age. Only occurs in male dogs. Caused by a defect in cytine metabolism. Nitroprusside test is unreliable to diagnose the disorder. Some dogs with stones will test negative. Unknown mode of inheritance.[16]

Ocular Disorders: The frequency of inherited ocular disorders in the breed cannot be determined because too few Scottish Deerhounds have undergone a CERF examination.[17]

Cataracts, and **Exocrine Pancreatic Insufficiency** are reported.[18]

Isolated Case Studies

Osteochondrodysplasia: The disorder was identified in 5 related Scottish Deerhound pups from 2 litters. At approximately 4 or 5 weeks, exercise intolerance and retarded growth were observed. Kyphosis, limb deformities, and joint laxity gradually developed. Radiograph findings included short long bones and vertebrae, and irregular and delayed epiphyseal ossification. In skeletally mature dogs, osteopenia and severe deformities were seen. A single autosomal recessive mode of inheritance was suspected.[19]

Congenital Hypothyroidism: Two Scottish Deerhound full-siblings had clinical and pathological features of congenital non-goitrous hypothyroidism. The puppies were smaller, had shorter limbs and shorter, broader heads than their littermates. They also had histories of weakness, difficulty in walking and somnolence. Radiographically, epiphyseal growth centers were absent. Both had depressed serum thyroxine (T4) levels and one did not respond to exogenous thyroid stimulating hormone.[20]

Orthostatic Tremor: A four-year-old male Scottish deerhound was presented with a two-year history of pelvic limb tremors, which progressed to the thoracic limbs. Primary OT was diagnosed from the clinical signs, typical electrophysiological findings and the absence of other identifiable disease.[21]

Genetic Tests

Tests of Genotype: Direct genetic test for Factor VII deficiency is available from PennGen and VetGen.

Tests of Phenotype: CHIC Certification: Required testing includes a congenital cardiac evaluation by a cardiologist with echocardiography, and direct test for Factor VII deficiency. Optional recommended test is serum bile acid test at Texas A&M. (See CHIC website; www.caninehealthinfo.org).

Recommend hip and elbow radiographs, CERF eye examination, patella evaluation, and thyroid profile including autoantibodies.

Miscellaneous

- **Breed name synonyms:** Royal Dog of Scotland, Rough Greyhound, Highland Deerhound (all historical), Deerhound, Scotch Greyhound.
- **Registries:** AKC, UKC, CKC, KCGB (Kennel Club of Great Britain), ANKC (Australian National Kennel Club), NKC (National Kennel Club).
- **AKC rank (year 2008):** 133 (153 dogs registered)
- **Internet resources: Scottish Deerhound Club of America:** www.deerhound.org
  The Deerhound Club (UK): www.deerhound.co.uk

References

1. Kintzer PP & Peterson ME: Progress in the Diagnosis and Treatment of Canine Hypothyroidism. 2007. Proceedings, ACVIM 2007

2. Vollmar, A: Echocardiographic examinations in Deerhounds, reference values for echocardiography. *Kleintierpraxis.* 1998. 43: 7, 497-508.

3. Evans KM & Adams VJ: Proportion of litters of purebred dogs born by caesarean section. J Small Anim Pract. 2010 Feb;51(2):113-8.

4. Court MH: Anesthesia of the sighthound. Clin Tech Small Anim Pract 1999 Feb;14(1):38-43.

5. Huff A, Seng A, Tuneva J, et. al.: Molecular, Metabolic, and Hematologic Screening for Hereditary Diseases at the University of Pennsylvania (PennGen). Proceedings, 2007 Tufts' Canine and Feline Breeding and Genetics Conference. 2007.

6. OFA Website breed statistics: www.offa.org Last accessed July 1, 2010.

7. Dillberger J: SDCA Health Survey. Scottish Deerhound Club of America. 2000.

8. Phillips J: Genetic analysis of osteosarcoma in the Scottish Deerhound. Proceedings Veterinary Cancer Society Meeting. 2003.

9. Phillips JC, Stephenson B, Hauck M, et. al.: Heritability and segregation analysis of osteosarcoma in the Scottish deerhound. Genomics. 2007 Sep;90(3):354-63.

10. Phillips JC, Lembcke L & Chamberlin T: A novel locus for canine osteosarcoma (OSA1) maps to CFA34, the canine orthologue of human 3q26. Genomics. 2010 Oct;96(4):220-7.

11. Meurs K: Inherited Heart Disease in the Dog. Proceedings Tufts' Canine and Feline Breeding and Genetics Conference, 2003.

12. Nachreiner RF, Refsal KR, Graham PA, et. al.: Prevalence of serum thyroid hormone autoantibodies in dogs with clinical signs of hypothyroidism. J Am Vet Med Assoc 2002 Feb 15;220(4):466-71.

13. Nachreiner R & Refsal K: Personal communication, Diagnostic Center for Population and Animal Health, Michigan State University. April, 2007.

14. Maxwell A, Hurley K, Burton C, et. al.: Reduced Serum Insulin-Like Growth Factor (IGF) and IGF-Binding Protein-3 Concentrations in Two Deerhounds with Congenital Portosystemic Shunts. J Vet Internal Med. 2000: 14 (5) : 542-545.

15. Kinzel S, Hein S, Buecker A, et. al.: Diagnosis and Treatment of Arthrosis of Cervical Articular Facet Joints in Scottish Deerhounds: 9 Cases (1998-2002). J Am Vet Med Assoc. Nov 1'03; 223[9]:1311-1315.

16. Osborne CA, Sanderson SL, Lulich JP, et. al.: Canine cystine urolithiasis. *Vet. Clinics of North America: Small Animal Practice.* 1999:29:193-211.

17. *Ocular Disorders Presumed to be Inherited in Purebred Dogs.* American College of Veterinary Ophthalmologists. ACVO, 2007.

18. *The Genetic Connection: A Guide to Health Problems in Purebred Dogs.* L Ackerman. p. 238. AAHA Press, 1999.

19. Breur GJ, Zerbe CA, Slocombe RF, et. al.: Clinical, radiographic, pathologic, and genetic features of osteochondrodysplasia in Scottish deerhounds. J Am Vet Med Assoc. 1989 Sep 1;195(5):606-12.

20. Robinson WF, Shaw SE, Stanley B, et. al.: Congenital hypothyroidism in Scottish Deerhound puppies. *Aust Vet J.* 1988 Dec;65(12):386-9.

21. Platt SR, De Stefani A, & Wieczorek L: Primary orthostatic tremor in a Scottish deerhound. Vet Rec. 2006 Oct 7;159(15):495-6.

22. *The Complete Dog Book, 20th Ed.* The American Kennel Club. Howell Book House, NY 2006. p. 218-222.

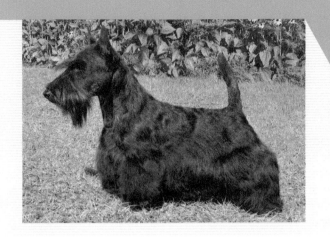

The Breed History

This breed has common roots with other Highland Terriers including the Skye, Dandie Dinmont, and Cairn terrier group. Early writings in the 1500s from Aberdeen Scotland refer to a dog of Scottie type, but the first time the breed was shown was in 1860 in England. In 1882, the first club was formed in the British Isles, and in 1883, the first specimens were imported to the USA. AKC recognition occurred in 1885. President Franklin Roosevelt chose a Scottie and this brought the breed into the limelight.

Breeding for Function

This compact terrier is built to withstand harsh weather and to be agile and work long days under rough conditions. Although bred to do terrier work such as ratting and hunting otter, badger, fox and rabbits, this breed of dog also makes a very good companion.

Physical Characteristics

Height at Withers: female 10" (25.4 cm), male 10" (25.4 cm)

Weight: females 18-21 lb (8-9.5 kg), males 19-22 lb(8.5-10 kg).

Coat: The colors of these double-coated dogs include brindle, black and wheaten. The outer haircoat is long, wiry and wavy.

Longevity: 12-15 years.

Points of Conformation: This plucky terrier has a very alert demeanor and is noted for pricked up small, fine ears and tail, long head in proportion to body, and stocky build with short and heavy legs. The nose should be black and large and the stop should be moderate. Eyes are deep-set and almond shaped, set under a distinct brow that is black or dark-brown in color. Their beard is also well developed. They possess a somewhat short thick neck and very muscular hindquarters, joined by a level topline. The tail is never docked, and it tapers towards the tip. Feet are compact; a slight toe-out is accepted, and the dewclaws can be removed.

Recognized Behavior Issues and Traits

This terrier is equally at home in country or town, and is a loyal dog, but quite spirited and independent minded. He is sometimes called the "Diehard" because of his stamina. They may become one-man dogs. They are suitable for homes with calm, older children. Some care should be taken with other dogs since Scotties may show

aggression. This is also a protective dog for the home, being a keen alarm barker. The Scottie needs firm, gentle training at an early age. Scotties are considered a low shedder and require regular grooming and periodic clipping. They require moderate exercise.

Normal Physiologic Variations

Hyperphosphatasemia: Benign elevations of alkaline phosphatase can occur in Scottish Terriers without any liver, adrenal, or skeletal abnormalities. These levels can be 1.7 to 17 time the reference range, occasionally going over 1,000 U/L. However, Scottish Terriers are also prone to liver and adrenal diseases that can raise AlkP, so they should be worked up.[1,2,3]

In a UK study, 59.8% of litters were born via **Cesarean section.**[4]

Drug Sensitivities

None reported

Inherited Diseases

Hip Dysplasia: Polygenically inherited trait causing degenerative joint disease and hip arthritis. OFA reports 15.8% affected.[5]

Patella Luxation: Polygenically inherited laxity of patellar ligaments, causing luxation, lameness, and later degenerative joint disease. Treat surgically if causing clinical signs. OFA reports 6.9% affected.[5]

Cerebellar Abiotrophy (CA, Cerebellar Ataxia): Autosomal recessive disorder causing cerebellar hypermetria, and an uncoordinated high stepping gait. Mild clinical signs are usually recognized from three months to one year of age; however some affected dogs with mild clinical signs may not be recognized for several years. The clinical signs usually progress slowly throughout the life of the dog; however some can progress more rapidly to constant stumbling. Diagnosis by clinical signs, CSF, MRI/CT, or post-mortem. Occurs at a low frequency, with a wide pedigree spread worldwide. Reported at a frequency of 1.6% in the 2005 STCA Health Survey. No genetic test is available.[6,7,8]

Scotty Cramp: An autosomal recessive inherited disorder of muscle cramping, spasticity, and limb hyperflexion or extension, most often in the pelvic limbs. Clinical signs usually appear after a stressful event or during exercise, and can last from 1-30 minutes. The age of first episode can be 6 weeks to 18 months. Scotty cramp is thought to be caused by a disorder in serotonin metabolism. Medical treatment is usually not necessary although fluoxetene can help in severe cases. Reported at a frequency of 1.2% in the 2005 STCA Health Survey. No genetic test is available.[8,9,10,11,12]

von Willebrand's Disease (vWD): Type III vWD in the Scottish Terrier is a serious, sometimes fatal, autosomal recessive bleeding disorder. Cryoprecipitate is more effective, with less side effects, than fresh frozen plasma in controlling bleeding episodes. A genetic test is available through VetGen, and shows 0.2% of Scottish

Terriers affected, and 10.0% are carriers.[13,14]

Craniomandibular Osteopathy (CMO): Autosomal recessive, painful non-neoplastic proliferation of bone on the ramus of the mandible and/or the tympanic bulla. Affected dogs present between 3-10 months of age, with varying degrees of difficulty prehending and chewing food, secondary weight loss and atrophy of the temporal and masseter muscles. In most cases, affected dogs are normal after bony remodeling. No genetic test is available.[15]

Elbow Dysplasia: Polygenically inherited trait causing elbow arthritis. Too few Scottish Terriers have been screened by OFA to determine an accurate frequency.[5]

Disease Predispositions

Persistent Pupillary Membranes: Strands of fetal remnant connecting; iris to iris, cornea, lens, or involving sheets of tissue. The later three forms can impair vision, and dogs affected with these forms should not be bred. Iris to lens strands are prevalent in the breed, and can be associated with punctate cataracts. Identified in 19.89% of Scottish Terriers CERF examined by veterinary ophthalmologists between 2000-2005. Reported at a frequency of 1.6% in the 2005 STCA Health Survey.[8,16]

Dystocia (difficulty whelping): A Swedish study reports 12.7% of Scottish Terrier pregnancies result in dystocia, often requiring a Caesarian section. It is hypothesized that this is due to some Scottish terriers having a dorso-ventrally flattened pelvic canal that increases the risk of obstruction.[4,17]

Cataracts: Anterior, posterior, intermediate and punctate cataracts are seen in the breed. Identified in 6.99% of Scottish Terriers CERF examined by veterinary ophthalmologists between 2000-2005. Reported at a frequency of 1.4% in the 2005 STCA Health Survey. CERF does not recommend breeding any Scottish Terrier with a cataract.[8,16]

Hypothyroidism: Inherited autoimmune thyroiditis. 6.7% positive for thyroid autoantibodies based on testing at Michigan State University. (Ave. for all breeds is 7.5%). Reported at a frequency of 3.9% in the 2005 STCA Health Survey.[8,18,19]

Transitional Cell Carcinoma (TCC, Bladder Cancer): Scottish Terriers have an 18x greater risk of developing TCC versus other breeds. Glickman et. al. found an increased risk for TCC in Scottish Terriers exposed to phenoxy-based lawn herbicides, and a decreased risk for TCC in Scottish Terriers that consumed green leafy or yellow-orange vegetables three times a week. TCC is a malignant cancer that can be controlled with surgery and piroxicam treatment. Reported at a frequency of 4.6% in the 2005 STCA Health Survey.[8,20,21,22,23]

Hyperadrenocorticism (Cushing's disease): Hyperfunction of the adrenal gland caused by a pituitary or adrenal tumor. Clinical signs may include increased thirst and urination, symmetrical truncal alopecia, and abdominal distention. Dorn reports a 3.97x odds ratio versus other breeds. Reported at a frequency of 3.5% in the 2005 STCA Health Survey.[8,24]

Vitreous Degeneration: Liquefaction of the vitreous gel which may predispose to retinal detachment. Identified in 2.15% of Scottish Terriers CERF examined by veterinary ophthalmologists between 2000-2005.[16]

Idiopathic Epilepsy: Inherited seizures can be generalized or partial seizures. Control with anticonvulsant medication. Reported at a frequency of 2.1% in the 2005 STCA Health Survey. Unknown mode of inheritance.[8]

Vacuolar Hepatopathy: Breed related liver condition characterized by hepatocyte swelling (vacuolar hepatopathy) and at different stages associated with variable inflammatory activity and fibrosis. All affected dogs have elevated alkaline phosphatase activity. It is not determined if this condition is primary or secondary to the AlkP elevation.[25]

Retinal Dysplasia: Focal retinal dysplasia and retinal folds are recognized in the breed. Can progress to retinal detachment and blindness. Identified in 1.61% of Scottish Terriers CERF examined by veterinary ophthalmologists between 2000-2005.[16]

Allergic Dermatitis: Inhalant or food allergy presents with pruritis and pyotraumatic dermatitis (hot spots). Reported at a frequency of 1.4% in the 2005 STCA Health Survey.[3]

Aggression: Reported at a frequency of 1.4% in the 2005 STCA Health Survey.[8]

Kinked Tails: Congenital disorder caused by caudal hemivertebra. Reported at a frequency of 1.3% in the 2005 STCA Health Survey.[8]

Demodicosis: Overgrowth of demodex mites in hair follicles due to an underlying immunodeficiency. Dorn reports a 1.73x odds ratio of developing demodectic mange versus other breeds. Reported at a frequency of 1.1% in the 2005 STCA Health Survey.[8,24]

Corneal Dystrophy: Either the epithelial/stromal, or endothelial form of corneal dystrophy can be seen in the breed. Identified in 1.08% of Scottish Terriers CERF examined by veterinary ophthalmologists between 2000-2005.[16]

Distichiasis: Abnormally placed eyelashes that irritate the cornea and conjunctiva. Can cause secondary corneal ulceration. Identified in 1.08% of Scottish Terriers CERF examined by veterinary ophthalmologists between 2000-2005.[16]

Acquired Myasthenia Gravis: Scottish Terriers are a breed at increased risk of developing generalized or focal acquired myasthenia gravis. The most common presenting signs were generalized weakness, with or without megaesophagus. Diagnosis is by identifying acetylcholine receptor antibodies. Undetermined mode of inheritance.[26]

Superficial Necrolytic Dermatitis (Hepatocutaneous syndrome): Three Scottish Terriers were identified in a study of 36 dogs with diagnoses of superficial necrolytic dermatitis, suggesting a breed prevalence. Affected dogs present with erythema, crusting, exudation, ulceration and alopecia involving footpads, peri-ocular or peri-oral regions, anal–genital regions, and pressure points on the trunk and limbs. Average age of presentation is 10 years. Diagnosis is by biopsy.[27]

Brachygnathism, Copper Toxicosis, Cystinuria, Fibrinoid Leukodystrophy, Lens Luxation, Progressive Retinal Atrophy, Renal Glycosuria, Seasonal Flank Alopecia, and Sebaceous Adenitis are reported.[28]

Isolated Case Studies

Idiopathic Multifocal Osteopathy: Fatal disease identified in four related Scottish Terriers between 16 months and 4.5 years of age presented with reluctance to move, stiff/stilted gait, carpal valgus/laxity, and drooling/dysphagia. Histopathology showed osteoclastic osteolysis and replacement of bone with fibrous tissue in the skull, cervical spine, and proximal radii, ulna, and femora.[29]

Central Axonopathy with Tremors: Three related Scottish Terrier puppies presented at 10 to 12 weeks with signs of severe whole-body tremors, ataxia, and paraparesis that worsened with activity and excitement and diminished during rest or sleep. Widespread CNS white matter axonal changes, vacuolation, and gliosis were found pathologically.[30]

Quadricuspid Aortic Valve: An 11-month-old, female Scottish terrier with a heart murmur was found to have four equally sized aortic valve cusps, a ventricular septal defect, with systolic left-to-right shunting, and aortic regurgitation into both ventricles. The dog was free of clinical signs 1 year after diagnosis.[31]

Suprasellar Cystic Papillary Meningioma: An 8-year-old spayed Scottish Terrier presented with intermittent abnormal behavior that progressed to hind limb ataxia and eventually to recumbency with opisthotonos. CT revealed a radiolucent mass in the area of the hypothalamus, pathologically identified as a cystic papillary meningioma in the sella turcica.[32]

Multiple Cartilaginous Exostoses: Case study of a 3 month old female Scottish terrier with multiple cartilaginous exostoses involving the right and left metatarsals and phalanges, left scapula, ends of several distal ribs, and the spinous processes of several thoracic and lumbar vertebrae. Neurological deficits were due to spinal cord compression at several thoracolumbar vertebrae.[33]

Factor IX Deficiency (Hemophilia B): X-linked recessive bleeding disorder identified in a male Scottish Terrier.[34]

Myeloencephalopathy (Alexander's Disease): Case study of a 9 month-old Scottish Terrier with progressive tetraparesis. Pathology revealed myeloencephalopathy with diffuse Rosenthal fiber formation.[35]

Genetic Tests

Tests of Genotype: Direct test for von Willebrand's disease (vWD) is available from Vetgen.

Direct test for brindle and wheaten coat color is available from VetGen.

Tests of Phenotype: CHIC Certification: Required testing includes direct genetic test for vWD, patella evaluation, and either a thyroid profile including autoantibodies or a CERF eye examination. (See CHIC website; www.caninehealthinfo.org).

Recommend hip and elbow radiographs, and cardiac examination.

Miscellaneous

- **Breed name synonyms:** Scottie, Aberdeen Terrier (historical)
- **Registries:** CKC, AKC, UKC,, KCGB (Kennel Club of Great Britain), ANKC(Australian National Kennel Club), NKC (National Kennel Club)
- **AKC rank (year 2008):** 49 (2,429 dogs registered)
- **Internet resources:** Scottish Terrier Club of America: http://clubs.akc.org/stca
  The Scottish Terrier Club (England): www.stcengland.co.uk
  The Canadian Scottish Terrier Club: www.canadianscottishterrierclub.org

References

1. Gallagher AE, Panciera DL, & Panciera RJ: Hyperphosphatasemia in Scottish terriers: 7 cases. J Vet Intern Med. 2006 Mar-Apr;20(2):418-21.
2. Nestor DD, Holan KM, Johnson CA, et. al.: Serum alkaline phosphatase activity in Scottish Terriers versus dogs of other breeds. J Am Vet Med Assoc. 2006 Jan 15;228(2):222-4.
3. Zimmerman KL, Panciera DL, Panciera RJ, et. al.: Hyperphosphatasemia and concurrent adrenal gland dysfunction in apparently healthy Scottish Terriers. J Am Vet Med Assoc. 2010 Jul 15;237(2):178-86.
4. Evans KM & Adams VJ: Proportion of litters of purebred dogs born by caesarean section. J Small Anim Pract. 2010 Feb;51(2):113-8.
5. OFA Website breed statistics: www.offa.org Last accessed July 1, 2010.
6. van der Merwe LL, Lane E: Diagnosis of cerebellar cortical degeneration in a Scottish terrier using magnetic resonance imaging. J Small Anim Pract. 2001 Aug;42(8):409-12.
7. Urkasemsin G, Linder KE, Bell JS, et. al.: Hereditary cerebellar degeneration in Scottish terriers. J Vet Intern Med. 2010 May-Jun;24(3):565-70.
8. Scottish Terrier Club of America: 2005 STCA Health Survey. Dec. 22, 2005.
9. Meyers KM, Lund JE, Padgett G, et. al.: Hyperkinetic episodes in Scottish Terrier dogs. J Am Vet Med Assoc. 1969 Jul 15;155(2):129-33.
10. Meyers KM, Padgett GA, Dickson WM: The genetic basis of a kinetic disorder of Scottish terrier dogs. J Hered. 1970 Sep-Oct;61(5):189-92.
11. Meyers KM, Schaub RG: The relationship of serotonin to a motor disorder of Scottish terrier dogs. Life Sci. 1974 May 16;14(10):1895-906.
12. Geiger KM & Klopp LS: Use of a selective serotonin reuptake inhibitor for treatment of episodes of hypertonia and kyphosis in a young adult Scottish Terrier. J Am Vet Med Assoc. 2009 Jul 15;235(2):168-71.
13. Venta PJ, Li J, Yuzbasiyan-Gurkan V, et. al.: Mutation causing von Willebrand's disease in Scottish Terriers. J Vet Intern Med. 2000 Jan-Feb;14(1):10-9.
14. Stokol T, Parry B: Efficacy of fresh-frozen plasma and cryoprecipitate in dogs with von Willebrand's disease or hemophilia A. J Vet Intern Med. 1998 Mar-Apr;12(2):84-92.
15. Padgett GA, Mostosky UV: The mode of inheritance of craniomandibular osteopathy in West Highland White terrier dogs. Am J Med Genet. 1986 Sep;25(1):9-13.
16. *Ocular Disorders Presumed to be Inherited in Purebred Dogs.* American College of Veterinary Ophthalmologists. ACVO, 2007.
17. Bergström A, Nødtvedt A, Lagerstedt AS, et. al.: Incidence and breed predilection for dystocia and risk factors for cesarean section in a Swedish population of insured dogs. Vet Surg. 2006 Dec;35(8):786-91.
18. Nachreiner RF, Refsal KR, Graham PA, et. al.: Prevalence of serum thyroid hormone autoantibodies in dogs with clinical signs of hypothyroidism. J Am Vet Med Assoc 2002 Feb 15;220(4):466-71.
19. Nachreiner R & Refsal K: Personal communication, Diagnostic Center for Population and Animal Health, Michigan State University. April, 2007.
20. Glickman LT, Raghavan M, Knapp DW, et. al.: Herbicide exposure and the risk of transitional cell carcinoma of the urinary bladder in Scottish Terriers. J Am Vet Med Assoc. 2004 Apr 15;224(8):1290-7.

21. Norris AM, Laing EJ, Valli VE, et. al.: Canine bladder and urethral tumors: a retrospective study of 115 cases (1980-1985). J Vet Intern Med. 1992 May-Jun;6(3):145-53.

22. Raghavan M, Knapp DW, Bonney PL, et. al.: Evaluation of the effect of dietary vegetable consumption on reducing risk of transitional cell carcinoma of the urinary bladder in Scottish Terriers. J Am Vet Med Assoc. 2005 Jul 1;227(1):94-100.

23. Raghavan M, Knapp DW, Dawson MH, et. al.: Topical flea and tick pesticides and the risk of transitional cell carcinoma of the urinary bladder in Scottish Terriers. J Am Vet Med Assoc. 2004 Aug 1;225(3):389-94.

24. Dorn CR: Canine breed-specific risks of frequently diagnosed diseases at veterinary teaching hospitals. Monograph. AKC Canine Health Foundation. 2000.

25. Lecoindre P, Toulza O, Hernandez J, et. al.: Vacuolar Hepatopathy in Scottish Terriers: Clinical, Biochemical, Ultrasonographic and Histological Findings in 13 Cases. Proceedings, 19th ECVIM-CA Congress. 2009.

26. Shelton GD, Schule A, Kass PH: Risk factors for acquired myasthenia gravis in dogs: 1,154 cases (1991-1995). J Am Vet Med Assoc. 1997 Dec 1;211(11):1428-31.

27. Outerbridge CA, Marks SL, Rogers QR: Plasma amino acid concentrations in 36 dogs with histologically confirmed superficial necrolytic dermatitis. Vet Dermatol. 2002 Aug;13(4):177-86.

28. *The Genetic Connection: A Guide to Health Problems in Purebred Dogs.* L Ackerman. p.238, AAHA Press, 1999.

29. Hay CW, Dueland RT, Dubielzig RR, et. al.: Idiopathic multifocal osteopathy in four Scottish terriers (1991-1996). J Am Anim Hosp Assoc. 1999 Jan-Feb;35(1):62-7.

30. Van Ham L, Vandevelde M, Desmidt M, et. al.: A tremor syndrome with a central axonopathy in Scottish terriers. J Vet Intern Med. 1994 Jul-Aug;8(4):290-2.

31. Kettner F, Cote E, Kirberger RM: Quadricuspid aortic valve and associated abnormalities in a dog. J Am Anim Hosp Assoc. 2005 Nov-Dec;41(6):406-12.

32. Schulman FY, Carpenter JL, Ribas JL, et. al.: Cystic papillary meningioma in the sella turcica of a dog. J Am Vet Med Assoc. 1992 Jan 1;200(1):67-9.

33. Liu SK, Thacher C: Case report 622. Multiple cartilaginous exostoses. Skeletal Radiol. 1990;19(5):383-5.

34. Campbell KL, Greene CE, Dodds WJ: Factor IX deficiency (hemophilia B) in a Scottish terrier. J Am Vet Med Assoc. 1983 Jan 15;182(2):170-1.

35. Sorjonen DC, Cox NR, Kwapien RP: Myeloencephalopathy with eosinophilic refractile bodies (Rosenthal fibers) in a Scottish terrier. J Am Vet Med Assoc. 1987 Apr 15;190(8):1004-6.

36. *The Complete Dog Book, 20th Ed.* The American Kennel Club. Howell Book House, NY 2006. pp 419-423.

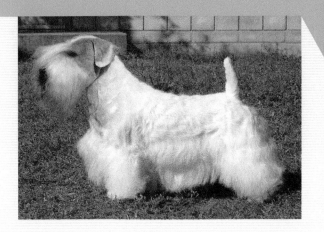

The Breed History

A small town in Wales called Sealyham was the first recorded home of the breed. In the late 1800s, crosses to breeds such as Dandie Dinmont, Corgi, Westie, and perhaps Wirehaired Fox Terriers were done to develop this hardy athletic stock. AKC registration first occurred in 1911, and it was about that time also that the breed was first brought to North America.

Breeding for Function

Hunting, defense, tracking of mid-sized quarry such as otter, badger and fox were some of the tasks these dogs were bred for. Digging and endurance, combined with lightning speed contributed to the success of the hunt.

Physical Characteristics

Height at Withers: ideal is 10.5" (26.5 cm)

Weight: females 22 lb (10 kg), males 23-24 lb (10.5-11 kg).

Coat: White to creamy white, the coarse haircoat is variably marked with small areas of beige or so-called lemon or badger distributed mostly around the head.

Longevity: 14-16 years.

Points of Conformation: Their slightly convex skulls, moderate stop and strong jaws contribute to the tough terrier image. Dark, deep and widely set oval eyes, black nose, and small triangular ears folded down with fine leather characterize their faces. Tails may be docked, and are carried vertical. A medium neck, large compact feet with arched toes and short-coupled stocky muscular body with a deep chest, level topline, and powerful build behind complete the image. Their way of going is quick, agile, and straight.

Recognized Behavior Issues and Traits

Reported breed traits include: Alert intelligence, a calculating stubborn streak, loyalty and adaptability to both country and city living make them a great companion. Their fanciers sometimes attribute to them a sense of humor. They thrive on close human contact and lots of attention. They enjoy barking, and are of medium trainability. They need moderate exercise and are considered low activity dogs and low shedders. Regular clipping, grooming or plucking will keep the coat in top form.

Sealyham Terrier

Normal Physiologic Variations
None reported

Drug Sensitivities
None reported

Inherited Diseases

Patella Luxation: Polygenically inherited laxity of patellar ligaments, causing luxation, lameness, and later degenerative joint disease. Treat surgically if causing clinical signs. Too few Sealyham Terriers have been screened by OFA to determine an accurate frequency.[1]

Primary Lens Luxation (PLL) and Secondary Glaucoma: An autosomal recessive gene causes primary lens luxation. Homozygous affected dogs usually develop lens luxation between 3-5 years of age. Rarely, heterozygous carriers can develop lens luxation, but at a later age. Lens luxation can lead to secondary glaucoma and blindness. A genetic mutation has been identified, and a genetic test is available. OFA testing shows 38% carrier, and 5% affected. Identified in 1.79% of Sealyham Terriers CERF examined by veterinary ophthalmologists between 2000-2005. CERF does not recommend breeding any Sealyham Terrier with lens luxation.[1,2,7]

Retinal Dysplasia: Autosomal recessive inheritance. Congenital retinal folds, geographic, and generalized retinal dysplasia with detachment is seen in Sealyham Terriers. Can progress to blindness. Identified in 2.98% of Sealyham Terriers CERF examined by veterinary ophthalmologists between 2000-2005. CERF does not recommend breeding any Sealyham Terrier with retinal dysplasia. There is no genetic test.[2,3]

Hip Dysplasia: Polygenically inherited trait causing degenerative joint disease and hip arthritis. Too few Sealyham Terriers have been screened by OFA to determine an accurate frequency.[1]

Elbow Dysplasia: Polygenically inherited trait causing elbow arthritis. Too few Sealyham Terriers have been screened by OFA to determine an accurate frequency.[1]

Disease Predispositions

Persistent Pupillary Membranes: Strands of fetal remnant connecting; iris to iris, cornea, lens, or involving sheets of tissue. The later three forms can impair vision, and dogs affected with these forms should not be bred. Identified in 5.95% of Sealyham Terriers CERF examined by veterinary ophthalmologists between 2000-2005.[2]

Cataracts: Anterior cortex punctate, and anterior or posterior cortex intermediate cataracts predominate in the breed. Identified in 3.57% of Sealyham Terriers CERF examined by veterinary ophthalmologists between 2000-2005. CERF does not recommend breeding any Sealyham Terrier with a cataract.[2]

Distichiasis: Abnormally placed eyelashes that irritate the cornea and conjunctiva. Can cause secondary corneal ulceration. Identified in 3.57% of Sealyham Terriers CERF examined by veterinary ophthalmologists between 2000-2005.[2]

Allergic Dermatitis (Atopy): Inhalant or food allergy presents with pruritis and pyotraumatic dermatitis (hot spots). Sealyham Terriers are over-represented with atopy versus other breeds.[4]

Hypothyroidism: Inherited autoimmune thyroiditis. 2.0% positive for thyroid autoantibodies based on testing at Michigan State University. (Ave. for all breeds is 7.5%).[5,6]

Vitreous Degeneration: A liquefaction of the vitreous gel which may predispose to retinal detachment resulting in blindness. Identified in 1.90% of Sealyham Terriers CERF examined by veterinary ophthalmologists between 2000-2005.[2]

Deafness: Congenital sensorineural deafness is reported in the breed. Can be unilateral of bilateral. Diagnosed by BAER testing. Unknown mode of inheritance.[8]

Chronic otitis externa, and **disk disease** are reported on the American Sealyham Terrier Club website.

Brachygnathism, Keratoconjunctivitis Sicca, Prognathism and **Progressive Retinal Atrophy** are reported.[9]

Isolated Case Studies
None reported

Genetic Tests
Tests of Genotype: Direct genetic test for lens luxation is available from OFA.

Tests of Phenotype: CHIC Certification: Required testing includes CERF eye examination and direct test for lens luxation. (See CHIC website: www.caninehealthinfo.org).

Recommend patella evaluation, hip and elbow radiographs, thyroid profile including autoantibodies, and cardiac examination.

Miscellaneous
- **Breed name synonyms:** Sealyham
- **Registries:** AKC, CKC, UKC, KCGB (Kennel Club of Great Britain), ANKC (Australian National Kennel Club), NKC (National Kennel Club)
- **AKC rank (year 2008):** 152 (56 dogs registered)
- **Internet resources: American Sealyham Terrier Club:**
  http://clubs.akc.org/sealy
  Sealyham Terrier Club of Canada:
  www.sealyhamcanada.com
  Sealyham Terrier Breeders Association (UK):
  www.davmar.freeuk.com/sealyhambreedersassoc.html

References
1. OFA Website breed statistics: www.offa.org Last accessed July 1, 2010.
2. *Ocular Disorders Presumed to be Inherited in Purebred Dogs.* American College of Veterinary Ophthalmologists. ACVO, 2007.
3. Dietz HH: Retinal dysplasia in dogs—a review. *Nord Vet Med.* 1985 Jan-Feb;37(1):1-9.
4. Ackerman L: Managing Inhalant Allergies. Proceedings, Tufts Animal Expo 2002.
5. Nachreiner RF, Refsal KR, Graham PA, et. al.: Prevalence of serum thyroid hormone autoantibodies in dogs with clinical signs of hypothyroidism. J Am Vet Med Assoc 2002 Feb 15;220(4):466-71.
6. Nachreiner R & Refsal K: Personal communication, Diagnostic Center for Population and Animal Health, Michigan State University. April, 2007.
7. Nasisse MP: Diseases of the Lens and Cataract Surgery. Proceedings, Waltham/OSU Symposium, Small Animal Ophthalmology, 2001.
8. Strain GM: Deafness prevalence and pigmentation and gender associations in dog breeds at risk. *Vet J.* 2004 Jan;167(1):23-32.
9. *The Genetic Connection: A Guide to Health Problems in Purebred Dogs.* L Ackerman. p 238, AAHA Press, 1999.
10. *The Complete Dog Book, 20th Ed.* The American Kennel Club. Howell Book House, NY 2006. p 424-427.

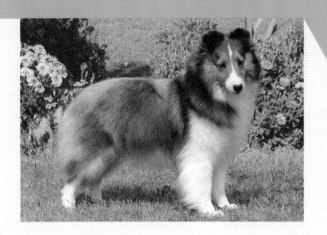

Shetland Sheepdog

The Breed History

This small rough collie-type dog is likely related to the collie (which in turn originated from the Border collie of Scotland), but though some sources report that shelties were collies selected for progressively smaller body stature, others claim the breed is distinct. The Sheltie, as the Shetland sheepdog is often called traces back to the Shetland Islands off of the coast of Scotland where *small* and *hardy* are the trademark of all species able to survive that harsh environment. The first AKC registration was in 1911.

Breeding for Function

These dogs were bred for sheep herding work in rough environments, and they are cherished for both their herding ability and their companionship. They excel in obedience trials due to their high intelligence, trainability, and willingness. Newer sports such as agility, tracking and performing tricks suit their talents as well.

Physical Characteristics

Height at Withers: 13-16" (33-40.5 cm)

Weight: females 12-16 lb (5.5-7 kg), males 14-18 lb (6-8 kg).

Coat: The double coat is thick and smooth, with a very full mane in males. Some feathering on limbs occurs, and coat volume thickens over the tail. Colors range from sable (golden brown to mahogany) marked with white or tan to black, and blue merle. Bi-black and bi-blue are accepted. Brindle or white-predominant coats are disqualified.

Longevity: 12-15 years.

Points of Conformation: The dog is compact, with a dolichocephalic skull, slight stop—overall forming a long blunt tapering profile. Eyes are oblique, almond-shaped and pigmented dark except in merle coated dogs, where blue or merle is permitted. The ears are small, and break about three quarters of the way up. Black nose pigmentation is standard. The neck is muscular, arched and of moderate length. The topline is level, and the chest is deep but narrows underneath, with moderate abdomen tuck. The tail when resting reaches the tarsus. Dewclaws may be removed. Compact arched toes in a small foot, and straight limbs contribute to a low, smooth gait and agility on rough ground.

Recognized Behavior Issues and Traits

Reported breed attributes include: Their alert intelligence means that they learn quickly, and they are also docile and quick to obey. They are loyal and very affectionate, love to please and need contact with their owners. An aloof attitude to strangers is expected, but timid or snappy behavior is unacceptable. They are alarm barkers, and noble defenders. Their training should start early, and socialization is important. As a minimum, they require a careful weekly grooming with prompt removal of any matting. They need daily exercise, and for mental stimulation, active playtime should be integrated.

Normal Physiologic Variations

Merle Coat Color: Caused by a dominant mutation in the SILV gene. Breeding two merle dogs together should be avoided, as homozygous dogs can be born with multiple defects, including blindness, deafness, and heart anomalies.[1]

Hyperlipidemia: Shetland Sheepdogs can have a non-pathological hyperlipidemia and hypercholesterolemia, that can increase with age. This can also progress to hypertriglyceridemia.[2]

Drug Sensitivities

MDR1 Mutation (Ivermectin/Drug Toxicity): Autosomal recessive disorder in the MDR1 gene allows high CNS drug levels of ivermectin, doramectin, loperamide, vincristine, moxidectin, and other drugs. Causes neurological signs, including tremors, seizures, and coma. A genetic test is now available for the mutated gene, showing 1.3% of Shetland sheepdogs are affected, and 10.5% carrier. In Germany, 8% test homozygous affected, and 43% test as carriers.[3,4,5]

Inherited Diseases

Collie Eye Anomaly/Choroidal Hypoplasia/Coloboma (CEA/CH): Autosomal recessive disorder of eye development that can lead to retinal detachment and blindness. Reported in 0.79% of Shetland sheepdogs CERF-examined by veterinary ophthalmologists between 1991-1999. A Swiss study showed 13.1% with CH, and 1.8% with CH and coloboma. A genetic test is available through Optigen, which reports 11% of Shetland sheepdogs test as affected, and 34% test as carriers. CERF does not recommend breeding any Shetland Sheepdogs affected with CEA/CH.[6,7,8,9]

Hip Dysplasia: Polygenically inherited trait causing degenerative joint disease and hip arthritis. OFA reports 4.7% affected. Listed as a significantly reported disorder in the 2000 ASSA Health Survey.[10,11]

Elbow Dysplasia: Polygenically inherited trait causing elbow arthritis. OFA reports 3.1% affected.[10]

Patella Luxation: Polygenically inherited laxity of patellar ligaments, causing luxation, lameness, and later degenerative joint disease. Treat surgically if causing clinical signs. Reported at a high frequency of Shetland sheepdogs screened by OFA, but too few have been examined for statistical accuracy.[10]

Von Willebrand's Disease (vWD): Shetland sheepdogs can have the severe bleeding Type III form of autosomal recessive vWD. A genetic test is available that shows 0.3% affected and 7.7% carrier in the breed.[12,13,14]

Disease Predispositions

Hypothyroidism: Inherited autoimmune thyroiditis. 12.7% positive for thyroid autoantibodies based on testing at Michigan State University. (Ave. for all breeds is 7.5%). Dorn reports a 1.32x odds ratio versus other breeds. Listed as a significantly reported disorder in the 2000 ASSA Health Survey.[11,15,16,17]

Dermatomyositis: Inherited disorder causing patches of scaling, crusting and alopecia over the muzzle, periorbital skin and distal limbs, and an associated myositis especially affecting the masticatory muscles. Onset between 3-6 months of age. Thought to be immune mediated, however specific autoantibodies have not been identified. Mode of inheritance is unknown, though some researchers suspect autosomal dominant with incomplete penetrance. Listed as a significantly reported disorder in the 2000 ASSA Health Survey.[11,18,19,20]

Distichiasis: Abnormally placed eyelashes that irritate the cornea and conjunctiva. Can cause secondary corneal ulceration. In Shelties, usually involves stiff lashes which require permanent epilation. Identified in 5.51% of Shetland Sheepdogs CERF examined by veterinary ophthalmologists between 2000-2005.[7]

Persistent Pupillary Membranes: Strands of fetal remnant connecting; iris to iris, cornea, lens, or involving sheets of tissue. The later three forms can impair vision, and dogs affected with these forms should not be bred. Identified in 5.01% of Shetland sheepdogs CERF-examined by veterinary ophthalmologists between 2000-2005.[7]

Corneal Dystrophy: Shetland sheepdogs can have an ulcerative stromal epithelial form of corneal dystrophy. Identified in 2.45% of Shetland sheepdogs CERF-examined by veterinary ophthalmologists between 2000-2005.[7,21]

Cataracts: Anterior and posterior cortex intermediate and punctate cataracts predominate in the breed. Identified in 1.05% of Shetland sheepdogs CERF examined by veterinary ophthalmologists between 2000-2005. CERF does not recommend breeding any Shetland sheepdog with a cataract.[7]

Uveodermatologic (VKH-Like) Syndrome: This is an autoimmune disease manifested by progressive uveitis and depigmenting dermatitis that closely resembles the human Vogt-Koyanagi-Harada syndrome. The disease presents between 1-1/2 and 4 years of age, and can progress to blindness. Treatment is with steroids. CERF does not recommend breeding any Shetland Sheepdog with the condition.[7]

Kidney Disease: No specific kidney diseases are documented in the literature, but Dorn reports a 17.82x odds ratio versus other breeds.[15]

Autoimmune Hemolytic Anemia (AIHA): Autoimmune destruction of red blood cells. Shetland sheepdogs have a 4.8x risk of developing AIHA versus other breeds. Females are more frequently affected than males. Clinical features included pale mucous membranes, weakness, lethargy and collapse. Treatment with prednisone is successful in most cases.[22]

Vesicular Cutaneous Lupus Erythematosus: Adult onset vesicular form of lupus that causes annular, polycyclic and serpiginous ulcerations distributed over sparsely haired areas of the body. These especially occur during the summer months due to ultraviolet exposure. Treatment is with immunosuppressive drugs and sunscreen. Shetland Sheepdogs are a breed at increased risk.[23]

Idiopathic Epilepsy: The breed has a form of frontal lobe epilepsy with an onset between 2-5 years of age, often progressing to status epilepticus. Control with anticonvulsant medication. Frequency and mode of inheritance not known.[24,25]

Gall Bladder Mucoceles: Gall bladder mucoceles and concurrent dyslipidemia or dysmotility are reported at a 7.2x odds ratio versus other breeds at a median age of 9 years. Treatment is surgery, and a more successful outcome is found in Shetland Sheepdogs who undergo surgery prior to the onset of clinical signs. In case studies, 9.3% of dogs diagnosed with gall bladder mucoceles were Shetland Sheepdogs. The disease is associated with a heterozygous mutation in the ABCB4 gene.[26,27]

Patent Ductus Arteriosus (PDA): Inherited congenital heart disorder; affected dogs are usually stunted, and have a loud heart murmur. Diagnosis is via Doppler ultrasound. Treatment is surgical. Shetland sheepdogs have an increased incidence versus other breeds.[28]

Rostally Displaced Maxillary Canine Teeth: Shetland Sheepdogs can have this abnormal dentition occur. They can also have **abnormal (small) upper third incisors**. Undetermined mode of inheritance. Reported on the ASSA website.

Superficial Necrolytic Dermatitis: Inherited skin disorder caused by a metabolic hepatopathy causing increased hepatic catabolism of amino acids and hypoaminoacidaemia.[29]

Distal Tibial Valgus Deformity: Distal hind limb deformity possibly due to premature closure of the lateral aspect of the distal tibial physis. Correct surgically. Reported at a 12.3x odds ratio versus other breeds.[30]

Lateral Luxation of The Superficial Digital Flexor Tendon: This disorder occurs with increased frequency in Shetland sheepdogs. Breeding studies suggest an autosomal recessive mode of inheritance.[31,32]

Brachygnathism, Central PRA, Color Dilution Alopecia, Cryptorchidism, Factor VII Deficiency, Factor IX Deficiency, Fanconi Syndrome, Mucinosis, Muscular Dystrophy, Oligodontia, Optic Nerve Hypoplasia, Peripheral Vestibular Disease, Posterior Crossbite, Progressive Retinal Atrophy, and **Uveal Hypopigmentation** are reported.[33]

Isolated Case Studies

Leukodystrophy: Rare, inherited mitochondrial disorder, where affected dogs develop tremors at two to nine weeks of age followed by progressive neurological worsening with ataxia, paresis, paralysis, spasticity, and cranial nerve dysfunction. Affected dogs had severe diffuse spongy degeneration of the white matter of the brain and spinal cord.[34,35]

Gastric Leiomyosarcoma: A 7-1/2 year old female Shetland Sheepdog presented with weight loss and bloody vomiting and diarrhea. A pleomorphic leiomyosarcoma was found in the pyloric stomach.[36]

Renal Agenesis: Two cases of bilateral renal agenesis were identified from related litters.[37]

Erythrocyte Fragility with Pigmenturia: A two year-old spayed female Shetland sheepdog had recurrent episodes of discolored urine correlating with stressful situations or excessive activity. Alkaline and osmotic fragility tests determined that an increase in erythrocyte fragility was the underlying cause of the recurrent pigmenturia.[38]

Genetic Tests

Tests of Genotype: Direct test for CEA/CH is available from Optigen.

Direct test for MDR1 (ivermectin sensitivity) gene is available from Washington State Univ.-VCPL.

Direct test for vWD is available from VetGen.

Direct test for bicolor, tricolor and sable colors is available from Health Gene and VetGen.

Tests of Phenotype: CHIC Certification: Required testing includes hip radiographs, CERF eye examination (annually until age 5, then every 2 years until age 9), and two of the following: Direct gene tests for vWD and MDR1, thyroid profile including autoantibodies (at 2, 4, and 7 years), direct gene test for CEA/CH, and elbow radiographs. Optional recommended tests include cardiac evaluation by a specialist and temperament test. (See CHIC website; www.caninehealthinfo.org).

Recommend patella examination.

Miscellaneous

- **Breed name synonyms:** Sheltie, Miniature Collie, Toy Collie
- **Registries:** AKC, CKC, UKC, KCGB (Kennel Club of Great Britain), ANKC (Australian National Kennel Club), NKC (National Kennel Club)
- **AKC rank (year 2008):** 19 (10,188 dogs registered)
- **Internet resources: American Shetland Sheepdog Association:** www.assa.org
  Canadian Shetland Sheepdog Association: www.canadianshelties.ca
  The English Shetland Sheepdog Club: www.essc.org.uk

References

1. Clark LA, Wahl JM, Rees CA, et. al.: Retrotransposon insertion in SILV is responsible for merle patterning of the domestic dog. Proc Natl Acad Sci U S A. 2006 Jan 31;103(5):1376-81.

2. Mori N, Lee P, Muranaka S, et. al.: Predisposition for primary hyperlipidemia in Miniature Schnauzers and Shetland sheepdogs as compared to other canine breeds. Res Vet Sci. 2010 Jun;88(3):394-9.

3. Neff MW, Robertson KR, Wong AK, et. al.: Breed distribution and history of canine mdr1-1Delta, a pharmacogenetic mutation that marks the emergence of breeds from the collie lineage. Proc Natl Acad Sci U S A. 2004 Aug 10;101(32):11725-30.

4. Mealey KL & Meurs KM: Breed distribution of the ABCB1-1Delta (multidrug sensitivity) polymorphism among dogs undergoing ABCB1 genotyping. J Am Vet Med Assoc. 2008 Sep 15;233(6):921-4.

5. Gramer I, Leidolf R, Döring B, et. al.: Breed distribution of the nt230(del4) MDR1 mutation in dogs. Vet J. 2011 Jul;189(1):67-71.

6. Bedford PG: Collie eye anomaly in the United Kingdom. Vet Rec. 1982 Sep 18;111(12):263-70.

7. *Ocular Disorders Presumed to be Inherited in Purebred Dogs.* American College of Veterinary Ophthalmologists. ACVO, 2007.

8. Lowe JK, Kukekova AV, Kirkness EF, et. al.: Linkage mapping of the primary disease locus for collie eye anomaly. Genomics. 2003 Jul;82(1):86-95.

9. Walser-Reinhardt L, Hässig M & Spiess B: Collie Eye Anomaly in Switzerland. Schweiz Arch Tierheilkd. 2009 Dec;151(12):597-603.

10. OFA Website breed statistics: www.offa.org Last accessed July 1, 2010.

11. American Shetland Sheepdog Association: 2000 ASSA Health Survey Results. 2000.

12. Pathak EJ: Type 3 von Willebrand's disease in a Shetland sheepdog. Can Vet J. 2004 Aug;45(8):685-7.

13. Raymond SL, Jones DW, Brooks MB, et. al.: Clinical and laboratory features of a severe form of von Willebrand disease in Shetland sheepdogs. J Am Vet Med Assoc. 1990 Nov 15;197(10):1342-6.

14. Loechel RH, Springer K, & Brewer GJ: VWD and VetGen: Ten Years of Genetic Test Results. Proceedings, 2007 Tufts' Canine and Feline Breeding and Genetics Conference. 2007.

15. Dorn CR: Canine breed-specific risks of frequently diagnosed diseases at veterinary teaching hospitals. Monograph. AKC Canine Health Foundation. 2000.

16. Nachreiner RF, Refsal KR, Graham PA, et. al.: Prevalence of serum thyroid hormone autoantibodies in dogs with clinical signs of hypothyroidism. *J Am Vet Med Assoc* 2002 Feb 15;220(4):466-71.

17. Nachreiner R & Refsal K: Personal communication, Diagnostic Center for Population and Animal Health, Michigan State University. April, 2007.

18. Ferguson EA, Cerundolo R, Lloyd DH, et. al.: Dermatomyositis in five Shetland sheepdogs in the United Kingdom. Vet Rec. 2000 Feb 19;146(8):214-7.

19. Clark LA, Credille KM, Murphy KE, et. al.: Linkage of dermatomyositis in the Shetland Sheepdog to chromosome 35. Vet Dermatol. 2005 Dec;16(6):392-4.

20. Wahl JM, Clark LA, Skalli O, et. al.: Analysis of gene transcript profiling and immunobiology in Shetland sheepdogs with dermatomyositis. Vet Dermatol. 2008 Apr;19(2):52-8.

21. Cooley PL, Dice PF 2nd: Corneal dystrophy in the dog and cat. Vet Clin North Am Small Anim Pract. 1990 May;20(3):681-92.

22. Miller SA, Hohenhaus AE, Hale AS: Case-control study of blood type, breed, sex, and bacteremia in dogs with immune-mediated hemolytic anemia. J Am Vet Med Assoc. 2004 Jan 15;224(2):232-5.

23. Jackson HA: Eleven cases of vesicular cutaneous lupus erythematosus in Shetland sheepdogs and rough collies: clinical management and prognosis. Vet Dermatol. 2004 Feb;15(1):37-41.

24. Morita T, Shimada A, Takeuchi T, et. al.: Cliniconeuropathologic findings of familial frontal lobe epilepsy in Shetland sheepdogs. Can J Vet Res. 2002 Jan;66(1):35-41.

25. Morita T, Takahashi M, Takeuchi T, et. al.: Changes in extracellular neurotransmitters in the cerebrum of familial idiopathic epileptic shetland sheepdogs using an intracerebral microdialysis technique and immunohistochemical study for glutamate metabolism. J Vet Med Sci. 2005 Nov;67(11):1119-26.

26. Aguirre AL, Center SA, Randolph JF, et. al.: Gallbladder disease in Shetland Sheepdogs: 38 cases (1995-2005). J Am Vet Med Assoc. 2007 Jul 1;231(1):79-88.

27. Mealey KL, Minch JD, White SN, et. al.: An insertion mutation in ABCB4 is associated with gallbladder mucocele formation in dogs. Comp Hepatol. 2010 Jul 3;9:6.

28. Ackerman N, Burk R, Hahn AW, et. al.: Patent ductus arteriosus in the dog: a retrospective study of radiographic, epidemiologic, and clinical findings. Am J Vet Res. 1978 Nov;39(11):1805-10.

29. Outerbridge CA, Marks SL, Rogers OR: Plasma amino acid concentrations in 36 dogs with histologically confirmed superficial necrolytic dermatitis. Vet Dermatol. 2002 Aug;13(4):177-86.

30. Jaeger GH, Marcellin-Little DJ, & Ferretti A: Morphology and correction of distal tibial valgus deformities. J Small Anim Pract. 2007 Dec;48(12):678-82.

31. Solanti S, Laitinen O, Atroshi F: Hereditary and clinical characteristics of lateral luxation of the superficial digital flexor tendon in Shetland sheepdogs. Vet Ther. 2002 Spring;3(1):97-103.

32. Mauterer JV Jr, Prata RG, Carberry CA, et. al.: Displacement of the tendon of the superficial digital flexor muscle in dogs: 10 cases (1983-1991). J Am Vet Med Assoc. 1993 Oct 15;203(8):1162-5.

33. *The Genetic Connection: A Guide to Health Problems in Purebred Dogs.* L Ackerman. p.238-9, AAHA Press, 1999.

34. Wood SL, Patterson JS: Shetland Sheepdog leukodystrophy. J Vet Intern Med. 2001 Sep-Oct;15(5):486-93.

35. Li FY, Cuddon PA, Song J, et. al.: Canine spongiform leukoencephalomyelopathy is associated with a missense mutation in cytochrome b. Neurobiol Dis. 2006 Jan;21(1):35-42.

36. Park CH, Ishizuka Y, Tsuchida Y, et. al.: Gastric pleomorphic leiomyosarcoma in a Shetland sheepdog. J Vet Med Sci. 2007 Aug;69(8):873-6.

37. Brownie CF, Tess MW, Prasad RD: Bilateral renal agenesis in two litters of Shetland sheepdogs. Vet Hum Toxicol. 1988 Oct;30(5):483-5.

38. LeGrange SN, Breitschwerdt EB, Grindem CB, et. al.: Erythrocyte fragility and chronic intermittent pigmenturia in a dog. J Am Vet Med Assoc. 1995 Apr 1;206(7):1002-6

39. *The Complete Dog Book, 20th Ed.* The American Kennel Club. Howell Book House, NY 2006. p. 688-693.

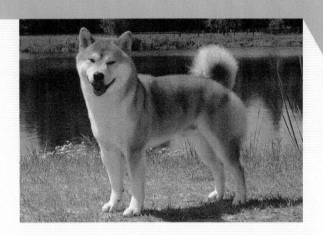

The Breed History

This is an ancient breed, thought to have its origins in the rugged mountains of Japan over 5000 years ago. The Shiba Inu was formally named and recognized in 1920. The smallest of the Japanese dog breeds, they are named accordingly; small (shiba) dog (inu). Another theory is that shiba refers to the red color of the brushwood bushes in which they often hunted; many of the breed specimens are also red in color. In the 1940s Shiba became very rare, such that only three lines remained in Japan. These were used to diligently revive the breed. First dogs were exported to America in 1954. The breed was registered in AKC first in 1992.

Breeding for Function

Historically the Shiba dog was used for hunting, especially in low dense brush. They were widely used for small game hunting. Today, they are primarily companion and show dogs, though they are also widely valued as watchdogs.

Physical Characteristics

Height at Withers: female 13.5-15.5" (34-39 cm), male 14.5-16.5" (36.83-42 cm).

Weight: females 17 lb (7.5 kg), males 23 lb (10.5 kg).

Coat: The double coat has a thick, dense, short undercoat of buff, grey or cream pigmentation; outer coat is straight and hard, with white to cream in specified pattern. This light outer coat pigment pattern is present with all three primary coat colors: Red, Sesame, and Black and Tan. Sesame is a black tipped coat with red as primary hair shaft color.

Longevity: 12-13 years

Points of Conformation: The Shiba Inu is a compact Spitz-type dog, with moderate bone and muscling and an almost square conformation. Slanting dark brown eyes are rimmed by tight black palpebral margins. Eyes are triangular in shape, and are deep and wide set. Upright pricked ears are forward tilting, and are small and triangular. The skull is flat and broad, the stop moderate, and the muzzle is straight, round in cross section, and pointed. The cheeks are prominent. Nose and lip margins are black, the neck is thick and the topline level. The thorax is deep with moderately sprung ribs, the abdomen tucked up, and the tail is high set and reaches the

tarsus when straightened; normal carriage is over the back curled or sickled. Limbs are straight boned and the feet are compact, with toes well knuckled up. Front dewclaws may be removed; there are no rear declaws. They possess an athletic, agile, springy gait.

Recognized Behavior Issues and Traits

Reported characteristics of the breed include: Loyal, a good watchdog, bold, independent, often have inter-dog aggression; especially inter-male, possessing a dominant personality, good at escaping fences by digging or jumping, aloof with strangers, low barking tendency (high pitched sound), and early socialization and obedience training is essential. They are considered good with children if raised with them. They tolerate heat and cold well, have moderate exercise needs, are easily housetrained, and are not keen on restraint. They may require patience for leash training. They are considered to have low grooming needs, and have moderate shedding tendency overall.

Normal Physiologic Variations

Microcytosis: Small red blood cells can be a typical finding in Shibas. Erythrocyte mean corpuscular volume in Shibas ranged from 55.6 to 69.1 fl (mean +/- SD, 61.2 +/- 4.3 fl; median, 60.6 fl; reference range, 63 to 73 fl).[1]

Hyperkalemia: Shiba Inu have a benign autosomal recessive inherited condition of high red blood cell potassium. A survey in Japan showed one-quarter to one-third of Shiba Inu were affected.[2,3]

Drug Sensitivities

None reported

Inherited Diseases

Patella Luxation: Polygenically inherited laxity of patellar ligaments, causing luxation, lameness, and later degenerative joint disease. Treat surgically if causing clinical signs. OFA reports 6.9% affected.[4]

Hip Dysplasia: Polygenically inherited trait causing degenerative joint disease and hip arthritis. OFA reports 5.6% affected.[4]

Elbow Dysplasia: Polygenically inherited trait causing elbow arthritis. OFA reports 3.6% affected.[4]

GM1-Gangliosidosis: A rare, fatal autosomal recessive storage disease causing loss of balance, intermittent lameness, ataxia, dysmetria and intention tremor around 5 to 6 months of age. Affected dogs can also form corneal opacities. The disorder is primarily seen in Japan where a genetic test is available, showing 2.9% carriers.[5,6,7,8,9]

Disease Predispositions

Glaucoma: Primary angle closure with pectinate ligament dysplasia occurs in the breed. Onset 10 weeks to 10 years. Can also predispose to **lens luxation**. Screen with gonioscopy and tonometry. Reported at a frequency of 33% in Japan. CERF Does not recommend breeding any Shiba Inu with primary angle closure.[10,11]

Persistent Pupillary Membranes: Strands of fetal remnant connecting; iris to iris, cornea, lens, or involving sheets of tissue. The later three forms can impair vision, and dogs affected with these forms should not be bred. Identified in 4.04% of Shiba Inu CERF examined by veterinary ophthalmologists between 2000-2005.[12]

Allergic Dermatitis (Atopy): Inhalant or food allergy, presents with pruritis and pyotraumatic dermatitis (hot spots). Reported as a significant problem on the NSCA website.[13]

Distichiasis: Abnormally placed eyelashes that irritate the cornea and conjunctiva. Can cause secondary corneal ulceration. Identified in 2.86% of Shiba Inu CERF examined by veterinary ophthalmologists between 2000-2005.[12]

Hypothyroidism: Inherited autoimmune thyroiditis. 2.3% positive for thyroid autoantibodies based on testing at Michigan State University. (Ave. for all breeds is 7.5%).[14,15]

Cataracts: Posterior suture punctate cataracts predominate in the breed. Identified in 2.27% of Shiba Inu CERF examined by veterinary ophthalmologists between 2000-2005. CERF does not recommend breeding any Shiba Inu with a cataract.[12]

Ventricular Septal Defect: Shiba Inu are over-represented in cases of ventricular septal defect; a congenital disorder causing a hole in the heart wall between the ventricles. Clinical signs can vary from heart failure to subclinical.[16]

Base Narrow Canines, Oligodontia, Rostrally Displaced Maxillary Canine, Uveodermatological Syndrome, von Willebrand's Disease, and **Wry Mouth** are reported.[17]

Isolated Case Studies

Congenital Nephrogenic Diabetes Insipidus: A two-year-old intact male Shiba Inu dog with excessive polyuria and polydipsia (PU-PD) was diagnosed as having congenital nephrogenic diabetes insipidus based on clinical findings, urinalysis, blood chemistry, a modified water deprivation test and a low dose dexamethasone suppression test.[18]

Congenital Esophageal Stricture: An 11-week-old female Shiba Inu with a history of intermittent regurgitation since birth had a partial obstruction of the caudal cervical esophagus ue to a narrow, transverse tissue band. Surgical ligation was curative.[19]

Cor Triatriatum Dexter: A Shiba Inu dog with marked abdominal distension was diagnosed with cor triatriatum dexter. Surgical correction was performed, postoperative contrast radiography of the caudal vena cava revealed normal flow into the right heart.[20]

Collagenofibrotic Glomerulonephropathy: A 3 year old Shiba Inu presented with anorexia, high BUN, creatinine, and proteinuria. A collagenofibrotic glomerulonephropathy was identified pathologically, with massive accumulation of type III collagenous fibrils.[21]

Genetic Tests

Tests of Genotype: Direct test for GM-1 gangliosidosis is available in Japan.

Tests of Phenotype: CHIC Certification: Required testing includes hip radiographs, CERF eye examination, and patella evaluation. (See CHIC website; www.caninehealthinfo.org).

Recommend elbow radiographs, thyroid profile including autoantibodies, and cardiac examination.

Miscellaneous

- **Breed name synonyms:** Brushwood dog, Small Brushwood dog, Shiba, Japanese Small-sized Dog.
- **Registries:** AKC, UKC (called Shiba in this registry), CKC, ANKC (Australian National Kennel Club), NKC (National Kennel Club), called Shiba in this registry.
- **AKC rank (year 2008):** 65 (1,376 dogs registered)
- **Internet resources: National Shiba Club of America:** www.shibas.org
  Shiba Inu Canada: www.shibainucanada.com

References

1. Gookin JL, Bunch SE, Rush LJ: Evaluation Of Microcytosis In 18 Shibas. J Am Vet Med Assoc 1998: 212[8]:1258-1259.
2. Fujise H, Hishiyama N, Ochiai H: Heredity of red blood cells with high K and low glutathione (HK/LG) and high K and high glutathione (HK/HG) in a family of Japanese Shiba Dogs. *Exp Anim.* 1997 Jan;46(1):41-6.
3. Fujise H, Higa K, Nakayama T, et. al.: Incidence of dogs possessing red blood cells with high K in Japan and East Asia. *J Vet Med Sci.* 1997 Jun;59(6):495-7.
4. OFA Website breed statistics: www.offa.org Last accessed July 1, 2010.
5. Yamato O, Masuoka Y, Yonemura M, et. al.: Clinical and clinico-pathologic characteristics of Shiba dogs with a deficiency of lysosomal acid beta-galactosidase: a canine model of human GM1 gangliosidosis. *J Vet Med Sci* 2003: 65[2]:213-7.
6. Yamato O, Jo EO, Shoda T, et. al.: Rapid and simple mutation screening of G(M1) gangliosidosis in Shiba dogs by direct amplification of deoxyribonucleic acid from various forms of canine whole-blood specimens. *J Vet Diagn Invest* 2004: 16[5]:469-72.
7. Yamato O, Jo EO, Chang HS, et. al.: Molecular screening of canine GM1 gangliosidosis using blood smear specimens after prolonged storage: detection of carriers among shiba dogs in northern Japan. J Vet Diagn Invest. 2008 Jan;20(1):68-71.
8. Chang HS, Arai T, Yabuki A, et. al.: Rapid and reliable genotyping technique for GM1 gangliosidosis in Shiba dogs by real-time polymerase chain reaction with TaqMan minor groove binder probes. J Vet Diagn Invest. 2010 Mar;22(2):234-7.
9. Nagayasu A, Nakamura T, Yamato O, et. al.: Morphological analysis of corneal opacity in Shiba dog with GM1 gangliosidosis. J Vet Med Sci. 2008 Sep;70(9):881-6.
10. Kato K, Sasaki N, Matsunaga S, et. al.: Incidence of canine glaucoma with goniodysplasia in Japan : a retrospective study. J Vet Med Sci. 2006 Aug;68(8):853-8.
11. Kato K, Sasaki N, Matsunaga S, et. al.: Possible association of glaucoma with pectinate ligament dysplasia and narrowing of the iridocorneal angle in Shiba Inu dogs in Japan. Vet Ophthalmol. 2006 Mar-Apr;9(2):71-5.
12. *Ocular Disorders Presumed to be Inherited in Purebred Dogs.* American College of Veterinary Ophthalmologists. ACVO, 2007.
13. Griffies JD: Atopic Disease–Clinical Presentation. Proceedings, 2002 Western Veterinary Conference. 2002.

14. Nachreiner RF, Refsal KR, Graham PA, et. al.: Prevalence of serum thyroid hormone autoantibodies in dogs with clinical signs of hypothyroidism. *J Am Vet Med Assoc* 2002 Feb 15;220(4):466-71.

15. Nachreiner R & Refsal K: Personal communication, Diagnostic Center for Population and Animal Health, Michigan State University. April, 2007.

16. Abbott JA, Hawkes K, Small MT, et. al.: Retrospective Description of Canine Ventricular Septal Defect. Proceedings, 2008 ACVIM Forum. 2008.

17. *The Genetic Connection: A Guide to Health Problems in Purebred Dogs.* L Ackerman. p 239. AAHA Press, 1999.

18. Takemura N: Successful long-term treatment of congenital nephrogenic diabetes insipidus in a dog. *J Small Anim Pract.* 1998 Dec;39(12):592-4.

19. Fox E, Lee K, Lamb CR, et. al.: Congenital oesophageal stricture in a Japanese shiba inu. J Small Anim Pract. 2007 Dec;48(12):709-12.

20. Tanaka R, Hoshi K, Shimizu M, et. al.: Surgical correction of cor triatriatum dexter in a dog under extracorporeal circulation. *J Small Anim Pract.* 2003 Aug;44(8):370-3.

21. Kamiie J, Yasuno K, Ogihara K, et. al.: Collagenofibrotic glomerulonephropathy with fibronectin deposition in a dog. Vet Pathol. 2009 Jul;46(4):688-92.

22. *The Complete Dog Book, 20th Ed.* The American Kennel Club. Howell Book House, NY 2006. p 593-596.

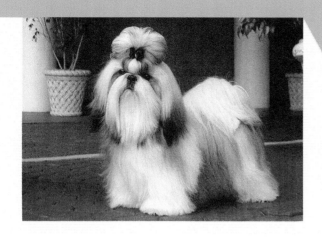

They are moderate shedders, and some owners prefer to have them clipped once to twice annually. They do well with children in the household. They enjoy close human contact, and have low to moderate exercise needs. They tolerate heat poorly.

Normal Physiologic Variations
None reported

Drug Sensitivities
None reported

Inherited Diseases
Renal Dysplasia: Autosomal dominant disease with incomplete penetrance causing renal failure. Affected dogs can succumb to renal failure from birth to two years of age. Mildly affected dogs can live with compensated renal insufficiency. Biopsy studies suggest that a majority of the breed is affected, although only a small percentage die from the condition. Dorn reports a 12.10x odds ratio for kidney disease in Shih Tzus versus other breeds. A direct genetic test for a susceptibility gene is available. (Affected dogs all have one copy of the gene, but most dogs with the gene will not develop kidney failure.)[1,2,3,4]

Hip Dysplasia and Legg–Calve–Perthes Disease: Polygenically inherited traits causing degenerative hip joint disease and arthritis. OFA reports 19.4% affected.[5]

Patella Luxation: Polygenically inherited laxity of patellar ligaments, causing luxation, lameness, and later degenerative joint disease. Treat surgically if causing clinical signs. OFA reports 2.4% affected.[5]

Elbow Dysplasia: Polygenically inherited trait causing elbow arthritis. Too few Shih Tzus have been screened by OFA to determine an accurate frequency.[5]

Disease Predispositions
Distichiasis: Abnormally placed eyelashes that irritate the cornea and conjunctiva. Can cause secondary corneal ulceration. Identified in 15.59% of Shih Tzus CERF-examined by veterinary ophthalmologists between 2000-2005. Dorn reports a 3.13x odds ratio in Shih Tzus versus other breeds.[1,6]

Primary (Narrow Angle) Glaucoma: Ocular condition causing increased pressure within the eyeball, and secondary blindness due to damage to the retina. Can also predispose to lens luxation. Screen with gonioscopy and tonometry. Reported at a frequency of 16.5% in Japan. Diagnosed in 1.58% of Shih Tzus presented to veterinary teaching hospitals.[7,8]

Brachycephalic Complex: The brachycephalic complex includes **Stenotic Nares, Elongated Soft Palate, Everted Laryngeal Saccules, Laryngeal Collapse,** and occasionally **Hypoplastic Trachea.** Can cause respiratory distress, apnea, and hypoxia. Early surgical correction of severe stenotic nares is recommended.[9,10]

The Breed History
The name means "lion" in Chinese. This dog perhaps originated in the Byzantine Empire or Tibet, though they are known to have reached China in the Tang Dynasty. Earliest records go back to about the year 625. Though they were brought to North America during World War II, they did not join AKC registry until 1969. It is possible the modern breed originated from Pekingese and Pug crossed with Tibetan dogs such as Lhasa Apso. Only 14 foundation dogs are thought to have been the source of the breed outside China since the 1900s.

Breeding for Function
They were bred for companionship and as a lapdog for the Chinese and Tibetan royalty.

Physical Characteristics
Height at Withers: female 9-10.5" (23-26.5 cm), male 9-10.5" (23-26.5 cm),

Weight: females 9-16 lb (4-7 kg), males 9-16 lb (4-7 kg).

Coat: Their dense, long, straight double coat can be any color.

Longevity: 13-15 years.

Points of Conformation: In these toy dogs, the tail is carried over the back, head carriage is high and the topline is straight. Though a toy breed, the Shih Tzu is built with solid stature and they are longer than high. The large dark round eyes are not prominent, eyelid and lip margins are pigmented darkly. Skull is brachycephalic and the small muzzle is about one inch long. The nose is black except for the liver and blue dogs, where they are liver and blue to match. They have large pendulous ears, a definite stop and a prognathic jaw. The abdomen has no waist, and the chest consists of a deep moderately sprung ribcage. Dewclaws may be taken off, and the legs are straight. Their gait is powerful and straight.

Recognized Behavior Issues and Traits
These dogs are reported to be intelligent, very alert, and friendly. Their docile nature is a high priority in breeding programs because they are used solely as companion dog. They are alarm barkers. Their profuse coat should be groomed daily and may require a regular bath. Hair above the eyes is either trimmed or tied up.

Epiphora: Ocular tear drainage with hair staining. Can occur secondary to medial canthal trichiasis and/or entropion. Shih Tzu are listed as the most frequently affected breed. Treat by keeping hair clipped short, and daily cleaning. Medial canthoplasty is curative in severe cases.[11]

Entropion: Rolling in of eyelids, often causing corneal irritation or ulceration. Identified in 7.88% of Shih Tzus CERF examined by veterinary ophthalmologists between 2000-2005.[6]

Vitreous Degeneration: Liquefaction of the vitreous gel which may predispose to retinal detachment. Identified in 7.36% of Shih Tzus CERF-examined by veterinary ophthalmologists between 2000-2005.[6]

Cataracts: Juvenile and adult onset. Anterior or posterior intermediate cataracts predominate in the breed. Median age of 6.5 +/- 3.4 years. In one large study, 4.14% of Shih Tzus had cataracts. Identified in 5.43% of Shih Tzus CERF-examined by veterinary ophthalmologists between 2000-2005. CERF Does not recommend breeding any Shih Tzu with a cataract.[6,12,13]

Eury/Macroblepharon: An exceptionally large palpebral fissure. With laxity, may lead to lower lid ectropion and upper lid entropion. Either of these conditions may lead to severe ocular irritation. Identified in 3.50% of Shih Tzus CERF-examined by veterinary ophthalmologists between 2000-2005.[6]

Exposure Keratopathy Syndrome/Pigmentary Keratitis: Corneal reactivity and drying from ocular exposure secondary to shallow orbits, exophthalmos, and lagophthalmos. Identified in 3.50% of Shih Tzus CERF-examined by veterinary ophthalmologists between 2000-2005.[6]

Hypothyroidism: Inherited autoimmune thyroiditis. 3.0% positive for thyroid autoantibodies based on testing at Michigan State University. (Ave. for all breeds is 7.5%).[14,15]

Ectopic Cilia: Hair emerging through the eyelid conjunctiva. Ectopic cilia can cause discomfort and corneal disease. Identified in 1.93% of Shih Tzus CERF-examined by veterinary ophthalmologists between 2000-2005.[6]

Corneal Dystrophy: Shih Tzus can have an epithelial/stromal form of corneal dystrophy. Identified in 1.75% of Shih Tzus CERF-examined by veterinary ophthalmologists between 2000-2005.[6]

Umbilical Hernia: Inherited umbilical hernias occur at an increased frequency in Shih Tzus versus other breeds. Correct surgically if large.[16]

Prolapsed Gland of the Nictitans (Cherry Eye): This condition occurs secondary to inflammation of the gland. Reported at an increased frequency in the breed.[17]

Progressive Retinal Atrophy (PRA): Progressive degeneration of the retina leading to blindness. Mode of inheritance not defined. Reported in 1.23% of Shih Tzus CERF examined by veterinary ophthalmologists between 2000-2005. CERF does not recommend breeding any Shih Tzu with PRA.[6]

Chronic Superficial Keratitis (Pannus): Chronic corneal inflammatory process that can cause vision problems due to corneal pigmentation. Treatment with topical ocular lubricants and anti-inflammatory medication. Identified in 1.05% of Shih Tzus CERF-examined by veterinary ophthalmologists between 2000-2005.[6]

Intervertebral Disc Disease (IVDD): Shih Tzus have an increased risk of developing spinal cord disease due to prolapsed disk material. Clinical signs include back pain, scuffing of paws, spinal ataxia, limb weakness, and paralysis. In a Japanese study, 11.4% of dogs with IVDD were Shih Tzus, primarily affecting the cervical spinal cord at an average age of 10 years.[18,19]

Portosystemic Shunt (PSS, Liver Shunt): Can be intrahepatic, extrahepatic or microvascular dysplasia. Causes stunting, abnormal behavior, possible seizures, and secondary ammonium urate urinary calculi. Diagnose with paired fasted and feeding serum bile acid and/or ammonia levels, and abdominal ultrasound. 0.78% of Shih Tzus (odds ratio of 15.4x) presented to veterinary teaching hospitals had PSS.[20,21,22]

Keratoconjunctivitis Sicca (KCS, Dry Eye): Ocular condition causing lack of tear production and secondary conjunctivitis, corneal ulcerations, and vision problems. In one study, 4.8% of dogs with KCS were Shih Tzus. Usually presents in the breed at 0-2 years of age, or 4-6 years of age. Treat with ocular lubricants and anti-inflammatory medications. CERF does not recommend breeding any Shih Tzu with KCS.[6,23]

Urinary Calculi: The breed is found to be at an increased risk of developing **struvite** and **oxalate** calculi. Dorn reports a 2.74x odds ratio in Shih Tzus versus other breeds.[1,24,25]

Optic Nerve Hypoplasia: Congenital malformation of the optic nerve causing blindness. 23% of reported cases are Shih Tzus. CERF does not recommend breeding any Shih Tzu with the condition.[6,26]

Allergic Inhalant Dermatitis, Cleft Lip/Palate, Dermoid Sinus, Hydrocephalus, Malassezia Dermatitis, Oligodontia, Prognathism, Sebaceous Adenitis, Tricuspid Valve Dysplasia, and **von Willebrand's Disease** are reported.[27]

Isolated Case Studies

Pancreatic Gastrinoma: Several cases of Shih Tzus with pancreatic gastinoma have been documented. Affected dogs present with vomiting, diarrhea and anorexia. Serum gastrin levels are elevated.[28,29]

Spinal Arachnoid Cyst: Two Shih Tzu littermates presenting with progressive ataxia and quadriparesis due to cranial cervical spinal arachnoid cysts. Treatment was surgical.[30]

Atlantoaxial Subluxation: An eight month-old male Shih Tzu with symmetric ataxia, tetraparesis, and neck pain was diagnosed with atlantoaxial subluxation due to absence of the transverse ligament of the atlas and malformation of the dens and atlas. The pup was euthanized.[31]

Polioencephalomyelopathy: A 17-month-old Shih Tzu presented with a 3 month history of progressive thoracic limb weakness consistent with a lesion affecting the cervicothoracic (C6 through T2) spinal cord. MRI identified symmetric lesions in the C5-C7 spinal cord, caudal colliculi, and vestibular and cerebellar nuclei. Pathology revealed polioencephalomyelopathy, similar to that seen in the mitochondrial disorder in Australian Cattle Dogs, and humans with Leigh disease.[32]

Genetic Tests

Tests of Genotype: Direct test for a renal dysplasia susceptibility gene is available from Dogenes (www.dogenes.com).

Direct test for coat color is available from VetGen.

Tests of Phenotype: Recommended tests are; CERF eye examination, hip and elbow radiographs, patella examination, thyroid profile including autoantibodies, cardiac examination, and genetic test for renal dysplasia susceptibility.

Miscellaneous

- **Breed name synonyms:** Chrysanthemum-faced Dog, Shi Tzu, Lion dog
- **Registries:** AKC, CKC, UKC, KCGB (Kennel Club of Great Britain), ANKC (Australian National Kennel Club), NKC (National Kennel Club)
- **AKC rank (year 2008):** 10 (20,219 dogs registered)
- **Internet resources: American Shih Tzu Club:** www.shihtzu.org **The Canadian Shih Tzu Club:** www.canadianshihtzuclub.ca **Shih Tzu Club (UK):** www.theshihtzuclub.co.uk

References

1. Dorn CR: Canine breed-specific risks of frequently diagnosed diseases at veterinary teaching hospitals. Monograph. AKC Canine Health Foundation. 2000.
2. O'Brien TD, Osborne CA, Yano BL, et. al.: Clinicopathologic manifestations of progressive renal disease in Lhasa Apso and Shih Tzu dogs. J Am Vet Med Assoc. 1982 Mar 15;180(6):658-64
3. Vannevel J: Familial renal disease in Shih Tzu puppies. Can Vet J. 1995 Jan;36(1):44.
4. Bovee KC: Renal Dysplasia in Shih Tzu Dogs. Proceedings, 2003 World Small Animal Veterinary Association World Congress, 2003.
5. OFA Website breed statistics: www.offa.org Last accessed July 1, 2010.
6. *Ocular Disorders Presumed to be Inherited in Purebred Dogs.* American College of Veterinary Ophthalmologists. ACVO, 2007.
7. Kato K, Sasaki N, Matsunaga S, et. al.: Incidence of canine glaucoma with goniodysplasia in Japan : a retrospective study. J Vet Med Sci. 2006 Aug;68(8):853-8.
8. Gelatt KN, MacKay EO: Prevalence of the breed-related glaucomas in pure-bred dogs in North America. Vet Ophthalmol. 2004 Mar-Apr;7(2):97-111.
9. Koch DA, Arnold S, Hubler M, et. al.: Brachycephalic Syndrome in Dogs. Compend Contin Educ Pract Vet. January 2003;25(1):48-55.
10. Huck JL, Stanley BJ, Hauptman JG, et. al.: Technique and outcome of nares amputation (Trader's technique) in immature shih tzus. J Am Anim Hosp Assoc. 2008 Mar-Apr;44(2):82-5.
11. Yi NY, Park SA, Jeong MB, et. al.: Medial canthoplasty for epiphora in dogs: a retrospective study of 23 cases. J Am Anim Hosp Assoc. 2006 Nov-Dec;42(6):435-9.
12. Gelatt KN, Mackay EO: Prevalence of primary breed-related cataracts in the dog in North America. Vet Ophthalmol. 2005 Mar-Apr;8(2):101-11.
13. Park SA, Yi NY, Jeong MB, et. al.: Clinical manifestations of cataracts in small breed dogs. Vet Ophthalmol. 2009 Jul-Aug;12(4):205-10.
14. Nachreiner RF, Refsal KR, Graham PA, et. al.: Prevalence of

serum thyroid hormone autoantibodies in dogs with clinical signs of hypothyroidism. *J Am Vet Med Assoc* 2002 Feb 15;220(4):466-71.
15. Nachreiner R & Refsal K: Personal communication, Diagnostic Center for Population and Animal Health, Michigan State University. April, 2007.
16. Young MD: Umbilical hernias in shih tzus. Vet Rec. 1991 Aug 31;129(9):204.
17. Herrera D: Surgery of the Eyelids. 2005. Proceedings, World Small Animal Veterinary Association Congress, 2005.
18. LeCouteur RA: Spinal Cord Diseases of Small Breed Dogs. 2006. Proceedings, Western Veterinary Conference.
19. Itoh H, Hara Y, Yoshimi N, et. al.: A retrospective study of intervertebral disc herniation in dogs in Japan: 297 cases. J Vet Med Sci. 2008 Jul;70(7):701-6.
20. Hunt GB: Effect of breed on anatomy of portosystemic shunts resulting from congenital diseases in dogs and cats: a review of 242 cases. Aust Vet J. 2004 Dec;82(12):746-9.
21. Tobias KM, Rohrbach BW: Association of breed with the diagnosis of congenital portosystemic shunts in dogs: 2,400 cases (1980-2002). J Am Vet Med Assoc. 2003 Dec 1;223(11):1636-9.
22. Center SA: Portosystemic Vascular Anomalies & Hepatic MVD: Evidence of Common Genetics in Small Dogs. Proceedings, 2008 ACVIM Forum. 2008.
23. Sanchez RF, Innocent G, Mould J, et. al.: Canine keratoconjunctivitis sicca: disease trends in a review of 229 cases. J Small Anim Pract. 2007 Apr;48(4):211-7.
24. Houston DM & Moore AE: Canine and feline urolithiasis: examination of over 50 000 urolith submissions to the Canadian veterinary urolith centre from 1998 to 2008. Can Vet J. 2009 Dec;50(12):1263-8.
25. Lekcharoensuk C, Lulich JP, Osborne CA, et. al.: Patient and environmental factors associated with calcium oxalate urolithiasis in dogs. J Am Vet Med Assoc. 2000 Aug 15;217(4):515-
26. da Silva EG, Dubielzig R, Zarfoss MK, et. al.: Distinctive histopathologic features of canine optic nerve hypoplasia and aplasia: a retrospective review of 13 cases. Vet Ophthalmol. 2008 Jan-Feb;11(1):23-9.
27. *The Genetic Connection: A Guide to Health Problems in Purebred Dogs.* L Ackerman. p 239, AAHA Press, 1999.
28. Fukushima R, Ichikawa K, Hirabayashi M, et. al.: A case of canine gastrinoma. J Vet Med Sci. 2004 Aug;66(8):993-5.
29. Fukushima U, Sato M, Okano S, et. al.: A case of gastrinoma in a Shih-Tzu dog. J Vet Med Sci. 2004 Mar;66(3):311-3.
30. Ness MG: Spinal arachnoid cysts in two shih tzu littermates. Vet Rec. 1998 May 9;142(19):515-6.
31. Watson AG, de Lahunta A: Atlantoaxial subluxation and absence of transverse ligament of the atlas in a dog. J Am Vet Med Assoc. 1989 Jul 15;195(2):235-7.
32. Kent M, Platt SR, Rech RR, et. al.: Clinicopathologic and magnetic resonance imaging characteristics associated with polioencephalomyel-opathy in a Shih Tzu. J Am Vet Med Assoc. 2009 Sep 1;235(5):551-7.
33. *The Complete Dog Book, 20th Ed.* The American Kennel Club. Howell Book House, NY 2006. p. 510-513.

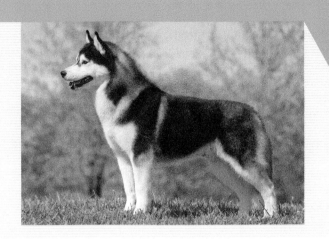

The Breed History

The origins of this breed are easily traced from the 19th century forward in Siberia. The Chukchi people in northeastern Asia were likely the original breeders of these hardy dogs. In Alaska, imports were used for sled dog racing in 1909. One of the famed serum dog teams that delivered life-saving serum from Neoma to Nome Alaska during the diphtheria outbreak of 1925 consisted of Siberians. The AKC recognized the breed in 1930.

Breeding for Function

The Chukchi people of Northeast Asia developed this breed for use as a sled dog. Emphasis was on endurance and tolerance of cold but selection also focused on those dogs requiring minimal food intake. They have been used extensively in Antarctic expeditions, and in search and rescue units during the Second World War. Today, they are most commonly seen in a companionship role, but they are still found out on the trail, ski-joring and pulling sleds.

Physical Characteristics

Height at Withers: female 20-22" (51-56 cm), male 21-23.5" (53-59.5 cm).

Weight: females 35-50 lb (16-22.5 kg), males 45-60 lb (20.5-27 kg).

Coat: Medium-length, double coat is very dense, soft and wooly in the undercoat, and outer coat hairs are straight. Markings on the head are variable, and the base color varies widely from black through white, and white legs and chest are common.

Longevity: 11-14 years

Points of Conformation: The Siberian Husky is medium in size, compact in conformation, with a very dense fur. Gait is agile and quick, smooth and ground covering with little apparent effort. His bushy tail is erect when alert, carried over the back in a sickle shape, but not deviated to the sides. The muzzle is straight in profile, gradually tapering, with a well-defined stop. Almond-shaped eyes are blue, brown, parti-colored or odd-eyed (one of each). They are slightly slanted upwards laterally, and are moderately wide-set. Ears are set high, triangular and medium in size, standing erect, and have semi-pointed tips and thick leather. Lips are tight and close, and the nose can have variable pigmentation as long as it is synchronized with coat color. The neck is medium in length and

Siberian Husky

muscling with a slight arch. The thorax is deep and somewhat laterally flattened; ribs are well sprung. The topline is level. They possess straight limbs which are moderately boned and muscled. Foreleg dewclaws may be removed, while the rear ones are usually removed. Feet are oval, medium sized and possess plenty of fur between the toes. Pads are thick.

Recognized Behavior Issues and Traits

Reported breed characteristics include: Independent streak, alert, gentle, friendly, not possessing watchdog tendencies. Very fastidious and thus low odor, tend to roam so should always be exercised off leash in a fenced area. Good in both rural and urban settings. Eager to work, fairly good with other dogs, intelligent, high energy and exercise needs, communal howlers but low barking tendency. Their bark is high pitched. Good with children. Low shedding except during the period in spring and fall when they are blowing the coat. Grooming needs are moderate. May dig and chew. This is a breed that needs close human contact.

Normal Physiologic Variations

Benign Familial Hyperphosphatasemia: This is a familial condition recognized from 11 weeks of age in families of Siberian huskies. Alkaline phosphatase levels average 5x normal due to an elevated bone isoenzyme. There are no clinical signs, and the elevation persists throughout life.[1]

Drug Sensitivities

None reported

Inherited Diseases

Juvenile Cataract: Autosomal recessive inherited lens opacity in the axial posterior cortex, developing between nine months to two years of age. Reported at a frequency of 6.6% in the 2006 Siberian Husky Health Survey. Reported in 4.7% of Siberian huskies presented to veterinary teaching hospitals. Dorn reports a 1.88x odds ratio versus other breeds. Cataracts are reported in 5.57% of Siberian huskies CERF-examined by veterinary ophthalmologists between 2000-2005. CERF does not recommend breeding any Siberian Husky with a cataract.[2,3,4,5]

Corneal Dystrophy: Autosomal recessive disorder causing bilaterally symmetrical white to grey oval or ring shaped opacities in the corneas. Affected dogs develop the opacities between six months to two years of age. Reported in 2.47% of Siberian huskies CERF-examined by veterinary ophthalmologists between 2000-2005. CERF does not recommend breeding any Siberian Husky with corneal dystrophy.[5,6]

Patella Luxation: Polygenically inherited laxity of patellar ligaments, causing luxation, lameness, and later degenerative joint disease. Treat surgically if causing clinical signs. Reported at a high frequency by the OFA, but too few Siberian Huskies have been screened to determine an accurate frequency.[7]

Hip Dysplasia: Polygenically inherited trait causing degenerative joint disease and hip arthritis. OFA reports 2.0% affected. Reported at a frequency of 3.9% in France.[7,8]

X-linked Progressive Retinal Atrophy (XLPRA): X-linked recessive degeneration of the retina causes blindness between one and three years of age. Reported in 0.28% of Siberian huskies CERF-examined by veterinary ophthalmologists between 2000-2005. CERF does not recommend breeding any Siberian Husky with XLPRA. A genetic test is available. [5,9,10,11]

Disease Predispositions

Hypothyroidism: Inherited autoimmune thyroiditis. 11.7% positive for thyroid autoantibodies based on testing at Michigan State University. (Ave. for all breeds is 7.5%).[12,13]

Cryptorchidism (Retained Testicles): Can be unilateral or bilateral. Reported at a frequency of 11.2% in the 2006 Siberian Husky Health Survey. Late descending testes was reported at a frequency of 6.5%.[3,14]

Epilepsy: Dorn reports a 29.32x odds ratio for epileptic seizures in Siberian huskies versus other breeds. Reported at an increased frequency in the 2006 Siberian Husky Health Survey.[2,3]

Bronchiectasis: Clinical signs of chronic cough with excessive airway mucous. Diagnosis with radiographs. Reported at a frequency of 3.1% and an odds ratio of 2.86x versus other breeds. Treatment is with bronchodilators and possibly corticosteroids.[15]

Primary (Narrow Angle) Glaucoma: Ocular condition causing increased pressure within the eyeball, and secondary blindness due to damage to the retina. Diagnose with tonometry and gonioscopy. Average age of diagnosis 5.3 +/- 1.7 years. Diagnosed in 1.88% of Siberian huskies presented to veterinary teaching hospitals. Dorn reports a 2.17x risk versus other breeds. CERF does not recommend breeding any Siberian Husky with glaucoma.[2,5,16,17]

Persistent Pupillary Membranes: Strands of fetal remnant connecting; iris to iris, cornea, lens, or involving sheets of tissue. The later three forms can impair vision, and dogs affected with these forms should not be bred. Identified in 1.48% of Siberian huskies CERF-examined by veterinary ophthalmologists between 2000-2005.[5]

Zinc Responsive Dermatosis: Breed specific condition with an unknown mode of inheritance. Affected dogs present with periocular crusts. Parakeratosis is found on skin biopsy. Treatment with oral zinc is curative in most affected dogs, but some may require parenteral zinc or retinoids.[18]

Eosinophilic Disease: The breed is predisposed to disorders that involve the buildup of eosinophilic tissue, including eosinophilic gastroenterocolitis, and eosinophilic granulomas of the eyelid and oral cavity.[19,20,21,22]

Uveodermatologic (VKH-Like) Syndrome: This is an autoimmune disease manifested by progressive uveitis and depigmenting dermatitis that closely resembles the human Vogt-Koyanagi-Harada syndrome. The disease presents between 1-1/2 - 4 years of age, and can progress to blindness. Treatment is with steroids. CERF does not recommend breeding any Siberian Husky with the disorder.[5,23,24]

Alopecia-X (Coat Cycle Arrest): Progressive, symmetrical, non-pruritic, truncal hair loss usually beginning in early adulthood. ACTH, LDDS, and thyroid panel results are normal. Elevated blood concentrations of 17-hydroxyprogesterone (17-OHP) have been seen post-ACTH stimulation. Treatment can include melatonin, mitotane, or oral trilostane. The disorder appears to be familial.[25,26]

Ectopic Ureters: Siberian huskies are an over-represented breed for ectopic ureters. Clinical signs are urinary incontinence and dribbling. Affected dogs can also have hydro-ureter, hydronephrosis, pyelonephritis, bladder hypoplasia or congenital incompetence of the urethral sphincter. Most affected dogs are female. Unknown mode of inheritance.[27]

Spontaneous Pneumothorax: Air release into the chest cavity causing collapsed lung lobes. Siberian huskies are found to be overrepresented compared to other breeds.[28]

Chronic Superficial Keratitis (Pannus): Chronic corneal inflammatory process that can cause vision problems due to corneal pigmentation. Treatment with topical ocular lubricants and anti-inflammatory medication. One study found Siberian huskies to be a breed at increased risk.[29]

Thyroid Cancer: Siberian Huskies have a 2.5 odds ratio versus other breeds of developing thyroid cancer. Affected dogs are usually between 10-15 years of age with a thyroid mass, and a diagnosis of carcinoma, or less frequently adenocarcinoma.[30]

Uveal Spindle Cell Tumor: Rare tumor of the anterior uveal tract of blue-eyed dogs. Median age of onset 10 years. Morphologically and immunohistochemically most consistent with schwannoma. Seen almost exclusively in Siberian Huskies and their crosses.[31]

Cutaneous Lupus Erythematosus, Deafness, Demodicosis, Entropion, Factor VIII Deficiency, Follicular Dysplasia, Hypertension, Laryngeal Paralysis, Microphthalmia, Myelodysplasia, Retinal Dysplasia, Tetralogy of Fallot, Ventricular Septal Defect, and **von Willebrand's Disease** are reported.[32]

Isolated Case Studies

Persistent Hyperplastic Primary Vitreous (PHPV): Two Siberian huskies were described with posterior lens capsule opacities secondary to abnormalities of development and regression of the hyaloid artery.[33]

Degenerative Myelopathy: Three related Siberian husky dogs had chronic progressive paresis and ataxia with muscle atrophy in the hind limbs. Pathology demonstrated disseminated degeneration of the spinal cord white matter. A direct genetic test for an autosomal recessive DM susceptability gene is available from the OFA.[34,35]

Genetic Tests

Tests of Genotype: Direct test for XLPRA is available from Optigen.

Direct test for coat color is available from VetGen.

Tests of Phenotype: CHIC Certification: Required tests are; CERF eye examination (minimum of 1 year of age), and hip dysplasia radiograph. (See CHIC website: www.caninehealthinfo.org)

Recommend elbow radiograph, patella evaluation, thyroid profile including autoantibodies, and cardiac examination.

Miscellaneous

- **Breed name synonyms:** Husky, Arctic Husky.
- **Registries:** AKC, UKC, CKC, KCGB (Kennel Club of Great Britain), ANKC (Australian National Kennel Club), NKC (National Kennel Club).
- **AKC rank (year 2008):** 23 (8,465 dogs registered)
- **Internet resources: Siberian Husky Club of America:**
  www.shca.org
  Siberian Husky Club of Canada:
  www.siberianhuskyclubofcanada.com
  Siberian Husky Club of Great Britain:
  www.siberianhuskyclub.com

References

1. Lawler DF, Keltner DG, Hoffman WE et. al.: Benign familial hyperphosphatasemia in Siberian huskies. *Am J Vet Res.* 1996 May;57(5):612-7.

2. Dorn CR: Canine breed-specific risks of frequently diagnosed diseases at veterinary teaching hospitals. Monograph. AKC Canine Health Foundation. 2000.

3. Siberian Husky Club of America: 2006 Siberian Husky Health Survey. 2006.

4. Gelatt KN, Mackay EO: Prevalence of primary breed-related cataracts in the dog in North America. *Vet Ophthalmol.* 2005 Mar-Apr;8(2):101-11.

5. *Ocular Disorders Presumed to be Inherited in Purebred Dogs.* American College of Veterinary Ophthalmologists. ACVO, 2007.

6. MacMillan AD, Waring GO 3rd, Spangler WL, et. al.: Crystalline corneal opacities in the Siberian Husky. *J Am Vet Med Assoc.* 1979 Oct 15;175(8):829-32.

7. OFA Website breed statistics: www.offa.org Last accessed July 1, 2010.

8. Genevois JP, Remy D, Viguier E, et. al.: Prevalence of hip dysplasia according to official radiographic screening, among 31 breeds of dogs in France. Vet Comp Orthop Traumatol. 2008;21(1):21-4.

9. Zangerl B, Zhang Q, Acland GM, et. al.: Characterization of three microsatellite loci linked to the canine RP3 interval. *J Hered.* 2002 Jan-Feb;93(1):70-3.

10. Acland GM, Blanton SH, Hershfield B, et. al.: XLPRA: a canine retinal degeneration inherited as an X-linked trait. *Am J Med Genet.* 1994 Aug 1;52(1):27-33.

11. Zangerl B, Johnson JL, Acland GM, et. al.: Independent origin and restricted distribution of RPGR deletions causing XLPRA. J Hered. 2007;98(5):526-30.

12. Nachreiner RF, Refsal KR, Graham PA, et. al.: Prevalence of serum thyroid hormone autoantibodies in dogs with clinical signs of hypothyroidism. *J Am Vet Med Assoc* 2002 Feb 15;220(4):466-71.

13. Nachreiner R & Refsal K: Personal communication, Diagnostic Center for Population and Animal Health, Michigan State University. April, 2007.

14. Zhao X, Du ZQ & Rothschild MF: An association study of 20 candidate genes with cryptorchidism in Siberian Husky dogs. J Anim Breed Genet. 2010 Aug;127(4):327-31.

15. Hawkins EC, Basseches J, Berry CR, et. al.: Demographic, clinical, and radiographic features of bronchiectasis in dogs: 316 cases (1988-2000). J Am Vet Med Assoc. 2003 Dec 1;223(11):1628-35.

16. Gelatt KN, MacKay EO: Prevalence of the breed-related glaucomas in pure-bred dogs in North America. *Vet Ophthalmol.* 2004 Mar-Apr;7(2):97-111.

17. Slater MR, Erb HN: Effects of risk factors and prophylactic treatment on primary glaucoma in the dog. *J Am Vet Med Assoc.* 1986 May 1;188(9):1028-30.

18. White SD, Bourdeau P, Rosychuk RA et. al.: Zinc-responsive dermatosis in dogs: 41 cases and literature review. *Vet Dermatol.* 2002 Feb;13(1):63.

19. Brellou GD, Kleinschmidt S, Meneses F, et. Al.: Eosinophilic Granulomatous Gastroenterocolitis and Hepatitis in a 1-year-old Male Siberian Husky. Vet Pathol. 2006 Nov;43(6):1022-5.

20. Vercelli A, Cornegliani L, Portigliotti L: Eyelid eosinophilic granuloma in a Siberian husky. *J Small Anim Pract.* 2005 Jan;46(1):31-3.

21. Lilliehook I, Tvedten H: Investigation of hypereosinophilia and potential treatments. *Vet Clin North Am Small Anim Pract.* 2003 Nov;33(6):1359-78, viii.

22. Madewell BR, Stannard AA, Pulley LT, et. al.: Oral eosinophilic granuloma in Siberian husky dogs. *J Am Vet Med Assoc.* 1980 Oct 15;177(8):701-3.

23. Glaze MB: Canine and Feline Uveitis. Proceedings, 2004 Northeast Veterinary Conference. 2004.

24. Sigle KJ, McLellan GJ, Haynes JS, et. al.: Unilateral uveitis in a dog with uveodermatologic syndrome. *J Am Vet Med Assoc.* 2006 Feb 15;228(4):543-8.

25. Frank LA, Hnilica KA, Oliver JW: Adrenal steroid hormone concentrations in dogs with hair cycle arrest (Alopecia X) before and during treatment with melatonin and mitotane. *Vet Dermatol.* 2004 Oct;15(5):278-84.

26. Frank LA, Hnilica KA, Rohrbach BW, et. al.: Retrospective evaluation of sex hormones and steroid hormone intermediates in dogs with alopecia. *Vet Dermatol.* 2003 Apr;14(2):91-7.

27. McLaughlin R Jr, Miller CW: Urinary incontinence after surgical repair of ureteral ectopia in dogs. *Vet Surg.* 1991 Mar-Apr;20(2):100-3.

28. Puerto DA, Brockman DJ, Lindquist C, et. al.: Surgical and nonsurgical management of and selected risk factors for spontaneous pneumothorax in dogs: 64 cases (1986-1999). *J Am Vet Med Assoc.* 2002 Jun 1;220(11):1670-4.

29. Chavkin MJ, Roberts SM, Salman MD, et. al.: Risk factors for development of chronic superficial keratitis in dogs. *J Am Vet Med Assoc.* 1994 May 15;204(10):1630-4.

30. Wucherer KL & Wilke V: Thyroid cancer in dogs: an update based on 638 cases (1995-2005). J Am Anim Hosp Assoc. 2010 Jul-Aug;46(4):249-54.

31. Zarfoss MK, Klauss G, Newkirk K, et. al.: Uveal spindle cell tumor of blue-eyed dogs: an immunohistochemical study. Vet Pathol. 2007 May;44(3):276-84.

32. *The Genetic Connection: A Guide to Health Problems in Purebred Dogs.* L Ackerman. p. 239-40. AAHA Press, 1999.

33. Ori J, Yoshikai T, Yoshimura S, et. al.: Persistent hyperplastic primary vitreous (PHPV) in two Siberian husky dogs. *J Vet Med Sci.* 1998 Feb;60(2):263-5.

34. Bichsel P, Vandevelde M, Lang J, et. al.: Degenerative myelopathy in a family of Siberian Husky dogs. *J Am Vet Med Assoc.* 1983 Nov 1;183(9):998-1000, 965.

35. Coates JR, Zeng R, Awano T, et. al.: An SOD1 Mutation Associated with Degenerative Myelopathy Occurs in Many Dog Breeds. Proceedings 2009 ACVIM Forum. 2009.

36. *The Complete Dog Book, 20th Ed.* The American Kennel Club. Howell Book House, NY 2006. p. 330-334.

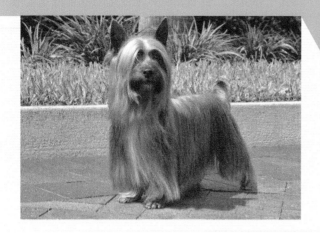

Silky Terrier

The Breed History

The breed origins trace to Australia in the late 1800s and early 1900s. They were developed as a result of crosses between Yorkshire terriers and native Australian terriers. The AKC recognized the breed in 1955.

Breeding for Function

Early in breed development, the Silky terriers were used for vermin control, but this breed was primarily developed for companionship.

Physical Characteristics

Height at Withers: 9-10 " (23-25.5 cm)

Weight: 8-11 lb (4-5 kg)

Coat: Single coated, the hairs are long, silky and glossy but not so long as to reach the ground. The topknot is prominent. Breed colors are blue and tan, though the blue varies considerably from so-called silver blue to a slate blue. The topknot is the lightest colored part of the coat and the tan markings have a set distribution.

Longevity: 11-14 years

Points of Conformation: This toy terrier has a fine bone structure, silky coat, and the hair is normally parted from the muzzle to the tail base, and in overall conformation they are low-set and longer than tall. The head is wedge-shaped, and the small dark eyes are almond shaped and lined with dark palpebral rims. Ears are triangular and small and carried pricked. The stop is shallow, the nose is black, and the neck is moderately curving and long. The topline is level, and the tail is usually docked and is carried upright. Limbs are straight, fine boned and the feet are small and compact; nails are dark. Dewclaws usually removed. The gait is springy and straight.

Recognized Behavior Issues and Traits

Reported breed characteristics include: Typical terrier personality; feisty, active, loves to dig, and prone to boredom vices if left alone, keenly alert, friendly and curious. They like to be included in all family activities. Good alert barker with moderate to high barking tendency. Good with gentle children. Low exercise needs. Grooming needs are high, with regular bathing recommended.

Normal Physiologic Variations

None reported

Drug Sensitivities

None reported

Inherited Diseases

Patella Luxation: Polygenically inherited laxity of patellar ligaments, causing luxation, lameness, and later degenerative joint disease. Treat surgically if causing clinical signs. Reported 16.0x odds ratio versus other breeds. OFA reports 1.6% affected. Reported at a frequency of 1.1% in the 2002 STCA Health Survey.[1,2,3]

Legg-Perthes Disease and Hip Dysplasia: Polygenically inherited traits causing degenerative hip joint disease and arthritis. Too few Silky Terriers have been screened by OFA to determine an accurate frequency. Legg-Perthes disease is reported at a frequency of 0.8% in the 2002 STCA Health Survey.[1,2]

Elbow Dysplasia: Polygenically inherited trait causing elbow arthritis. Too few Silky Terriers have been screened by OFA to determine an accurate frequency.[1]

Disease Predispositions

Persistent Pupillary Membranes: Strands of fetal remnant connecting; iris to iris, cornea, lens, or involving sheets of tissue. The later three forms can impair vision, and dogs affected with these forms should not be bred. Identified in 10.56% of Silky Terriers CERF examined by veterinary ophthalmologists between 2000-2005.[4]

Cataracts: Anterior, posterior, intermediate and punctate cataracts occur in the breed. Age of onset 4-5 years. Dorn reports a 1.76x odds ratio of developing cataracts versus other breeds. One study estimated the frequency of cataracts in the breed at 10.29%. Identified in 9.94% of Silky Terriers CERF examined by veterinary ophthalmologists between 2000-2005. Reported at a frequency of 4.2% in the 2002 STCA Health Survey. CERF does not recommend breeding any Silky Terrier with a cataract.[2,4,5,6]

Aggression: Food, dog-dog, or people aggression. Reported at a frequency of 3.8% in the 2002 STCA Health Survey.[2]

Cryptorchidism (Retained Testes): Can be bilateral or unilateral, and seen at an increased frequency in the breed. Reported at a frequency of 3.7% in the 2002 STCA Health Survey.[2]

Allergies: Inhalant or food allergy. Presents with pruritis and pyotraumatic dermatitis (hot spots). Reported at a frequency of 3.4% in the 2002 STCA Health Survey.[2]

Hypothyroidism: Inherited autoimmune thyroiditis. 3.0% positive for thyroid autoantibodies based on testing at Michigan State University. (Ave. for all breeds is 7.5%). Reported at a frequency of 1.3% in the 2002 STCA Health Survey.[2,7,8]

Vitreous Degeneration: Liquefaction of the vitreous gel which may predispose to retinal detachment. Identified in 2.48% of Silky Terriers CERF examined by veterinary ophthalmologists between 2000-2005.[4]

Focal Alopecia: Silky Terriers can develop focal areas of hair loss secondary to injections or vaccinations. Dorn reports a 8.98x odds ratio of alopecia versus other breeds.[5]

Progressive Retinal Atrophy (PRA): A late onset PRA occurs in the breed. Clinically evident at 5-11 years of age. Identified in 1.24% of Silky Terriers CERF examined by veterinary ophthalmologists between 2000-2005. Undetermined mode of inheritance.[4]

Retinal Dysplasia: Retinal folds, geographic, and detachment are recognized in the breed. Can progress to blindness. Identified in 1.24% of Silky Terriers CERF examined by veterinary ophthalmologists between 2000-2005.[4]

Hyperadrenocorticism (Cushing's Disease): Hyperfunction of the adrenal gland caused by a pituitary or adrenal tumor. Clinical signs may include increased thirst and urination, symmetrical truncal alopecia, and abdominal distention. Dorn reports a 2.17x odds ratio versus other breeds. Reported at a frequency of 0.9% in the 2002 STCA Health Survey.[2,5]

Idiopathic Epilepsy: Inherited seizures can be generalized or partial seizures. Control with anti-seizure medication. Reported at a frequency of 0.8% in the 2002 STCA Health Survey.[2]

Diabetes Mellitus: Caused by a lack of insulin production by the pancreas. Controlled by insulin injections, diet, and glucose monitoring. Dorn reports a 3.76x odds ratio of developing diabetes versus other breeds. Reported at a frequency of 0.4% in the 2002 STCA Health Survey.[2,5]

Collapsing Trachea: Caused by diminished integrity of the cartilage rings in the trachea and can produce increased coughing, stridor, and respiratory distress. Dorn reports a 3.53x odds ratio versus other breeds.[5]

Portosystemic Shunt (PSS, Liver Shunt): Abnormal blood vessels connecting the systemic and portal blood flow. Vessels can be intrahepatic, extrahepatic or microvascular dysplasia. Causes stunting, abnormal behavior and possible seizures. Diagnose with paired fasted and feeding serum bile acid and/or ammonia levels, and abdominal ultrasound. The Silky Terrier is a breed at increased risk of having PSS. Undetermined mode of inheritance.[9]

Cystine Urinary Calculi: Silky Terriers are a breed with increased risk of developing cystine calculi. Caused by a defect in cystine metabolism.[10]

Glucocerebrosidosis (Gaucher Disease): Rare, fatal lysosomal storage disease causing neurological deterioration and seizures at 4-6 months of age. Undetermined mode of inheritance.[11]

Brachygnathism, Color Dilution Alopecia, Hydrocephalus, Prognathism, and **Spongiform Leukodystrophy** are reported.[12]

Isolated Case Studies

Myopathy: A young female Silky Terrier presented with severe, progressive weakness caused by an underlying subacute skeletal myopathy. Muscle degeneration appeared to involve extensive segmental disarray of sarcomeres with formation of nemaline rod-like bodies. The clinicopathologic features suggested that there was a primary myopathy with a probable genetic basis. Dystrophinopathy was excluded on the basis of immunostaining.[13]

Genetic Tests

Tests of Genotype: none

Tests of Phenotype: CHIC Certification: CERF eye examination and patella evaluation. (See CHIC website; www.caninehealthinfo.org).

Recommend hip and elbow radiographs, thyroid profile including autoantibodies, and cardiac examination.

Miscellaneous

- **Breed name synonyms:** Sydney Silky terrier (historical), Australian Silky Terrier (historical), Silky Toy Terrier, Silky.
- **Registries:** AKC, UKC, CKC, NKC (National Kennel Club).
- **AKC rank (year 2008):** 77 (968 dogs registered)
- **Internet resources: Silky Terrier Club of America:** www.silkyterrierclubofamerica.org
  Maple Leaf Silky Terrier Club (Canada): http://silkyterrier-canada.org/
  Australian Silky Terrier Club of Great Britain: http://79.170.44.132/australiansilkyterriers.co.uk/

References

1. OFA Website breed statistics: www.offa.org Last accessed July 1, 2010.
2. Silky Terrier Club of America: 2002 STCA Health Survey. 2002.
3. LaFond E, Breur GJ & Austin CC: Breed susceptibility for developmental orthopedic diseases in dogs. J Am Anim Hosp Assoc. 2002 Sep-Oct;38(5):467-77.
4. *Ocular Disorders Presumed to be Inherited in Purebred Dogs.* American College of Veterinary Ophthalmologists. ACVO, 2007.
5. Dorn CR: Canine breed-specific risks of frequently diagnosed diseases at veterinary teaching hospitals. Monograph. AKC Canine Health Foundation. 2000.
6. Gelatt KN, Mackay EO: Prevalence of primary breed-related cataracts in the dog in North America. *Vet Ophthalmol.* 2005 Mar-Apr;8(2):101-11.
7. Nachreiner RF, Refsal KR, Graham PA, et. al.: Prevalence of serum thyroid hormone autoantibodies in dogs with clinical signs of hypothyroidism. J Am Vet Med Assoc 2002 Feb 15;220(4):466-71.
8. Nachreiner R & Refsal K: Personal communication, Diagnostic Center for Population and Animal Health, Michigan State University. April, 2007.
9. Hunt GB: Effect of breed on anatomy of portosystemic shunts resulting from congenital diseases in dogs and cats: a review of 242 cases. *Aust Vet J.* 2004 Dec;82(12):746-9.
10. Case LC, Ling GV, Franti CE, et. al.: Cystine-containing urinary calculi in dogs: 102 cases (1981-1989). *J Am Vet Med Assoc.* 1992 Jul 1;201(1):129-33.
11. Hartley WJ, Blakemore WF: Neurovisceral glucocerebroside storage (Gaucher's disease) in a dog. Vet Pathol 1973: 10:191.
12. *The Genetic Connection: A Guide to Health Problems in Purebred Dogs.* L Ackerman. p. 240. AAHA Press, 1999.
13. Huxtable CR, Chadwick B, Eger C: Severe Subacute Progressive Myopathy in a Young Silky Terrier. *Prog Vet Neurol* 1994: 5[1]:21-27.
14. *The Complete Dog Book, 20th Ed.* The American Kennel Club. Howell Book House, NY 2006. p. 514-516

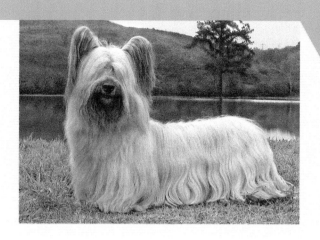

The Breed History

Sky Terriers are considered to be one of the most ancient of terriers. This type can be traced back to records dating four centuries ago in the Isle of Skye in the Hebrides region of Scotland. Popular with English Royalty in the 1600s, they remain popular today in the British Isles. The AKC first registered this breed in 1887. The breed reputation for loyalty was advanced by the story of Bobby, a Skye terrier who was featured in Disney's story of "Greyfriar's Bobby".

Breeding for Function

Agility, strength, versatility and a tenacious pursuit of vermin, badgers, otter and foxes were bred into them. These dogs are adept at going to ground, and display unusual courage and agility.

Physical Characteristics

Height at Withers: female 9.5" (24 cm), male 10" (25.5 cm)

Weight: 19-23 lb (8.5-10.5 kg)

Coat: The double haircoat consists of a short soft wooly undercoat and a hard long straight outer coat. Coat length is about 5 1/2". They are normally groomed with a part that extends along the topline from head to tail. The hair cover on the head historically served to protect against thorns and foe since the hair normally covers the eyes. The coat is essentially one color, and options include black, fawn, cream, silver platinum, blue, or varying shades of gray. Points may be dark to black, and a small (< 2") white marking on the chest is tolerated. Until the mature coat finalizes at 1 1/2 years, the color may vary from the standard and is not penalized in show.

Longevity: 13-15 years.

Points of Conformation: Skye Terriers are twice as long as high, and a long flowing silky coat that hangs to the ground is a key breed characteristic. Well boned and muscled, they are sturdy and possess high head carriage. They have medium-sized eyes which are usually darkly colored, close set and have a very bright expression. The head is long, ears are feathered and either carried pricked up or dropped depending on the type. The drop ear breed variety has larger low set pendulous ears that hang against the head. The stop is slight, the muzzle strong and it tapers slightly. The nose is black. Other nose colors disqualify the dog. The neck is arched and

moderate in length. The topline is level. The thorax is fairly deep and oval in cross section. A well-feathered tail is carried below the topline and is long and slightly curved. The limbs described in the standard can have a slight curvature, and are notably short. Feet are hare in shape, nails short and strong and preferred black in color. The gait is long, low, fast and smooth.

Recognized Behavior Issues and Traits

Descriptors of the breed include: Exceptionally loyal, intelligent, independent streak, friendly with family, though they can be snappy especially with children.

They are aloof with strangers, and may fight with other dogs. They have medium grooming needs. These are high activity, high barking dogs, and good for country or city living (even apartments). They can be one-man dogs. Early socialization to people, pets and places is important. Early obedience training is also recommended. They like to dig, especially if bored.

Normal Physiologic Variations

None Reported

Drug Sensitivities

There are reports of Skye Terriers having serious, and sometimes fatal reactions to high doses of ivermectin (not the low dose found in heartworm preventatives). The Skye Terrier Foundation (see below) is offering free testing for the recently discovered MDR1 (ivermectin/drug toxicity) mutation to see if it exists in the breed. The mutation was not found in 5 Skye Terriers tested by the original researchers.[1]

Inherited Diseases

Patella Luxation: Polygenically inherited laxity of patellar ligaments, causing luxation, lameness, and later degenerative joint disease. Treat surgically if causing clinical signs. Reported at a high frequency by OFA, but too few Skye Terriers have been screened to determine an accurate frequency.[2]

Hip Dysplasia: Polygenic trait causing degenerative joint disease and hip arthritis. Too few Skye Terriers have been screened by OFA to determine an accurate frequency.[2]

Elbow Dysplasia: Polygenic trait causing elbow arthritis. Too few Skye Terriers have been screened by OFA to determine an accurate frequency.[2]

Disease Predispositions

Hypothyroidism: Inherited autoimmune thyroiditis. 16.99% of Skye Terriers test positive for thyroid autoantibodies, with a 3.04x odds ratio versus other breeds. (Average for all breeds in this study was 6.40%).[3,4]

Copper Toxicosis (Copper Hepatopathy): Signs include anorexia, depression, and jaundice. Can lead to chronic hepatitis, cirrhosis, and acquired portosystemic shunt. Treat with copper chelating agents and liver support medications. The disease can be diagnosed by a liver biopsy. Thought to be caused by a disorder of intracellular bile metabolism. Unknown mode of inheritance.[5,6,7]

Ectopic Ureters: Skye Terriers are an over-represented breed for ectopic ureters. Clinical signs are urinary incontinence and dribbling. Affected dogs can also have hydro-ureter, hydronephrosis, pyelonephritis, bladder hypoplasia or congenital incompetence of the urethral sphincter. Most affected dogs are female. Unknown mode of inheritance.[8]

Ocular Disorders: Too few Skye Terriers have been CERF examined to determine accurate frequencies for inherited ocular disorders. All Skye Terriers considered for breeding should have a CERF examination.[9]

Renal Dysplasia and **Polycystic Kidney Disease** are reported on the Skye Terrier Club (UK) website.

Allergic inhalant dermatitis, Lens luxation, Oligodontia, Tracheal collapse, and **von Willebrand's Disease** are reported.[10]

Genetic Tests

Tests of Genotype: none

Tests of Phenotype: Recommend patella evaluation, hip and elbow radiographs, CERF eye examination, thyroid profile including autoantibodies, cardiac examination, and kidney ultrasound.

Miscellaneous

- **Breed name synonyms:** Skye
- **Registries:** AKC, UKC, CKC, KCGB (Kennel Club of Great Britain), ANKC (Australian National Kennel Club), NKC (National Kennel Club)
- **AKC rank (year 2008):** 143 (88 dogs registered)
- **Internet resources: The Skye Terrier Club of America:** http://clubs.akc.org/skye/
  Skye Canada: www.skyecanada.ca
  The Skye Terrier Club (UK): www.skyeterrierclub.org.uk
  The Skye Terrier Foundation: www.skyeterrier.org

References

1. Neff MW, Robertson KR, Wong AK, et. al.: Breed distribution and history of canine mdr1-1Delta, a pharmacogenetic mutation that marks the emergence of breeds from the collie lineage. Proc Natl Acad Sci U S A. 2004 Aug 10;101(32):11725-30.
2. OFA Website breed statistics: www.offa.org Last accessed July 1, 2010.
3. Nachreiner RF, Refsal KR, Graham PA, et. al.: Prevalence of serum thyroid hormone autoantibodies in dogs with clinical signs of hypothyroidism. *J Am Vet Med Assoc.* 2002 Feb 15;220(4):466-71.
4. Nachreiner R & Refsal K: Personal communication, Diagnostic Center for Population and Animal Health, Michigan State University. April, 2007.
5. McGrotty YL, Ramsey IK, Knottenbelt CM: Diagnosis and management of hepatic copper accumulation in a Skye terrier. *J Small Anim Pract.* 2003 Feb;44(2):85-9.
6. Haywood S, Rutgers HC, Christian MK: Hepatitis and copper accumulation in Skye terriers. *Vet Pathol.* 1988 Nov;25(6):408-14.
7. Fuentealba IC, Aburto EM: Animal models of copper-associated liver disease. *Comp Hepatol.* 2003 Apr 3;2(1):5.
8. Holt PE, Moore AH: Canine ureteral ectopia: an analysis of 175 cases and comparison of surgical treatments. *Vet Rec.* 1995 Apr 8;136(14):345-9.
9. *Ocular Disorders Presumed to be Inherited in Purebred Dogs.* American College of Veterinary Ophthalmologists. ACVO, 2007.
10. *The Genetic Connection: A Guide to Health Problems in Purebred Dogs.* L Ackerman. p. 240. AAHA Press, 1999.
11. *The Complete Dog Book, 20th Ed. The American Kennel Club.* Howell Book House, NY 2006. p. 428-431.

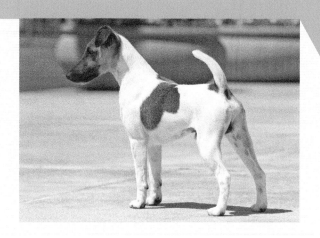

The Breed History

Originally, smooth and wire fox terriers were coat varieties of a single breed. In 1985, they were split in the AKC registry. First records date to the late 1700s in Britain (about 20 years after the wire variety records started), but a formal breeding program didn't begin until the mid 1800s. The now extinct smooth Black and Tan Terrier may have been the smooth fox terrier progenitor. Other breeds that are purported to have influenced this variety are the Greyhound and Beagle. This breed image became widely known as the dog in the gramophone logo for RCA.

Breeding for Function

As their name implies these were originally bred for fox hunting, and excelled at going to ground, or following their quarry into the burrow. They were successfully used as small game hunters and to clear vermin. Now, commonly used for bench showing and companionship. They also have an affinity for tricks.

Physical Characteristics

Height at Withers: Less than 15.5" (39.5 cm)

Weight: male 18 lb (8 kg), female 16 lb (7 kg)

Coat: Short, hard hairs are dense. These predominantly white dogs have well demarcated color patches. Brindle and red-liver are not favored as the second color. Black and tan is most common.

Longevity: 13-14 years.

Points of Conformation: An alert expression, high head and tail carriage, and sturdy square athletic build characterize this breed. The back is short, and the head has a measured standard length of 7-7.25 inches. Their small, round dark colored eyes are fairly close and deep set, with an intense expression. The top of the folded ear should be above skull level; ears are medium-leathered, triangular and hang forward. The skull is of defined width between the eyes and a minimal stop is present. The nose is black, the neck moderately long and fine, and is not throaty. The topline is level. The thorax is deep and oval in cross-section, and the caudal ribs are deep. The high set thick tail (if docked) is 3/4 of the natural length. Limbs are straight, metatarsals and metacarpals heavy and short, feet small and compact with tough pads, toes moderately arched. In body type, in all respects this breed is the same as the Wire Fox

Terrier. Gait is quick and agile, springy, with a ground-covering stride.

Recognized Behavior Issues and Traits

Reported attributes of this breed include: Digger, can be snappy, don't tend to get along with other dogs. Though loyal, not demonstrative; in general, rather reserved. Need early obedience training to counteract independent streak. These are very active dogs that need activities and exercise so they do not become bored. They are friendly, playful and extroverted with family, and good with children especially if early socialization is carried out. Easy grooming care, a low shedding tendency, and may tend to bark.

Normal Physiologic Variations

None reported

Drug Sensitivities

None reported

Inherited Diseases

Hip Dysplasia and Legg-Calve Perthe's Disease: Polygenic trait causing degenerative hip joint disease and arthritis. OFA reports 12.2% affected.[1]

Patella Luxation: Polygenically inherited laxity of patellar ligaments, causing luxation, lameness, and later degenerative joint disease. Treat surgically if causing clinical signs. OFA reports 2.0% affected.[1]

Elbow Dysplasia: Polygenic trait causing elbow arthritis. Too few Smooth Fox Terriers have been screened by OFA to determine an accurate frequency.[1]

Congenital Myasthenia Gravis: A lethal, autosomal recessive disorder in the breed. Presents within 5 weeks of birth with muscle weakness, megaesophagus, and secondary aspiration pneumonia.[2,3,4]

Disease Predispositions

Cataracts: Posterior subcapsular progressive cataracts predominate in the breed. Unknown mode of inheritance. 11.70% of Smooth Fox Terriers presented to veterinary teaching hospitals had cataracts. CERF does not recommend breeding any Smooth Fox Terrier with a cataract.[5,6]

Persistent Pupillary Membranes: Strands of fetal remnant connecting; iris to iris, cornea, lens, or involving sheets of tissue. The later three forms can impair vision, and dogs affected with these forms should not be bred. Identified in 5.66% of Smooth Fox Terriers CERF examined by veterinary ophthalmologists between 2000-2005.[6]

Hypothyroidism: Inherited autoimmune thyroiditis. 4.3% positive for thyroid autoantibodies based on testing at Michigan State University. (Ave. for all breeds is 7.5%).[7,8]

Vitreous Degeneration: A liquefaction of the vitreous gel which may predispose to retinal detachment resulting in blindness. Identified in 2.83% of Smooth Fox Terriers CERF examined by veterinary ophthalmologists between 2000-2005.[6]

Glaucoma and Lens Luxation: Glaucoma is an increased intraocular pressure, that can predispose to lens luxation and retinal degeneration. An inherited predisposition towards glaucoma and secondary lens luxation occurs in the breed. CERF does not recommend breeding any Smooth Fox Terrier with glaucoma or lens luxation.[6,9]

Pulmonic Stenosis: The breed is reported with a higher frequency of the disorder. Affected dogs present with exercise intolerance, stunting, dyspnea, syncope and ascites due to a malformed pulmonic valve, stricture of the right ventricular outflow tract or stricture of the pulmonary artery. Polygenic mode of inheritance.[10]

Deafness: Congenital deafness can be unilateral or bilateral. Diagnosed by BAER testing. Unknown mode of inheritance. OFA reports a high frequency, but too few have been screened for an accurate frequency.[1,11]

Cystinuria/Cystine Bladder Stones: Smooth Fox Terriers have an increased risk for developing cystine bladder stones. Caused by a defect in cystine metabolism. Treat with surgical removal and life-long medical therapy. Unknown mode of inheritance in this breed.[12]

Hereditary Ataxia: Rare disease, where affected puppies develop progressive ataxia and hypermetria at approximately four months of age, with a variable course of progression. Pathology reveals bilaterally symmetrical demyelination of dorsal spinocerebellar tracts in the cervical, thoracic and lumbar regions of the spinal cord. An autosomal recessive mode of inheritance is suspected.[13]

Brachygnathism, Cervical Vertebral Instability, Epilepsy, Mitral Valve Disease, Oigodontia, Prognathism, Progressive Retinal Atrophy, and **von Willebrand's Disease** are reported.[14]

Genetic Tests

Tests of Genotype: Direct test for coat color is available from VetGen.

Tests of Phenotype: CHIC Certification: Required testing includes cardiac evaluation and patella evaluation. (See CHIC website; www.caninehealthinfo.org).

Recommend hip and elbow radiographs, CERF eye examination, thyroid profile including autoantibodies, and BAER hearing test.

Miscellaneous

- **Breed name synonyms:** Fox Terrier, Smooth Fox, Smooth-haired Fox Terrier
- **Registries:** AKC, UKC, CKC, KCGB (Kennel Club of Great Britain), ANKC (Australian National Kennel Club), NKC (National Kennel Club)
- **AKC rank (year 2008):** 106 (415 dogs registered)
- **Internet resources: American Fox Terrier Club:** www.aftc.org
  The Smooth Fox Terrier Association (UK):
  www.smoothfoxterrierassociation.co.uk

The Fox Terrier Club (UK): www.thefoxterrierclub.co.uk

References

1. OFA Website breed statistics: www.offa.org Last accessed July 1, 2010.
2. Miller LM, Hegreberg GA, Prieur DJ, et. al.: Inheritance of congenital myasthenia gravis in smooth fox terrier dogs. *J Hered.* 1984 May-Jun;75(3):163-6.
3. Jenkins WL, van Dyk E, McDonald CB: Myasthenia gravis in a Fox Terrier litter. *J S Afr Vet Assoc.* 1976 Mar;47(1):59-62.
4. Miller LM, Lennon VA, Lambert EH, et. al.: Congenital myasthenia gravis in 13 smooth fox terriers. *J Am Vet Med Assoc.* 1983 Apr 1;182(7):694-7.
5. Gelatt KN, Mackay EO: Prevalence of primary breed-related cataracts in the dog in North America. *Vet Ophthalmol.* 2005 Mar-Apr;8(2):101-11.
6. *Ocular Disorders Presumed to be Inherited in Purebred Dogs.* American College of Veterinary Ophthalmologists. ACVO, 2007.
7. Nachreiner RF, Refsal KR, Graham PA, et. al.: Prevalence of serum thyroid hormone autoantibodies in dogs with clinical signs of hypothyroidism. *J Am Vet Med Assoc* 2002 Feb 15;220(4):466-71.
8. Nachreiner R & Refsal K: Personal communication, Diagnostic Center for Population and Animal Health, Michigan State University. April, 2007.
9. Gelatt KN & MacKay EO: Prevalence of the breed-related glaucomas in pure-bred dogs in North America. *Vet Ophthalmol.* 2004 Mar-Apr;7(2):97-111.
10. McCaw D, Aronson E: Congenital cardiac disease in dogs. *Mod Vet Pract.* 1984 Jul;65(7):509-12.
11. Strain GM: Deafness prevalence and pigmentation and gender associations in dog breeds at risk. *Vet J.* 2004 Jan;167(1):23-32.
12. Jones BR, Kirkman JH, Hogan J, et. al.: Analysis of uroliths from cats and dogs in New Zealand, 1993-96. *N Z Vet J.* 1998 Dec;46(6):233-6.
13. Rohdin C, Lüdtke L, Wohlsein P, et. al.: New aspects of hereditary ataxia in smooth-haired fox terriers. *Vet Rec.* 2010 May 1;166(18):557-60.
14. *The Genetic Connection: A Guide to Health Problems in Purebred Dogs.* L. Ackerman. p. 217. AAHA Press, 1999.
15. *The Complete Dog Book, 20th Ed.* The American Kennel Club. Howell Book House, NY 2006. p. 370-373.

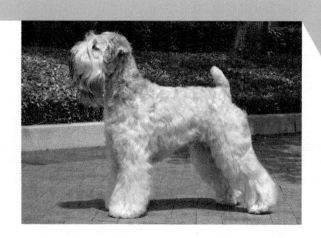

Soft Coated Wheaten Terrier

The Breed History

Breed records dating back to the 1700s in Ireland (counties Kerry and Cork) may not reflect the earliest days of the breed. They are closely related to Irish terriers and contributed to the development of the Kerry Blue terrier. Wheatens were first brought to America in 1946, and first registered in the AKC studbook in 1973.

Breeding for Function

These dogs were widely used for hunting small game and vermin, herding, and as a guard dog for the home and livestock. Today, they are primarily companion dogs.

Physical Characteristics

Height at Withers: female 17-18" (43-45.5 cm), male 18-19" (45.5-48 cm).

Weight: females 30-35 lb (13.5-16 kg), males 35-40 lb (16-18 kg).

Coat: As the name suggests, the coat is very soft and is wheaten in coloration. On some dogs, the ears and muzzle have blue-gray shading. The hairs of the coat are silky and slightly wavy. The color and texture does not fully set until 1 1/2 to 2 years of age. From sexual maturity on, the coat is lighter wheaten. Puppies are often dark wheaten and some puppies have black tips. This is a silky shiny single coat.

Longevity: 13-15 years

Points of Conformation: They are a square, medium-sized terrier with moderate bone and muscling. They move with smooth ground covering strides. They are to move with tails held erect. The head has a moderately long rectangular conformation, the muzzle is block and there is a defined stop. The nose is large and both lip margins and nose are pigmented black. Eyes are almond shaped and medium in size, brown, the palpebral margins are pigmented black and the eyes are fairly wide set. Hair falls over the eyes to a significant extent. Ears are triangular and fold to hang parallel to the head. The neck is medium in length, muscular and not throaty. The topline is level, and the back short. The thorax is deep and ribs are well sprung. The tails are usually docked, and are set high. Legs straight boned and feet are compact and round in shape with black nails. Dewclaws are removed in North America. Rear dewclaws are penalized.

Recognized Behavior Issues and Traits

Reported breed characteristics include: Intelligent, responsive, a merry disposition, and loving. They are considered more even-tempered and obedient than some of the other terrier breeds. Grooming needs are high. The Wheaten needs moderate exercise. They are energetic, but less so than some of the terriers. Good with children, good alarm barkers. Some suggest this dog is better for older children (not toddlers) because of the high energy level. If off leash, they should be in a fenced enclosure. It is recommended that obedience training be started early, and some dogs are headstrong. They like to jump vertically in place, they can also tend to be leash pullers. If bored, the Wheaten Terrier may dig or chew. Considered good with other dogs and cats if raised together, but as a terrier, they may chase small pets. They tend to keep their puppy-like exuberance well into middle age (5-7 yrs).

Normal Physiologic Variations

None reported

Drug Sensitivities

None reported

Inherited Diseases

Elbow Dysplasia: Polygenically inherited trait causing elbow arthritis. OFA reports 9.2% affected.[1]

Hip Dysplasia: Polygenically inherited trait causing degenerative joint disease and hip arthritis. OFA reports 4.8% affected.[1]

Patella Luxation: Polygenically inherited laxity of patellar ligaments, causing luxation, lameness, and later degenerative joint disease. Treat surgically if causing clinical signs. OFA reports 4.0% affected.[1]

Disease Predispositions

Protein-Losing Nephropathy (PLN): Inherited disease causing protein loss through the kidneys. General clinical signs include vomiting, diarrhea, weight loss, and pleural and peritoneal effusions. Laboratory findings include hypoalbuminemia, proteinuria, hypercholesterolemia, and azotemia. Renal lesions typically showed chronic glomerulonephritis and glomerulosclerosis, and less commonly end-stage renal disease. Average age of diagnosis is 6.3 years. Food hypersensitivity may play a role in the disorder. This disease can present concurrently with PLE, and may share a genetic basis. Estimated to affect 10-15% of the breed. Reported at a frequency of 2.7% in the 2000 General Health Survey on Soft Coated Wheaten Terriers. Unknown mode of inheritance. Fecal perinuclear antineutrophilic cytoplasmic antibody (PANCA) can be used as a phenotypic screening test.[2,3,4,5,6]

Allergies: Food Allergy was identified in 7.0% of dogs, and Inhalant allergies were identified in 5.7% in the 2000 General Health Survey on Soft Coated Wheaten terriers. Dorn reports a 1.34x odds ratio for allergic dermatitis versus other breeds.[5,7]

Persistent Pupillary Membranes: Strands of fetal remnant connecting; iris to iris, cornea, lens, or involving sheets of tissue. The later three forms can impair vision, and dogs affected with these forms should not be bred. Identified in 3.96% of Soft-coated Wheaten terriers CERF-examined by veterinary ophthalmologists between 2000-2005.[8]

Dental Issues: The 2000 General Health Survey on Soft Coated Wheaten terriers reports 3.9% with **missing teeth**, and 2.1% with **undershot bites**.[5]

Protein-Losing Enteropathy (PLE): Inherited disease causing protein loss through the intestines. General clinical signs include vomiting, diarrhea, weight loss, and pleural and peritoneal effusions. Laboratory findings include panhypoproteinemia and hypocholesterolemia. Intestinal lesions include inflammatory bowel disease, dilated lymphatics, and lipogranulomatous lymphangitis. Average age of diagnosis is 4.7 years. Food hypersensitivity may play a role in the disorder. This disease can present concurrently with PLN, and may share a genetic basis. Reported at a frequency of 2.6% in the 2000 General Health Survey on Soft Coated Wheaten terriers. Unknown mode of inheritance. Perinuclear antineutrophilic cytoplasmic antibody (pANCA) can be used as a pre-clinical phenotypic screening test.[2,3,6,9]

Cataracts: Anterior cortex punctate cataracts predominate in the breed. Identified in 2.40% of Soft-coated Wheaten terriers CERF examined by veterinary ophthalmologists between 2000-2005. CERF does not recommend breeding any Soft-coated Wheaten terrier with a cataract.[8]

Renal Dysplasia (RD): Affected Soft Coated Wheaten terriers present between 4.5 to 30 weeks of age with polyuria, polydipsia, isosthenuria, azotemia, and small kidneys. Proteinuria is not a hallmark of the disease. Affected dogs die of progressive renal failure by three years of age. Histopathologic changes include immature (fetal) glomeruli, persistent fetal mesenchyme, and tubular dilatation. There is no sex predilection. Some researchers postulate an autosomal recessive mode of inheritance. A genetic test for a dominant susceptibility gene is available. (Affected dogs all have one copy of the gene, but most dogs with the gene will not develop kidney failure.)[4,10]

Hypothyroidism: Inherited autoimmune thyroiditis. 1.7% positive for thyroid autoantibodies based on testing at Michigan State University. (Ave. for all breeds is 7.5%). Reported at a frequency of 2.5% in the 2000 General Health Survey on Soft Coated Wheaten Terriers.[5,11,12]

Distichiasis: Abnormally placed eyelashes that irritate the cornea and conjunctiva. Can cause secondary corneal ulceration. Identified in 1.20% of Soft-coated Wheaten terriers CERF-examined by veterinary ophthalmologists between 2000-2005.[8]

Hypoadrenocorticism (Addison's Disease): Typical presentation of lethargy, poor appetite, vomiting, weakness, and dehydration can occur from 4 months to several years of age. Cited as a breed at significantly higher risk. Treatment with DOCA injections or oral fludrocortisone. Unknown mode of inheritance.[13]

Persistent Hyaloid Artery (PHA): A congenital defect resulting from abnormalities in the development and regression of the hyaloid artery. Identified in 1.09% of Soft-coated Wheaten terriers CERF-examined by veterinary ophthalmologists between 2000-2005.[8]

Ectopic Ureter: Congenital disorder where the ureters do not enter the urinary bladder, but instead deposit urine in the urethra or vestibule. Causes urinary incontinence, especially in females. Reported at an increased incidence in the breed. Undetermined mode of inheritance.[14]

XX-Sex Reversal: Sry-negative XX-sex reversal causes external make characteristics of a prepuce and an enlarged clitoris, in genetically female dogs. A uterus is usually present. Reported as a rare disorder in the breed. Presumed autosomal recessive mode of inheritance.[15]

Anterior Crossbite, Brachygnathism, Cutaneous Asthenia, Microphthalmia, Optic Nerve Hypoplasia, Prognathism, Progressive Retinal Atrophy, and **von Willebrand's Disease** are reported.[16]

Isolated Case Studies

Multiple Ocular Anomalies: Two related litters of wheaten terriers had various combinations abnormalities including; lens luxation, persistent pupillary membranes, distichiasis, persistent right aortic arch, hydronephrosis, atypical coloboma of the posterior segment, choroid hypoplasia, scleral thinning, posterior cortical cataract, anterior iris adhesion to the cornea, microphthalmia, strabismus, limbic corneal edema, abnormal scleral outgrowth, and dermoid.[17]

Pilomatricoma: Reported case studies of pilomatricona have been published in the breed. These are usually subcutaneous calcifying tumors of the skin, usually over the shoulders or extremeties. Surgical removal is usually curative, although one case report was on a malignant form in the pelvis that had spread to the lungs.[18,19]

Segmental Aplasia of the Caudal Vena Cava: A two year-old wheaten terrier with lethargy, exercise intolerance, and ascites was diagnosed with segmental aplasia of the caudal vena cava with azygos continuation, complicated by thrombus formation.[20]

Ichthyosiform Dermatosis: A wheaten terrier had patches of thick, scaly skin from birth. By three months of age, the scaling was generalized and was accompanied by a greasy exudation which matted the haircoat. Microscopically, the skin had patchy areas of ortho- and parakeratotic hyperkeratosis, follicular keratosis, superficial perivascular dermatitis, and variable hypergranulosis.[21]

Genetic Tests

Tests of Genotype: Direct test for a renal dysplasia susceptibility gene is available from Dogenes (www.dogenes.com).

Tests of Phenotype: CHIC Certification: Required testing includes CERF eye examination and hip radiograph. (See CHIC website; www.caninehealthinfo.org).

Recommend patella examination, elbow radiographs, thyroid profile including autoantibodies, cardiac examination, and annual screening for PLE/PLN (urine protein:creatinine ratios, fecal alpha[1]-protease inhibitor concentrations and serum globulin, albumin and creatinine levels).

An open registry and DNA bank for Soft Coated Wheaten Terriers exists at the University of Pennsylvania Veterinary School.[22]

Miscellaneous

- **Breed name synonyms:** Wheaten.
- **Registries:** AKC, UKC, CKC, KCGB (Kennel Club of Great Britain), ANKC (Australian National Kennel Club), NKC (National Kennel Club).
- **AKC rank (year 2008):** 60 (1,481 dogs registered)
- **Internet resources: Soft Coated Wheaten Terrier Club of America:** www.scwtca.org
  Soft Coated Wheaten Terrier Association of Canada: www.scwtac.com
  Soft Coated Wheaten Terrier Club of Great Britain: www.wheaten.org.uk
  Wheaten Health Initiative: www.wheatenhealthinitiative.com

References

1. OFA Website breed statistics: www.offa.org Last accessed July 1, 2010.
2. Littman MP, Dambach DM, Vaden SL, et. al.: Familial protein-losing enteropathy and protein-losing nephropathy in Soft Coated Wheaten Terriers: 222 cases (1983-1997). *J Vet Intern Med.* 2000 Jan-Feb;14(1):68-80.
3. Vaden SL, Hammerberg B, Davenport DJ, et. al.: Food hypersensitivity reactions in Soft Coated Wheaten Terriers with protein-losing enteropathy or protein-losing nephropathy or both: gastroscopic food sensitivity testing, dietary provocation, and fecal immunoglobulin E. *J Vet Intern Med.* 2000 Jan-Feb;14(1):60-7
4. Lees, GE: Inherited Kidney Diseases in Dogs and Cats. Proceedings, 2005 Tufts' Canine and Feline Breeding and Genetics Conference. 2005.
5. Slater MR & Harbison J: General Health Survey on Soft Coated Wheaten Terriers. Soft Coated Wheaten Terrier Club of America. 2000.
6. Allenspach K, Lomas B, Wieland B, et. al.: Evaluation of perinuclear anti-neutrophilic cytoplasmic autoantibodies as an early marker of protein-losing enteropathy and protein-losing nephropathy in Soft Coated Wheaten Terriers. Am J Vet Res. 2008 Oct;69(10):1301-4.
7. Dorn CR: Canine breed-specific risks of frequently diagnosed diseases at veterinary teaching hospitals. Monograph. AKC Canine Health Foundation. 2000.
8. *Ocular Disorders Presumed to be Inherited in Purebred Dogs.* American College of Veterinary Ophthalmologists. ACVO, 2007.
9. Luckschander N, Allenspach K, Hall J, et. al.: Perinuclear antineutrophilic cytoplasmic antibody and response to treatment in diarrheic dogs with food responsive disease or inflammatory bowel disease. J Vet Intern Med. 2006 Mar-Apr;20(2):221-7.
10. Nash AS, Creswick JA: Familial nephropathy in soft-coated wheaten terriers. *Vet Rec.* 1988 Dec 17;123(25):654-5.
11. Nachreiner RF, Refsal KR, Graham PA, et. al.: Prevalence of serum thyroid hormone autoantibodies in dogs with clinical signs of hypothyroidism. *J Am Vet Med Assoc* 2002 Feb 15;220(4):466-71.
12. Nachreiner R & Refsal K: Personal communication, Diagnostic Center for Population and Animal Health, Michigan State University. April, 2007.
13. Peterson ME, Kintzer PP, Kass PH: Pretreatment clinical and laboratory findings in dogs with hypoadrenocorticism: 225 cases (1979-1993). *J Am Vet Med Assoc.* 1996 Jan 1;208(1):85-91.
14. Chew DJ & DiBartola SP: Urinary Incontinence in Dogs--Diagnosis and Treatment. Proceedings, 2008 Atlantic Coast Veterinary Conference. 2008.
15. De Lorenzi L, Groppetti D, Arrighi S, et. al.: Mutations in the RSPO1 coding region are not the main cause of canine SRY-negative XX sex

reversal in several breeds. Sexual Development. 2008;2(2):84-95.
16. *The Genetic Connection: A Guide to Health Problems in Purebred Dogs.* L Ackerman. p. 240. AAHA Press, 1999.
17. van der Woerdt A, Stades FC, van der Linde-Sipman JS: Multiple Ocular Anomalies in Two Related Litters of Soft Coated Wheaten Terriers. *Vet Comp Ophthalmol* 1995: 5[2]:78-82. *The Complete Dog Book, 19th Ed.* The American Kennel Club. Howell Book House, NY 1998. p. 392-95.
18. Jackson K, Boger L, Goldschmidt M, et. al.: Malignant pilomatricoma in a soft-coated Wheaten Terrier. Vet Clin Pathol. 2010 Jun;39(2):236-40.
19. Holt TL & Mann FA: Carbon dioxide laser resection of a distal carpal pilomatricoma and wound closure using swine intestinal submucosa in a dog. J Am Anim Hosp Assoc. 2003 Sep-Oct;39(5):499-505.
20. Harder MA, Fowler D, Pharr JW, et. al.: Segmental aplasia of the caudal vena cava in a dog. *Can Vet J.* 2002 May;43(5):365-8.
21. Helman RG, Rames DS, Chester DK: Ichthyosiform Dermatosis in a Soft-Coated Wheaten Terrier. *Vet Dermatol* 1997: 8[1]:53-58.
22. Littman MP & Smagala AJ: The Open Registry and DNA Bank for Soft-Coated Wheaten Terriers at the University of Pennsylvania School of Veterinary Medicine. Proceedings, 2009 Tufts' Canine and Feline Breeding and Genetics Conference. 2009.
23. *The Complete Dog Book, 20th Ed.* The American Kennel Club. Howell Book House, NY 2006. p. 432-435.

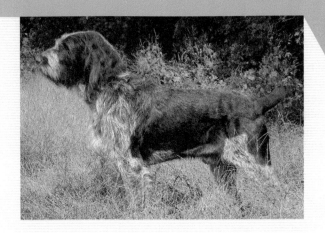

The Breed History

The breed harkens from the Piedmont region of Northern Italy. A rare breed, this is a bird gundog in the AKC Sporting Dog group. It is one of the most ancient of the Italian hunting dog breeds, with very early records of a tough, bristly pointer meeting the description of the Spinone dating to a work in 500 BC. Works from the 13th to 15th century describe very closely such a dog—then termed bristled hound, bacco Spinoso or the rough-coated hound. AKC recognition occurred in 2000.

Breeding for Function

This dog was bred for hunting at an easy pace, built to last all day long. An easy-going temperament makes this an ideal companion dog as well. All terrain dogs, they can handle temperature extremes and water—with topnotch retriever and pointing skills and strong swimming ability. They are versatile in their working abilities. Tracking and obedience are also areas in which they excel. Some of these dogs have proven themselves as therapy dogs. Excellent tolerance of cold water and thorny dense underbrush is characteristic. This dog waves his tail back and forth while working. The Spinone prefers to maintain close communication—they say he hunts for the hunter not himself.

Physical Characteristics

Height at Withers: female 22-25" (56-63.5 cm), male 23-27" (58.5-68.5 cm)

Weight: females 62-70 lb (28-32 kg) males 70-84 lb (32-38 kg)

Coat: Harsh dense wired texture of haircoat and thick skin keep this dog warm and comfortable in the field. Single-coated, with straight to crimped hairs. Length is closely controlled, with 1.5-2.5" being the breed standard, with a 0.5" tolerance outside the standard. Not feathered but face is embellished with moustache, eyebrows and beard to protect the dog from rough going. Colors are limited to Capuchin Friar's Frock, also called "monk's habit" (a chestnut brown), white with brown markings, white, orange roan +/- orange markings, brown roan, +/- brown markings.

Longevity: 12-14 years

Points of Conformation: These large dogs have a very people-like expression. Skull is long, and expression is of gentle intelligence.

Spinone Italiano

Eyes are yellow brown, with the depth of color well matched to the coat. Wide-set, the eyes have tight fitting lids and eyes are closest to round in shape and neither protrude or recess. Eyelid margins match the coat, ranging from brown through flesh tone. The nose is large and protrudes forward of the front lip profile. A scissors or level bite is accepted. Occipital protuberance is prominent. The muzzle is square, the stop is subtle. The profile is straight to slightly Roman-nosed. The triangular fine-leathered ears with rounded tip hang particularly low and back on the skull. The neck has a double dewlap and is thick. A broad, deep thorax is evident, and the topline drops down except for an arch over the loin area, with minimal abdominal tuck up. A square conformation and good solid bone characterize this strong hunter.

The tail is thicker at the base, and carried below back level. Can be docked to 5.5-8" in length. The feet are large but well knuckled up—nails are dark but not black and the front and rear dewclaws may be removed. The rear feet are more oval than the front feet. The gait is a long easy trot that covers a great deal of ground with each stride.

Grooming: Periodic bathing on an as-needed basis. Periodic coat stripping as needed. Weekly brushing will usually suffice.

Recognized Behavior Issues and Traits

Breed attributes ascribed include: Docile, easy-going, very patient, excellent stamina, courageous, loyal, playful until late in life, sociable, though some are cautious with strangers and should be socialized early. Early obedience training will ensure a good transition to maturity. Learns quickly, very intelligent, can be somewhat independent and stubborn. Needs lots of human interaction, especially in late puppyhood. Needs to be handled from 4-10 months of age with good gentle environment to prevent shyness or timidity. Not a barky breed, but will alarm for family—not a protection dog though. Can jump very high, and some will dig, so a proper fence is needed to keep him in the yard. Requires less exercise than most of the other hunting breeds.

Normal Physiologic Variations
None reported

Drug Sensitivities
None reported

Inherited Diseases

Hip Dysplasia: Polygenic trait causing degenerative joint disease and hip arthritis. OFA reports 15.5% affected.[1]

Elbow Dysplasia: Polygenic trait causing elbow arthritis. OFA reports 5.8% affected.[1]

Patella Luxation: Polygenically inherited laxity of patellar ligaments, causing luxation, lameness, and later degenerative joint disease. Treat surgically if causing clinical signs. Too few Spinone Italianos have been screened by OFA to determine an accurate frequency.[1]

Cerebellar Ataxia (CA, Cerebellar Abiotrophy): Autosomal recessive disease of progressive incoordination. Onset of hypermetria and ataxia about 4-8 months of age. No affected dogs survive past 1 year of age. Identified in Spinone in Italy, Great Britain, Denmark, Holland, and the US. All affected dogs trace back to a common family. A linked-marker based genetic test is available.[2,3]

Disease Predispositions

Ectropion: A rolling out of the eyelids, can cause frequent conjunctivitis, and ocular discharge. Often with a medial canthus pocket. Reported in 17.5% of Spinones in the 1999 SCA Health Survey Report.[4]

Allergies: Inhalent or food. Presents with pruritis and pyotraumatic dermatitis (hot spots). Reported in 15.6% of Spinones in the 1999 SCA Health Survey Report.[4]

Hypothyroidism: 8.0% positive for thyroid autoantibodies based on testing at Michigan State University. (Ave. for all breeds is 7.5%).[5,6]

Otitis Externa: Recurrent Ear Infection. Reported in 5.8% of Spinones in the 1999 SCA Health Survey Report.[4]

Cataracts: Anterior cortex intermediate and nuclear punctate cataracts predominate in the breed. Identified in 3.87% of Spinone Italiani CERF examined by veterinary ophthalmologists between 2000-2005. CERF does not recommend breeding any Spinone Italiano with a cataract.[7]

Inherited Epilepsy: Grand-mal or petit-mal seizures. Control with anticonvulsant medication. Reported in 3.4% of Spinones in the 1999 SCA Health Survey Report.[4,8]

Persistent Pupillary Membranes: Strands of fetal remnant connecting; iris to iris, cornea, lens, or involving sheets of tissue. The later three forms can impair vision, and dogs affected with these forms should not be bred. Identified in 3.03% of Spinone Italiani CERF examined by veterinary ophthalmologists between 2000-2005.[7]

Entropion: A rolling in of the eyelids that can cause corneal irritation and ulceration. Identified in 2.53% of Spinone Italiani CERF examined by veterinary ophthalmologists between 2000-2005.[7]

Gastric Dilatation–Volvulus (Bloat, GDV): Polygenically inherited, life-threatening twisting of the stomach within the abdomen. Requires immediate veterinary attention. Reported in 1.9% of Spinones in the 1999 SCA Health Survey Report.[4]

Portosystemic Shunt is reported.[9]

Isolated Case Studies

Myxoid Liposarcoma: Case report of a non-resectable thoracic mass in a 5-year-old, intact male Italian Spinone.[10]

Genetic Tests

Tests of Genotype: A linked-marker test is available for cerebellar ataxia from the Animal Health Trust.

Tests of Phenotype: CHIC Certification: Required testing includes hip and elbow radiographs, and CERF eye examination (beginning at 2 years of age). Optional recommended testing includes congenital cardiac examination, and thyroid profile including autoantibodies (annually until year 6, then every other year until 10). (See CHIC website; www.caninehealthinfo.org).

Recommend patella evaluation.

Miscellaneous

- **Breed name synonyms:** Spinone, Spinoni Italiani (pl), Italian Griffon, Italian Spinone.
- **Registries:** AKC, CKC, KCGB (Kennel Club of Great Britain), NKC (National Kennel Club).
- **AKC rank (year 2008):** 114 (318 dogs registered)
- **Internet Resources: Spinone Club of America:** www.spinonecluboffamerica.com
  Italian Spinone Club of Great Britain: www.italianspinone.co.uk

References

1. OFA Website breed statistics: www.offa.org Last accessed July 1, 2010.
2. Bianchi E, Corradi A, Dondi M, et. al.: Two Cases of Cerebellar Cortical Abiotrophy in Italian Spinone. Proceedings World Small Animal Veterinary Association Congress 2002.
3. Wheeler S & Rusbridge C: Neurological syndrome in Italian spinones. Vet Rec. 1996 Mar 2;138(9):216.
4. Spinone Club of America: 1999 Spinone Club of America Health Survey Report. January, 2000.
5. Nachreiner RF, Refsal KR, Graham PA, et. al.: Prevalence of serum thyroid hormone autoantibodies in dogs with clinical signs of hypothyroidism. J Am Vet Med Assoc 2002 Feb 15;220(4):466-71.
6. Nachreiner R & Refsal K: Personal communication, Diagnostic Center for Population and Animal Health, Michigan State University. April, 2007.
7. *Ocular Disorders Presumed to be Inherited in Purebred Dogs.* American College of Veterinary Ophthalmologists. ACVO, 2007.
8. Hill C: Primary epilepsy in the Italian spinone. Vet Rec. 2006 Sep 9;159(11):368.
9. The Genetic Connection: A Guide to Health Problems in Purebred Dogs. L Ackerman. AAHA Press, p. 240, 1999.
10. Boyd SP, Taugner FM, Serrano S, et. al.: Matrix "blues": clue to a cranial thoracic mass in a dog. Vet Clin Pathol. 2005 Sep;34(3):271-4.
11. *The Complete Dog Book, 20th Ed.* The American Kennel Club. Howell Book House, NY 2006. p. 115-119.

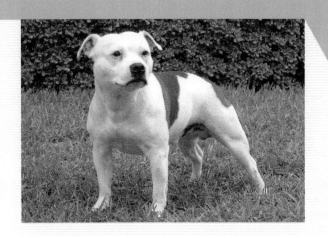

The Breed History

Ancient lineage of all fighting dogs traces back to Roman war dogs, from which the Mastiff lines arose. The early Staffordshire arose from Bulldog and Mastiff crosses, and were used for bull and bear baiting. These were called Old Pit Bulls, or Pit Dogs. Manchester terrier and English White terrier (now extinct) crosses were done to make the dog smaller and quicker when dog fighting replaced baiting. These terrier crosses were termed Bull and Terrier, and eventually became known as Staffordshire Bull Terriers. The first dogs to reach North America arrived in the 1880s. It was from these American imports that the American Staffordshire Terriers originated, which are taller and heavier in stature than the Staffordshire bull. First AKC registry for Staffordshire Bull Terriers occurred in 1974.

Breeding for Function

Originally bred for bull and bear baiting, they were later bred for dog fighting. They were also highly prized as ratters. Staffordshire Bull Terriers were sometimes called Nanny Dogs in Britain because of their role as guardians of the home and family.

Physical Characteristics

Height at Withers: 14-16" (35.5-40.5 cm)

Weight: females 24-34 lb (11-15.5 kg), males 28-38 lb (12.5-17 kg).

Coat: The short, smooth glossy coat lies flat and colors accepted include brindle, brindle and white, black, red, white, fawn or blue. Liver or Black and Tan are disqualifying colors.

Longevity: 11-12 years

Points of Conformation: The breed is characterized by a compact, muscular square conformation. They possess a broad skull with prominent masseter muscles, a black nose, and short blocky muzzle. The stop is distinct. The eyes are front facing and moderate in size, round and variable in color. Ears are small to medium in size, half pricked or rose. They have a short well-muscled neck, level topline, and are broad through the chest. The thorax is barrel shaped and the abdomen mildly tucked up. The low set tapering tail is carried low. Limbs are straight-boned, the feet are compact and medium in size. Dewclaws may be removed. The hindquarters are well muscled. The gait is strong, quick, moderate in stride length, and agility is evident.

Staffordshire Bull Terrier

Recognized Behavior Issues and Traits

Reported breed attributes include: Good with family, gentle, loyal, playful, intelligent, low shedding and grooming needs, good for city or country, and have moderate exercise needs.

They may see small pets or children as prey, may fight with other dogs, will not back down in a fight and have a tenacious crushing bite. They should be on leash unless in a fenced enclosure. Electric fencing will not deter them. They are good diggers. They need human companionship, and do not do well if left alone or kenneled. They do not tolerate temperature extremes well. At least a basic level obedience training course is strongly advised. Early socialization to children and other pets should be done. They are generally tolerant, but should be supervised. They will guard family, but not the home. They may snore.

Normal Physiologic Variations

None reported

Drug Sensitivities

None reported

Inherited Diseases

Hip Dysplasia: Polygenically inherited trait causing degenerative joint disease and hip arthritis. OFA reports 17.4% affected.[1]

Elbow Dysplasia: Polygenically inherited trait causing elbow arthritis. OFA reports 16.4% affected.[1]

Juvenile Cataracts (Hereditary Cataracts, HC): Autosomal recessive disorder causing bilateral nuclear and cortical cataracts with an onset around 3 months of age. Identified in 2.05% of Staffordshire Bull Terriers CERF examined by veterinary ophthalmologists between 2000-2005. A genetic test is available. CERF does not recommend breeding any Staffordshire Bull Terrier with a cataract.[2,3]

L-2-Hydroxyglutaric Aciduria (L2-HGA): Autosomal recessive disorder. Affected Staffordshire Bull Terriers present with seizures, ataxia, dementia, and tremors. Levels of L-2-hydroxyglutaric acid are elevated in all body fluids evaluated (urine, plasma, and CSF). A genetic test is available.[4,5]

Patella Luxation: Polygenically inherited laxity of patellar ligaments, causing luxation, lameness, and later degenerative joint disease. Treat surgically if causing clinical signs. Too few Staffordshire Bull Terriers have been screened by OFA to determine an accurate frequency.[1]

Disease Predispositions

Distichiasis: Abnormally placed eyelashes that irritate the cornea and conjunctiva. Can cause secondary corneal ulceration. Identified in 10.25% of Staffordshire Bull Terriers CERF examined by veterinary ophthalmologists between 2000-2005.[2]

Brachycephalic Complex: Includes **Elongated Soft Palate, Stenotic Nares, Hypoplastic Trachea, and Everted Laryngeal Saccules**. Causes dyspnea, and can cause collapse and death with extreme stress. Identified in 5.5% of Staffordshire Bull Terriers in an Australian study. Surgery is indicated in severe cases.[6]

Hypothyroidism: Inherited autoimmune thyroiditis. Too few Staffordshire Bull Terriers have been tested for thyroid autoantibodies at Michigan State University to determine an accurate frequency. (Ave. for all breeds is 7.5%).[7,8]

Tibial Tuberosity Avulsion Fracture: Traumatic avulsion seen in immature dogs, usually between 4-6 months of age. Requires surgical repair. Occurs in 3.3% of Staffordshire Bull Terriers, who account for 85% of all cases seen.[9]

Persistent Pupillary Membranes: Strands of fetal remnant connecting; iris to iris, cornea, lens, or involving sheets of tissue. The later three forms can impair vision, and dogs affected with these forms should not be bred. Identified in 1.23% of Staffordshire Bull Terriers CERF examined by veterinary ophthalmologists between 2000-2005.[2]

Demodicosis, Juvenile Generalized: Overgrowth of demodex mites in hair follicles due to an underlying immunodeficiency. Causes hair loss and inflammation. Reported 17.1 odds ratio versus other breeds.[10]

Gastric Carcinoma: A breed predisposition is identified for this stomach cancer. The most frequent clinical features are vomiting, polydipsia and weight loss, with endoscopic findings of a large deep ulcer with thickened, irregular rims and walls.[11]

Mast Cell Tumor: Subcutaneous skin tumors that produce histamine and cause inflammation and ulceration. An increased incidence of mast cell tumors is identified in Staffordshire Bull Terriers versus other breeds.[12]

Persistent Hyperplastic Primary Vitreous (PHPV): Congenital ocular disorder affecting the development and regression of the hyaloid artery (the primary vitreous). It can progress to secondary cataracts or intra-lenticular hemorrhage. Unknown mode of inheritance. CERF does not recommend breeding any Staffordshire Bull Terrier with PHPV.[2,13]

Cystinuria/Cystine bladder stones: A study in the UK showed that 21.6% of cases of cystine bladder stone cases were Staffordshire Bull Terriers. Caused by an error in cystine metabolism. Treat with surgical removal and life-long medical therapy. Unknown mode of inheritance in this breed.[14]

Inverted Canines: In affected Staffordshire Bull Terriers, the mandibular canine teeth are tipped (curved) caudally and impact at the mesio-palatal gingival margin of the maxillary canine teeth.[15]

Chronic Pulmonary Fibrosis: Causes progressive chronic cough, dyspnea, and tachypnea over months to years. Response to prednisolone, with or without bronchodilators, is variable. Reported at an increased frequency in young to middle aged Staffordshire Bull Terriers. Undetermined mode of inheritance.[16]

Congenital Laryngeal Paralysis: Reported at an increased frequency in the breed in the UK, with an average age of onset of 4 to 6 months. Causes voice change or hoarse bark, exercise intolerance, gagging, coughing, stridor, dyspnea, cyanosis, collapse, and vomiting. Undetermined mode of inheritance.[17]

Compulsive Tail Chasing, Epilepsy, Osteochondritis Dessicans-Stifle, and **Prognathism** are reported.[18]

Isolated Case Studies

Ciliary Dyskinesia: Primary ciliary dyskinesia was diagnosed in a 14-week old Staffordshire bull terrier that had a history of respiratory disease from 7 weeks of age. Pneumonia was diagnosed based on thoracic radiographs and trans-tracheal aspirate. Transmission electron microscopy of the bronchi and trachea indicated the presence of both primary and secondary ciliary dyskinesia.[19]

Ocular Mixed Germ Cell Tumor: A 3-year-old female neutered Staffordshire Bull Terrier presented with a mixed germ cell tumor involving the base of the iris and the ciliary body of the right eye.[20]

Rhabdomyoma/Myxosarcoma: Separate case reports of; a six-year-old Staffordshire bull terrier with right atrial rhabdomyoma, a six-year-old Staffordshire bull terrier with a lingual rhabdomyosarcoma, and a case of right atrial myxosarcoma in a Staffordshire bull terrier.[21,22,23]

Genetic Tests

Tests of Genotype: Direct test for L2-HGA is available from the Animal Health Trust.

Direct test for HC is available from the Animal Health Trust.

Direct test for black color, tan points and mask is available from Health Gene.

Tests of Phenotype: Recommend patella evaluation, hip and elbow radiographs, CERF eye examination, and thyroid profile including autoantibodies.

Miscellaneous

- **Breed name synonyms:** Stafford
- **Registries:** AKC, UKC, CKC, KCGB (Kennel Club of Great Britain), ANKC (Australian National Kennel Club), NKC (National Kennel Club)
- **AKC rank (year 2008):** 78 (958 dogs registered)
- **Internet resources:** Staffordshire Bull Terrier Club of America: www.sbtca.com
  Staffordshire Bull Terrier Club of Canada: www.staffordcanada.com
  Staffordshire Bull Terrier Club (UK): www.thesbtc.com

References

1. OFA Website breed statistics: www.offa.org Last accessed July 1, 2010.
2. *Ocular Disorders Presumed to be Inherited in Purebred Dogs.* American College of Veterinary Ophthalmologists. ACVO, 2007.
3. Mellersh CS, Pettitt L, Forman OP, et. al.: Identification of mutations in HSF4 in dogs of three different breeds with hereditary cataracts. Vet Ophthalmol. 2006 Sep-Oct;9(5):369-78.
4. Abramson CJ, Platt SR, Jakobs C, et. al.: L-2-Hydroxyglutaric aciduria in

Staffordshire Bull Terriers. *J Vet Intern Med.* 2003 Jul-Aug;17(4):551-6.

5. Scurrell E, Davies E, Baines E, et. al.: Neuropathological findings in a Staffordshire bull terrier with l-2-hydroxyglutaric aciduria. J Comp Pathol. 2008 Feb-Apr;138(2-3):160-4.

6. Torrez CV & Hunt GB: Results of surgical correction of abnormalities associated with brachycephalic airway obstruction syndrome in dogs in Australia. J Small Anim Pract. 2006 Mar;47(3):150-4.

7. Nachreiner RF, Refsal KR, Graham PA, et. al.: Prevalence of serum thyroid hormone autoantibodies in dogs with clinical signs of hypothyroidism. *J Am Vet Med Assoc* 2002 Feb 15;220(4):466-71.

8. Nachreiner R & Refsal K: Personal communication, Diagnostic Center for Population and Animal Health, Michigan State University. April, 2007.

9. Gower JA, Bound NJ, Moores AP, et. al.: Tibial tuberosity avulsion fracture in dogs: a review of 59 dogs. J Small Anim Pract. 2008 Jul;49(7):340-3.

10. Plant JD, Lund EM & Yang M: A case-control study of the risk factors for canine juvenile-onset generalized demodicosis in the USA. Vet Dermatol. 2011 Feb;22(1):95-9.

11. Sullivan M, Lee R, Fisher EW, et. al.: A study of 31 cases of gastric carcinoma in dogs. Vet Rec. 1987 Jan 24;120(4):79-83.

12. Baker-Gabb M, Hunt GB, France MP: Soft tissue sarcomas and mast cell tumours in dogs; clinical behaviour and response to surgery. *Aust Vet J.* 2003 Dec;81(12):732-8.

13. Curtis R, Barnett KC, Leon A: Persistent hyperplastic primary vitreous in the Staffordshire bull terrier. *Vet Rec.* 1984 Oct 13;115(15):385.

14. Allen LBA, Pratt A, Lulich J, et. al.: Canine Cystine Urolithiasis: Investigation of Cases Identified in the United Kingdom. Proceedings, 2008 British Small Animal Veterinary Congress. 2008.

15. Wilson GJ: Inverted Canines in the Staffordshire Bull Terrier - A New Clinical Condition. *Aust Vet Pract* 2003: 33[2]:83-85.

16. Clercx C: Chronic Non-Cardiac Cough in Dogs. Proceedings, 2010 World Small Animal Veterinary Association World Congress. 2010.

17. Kirby BM: Laryngeal Paralysis Diagnosis and Management. Proceedings, 2008 World Small Animal Veterinary Association World Congress. 2008.

18. *The Genetic Connection: A Guide to Health Problems in Purebred Dogs.* L Ackerman. p. 207 AAHA Press, 1999.

19. De Scally M, Lobetti RG, Van Wilpe E: Primary ciliary dyskinesia in a Staffordshire bull terrier. *J S Afr Vet Assoc.* 2004 Sep;75(3):150-2.

20. Patterson-Kane JC, Schulman FY, Santiago N, et. al.: Mixed germ cell tumor in the eye of a dog. *Vet Pathol.* 2001 Nov;38(6):712-4.

21. Mansfield CS, Callanan JJ, McAllister H: Intra-atrial rhabdomyoma causing chylopericardium and right-sided congestive heart failure in a dog. *Vet Rec.* 2000 Sep 2;147(10):264-7.

22. Lascelles BD, McInnes E, Dobson JM, et. al.: Rhabdomyosarcoma of the tongue in a dog. *J Small Anim Pract.* 1998 Dec;39(12):587-91.

23. Briggs OM, Kirberger RM, Goldberg NB: Right atrial myxosarcoma in a dog. *J S Afr Vet Assoc.* 1997 Dec;68(4):144-6.

24. *The Complete Dog Book, 20th Ed.* The American Kennel Club. Howell Book House, NY 2006. p. 436-438.

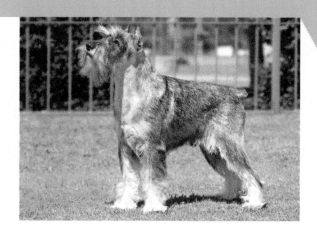

Standard Schnauzer

toes are well arched, with thick pads and black nails. Rear dewclaws are generally taken off. The gait is quick, smooth and true.

The Breed History

This breed is the original Schnauzer dog from which the Giant and Miniature were developed. The records of origin trace back to Germany in the year 1500, though they are depicted in artwork around the mid 1400s. Bavaria and Wurtemmburg are regions that provide earliest records of the breed type. The genealogy of the breed is thought to include Dog de Bologne, Wirehaired Pincher, black German Poodle, and gray Wolf Spitz. The first breed standard was published in 1880. AKC recognition occurred in 1904.

Breeding for Function

Vermin control and guard dog were the original functions that this breed was developed for. A fearless temperament was valued highly. Because of their obedience and tenacity, they were widely used in war for dispatch and aides, as well as for police work. Versatile, they have even been used for water retrieving work and sheep herding.

Physical Characteristics

Height at Withers: female 17.5-18.5" (44.5-47 cm), male 18.5-19.5" (47-49.5 cm).

Weight: males 40-45 lb (18-20.5 kg), females 35-40 lb (16-18 kg).

Coat: They possess a double coat consisting of a soft undercoat and outer hairs that are stiff, wiry and tight. The coat is ideally maintained by stripping not clipping. Salt and pepper is most common (mixture of hairs with bands of white and black mixed with black hairs and white hairs) but solid black is also sometimes seen.

Longevity: 12-14 years

Points of Conformation: Bushy bristling brows, substantial beard, wiry coat, a compact, square conformation, and abundant whiskers characterize the Standard Schnauzer. Heavy muscling and bone, and alert, high head carriage is also characteristic. The head is rectangular in shape. There is a flat moderately broad skull, and a slight stop. The eyes are medium in size, oval, and dark brown in color. Medium-sized ears are triangular, high set and the leather is moderate. Sometimes the ears are cropped. The nose is black and large. The neck is of moderate length and arched, and no throatiness should be evident. The topline is straight, descending very slightly towards the rear. The thorax is medium in depth, and ribs are well sprung. Moderate abdominal tuck up is present and the tail is short, usually docked to 1-2" (2.5-5 cm) length. Limbs are straight boned, moderately muscled, and forelimb dewclaws may be removed. Feet are small, and

Recognized Behavior Issues and Traits

Reported breed characteristics include: High intelligence, a good guard dog, devoted, reliable, sociable, good trainability, excellent endurance. High grooming needs, including at least a twice yearly stripping and daily grooming of whiskers and legs is necessary. The stripped coat is low shedding. Good for city or country settings, and generally good with children. Spirited temperament may result in an effort to dominate the household. Active dogs, they are in need of moderate exercise. These dogs do not do well in kennel situations; needing mental stimulation to prevent boredom. They have a moderate barking tendency. Early socialization and obedience training is important.

Normal Physiologic Variations

None reported

Drug Sensitivities

None reported

Inherited Diseases

Hip Dysplasia: Polygenically inherited trait causing degenerative joint disease and hip arthritis. OFA reports 8.6% affected.[1]

Elbow Dysplasia: Polygenically inherited trait causing elbow arthritis. OFA reports 6.1% affected.[1]

Patella Luxation: Polygenically inherited laxity of patellar ligaments, causing luxation, lameness, and later degenerative joint disease. Treat surgically if causing clinical signs. Too few Standard Schnauzers have been screened by OFA to determine an accurate frequency.[1]

Disease Predispositions

Hypothyroidism: Inherited autoimmune thyroiditis. 7.0% positive for thyroid autoantibodies based on testing at Michigan State University. (Ave. for all breeds is 7.5%).[2,3]

Pancreatitis: Inflammation of the pancreas causing vomiting. In extreme cases, can cause peritonitis and require hospitalization. Dorn reports a 55.06x odds ratio versus other breeds.[4]

Diabetes Mellitus: Sugar diabetes. Treat with insulin injections, diet, and glucose monitoring. Dorn reports a 10.01x odds ratio versus other breeds.[4]

Calcium Oxalate Urolithiasis: The Standard Schnauzer is a breed with a predisposition to develop calcium oxalate bladder stones, with an 18.06x odds ratio versus other breeds. Dorn reports a 55.06x odds ratio for bladder stones versus other breeds.[4,5]

Cataracts: Posterior polar and cortex cataracts predominate in the breed. Reported in 4.73% of Standard Schnauzers presented to veterinary teaching hospitals. Identified in 1.53% of Standard Schnauzers CERF examined by veterinary ophthalmologists between

2000-2005. CERF does not recommend breeding any Standard Schnauzer with a cataract.[6,7]

Hyperadrenocorticism: Hyperfunction of the adrenal gland caused by a pituitary or adrenal tumor. Clinical signs may include increased thirst and urination, symmetrical truncal alopecia, and abdominal distention. Dorn reports a 3.77x odds ratio versus other breeds.[4]

Distichiasis: Abnormally placed eyelashes that irritate the cornea and conjunctiva. Can cause secondary corneal ulceration. Identified in 1.65% of Standard Schnauzers CERF examined by veterinary ophthalmologists between 2000-2005.[6]

Retinal Dysplasia: Focal retinal dysplasia and retinal folds are recognized in the breed. Severe cases can progress to retinal detachment and blindness. Reported in 1.27% of Standard Schnauzers CERF examined by veterinary ophthalmologists between 2000-2005.[6]

Corneal Dystrophy: Epithelial/stromal form of corneal opacities. Identified in 1.02% of Standard Schnauzers CERF examined by veterinary ophthalmologists between 2000-2005.[6]

Portosystemic shunt (PSS, liver shunt): Congenital abnormal blood vessel connecting the portal and systemic circulation. Can be intrahepatic, extrahepatic, or microvascular dysplasia. Causes stunting, abnormal behavior, possible seizures, and secondary ammonium urate urinary calculi in the breed. Treatment of PSS includes partial ligation and/or medical and dietary control of symptoms. Tobias reports a 16.1x odds ratio versus other breeds.[8]

Progressive Retinal Atrophy (PRA): Inherited retinal degeneration resulting in blindness. Assumed autosomal recessive inheritance. CERF does not recommend breeding any Standard Schnauzers with PRA.[6]

Stomatocytosis: Occurs in Standard Schnauzers causing stomatocytes in blood, increased osmotic fragility, and possibly hemolytic anemia. Circulating stomatocytes, macrocytosis, anisocytosis, increased erythrocyte fragility and high intracellular sodium and potassium concentrations are found, although stomatin levels are normal.[9,10]

Liver Cancer, Epilepsy, and **Dilated Cardiomyopathy** are identified at an increased frequency in the Standard Schnauzer Club of America Health Survey of 2008.[11]

Anterior Crossbite, Base Narrow Canines, Persistent Primary Vitreous, Prognathism, Pulmonic Stenosis, and **Wry Mouth** are reported.[12]

Isolated Case Studies

Orbital Adenoma: A case of adenoma involving the orbit in a 13-year-old, female, standard Schnauzer is reported. Excision was curative.[13]

Corticotrophic Tumor and Phaeochromocytoma: A 10 year old spayed female Standard schnauzer was treated for pituitary dependent hyperadrenocorticism by bilateral adrenalectomy. She was euthanized 3-1/2 years later due to neurological signs from a pituitary tumor, and was diagnosed with both a corticotrophic tumor and a phaeochromocytoma on necropsy.[14]

Microgliomatosis: A 7-year-old male Standard Schnauzer presented with neurological signs, and deteriorated over an 8 week period. Necropsy of the brain revealed microgliomatosis.[15]

Genetic Tests

Tests of Genotype: None.

Tests of Phenotype: CHIC Certification: Required testing includes hip radiographs, CERF eye examination (at 2 years of age, and then every other year until age 7), and one of the following: Cardiac evaluation by a cardiologist, thyroid profile including autoantibodies (every other year until age 7), or a blood sample in the CHIC DNA repository. (See CHIC website; www.caninehealthinfo.org).

Recommend elbow radiographs and patella evaluation.

Miscellaneous

- **Breed name synonyms:** Mittelschnauzer, nicknamed "the dog with the human brain", Wire-haired Pinscher (historical).
- **Registries:** AKC, UKC, CKC, ANKC (Australian National Kennel Club), NKC (National Kennel Club).
- **AKC rank (year 2008):** 99 (552 dogs registered)
- **Internet resources:** The Standard Schnauzer Club of America: www.standardschnauzer.org
  Standard Schnauzer Club of Canada: http://standardschnauzerclub.com
  The Schnauzer Club of Great Britain: www.schnauzerclub.co.uk

References

1. OFA Website breed statistics: www.offa.org Last accessed July 1, 2010.
2. Nachreiner RF, Refsal KR, Graham PA, et. al.: Prevalence of serum thyroid hormone autoantibodies in dogs with clinical signs of hypothyroidism. J Am Vet Med Assoc 2002 Feb 15;220(4):466-71.
3. Nachreiner R & Refsal K: Personal communication, Diagnostic Center for Population and Animal Health, Michigan State University. April, 2007.
4. Dorn CR: Canine breed-specific risks of frequently diagnosed diseases at veterinary teaching hospitals. Monograph. AKC Canine Health Foundation. 2000.
5. Lekcharoensuk C, Lulich JP, Osborne CA, et. al.: Patient and environmental factors associated with calcium oxalate urolithiasis in dogs. *J Am Vet Med Assoc.* 2000 Aug 15;217(4):515-9.
6. *Ocular Disorders Presumed to be Inherited in Purebred Dogs.* American College of Veterinary Ophthalmologists. ACVO, 2007.
7. Gelatt KN, Mackay EO: Prevalence of primary breed-related cataracts in the dog in North America. Vet Ophthalmol. 2005 Mar-Apr;8(2):101-11.
8. Tobias KM, Rohrbach BW: Association of breed with the diagnosis of congenital portosystemic shunts in dogs: 2,400 cases (1980-2002). J Am Vet Med Assoc. 2003 Dec 1;223(11):1636-9.
9. Paltrinieri S, Comazzi S, Ceciliani F, et. al.: Stomatocytosis of Standard Schnauzers is not associated with stomatin deficiency. *Vet J.* 2007 Jan;173(1):200-3.
10. Bonfanti U, Comazzi S, Paltrinieri S, et. al.: Stomatocytosis in 7 related Standard Schnauzers. *Vet Clin Pathol.* 2004;33(4):234-9.
11. Mohrenweiser H & Standard Schnauzer Club of America: Standard Schnauzer Club of America Health Survey of 2008 – Final Report. 2008.
12. *The Genetic Connection: A Guide to Health Problems in Purebred Dogs.* L. Ackerman. p. 237-38. AAHA Press, 1999.
13. Giudice C, Marco R, Mirko R, et. al.: Zygomatic gland adenoma in a dog: histochemical and immunohistochemical evaluation. *Vet Ophthalmol.* 2005 Jan-Feb;8(1):13-6.
14. Thuroczy J, van Sluijs FJ, Kooistra HS, et. al.: Multiple endocrine neoplasias in a dog: corticotrophic tumour, bilateral adrenocortical tumours, and pheochromocytoma. *Vet Q.* 1998 Apr;20(2):56-61.
15. Willard MD, Delahunta A: Microgliomatosis in a Schnauzer dog. *Cornell Vet.* 1982 Apr;72(2):211-9.
16. *The Complete Dog Book, 20th Ed.* The American Kennel Club. Howell Book House, NY 2006. p. 335-339.

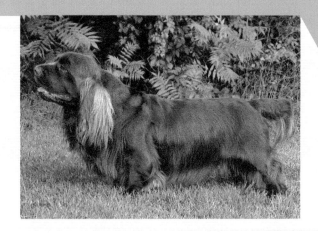

Sussex Spaniel

The Breed History

In county Sussex in England during the 1800s, the breed was established and offspring were consistently selected for the distinctive golden liver colored haircoat. The AKC admitted the breed in 1884. Over the next century, the population declined to critically low levels and it is still a very rare breed.

Breeding for Function

A hunting companion for upland game for the hunter on foot, he was renowned for excellent scent tracking and possessed the resolve to find and flush the quarry.

Like hounds, these spaniels bay, or give tongue when game is scented. They move slowly and deliberately on the trail unlike most other hunting dogs. This slow pace should not be confused with poor function.

Physical Characteristics

Height at Withers: 13-15" (33-38 cm)

Weight: 35-45 lb (16-20.5 kg)

Coat: The thick golden liver coat is double, with flat silky or slightly wavy outer hairs. The ears, tail and neck have furnishings, and only small white chest markings are acceptable. The tips of the hairs are golden. The haircoat is medium long, and the feathers around the feet (a breed characteristic) are long.

Longevity: 12-13 years

Points of Conformation: Unlike other members of the spaniel group, Sussex Spaniels are quite short limbed and possess a massive constitution, are longer than tall, and low slung. Large eyes are hazel, and the heavy brows and wrinkled forehead produce a serious looking expression. Large pendulous ears are thick leathered and set fairly low. Some lower eyelid eversion is common. The skull is wide and the stop prominent, the muzzle is square, and the nose is liver colored. The lips are pendulous, the neck is short and well muscled. The topline is level, the thorax is barrel shaped, and the rib cage extends well back. The low set tail is usually docked to 5-7" in length and is carried level or below the back. The limbs are strong and short, and may be slightly bowed. The metacarpals and metatarsals are short. The gait is rolling, and low.

Recognized Behavior Issues and Traits

Reported breed characteristics include: Friendly, happy, not heat tolerant, likes to please and is easily trained, though not generally seen at high levels in obedience training. Tolerate other dogs sometimes. They have moderate exercise needs. They have a high barking tendency, especially alarm barking. Moderate coat care is required and they adapt well to country or city.

Normal Physiologic Variations

None reported

Drug Sensitivities

None reported

Inherited Diseases

Hip Dysplasia: Polygenically inherited trait causing degenerative joint disease and hip arthritis. OFA reports 40.9% affected.[1]

Elbow Dysplasia: Polygenically inherited trait causing elbow arthritis. OFA reports 17.4% affected.[1]

Pyruvate Dehydrogenase Deficiency/Mitochondrial Myopathy (PDP1): Autosomal recessive metabolic disorder, where affected dogs show exercise intolerance, collapse, and severe metabolic acidosis. Affected dogs have high serum lactate and pyruvate concentrations and urinary organic acids. Dietary therapy may control clinical signs. Affected dogs have also been treated with human recombinant PDP1. One study reported a worldwide spread of the mutation with a 20% carrier frequency. A genetic test is available.[2,3,4,5]

Patella Luxation: Polygenically inherited laxity of patellar ligaments, causing luxation, lameness, and later degenerative joint disease. Treat surgically if causing clinical signs. Too few Sussex Spaniels have been screened by OFA to determine an accurate frequency.[1]

Disease Predispositions

Ectropion: Rolling out of eyelids, often with a medial canthal pocket. Can be secondary to **Macroblepharon**; an abnormally large eyelid opening. Can also cause conjunctivitis. Ectropion is reported in 3.96%, and macroblepharon in 11.88% of Sussex Spaniels CERF examined by veterinary ophthalmologists between 2000-2005.[6]

Retinal Dysplasia: Retinal folds, geographic, and detachment are recognized in the breed. Can lead to blindness. Identified in 10.89% of Sussex Spaniels CERF examined by veterinary ophthalmologists between 2000-2005.[6]

Persistent Hyaloid Artery (PHA): Congenital defect resulting from abnormalities in the development and regression of the hyaloid artery. Identified in 7.92% of Sussex Spaniels CERF examined by veterinary ophthalmologists between 2000-2005.[6]

Hypothyroidism: Inherited autoimmune thyroiditis. Too few Sussex Spaniels have been tested for thyroid autoantibodies at Michigan State University to determine an accurate frequency. (Ave. for all breeds is 7.5%). Reported as a breed problem on the SSCA website.[7,8]

Allergies: Inhalant or food allergy. Presents with pruritis (itching) and pyotraumatic dermatitis (hot spots). Reported as a breed problem on the SSCA website.

Cataracts: Anterior, posterior, intermediate and punctate cataracts occur in the breed. Identified in 2.97% of Sussex Spaniels CERF examined by veterinary ophthalmologists between 2000-2005. CERF does not recommend breeding any Sussex Spaniel with a cataract.[6]

Persistent Pupillary Membranes: Strands of fetal remnant connecting; iris to iris, cornea, lens, or involving sheets of tissue. The later three forms can impair vision, and dogs affected with these forms should not be bred. Identified in 1.98% of Sussex Spaniels CERF examined by veterinary ophthalmologists between 2000-2005.[6]

Distichiasis: Abnormally placed eyelashes that irritate the cornea and conjunctiva. Can cause secondary corneal ulceration. Identified in 1.11% of Sussex Spaniels CERF examined by veterinary ophthalmologists between 2000-2005.[6]

Iris Coloboma: A coloboma is a congenital defect which may affect the iris, choroid or optic disc. Identified in 0.99% of Sussex Spaniels CERF examined by veterinary ophthalmologists between 2000-2005. CERF does not recommend breeding any Sussex Spaniel with an iris coloboma.[6]

Congenital Heart Disease: The SSCA reports an increased incidence of **Pulmonic Stenosis, Patent Ductus Arteriosus (PDA),** and **Tetralogy of Fallot.** (See SSCA website.)

Deafness: Congenital deafness can be unilateral of bilateral. Diagnosed by BAER testing.[9]

Gastric Dilatation-Volvulus (bloat, GDV): Polygenically inherited, life-threatening twisting of the stomach within the abdomen. Requires immediate treatment. Reported to occur in the breed on the Sussex Spaniel Association (UK) website.

Prognathism is reported.[10]

Isolated Case Studies
None reported

Genetic Tests
Tests of Genotype: Direct genetic test for PDP1 is available at the University of Missouri and the Animal Health Trust.

Tests of Phenotype: Recommend hip and elbow radiographs, CERF eye examination, cardiac evaluation, patella evaluation, and thyroid profile including autoantibodies.

Miscellaneous
- **Breed name synonyms:** Sussex
- **Registries:** AKC, UKC, CKC, KCGB (Kennel Club of Great Britain),

ANKC (Australian National Kennel Club), NKC (National Kennel Club)
- **AKC rank (year 2008):** 147 (74 dogs registered)
- **Internet resources: Sussex Spaniel Club of America:** www.sussexspaniels.org
- **Sussex Spaniel Association (UK):** www.sussexspaniels.org.uk

References

1. OFA Website breed statistics: www.offa.org Last accessed July 1, 2010.
2. Abramson CJ, Platt SR, Shelton GD: Pyruvate dehydrogenase deficiency in a Sussex spaniel. *J Small Anim Pract.* 2004 Mar;45(3):162-5.
3. Houlton JE, Herrtage ME: Mitochondrial myopathy in the Sussex spaniel. Vet Rec. 1980 Mar 1;106(9):206.
4. Shelton GD: Inherited Neuromuscular Disease. Proceedings, 2002 ACVIM Forum. 2002.
5. Cameron JM, Maj MC, Levandovskiy V, et. al.: Identification of a canine model of pyruvate dehydrogenase phosphatase 1 deficiency. Mol Genet Metab. 2007 Jan;90(1):15-23.
6. *Ocular Disorders Presumed to be Inherited in Purebred Dogs.* American College of Veterinary Ophthalmologists. ACVO, 2007.
7. Nachreiner RF, Refsal KR, Graham PA, et. al.: Prevalence of serum thyroid hormone autoantibodies in dogs with clinical signs of hypothyroidism. *J Am Vet Med Assoc* 2002 Feb 15;220(4):466-71.
8. Nachreiner R & Refsal K: Personal communication, Diagnostic Center for Population and Animal Health, Michigan State University. April, 2007.
9. Strain GM: Deafness prevalence and pigmentation and gender associations in dog breeds at risk. *The Veterinary Journal* 2004; 167(1):23-32.
10. *The Genetic Connection: A Guide to Health Problems in Purebred Dogs.* L Ackerman. p. 241. AAHA Press, 1999.
11. *The Complete Dog Book, 20th Ed.* The American Kennel Club. Howell Book House, NY 2006. p. 106-110.

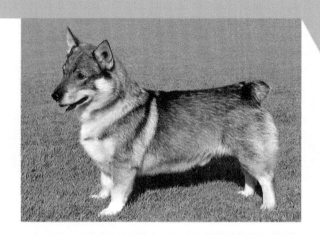

Swedish Vallhund

Recognized Behavior Issues and Traits

The breed is watchful, energetic, fearless, alert, intelligent, friendly, eager to please, active, and steady, making a good herding and companion dog. Sound temperament, neither vicious or shy.

Normal Physiologic Variations

In a UK study, 30% of litters were born via **Cesarean section.**[1]

Drug Sensitivities

None Reported

Inherited Diseases

Patella Luxation: Polygenically inherited laxity of patellar ligaments, causing luxation, lameness, and later degenerative joint disease. Treat surgically if causing clinical signs. Reported at a high frequency, however, too few Swedish Vallhunds have been screened by OFA to determine an accurate frequency. Reported as a breed problem on the SVCA website.[2]

Hip Dysplasia: Polygenically inherited trait causing degenerative joint disease and hip arthritis. OFA reports 10.2% affected.[2]

Elbow Dysplasia: Polygenically inherited trait causing elbow arthritis. OFA reports 2.4% affected.[2]

Disease Predispositions

Persistent Pupillary Membranes: Strands of fetal remnant connecting; iris to iris, cornea, lens, or involving sheets of tissue. The later three forms can impair vision, and dogs affected with these forms should not be bred. Identified in 15.15% of Swedish Vallhunds CERF examined by veterinary ophthalmologists between 2000-2005.[3]

Cataracts: Punctate cataracts predominate in the breed. Identified in 4.85% of Swedish Vallhunds CERF examined by veterinary ophthalmologists between 2000-2005. CERF does not recommend breeding any Swedish Vallhund with a cataract.[3]

Vitreous Degeneration: Liquefaction of the vitreous gel which may predispose to retinal detachment. Identified in 3.64% of Swedish Vallhunds CERF examined by veterinary ophthalmologists between 2000-2005.[3]

Distichiasis: Abnormally placed eyelashes that irritate the cornea and conjunctiva. Can cause secondary corneal ulceration. Identified in 3.03% of Swedish Vallhunds CERF examined by veterinary ophthalmologists between 2000-2005.[3]

Retinal Dysplasia: Focal retinal dysplasia/folds, and geographic retinal dysplasia are recognized in the breed. The later can progress to retinal detachment and blindness. Reported in 2.42% of Swedish Vallhunds CERF-examined by veterinary ophthalmologists between 2000-2005.[3]

The Breed History

It is believed that the Swedish Vallhund goes back more than 1000 years to the days of the Vikings. During the eighth or ninth century, historians state, either the Swedish Vallhund was brought to Wales or the Corgi was taken to Sweden, hence the similarities between the two breeds. By 1942, the breed was almost extinct, and a breeding program was started. In 1948, the Swedish Kennel Club recognized the breed. In 1974, the first Swedish Vallhund came to England, and the Swedish Vallhund Society received approval from the UK Kennel Club in 1980. The first litter was born in the US in 1986. The breed received AKC recognition in 2007.

Breeding for Function

The Swedish Vallhund is a small, powerful, fearless, sturdily built Spitz herding dog. Swedish Vallhunds are bred to work on farms and ranches as a cattle/sheep herder. Their herding style is low to the ground and they herd by rounding up and nipping at the hocks.

Physical Characteristics

Height at Withers: female 11.5 - 12.5" (29-32 cm), male 12.5 - 13.5" (32-34.5 cm)

Weight: 25-35 lbs. (11.5-16 kg).

Coat: Medium length hair, harsh; topcoat close and tight. Undercoat is soft and dense. Hair is short on the head and the foreparts of the legs and slightly longer on the neck, chest and back parts of the hind legs. A sable pattern is seen in colors of grey through red. Dark muzzle/mask. White is permitted as a narrow blaze, neck spot, slight necklace, and white markings on the legs, and chest. White can not be in excess of one third of the dog's total color.

Longevity: 12-14 years.

Points of Conformation: The relationship of height to length of body should be 2:3. Viewed from above, the head forms an even wedge from skull to tip of the nose and is well filled-in under the eyes. The eyes are medium size, oval in shape and dark brown with black eye rims. Prick ears. Viewed from the side, the muzzle should look rather square, slightly shorter than the skull. Scissors bite. Tails may be long, stub, or bob. Dewclaws may be removed. The gait is sound with strong reach and drive.

Hypothyroidism: Inherited autoimmune thyroiditis. Too few Swedish Vallhunds have been tested for thyroid autoantibodies at Michigan State University to determine an accurate breed frequency. (Ave. for all breeds is 7.5%).[4,5]

Cryptorchidism (Retained Testicles): Can be bilateral or unilateral. Reported as a breed problem on the SVCA website.

Missing Teeth: Congenital absence of teeth, usually involving premolars. Reported as a breed problem on the SVCA website.

Isolated Case Studies
None Reported

Genetic Tests
Tests of Genotype: none

Tests of Phenotype: CHIC Certification: Hip radiograph and CERF eye examination. (See CHIC website; www.caninehealthinfo.org).

Recommend elbow radiographs, patella evaluation, thyroid profile including autoantibodies, and cardiac examination.

Miscellaneous
- **Breed name synonyms:** Vasgotaspets, Swedish Cattle Dog, Viking Dog, Spitz of the West Goths
- **Registries:** AKC, CKC, UKC, KCGB (Kennel Club of Great Britain), ANKC (Australian National Kennel Club), NKC (National Kennel Club), FCI.
- **AKC rank (year 2008):** 149 (67 dogs registered)
- **Internet resources: Swedish Vallhund Club of America:** http://swedishvallhund.com
  Swedish Vallhund Club of Canada: www.swedishvallhundclubofcanada.com
  Swedish Vallhund Society (UK): www.swedishvallhunds.co.uk

References
1. Evans KM & Adams VJ: Proportion of litters of purebred dogs born by caesarean section. J Small Anim Pract. 2010 Feb;51(2):113-8.
2. OFA Website breed statistics: www.offa.org Last accessed July 1, 2010.
3. *Ocular Disorders Presumed to be Inherited in Purebred Dogs.* American College of Veterinary Ophthalmologists. ACVO, 2007.
4. Nachreiner RF, Refsal KR, Graham PA, et. al.: Prevalence of serum thyroid hormone autoantibodies in dogs with clinical signs of hypothyroidism. *J Am Vet Med Assoc* 2002 Feb 15;220(4):466-71.
5. Nachreiner R & Refsal K: Personal communication, Diagnostic Center for Population and Animal Health, Michigan State University. April, 2007.
6. *The Complete Dog Book, 20th Ed.* The American Kennel Club. Howell Book House, NY 2006. p. 706-709.

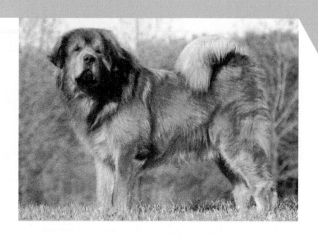

Tibetan Mastiff

is embellished by a mane. The head is held high. The stop is prominent. A curved tail is carried high over the dorsum, and is not longer than the hock when measured. Moderate flews are acceptable, and the facial skin may be somewhat wrinkled in the mature animal. Wide set almond shaped eyes are pigmented brown, and not prominent. Ears are triangular, covered with short hair, with thick leather, and hanging to the head when resting, but high set and carried high when active. A scissor or level bite is acceptable. Some dewlap may be present. Straight level back, and thorax deep and broad but not barrel. The abdomen is tucked up. The dog has low set hocks, and tight large strong compact feet. A TM may single track during motion. Single dewclaws are present on the forefeet, single or double may be present on the hind feet. Rear dewclaw removal is optional.

The Breed History
These massive quintessential guardians originated in Tibet, and were traditional guards of home and monastery. Though used for livestock defense, they are territory guardians first and foremost. Some consider these dogs to have been the original Mastiff-type dog which was exported to develop other versions of the mastiff in Europe and the various mountain dogs. The first Mastiff is thought to have arrived in England around 1847, with a pair arriving around 1874. The year 1931 marked the first recognition of the breed in the UK kennel club. In the early 1970s, breeding stock was introduced to the US. Because of the nomadic life style of the Tibetans, regional variations in type occurred, so variation in conformation and size is a hallmark of the native stock. The AKC accepted the breed as its 155th in 2006. DNA analysis suggests that the breed is more ancient than other domestic dog breeds, diverging from the grey wolf lineage approximately 58,000 years ago.[1]

Breeding for Function
The Himalayas are a harsh mountainous region, with extremes of temperature and terrain. These hardy strong dogs were bred exclusively for guardian function and to withstand the rigors of their environment.

Physical Characteristics
Height at Withers: males 26-30in." (66-76cm), females 24-28 in. (61-71 cm)

Weight: males 100-165 lbs. (45-72.5 kg) females 75-120 lbs. (34-54.5 kg)

Coat: Haircoat is thick, double, with wooly undercoat and stiff outer hairs that are not curly. Feathering is present on the tail and breeches. Colors accepted include black, black and tan, chocolate brown, gray or dilutes. White markings OK in specified locations.

Longevity: Lifespan is long for a giant breed (10+ years).

Points of Conformation: Only slightly longer than tall this is an extremely agile dog, powerful and impressive for its' size and substance. The massive broad skull has a prominent massive occipital protuberance, typical of a heavily boned animal. The muzzle is broad and square, and the well muscled neck

Recognized Behavior Issues and Traits
Loyal to family and home, these dogs are generally aloof with strangers. Dogs of this breed need plenty of exercise and some people contact. They are too intelligent to be left alone and can be very destructive if bored and lonely. Lots of room in the home to accommodate their large stature, and plenty of room outdoors to run are essential. Can night bark. Instinct for protection of home is strong. Socialize with children early. High intelligence and strong independence makes them a tougher dog to train than some. Some refer to them as having a strong stubborn streak. Early socialization and plenty of training is essential. Crate training is important so the dog learns to be alone and comfortable in a safe "den". Highly territorial, these dogs will defend vigorously. May be quite dominant with other dogs, and must be supervised when introduced to new people or animals to prevent possible mishaps. They are capable climbers, so a high sturdy fence is necessary. Not for off leash, these independent dogs may not come when called. A dog may not allow visitors into a home without introduction so caution is needed if children come to play. Can be destructive, especially when young; with their strong jaws, they can chew extensively. Needs daily brushing while blowing their coat using a rake, otherwise a weekly slicker brush is usually adequate. Moderate exercise requirements—are less active indoors, more active outdoors.

Normal Physiologic Variations
Females have a once yearly estrus, usually in fall.

They shed once a year in the spring (4-8 weeks).

Drug Sensitivities
None reported

Inherited Diseases
Hip Dysplasia: Polygenically inherited trait causing degenerative joint disease and hip arthritis. OFA reports 14.2% affected.[2]

Elbow Dysplasia: Polygenically inherited trait causing elbow arthritis. OFA reports 11.9% affected.[2]

Patella Luxation: Polygenically inherited laxity of patellar ligaments, causing luxation, lameness, and later degenerative joint disease. Treat surgically if causing clinical signs. Too few Tibetan Mastiffs have been screened by OFA to determine an accurate frequency.[2]

Progressive Retinal Atrophy (PRA): Autosomal recessive progressive degeneration of the retina leading to blindness. There is no test for carriers.[3]

Hypertrophic Neuropathy (Canine Inherited Demyelinative Neuropathy (CIDN)): An autosomal recessive neurological disorder causing generalized weakness with hyporeflexia between 6-10 weeks of age. Most affected dogs die by nine months, although some that do not develop limb contractures can became clinically stable for long periods. There is no test for carriers.[4,5]

Disease Predispositions

Hypothyroidism: Inherited autoimmune thyroiditis is reported in the breed. 10.2% positive for thyroid autoantibodies based on testing at Michigan State University. (Ave. for all breeds is 7.5%).[6,7]

Osteochondrosis Dessicans (OCD) of the Shoulder: Inherited cartilage defect of the shoulder joint, causes lameness in young growing dogs. More prevalent in males. Mild cases may heal on own with rest. Severe cases require surgery. Reported on the Tibetan Mastiff Club of America website.

Panosteitis: A self-limiting disease involving the diaphyseal and metaphyseal areas of the tubular long bones, characterized by medullary fibrosis and both endosteal and subperiosteal new bone deposition. Affected dogs show intermittent lameness. Reported on the Tibetan Mastiff Club of America website.

Idiopathic Epilepsy: Inherited seizures can be generalized or partial seizures. Unknown mode of inheritance. Reported on the Tibetan Mastiff Club of America website.

Cataracts: Cataracts are reported in the breed. Location and age of onset are not reported. Undetermined mode of inheritance. Do not breed a Tibetan Mastiff with a cataract.[8]

Ocular Disorders: Too few Tibetan Mastiffs have been DERF examined to determine accurate frequencies for inherited ocular disorders.[9]

Demodicosis and **Factor VIII Deficiency** are reported.[10]

Isolated Case Studies
None Reported

Genetic Tests

Tests of Genotype: Direct tests for coat color are available from VetGen.

Tests of Phenotype: CHIC Certification: Required tests are; CERF eye examination, hip radiographs, and thyroid profile, including autoantibodies. Optional recommended test is elbow radiographs. (See CHIC website: www.caninehealthinfo.org)

Recommend patella evaluation and cardiac examination.

Miscellaneous

- **Breed name synonyms:** Do-Khyi, for the smaller herding type, the name Tsang-Khyi is used for the most massive type. TM.
- **Registries:** UKC, AKC, CKC, FCI, KCGB (Kennel Club of Great Britain)
- **AKC rank (year 2008):** 128 (210 registered)
- **Internet resources: American Tibetan Mastiff Association:** www.tibetanmastiff.org
  Canadian Tibetan Mastiff Society: www.canadatms.org
  Tibetan Mastiff Club of Great Britian: www.tmcgb.net

References

1. Li Q, Liu Z, Li Y, et. al.: Origin and phylogenetic analysis of Tibetan Mastiff based on the mitochondrial DNA sequence. J Genet Genomics. 2008 Jun;35(6):335-40.
2. OFA Website breed statistics: www.offa.org Last accessed July 1, 2010.
3. Dekomien G, Epplen JT: Exclusion of the PDE6A gene for generalised progressive retinal atrophy in 11 breeds of dog. Anim Genet. 2000 Mar;31(2):135-9.
4. Cummings JF, Cooper BJ, de Lahunta A, et. al.: Canine inherited hypertrophic neuropathy. Acta Neuropathol (Berl). 1981;53(2):137-43.
5. Sponenberg DP, deLahunta A: Hereditary hypertrophic neuropathy in Tibetan Mastiff dogs. J Hered. 1981 Jul-Aug;72(4):287.
6. Nachreiner RF, Refsal KR, Graham PA, et. al.: Prevalence of serum thyroid hormone autoantibodies in dogs with clinical signs of hypothyroidism. J Am Vet Med Assoc 2002 Feb 15;220(4):466-71.
7. Nachreiner R & Refsal K: Personal communication, Diagnostic Center for Population and Animal Health, Michigan State University. April, 2007.
8. Mellersh C: Identifying Mutations Associated with HC in the Dog. Proceedings, 2009 Tufts' Canine and Feline Breeding and Genetics Conference. 2009.
9. *Ocular Disorders Presumed to be Inherited in Purebred Dogs.* American College of Veterinary Ophthalmologists. ACVO, 2007.
10. *The Genetic Connection: A Guide to Health Problems in Purebred Dogs.* L Ackerman. p. 221. AAHA Press, 1999.
11. *The Complete Dog Book, 20th Ed.* The American Kennel Club. Howell Book House, NY 2006. p.710-714.

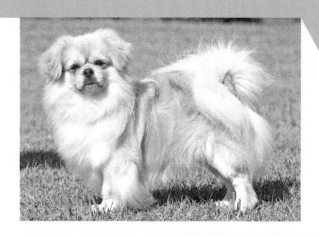

The Breed History

Tibetan Spaniels can be found in over 2000 years of recorded history. This breed was highly esteemed in the Tibetan Monasteries, and these dogs nicknamed "Lion dog" were frequently given as gifts—never sold to visiting dignitaries. The Pekingese and Japanese Chin may be relatives of this dog. First exports to England occurred in the late 1800s, and export to America occurred in the year 1965. Breed registry with the AKC was established in 1984.

Breeding for Function

These dogs functioned as monastery watchdogs and companions. These are not true hunting spaniels.

Physical Characteristics

Height at Withers: 10" (25.4 cm)

Weight: 9-15 lb (4-7 kg)

Coat: The double coat is flat, silky, of moderate length and furnishings are present. Males have a more pronounced ruff. White markings are accepted on the feet and all colors and color mixes are allowed.

Longevity: 13-15 years

Points of Conformation: The Tibetan spaniels are longer than tall, have very high head carriage, and a small head. The oval eyes are dark brown and medium-sized, wide set and set facing forward, and the palpebral margins are black. The ears are pendulous, high set, well feathered and medium in size. The skull is lightly domed, the stop defined, muzzle blunt and moderate in length, and the nose should be pigmented black. The normal bite is somewhat prognathic, and the neck is short and strong. The topline is level, and thorax deep and round. The tail is plumed, high set, and when active sits curled over the back. The bone is moderately heavy, muscling moderate, and the forelimbs are slightly bowed. Dewclaws may be taken off. They move with quick strides and low elastic movement.

Recognized Behavior Issues and Traits

Reported breed attributes include: Alarm barkers, friendly, active-high energy, cat-like disposition, loyal, intelligent, good temperament but assertive and aloof with strangers. They need close human companionship. Noted for being calm and easily trained. They have low grooming needs.

Normal Physiologic Variations

None reported

Drug Sensitivities

None reported

Inherited Diseases

Patella Luxation: Polygenically inherited laxity of patellar ligaments, causing luxation, lameness, and later degenerative joint disease. Treat surgically if causing clinical signs. OFA reports 9.4% affected. Reported at a frequency of 3.1% in the 2006 TSCA Health Survey.[1,2]

Elbow Dysplasia: Polygenically inherited trait causing elbow arthritis. OFA reports 7.9% affected.[1]

Hip Dysplasia: Polygenically inherited trait causing degenerative joint disease and hip arthritis. OFA reports 7.9% affected.[1]

Progressive Retinal Atrophy (PRA): Autosomal recessive degeneration of the retina causing blindness, usually between 1.5 to 4 years of age, but as late as 7 years of age. Ophthalmoscopic diagnosis can be difficult due to the partial or total lack of the tapetum in some dogs. Identified in 0.45% of Tibetan Spaniels CERF examined by veterinary ophthalmologists between 2000-2005. CERF does not recommend breeding any Tibetan Spaniel with PRA. There is no genetic test.[3,4]

Disease Predispositions

Hernias: Congenital abdominal wall opening. Requires surgery if large. Umbilical hernia is reported at a frequency of 25.5%, and Inguinal hernia 4.25% in the 2006 TSCA Health Survey.[2]

Prolapsed Gland of the Nictitans (Cherry Eye): This condition occurs secondary to inflammation of the gland. Reported at a frequency of 16.0% in the 2006 TSCA Health Survey.[2]

Retained Deciduous Teeth: Failure to lose deciduous teeth on eruption of permanent teeth. Canines are most frequently affected. Reported at a frequency of 11.0% in the 2006 TSCA Health Survey.[2]

Distichiasis: Abnormally placed eyelashes that irritate the cornea and conjunctiva. Can cause secondary corneal ulceration. Identified in 6.97% of Tibetan Spaniels CERF examined by veterinary ophthalmologists between 2000-2005. Reported at a frequency of 6.0% in the 2006 TSCA Health Survey.[2,4]

Hypothyroidism: Inherited autoimmune thyroiditis. 6.0% positive for thyroid autoantibodies based on testing at Michigan State University. (Ave. for all breeds is 7.5%).[5,6]

Entropion: Rolling in of eyelids, often causing corneal irritation or ulceration. Entropion is reported in 4.82% of Tibetan Spaniels CERF examined by veterinary ophthalmologists between 2000-2005.[4]

Intervertebral Disc Disease (IVDD): Spinal cord disease due to prolapsed disk material. Requires immediate veterinary attention. Clinical signs include back pain, scuffing of paws, spinal ataxia, limb weakness, and paralysis. Reported at a frequency of 2.8% in the 2006 TSCA Health Survey.[2]

Portosystemic Shunt (PSS, Liver Shunt): Undetermined mode of inheritance. Abnormal blood vessels connecting the systemic and portal blood flow. Vessels can be intrahepatic, extrahepatic, or microvascular dysplasia. Causes stunting, abnormal behavior and possible seizures. Diagnose with paired fasting and post-meal bile acids +/- blood ammonia, and abdominal ultrasound. Reported at a frequency of 2.5% in the 2006 TSCA Health Survey.[2]

Allergic Dermatitis: Inhalant or food allergy. Presents with pruritis and pyotraumatic dermatitis (hot spots). Reported at a frequency of 2.4% in the 2006 TSCA Health Survey.[2]

Cataracts: Anterior cortex intermediate and punctate cataracts predominate in the breed. Identified in 2.25% of Tibetan Spaniels CERF examined by veterinary ophthalmologists between 2000-2005. CERF does not recommend breeding any Tibetan Spaniel with a cataract.[4]

Brachycephalic Complex: Can cause dyspnea, and collapse. Includes Elongated Soft Palate, Stenotic Nares, Hypoplastic Trachea, and Everted Laryngeal Saccules. Surgery is indicated in severe cases. Reported at a frequency of 1.65% in the 2006 TSCA Health Survey.[2]

Persistent Pupillary Membranes: Strands of fetal remnant connecting; iris to iris, cornea, lens, or involving sheets of tissue. The later three forms can impair vision, and dogs affected with these forms should not be bred. Identified in 1.54% of Tibetan Spaniels CERF examined by veterinary ophthalmologists between 2000-2005.[4]

Cryptorchidism (Retained Testicles): Can be unilateral or bilateral. Reported at a frequency of 1.45% in the 2006 TSCA Health Survey.[2]

Cystinuria/Cystine Bladder Stones: Tibetan Spaniels have an increased risk for developing cystine bladder stones due to a defect in cystine metabolism. Treat with surgical removal and life-long medical therapy. Unknown mode of inheritance in this breed.[7]

Demodicosis: Case studies suggest a breed predisposition for demodex mite dermatitis. The generalized disorder has an underlying immunodeficiency in its pathogenesis. Unknown mode of inheritance.[8,9]

Brachygnathism, Epilepsy, Micropapilla, Microphthalmia, Optic nerve hypoplasia, PDA, Prognathism, and **Retinal Dysplasia** are reported.[10]

Isolated Case Studies

Oxalate Nephropathy: Severe oxalate nephropathy with end-stage kidney lesions was found in two pups of a litter of three Tibetan Spaniels. This histopathologic finding strongly suggests a primary hyperoxaluria since there was no exposure to agents capable of producing secondary hyperoxaluria.[11]

Genetic Tests
Tests of Genotype: none

Tests of Phenotype: CHIC Certification: CERF eye examination and patella evaluation. (See CHIC website; www.caninehealthinfo.org).

Recommend hip and elbow radiographs, thyroid profile including autoantibodies, and cardiac examination.

Miscellaneous
- **Breed name synonyms:** Tibbie, Tibby
- **Registries:** AKC, UKC, CKC, KCGB (Kennel Club of Great Britain), ANKC (Australian National Kennel Club)
- **AKC rank (year 2008):** 104 (432 dogs registered)
- **Internet resources: Tibetan Spaniel Club of America:** www.tsca.ws
  Tibetan Spaniel Association (UK): www.tsauk.freeserve.co.uk

References

1. OFA Website breed statistics: www.offa.org Last accessed July 1, 2010.
2. De A & Tibetan Spaniel Club of America: 2006 Tibetan Spaniel Club of America Health Survey. October 8, 2006.
3. Bjerkas E, Narfstrom K: Progressive retinal atrophy in the Tibetan spaniel in Norway and Sweden. *Vet Rec.* 1994 Apr 9;134(15):377-9.
4. *Ocular Disorders Presumed to be Inherited in Purebred Dogs.* American College of Veterinary Ophthalmologists. ACVO, 2007.
5. Nachreiner RF, Refsal KR, Graham PA, et. al.: Prevalence of serum thyroid hormone autoantibodies in dogs with clinical signs of hypothyroidism. *J Am Vet Med Assoc* 2002 Feb 15;220(4):466-71.
6. Nachreiner R & Refsal K: Personal communication, Diagnostic Center for Population and Animal Health, Michigan State University. April, 2007.
7. Hoppe A, Denneberg T: Cystinuria in the dog: clinical studies during 14 years of medical treatment. *J Vet Intern Med.* 2001 Jul-Aug;15(4):361-7.
8. Knottenbelt MK: Chronic otitis externa due to Demodex canis in a Tibetan spaniel. Vet Rec. 1994 Oct 22;135(17):409-10.
9. Nayak DC, Tripathy SB, Dey PC, et. al.: Prevalence of canine demodicosis in Orissa (India). *Vet Parasitol.* 1997 Dec 31;73(3-4):347-52.
10. *The Genetic Connection: A Guide to Health Problems in Purebred Dogs.* L Ackerman. p. 241-42. AAHA Press, 1999.
11. Jansen JH, Arnesen K: Oxalate nephropathy in a Tibetan spaniel litter. A probable case of primary hyperoxaluria. *J Comp Pathol.* 1990 Jul;103(1):79-84.
12. *The Complete Dog Book, 20th Ed.* The American Kennel Club. Howell Book House, NY 2006. p. 597-601.

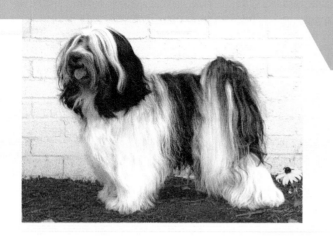

The Breed History

History records that this breed has existed for about 2000 years and that they were monastery dogs for most of this time. Considered good luck, they were given as gifts—never sold. The first dogs arrived in America in 1956. They are not terriers, but this term was applied because they were in the terrier range for size. Common names used in Tibet included "Holy dog" or "luck bringer dog", and because of their highly esteemed position as a lucky charm, outbreeding was unheard of. First registration in the AKC occurred in 1973. In general type, they resemble the Llasa Apso.

Breeding for Function

These dogs were bred for companionship and as monastery watchdogs. They may have been used to herd, though this was not their primary function.

Physical Characteristics

Height at Withers: female 14-15" (35.5-38 cm), male 15-16" (38-40.5 cm)

Weight: 20-24 lb (9-11 kg) ideally, though can range from 18-30 lb (8-13.5 kg)

Coat: It is a profuse double coat, the feet are well haired (snowshoe feet), and lots of hair falls over eyes and face. The undercoat is wooly and soft, the outer coat hairs are straight or wavy, fine in texture, and though long, the coat should not reach the ground. Colors include golden, sable, cream, silver, white and black in solid and parti-color.

Longevity: 13-15 years

Points of Conformation: Compact and squarely built, their high set medium length tail curls over the back and is well feathered. It is acceptable for the tail to be kinked at the tip. The feet are large and flat, with long hair between toes and over the feet. The skull is domed and moderate in width with a well-defined stop. The nose is black, eyes are dark brown and moderately deep-set, palpebral margins are dark and the eyelashes long. Ears are pendulous, triangular and well feathered. The topline is level, and heavy furnishings occur on the chest and legs. The ribs are well sprung, thorax is of moderate depth, limbs straight boned, and dewclaws may be removed. The gait is agile and smooth, with good drive.

Tibetan Terrier

Recognized Behavior Issues and Traits

Reported attributes of the breed include: Intelligent, friendly, very good with children, can be aloof with strangers, loyal, low exercise needs, fairly easily trained, and a good alert barker. They have moderate grooming requirements and low doggy odor and they are considered low shedders. Tibetan terriers are adaptable to country or city living, including apartments. They have calm personalities but enjoy play activities.

Normal Physiologic Variations

None reported

Drug Sensitivities

None reported

Inherited Diseases

Patella Luxation: Polygenically inherited laxity of patellar ligaments, causing luxation, lameness, and later degenerative joint disease. Treat surgically if causing clinical signs. OFA reports 7.8% affected.[1]

Hip Dysplasia: Polygenically inherited trait causing degenerative joint disease and hip arthritis. OFA reports 5.8% affected.[1]

Elbow Dysplasia: Polygenically inherited trait causing elbow arthritis. OFA reports 3.9% affected.[1]

Ceroid Lipofuscinosis (CL, Neuronal Ceroid Lipofuscinosis, NCL): Autosomal recessive, slowly progressive disorder beginning with retinal degeneration and nyctalopia from 3-6 years of age. Affected dogs then progress to cerebellar ataxia and dementia. Reported at a frequency of 1.0% in the 2003 TTCA Health Survey. A genetic test is available.[2,3,4,5,6]

Primary Lens Luxation (PLL) and Secondary Glaucoma: An autosomal recessive primary lens luxation occurs in the breed due to abnormalities of the suspensory apparatus of the lens (zonule). Homozygous affected dogs usually develop lens luxation between 3 to 8 years of age, but has been seen as early as 14 months. Rarely, heterozygous carriers can develop lens luxation, but at a later age. Often progresses to secondary glaucoma. Relative risk of 3.69x versus other breeds. Identified in 0.32% of Tibetan Terriers CERF examined by veterinary ophthalmologists between 2000-2005. CERF does not recommend breeding any Tibetan Terrier with lens luxation. A genetic mutation has been identified, and a genetic test is available. OFA testing shows 27% carrier, and 1% affected.[5,7,8,9,10,11]

Progressive Retinal Atrophy (PRA): An autosomal recessive, early onset form of PRA occurs in the breed. Causes progressive blindness, beginning with night blindness at approximately 1 year of age. Identified in 0.49% of Tibetan Terriers CERF examined by veterinary ophthalmologists between 2000-2005. CERF does not recommend breeding any Tibetan Terrier with PRA. There is no genetic test.[8,12,13]

Disease Predispositions

Hypothyroidism: Inherited autoimmune thyroiditis. 17.7% positive for thyroid autoantibodies based on testing at Michigan State University. (Ave. for all breeds is 7.5%).[14,15]

Allergic Dermatitis: Inhalant or food allergy. Presents with pruritis and pyotraumatic dermatitis (hot spots). Reported at an increased frequency versus other breeds. Reported at a frequency of 7.9% in the 2003 TTCA Health Survey.[15,16]

Umbilical Hernia: Congenital opening of the body wall at the umbilicus. Requires surgical closure if large. Reported at a frequency of 5.5% in the 2003 TTCA Health Survey. Unknown mode of inheritance.[5]

Persistent Pupillary Membranes: Strands of fetal remnant connecting; iris to iris, cornea, lens, or involving sheets of tissue. The later three forms can impair vision, and dogs affected with these forms should not be bred. Identified in 4.91% of Tibetan Terriers CERF examined by veterinary ophthalmologists between 2000-2005.[8]

Deafness: Congenital sensorineural deafness can be unilateral of bilateral. Diagnosed by BAER testing. Reported at a frequency of 3.1% in the 2003 TTCA Health Survey. Unknown mode of inheritance.[5,17]

Missing Teeth: Reported at a frequency of 2.6% in the 2003 TTCA Health Survey. Unknown mode of inheritance.[5]

Cataracts: Anterior cortex punctate cataracts predominate in the breed. Non-congenital cataracts have a heritability of 0.13, and are 76% correlated to PRA in the breed. Reported in 5.92% of Tibetan Terriers presented to veterinary teaching hospitals. Cataracts between 2-7 years of age are reported at a frequency of 2.2% in the 2003 TTCA Health Survey. Identified in 2.39% of Tibetan Terriers CERF examined by veterinary ophthalmologists between 2000-2005. Unknown mode of inheritance. CERF does not recommend breeding any Tibetan Terrier with a cataract.[5,8,18,19]

Distichiasis: Abnormally placed eyelashes that irritate the cornea and conjunctiva. Can cause secondary corneal ulceration. Identified in 1.47% of Tibetan Terriers CERF examined by veterinary ophthalmologists between 2000-2005.[8]

Corneal Dystrophy: Epithelial/stromal form of corneal opacities. Identified in 1.47% of Tibetan Terriers CERF examined by veterinary ophthalmologists between 2000-2005.[8]

Diabetes Mellitus: Sugar diabetes due to immune mediated destruction of the pancreatic beta cells. Treat with insulin injections, diet, and glucose monitoring. Identified as a breed at increased risk of developing diabetes.[20,21]

Idiopathic Epilepsy: Inherited seizures can be generalized or partial seizures. Control with anticonvulsant medication. Reported at a frequency of 0.5% in the 2003 TTCA Health Survey.[5]

Renal Dysplasia: Affected dogs can succumb to renal failure from birth to two years of age. Mildly affected dogs can live with compensated renal insufficiency. A direct genetic test for a dominant susceptibility gene is available. (Affected dogs all have one copy of the gene, but most dogs with the gene will not develop kidney failure.)

Vestibular Disease: An inherited, congenital unilateral peripheral vestibular syndrome occurs in the breed. Clinical signs include head tilt, circling, and ataxia. Unknown mode of inheritance.[22,23]

Hemophagocytic Syndrome: Proliferative disorder of activated macrophages that is associated with multiple blood cytopenias. Can be idiopathic, or secondary to infectious, neoplastic, or immune-mediated diseases. Can be fatal depending on the underlying disease. The Tibetan Terrier breed is overrepresented in dogs with the condition.[24]

Brachygnathism, Polydontia, Prognathism, Retinal Dysplasia, and **von Willebrand's Disease** are reported.[25]

Isolated Case Studies

Recurrent Flank Alopecia (Seasonal Flank Alopecia): Case report of a 2-year-old, male, neutered Tibetan Terrier with winter flank alopecia. The disorder is characterized by episodes of truncal non-scarring alopecia (and often hyperpigmentation) that usually occur on a recurrent, seasonal basis. Diagnosis is by clinical signs and biopsy.[26]

Malignant Histiocytosis: An 8-year-old male Tibetan Terrier showed prolonged astasia, complete paralysis, tic-like signs, and seizure and died 2 months after the onset of symptoms. Histopathologic diagnosis was diffuse leptomeningeal malignant histiocytosis of the brain and spinal cord.[27]

Genetic Tests

Tests of Genotype: A direct test for NCL is available from the OFA.

A direct test for PLL is available from the OFA and Animal Health Trust.

A direct test for a dominant renal dysplasia susceptibility gene is available from Dogenes.

Tests of Phenotype: CHIC Certification: Required testing includes hip radiographs, annual CERF eye examination and BAER testing for deafness. Recommended tests include patella evaluation, elbow radiographs, and thyroid profile including autoantibodies. (See CHIC website; www.caninehealthinfo.org).

Recommended cardiac examination.

Miscellaneous

- **Breed name synonyms:** Dhokhi Apso
- **Registries:** AKC, UKC, CKC, KCGB (Kennel Club of Great Britain), ANKC (Australian National Kennel Club)
- **AKC rank (year 2008):** 96 (626 dogs registered)
- **Internet resources:** Tibetan Terrier Club of America: www.ttca-online.org
  Tibetan Terrier Club of Canada: www.tibetanterriercanada.com
  Tibetan Terrier Association of the U.K.: www.the-tta.org.uk

References

1. OFA Website breed statistics: www.offa.org Last accessed July 1, 2010.

2. Katz ML, Narfstrom K, Johnson GS, et. al.: Assessment of retinal function and characterization of lysosomal storage body accumulation in the retinas and brains of Tibetan Terriers with ceroid-lipofuscinosis. *Am J Vet Res.* 2005 Jan;66(1):67-76.

3. Riis RC, Cummings JF, Loew ER, et. al.: Tibetan terrier model of canine ceroid lipofuscinosis. *Am J Med Genet.* 1992 Feb 15;42(4):615-21.

4. Alroy J, Schelling SH, Thalhammer JG, et. al.: Adult onset lysosomal storage disease in a Tibetan terrier: clinical, morphological and biochemical studies. *Acta Neuropathol (Berl).* 1992;84(6):658-63.

5. Tibetan Terrier Club of America: 2003 TTCA Health Survey. 2004.

6. Katz ML, Sanders DN, Mooney BP, et. al.: Accumulation of glial fibrillary acidic protein and histone H4 in brain storage bodies of Tibetan terriers with hereditary neuronal ceroid lipofuscinosis. J Inherit Metab Dis. 2007 Nov;30(6):952-63.

7. Curtis R, Barnett KC, Lewis SJ: Clinical and pathological observations concerning the aetiology of primary lens luxation in the dog. *Vet Rec.* 1983 Mar 12;112(11):238-46.

8. *Ocular Disorders Presumed to be Inherited in Purebred Dogs.* American College of Veterinary Ophthalmologists. ACVO, 1999.

9. Curtis R: Lens luxation in the dog and cat. *Vet Clin North Am Small Anim Pract.* 1990 May;20(3):755-73.

10. Curtis R: Aetiopathological aspects of inherited lens dislocation in the Tibetan Terrier. *J Comp Pathol.* 1983 Jan;93(1):151-63.

11. Sargan DR, Withers D, Pettitt L, et. al.: Mapping the mutation causing lens luxation in several terrier breeds. J Hered. 2007;98(5):534-8.

12. Akhmedov NB, Baldwin VJ, Zangerl B, et. al.: Cloning and characterization of the canine photoreceptor specific cone-rod homeobox (CRX) gene and evaluation as a candidate for early onset photoreceptor diseases in the dog. *Mol Vis.* 2002 Mar 22;8:79-84.

13. Millichamp NJ, Curtis R, Barnett KC: Progressive retinal atrophy in Tibetan terriers. *J Am Vet Med Assoc.* 1988 Mar 15;192(6):769-76.

14. Nachreiner RF, Refsal KR, Graham PA, et. al.: Prevalence of serum thyroid hormone autoantibodies in dogs with clinical signs of hypothyroidism. *J Am Vet Med Assoc* 2002 Feb 15;220(4):466-71.

15. Nachreiner R & Refsal K: Personal communication, Diagnostic Center for Population and Animal Health, Michigan State University. April, 2007.

16. White SD: Update on Allergies: Atopic Dermatitis. Proceedings, Northeast Veterinary Conference 2004.

17. Strain GM: Deafness prevalence and pigmentation and gender associations in dog breeds at risk. *Vet J.* 2004 Jan;167(1):23-32.

18. Ketteritzsch K, Hamann H, Brahm R, et. al.: Genetic analysis of presumed inherited eye diseases in Tibetan Terriers. *Vet J.* 2004 Sep;168(2):151-9.

19. Gelatt KN, Mackay EO: Prevalence of primary breed-related cataracts in the dog in North America. Vet Ophthalmol. 2005 Mar-Apr;8(2):101-11.

20. Catchpole B, Ristic JM, Fleeman LM, et. al.: Canine diabetes mellitus: can old dogs teach us new tricks? *Diabetologia.* 2005 Oct;48(10):1948-56.

21. Catchpole B, Kennedy LJ, Davison LJ, et. al.: Canine diabetes mellitus: from phenotype to genotype. J Small Anim Pract. 2008 Jan;49(1):4-10.

22. Ter Haar G: Diseases of the Middle and Inner Ear. Proceedings, 2005 World Small Animal Veterinary Association Congress. 2005.

23. Bower JM: Head tilt in Tibetan terrier puppies. *Vet Rec.* 1983 Jan 8;112(2):46.

24. Weiss DJ: Hemophagocytic syndrome in dogs: 24 cases (1996-2005). J Am Vet Med Assoc. 2007 Mar 1;230(5):697-701.

25. *The Genetic Connection: A Guide to Health Problems in Purebred Dogs.* L Ackerman. p. 242. AAHA Press, 1999.

26. Bassett RJ, Burton GG, Robson DC: Recurrent flank alopecia in a Tibetan Terrier. *Aust Vet J.* 2005 May;83(5):276-9.

27. Uchida K, Morozumi M, Yamaguchi R, et. al.: Diffuse leptomeningeal malignant histiocytosis in the brain and spinal cord of a Tibetan Terrier. *Vet Pathol.* 2001 Mar;38(2):219-22.

28. *The Complete Dog Book, 20th Ed.* The American Kennel Club. Howell Book House, NY 2006. p. 602-605.

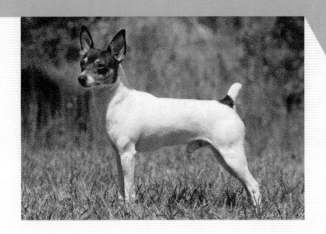

The Breed History

The breed was developed in the US by crossing a number of toy breed dogs. Foundation breeds include Manchester terrier, Miniature Pinschers, Chihuahua, and obviously, a fox terrier (Smooth Fox). Beginning in the 1930's, breeders carefully crossed to a number of toy breeds to calm the personality a bit, but keep the touch of spunk, and the look of the Smooth fox.

The AKC fully recognized the Toy Fox Terrier breed in 2003, as its 148th breed, in the Toy division.

Breeding for Function

The goal of breed development was to produce a small fox terrier, with temperament well suited for a close companion, house dog. The terrier base of the breed makes them well suited to trials of agility and they are well suited to obedience, and even retain their love of hunting and will flush targets out of holes. Animated movement, fit and agile, strong and excellent endurance characterize these spunky little dogs.

Physical Characteristics

Height at Withers: Ideal 9-11" (23-28 cm), 8.5-11.5 in. (21.5-29 cm) accepted.

Weight: 3.5-7 lbs. (1.5-3 kg.)

Coat: A short, shiny coat which may be a bit longer at the ruff. Soft hair texture. Patterns vary, but body is mostly white and head is mostly solid. Tricolor black, tan and white with defined marking size and location described by the breed standard. Other tri-colors include chocolate/tan/white. Bi-colors include white and tan, white and chocolate, and white and black.

Longevity: 13-14 years

Points of Conformation: Square conformation, strong bone but not coarse. A soft wedge, the skull is moderate in size, stop is moderate, muzzle parallel to top of skull. Head is refined, with an alert expression, ears are prick and close/high set, with a v-shaped pinna. Ears can take up to 6 months to fully prick. Palpebral margins are black or self in chocolates, round prominent wide set eyes are dark in color. Nose also black or self in chocolates. Teeth scissors bite. High head carriage, the neck is tapered towards the head, and

Toy Fox Terrier

is not throaty. Well sloped shoulder and front of chest prominent. Level topline smoothly merges with tail, thorax is deep and ribs well sprung, abdomen has moderate tuck up. Limbs straight, the feet are compact and small, with oval shape and well knuckled up, dewclaws will usually be removed from rear limbs. Gait is long, low and smooth—topline remains straight. The tail is high set and usually docked to the 3-4th vertebra joint.

Recognized Behavior Issues and Traits

Reported characteristics include: Active, game and courageous, playful, high intelligence, a bit of toy - bit of terrier mixed in for personality and activity level, these little dogs stay playful late in life. Loving, with typical terrier devotion they are also adaptable, spirited and determined.

Normal Physiologic Variations

None Reported

Drug Sensitivities

None Reported

Inherited Diseases

Patella Luxation: Polygenically inherited laxity of patellar ligaments, causing luxation, lameness, and later degenerative joint disease. Treat surgically if causing clinical signs. Reported 12.8x odds ratio versus other breeds. OFA reports 4.2% affected. Reported as "commonly identified" in the TFT Health Survey.[1,2,3]

Hip Dysplasia and Legg-Calve Perthes Disease: Polygenically inherited traits causing degenerative hip joint disease and arthritis. Too few Toy Fox Terriers have been screened by OFA to determine an accurate frequency.[1]

Congenital Hypothyroidism with Goiter: An autosomal recessive disorder in Toy Fox Terriers. Neonatal affected pups exhibit inactivity, abnormal hair coat, stenotic ear canals, and delayed eye opening. Goiterous ventrolateral cervical swellings are evident by 1 week of age. Serum thyroid hormone and thyroid-stimulating hormone concentrations were low and high, respectively. Oral thyroid hormone replacement therapy restores near-normal growth and development. A nonsense mutation in the thyroid peroxidase gene causes the disorder. Reported as "commonly identified" in the TFT Health Survey. A genetic test is available.[2,4]

Primary Lens Luxation (PLL) and Secondary Glaucoma: An autosomal recessive gene causes primary lens luxation. Homozygous affected dogs usually develop lens luxation between 4-8 years of age. Rarely, heterozygous carriers can develop lens luxation, but at a later age. Lens luxation can lead to secondary glaucoma and blindness. A genetic mutation has been identified, and a genetic test is available. OFA testing shows 28% carrier, and 2% affected.[5]

Elbow Dysplasia: Polygenic trait causing elbow arthritis. Too few Toy Fox Terriers have been screened by OFA to determine an accurate frequency.[1]

Disease Predispositions

Cataracts: Too few Toy Fox Terriers have been CERF eye examined to determine an accurate frequency in the breed. Reported in 3.78% of Toy Fox Terriers presented to veterinary teaching hospitals.[6,7]

Hypothyroidism: Inherited autoimmune thyroiditis. 3.0% positive for thyroid autoantibodies based on testing at Michigan State University. (Ave. for all breeds is 7.5%).[8,9]

Food Allergies: Reported as "commonly identified" in the TFT Health Survey.[2]

Heart Valve Problems: Can cause congestive heart disease. Identified by auscultation or echocardiogram. Reported as "commonly identified" in the TFT Health Survey.[2]

von Willebrand's Disease (vWD): Mild bleeding disorder. Reported as "commonly identified" in the TFT Health Survey. A genetic test is not available for this breed.[2]

Cryptorchidism (Retained Testicles): Can be unilateral or bilateral. Reported as "commonly identified" in the TFT Health Survey.[2]

Eye Disorders: Too few Toy Fox Terriers have been CERF eye examined to determine accurate frequencies for eye disorders.[6]

Deafness: Congenital deafness can be unilateral of bilateral. Diagnosed by BAER testing. Unknown mode of inheritance.[10]

Demodicosis is also reported on the ATFTC website.

Isolated Case Studies

Immune-Mediated Diabetes Mellitus/Hemolytic Anemia:
A four-year-old, spayed female toy fox terrier presented with hyperglycemia and severe anemia. A diagnosis of immune-mediated diabetes mellitus was made based upon the finding of beta-cell specific antibodies. Immune-mediated hemolytic anemia was diagnosed based on findings of a regenerative anemia, spherocytosis, hyperbilirubinemia, hemoglobinuria, and bilirubinuria. The anemia resolved following two months of immunosuppressive therapy. The diabetes was treated with insulin for four months, after which time treatment was no longer necessary.[11]

Genetic Tests

Tests of Genotype: Direct test for Congenital Hypothyroidism is available from the Fyfe laboratory at Michigan State University: http://mmg.msu.edu/faculty/fyfe.htm (517-355-6463 x1559), HealthGene, and PennGen.

Direct test for PLL is available from the OFA and Animal Health Trust.

Tests of Phenotype: Recommend patella evaluation, hip and elbow radiographs, CERF eye examination, cardiac evaluation, and thyroid profile including autoantibodies.

Miscellaneous

- **Breed name synonyms:** American Toy
- **Registries:** AKC, UKC, CKC, NKC (National Kennel Club).
- **AKC rank (year 2008):** 88 (731 dogs registered)
- **Internet resources: American Toy Fox Terrier Club:** www.atftc.com
  Toy Fox Terrier Club of Canada: www.tftcc.ca

References

1. OFA Website breed statistics: www.offa.org Last accessed July 1 2010.
2. American Toy Fox Terrier Club: TFT Health Survey Results: Most Commonly Identified Problems. 2007.
3. LaFond E, Breur GJ & Austin CC: Breed susceptibility for developmental orthopedic diseases in dogs. J Am Anim Hosp Assoc. 2002 Sep-Oct;38(5):467-77.
4. Fyfe JC, Kampschmidt K, Dang V, et. al.: Congenital hypothyroidism with goiter in toy fox terriers. *J Vet Intern Med.* 2003 Jan-Feb;17(1):50-7.
5. Sargan DR, Withers D, Pettitt L, et. al.: Mapping the mutation causing lens luxation in several terrier breeds. J Hered. 2007;98(5):534-8.
6. *Ocular Disorders Presumed to be Inherited in Purebred Dogs.* American College of Veterinary Ophthalmologists. ACVO, 2007.
7. Gelatt KN, Mackay EO: Prevalence of primary breed-related cataracts in the dog in North America. Vet Ophthalmol. 2005 Mar-Apr;8(2):101-11.
8. Nachreiner RF, Refsal KR, Graham PA, et. al.: Prevalence of serum thyroid hormone autoantibodies in dogs with clinical signs of hypothyroidism. J Am Vet Med Assoc 2002 Feb 15;220(4):466-71.
9. Nachreiner R & Refsal K: Personal communication, Diagnostic Center for Population and Animal Health, Michigan State University. April, 2007.
10. Strain GM: Deafness prevalence and pigmentation and gender associations in dog breeds at risk. *Vet J.* 2004 Jan;167(1):23-32.
11. Elie M, Hoenig M: Canine immune-mediated diabetes mellitus: a case report. *J Am Anim Hosp Assoc.* 1995 Jul-Aug;31(4):295-9.
12. *The Complete Dog Book, 20th Ed.* The American Kennel Club. Howell Book House, NY 2006. p.517-520.

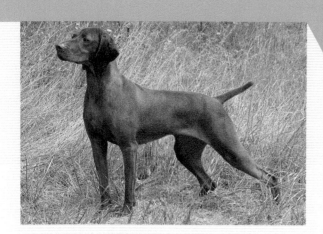

Vizsla

very straight, the feet are small and very compact and the toes are well arched. Dewclaws usually are removed if present. Gait is easy, long-strided, very animated and elastic, and they are nimble-footed. They will single track at a fast trot.

The Breed History

The Maygars who originally bred the ancestors of these dogs a millennium ago were a Central European people. They eventually colonized Hungary. The Vizsla first entered the history record formally in the 1200s, and the name in Hungarian means "pointer". It is thought that breeds such as the German Shorthaired Pointer, Pointer, Transylvanian Hound and perhaps others contributed to the bloodlines. During the World Wars, these dogs were almost rendered extinct. A few were exported out of the country and served to perpetuate the breed. They were brought to North America in the 50's and were admitted to the AKC in 1960.

Breeding for Function

Hunting dogs of exceptional speed, agility, good nose and stealth, they were bred for close work for bird and upland game hunting, and for waterfowl retrieving. They perform well in obedience trials and agility.

Physical Characteristics

Height at Withers: female 21-23" (53-58.5 cm), male 22-24" (56-61 cm)

Weight: females 40-55 lb (18-25 kg), males 45-60 lb (20.5-27 kg).

Coat: Their distinctively colored russet gold (golden rust) short dense glossy coat is the only color of the breed, though a narrow spectrum of shades is acceptable. Only very limited small white marking of chest or toes is acceptable. In Europe, a longhaired variety exists, and this haircoat is similar to the German Wirehaired Pointer coat. The longhaired variety is also recognized by the Canadian Kennel Club.

Longevity: 12-14 years.

Points of Conformation: These lithe dogs are medium-sized and regal in their carriage, the chiseled skull is of moderate conformation (mesocephalic), with moderate stop, square muzzle, brown nose, and long pendulous silky ears with very fine leather. Eyes should blend with the coat, but not be yellow. Moderate length and arch define the neck, and the back is short, and only towards the hind end does it gently round. A deep chest and well-sprung ribs meld into a lightly tucked loin. The tail is often docked to one-third length and is carried horizontally. The legs are

Recognized Behavior Issues and Traits

Reported breed characteristics include: Very active dogs, but they are also very gentle and affectionate and they make an excellent companion dog for an active outdoorsy family. They are considered highly trainable, but can be distracted more easily than some. They are naturally protective and crave close social contact with people. They are good alarm barkers and should be socialized early. They have very high exercise needs, and must be provided with regular exercise sessions to prevent boredom vices such as chewing. Avoid lines that are high strung or tend to dominance. Some dogs are prone to separation anxiety and thunderstorm anxiety. The coat needs minimal brushing, and shedding is low to average.

Normal Physiologic Variations
None reported

Drug Sensitivities
None reported

Inherited Diseases

Hip Dysplasia: Polygenically inherited trait causing degenerative joint disease and hip arthritis. OFA reports 7.1% affected.[1]

Elbow Dysplasia: Polygenically inherited trait causing elbow arthritis. OFA reports 2.2% affected.[1]

Patella Luxation: Polygenically inherited laxity of patellar ligaments, causing luxation, lameness, and later degenerative joint disease. Treat surgically if causing clinical signs. Too few Vizslas have been screened by OFA to determine an accurate frequency.[1]

Fibrinogen (Factor I) Deficiency: A rare, autosomal recessive fibrinogen deficiency occurs in the breed, producing severe bleeding early in life.[2]

Disease Predispositions

Anxiety: In the 2008 Vizsla Health Survey, 8.22% were reported with Storm Anxiety, 5.35% with Separation Anxiety, and 4.71% with Noise Anxiety.[5]

Hypothyroidism: Inherited autoimmune thyroiditis. 7.9% positive for thyroid autoantibodies based on testing at Michigan State University. (Ave. for all breeds is 7.5%).[3,4]

Allergies: Inhalant or food allergy. Presents with pruritis (itching) and pyotraumatic dermatitis (hot spots). Reported as a breed at increased risk in a Hungarian study. 6.99% were reported with Seasonal Allergies at a mean age of 1.9 years, and 4.79% with

Food Allergies at a mean age of 1.7 years in the 2008 Vizsla Health Survey.[5,6]

Demodicosis, Juvenile: Demodectic mange has an underlying immunodeficiency in its pathogenesis. Reported at a frequency of 6.27% in the the 2008 Vizsla Health Survey.[5]

Mast Cell Tumor (MCT): Skin tumors that produce histamine, causing inflammation and ulceration. They can reoccur locally or with distant metastasis. Reported at a frequency of 5.91% at a mean age of 6.4 years in the 2008 Vizsla Health Survey.[5]

Arthritis: 3.95% of Vizslas are reported with arthritis at a mean age of 8.3 years in the 2008 Vizsla Health Survey.[5]

Idiopathic Epilepsy: In Vizslas, epilepsy appears to be primarily (73% of affected dogs) a partial onset seizure disorder that can present with clinical signs of; limb tremors, staring, pupillary dilatation, or salivation without loss of consciousness. Average age of onset is 3 years. One study suggests a possible autosomal recessive mode of inheritance. Control with anticonvulsant medication. Reported at a frequency of 3.07% at a mean age of 2.8 years in the 2008 Vizsla Health Survey.[5,7]

Umbilical Hernia: Congenital opening of the body wall at the umbilicus. Should be closed surgically if large. Reported at a frequency of 3.03% in the 2008 Vizsla Health Survey.[5]

Persistent Pupillary Membranes: Strands of fetal remnant connecting; iris to iris, cornea, lens, or involving sheets of tissue. The later three forms can impair vision, and dogs affected with these forms should not be bred. Identified in 3.03% of Vizslas CERF-examined by veterinary ophthalmologists between 2000-2005.[8]

Hemangiosarcoma: Malignant cancer of red blood cells, usually involving the spleen, liver, heart, or bone marrow. Reported at a frequency of 2.91% at a mean age of 9.1 years in the 2008 Vizsla Health Survey.[5]

Cataracts: Anterior, posterior, intermediate and punctate cataracts occur in the breed. Identified in 2.84% of Vizslas CERF-examined by veterinary ophthalmologists between 2000-2005. CERF does not recommend breeding any Vizsla with a cataract.[8]

Heart Murmur: According to the 2008 Vizsla Health Survey, 1.84% of Vizsla are identified with a heart murmur at a mean age of 5.4 years. The valvular location of the murmur is not indicated.[5]

Lymphoma/Lymphosarcoma: Malignant cancer of lymphoid tissue. Can present as B-cell or T-cell (mycosis fungoides) type. Reported at a frequency of 1.84% at a mean age of 8.3 years in the 2008 Vizsla Health Survey.[5]

Primary Glaucoma: The breed is predisposed to primary glaucoma due to goniodysplasia. Screen with gonioscopy and tonometry. Unknown mode of inheritance.[9]

Cryptorchidism (Retained Testicles): Can be unilateral or bilateral. Reported at a frequency of 1.40% of males in the 2008 Vizsla Health Survey.[5]

Corneal Dystrophy: Epithelial/stromal form of corneal opacities. Identified in 1.33% of Vizslas CERF-examined by veterinary ophthalmologists between 2000-2005.[8]

Distichiasis: Abnormally placed eyelashes that irritate the cornea and conjunctiva. Can cause secondary corneal ulceration. Identified in 1.14% of Vizslas CERF-examined by veterinary ophthalmologists between 2000-2005.[8]

Sebaceous Adenitis: A condition leading to destruction of the sebaceous glands. The focal form occurs in the Vizsla, with localized areas of alopecia, erythema, and excessive scaling. The head and extremities appear to be more consistently involved. Unknown mode of inheritance.[10]

Immune-Mediated Hemolytic Anemia (IMHA): Autoimmune destruction of blood cells. IMHA is reported at an increased frequency versus other breeds. An Australian study showed a 10x odds ratio versus other breeds. There is a female preponderance.[11,12]

Polymyositis: Affected Vizslas present with with clinical signs of dysphagia, regurgitation, excessive salvation, masticatory muscle atrophy and pain on opening the jaw between 1-9 years of age. The majority of affected dogs are male. The condition is poorly responsive to prednisone or azathioprine. Undetermined mode of inheritance.[13]

Entropion, Factor VII Deficiency, Osteochondritis Dessicans of the Shoulder, Progressive Retinal Atrophy, and **von Willebrand's Disease** are reported.[14]

Isolated Case Studies

Myasthenia Gravis and Masticatory Muscle Myositis: A 21-month-old, castrated male Vizsla was presented for pelvic limb weakness, difficulty opening his mouth, ptyalism, voice change, and urinary incontinence. Myasthenia gravis and masticatory myositis were diagnosed.[15]

ACTH-independent Hyperadrenocorticism: A 6 year old Vizsla dog was diagnosed with ACTH-independent hyperadrenocorticism associated with meal-induced hypercortisolemia. Treatment was with trilostane.[16]

Genetic Tests

Tests of Genotype: None

Tests of Phenotype: CHIC Certification: Hip radiographs, CERF eye examination, and thyroid profile including autoantibodies (annually until 8 years). Optional tests include cardiac evaluation (with a specialist), elbow radiographs, skin biopsy for sebaceous adenitis, and von Willebrand's assay test. (See CHIC website; www.caninehealthinfo.org).

Recommend patella evaluation.

Miscellaneous

- **Breed name synonyms:** Magyar Vizsla (historical), Hungarian Vizsla, Hungarian Pointer, Drotszoro Magyar Vizsla (historical), Viszla

- **Registries:** AKC, CKC, KCGB (Kennel Club of Great Britain)
- **AKC rank (year 2008):** 44 (3,010 dogs registered)
- **Internet resources: Vizsla Club of America:** www.vcaweb.org
  Vizsla Canada: www.vizslacanada.ca
  Hungarian Vizsla Club (UK): www.hungarianvizslaclub.org.uk

References

1. OFA Website breed statistics: www.offa.org Last accessed July 1, 2010.

2. Dodds WJ: Bleeding Disorders in Animals. Proceedings, 2005 World Small Animal Veterinary Association Congress. 2005.

3. Nachreiner RF, Refsal KR, Graham PA, et. al.: Prevalence of serum thyroid hormone autoantibodies in dogs with clinical signs of hypothyroidism. J Am Vet Med Assoc 2002 Feb 15;220(4):466-71.

4. Nachreiner R & Refsal K: Personal communication, Diagnostic Center for Population and Animal Health, Michigan State University. April, 2007.

5. Gibbons TA, Ruffini L, & Rieger RH: The 2008 Vizsla Health Survey. West Chester Statistics Institute, West Chester, PA: 2009.

6. Tarpataki N, Pápa K, Reiczigel J, et. al.: Prevalence and features of canine atopic dermatitis in Hungary. Acta Vet Hung. 2006 Sep;54(3):353-66.

7. Patterson EE, Mickelson JR, Da Y, et. al.: Clinical characteristics and inheritance of idiopathic epilepsy in Vizslas. *J Vet Intern Med.* 2003 May-Jun;17(3):319-25.

8. *Ocular Disorders Presumed to be Inherited in Purebred Dogs.* American College of Veterinary Ophthalmologists. ACVO, 2007.

9. Bedford P: Inherited Disease of the Canine Eye. Proceedings, 2001 World Small Animal Veterinary Association Congress. 2001.

10. White SD: When Hair Loss Isn't an Infection: Sebaceous Adenitis and Ischemic Dermatitis. Proceedings, 2004 Northeast Veterinary Conference. 2004.

11. Macklin, A: Immune-Mediated Hemolytic Anemia: Pathophysiology & Diagnosis. Proceedings, 2009 Western Veterinary Conference. 2009.

12. McAlees TJ: Immune-mediated haemolytic anaemia in 110 dogs in Victoria, Australia. Aust Vet J. 2010 Jan;88(1-2):25-8.

13. Haley AC, Platt SR, Kent R, et. al.: Breed Specific Polymyositis in the Hungarian Vizsla Dog. Proceedings, 2009 ACVIM Forum. 2009.

14. *The Genetic Connection: A Guide to Health Problems in Purebred Dogs.* L Ackerman. p 242, AAHA Press, 1999

15. Clooten JK, Woods JP, Smith-Maxie LL: Myasthenia gravis and masticatory muscle myositis in a dog. *Can Vet J.* 2003 Jun;44(6):480-3.

16. Galac S, Kars VJ, Voorhout G, et. al.: ACTH-independent hyperadreno-corticism due to food-dependent hypercortisolemia in a dog: a case report. Vet J. 2008 Jul;177(1):141-3.

17. *The Complete Dog Book, 20th Ed.* The American Kennel Club. Howell Book House, NY 2006. p 120-123.

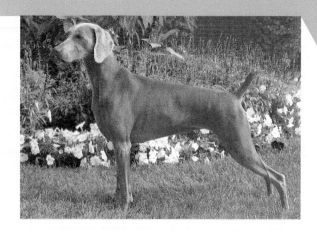

Weimaraner

chest and well-sprung rib cage, level loins, and a moderately tucked waist. They possess fine long straight limbs, with small compact feet well knuckled up and webbed. The tail is medium and tapering, but often cropped to 6" (15 cm) adult length. Their gait is long and straight, smooth but elastic.

The Breed History

Weimaraners were developed by aristocrats in the 17th century in Germany; the best known was Grand Duke Karl August of Weimer. Breed ancestors are thought to include Pointers, German Schweisshunds, red Haidbracke, and red Hanoverian Bloodhound (the latter is traced back to the gray Leithunder dog of French deer hunting stock). Weimaraners stayed exclusively owned by the German Weimaraner club members for many years. Official breed recognition in Germany came in 1896, and registration by the AKC occurred in 1943. The first dogs arrived in the US in 1929.

Breeding for Function

This breed was originally selected to be an all-purpose high-endurance hunting dog (fur and feather), bred to hunt, point and retrieve. The most popular use for this dog in modern times is as an obedience dog or hunting dog. They also enjoy flyball and agility sports.

Physical Characteristics

Height at Withers: females 23-25" (58-64 cm), males 25-27" (64-69.5 cm)

Weight: females 70-80 lb (31.8-36.4 kg), males 75-88 lb (34.1-40 kg)

Coat: The short single-layered glossy haircoat is only recognized in the color of silver-gray to mouse-gray with a "metallic sheen"; only one small spot of white is tolerated on the chest. Over the head, and particularly the ears, a lighter metallic gray color is noted.

Though the longhaired Weimaraner is not recognized, this subtype was used for waterfowl hunting. This double-coated, medium length water resistant coat is feathered on legs and tail. There are variations in the length, texture and volume of undercoat. A genetic test is available.

Longevity: 10-14 years.

Points of Conformation: This aristocratic, muscular athletic large dog possesses a medium weight mesocephalic skull with a moderate stop and slight median line over the forehead, amber nose, light gray, gray-blue or amber eyes, and fine leathered pendulous large and high-set ears. Note that puppies are born with intense sky blue eyes. They have a medium muscular neck, deep

Recognized Behavior Issues and Traits

Reported to be: Affectionate, keen, gentle and very obedient, but protective. A high amount of exercise should be provided (one hour per day minimum is recommended). High intelligence and fairly high social needs make this dog unsuitable for kenneled life. They should be kept busy to prevent boredom vices such as chewing. Due to their strong chase instinct, they should be raised with, or carefully introduced to smaller pets. They need close contact with their owners, and are devoted, sensitive and loyal. They have low grooming needs and are low to medium shedders. They are loud alarm barkers.

Normal Physiologic Variations

Autosomal recessive longhaired Weimaraners occur. A genetic test is available.

Drug Sensitivities

The breed is predisposed to vaccine-induced HOD (see below). Recommend only using core vaccines, preferring recombinant DNA vaccines when available, especially during puppy vaccinations.

Inherited Diseases

Hip Dysplasia: Polygenically inherited trait causing degenerative joint disease and hip arthritis. OFA reports 8.5% affected.[1]

Elbow Dysplasia: Polygenically inherited trait causing elbow arthritis. OFA reports 1.8% affected.[1]

Patella Luxation: Polygenically inherited laxity of patellar ligaments, causing luxation, lameness, and later degenerative joint disease. Treat surgically if causing clinical signs. Reported at a high frequency by the OFA, but too few Weimaraners have been screened to determine an accurate frequency.[1]

Hyperuricosuria (HUU)/Urate Bladder Stones: An autosomal recessive mutation in the SLC2A9 gene causes urate urolithiasis and can predispose male dogs to urinary obstruction. Weimaraners have a computed 0.15 frequency of the defective gene. A genetic test is available.[38]

Disease Predispositions

Distichiasis: Abnormally placed eyelashes that irritate the cornea and conjunctiva, more seriously in Weimaraners than other breeds. Can cause secondary corneal ulceration. Dorn reports a 1.76x odds ratio versus other breeds. Identified in 26.67% of Weimaraners CERF-examined by veterinary ophthalmologists between 2000-2005. CERF discourages breeding affected Weimaraners.[2]

Hypothyroidism: Inherited autoimmune thyroiditis. 6.9% positive for thyroid autoantibodies based on testing at Michigan State University. (Ave. for all breeds is 7.5%).[3,4]

Cataracts: Anterior cortex intermediate cataracts predominate in the breed. Identified in 5.60% of Weimaraners CERF-examined by veterinary ophthalmologists between 2000-2005. CERF does not recommend breeding any Weimaraner with a cataract.[2]

Gastric Dilation/Volvulus (GDV, Bloat): Life-threatening twisting of the stomach within the abdomen. Requires immediate veterinary attention. There is a 9.1% lifetime risk of developing GDV, with 4.8% of all Weimaraners dying from the condition. Odds ratios of 4.6x to 6.2x for developing bloat versus other breeds have been computed. A UK study shows a 5% prevalence of GVD, with it being the cause of death of 11.6% of Weimaraners.[5,6,7,8]

Hypertrophic Osteodystrophy (HOD): Immune-mediated disorder causing fever, and painful, swollen joints and bones in young Weimaraners. Occurs mostly within 3-14 days post-vaccination. The disorder is not linked to a specific type of vaccine. Age of onset is 8-16 weeks. Risk factor is 21x that of other breeds, with an incidence of 5.4%. Reported 21.4x odds ratio versus other breeds. One study found distemper virus contained in the affected growth plates. This breed is prone to a severe variant of HOD that can result in death without steroid therapy. Unknown mode of inheritance, but the heritability of HOD in the breed is 0.68. Occurs as a widespread disorder in the breed, with no familial line having a greater risk.[9,10,11,12,13]

Hormonal Urinary Incontinence: Weimaraners are found to be a breed with increased risk for spayed females to develop urinary incontinence. Treat with phenylpropanolamine.[14]

Corneal Dystrophy: Epithelial/stromal form of corneal opacities. Identified in 2.40% of Weimaraners CERF-examined by veterinary ophthalmologists between 2000-2005.[2]

Persistent Pupillary Membranes: Strands of fetal remnant connecting; iris to iris, cornea, lens, or involving sheets of tissue. The later three forms can impair vision, and dogs affected with these forms should not be bred. Identified in 2.13% of Weimaraners CERF-examined by veterinary ophthalmologists between 2000-2005.[2]

Mast Cell Tumor (MCT): Skin tumors that produce histamine, and can cause inflammation and ulceration. They can reoccur locally or with distant metastasis. Weimaraners have a 4-8 times greater risk for developing cutaneous mast cell tumors than other breeds.[15]

Everted Cartilage of the Third Eyelid: A scroll-like curling of the cartilage of the third eyelid, usually everting the margin. Can be unilateral or bilateral, and cause ocular irritation. Identified in 1.07% of Weimaraners CERF-examined by veterinary ophthalmologists between 2000-2005.[2,16]

Follicular Dysplasia: Affected young adult Weimaraners show progressive alopecia of the trunk (head and limbs are spared) associated with recurrent folliculitis/furunculosis. Diagnosis by histopathology. The lesions are similar to mild cases of color dilution alopecia.[17]

Spinal Dysraphism (Syringomyelia, Myelodysplasia): Congenital spinal cord disorder seen in Weimaraners beginning at 6-8 weeks of age. Presents as a bunny hopping gait with loss of reciprocal hind limb movement. There can be varying degrees of loss of proprioception and postural reactions in the pelvic limbs, with a wide based stance. Pain perception is unaffected. Unknown mode of inheritance. In matings between two severely affected dogs, 80% of the offspring were affected.[18,19]

Exocrine Pancreatic Insufficiency: The Weimaraner breed has a predisposition to maldigestion from exocrine pancreatic insufficiency based on cPLI testing.[20]

Cervical Spondylomyelopathy (Wobbler Syndrome): Presents with neck pain, UMN spasticity and ataxia. Imaging studies suggest that the primary lesion is spinal cord compression at C5-6 or C6-7. MRI is superior to myelography in determining site, severity, and nature of the spinal cord compression. Seen at an increased incidence in the breed. Undetermined mode of inheritance.[21]

Immunodeficiency: Rare, familial disorder expressed as low IgA, IgG, IgM and leading to recurrent infections of skin, GIT, and CNS. Unknown mode of inheritance.[22,23,24]

XX-Sex Reversal: Sry-negative XX-sex reversal causes external make characteristics of a prepuce and an enlarged clitoris, in genetically female dogs. A uterus is usually present. Reported as a rare disorder in the breed. Presumed autosomal recessive mode of inheritance.[25]

Immunodeficient Dwarfism: Immunodeficient dwarfism in an inbred line of Weimaraner dogs was characterized by failure to grow, emaciation, growth hormone (GH) deficiency, decreased lymphocyte blastogenic responsiveness to mitogens, lack of thymus cortex, and recurrent infections usually resulting in death.[26,27]

Corneal Dystrophy, Factor XI Deficiency, Lupoid Onychopathy, Prognathism, and **Tricuspid Valve Dysplasia** are reported.[28]

Isolated Case Studies

Factor VII Deficiency/Hemophilia A: Two males from a litter of Weimaraners were diagnosed with hemophilia A. No other relatives tested as affected or carrier, indicating a recent mutation.[29]

Muscular Dystrophy: A 2-year-old, male Weimaraner presented with a slowly progressive form of muscular dystrophy with organ agenesis. He showed generalized muscle atrophy of the limbs; hypertrophy of the neck, infraspinatus, and lingual muscles; dysphagia; regurgitation; and unilateral renal agenesis, and hiatal hernia.[30]

Immune-Complex (Arthus-Type) Vasculitis: A 7-year-old Weimaraner dog with multiple episodes of neurological illness was euthanatized and submitted for postmortem examination. Lesions in the white matter of the cerebral cortex and cervical spinal cord showed necrotizing vasculitis. More chronic changes consisted of perivascular demyelination.[31]

Pansteatitis: Three unrelated Weimaraners were identified with pyrexia and multiple subcutaneous nodules. Clinical investigation revealed inflammation of subcutaneous, mesenteric and falciform fat, with histopathological findings of sterile pansteatitis. Unknown mode of inheritance.[32]

Hypomyelination: Two litters of Weimaraners developed tremors by 3 weeks of age. Many axons in the brain and spinal cord were either thinly myelinated or nonmyelinated relative to controls, while the peripheral nervous system was normally myelinated. In all areas of white matter evaluated, astrocytes subjectively outnumbered oligodendrocytes, suggesting an abnormality in glial differentiation. Clinical signs in two dogs resolved.[33]

Juvenile Nephropathy: A two-year-old Weimaraner bitch presented in renal failure. Renal pathology consisted of tubular as well as glomerular lesions. There was also an inflammatory left atrial wall necrotizing arteritis.[34]

Endocardial Fibroelastosis: A 9-week-old Weimaraner presented with left-sided heart failure. On necropsy, diffuse fibroplasia over the left ventricular endocardium; small, deformed papillary muscles; and pulmonary congestion were evident, consistent with congenital endocardial fibroelastosis.[35]

Narcolepsy: A 3-year-old male neutered Weimaraner dog presented with acute onset cataplectic attacks, triggered by emotional events such as playing or eating. The diagnosis of narcolepsy and cataplexy was made based on clinical signs and evaluation of cerebrospinal fluid (CSF) that contained a dramatically decreased hypocretin-1 concentration.[36]

Genetic Tests

Tests of Genotype: Direct genetic test for HUU is available from UC-Davis VGL and the Animal Health Trust.

Direct genetic test for long coat is available from the Animal Health Trust and VetGen.

Tests of Phenotype: CHIC Certification: Required testing includes hip radiographs, CERF eye examination, and thyroid profile including autoantibodies. Optimal testing includes genetic test for HUU. (See CHIC website; www.caninehealthinfo.org).

Recommend elbow radiographs, patella evaluation, and cardiac examination.

Miscellaneous

- **Breed name Synonyms:** Vorsthund, Vorstenhund, Weimar Pointer, Grey Ghost
- **Registries:** AKC, CKC, UKC, KCGB (Kennel Club of Great Britain), ANKC (Australian National Kennel Club), NKC (National Kennel Club)
- **AKC rank (year 2008):** 31 (8,732 dogs registered)
- **Internet resources: Weimaraner Club of America:** www.weimclubamerica.org
  Weimaraner Association of Canada: www.weims.ca
  Weimaraner Club of Great Britain: www.weimaranerclubofgreatbritain.org.uk

References

1. OFA Website breed statistics: www.offa.org Last accessed July 1, 2010.
2. *Ocular Disorders Presumed to be Inherited in Purebred Dogs.* American College of Veterinary Ophthalmologists. ACVO, 2007.
3. Nachreiner RF, Refsal KR, Graham PA, et. al.: Prevalence of serum thyroid hormone autoantibodies in dogs with clinical signs of hypothyroidism. *J Am Vet Med Assoc* 2002 Feb 15;220(4):466-71.
4. Nachreiner R & Refsal K: Personal communication, Diagnostic Center for Population and Animal Health, Michigan State University. April, 2007.
5. Ward MP, Patronek GJ, Glickman LT: Benefits of prophylactic gastropexy for dogs at risk of gastric dilatation-volvulus. *Prev Vet Med.* 2003 Sep 12;60(4):319-29.
6. Dorn CR: Canine breed-specific risks of frequently diagnosed diseases at veterinary teaching hospitals. Monograph. AKC Canine Health Foundation. 2000
7. Glickman LT, Glickman NW, Perez CM, et. al.: Analysis of risk factors for gastric dilatation and dilatation-volvulus in dogs. *J Am Vet Med Assoc.* 1994 May 1;204(9):1465-71.
8. Evans KM & Adams VJ: Mortality and morbidity due to gastric dilatation-volvulus syndrome in pedigree dogs in the UK. J Small Anim Pract. 2010 Jul;51(7):376-81.
9. Mee AP, Gordon, MT,May, C, Benett, D, Anderson, DC, and sharpe, PT (1983). Canine distemper virus transcripts detected in the bone cells of dogs with metaphysical osteopathy. Bone Vol. 14:59-67.
10. Munjar, TA, Austin, CC, and Bruer, GJ (1998). Comparison risk factors for Hypertrophic Osteodystrophy, Craniomandibular Osteopathy and Canine Distemper Virus Infection. Veterinary Comparative Orthopedic Traumatology, Vol. 11:37-437.
11. Malik, R, Dowden, M, Davis, PE, Allan, GS, Barrs, VR, Canfield, PJ, and Love, DN. (1995) Concurrent juvenile cellulites and metaphyseal osteopathy: An atypical canine Distemper virus syndrome. Aust. Vet. Pract. Vol. 25:62-67.
12. Crumlish PT, Sweeney T, Jones B, et. al.: Hypertrophic osteodystrophy in the Weimaraner dog: lack of association between DQA1 alleles of the canine MHC and hypertrophic osteodystrophy. Vet J. 2006 Mar;171(2):308-13.
13. LaFond E, Breur GJ & Austin CC: Breed susceptibility for developmental orthopedic diseases in dogs. J Am Anim Hosp Assoc. 2002 Sep-Oct;38(5):467-77.
14. Holt PE, Thrusfield MV: Association in bitches between breed, size, neutering and docking, and acquired urinary incontinence due to incompetence of the urethral sphincter mechanism. *Vet Rec.* 1993 Aug 21;133(8):177-80.
15. Moore AS: Cutaneous Mast Cell Tumors in Dogs. Proceedings, 2005 World Small Animal Veterinary Association Congress. 2005.
16. Herrera D: Surgery of the Eyelids. Proceedings, 2005 World Small Animal Veterinary Association Congress. 2005.
17. Laffort-Dassot C, Beco L, Carlotti DN: Follicular dysplasia in five Weimaraners. *Vet Dermatol.* 2002 Oct;13(5):253-60.
18. Confer AW, Ward, BC: Spinal Dysraphism: A Congenital Myelodysplasia in the Weimaraner. J Am Vet Med Assoc. 1972 May 15;160(10):1423-6.
19. Engel HN, Draper DD: Comparative prenatal development of the spinal cord in normal and dysraphic dogs: embryonic stage. *Am J Vet Res.* 1982 Oct;43(10):1729-34.
20. Williams DA, Minnich F: Canine exocrine pancreatic insufficiency--A survey of 640 cases diagnosed by assay of serum trypsin-like immunoreactivity. *J Vet Intern Med* 1990: 4[2]:123
21. da Costa RC & Parent J: Magnetic Resonance Imaging Findings in 60 Dogs with Cervical Spondylomyelopathy. Proceedings, 2009 ACVIM Forum. 2009.
22. Couto, CG, Krakowka, S, Johnson, G, Ciekot, P, Hill, R, Lafrado, L and Kociba, G (1989),. In vitro immunologic features of Weimaraner dogs with neutrophil abnormalities and recurrent infections. Vet. Immunology and Pathology, Vol. 23:103-112.

23. Day, MJ, Power, C, Oleshenko, J, and Rose, M (1997) Low serum immunoglobulin concentrations in related Weimaraner dogs. Journal of Small Animal Practice, Vol. 38:311-315.

24. Hansen, P, Clerex, Henroteaux, M, Ritten, VPMG, and Bernadina, WE (1995). Neutrophil phagocyte dysfunction in a Weimaraner with recurrent infections. Journal Small Animal Practice Vol. 17:721-735.

25. Meyers-Wallen VN: Inherited Disorders of Sexual Development in Dogs and Cats. Proceedings, 2007 Tufts' Canine and Feline Breeding and Genetics Conference. 2007.

26. Roth JA, Lomax LG, Altszuler N, et. al.: Thymic abnormalities and growth hormone deficiency in dogs. *Am J Vet Res.* 1980 Aug;41(8):1256-62

27. Roth JA, Kaeberle ML, Grier RL, et. al.: Improvement in clinical condition and thymus morphologic features associated with growth hormone treatment of immunodeficient dwarf dogs. *Am J Vet Res.* 1984 Jun;45(6):1151-5.

28. *The Genetic Connection: A Guide to Health Problems in Purebred Dogs.* L Ackerman. p. 242, AAHA Press, 1999.

29. Dunning MD, Averis GF, Pattinson H, et. al.: Haemophilia A (factor VIII deficiency) in a litter of Weimaraners. J Small Anim Pract. 2009 Jul;50(7):357-9.

30. Baltzer WI, Calise DV, Levine JM, et. al.: Dystrophin-deficient muscular dystrophy in a Weimaraner. J Am Anim Hosp Assoc. 2007 Jul-Aug;43(4):227-32.

31. Berrocal A, Montgomery DL, Pumarola M: Leukoencephalitis and vasculitis with perivascular demyelination in a Weimaraner dog. *Vet Pathol.* 2000 Sep;37(5):470-2.

32. German AJ, Foster AP, Holden D, et. al.: Sterile nodular panniculitis and pansteatitis in three weimaraners. *J Small Anim Pract.* 2003 Oct;44(10):449-55.

33. Kornegay JN, Goodwin MA, Spyridakis LK: Hypomyelination in Weimaraner dogs. *Acta Neuropathol (Berl).* 1987;72(4):394-401.

34. Roels S, Schoofs S, Ducatelle R: Juvenile nephropathy in a Weimaraner dog. *J Small Anim Pract.* 1997 Mar;38(3):115-8.

35. Bentley DM: Congenital endocardial fibroelastosis in a dog. *Can Vet J.* 1999 Nov;40(11):805-7.

36. Schatzberg SJ, Cutter-Schatzberg K, Nydam D, et. al.: The effect of hypocretin replacement therapy in a 3-year-old Weimaraner with narcolepsy. *J Vet Intern Med.* 2004 Jul-Aug;18(4):586-8.

37. *The Complete Dog Book, 20th Ed.* The American Kennel Club. Howell Book House, NY 2006. P 124-127.

38. Karmi N, Brown EA, Hughes SS, et. al.: Estimated frequency of the canine hyperuricosuria mutation in different dog breeds. J Vet Intern Med. 2010 Nov-Dec;24(6):1337-42.

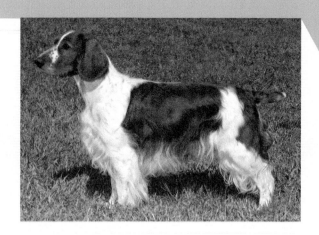

Welsh Springer Spaniel

The gait is smooth, long, and ground covering.

The Breed History

The origins of this ancient breed trace back to the British Isles, where records describe a "springing" type dog. This refers to their talent of springing or flushing hidden game. Concise breed records date from the 1600s. The English Springer Spaniel may be closely related to the Welsh Springer Spaniel. First AKC recognition came in 1906.

Breeding for Function

A solid retriever valued for gun and bow hunting, they were tireless in the field, and particularly excelled at water work. They also excelled in scent tracking and springing game. They were also used to drive cattle and to herd sheep.

Physical Characteristics

Height at Withers: female 17-18" (43-45.5 cm), male 18-19" (45.5-48 cm)

Weight: 35-45 lb (16-20 kg)

Coat: The red and white silky haircoat is flat, straight and soft, and feathering is moderate. Note that the white areas may be flecked with red.

Longevity: 12-14 years

Points of Conformation: They possess a compact build and are sized between larger English Springer Spaniels and smaller English Cocker Spaniels. The head is more long and refined than other spaniels and is a distinctive characteristic for the breed. The skull is slightly domed, stop is distinct, muzzle is square, nose is black or brown. The neck is long, not throaty, and is slightly arched. The face is well chiseled, the eyes soft in expression and darker colored eyes are preferred (range is from medium to dark brown). Dark palpebral margins are preferred and the nictitans should not show. The eyes are moderately deep set and medium in size. Ears are pendulous and they narrow towards the lightly feathered tip. They are shorter and narrower than English Springer ears. The topline is level, the thorax is deep and ribs are well sprung. The tail is high set, carried approximately level to the back and may be docked. Limbs are medium in length, straight boned and possess good muscling. Dewclaws may be removed in front, and are usually removed on the hind limbs. Feet are compact and round with well knuckled up toes and thick pads. The limbs have short metacarpals and metatarsals.

Recognized Behavior Issues and Traits

Breed attributes include: Good bark alert dog, good with children, loyal and tireless worker, good with other animals, good at obedience training, and a high activity dog. They are friendly with family, but aloof with strangers. They generally possess a steady temperament, and need close human companionship. Early socialization is important. They have high exercise needs, and if off leash, need to be in a fenced enclosure. They have a moderate shedding tendency and moderate grooming needs.

Normal Physiologic Variations

None reported

Drug Sensitivities

None reported

Inherited Diseases

Hip Dysplasia: Polygenically inherited trait causing degenerative joint disease and hip arthritis. OFA reports 11.9% affected.[1]

Elbow Dysplasia: Polygenically inherited trait causing elbow arthritis. OFA reports 2.6% affected.[1]

Patella Luxation: Polygenically inherited laxity of patellar ligaments, causing luxation, lameness, and later degenerative joint disease. Treat surgically if causing clinical signs. Too few Welsh Springer Spaniels have been screened by OFA to determine an accurate frequency.[1]

Shaking Pup/Dysmyelinogenesis: Rare, X-linked recessive disorder, where affected males begin with tremors between 5-14 days of age. If maintained, affected dogs develop seizures between 4-6 months, and extensor rigidity and spasticity between 9-12 months. None survive by 2 years of age. Caused by a lack of myelin in the brain and CNS white matter.[2]

Disease Predispositions

Persistent Pupillary Membranes: Strands of fetal remnant connecting; iris to iris, cornea, lens, or involving sheets of tissue. The later three forms can impair vision, and dogs affected with these forms should not be bred. Identified in 20.24% of Welsh Springer Spaniels CERF examined by veterinary ophthalmologists between 2000-2005.[3]

Hypothyroidism: Inherited autoimmune thyroiditis. 13.9% positive for thyroid autoantibodies based on testing at Michigan State University. (Ave. for all breeds is 7.5%).[4,5]

Distichiasis: Abnormally placed eyelashes that irritate the cornea and conjunctiva. Can cause secondary corneal ulceration. Identified in 11.08% of Welsh Springer Spaniels CERF examined by veterinary ophthalmologists between 2000-2005.[3]

Inherited Epilepsy: Inherited seizures can be generalized or partial seizures. Control with anticonvulsant medication. Average onset 3 years of age. Male predominance, with possibly a major autosomal recessive gene involved in its inheritance. (See WSSCA website.)

Cataracts: Anterior cortex punctate and generalized cataracts predominate in the breed. Onset 8-12 weeks, with complete cataract by 1-2 years. Suggested autosomal recessive inheritance. Identified in 2.22% of Welsh Springer Spaniels CERF examined by veterinary ophthalmologists between 2000-2005. CERF does not recommend breeding any Welsh Springer Spaniel with a cataract.[3,6]

Corneal Dystrophy: Epithelial/stromal form causes a bilateral non-inflammatory corneal opacity (white to gray). Identified in 1.77% of Welsh Springer Spaniels CERF-examined by veterinary ophthalmologists between 2000-2005.[3]

Retinal Dysplasia: Retinal folds, geographic, and detachment are recognized in the breed. Reported in 1.77% of Welsh Springer Spaniels CERF-examined by veterinary ophthalmologists between 2000-2005. CERF does not recommend breeding any Welsh Springer Spaniel with retinal dysplasia.[3]

Entropion: A rolling in of the eyelids that can cause corneal irritation and ulceration. Entropion is reported in 1.33% of Welsh Springer Spaniels CERF examined by veterinary ophthalmologists between 2000-2005.[3]

Glaucoma: Primary angle closure occurs in the breed. Onset 10 weeks to 10 years. Can also predispose to lens luxation. A female predominance is seen in Welsh Springer Spaniels. Screen with gonioscopy and tonometry. Suggested autosomal dominant inheritance. CERF Does not recommend breeding any Welsh Springer Spaniel with primary angle closure.[3,7]

Prognathism, and **Progressive Retinal Atrophy** are reported.[8]

Isolated Case Studies

Juvenile Polyarteritis Syndrome: Two full-sibling Welsh springer spaniels presented at 8 and 18 mo of age with rapidly progressive ataxia, recumbency, and pyrexia. The spinal cord contained extensive subdural hemorrhage and, in one dog, suppurative and necrotizing arteritis in the dura. The findings suggest a familial form of canine juvenile polyarteritis syndrome.[9]

Azoospermia: Case report of two intact male Welsh Springer Spaniels with an absence of sperm production.[10]

Genetic Tests

Tests of Genotype: None

Tests of Phenotype: CHIC Certification: Required testing includes hip and elbow radiographs, CERF eye examination (at 2, 5, and 7 years of age), and thyroid profile including autoantibodies (at 2, 3, 5, and 7 years of age). (See CHIC website; www.caninehealthinfo.org).

Recommend patella examination and cardiac examination.

Miscellaneous

- **Breed name synonyms:** Springer Spaniel, Welsh, Land Spaniel (historical), Welsh Cocker (historical)
- **Registries:** AKC, UKC, CKC, KCGB (Kennel Club of Great Britain), ANKC (Australian National Kennel Club), NKC (National Kennel Club)
- **AKC rank (year 2008):** 122 (240 dogs registered)
- **Internet resources:** Welsh Springer Spaniel Club of America: www.wssca.com
  Welsh Springer Springer Spaniel Club (UK): www.wssc.org.uk

References

1. OFA Website breed statistics: www.offa.org Last accessed July 1, 2010.
2. Duncan ID: Inherited and Acquired Disorders of Myelin in the Dog and Cat. Proceedings, 2010 World Small Animal Veterinary Association World Congress. 2010.
3. *Ocular Disorders Presumed to be Inherited in Purebred Dogs.* American College of Veterinary Ophthalmologists. ACVO, 2007.
4. Nachreiner RF, Refsal KR, Graham PA, et. al.: Prevalence of serum thyroid hormone autoantibodies in dogs with clinical signs of hypothyroidism. J Am Vet Med Assoc 2002 Feb 15;220(4):466-71.
5. Nachreiner R & Refsal K: Personal communication, Diagnostic Center for Population and Animal Health, Michigan State University. April, 2007.
6. Barnett KC: Hereditary cataract in the Welsh Springer spaniel. *J Small Anim Pract.* 1980 Nov;21(11):621-5.
7. Cottrell BD, Barnett KC: Primary Glaucoma in the Welsh springer spaniel. *J Small Anim Pract* 1988, 29: 185-199.
8. *The Genetic Connection: A Guide to Health Problems in Purebred Dogs.* L Ackerman. p. 241, AAHA Press, 1999.
9. Caswell JL, Nykamp SG: Intradural vasculitis and hemorrhage in full sibling Welsh springer spaniels. *Can Vet J.* 2003 Feb;44(2):137-9.
10. Hadley JC: Spermatogenic arrest with azoospermia in two Welsh Springer Spaniels. *J Small Anim Pract.* 1972 Mar;13(3):135-8.
11. *The Complete Dog Book, 20th Ed.* The American Kennel Club. Howell Book House, NY 2006. p 111-114.

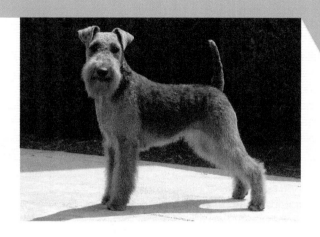

Welsh Terrier

The Breed History
This breed is likely an early offshoot of the Old English Black and Tan Wire (or Coarse) Haired Terrier and as the name implies, Wales is their place of origin. Records there date back 1000 years. In the year 1855 the breed was given this official name. They were first brought to America in the late 1880s and AKC registered in 1888. They are similar in appearance to Lakeland Terriers, though the latter dogs lack the distinctive coloring.

Breeding for Function
In Wales these dogs were valued hunters, successful with foxes, badgers and otter, and also excelled as vermin control dogs. Today, these dogs generally serve as companion animals.

Physical Characteristics
Height at Withers: female 14-15" (35.5-38cm), male 15-15.5" (38-39 cm)

Weight: Average 20-21 lb (9-10 kg)

Coat: They possess a wiry coarse outer coat with distinctive black and tan coloring. The undercoat is short, dense and wooly. Tan is found on the head, legs and belly. The black jacket can be grizzled. Puppies are often born almost all black.

Longevity: 10-14 years

Points of Conformation: The Welsh Terrier has a compact square conformation, is medium sized, and the head is square. In overall type, they appear similar to a scaled down Airedale. The eyes are small, dark and almond-shaped, deep and fairly wide set. The ears are triangular and small, and the fold sits above the top of the skull and fold forwards. The stop is slight, and the muzzle is square; nose is black, lips are pigmented black also. The neck is moderate in muscling and thickness; slightly arching without throatiness. The topline is level, the thorax deep and ribs are well sprung. The foreface furnishings include a well-developed moustache, brows and beard. The high set tail is usually docked and is held high. The limbs are straight boned and the feet are round and small; nails are black. The stride is longer than with most terriers, and movement projects an effortless appearance.

Recognized Behavior Issues and Traits
Reported breed characteristics include: Well mannered, gregarious, good with other dogs; better than most terriers, though may see small pets as prey. An extroverted personality, high activity levels, high exercise needs and high intelligence characterize the Welsh Terrier breed. The beard may need cleaning after meals. May tend to dig, especially if bored. Should not be off leash unless in a fenced enclosure. Low shedding dogs but the haircoat needs regular grooming and stripping twice a year.

Known to persevere in a dog fight, and some dogs have a stubborn streak. They are generally good with children. Some report that females can be a bit more difficult to housetrain.

Normal Physiologic Variations
None reported

Drug Sensitivities
None reported

Inherited Diseases
Hip Dysplasia: Polygenically inherited trait causing degenerative joint disease and hip arthritis. OFA reports 17.8% affected.[1]

Patella Luxation: Polygenically inherited laxity of patellar ligaments, causing luxation, lameness, and later degenerative joint disease. Treat surgically if causing clinical signs. Too few Welsh Terriers have been screened by OFA to determine an accurate frequency.[1]

Elbow Dysplasia: Polygenically inherited trait causing elbow arthritis. Too few Welsh Terriers have been screened by OFA to determine an accurate frequency.[1]

Primary Lens Luxation (PLL) and Secondary Glaucoma: An autosomal recessive gene causes primary lens luxation. Homozygous affected dogs usually develop lens luxation between 4-8 years of age. Rarely, heterozygous carriers can develop lens luxation, but at a later age. Lens luxation can lead to secondary glaucoma and blindness. Relative risk of 7.20x versus other breeds. Reported in 0.58% of Welsh Terriers CERF-examined by veterinary ophthalmologists between 2000-2005. CERF does not recommend breeding any Welsh Terrier with lens luxation. A genetic mutation has been identified, and a genetic test is available. OFA testing shows 36% carrier, and 1% affected.[1,2,3]

Disease Predispositions
Persistent Pupillary Membranes: Strands of fetal remnant connecting; iris to iris, cornea, lens, or involving sheets of tissue. The later three forms can impair vision, and dogs affected with these forms should not be bred. Identified in 10.40% of Welsh Terriers CERF-examined by veterinary ophthalmologists between 2000-2005.[2]

Allergic Dermatitis: Inhalant or food allergy. Presents with pruritis and pyotraumatic dermatitis (hot spots). Welsh Terriers are significantly over-represented with atopy versus other breeds.[4]

Glaucoma: Primary, narrow angle glaucoma occurs in the breed. Can cause **secondary lens luxation**. Age of onset 4-6 years. Screen with gonioscopy. There is a 2.6 to 1 female to male prevalence in the breed, with an affected frequency of 3.6%. CERF does not recommend breeding any Welsh Terrier with narrow angles.[2,5,6]

Hypothyroidism: Inherited autoimmune thyroiditis. 2.3% positive for thyroid autoantibodies based on testing at Michigan State University. (Ave. for all breeds is 7.5%).[7,8]

Cataracts: Anterior, Posterior, intermediate and punctate cataracts occur in the breed. Reported in 5.14% of Welsh Terriers presented to veterinary teaching hospitals. Identified in 1.73% of Welsh Terriers CERF examined by veterinary ophthalmologists between 2000-2005. CERF does not recommend breeding any Welsh Terrier with a cataract.[2,9]

Corneal Dystrophy: Epithelial/stromal form causes a bilateral non-inflammatory corneal opacity (white to gray). Identified in 1.73% of Welsh Terriers CERF-examined by veterinary ophthalmologists between 2000-2005.[2]

Distichiasis: Abnormally placed eyelashes that irritate the cornea and conjunctiva. Can cause secondary corneal ulceration. Reported in 1.30% of Welsh Terriers CERF-examined by veterinary ophthalmologists between 2000-2005.[2]

Idiopathic Epilepsy: Inherited seizures can be generalized or partial seizures. Control with anticonvulsant medication. Seizures generally appear between 1-3 years of age. Reported on the WTCA website.

von Willebrand's Disease is reported.[10]

Isolated Case Studies

Pectus Excavatum: Two six-week-old intact Welsh terrier littermates were presented for funnel-like depressions of the cranial sternum associated with inversion of the rib cage. Thoracic radiographic examination revealed a significant dorsal deviation of the first to the fifth sternebrae. At 12 weeks of age, there was complete radiographic resolution of the sternal deformity.[11]

Medullary Thyroid Carcinoma: A 14-year-old female Welsh Terrier was presented with a paratracheal mass. Cytology demonstrated round to polygonal cells with distinct cell borders, mild to moderate anisocytosis, round to oval eccentric nuclei with prominent nucleoli, and a variable amount of finely granular, eosinophilic cytoplasm. Histopathology and immunohistochemistry diagnosed a medullary thyroid carcinoma.[12]

Genetic Tests

Tests of Genotype: Direct test for Lens Luxation is available from OFA and Animal Health Trust.

Tests of Phenotype: Recommend patella evaluation, hip and elbow radiographs, CERF eye examination, thyroid profile including autoantibodies, and cardiac examination.

Miscellaneous
- **Breed name synonyms:** none
- **Registries:** AKC, UKC, CKC, KCGB (Kennel Club of Great Britain), ANKC (Australian National Kennel Club), NKC (National Kennel Club).
- **AKC rank (year 2008):** 101 (534 registered)
- **Internet resources:** Welsh Terrier Club of America: http://clubs.akc.org/wtca/
  Welsh Terrier Club of Great Britain: www.welshterrierclub.co.uk

References

1. OFA Website breed statistics: www.offa.org Last accessed July 1, 2010.
2. *Ocular Disorders Presumed to be Inherited in Purebred Dogs.* American College of Veterinary Ophthalmologists. ACVO, 2007.
3. Sargan DR, Withers D, Pettitt L, et. al.: Mapping the mutation causing lens luxation in several terrier breeds. J Hered. 2007;98(5):534-8.
4. Nødtvedt E, Egenvall A, Holm L: Estimating the Incidence of Canine Atopic Dermatitis Based on Insurance Claims. Proceedings, 13th ECVIM-CA Congress. 2003.
5. Bedford P: Inherited Disease of the Canine Eye. Proceedings, 2001 WSAVA Congress. 2001.
6. Gelatt KN & MacKay EO: Prevalence of the breed-related glaucomas in pure-bred dogs in North America. Vet Ophthalmol. 2004 Mar-Apr;7(2):97-111.
7. Nachreiner RF, Refsal KR, Graham PA, et. al.: Prevalence of serum thyroid hormone autoantibodies in dogs with clinical signs of hypothyroidism. J Am Vet Med Assoc 2002 Feb 15;220(4):466-71.
8. Nachreiner R & Refsal K: Personal communication, Diagnostic Center for Population and Animal Health, Michigan State University. April, 2007.
9. Gelatt KN, Mackay EO: Prevalence of primary breed-related cataracts in the dog in North America. Vet Ophthalmol. 2005 Mar-Apr;8(2):101-11.
10. *The Genetic Connection: A Guide to Health Problems in Purebred Dogs.* L Ackerman. p. 243. AAHA Press, 1999.
11. Ellison G, Halling KB: Atypical pectus excavatum in two Welsh terrier littermates. *J Small Anim Pract.* 2004 Jun;45(6):311-4.
12. Bertazzolo W, Giudice C, Dell'Orco M, et. al.: Paratracheal cervical mass in a dog. *Vet Clin Pathol.* 2003;32(4):209-12.
13. *The Complete Dog Book, 20th Ed.* The American Kennel Club. Howell Book House, NY 2006. p. 439-441.

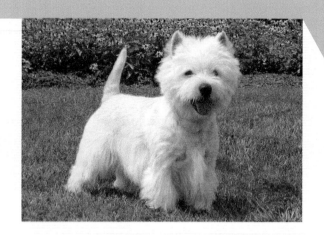

The Breed History

The Scottish terrier group all likely arose from the same ancestors (this includes the Scotties, Dandie Dinmonts, Skye, and Cairn terriers). This breed arose in Poltalloch, Scotland perhaps in the times of King James I and may have been previously known as the Dog of Argyleshire. The family of Colonel Malcolm of Poltalloch is considered to have developed the main lineage up through the early 20th century. It may be that the earliest stock was primarily white Cairn in origin. AKC registration was first recorded in 1908.

Breeding for Function

These dogs were originally bred to be vermin, fox and otter hunters; bred for exceptional spunk, speed and intelligence. Sporty and agile, they can work a long day. They are now enjoying success in earthdog trials, obedience and agility. They are excellent companions.

Physical Characteristics

Height at Withers: female 10" (25.5 cm), male 11" (28 cm)

Weight: females 13-16 lb (6-7 kg), males 15-22 lb (7-10 kg).

Coat: Their outer coat is harsh and dense and the undercoat is fine and wooly. They are all white, and the coat is about 2" in length.

Longevity: 15 years.

Points of Conformation: The Westie is a compact, short coupled dog, and has well developed musculature. Deep in the chest, they are characterized by a straight topline. Dark brown eyes with dark palpebral margins, small erect ears with thick leather, heavy eyebrows, black nose and lips and a defined stop with blunt muzzle characterize their head. The tail is short and carried high, and incidentally, is tough enough so that the handler can pull the dog out of the burrow by the tail if needed.

Recognized Behavior Issues and Traits

These dogs are reported to be very alert, intelligent, devoted, independent and fun-loving. They thrive on close human contact. They are game to learn, courageous, and are fairly tolerant of strangers. They are high activity dogs. They like to dig and bark especially if bored, and are a good watchdog. As with any of the terrier type breeds, they can nip when irritated and need to be

socialized early to other pets and children. Training should be gentle but firm and also start early. The coat should be periodically clipped or stripped to remove dead undercoat hairs.

Normal Physiologic Variations

None Reported

Drug Sensitivities

None Reported

Inherited Diseases

Hip Dysplasia and Legg-Calve Perthes Disease: Polygenically inherited traits causing degenerative hip joint disease and arthritis. Reported 33.2x odds ratio for Legg-Calve-Perthes versus other breeds. OFA reports 12.4% affected. Legg-Calve Perthes is reported at a frequency of 1.2% in the 2005 WHTCA Health Survey.[1,2,3]

Patella Luxation: Polygenically inherited laxity of patellar ligaments, causing luxation, lameness, and later degenerative joint disease. Treat surgically if causing clinical signs. OFA reports 3.8% affected. Reported at a frequency of 6.6% in the 2005 WHTCA Health Survey.[1,2]

Elbow Dysplasia: Polygenically inherited trait causing elbow arthritis. Reported at a high frequency, however too few West Highland White Terriers have been screened by OFA to determine an accurate frequency.[1]

Craniomandibular Osteopathy (CMO): Autosomal recessive, painful non-neoplastic proliferation of bone on the ramus of the mandible and/or the tympanic bulla. Affected dogs present between 3-10 months of age, with varying degrees of difficulty prehending and chewing food, secondary weight loss and atrophy of the temporal and masseter muscles. In most cases, affected dogs are normal after bony remodeling. Reported 1,313x odds ratio versus other breeds. Reported at a frequency of 0.9% in the 2005 WHTCA Health Survey. No genetic test is available.[2,3,4]

Globoid Cell Leukodystrophy (Krabbe Disease): An autosomal recessive lysosomal storage disease causing severe neurological symptoms including seizures, hypotonia, blindness, and death in young affected dogs. Reported at a frequency of 0.6% in the 2005 WHTCA Health Survey. A genetic test is available.[2,5]

Pyruvate Kinase Deficiency (PK): A rare, autosomal recessive disease of red blood cells causing exercise intolerance with a persistent, severe, and highly regenerative anemia, splenomegaly, and progressive osteosclerosis. A genetic test is available.[6]

Disease Predispositions

Atopic Dermatitis (Allergies): Presents with pruritis (itching) and pyotraumatic dermatitis (hot spots). Reported increased risk versus other breeds in multiple studies. Food allergy was identified in

24% of West Highland White Terriers, and Inhalant allergies were identified in 20% in one study. Reported at a frequency of 31.1% in the 2005 WHTCA Health Survey.[2,7,8,9]

Chronic Interstitial Lung Disease: Progressive respiratory failure, **Pulmonary Fibrosis/Bronchiectasis**, and **Pulmonary Hypertension** in West Highland White Terriers is an inherited disorder of aberrant collagen regulation. Affected dogs have chronic cough, dyspnea, and tachypnea over months to years. The mean survival time from onset of clinical signs is 17.9 months. Response to prednisolone, with or without bronchodilators, is variable. Reported at a frequency of 2.8% and an odds ratio of 4.45x versus other breeds. Reported at a frequency of 10.5% in the 2005 WHTCA Health Survey. Undetermined mode of inheritance.[2,10,11,12,13]

Lymphoma/Lymphosarcoma: Malignant cancer of lymphoid tissue. Reported at a frequency of 9.1% in the 2005 WHTCA Health Survey.[2]

Mitral Valvular Disease/Congestive Heart Failure: Mitral regurgitation that can eventually lead to congestive heart disease, cardiac arrhythmias (irregular heart beats) and cardiac failure. Diagnose with auscultation and echocardiography. Treat medically. Reported at a frequency of 9.1% in the 2005 WHTCA Health Survey.[2]

Persistent Pupillary Membranes: Strands of fetal remnant connecting; iris to iris, cornea, lens, or involving sheets of tissue. The later three forms can impair vision, and dogs affected with these forms should not be bred. Identified in 8.75% of West Highland White Terriers CERF examined by veterinary ophthalmologists between 2000-2005.[14]

Cataracts: A posterior Y suture cataract predominates, with an onset of less than 6 months of age. An autosomal recessive mode of inheritance is suggested. Identified in 8.75% of West Highland White Terriers CERF examined by veterinary ophthalmologists between 2000-2005. Juvenile cataracts are reported at a frequency of 1.8% in the 2005 WHTCA Health Survey. CERF does not recommend breeding any West Highland White Terrier with a cataract.[2,14,15]

Diabetes Mellitus: Sugar diabetes. Research shows mutations in the CTLA4 promoter gene. Treat with insulin injections, diet, and glucose monitoring. Reported at a frequency of 8.7% in the 2005 WHTCA Health Survey.[2,16]

Keratoconjunctivitis Sicca (KCS, Dry Eye): A familial incidence in the West Highland White has been demonstrated. One study showed one-third of all cases occurring in this breed, with the majority being females between 4 and 7 years of age. Conjunctival hyperaemia and mucus discharge are the primary clinical signs in this breed. Reported at a frequency of 8.4% in the 2005 WHTCA Health Survey. CERF does not recommend breeding any West Highland White Terrier with KCS.[2,14,17,18]

Inflammatory Bowel Disease (IBD): Inflammatory GI disease resulting in vomiting, diarrhea, and weight loss. Affected dogs can usually be controlled with diet and/or medications. Reported at a frequency of 6.6% in the 2005 WHTCA Health Survey.[2]

Aggression: Reported at a frequency of 4.0% in the 2005 WHTCA Health Survey.[2]

Bladder Cancer: Reported at a frequency of 4.0% in the 2005WHTCA Health Survey.[2]

Copper Toxicosis: Inherited disorder causing up to 22x normal hepatic copper concentrations. The disorder can cause hepatitis, hepatic necrosis and cirrhosis. Zinc acetate is an effective and nontoxic treatment. Unknown mode of inheritance. Reported at a frequency of 4.0% in the 2005 WHTCA Health Survey.[2,19,20]

Hyperadrenocorticism (Cushing's Disease): Caused by a functional adrenal or pituitary tumor. Clinical signs may include increased thirst and urination, symmetrical truncal alopecia, and abdominal distention. Reported at a frequency of 3.7% in the 2005 WHTCA Health Survey.[2]

Hypothyroidism: Inherited autoimmune thyroiditis. 2.9% positive for thyroid autoantibodies based on testing at Michigan State University. (Ave. for all breeds is 7.5%).[21,22]

Malassezia Pachydermatis Infection: West Highland white terriers are significantly overrepresented versus other breeds. Affected dogs present with pruritus, alopecia and lichenification. Skin biopsy specimens show Epidermal Dysplasia, which may be an inflammatory or hypersensitivity reaction to the Malassezia infection. One case reports control with interferon-gamma therapy.[23,24,25]

Retinal Dysplasia: Retinal folds, geographic, and generalized retinal dysplasia with detachment are recognized in the breed. Can lead to blindness. Identified in 2.50% of West Highland White Terriers CERF examined by veterinary ophthalmologists between 2000-2005.[14]

Renal Dysplasia: Disorder of progressive renal failure in young dogs. Affected dogs are polyuric and polydipsic, uremic, and anemic. Unknown mode of inheritance. Reported at a frequency of 2.4% in the 2005 WHTCA Health Survey.[2]

Hypoadrenocorticism (Addison's Disease): Immune mediated destruction of the adrenal gland. Typical presentation of lethargy, poor appetite, vomiting, weakness, and dehydration can occur from 4 months to several years of age. Treatment with DOCA injections or oral fludrocortisone. Unknown mode of inheritance. Reported at a frequency of 2.1% in the 2005 WHTCA Health Survey.[2,26]

Progressive Retinal Atrophy: Degenerative disorder of the retinal causing progressive blindness. Presumed to be autosomal recessively inherited. No genetic test is available. CERF does not recommend breeding any West Highland White Terrier with PRA.[14]

White Shaker Dog Syndrome: Affected dogs present between 6 months to 5 years of age, with diffuse, fine, whole body tremor, and can also show nystagmus, menace response abnormalities, proprioceptive deficits, and seizures. CSF usually is abnormal containing a mild lymphocytic pleocytosis. Protein concentration may be normal or mildly increased. Treat with tapering doses of corticosteroid. Unknown mode of inheritance. Reported at a frequency of 1.8% in the 2005 WHTCA Health Survey.[2,27]

Sick Sinus Syndrome: Affected dogs present with episodic weakness and syncope. Electrocardiographic findings included sinus bradycardia, sinus arrest with or without escape complexes, disturbances of atrioventricular conduction, paroxysmal supraventricular tachycardia, or some combination of these dysrhythmias. Reported at a frequency of 1.8% in the 2005 WHTCA Health Survey.[2,28]

Portosystemic Shunt (PSS, Liver Shunt): Abnormal blood vessels connecting the systemic and portal blood flow. Can be intrahepatic extrahepatic or microvascular dysplasia. Causes stunting, abnormal behavior, possible seizures, and secondary ammonium urate urinary calculi. Diagnosis with paired fasted and feeding serum bile acid and/or ammonium levels, and abdominal ultrasound. Reported 6.0x odds ratio versus other breeds. Reported at a frequency of 1.5% in the 2005 WHTCA Health Survey. Undetermined mode of inheritance.[2,29]

Cystic Calculi (Bladder Stones): West Highland White Terriers are found to have a predisposition to forming bladder stones. Mineral composition is not reported.[30]

Superficial Necrolytic Dermatitis: A metabolic hepatopathy. Increased hepatic catabolism of amino acids is hypothesized to explain the hypoaminoacidaemia seen. Reported with at a higher frequency in the breed. In one report, the median age was 10 years, and 75% were male.[31]

Deafness, Glaucoma, Ichthyosis, IgA Deficiency, Microphthalmia, Oligodontia, Prognathism, Pulmonic Stenosis, and **Retained Deciduous Teeth** are reported.[32]

Isolated Case Studies

Polycystic Kidney and Liver Disease: Polycystic kidney and liver disease was present in four of six female and three of five male offspring born in two matings between the same pair of West Highland White Terriers. Clinical signs and serum biochemistry analysis consistent with liver failure was evident by 5 weeks of age. Affected pups were euthanized because of their disease. An autosomal recessive mode of inheritance is suggested.[33]

Congenital Angiomatous Cardiac Cysts: Two unrelated male 16 week old West Highland White Terriers presented with acute respiratory distress and heart failure. Postmortem examination showed multiple ventricular cysts, primarily toward the apex, and valvular malformation.[34]

Necrotizing Encephalitis: A 2 year old male West Highland White Terrier presented with seizures, depressed mentation, proprioceptive deficits and a decreased menace response. Post-mortem examination showed cerebral non-suppurative inflammation and large areas of cavitation, as well as anti-glomerular basement membrane positive glomerulonephritis.[35]

L-2-Hydroxyglutaric Aciduria: A 5 year old male West Highland White Terrier presented with seizures, moderate four limb ataxia, impaired vision, dementia, and recent episodes of severe head tremor when stressed. MRI demonstrated bilaterally symmetrical polioencephalopathy. Biochemical testing showed L-2-hydroxyglutaric aciduria.[36]

Ectrodactyly: A case of monomelic forelimb ectrodactyly (lobster-claw deformity) in a West Highland white terrier is reported. The dog was treated with a soft tissue reconstruction. This was the second report of ectrodactyly in this breed.[37]

Genetic Tests

Tests of Genotype: Direct test for Globoid Leukodystrphy is available from the Jefferson Medical College (215-955-1666) and HealthGene.

Direct test for Pyruvate Kinase Deficiency is available from HealthGene, PennGen, and VetGen.

Tests of Phenotype: CHIC Certification: CERF eye examination (annually until at least age 8 years), hip radiographs, and patella evaluation. (See CHIC website; www.caninehealthinfo.org).

Recommend elbow radiographs, chest (lung) radiographs, thyroid profile including autoantibodies, and cardiac examination.

Miscellaneous

- **Breed name synonyms:** Roseneath Terrier (historical), Poltalloch Terrier (historical), Westie.
- **Registries:** AKC, UKC, CKC, KCGB (Kennel Club of Great Britain), ANKC (Australian National Kennel Club), NKC (National Kennel Club)
- **AKC rank (year 2008):** 34 (4,755 dogs registered)
- **Internet resources: West Highland White Terrier Club of America:** www.westieclubamerica.com
  Canadian West Highland White Terrier Club: www.canadawestieclub.ca
  The West Highland White Terrier Club of England: www.thewesthighlandwhiteterrierclubofengland.co.uk
  Westie Health Foundation: www.westiefoundation.org

References

1. OFA Website breed statistics: www.offa.org Last accessed July 1, 2010.
2. West Highland White Terrier Club of America & Grayson JK: 2005 West Highland White Terrier Club of America Health Survey: Final Report. Feb 20, 2007.
3. LaFond E, Breur GJ & Austin CC: Breed susceptibility for developmental orthopedic diseases in dogs. J Am Anim Hosp Assoc. 2002 Sep-Oct;38(5):467-77.
4. Padgett GA, Mostosky UV: The mode of inheritance of craniomandibular osteopathy in West Highland White terrier dogs. Am J Med Genet. 1986 Sep;25(1):9-13.
5. Wenger DA, Victoria T, Rafi MA, et. al.: Globoid cell leukodystrophy in cairn and West Highland white terriers. J Hered. 1999 Jan-Feb;90(1):138-42.
6. Skelly BJ, Wallace M, Rajpurohit YR, et. al.: Identification of a 6 base pair insertion in West Highland White Terriers with erythrocyte pyruvate kinase deficiency. Am J Vet Res. 1999 Sep;60(9):1169-72.
7. Vroom MW: A retrospective study in 45 West Highland White Terriers with skin problems. Tijdschr Diergeneeskd. 1995 May 15;120(10):292-5.
8. Schick RO, Fadok VA: Responses of atopic dogs to regional allergens: 268 cases (1981-1984). J Am Vet Med Assoc. 1986 Dec 1;189(11):1493-6.
9. Nødtvedt A, Egenvall A, Bergvall K, et. al.: Incidence of and risk factors for atopic dermatitis in a Swedish population of insured dogs. Vet Rec. 2006 Aug 19;159(8):241-6.
10. Norris AJ, Naydan DK, Wilson DW: Interstitial lung disease in West Highland White Terriers. Vet Pathol. 2005 Jan;42(1):35-41.
11. Hawkins EC, Basseches J, Berry CR, et. al.: Demographic, clinical, and radiographic features of bronchiectasis in dogs: 316 cases (1988-2000). J

Am Vet Med Assoc. 2003 Dec 1;223(11):1628-35.

12. Corcoran BM, Cobb M, Martin MW, et. al.: Chronic pulmonary disease in West Highland white terriers. Vet Rec. 1999 May 29;144(22):611-6.

13. Schober KE & Baade H: Doppler echocardiographic prediction of pulmonary hypertension in West Highland white terriers with chronic pulmonary disease. J Vet Intern Med. 2006 Jul-Aug;20(4):912-20.

14. *Ocular Disorders Presumed to be Inherited in Purebred Dogs.* American College of Veterinary Ophthalmologists. ACVO, 2007.

15. Narfstrom K: Cataract in the West Highland white terrier. J Small Anim Pract. 1981 Jul;22(7):467-71.

16. Short AD, Saleh NM, Catchpole B, et. al.: CTLA4 promoter polymorphisms are associated with canine diabetes mellitus. Tissue Antigens. 2010 Mar;75(3):242-52.

17. Barnett KC, Sansom J: Dry eye in the dog and its treatment. Trans Ophthalmol Soc U K. 1985;104 (Pt 4):462-6.

18. Sanchez RF, Innocent G, Mould J, et. al.: Canine keratoconjunctivitis sicca: disease trends in a review of 229 cases. J Small Anim Pract. 2007 Apr;48(4):211-7.

19. Thornburg LP, Shaw D, Dolan M, et. al.: Hereditary copper toxicosis in West Highland white terriers. Vet Pathol. 1986 Mar;23(2):148-54.

20. Brewer GJ, Dick RD, Schall W, et. al.: Use of zinc acetate to treat copper toxicosis in dogs. J Am Vet Med Assoc. 1992 Aug 15;201(4):564-8.

21. Nachreiner RF, Refsal KR, Graham PA, et al.: Prevalence of serum thyroid hormone autoantibodies in dogs with clinical signs of hypothyroidism. J Am Vet Med Assoc 2002 Feb 15;220(4):466-71.

22. Nachreiner R & Refsal K: Personal communication, Diagnostic Center for Population and Animal Health, Michigan State University. April, 2007.

23. Nett CS, Reichler I, Grest P, et. al.: Epidermal dysplasia and Malassezia infection in two West Highland White Terrier siblings: an inherited skin disorder or reaction to severe Malassezia infection? Vet Dermatol. 2001 Oct;12(5):285-90.

24. Bond R, Ferguson EA, Curtis CF, et. al.: Factors associated with elevated cutaneous Malassezia pachydermatis populations in dogs with pruritic skin disease. J Small Anim Pract. 1996 Mar;37(3):103-7.

25. Nishifuji K, Park SJ, Iwasaki T, et. al.: A case of hyperplastic dermatosis of the West Highland White Terrier controlled by recombinant canine interferon-gamma therapy. J Vet Med Sci. 2007 Apr;69(4):455-7.

26. Peterson ME, Kintzer PP, Kass PH: Pretreatment clinical and laboratory findings in dogs with hypoadrenocorticism: 225 cases (1979-1993). J Am Vet Med Assoc. 1996 Jan 1;208(1):85-91.

27. Bagley RS: Differential Diagnosis of Animals with Peripheral Nervous System Disease. Proceedings, 2002 Atlantic Coast Veterinary Conference. 2002.

28. Moneva-Jordan A, Corcoran BM, French A, et. al.: Sick sinus syndrome in nine West Highland white terriers. Vet Rec. 2001 Feb 3;148(5):142-7.

29. Tobias KM & Rohrbach BW: Association of breed with the diagnosis of congenital portosystemic shunts in dogs: 2,400 cases (1980-2002). J Am Vet Med Assoc. 2003 Dec 1;223(11):1636-9.

30. Weichselbaum RC, Feeney DA, Jessen CR, et. al.: Evaluation of the morphologic characteristics and prevalence of canine urocystoliths from a regional urolith center. Am J Vet Res. 1998 Apr;59(4):379-87.

31. Outerbridge CA, Marks SL, Rogers QR: Plasma amino acid concentrations in 36 dogs with histologically confirmed superficial necrolytic dermatitis. Vet Dermatol. 2002 Aug;13(4):177-86.

32. *The Genetic Connection: A Guide to Health Problems in Purebred Dogs.* L Ackerman. p. 243, AAHA Press, 1999.

33. McAloose D, Casal M, Patterson DF, et. al.: Polycystic kidney and liver disease in two related West Highland White Terrier litters. Vet Pathol. 1998 Jan;35(1):77-81.

34. Kovacevic A, Little CJ, Lombard CW, et. al.: Heart failure in two West Highland white terriers caused by congenital angiomatous cardiac anomaly. Vet Rec. 2007 Aug 4;161(5):161-4.

35. Aresu L, D'Angelo A, Zanatta R, et. al.: Canine necrotizing encephalitis associated with anti-glomerular basement membrane glomerulonephritis. J Comp Pathol. 2007 May;136(4):279-82.

36. Garosi LS, Penderis J, McConnell JF, et. al.: L-2-hydroxyglutaric aciduria in a West Highland white terrier. Vet Rec. 2005 Jan 29;156(5):145-7.

37. Barrand KR: Ectrodactyly in a West Highland white terrier. J Small Anim Pract. 2004 Jun;45(6):315-8.

38. *The Complete Dog Book, 20th Ed.* The American Kennel Club. Howell Book House, NY 2006. p 442-445.

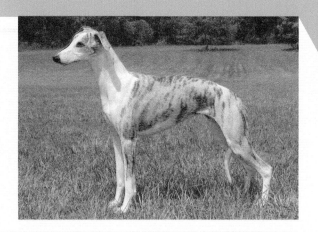

Whippet

back is broad and the loin is long. The topline is arched starting over the loin. The thorax is deep and ribs are well sprung. They possess a well tucked up abdomen. The tail is long, thin, tapering and carried low between the legs. It is gently curved upwards, reaching to the tarsus. Leg bones are straight, feet have hare-to-cat-like shape and the pads are hard and thick; toes well arched. Dewclaws may be removed. Metatarsals are short.

The Breed History

Whippets have been compared to the English Greyhound, in miniature. They originate from England, and were given official breed status there in 1891. The breed was derived from crosses of small English Greyhounds with both rough and smooth-coated terriers. Later, Italian Greyhound was added to the mix. AKC recognition occurred in 1888.

Breeding for Function

These medium-sized sight hounds were bred for function so their conformation development was focused on maximal speed and agility. Racing, including steeple chasing was a favored sport. Over a short stretch their speed was so great they could pass a Greyhound. Their speed is the fastest in this weight range of domesticated animal (35 mph or 56 km/hr). Rabbit coursing was another sport that the Whippet was tasked to; informal betting earned them the historical nickname *"poor man's racehorse"*. Other talents include ratter, lure coursing, agility, flyball, and obedience. Companion dog is a common purpose of this breed today.

Physical Characteristics

Height at Withers: female 18-21" (45.5-53.5cm), male 19-22" (48-56 cm).

Weight: females 14-25 lb (6-11 kg), males 17-28 lb (7.5-12.5 kg).

Coat: The very short coat is firm textured but not coarse, lays flat and hairs are straight. Any colors are accepted. A longhaired whippet association exists, though the breed standard for AKC or any other major registry does not mention these. They cannot compete as whippets in racing and coursing etc. In the longhaired standard, miniatures are described and for these dogs; the upper size limit is 10 lb (4.5 kg).

Longevity: 12-14 years

Points of Conformation: They have a long narrow skull and tapered muzzle, though the skull is wider between the eyes. The stop is minimal. Their gait is graceful and smooth. They possess light bone and lithe musculature. The nose is black, and eyes must be same color and large, and dark with pigmented palpebral margins. Small fine-leathered ears (rose ears) are carried back and folded. The neck is arched, long and fine, though well muscled. The

Recognized Behavior Issues and Traits

Reported breed characteristics include: Very active outdoors but quiet in the household, affectionate, intelligent, not barky, and generally tolerate visitors well, like to sleep on the couch or bed. Not biters or snappers, easy to handle though very excited while running around, gentle, good with children, low grooming needs but don't tolerate temperature extremes well. Love to chase. They need to be a house pet; not kenneled. Whippets need close human contact. Invisible fences are not good since they will lose a fight with intruding dogs, and may go through the boundary if quarry is sighted. Should not be allowed off leash in open areas. Puppies may chew, and early obedience training recommended. They have low shedding, and low doggy odor. Good for indoor living, but if in an apartment, should get a daily run.

Normal Physiologic Variations

Sight hounds have lower normal ranges for T4 and T3 concentrations compared to other breeds.[1,2]

The breed can be prone to having eccentrocytes; RBCs that appear in a peripheral blood smear to have their hemoglobin shifted to one side of the cell.[3]

Vertebral Heart Size: In lateral views, the VHS was 11.0 +/- 0.5 vertebrae (mean +/- SD) on right-to-left lateral and 11.3 +/- 0.5 vertebrae on left-to-right lateral radiographs, being larger than the 9.7 +/- 0.5 vertebrae proposed by Buchanan (P < 0.0001). The VHS was 10.5 +/- 0.6 vertebrae on dorsoventral radiographs and 11.1 +/- 0.6 vertebrae on ventrodorsal radiographs. Both values were larger than the 10.2 +/- 1.5 vertebrae (dorsoventral) (P < 0.0082) or 10.2 +/- 0.8 vertebrae (ventrodorsal) (P < 0.0001) proposed by Buchanan. Dogs out of racing pedigree lines had a significantly larger VHS than those out of show pedigree lines, and trained dogs had a significantly larger VHS than nontrained dogs.[4]

Electrocardiogram Normal Values: Whippets can have normal ECG values that fall outside of the normal range for other breeds, probably relating to their vertebral heart size. These include: P-amplitude (0.30 to 0.42), R-amplitude (3.02 to 4.32), ST-segment (0.06 to 0.20) and T-amplitude (0.42 to 0.84).[5]

Echocardiographic Normal Values[6]			
Parameter	Mean	Mean ±2SD	Range
Body weight (kg)	13.2	9.0-17.4	9.3-17.2
Body surface area (m²)	0.56	0.44-0.68	0.45-0.68
Heart rate (bpm)	93.9	48.5-139.3	54.0-158.0
M-mode (mm)			
IVSd	9.4	7.0-11.8	7.1-12.9
LVDd	37.3	29.7-44.8	25.7-47.5
LVWd	8.8	6.6-10.9	6.4-11.5
IVSs	12.0	9.0-15.1	9.0-15.5
LVDs	26.9	19.8-34.1	17.0-36.1
LVWs	12.4	9.3-15.4	8.6-17.2
EPSS	4.2	1.4-7.1	0.4-9.2
2D			
Ao(sa) (mm)	19.0	15.7-22.3	14.8-24.0
LA(sa) (mm)	26.5	20.2-32.8	18.4-33.7
LA/Ao	1.4	1.1-1.7	1.1-1.7
LA(la) (mm)	32.0	26.5-37.6	23.5-38.7

M-mode measurements: IVSd, interventricular septal thickness in diastole; LVDd, left ventricular internal diameter in diastole; LVWd, left ventricular wall thickness in diastole; IVSs, interventricular septal thickness in systole; LVDs, left ventricular internal diameter in systole; LVWs, left ventricular wall thickness in systole; EPSS, E-point to septal separation. **2D measurements:** Ao(sa), aortic root diameter from short-axis view; LA(sa), left atrial diameter from short-axis view; LA(la), left atrial diameter from long-axis view.

Drug Sensitivities

Anesthesia: Sight hounds require particular attention during anesthesia. Their lean body conformation with high surface-area-to-volume ratio predisposes them to hypothermia during anesthesia. Impaired biotransformation of drugs by the liver results in prolonged recovery from barbiturate and thiobarbiturate intravenous anesthetics. Propofol, and ketamine/diazepam combination are recommended induction agents.[7]

Drug Sensitivity: Longhaired Whippets can be homozygous for the autosomal recessive **MDR1 mutation** allowing toxicity due to high CNS drug levels of ivermectin, doramectin, loperamide, vincristine, moxidectin, and other drugs. Testing in the US shows 58% carriers and in Germany shows 60% carrier and 15% affected. A genetic test is available.[8,9]

Inherited Diseases

Hip Dysplasia: Polygenically inherited trait causing degenerative joint disease and hip arthritis. OFA reports 1.4% affected.[10]

Patella Luxation: Polygenically inherited trait causing stifle instability and arthritis. Too few Whippets have been screened by OFA to determine an accurate frequency.[10]

Elbow Dysplasia: Polygenically inherited trait causing elbow arthritis. Too few Whippets have been screened by OFA to determine an accurate frequency.[10]

Gross Muscle Hypertrophy (Bully Whippets): An incomplete dominant mutation in the myostatin gene produces gross muscle atrophy in the homozygous state, and increased muscle mass and athletic performance in the heterozygous state. Affected dogs can show intermittent cramping and stiffness. A genetic test is available.[11,12]

Disease Predispositions

Cryptorchidism (Retained Testicles): Can be bilateral or unilateral. Reported at a frequency of 19% in the Whippet Health Survey.[13]

Canine Pattern Baldness: Progressive alopecia developing at the post- and/or pre-auricular regions, along the ventral neck, thorax and abdomen, and on the caudomedial thighs. The hair loss starts around 6 months of age and gradually progresses over the following year, but remains restricted to the described areas. Reported at a frequency of 12% in the Whippet Health Survey, primarily affecting females.[13,14]

Demodicosis: Overgrowth of demodex mites causing hairloss and dermatitis. The condition has an underlying immunodeficiency in its pathogenesis. Reported at a frequency of 8% in the Whippet Health Survey. Unknown mode of inheritance.[13]

Vitreous Degeneration: A liquefaction of the vitreous gel which may predispose to retinal detachment resulting in blindness. Identified in 5.19% of Whippets CERF examined by veterinary ophthalmologists between 2000-2005.[15]

Allergic Dermatitis: Inhalant or food allergy. Presents with pruritis and pyotraumatic dermatitis (hot spots). Reported at a frequency of 3% in the Whippet Health Survey.[13]

Hypothyroidism: Inherited autoimmune thyroiditis. 2.9% positive for thyroid auto-antibodies based on testing at Michigan State University. (Ave. for all breeds is 7.5%).[16,17]

Deafness: Congenital sensorineural deafness can be unilateral of bilateral. Diagnosed by BAER testing. Not associated with a specific color variety in this breed. Strain reports 2.4% bilaterally deaf Whippets through BAER testing. Reported at a frequency of 1% in the Whippet Health Survey. Undetermined mode of inheritance.[13,18]

Cataracts: Anterior cortex and nuclear punctate cataracts predominate in the breed. Identified in 2.35% of Whippets CERF examined by veterinary ophthalmologists between 2000-2005. CERF does not recommend breeding any Whippet with a cataract.[15]

Persistent Pupillary Membranes: Strands of fetal remnant connecting; iris to iris, cornea, lens, or involving sheets of tissue. The later three forms can impair vision, and dogs affected with these forms should not be bred. Identified in 1.21% of Whippets CERF examined by veterinary ophthalmologists between 2000-2005.[15]

Primary Lens Luxation: Occurs at an increased frequency in the breed. Often progresses to secondary **glaucoma** and blindness. Reported relative risk of 4.57x versus other breeds.[19]

Color Dilution Alopecia: Associated with the blue (dilute) coat color in Whippets. Tardive alopecia occurs in areas covered by darkly pigmented diluted hairs, while the non-pigmented or lightly pigmented hairs remain unaffected.[20]

Hemangiosarcoma and Hemangioma: In one study, Whippets had an increased frequency of visceral and nonvisceral hemangiosarcoma and hemangiomas.[21]

Brachygnathism, Corneal Dystrophy, Ectodermal Defect, Gastric Dilatation-Volvulus, Micropapilla, Osteochondritis Dessicans-Shoulder, Prognathism, Progressive Retinal Atrophy, and **von Willebrand's Disease** are reported.[22]

Isolated Case Studies

Phosphofructokinase Deficiency: Two male Whippet littermates presented at 1 year of age with pallor, tachycardia, systolic heart murmur, dark yellow to orange feces, intermittent lethargy, pigmenturia, and muscle shivering or cramping after exercise. They were anemic, with increased serum creatine kinase activity and hyperkalemia. They were homozygous for the mutation in the PFK gene found in English Springer Spaniel dogs with PFK deficiency.[23]

Lung Lobe Torsion: A four-year-old, entire male whippet was presented with a three-day history of lethargy, inappetence, occasional retching, a soft cough and intermittent episodes of haemoptysis. Thoracic radiographs suggested a diagnosis of lung lobe torsion. A concurrent lung lobe torsion of the right cranial and right middle lung lobes was confirmed at exploratory thoracotomy. Management included resection of both of the affected lung lobes.[24]

Membranoproliferative Glomerulonephritis and Nephrotic Syndrome: A 2-year-old spayed female Whippet with proteinuria and decreased serum albumin was diagnosed by kidney biopsy to have membranoproliferative glomerulonephritis.[25]

Malignant Lymphoma: A 4-year-old Whippet was diagnosed with malignant lymphoma with cardiac and bone involvement, using radiography, histology, nuclear scintigraphy of the skeleton and heart, and cardiac ultrasonography.[26]

Genetic Tests

Tests of Genotype: Direct test for MDR1 (ivermectin sensitivity) is available from Washington State Univ. http://www.vetmed.wsu.edu/depts-VCPL/test.asp (Longhaired Whippets).

Direct test for CEA/CH (Collie Eye Anomoly/Choroidal Hypoplasia) is available from Optigen (Longhaired Whippets).

Direct test for coat length gene is available from VetGen.

Direct test for Bully Whippet gene is available from DDC Veterinary.

Tests of Phenotype: CHIC Certification: Required testing includes CERF eye examination, ECHOcardiogram by a cardiologist, BAER testing for deafness, and entry into the Whippet Health Foundation database. Optional testing includes hip radiographs and thyroid profile including autoantibodies. (See CHIC website; www.caninehealthinfo.org).

Recommend elbow radiographs and patella evaluation.

Miscellaneous

- **Breed name synonyms:** Snap-dog (historical).

- **Registries:** AKC, UKC, CKC, KCGB (Kennel Club of Great Britain), ANKC (Australian National Kennel Club), NKC (National Kennel Club).
- **AKC rank (year 2008):** 63 (1,435 dogs registered)
- **Internet resources: American Whippet Club:** www.americanwhippetclub.net
  National Whippet Club of Canada: www.whippetcanada.com
  The Whippet Club (UK): www.thewhippetclub.com
  Longhaired Whippet Association: http://home.ica.net/~westwood/
  Whippet Health Foundation: www.whippethealth.org

References

1. Kintzer PP & Peterson ME: Progress in the Diagnosis and Treatment of Canine Hypothyroidism. 2007. Proceedings, ACVIM 2007.
2. van Geffen C, Bavegems V, Duchateau L, et. al.: Serum thyroid hormone concentrations and thyroglobulin autoantibodies in trained and non-trained healthy whippets. Vet J. 2006 Jul;172(1):135-40.
3. Caldin M, Carli E, Furlanello T, et. al.: A retrospective study of 60 cases of eccentrocytosis in the dog. *Vet Clin Pathol.* 2005 Sep;34(3):224-31.
4. Bavegems V, Van Caelenberg A, Duchateau L, et. al.: Vertebral heart size ranges specific for whippets. *Vet Radiol Ultrasound.* 2005 Sep-Oct;46(5):400-3.
5. Bavegems V, Duchateau L, Ham LV, et. al.: Electrocardiographic reference values in whippets. Vet J. 2009 Oct;182(1):59-66.
6. Bavegems V, Duchateau L, Sys SU, De Rick A: Echocardiographic Reference Values in Whippets. Vet Radiol Ultrasound. 2007, 48(3):230-238.
7. Court MH: Anesthesia of the sighthound. Clin Tech Small Anim Pract 1999 Feb;14(1):38-43.
8. Mealey KL & Meurs KM: Breed distribution of the ABCB1-1Delta (multidrug sensitivity) polymorphism among dogs undergoing ABCB1 genotyping. J Am Vet Med Assoc. 2008 Sep 15;233(6):921-4.
9. Gramer I, Leidolf R, Döring B, et. al.: Breed distribution of the nt230(del4) MDR1 mutation in dogs. Vet J. 2011 Jul;189(1):67-71.
10. OFA Website breed statistics: www.offa.org Last accessed July 1, 2010.
11. Shelton GD & Engvall E: Gross muscle hypertrophy in whippet dogs is caused by a mutation in the myostatin gene. Neuromuscul Disord. 2007 Oct;17(9-10):721-2.
12. Mosher DS, Quignon P, Bustamante CD, et. al.: A mutation in the myostatin gene increases muscle mass and enhances racing performance in heterozygote dogs. PLoS Genet. 2007 May 25;3(5):e79.
13. Whippet Health Foundation, Inc.: 2000 Whippet Health Survey. 2000.
14. White SD: Update on Follicular Alopecias: "Pseudo-Endocrinopathies". Proceedings, 2005 ACVIM Forum. 2005.
15. *Ocular Disorders Presumed to be Inherited in Purebred Dogs.* American College of Veterinary Ophthalmologists. ACVO, 2007.
16. Nachreiner RF, Refsal KR, Graham PA, et. al.: Prevalence of serum thyroid hormone autoantibodies in dogs with clinical signs of hypothyroidism. J Am Vet Med Assoc 2002 Feb 15;220(4):466-71.
17. Nachreiner R & Refsal K: Personal communication, Diagnostic Center for Population and Animal Health, Michigan State University. April, 2007.
18. Strain GM: Deafness prevalence and pigmentation and gender associations in dog breeds at risk. *Vet J* 2004; Jan;167(1):23-32.
19. Sargan DR, Withers D, Pettitt L, et. al.: Mapping the mutation causing lens luxation in several terrier breeds. J Hered. 2007;98(5):534-8.
20. Miller WH: Alopecia Associated with Coat Color Dilution in Two Yorkshire Terriers, One Saluki, and One Mixed-Breed Dog. J Am Anim Hosp Assoc 1991: 27(1):39-43.
21. Schultheiss PC: A retrospective study of visceral and nonvisceral hemangiosarcoma and hemangiomas in domestic animals. *J Vet Diagn Invest.* 2004 Nov;16(6):522-6.
22. *The Genetic Connection: A Guide to Health Problems in Purebred Dogs.* L Ackerman. p. 243-44. AAHA Press, 1999.

23. Gerber K, Harvey JW, D'Agorne S, et. al.: Hemolysis, myopathy, and cardiac disease associated with hereditary phosphofructokinase deficiency in two Whippets. Vet Clin Pathol. 2009 Mar;38(1):46-51.

24. White RN, Corzo-Menendez N: Concurrent torsion of the right cranial and right middle lung lobes in a whippet. *J Small Anim Pract.* 2000 Dec;41(12):562-5.

25. Grauer GF, Frisbie DD, Snyder PS, et. al.: Treatment of membranopro-liferative glomerulonephritis and nephrotic syndrome in a dog with a thromboxane synthetase inhibitor. *J Vet Intern Med.* 1992 Mar-Apr;6(2):77-81.

26. Ogilvie GK, Brunkow CS, Daniel GB, et. al.: Malignant lymphoma with cardiac and bone involvement in a dog. *J Am Vet Med Assoc.* 1989 Mar 15;194(6):793-6.

27. *The Complete Dog Book, 20th Ed.* The American Kennel Club. Howell Book House, NY 2006. p. 223-226.

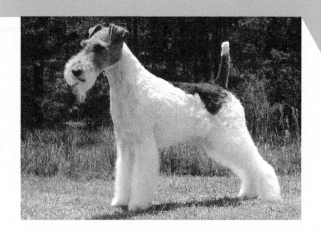

The Breed History

First breed records date to the 1700s in Britain. The extinct wire-haired Black and Tan Terrier may have been the wirehaired breed progenitor. Originally, the smooth and wire fox terriers were considered a single breed with AKC recognition in 1885. In 1984, they were split in the AKC registry. Normal Rockwell depicted this breed in some of his paintings.

Breeding for Function

As their name implies these were originally bred for fox hunting and excelled at going to ground (following their quarry into the burrow). They were also successfully used as small game hunters, and to clear vermin.

Physical Characteristics

Height at Withers: Less than 15.5" (39.5 cm)

Weight: male 18 lb (8 kg), female 16 lb (7 kg)

Coat: The dense, tough wiry non-curly hairs produce the effect of a broken coat, and overlay a dense soft undercoat. Outer coat hairs are sometimes a bit wavy. The overcoat length and texture varies over the surface of the dog, being between 0.5-1.5" long, and softer in texture on the sides and underside. The coat is mostly white with well-demarcated color patches. Brindle and red-liver are not favored as the second color. Markings on white are usually black and tan. A pure white dog is also acceptable. Ginger and white dogs can produce both tri-color and ginger colored offspring, whereas tri-color dogs bred together will only produce tri-color puppies.

Longevity: 13-14 years.

Points of Conformation: An alert expression, high head and tail carriage, and sturdy square athletic build characterize this breed. The back is short, the gait is a springy ground-covering stride, and the head has a measured standard length of 7-7.25". Small round darkly colored eyes are fairly close and deep set, with an intense expression. The top of the folded ear should be above skull level; ears are medium leathered, triangular and hang forward. The skull is of defined width between the eyes and shows minimal stop, the nose is black, neck moderately long and fine and not throaty. The topline is level. The thorax is deep and oval in cross section, and the caudal ribs are deep. The tail (if docked) is 3/4 of the natural

length. It is high set and thick. Limbs are straight, metatarsals and metacarpals heavy and short, feet small and compact and pads tough. The toes are moderately arched. In body type in all respects they are the same as the Smooth Fox Terrier.

Recognized Behavior Issues and Traits

Traits attributed to this breed include: These are diggers, can be snappy, may not tend to get along with other dogs, and are especially likely to have inter-male aggression. Though loyal, these dogs are not demonstrative; instead, rather reserved.

Like lots of attention and mentally stimulating activities, good alarm barkers, high trainability but early obedience training is recommended.

Have high energy and high exercise needs, good with children, and have moderate grooming needs. The breed has a low shedding tendency.

Normal Physiologic Variations

None reported

Drug Sensitivities

None reported

Inherited Diseases

Hip Dysplasia and Legg-Calve Perthes Disease: Polygenically inherited traits causing degenerative hip joint disease and arthritis. OFA reports 4.6% affected.[1]

Patella Luxation: Polygenically inherited laxity of patellar ligaments, causing luxation, lameness, and later degenerative joint disease. Treat surgically if causing clinical signs. Too few Wire Fox Terriers have been screened by OFA to determine an accurate frequency.[1]

Elbow Dysplasia: Polygenically inherited trait causing elbow arthritis. Too few Wire Fox Terriers have been screened by OFA to determine an accurate frequency.[1]

Primary Lens Luxation (PLL): An autosomal recessive gene causes primary lens luxation. Homozygous affected dogs usually develop lens luxation between 4-8 years of age. Rarely, heterozygous carriers can develop lens luxation, but at a later age. Lens luxation can lead to secondary **glaucoma** and blindness. A genetic mutation has been identified, and a genetic test is available.

Disease Predispositions

Persistent Pupillary Membranes: Strands of fetal remnant connecting; iris to iris, cornea, lens, or involving sheets of tissue. The later three forms can impair vision, and dogs affected with these forms should not be bred. Identified in 33.96% of Wire Fox Terriers CERF examined by veterinary ophthalmologists between 2000-2005.[2]

Cataracts: Posterior subcapsular progressive cataracts predominate in the breed. Unknown mode of inheritance. Identified in 7.55% of Wire Fox Terriers CERF examined by veterinary ophthalmologists between 2000-2005.CERF does not recommend breeding any Wire Fox Terrier with a cataract.[2]

Hypothyroidism: Inherited autoimmune thyroiditis. 4.2% positive for thyroid autoantibodies based on testing at Michigan State University. (Ave. for all breeds is 7.5%).[3,4]

Primary (Narrow Angle) Glaucoma: Ocular condition causing increased pressure within the eyeball, and secondary blindness due to damage to the retina. Diagnose with tonometry and gonioscopy. Can also predispose to lens luxation. Dorn reports a 5.47x odds ratio versus other breeds. Diagnosed in 2.28% of Wire Fox Terriers presented to veterinary teaching hospitals.[5,6,7]

Pulmonic Stenosis: Suspected polygenic mode of inheritance. The breed is reported with a higher than expected frequency of the disorder. Affected dogs present with exercise intolerance, stunting, dyspnea, syncope and ascites, due to a malformed pulmonic valve, stricture of the right ventricular outflow tract or stricture of the pulmonary artery.[8]

Demodicosis: Overgrowth of demodex mites in hair follicles due to an underlying immunodeficiency. Causes hair loss and inflammation. Also associated with sebaceous gland hyperplasia in this breed.[9]

Cystinuria/Cystine Bladder Calculi: Wire Fox Terriers have an increased risk for developing cystine bladder stones due to a defect in cystine metabolism. Treat with surgical removal and life-long medical therapy. Unknown mode of inheritance in this breed.[10]

Megaesophagus: Wire Fox Terriers are overrepresented in diagnoses of primary megaesophagus. Onset can be at weaning, or in adulthood. Clinical signs include regurgitation, excess salivation, and aspiration pneumonia.[11]

Allergic Inhalant Dermatitis, Brachygnathism, Cerebellar Hypoplasia, Deafness, Epilepsy, Lissencephaly, Mitral Valve Disease, Oligodontia, Prognathism, Retinal Pigmented Epithelium Dystrophy, and **von Willebrand's Disease** are reported.[12]

Isolated Case Studies

Ectopic Ureter: Urinary incontinence was associated with an ectopic ureter in a 5-month-old, male Wire Fox Terrier. The dog regained urinary continence after transplantation of the ureter from the urethra into the urinary bladder.[13]

Multiple Cardiac Anomalies: A 7-week-old Wire Fox Terrier was admitted with pulmonary atresia, with intact ventricular septum. The right ventricle and tricuspid valve were hypoplastic, and venous return to the right atrium reached the left side through an atrial septal defect. Oxygenation was via hyperplastic bronchial arteries. There was no evidence of ductus arteriosus.[14]

Aortic Body Tumor: An aortic body tumor in a 7-year-old wire-haired fox terrier with hind limb ataxia is described. A metastatic lesion in the dorsal arch of the eighth thoracic vertebra caused compression of the spinal cord.[15]

Genetic Tests

Tests of Genotype: Direct test for PLL is available from OFA and the Animal Health Trust.

Tests of Phenotype: CHIC Certification: Required testing includes cardiac and patella evaluations. (See CHIC website; www. caninehealthinfo.org)

Recommend hip and elbow radiographs, CERF eye examination, and thyroid profile including autoantibodies.

Miscellaneous

- **Breed name synonyms:** Wire-haired Fox Terrier, Fox Terrier, Wire Fox
- **Registries:** AKC, UKC, CKC, KCGB (Kennel Club of Great Britain), ANKC (Australian National Kennel Club), NKC (National Kennel Club)
- **AKC rank (year 2008):** 90 (708 dogs registered)
- **Internet resources: American Fox Terrier Club:** www.aftc.org **Wire Fox Terrier Association (UK):** www.wirefoxterrierassociation.co.uk The **Fox Terrier Club (UK):** www.thefoxterrierclub.co.uk

References

1. OFA Website breed statistics: www.offa.org Last accessed July 1, 2010.
2. *Ocular Disorders Presumed to be Inherited in Purebred Dogs.* American College of Veterinary Ophthalmologists. ACVO, 2007.
3. Nachreiner RF, Refsal KR, Graham PA, et. al.: Prevalence of serum thyroid hormone autoantibodies in dogs with clinical signs of hypothyroidism. J Am Vet Med Assoc 2002 Feb 15;220(4):466-71.
4. Nachreiner R & Refsal K: Personal communication, Diagnostic Center for Population and Animal Health, Michigan State University. April, 2007.
5. Gelatt KN, MacKay EO: Prevalence of the breed-related glaucomas in pure-bred dogs in North America. *Vet Ophthalmol.* 2004 Mar-Apr;7(2):97-111.
6. Nell B, Walde I: Primary glaucoma in two German hunting terriers and a wire-haired fox terrier. *Tierarztl Prax.* 1996 Apr;24(2):203-8.
7. Dorn CR: Canine breed-specific risks of frequently diagnosed diseases at veterinary teaching hospitals. Monograph. AKC Canine Health Foundation. 2000.
8. McCaw D, Aronson E: Congenital cardiac disease in dogs. *Mod Vet Pract.* 1984 Jul;65(7):509-12.
9. Ordeix L, Bardagi M, Scarampella F, et. al.: Demodex injai infestation and dorsal greasy skin and hair in eight wirehaired fox terrier dogs. Vet Dermatol. 2009 Aug;20(4):267-72.
10. Jones BR, Kirkman JH, Hogan J, et. al.: Analysis of uroliths from cats and dogs in New Zealand, 1993-96. *N Z Vet J.* 1998 Dec;46(6):233-6.
11. Marks, SL: Dysphagia and Regurgitation in Dogs Proceedings, 2010 Western Veterinary Conference. 2010.
12. *The Genetic Connection: A Guide to Health Problems in Purebred Dogs.* L Ackerman. p. 217-18. AAHA Press, 1999.
13. Osborne CA, Dieterich HF, Hanlon GF, et. al.: Urinary incontinence due to ectopic ureter in a male dog. *J Am Vet Med Assoc.* 1975 May 1;166(9):911-4.
14. Brown DJ, Patterson DF: Pulmonary atresia with intact ventricular septum and agenesis of the ductus arteriosus in a pup. *J Am Vet Med Assoc.* 1989 Jul 15;195(2):229-34.
15. Carlisle CH, Kelly WR, Samuel J, et. al.: Spinal cord compression caused by a metastatic lesion from an aortic body tumour. *Aust Vet J.* 1978 Jun;54(6):311-3.
16. *The Complete Dog Book, 20th Ed.* The American Kennel Club. Howell Book House, NY 2006. p. 374-377.

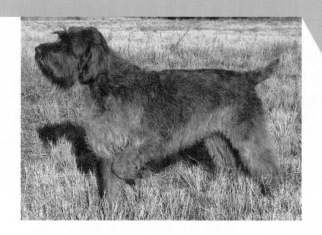

Wirehaired Pointing Griffon

The Breed History

In the Netherlands, initial breed development was undertaken by Eduard Korthals starting in 1873-1874. From there, breed fanciers in France continued to evolve the type. Otterhound, German Griffon, German shorthaired pointer, French pointer, Spaniel and Setter may have contributed genes. The Wirehaired Pointing Griffons look a lot like a German Wirehaired Pointer or the Czechoslovakian Cesky Fousek, but this latter breed is not closely related, and the other characteristics of the Fousek more closely approximate the German Wirehaired Pointer breed. When the Wirehaired Pointing Griffon is compared with the German Wirehaired Pointer, these pointing griffon dogs are smaller, less sharp in temperament, their coat is longer, and the pointing style is lower than the point seen in the German Wirehaired Pointer dog. AKC recognition occurred in 1887.

Breeding for Function

The Wirehaired Pointing Griffon is somewhat slow and deliberate in his way of going during the hunt since these dogs were developed to accompany a hunter on foot. They have an excellent nose and make an excellent pointer and retriever, particularly for upland birds. Their harsh coat was developed to provide protection in close bush, especially in thorns. A strong swimming talent and the endurance to withstand a long day in the field were selected for.

Physical Characteristics

Height at Withers: female 20-22" (51-56 cm), male 22-24" (56-61cm).

Weight: females 35-50 lb (16-23 kg) males 50-60 lb (23-27 kg).

Coat: The double coat consists of an undercoat of lighter colored soft dense hair overlaid by a very coarse wiry straight haircoat that is medium in length. Black is not allowed, but brown, steel gray with brown markings, roan and white, and orange or brown are accepted.

Longevity: 10-13 years

Points of Conformation: The Wirehaired Pointing Griffon is characterized by a very strong constitution, a medium size, and is built slightly longer than he is tall. The head is square in shape, the stop is not well pronounced, and eyebrows, moustache and beard are well developed. Eyes are rounded, large and have a friendly expression; many eye colors are accepted including brown and yellow. Ears are flat lying, medium sized and the nose is always brown with wide nostrils. The nictitans should not show. The neck is long and not throaty, and is slightly arched. The topline descends slightly towards the rear. The thorax is deep with moderately sprung ribs. The tail is carried horizontally or a bit higher when active, and may be docked to about 1/3 to 1/2 of the normal length. Limbs are straight boned, and the dewclaws are removed in America. The feet are round; the toes webbed. The gait is smooth with ground covering strides, and lots of natural agility.

Recognized Behavior Issues and Traits

Reported breed characteristics include: Devoted, low grooming needs, though even after brushing, the dog may appear somewhat unkempt. Need to hand strip twice a year for best coat condition. High trainability, even tempered, willing to please, and calm. Adult haircoat does not finish development until 24 to 36 months of age. Needs human contact, and a fenced yard if off leash. Moderate exercise needs. Fairly quiet around the household. Not considered suitable for apartment life. Good with children, may alert bark but not a guard dog. Need to carry out early obedience and socialization.

Normal Physiologic Variations

None reported

Drug Sensitivities

None reported

Inherited Diseases

Hip Dysplasia: Polygenically inherited trait causing degenerative joint disease and hip arthritis. OFA reports 7.8% affected. Reported at a frequency of 4.4% in the AWPGA National Health Survey 2002-2003.[1,2]

Elbow Dysplasia: Polygenically inherited trait causing elbow arthritis. OFA reports 4.6% affected.[1]

Patella Luxation: Polygenically inherited laxity of patellar ligaments, causing luxation, lameness, and later degenerative joint disease. Treat surgically if causing clinical signs. Too few Wirehaired Pointing Griffons have been screened by OFA to determine an accurate frequency.[1]

Disease Predispositions

Otitis Externa: Chronic or intermittent ear infections. Reported at a frequency of 22% in the AWPGA National Health Survey 2002-2003.[2]

Umbilical Hernia: Congenital opening of the body wall at the umbilicus. Should be closed surgically if large. Reported at a frequency of 3.3% in the AWPGA National Health Survey 2002-2003.[2]

Allergies: Inhalant or food. Presents with pruritis and pyotraumatic dermatitis (hot spots). Inhalant allergy is reported at a frequency of 2.2%, and food allergy at 2.7% in the AWPGA National Health Survey 2002-2003.[2]

Hypothyroidism: Inherited autoimmune thyroiditis. 2.4% positive for thyroid autoantibodies based on testing at Michigan State University. (Ave. for all breeds is 7.5%). Reported at a frequency of 2.2% in the AWPGA National Health Survey 2002-2003.[2,3,4]

Cataracts: Nuclear punctate and anterior cortex intermediate cataracts are reported in the breed. Identified in 1.39% of Wirehaired Pointing Griffons CERF examined by veterinary ophthalmologists between 2000-2005. Reported at a frequency of 1.6% at a mean age of 2.5 years in the AWPGA National Health Survey 2002-2003. CERF does not recommend breeding any Wirehaired Pointing Griffon with a cataract.[2,5]

Corneal Dystrophy: The endothelial form of corneal dystrophy is seen in the breed. An abnormal loss of the inner lining of the cornea causes progressive edema, keratitis and decreased vision. Identified in 1.39% of Wirehaired Pointing Griffons CERF examined by veterinary ophthalmologists between 2000-2005.[5]

Cryptorchidism (Retained Testicles): Can be unilateral or bilateral. Reported at a frequency of 1.1% of males in the AWPGA National Health Survey 2002-2003.[2]

Idiopathic Epilepsy: Inherited seizures can be generalized or partial seizures. Control with anticonvulsant medication. Unknown mode of inheritance. Reported at a frequency of 1.1% in the AWPGA National Health Survey 2002-2003.[2]

Entropion: A rolling in of the eyelids that can cause corneal irritation and ulceration. Reported at a frequency of 1.1% in the AWPGA National Health Survey 2002-2003.[2]

Recurrent Flank Alopecia (Seasonal Flank Alopecia): Characterized by episodes of truncal non-scarring alopecia (and often hyperpigmentation) that usually occurs on a recurrent, seasonal basis. Diagnosis is by clinical signs and biopsy. Responds to melatonin treatment, or waiting until the next season.[6]

Isolated Case Studies

Hypothalamic Hamartoma: Identified in a 10-month-old female, Wire-haired Pointing Griffon dog with a 7-month history of increasing episodes of sudden flaccid collapse.[7]

Genetic Tests

Tests of Genotype: Direct tests for coat and nose colors, nose are available from HealthGene and VetGen.

Tests of Phenotype: CHIC Certification: Required testing includes CERF eye examination (after 12 months), and hip and elbow radiographs. (See CHIC website; www.caninehealthinfo.org).

Recommend thyroid profile including autoantibodies, patella evaluation, and cardiac examination.

Miscellaneous

- **Breed name synonyms:** Korthals' Griffon, Griffon d'Arret a Poil Dur, Griffon d'Arret Korthals, Pointing Griffon, Griff.
- **Registries:** AKC, UKC, CKC, NKC (National Kennel Club).
- **AKC rank (year 2008):** 105 (419 registered)
- **Internet resources: The American Wirehaired Pointing Griffon:** Association www.awpga.com
  Wirehaired Pointing Griffon Club of America: www.wpgca.org

References

1. OFA Website breed statistics: www.offa.org Last accessed July 1, 2010.
2. Glickman L, Raghavan M, Glickman N: The American Wirehaired Pointing Griffon Association National Health Survey 2002-2003. Aug 2003. Purdue School of Veterinary Medicine.
3. Nachreiner RF, Refsal KR, Graham PA, et. al.: Prevalence of serum thyroid hormone autoantibodies in dogs with clinical signs of hypothyroidism. J Am Vet Med Assoc 2002 Feb 15;220(4):466-71.
4. Nachreiner R & Refsal K: Personal communication, Diagnostic Center for Population and Animal Health, Michigan State University. April, 2007.
5. Ocular Disorders Presumed to be Inherited in Purebred Dogs. American College of Veterinary Ophthalmologists. ACVO, 2007.
6. White SD: Update on Follicular Alopecias: "Pseudo-Endocrinopathies" 2005 Proceedings ACVIM 2005 Forum.
7. Cook RW: Hypothalamic hamartoma in a dog. Vet Pathol. 1977 Mar;14(2):138-45.
8. The Complete Dog Book, 20th Ed. The American Kennel Club. Howell Book House, NY 2006. p. 128-131.

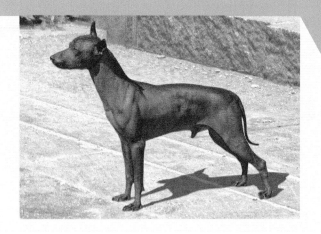

Xoloitzcuintli

The Breed History

Since the 1500s these unusual dogs have been reported, and are thought to have originated in Mexico. Their history perhaps goes back to ancient societies such as the Aztecs since dog skulls have been found that resemble this breed's in size and shape that date to 3300 years ago in Central America. The name derives from the Aztec word for God *"Xoloti"* and *"Itzcuintli"*, the Aztec word for dog. Commonly, these dogs are referred to as the **Mexican Hairless**. AKC recognition occurred in 2011.

Molecular genetic (mitochondrial DNA) results do not support a New World domestication of Xoloitzcuintli, or close association with other hairless breeds of dogs. Despite their phenotypic uniformity, the Xoloitzcuintli has a surprisingly high level of mtDNA sequence variation, suggesting that the breed was founded with a large number of dogs from outbred populations.[1]

Breeding for Function

Throughout their history, their prime purpose has been companionship; perhaps they were also the object of sacrifice in ancient Aztec, Toltec and Mayan civilizations. They were thought to have healing powers because of their warm skin temperature and were used by arthritis sufferers for that purpose.

Physical Characteristics

Toy
Height at Withers: 11-12" (28-31cm),
Weight: 9-18 lb (4-8 kg)

Miniature
Height at Withers: 12-15" (30-38 cm).
Weight: 13-22 lb (6-10kg)

Standard
Height at Withers: 16-22.5" (41-57 cm)
Weight: 20-31 lb (9-14 kg)

Coat: There are two haircoat types: Hairless and Powder Puff. The latter is not accepted for show purposes. Colors include orange, black, slate, liver, bronze, and charcoal.

Longevity: 12-15 years

Points of Conformation:

This is a small finely put together dog with a noble carriage, and similar to sight hounds in body structure. Limbs are straight boned. The somewhat almond-shaped eyes are wide set, dark brown, and moderate in size and depth of setting. The muzzle tapers to a point, nose is black, ears are erect and triangular with pointed tips, and sometimes traces of hair exist on the top of the skull, on the tip of the tail and around the toes in the hairless type. They have a moderately deep thorax, and the abdomen is well tucked up. The fine tail hangs down and tapers to a point at the tarsus. The long neck is slightly arched and finely built, and the feet are hare-like in conformation. Their gait is quick and elastic.

Recognized Behavior Issues and Traits

Reported breed characteristics include: Active, a good alarm barker and good in apartments. Only suitable as an indoor dog, and needs a winter sweater unless in a sub-tropical or tropical environment. The personality is similar to the terriers—like fox terriers particularly; also quite playful. It may be necessary to bathe a Xolo periodically and apply lotion to keep the skin moist. This is a type of dog that has low exercise needs. Xolo dogs are good with children, but children need to be very gentle so as not to injure these dogs, especially the smallest variety. Good for some allergy sufferers (hairless variety).

Normal Physiologic Variations

Hairlessness is caused by a autosomal semidominant mutation in the FOX13 gene that is lethal in utero in the homozygous state. This gene also produces variably expressed missing premolars in the heterozygous state. Because of the lethal homozygous state, breeding two heterozygous hairless dogs together produces a 2:1 ratio of hairless to (homozygous normal) powderpuff dogs. Breeding hairless to powderpuff dogs, produces a 1:1 ratio of hairless to powderpuff offspring.[2,3,4]

Xoloitzcuintli are very sensitive to heat and cold. The skin is thin, and prone to lacerations, and dryness. They sweat through their skin so they do not pant as much as other breeds.

Hairlessness is accompanied by early atrophy of the thymus after birth, and is followed by poor accumulation of lymphocytes in the thymus-dependent area of the spleen and the mesenteric lymph nodes. This presentation is different from that seen in athymic nude mice and rats. No immunodeficiency or diminished antibody response has been documented in the breed.[5]

Drug Sensitivities
None Reported

Inherited Disease

Incomplete Dentition: It is common to have variable expression of missing premolars with the autosomal dominant hairless phenotype.[3]

Patella Luxation: Polygenically inherited laxity of patellar ligaments, causing luxation, lameness, and later degenerative joint disease. Treat surgically if causing clinical signs. Too few Xoloitzcuintli have been evaluated by the OFA to determine an accurate frequency in the breed.[6]

Hip Dysplasia and Legg-Calve-Perthes Disease: Polygenically inherited traits causing degenerative hip joint disease and arthritis. Too few Xoloitzcuintli have been screened by the OFA to determine an accurate frequency in the breed.[6]

Elbow Dysplasia: Polygenically inherited trait causing elbow arthritis. Too few Xoloitzcuintli have been screened by the OFA to determine an accurate frequency in the breed.[6]

Disease Predispositions

Sunburn: Xoloitzcuintli are very sensitive to sunlight (ultraviolet radiation). Sun block should be used when exposed to direct sunlight.[7]

Comedomes (Blackheads): The skin of Xoloitzcuintli is prone to spontaneous comedome formation throughout the dorsal skin, on the limbs and prepuce. Plugged follicles containing abundant sebum and keratic substances resembles human acne.[8]

Cryptorchidism: Unilateral or bilateral retained testes reported in the breed. This is a sex-limited disorder with an unknown mode of inheritance.[9]

Hypothyroidism: Inherited autoimmune thyroiditis. Too few Xoloitzcuintli have been tested at Michigan State University to determine an accurate breed frequency. (Ave. for all breeds is 7.5%).[10,11]

Lawn Chemical Hypersensitivity: Reaction to lawn chemicals included epidermal degeneration, vasodilation, intradermal infiltration of inflammatory cells, and comedoes with well-developed pilosebaceous glands.[12]

Inherited Ocular Disorders: Too few Xoloitzcuintli have been CERF examined by veterinary ophthalmologists to determine an accurate frequency of inherited ocular disorders.[13]

Isolated Case Studies

None Reported

Genetic Tests

Tests of Genotype: None

Tests of Phenotype: Recommend hip and elbow radiographs, patella evaluation, CERF eye examination, thyroid profile including autoantibodies, cardiac examination, and examination for descended testes.

Miscellaneous

- **Breed name synonyms:** Mexican Hairless, Tepeizeuintli, Xolo
- **Registries:** UKC, CKC, KCGB (Kennel Club of Great Britain), AKC -provisional, NKC

AKC rank: (None) Became an AKC recognized breed Jan. 2011. Entire studbook registered.
- **Internet resources: Xoloitzcuintli Club of America:** www.xoloitzcuintliclubofamerica.com **Xoloitzcuintli Club USA:** www.xoloworld.com

References

1. Vila C, Maldonado JE, Wayne RK: Phylogenetic relationships, evolution, and genetic diversity of the domestic dog. *J Hered.* 1999 Jan-Feb;90(1):71-7.
2. Kimura T, Ohshima S, Doi K: The inheritance and breeding results of hairless descendants of Mexican hairless dogs. *Lab Anim.* 1993 Jan;27(1):55-8.
3. Goto N, Imamura K, Miura Y, et. al.: The Mexican hairless dog, its morphology and inheritance. *Jikken Dobutsu.* 1987 Jan;36(1):87-90.
4. Drögemüller C, Karlsson EK, Hytönen MK, et. al.: A mutation in hairless dogs implicates FOX13 in ectodermal development. Science. 2008 Sep 12;321(5895):1462.
5. Fukuta K, Koizumi N, Imamura K, et. al.: Microscopic observations of skin and lymphoid organs in the hairless dog derived from the Mexican hairless. *Jikken Dobutsu.* 1991 Jan;40(1):69-76.
6. OFA Website breed statistics: www.offa.org Last accessed July 1, 2010.
7. Kimura T, Doi K: Dorsal skin reactions to sunlight and artificial ultraviolet light in hairless descendants of Mexican hairless dogs. *Exp Anim.* 1995 Oct;44(4):293-9.
8. Kimura T, Doi K: Spontaneous comedones on the skin of hairless descendants of Mexican hairless dogs. *Exp Anim.* 1996 Oct;45(4):377-84.
9. Romagnoli SE: Canine cryptorchidism. *Vet Clin North Am Small Anim Pract.* 1991 May;21(3):533-44.
10. Nachreiner RF, Refsal KR, Graham PA, et. al.: Prevalence of serum thyroid hormone autoantibodies in dogs with clinical signs of hypothyroidism. *J Am Vet Med Assoc* 2002 Feb 15;220(4):466-71.
11. Nachreiner R & Refsal K: Personal communication, Diagnostic Center for Population and Animal Health, Michigan State University. April, 2007.
12. Kimura T, Kuroki K, Doi K: Dermatotoxicity of agricultural chemicals in the dorsal skin of hairless dogs. *Toxicol Pathol.* 1998 May-Jun;26(3):442-7.
13. *Ocular Disorders Presumed to be Inherited in Purebred Dogs.* American College of Veterinary Ophthalmologists. ACVO, 2007.
14. AKC Breed Website www.akc.org/breeds/xoloitzcuintli/ Last accessed July 1, 2010.

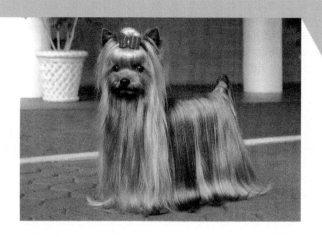

The Breed History

The Yorkie's origins trace from Scottish terrier lines in the Victorian era, specifically the Waterside terrier crossed with Paisley, Skye, Clydesdale, and rough coated Black and Tan English terriers. This terrier went to Yorkshire England from Scotland as a companion for immigrating weavers. They were brought to the USA in the late 1800s, and AKC recognition occurred in 1885.

Breeding for Function

This terrier was originally used to help control vermin. It was originally much larger, but was progressively bred for smaller body size, and as a companion dog, enjoys travel in purses and totes.

Physical Characteristics

Height at Withers: female 6" (15 cm), male 7" (18 cm)

Weight: females less than 7 lb (3 kg), males less than 7 lb (3 kg). They average 3-5 lb (1.5-2 kg)

Coat: The long silky, low-shed straight haircoat is colored the trademark blue and tan. Coats are parted over the topline and the forehead in the middle, or more commonly, the topknot is tied up. The body coat has a dark blue metallic highlight that develops at maturity. Puppies are born black and tan.

Longevity: 12-15 years.

Points of Conformation: Yorkies possess a small head, the eyes are prominent, large and dark, the nose is black and button shaped, ears are set high, V-shaped and held pricked up or semi-erect. The muzzle is tapering and trim. The tail is generally docked to one half length, and the compact body has a short, level topline. Dewclaws are usually removed, and nail color is black. They move with agility and straight, medium-length strides.

Recognized Behavior Issues and Traits

Reported breed characteristics include: Though very active, they make a suitable city pet. These little dogs are spunky, loyal and intelligent. They are sometimes aggressive to other animals, and may snap if alarmed or frightened. They should be introduced to children and other pets at an early age. They may prefer older quiet children. They will readily alarm bark. They need plenty of attention. They are low shedders that require regular grooming,

and are known not to tolerate temperature extremes well. They are considered of moderate trainability.

Normal Physiologic Variations

Cardiac Ventricular and Hemisphere Size: Ratio of cardiac ventricular to hemisphere size measured to 5.3 by low-field MRI.[1]

Radiographic Vertebral Heart Scale: Heart size was measured on right lateral recumbent thoracic radiographs. There was a trend for dogs with cardiac disease (but not respiratory disease) to have higher mean values on the scale than normal dogs of the same breed. This was most consistent in Yorkshire terriers with dilatative cardiac disease.[2]

Drug Sensitivities

None reported

Inherited Disease

Patella Luxation: Polygenically inherited congenital laxity of patellar ligaments, causing medial luxation, lameness, and later degenerative joint disease. OFA reports 23.8% affected. Dorn reports a 7.86x odds ratio versus other breeds. Another study reports a 8.3x odds ratio versus other breeds. Reported at a frequency of 6.2% in the 2006 YTCF Health Survey.[3,4,5,6]

Legg-Calvé-Perthes Disease: Polygenically inherited aseptic necrosis of the femoral neck. Can be unilateral or bilateral, with onset of degeneration usually under 9 months of age. Treat surgically if causing lameness or discomfort. Yorkshire terriers have a 35.8x odds ratio for developing the disease versus other breeds. OFA reports 5.0% affected. Reported at a frequency of 7.8% in the 2006 YTCF Health Survey.[3,5,6]

Hip Dysplasia: Polygenically inherited trait causing degenerative joint disease and hip arthritis. OFA reports 5.0% affected. Reported at a frequency of 2.2% in the 2006 YTCF Health Survey.[3,6]

Elbow Dysplasia: Polygenically inherited trait causing elbow arthritis. Too few Yorkshire Terriers have been evaluated by the OFA to determine an accurate frequency in the breed.[3]

Disease Predispositions

Tracheal Collapse: Causes persistent cough, especially when excited. Dorn reports a 36.73x odds ratio for tracheal collapse versus other breeds. Usually occurs in middle-aged to older dogs. Usually poorly responsive to surgery. Many cases can be controlled medically. Reported at a frequency of 17.4% in the 2006 YTCF Health Survey.[4,6,7]

Allergic Dermatitis: Inhalant or food allergy presents with pruritis and pyotraumatic dermatitis (hot spots). Reported at a frequency of 16.6% in the 2006 YTCF Health Survey.[6]

Hypoglycemia: Neonatal and young juvenile Yorkshire terriers can develop transient hypoglycemia when stressed. May be related to inadequate gluconeogenesis. Prevented by frequent feeding of a high-energy, protein-rich diet to both mother and pups. Reported at a frequency of 15.8% in the 2006 YTCF Health Survey.[6,8,9]

Valvular Heart Disease (Chronic Myxomatous Valvular Endocardiosis): Degenerative valvular thickening and regurgitation affecting primarily the mitral valve; though the tricuspid valve (34% of cases) and aortic valve (3% of cases) can also be involved. Secondary dilation of the left atrium and left ventricle develop, leading to congestive heart disease. Considered an age related change in small breeds, however seen in increased frequency at a younger age in this breed. Reported at a frequency of 12.6% in the 2006 YTCF Health Survey.[6,10]

Portosystemic Shunt (PSS, Liver Shunt): Congenital abnormal blood vessel connecting the portal and systemic circulation. Can be intrahepatic or extrahepatic. **Hepatic Microvascular Dysplasia** may also be genetically related to this condition. Causes stunting, abnormal behavior, possible seizures, and secondary ammonium urate urinary calculi in the breed (see below). Diagnose with paired fasted and feeding serum bile acid and/or ammonium levels, and abdominal ultrasound. Treatment of PSS includes partial ligation and/or medical and dietary control of symptoms. Studies show a 35.9x to 293x increased incidence in the breed over other breeds. Breeding studies rule out a simple (autosomal dominant, recessive, or x-linked) mode of inheritance. Reported in 3.2% of Yorkshire Terriers presented to veterinary teaching hospitals. PSS is reported at a frequency of 10.4%, and MVD at 3.2% in the 2006 YTCF Health Survey.[4,6,11,12,13]

Persistent Pupillary Membranes: Strands of fetal remnant connecting; iris to iris, cornea, lens, or involving sheets of tissue. The later three forms can impair vision, and dogs affected with these forms should not be bred. Identified in 9.86% of Yorkshire terriers CERF-examined by veterinary ophthalmologists between 2000-2005.[14]

Keratoconjunctivitis Sicca (KCS, Dry Eye): Ocular condition causing lack of tear production and secondary conjunctivitis, corneal ulcerations, and vision problems. Can be due to **Unilateral** or **Bilateral Aplasia** or **Hypoplasia of the Lacrimal Gland (Congenital Alacrima)** in the breed. KCS is reported at a frequency of 9.6% in the 2006 YTCF Health Survey. CERF does not recommend breeding any Yorkshire Terrier with KCS.[6,14,15,16,17]

Cryptorchidism (Retained Testicles): Can be unilateral or bilateral. Reported at a frequency of 8.0% in the 2006 YTCF Health Survey.[6]

Cataracts: Anterior cortex punctate and posterior cortex intermediate cataracts predominate in the breed. Primarily late onset with a mean age of 9.5 years. Identified in 7.08% of Yorkshire terriers CERF examined by veterinary ophthalmologists between 2000-2005. Unknown mode of inheritance. CERF does not recommend breeding any Yorkshire Terrier with a cataract.[14,18]

Hyperadrenocorticism (Cushing's Disease): Caused by a functional adrenal or pituitary tumor. Clinical signs may include increased thirst and urination, symmetrical truncal alopecia, and abdominal distention. Treat medically. Reported at a frequency of 5.4% in the 2006 YTCF Health Survey.[6,19]

Urinary Tract Calculi: Increased incidence of oxalate and ammonium urate bladder stones reported at a frequency of 7.4% in a UK study. Prevalence of ammonium urate stones is secondary to portosystemic liver shunts. Dorn reports a 2.21x incidence in the breed versus other breeds. Yorkshire terriers also have an increased propensity to develop kidney stones.[4,20,21,22,23]

Progressive Retinal Atrophy (PRA): Presumed autosomal recessive inherited retinal degeneration resulting in blindness. Identified in 3.76% of Yorkshire Terriers CERF examined by veterinary ophthalmologists between 2000-2005. CERF does not recommend breeding any Yorkshire Terrier with PRA. Reported at a frequency of 2.2% in the 2006 YTCF Health Survey.[6,14]

Distichiasis: Abnormally placed eyelashes that irritate the cornea and conjunctiva. Can cause secondary corneal ulceration. Identified in 2.82% of Yorkshire Terriers CERF-examined by veterinary ophthalmologists between 2000-2005.[14]

Hypothyroidism: Inherited autoimmune thyroiditis. 2.5% positive for thyroid autoantibodies based on testing at Michigan State University. (Ave. for all breeds is 7.5%).[24,25]

Diabetes Mellitus: Sugar diabetes. Associated with mutations in the CTLA4 promoter gene. Treat with insulin injections, diet, and glucose monitoring. Increased incidence seen in the breed. Dorn reports a 3.45x increased odds ratio versus other breeds. Reported at a frequency of 2.4% in the 2006 YTCF Health Survey.[4,6,26,27]

Corneal Dystrophy: Either the epithelial/stromal, or endothelial form of corneal dystrophy can be seen in the breed. Identified in 1.88% of Yorkshire Terriers CERF examined by veterinary ophthalmologists between 2000-2005.[14]

Protein Losing Enteropathy (PLE, Lymphangiectasia): Presents with diarrhea, weight loss, and/or abdominal effusion due to dilation of lymph vessels in the intestine. Inflammatory cell buildup blocks normal absorption of nutrients. Can occur at any age, but primarily affects middle-aged dogs. Yorkshire terriers are predisposed to this condition. Treatment consists of chronic anti-inflammatory medication and dietary restriction. Some dogs with severe cases have a poor prognosis.[28,29,30]

Retinal Dysplasia: Multifocal and geographic retinal dysplasia has been described in families of Yorkshire terriers. Can lead to retinal hemorrhage, retinal detachment, and blindness. Can also be related to subendothelial corneal opacities. Diagnosis by ophthalmoscopic examination. Identified in 0.94% of Yorkshire terriers CERF examined by veterinary ophthalmologists between 2000-2005. Unknown mode of inheritance.[14,31,32]

Necrotizing Meningoencephalitis: Rare disorder causing sterile, multifocal/diffuse encephalitis. Associated with a DLA haplotype. Can cause seizures, or focal neurological signs depending on the location of brain lesions. Age of onset 2-10 years of age. Diagnosis by CSF tap and MRI or CT, or post-mortem. No treatment is available.[33,34,35,36,37,38,39]

Cutaneous Plasmacytoma: Eight of 63 dogs diagnosed with cutaneous or mucocutaneous plasmacytoma were Yorkshire terriers. Prognosis was good with removal.[40]

Dermatophytosis (M. Canis): Ringworm. Increased incidence found in the breed. In one study, it was possibly secondary to immunosuppression from infection with leishmaniasis, ehrlichiosis, or with diabetes mellitus.[41,42]

Isolated Case Studies

Epitheliotropic Cutaneous (T-Cell) Lymphoma (Mycosis Fungoides): Case report of a 7 year old male Yorkshire Terrier with chronic skin and oral lesions.[43]

Renal Cortical Hypoplasia: Case report of a young Yorkshire terrier with congenital malformation of the kidneys causing juvenile renal disease and kidney failure.[44]

Dermoid Sinus and Spinal Malformations: Case report on one young Yorkshire terrier.[45]

Hypertrophic Cardiomyopathy (HCM): One case report of a 14 year old Yorkshire terrier with a cardiac murmur and syncope due to outflow obstruction, and one case report of occult HCM in a 6 year old female Yorkshire Terrier that died under anesthesia.[46,47]

Persistent Right Aortic Arch: A 5-year-old neutered male Yorkshire terrier first presented with regurgitation at 3 months of age, and was maintained on a modified diet and motility enhancing drugs. Megaesophagus was diagnosed at 2 years of age, and vascular ring anomaly was diagnosed at 4 years of age. Surgery was performed at 5 years of age.[48]

Lung Lobe Torsion: Case report of a 9 year old female Yorkshire Terrier with lung lobe torsion. Treatment was surgical removal.[49]

Color Dilution Alopecia, Hypotrichosis, Patent Ductus Arteriosus, Retained Primary Teeth, Shaker Syndrome, and **von Willebrand's Disease** are reported.[50]

Genetic Tests

Tests of Genotype: None

Tests of Phenotype: CHIC Certification: CERF eye examination (at 1, 3, and 6 years) and patella evaluation. Optional tests include hip radiograph (for Legg-Perthes or hip dysplasia), thyroid profile including autoantibodies (at 1, 3, and 6 years), blood donation to the Cornell DNA bank, or to the CHIC DNA repository. (See CHIC website; www.caninehealthinfo.org).

Recommend paired fasted and feeding serum bile acid and/or ammonium levels for PSS, cardiac examination and elbow radiographs.

Miscellaneous

- **Breed name synonyms:** Yorkie, Broken-haired Scotch terrier (historical)
- **Registries:** CKC, AKC, UKC, KCGB (Kennel Club of Great Britain), ANKC (Australian National Kennel Club), NKC (National Kennel Club)
- **AKC rank (year 2008):** 2 (41,914 dogs registered).
- **Internet resources: Yorkshire Terrier Club of America:** www.ytca.org
  Yorkshire Terrier Club Foundation: http://yorkiefoundation.org
  The Yorkshire Terrier Club (UK): www.the-yorkshire-terrier-club.co.uk
  The Canadian Yorkshire Terrier Association: www.cyta.ca

References

1. Esteve-Ratsch B, Kneissl S, Gabler C. Comparative evaluation of the ventricles in the Yorkshire Terrier and the German Shepherd dog using low-field MRI. *Vet Radiol Ultrasound.* 2001 Sep-Oct;42(5):410-3.
2. Lamb CR, Wikeley H, Boswood A, et. al.: Use of breed-specific ranges for the vertebral heart scale as an aid to the radiographic diagnosis of cardiac disease in dogs. *Vet Rec.* 2001 Jun 9;148(23):707-11.
3. OFA Website breed statistics: www.offa.org Last accessed July 1, 2010.
4. Dorn CR: Canine breed-specific risks of frequently diagnosed diseases at veterinary teaching hospitals. Monograph. AKC Canine Health Foundation. 2000.
5. LaFond E, Breur GJ, Austin CC: Breed susceptibility for developmental orthopedic diseases in dogs. *J Am Anim Hosp Assoc.* 2002 Sep-Oct;38(5):467-77.
6. Yorkshire Terrier Club Foundation, Inc.: 2006 Health Survey Data Report. 2007.
7. Longbottom GM. A case of tracheal collapse in the dog. *Vet Rec.* 1977 Jul 16;101(3):54-5.
8. Vroom MW and Slappendel RJ: Transient juvenile hypoglycaemia in a Yorkshire terrier and in a Chihuahua. *Vet Q.* 1987 Apr;9(2):172-6.
9. van Toor AJ, van der Linde-Sipman JS, van den Ingh TS, et. al.: Experimental induction of fasting hypoglycaemia and fatty liver syndrome in three Yorkshire terrier pups. *Vet Q.* 1991 Jan;13(1):16-23.
10. Bonagura J: Chronic Valvular Heart Disease in Dogs. *Proceedings World Small Animal Veterinary Association World Congress,* 2001.
11. Winkler JT, Bohling MW, Tillson DM, et. al.: Portosystemic Shunts: Diagnosis, Prognosis, and Treatment of 64 Cases (1993-2001). *J Am Anim Hosp Assoc* Mar-Apr'03; 39[2]:169-185.
12. Tobias KM And Rohrbach BW: Association of Breed with the Diagnosis of Congenital Portosystemic Shunts in Dogs: 2,400 Cases (1980-2002). *J Am Vet Med Assoc* Dec 1'03;223[11]:1636-1639.
13. Tobias KM: Determination of Inheritance of Single Congenital Portosystemic Shunts in Yorkshire Terriers. *J Am Anim Hosp Assoc* Jul-Aug'03;39[4]:385-389.
14. *Ocular Disorders Presumed to be Inherited in Purebred Dogs.* American College of Veterinary Ophthalmologists. ACVO, 2007.
15. Westermeyer HD, Ward DA & Abrams K: Breed predisposition to congenital alacrima in dogs. Vet Ophthalmol. 2009 Jan-Feb;12(1):1-5.
16. Herrera HD and Weichsler, N: Severe, Unilateral, and Non-Responsive Keratoconjunctivitis Sicca in Eleven Young Yorkshire Terriers. *Proceedings WSAVA 2002 Congress.* 2002.
17. Herrera HD, Weichsler N, Gómez JR, et. al.: Severe, unilateral, unresponsive keratoconjunctivitis sicca in 16 juvenile Yorkshire Terriers. Vet Ophthalmol. 2007 Sep-Oct;10(5):285-8.
18. Park SA, Yi NY, Jeong MB, Kim WT, et. al.: Clinical manifestations of cataracts in small breed dogs. Vet Ophthalmol. 2009 Jul-Aug;12(4):205-10.
19. Lee YM, Kang BT, Jung DI, et. al.: A case of adrenal gland dependent hyperadrenocorticism with mitotane therapy in a Yorkshire terrier dog. J Vet Sci. 2005 Dec;6(4):363-6.
20. Houston DM & Moore AE: Canine and feline urolithiasis: examination of over 50 000 urolith submissions to the Canadian veterinary urolith centre from 1998 to 2008. Can Vet J. 2009 Dec;50(12):1263-8.
21. Rogers KD, Jones B, Roberts L, et. al.: Composition of uroliths in small domestic animals in the United Kingdom. Vet J. 2011 May;188(2):228-30.
22. Lekcharoensuk C, Lulich JP, Osborne CA, et. al.: Patient and environmental factors associated with calcium oxalate urolithiasis in dogs.

J Am Vet Med Assoc. 2000 Aug 15;217(4):515-9.

23. Ling GV, Ruby AL, Johnson DL, et. al.: Renal Calculi in Dogs and Cats: Prevalence, Mineral Type, Breed, Age, and Gender Interrelationships (1981-1993). J Vet Intern Med. Jan/Feb'98;12[1]:11-21.

24. Nachreiner RF, Refsal KR, Graham PA, et. al.: Prevalence of serum thyroid hormone autoantibodies in dogs with clinical signs of hypothyroidism. J Am Vet Med Assoc 2002 Feb 15;220(4):466-71.

25. Nachreiner R & Refsal K: Personal communication, Diagnostic Center for Population and Animal Health, Michigan State University. April, 2007.

26. Davison LJ, Herrtage ME, Catchpole B: Study of 253 dogs in the United Kingdom with diabetes mellitus. Vet Rec 2005 Apr 9; 156[15]:467-71.

27. Short AD, Saleh NM, Catchpole B, et. al.: CTLA4 promoter polymorphisms are associated with canine diabetes mellitus. Tissue Antigens. 2010 Mar;75(3):242-52.

28. Melzer KJ and Sellon RK: Canine Intestinal Lymphangiectasia. Compend Contin Educ Pract Vet. Dec'02;24[12]:953-961.

29. Kimmel SE, Waddell LS, Michel KE: Hypomagnesemia and hypocalcemia associated with protein-losing enteropathy in Yorkshire terriers: five cases (1992-1998). J Am Vet Med Assoc. 2000 Sep 1;217(5):703-6.

30. Lecoindre P, Chevallier M & Guerret S: Protein-losing enteropathy of non neoplastic origin in the dog: a retrospective study of 34 cases. Schweiz Arch Tierheilkd. 2010 Mar;152(3):141-6.

31. Stades FC: Hereditary retinal dysplasia (RD) in a family of Yorkshire terriers. Tijdschr. Diergeneesk. 1978;103:1087.

32. Walde I: Retinal and corneal dysplasias in the Yorkshire terrier and other dog breeds in Austria. Tierarztl Prax. 1997 Jan;25(1):62-7.

33. Ducote JM, Johnson KE, Dewey CW, et. al.: Computed tomography of necrotizing meningoencephalitis in 3 Yorkshire Terriers. Vet Radiol Ultrasound. 1999 Nov-Dec;40(6):617-21.

34. Lotti D, Capucchio MT, Gaidolfi E, et. al.: Necrotizing encephalitis in a Yorkshire Terrier: clinical, imaging, and pathologic findings. Vet Radiol Ultrasound. 1999 Nov-Dec;40(6):622-6.

35. Kuwamura M, Adachi T, Yamate J, et. al.: Necrotising encephalitis in the Yorkshire terrier: a case report and literature review. J Small Anim Pract. 2002 Oct;43(10):459-63.

36. Lezmi S, Toussaint Y, Prata D, et. al.: Severe necrotizing encephalitis in a Yorkshire terrier: topographic and immunohistochemical study. J Vet Med A Physiol Pathol Clin Med. 2007 May;54(4):186-90.

37. von Praun F, Matiasek K, Grevel V, et. al.: Magnetic resonance imaging and pathologic findings associated with necrotizing encephalitis in two Yorkshire terriers. Vet Radiol Ultrasound. 2006 May-Jun;47(3):260-4.

38. Baiker K, Hofmann S, Fischer A, et. al.: Leigh-like subacute necrotising encephalopathy in Yorkshire Terriers: neuropathological characterisation, respiratory chain activities and mitochondrial DNA. Acta Neuropathol. 2009 Nov;118(5):697-709.

39. Pedersen NC, Vernau K, Dickinson P, et. al.: DLA Association in Various Toy Breeds with Immune Mediated Encephalopathies. Proceedings, 4th Tufts' Canine and Feline Breeding and Genetics Conference. 2009.

40. Cangul IT, Wijnen M, Van Garderen E, et. al.: Clinico-pathological aspects of canine cutaneous and mucocutaneous plasmacytomas. J Vet Med A Physiol Pathol Clin Med. 2002 Aug;49(6):307-12.

41. Cerundolo R: Generalized Microsporum canis dermatophytosis in six Yorkshire terrier dogs. Vet Dermatol. 2004 Jun;15(3):181-7.

42. Sparkes AH, Gruffydd-Jones TJ, Shaw SE, et. al.: Epidemiological and diagnostic features of canine and feline dermatophytosis in the United Kingdom from 1956 to 1991. Vet Rec. 1993 Jul 17;133(3):57-61.

43. Bhang DH, Choi US, Kim MK, et. al.: Epitheliotropic cutaneous lymphoma (mycosis fungoides) in a dog. J Vet Sci. 2006 Mar;7(1):97-9.

44. Klopfer U, Nobel TA, Kaminski R: A nephropathy similar to renal cortical hypoplasia in a Yorkshire Terrier. Vet Med Small Anim Clin. 1978 Mar;73(3):327-30.

45. Fatone G, Brunetti A, Lamagna F, et. al.: Dermoid sinus and spinal malformations in a Yorkshire terrier: diagnosis and follow-up. J Small Anim Pract. 1995 Apr;36(4):178-80.

46. Washizu M, Takemura N, Machida N, et. al.: Hypertrophic cardiomyopathy in an aged dog. J Vet Med Sci. 2003 Jun;65(6):753-6.

47. Pang D, Rondenay Y, Hélie P, et. al.: Sudden cardiac death associated with occult hypertrophic cardiomyopathy in a dog under anesthesia. Can Vet J. 2005 Dec;46(12):1122-5.

48. Loughin CA & Marino DJ: Delayed primary surgical treatment in a dog with a persistent right aortic arch. J Am Anim Hosp Assoc. 2008 Sep-Oct;44(5):258-61.

49. Choi J, & Yoon J: Lung lobe torsion in a Yorkshire terrier. J Small Anim Pract. 2006 Sep;47(9):557.

50. The Genetic Connection: A Guide to Health Problems in Purebred Dogs. L Ackerman. p. 244, AAHA Press, 1999.

51. The Complete Dog Book, 20th Ed. The American Kennel Club. Howell Book House, NY 2006. p. 521-523.

Introduction

As a practitioner, one sees many fascinating breeds of cats pass through the doors, but their rarity compared with the general domestic shorthair and longhair cat population makes it difficult for veterinarians to stay up-to-date and be fully informed about all cat breeds. The breeds themselves are evolving quickly, as they are under perpetual development. Breeders select for characteristics that evolve quite quickly as standards are updated or expanded, and the set of new provisional or now extinct breeds also changes.

Accessing relevant information not only about the abnormalities that may afflict each breed, but about what is normal for that breed can be a time consuming task since literature about cat breed-related problems is sparse, and very widely dispersed. Many reports are found in journals outside the normal spectrum of practitioner subscription journals. Reviews in clinical practice journals tend to be tables of conditions, with limited depth of coverage of the conditions.

The scope of this resource is to provide only breed-related information—not general medicine and surgery, or treatment and does not cover detailed coat color genetics. Resources are provided in the appendix and reference lists for those wishing to access detailed material.

Note that different cat registries have disparate standards, and geographic variation within these standards occurs. Generic breed descriptions in the chapters have therefore been loosely based on the CFA standard, with detailed comparisons between registries being absent due to space constraints. Due to the fact that if a reader is in a part of the world where other registry standards predominate, referring to the local registry standard is recommended. Variations between registry standards are very complex, and can be significant, even to the point of different breed names, different categories and varieties being recognized, different conformation accepted, and different details of coat color, texture, and pattern distribution preferred.

Likewise, as far as specific breed origins, many different "stories" can be found in published reports. The summaries supplied herein are aggregated from many sources, relaying what could to be the most widely accepted "theory". The interpretation of history may be flawed, and in many cases, it appears a lack of accurate historical documentation exists. This means that for some breed origins, we will never likely know the "real" story. New genetic tools are also changing the way we look at breed origins, and as new information accrues, it is likely some of the stories will give way to the new evidence.

The scope of this book encompasses the clinical signs and anticipated age of onset, progression, prognosis and cursory discussion of particularly helpful diagnostic tests. Where the scope of the tests is outside the standard minimum database, or selection or interpretation of those tests is non-standard, we have noted such.

Unfortunately for the cat world, support for research is sparse except when animal models of human disease apply. There is a dearth of studies reported since the 1980s, though recently with private funding bodies like the Winn Feline Foundation and American Association of Feline Practitioners supporting important projects, a new surge in research is now occurring. Advances in genetic technology provide new tools such as gene sequencing, with linkage and gene testing. These have inspired a new generation of researchers and provided new power for carrier detection. Still, when compared with dogs, there is very little available in the literature. Big holes are especially obvious in the rare breeds.

A weakness of reporting in the primary literature is the inconsistent definition of breed names. For example, Domestic Shorthair is sometimes used interchangeably with American Shorthair and British Shorthair if registration is not relayed in the signalment portion of the study. Since American Shorthair breed cats used to be called Domestic shorthair, older reports may actually refer to registered cats. If a study does not include "pedigreed" or "registered" in the content of the report, these were excluded from the present data gathering since the purebred and domestic population gene pool is now different because registries have been closed for quite a while. Some older references that dealt with American Shorthair (formerly Domestic Shorthair) will have thus been passed over. Breeds where color groups or hair coats have become breeds of their own in some registries also complicate study assignment to a breed. Scottish Fold/Highland Fold, Persian/Himalayan, Manx/Cymric are some examples.

Few formal breed-wide surveys have been done in cats, though recent efforts to gather breeder data into a larger database in the field have been carried out. Keeping data secure and protecting identity is often necessary for wide survey acceptance. Statistical significance which can be useful for management of breeding stock is still rarely generated. Breeder surveys are generally not statistically rigorous, and in evidence-based medicine not as high a level of significance, so results should be considered "getting a finger on the pulse" of a problem, rather than providing hard and fast data.

Another point to note is that much data from research colonies has been reported, with efforts at extrapolation; these populations are closed and do not necessarily reflect the wider picture in a breed. Establishing breed "normals" has just begun.

Many disorders have been documented in purebred or DSH/DLH cats. Some, like polycystic kidney disease in Persian and Persian-related cats, account for a major proportion of genetic disorders in the general registered cat population, others are only found in rare case reports. Rare conditions are often found in early literature, and may seemed to have apparently dropped out of existence since the report, but perhaps have undergone an insidious silent spread if not widely recognized.

If the veterinarian does not know about these rare cases, inevitably, the condition will not be widely recognized and diagnosed. The decision to place rare reports in our chapters was based on the need for the practitioner to be aware of their possible existence and to provide sources for research about these rarely reported conditions. Inclusion of these does not implicate it as a "breed problem" per se.

Lack of reported disorders in a chapter does not imply that those problems are not found in the breed, it just reflects the lack of reports—or the fact that is not a particularly breed-specific disorder. Conversely, a plethora of reports in a chapter does not necessarily correlate with an unhealthy breed, or a high prevalence of reported conditions, but may just reflect the reality that a breed is popular, therefore populous, and more literature reports are thus generated.

Many conditions are not breed specific and thus not covered in detail in this reference. Readers are referred to general feline and internal medicine texts to garner more information on those conditions.

The proportion of purebreds in the cat population is still lower than in dogs (cats are ratio of about 1 registered: 5 unregistered), so overall in practice one still sees more infectious and trauma cases than genetic disorders in cats. Nevertheless, newer studies are starting to point to genetically determined susceptibility to certain immune and infectious conditions (autoimmunity, FIP susceptibility, certain cancers) so inherited "disorders" are in fact, much more pervasive than was previously thought.

It remains difficult in some conditions to distinguish between congenital and inherited, versus environmental or acquired (nature versus nurture) etiologies. Thus, dividing these conditions by cause is somewhat arbitrary, and some breed conditions may need to be moved from the Disease Predispositions to the Inherited Diseases section or vice versa as further research elucidates these problems.

It is important to know about inherited disorders since many breeds of cats are genetically closed and suffer from reduced genetic diversity. It is important to identify and correctly manage these disorders in order to preserve genetic diversity without perpetuating harmful genetic conditions, and each veterinarian needs to understand and embrace proper genetic counseling.

Breeding closely to embed desirable genetic constitution can also co-select for rare mutations or polygenic traits that can be amplified within a line or a breed. Removal of undesirable genetic traits must be a gradual process so that strong genetic lines are not lost or compromised. Long-term commitment by breeders and the health care team is needed to properly manage such disorders from a population medicine point of view.

Newer advances in molecular biology allow linkage marker identification, definitive gene sequencing, and PCR-based genetic testing that can identify carriers at any age with non-invasive tests. These new advances are helping breeders and veterinarians make informed choices. This technology is a double edged sword though, and these powerful aids to selection must be applied intelligently. See the section from Dr. Bell on genetic counseling to review appropriate management recommendations for breeders.

Not every cat breed is included in the first edition, and as the book is updated, adjustments and additions will need to be made in order to keep the listing current. Readers are encouraged to send comments to help us update the cat breed section. Use the contact address provided in the book preface. Chapters are in alphabetical order.

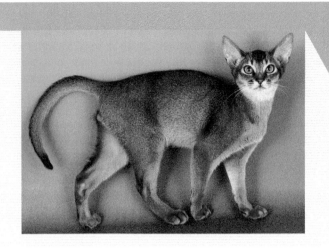

Abyssinian

Eyes: The large almond eyes are fairly wide set; may be green or gold in the CFA-approved colors. There are dark rims set within a lighter spectacle.

Points of Conformation: The Abby is a lithe, medium-sized cat with slender legs and long arched neck. The wide set moderately sized ears are tipped forward. The face and head has a distinct rounded-wedge shape, without flat planes. The English Abyssinian has a more elongated head when compared with the American cat. There is a slight break of the nose. Feet are small, compact, and oval. Chin hairs are light. Tail terminus is the ticking color and the tail is the same length as the body; fine and tapering from a thick base. Back is slightly arched.

Grooming: Low grooming requirements. A chamois cloth or hand grooming once weekly will usually suffice.

Recognized Behavior Issues and Traits
Reported breed characteristics include: Athletic, playful, very active, affectionate, curious, highly intelligent, independent, love to jump and be in high places. A few lines have high strung/nervous or independent temperament. They tend to become very attached to their caregivers and may demand attention and shadow. Highly social, they enjoy the company of other cats in the household; a busy-body. Quiet voiced cats. Play fetch and ride shoulders-recommended to have climbing trees. Many like water and will use their paws to drink and play in water.

Normal Breed Variations
Small litters

Quick to mature

Drug Sensitivities
None reported in the literature except anecdotal reports of sensitivity to griseofulvin.

Inherited Diseases
Systemic AA/Renal Amyloidosis: Amyloidosis can occur in chronic inflammatory diseases (secondary), or be inherited (primary). Amyloidosis is considered a primary condition in this breed (and the Somali). Glomerular and medullary interstitial amyloid (amyloid AA, an inert beta pleated fibrillar protein) deposits, with papillary necrosis and medullary interstitial fibrosis resulting. Renal amyloidosis is considered a subset of systemic amyloidosis; in most if not all cats, deposits occur in many organs (e.g., thyroid) but the primary clinical picture results from the renal deposits. Resulting chronic renal failure is typical in clinical presentation and occurs in young cats. Severe proteinuria is uncommon in the cat (compared with amyloidosis in dogs) because the most severe changes affect the medullary interstitium (rather than the glomeruli, as is the case in canines).[1]

The Breed History
As with many cat breeds, the true origins of this ancient breed have been lost. One theory is that it was in Abyssinia (now Ethiopia) that these distinctive cats originated. According to one source though, genetic studies have indicated their place of origin was in Southeast Asia and the Indian Ocean coast instead. The first reported export to Britain was *Zula*, in 1868. The Abyssinian maintains a distinctive wildcat look, closely resembling cats depicted in the Egyptian tombs. By the late 1800s, the Aby, as they are fondly termed, was well known as a distinct breed. Residual tabby markings are often visible along the topline, over the eyes, and faint broken bars may be visible on neck and legs. Note that the breed standard for this cat varies depending on the registry, with the European type being more extreme in shape, and a wider spectrum of colors accepted there. Foundation stock for the American Abyssinian arrived from Britain in the 1930s. Following WW II, only 12 registered cats remained in England. The CFA does not allow outcrossing.

Physical Characteristics
Weight: 9-12 lb (4-5.5 kg)

Coat: It is thought that the tabby pattern underlying the agouti ticked coat was originally much more prominent and that selective breeding for the ticking and against the tabby resulted in the modern coat. Chin and chest are white. The fine, short, shiny, firm but not harsh hairs have the distinctive agouti pattern. The agouti typically provides two to four color bands over the shaft of the hair, with the ticking color at the terminus of the hair and the base of the hair being the main coat color. Names below that are bolded are accepted in CFA. Others are accepted in European registries. Agouti is a dominant coat factor (A).
Ruddy: The most popular color, the **"Usual"** Abyssinian coloring is a rich medium honey brown (burnt sienna) ticked with dark brown/black.
Blue: Is a base coat of pale beige (oatmeal) with ticking of bluish-grey (slate blue).
Sorrel: The so-called **red** color is popular—it's a rich ginger red (also termed **apricot**); ticking is a dark rich chocolate brown. This is not a true red (red is a sex-linked recessive).
Fawn: A pale orange (rose beige) base color with warm milk chocolate (cocoa) ticking.
Lilac and silver: Not yet accepted in North America.

Typical age of presentation is 1-5 years old; the female to male ratio is 1.4:1, and first evidence of renal amyloid deposits in the kidney can be found at 9-24 months of age. An autosomal dominance inheritance with variable penetrance was proposed. In some cats, by one year later renal failure may be evident while in others, deposition of amyloid is slow and they may live a clinically normal full lifespan. A surgical biopsy of both renal medulla and cortex is most likely to be diagnostic. Apart from routine H&E, a Congo red stain is performed to highlight amyloid.[2]

In a summary of generalized AA amyloidosis in various cat breeds (especially Siamese and Oriental cats 1987-1994), amyloidosis was reported to be a familial trait in the Abyssinian.[3]

In a study of cats (1983-1997; Netherlands), 3.1% of 258 Abyssinian referrals were diagnosed with AA-amyloidosis. Affected cats were quite inbred. In 25% of the Abyssinian cats with amyloidosis, inflammatory conditions were present concurrently (e.g., rhinitis, FIP).[4]

The amyloidosis [apo-lipoprotein—serum amyloid A (AA)] propensity is still not clearly elucidated as a solely genetic problem; sequencing of the proteins shows amino acid shifts common to different breeds and this may mean that in addition to the presence of amyloid associated genes, other factors such as chronic inflammation or certain infections are involved in the genesis of phenotypic clinically significant amyloidosis. There may be three genes involved.[5]

Recessive Hereditary Rod–Cone Degeneration rdAc/Progressive Retinal Atrophy [PRA]: Age of onset is usually early adulthood (1.5-2 y), with slow progression to generalized retinal atrophy by middle age. A plasma lipid abnormality was found in conjunction with the eye problem—a reduced plasma level of docosahexanoic acid, an omega-3 fatty acid was documented. This fatty acid is the major fatty acid in outer segments of retina rods.[6] This condition is similar to retinitis pigmentosa in humans.[7]

It was determined that an **autosomal recessive** pattern of inheritance was occurring. In an early report of Swedish cats, indirect binocular ophthalmoscopic examination proved that of 205 cats assessed over 2 years old, 68 had bilateral disease (34%), while 45% were affected in one or both eyes. At 1.5-2 years of age, the first ophthalmoscopic changes were noted, and peripheral tapetal fundus was discolored brown to grey, along with retinal vessel attenuation. By about three years of age, tapetum color had changed to gray. Late stage, there was tapetal hyper-reflectivity, and severe vessel attenuation was noted; PLR was reduced or absent. Latest age of onset was at four years of age.[8]

It was reported that when homozygous for the trait, affected kittens had an abnormal ERG as early as eight weeks of age; the cat retina is considered fully developed at about 10 weeks of age. Ophthalmoscopic examination in those cats can remain normal until almost two years of age.[9] This study also confirmed an early drop in the levels of inter-photoreceptor retinoid-binding protein (IRBP) starting at four to six weeks of age in homozygous kittens. This protein also binds fatty acids at the retina.

The even distribution of retinal pathology during early phases changes to retention of function preferentially in the central retina, with loss of function peripherally in later stage disease.[10] Retina blood flow was found to be severely compromised in a study of cats with late stage PRA.[11] Antibodies against both green- and blue-sensitive cones were used to establish that early reduction of both of these cone types occurs, while the inner retina is mostly preserved. Late in disease, the ERG is not recordable and the retina is markedly thinned.[12]

Recent data using electron microscopy proves that the arterial walls of vessels in the iris are abnormal even though innervation is normal. The ciliary processes were also shorter and more compact than in normal cats.[13]

A closed colony was studied to further elucidate the correlation with phenotype and genotype. The rdAc allele was found in European and Australian cats with moderate frequency.[14]

Dominant Abyssinian Rod-cone Dysplasia (Rdy): A second type of retinal condition has been described in Abyssinians which has an autosomal dominant mode of inheritance.[7] Visual deficits are congenital, and horizontal nystagmus may also be noted. At four weeks of age mydriasis is noted, and significant visual deficits or blindness occur by 12-16 weeks of age. By two weeks of age, early retinal changes are occurring and the rods and cones are equally affected. Progressive loss occurs from central retina towards the periphery.[15] This condition has only been reported in the UK. This is a true dysplasia as rods and cones never fully develop.

A single mutation was identified as a single base pair deletion on the Exon 4 of the CRX peptide gene in the cat, which interferes with formation of the key protein.[16]

Arterial Thromboembolism: In one study of 127 affected cats, Abyssinian cats were one of three breeds overrepresented with arterial thromboembolism.[17]

Blood Type B: There may be geographic variation since in a small study of cats in Hungary, none of the cats tested were of B blood type.[18]

Prevalence of B blood type in the USA was 20% in one report.[19] In another study of blood type distribution in the USA, 230 Abyssinian cats had a prevalence of 13.5% blood type B,[20] and in a summary of studies 16% pooled prevalence of type B was reported.[21]

In Australia, all PK cats tested (n=36) were determined to be type A.[22] (See below for more about PK deficiency).

Neonatal Isoerythrolysis (NI): The reported proportion of matings at risk for NI is 0.12.[23]

Pyruvate Kinase Deficiency and Increased Osmotic Fragility of RBCs: The pyruvate kinase enzyme (PK) is involved in the anaerobic glycolytic pathway of erythrocytes. Lack of the enzyme function results in energy depletion, and premature red cell destruction. Cats with this condition may experience a range of severity of anemia, with some experiencing recurrent severe hemolytic anemia and splenomegaly.

In one study, osmotic fragility occurred in the absence of PK deficiency. Reported onset of anemia ranged from 6 months to 5 years of age (mean 23 months) and typical PCV ranged from

15%-25% (as low as 5%). Hepatic enzymes were elevated in some of the cats. Macrocytic anemia with reticulocytosis occurred. Macrocytosis persisted when the anemia resolved. Osmotic fragility tests indicated much higher fragility than normal. Some of the 18 affected cats with this primary erythrocyte fragility were closely related (both Somali, Abyssinian) and an autosomal recessive mode of inheritance was postulated.[24]

In another study of Abyssinian and Somali cats aged 1-10 years, chronic intermittent hypochromic regenerative hemolytic anemia and mild splenomegaly were reported. Pyruvate kinase activity ranged from 6%-20% of normal. Since parents were less severely affected, it was postulated to be an autosomal recessive condition—now confirmed. Osmotic fragility was normal to mildly increased.[25]

In a case report, a one year old male Abby cat presented with splenomegaly, mild exercise intolerance and severe regenerative hemolytic anemia (Coomb's negative). Splenectomy produced partial remission at 1.5 years of age; proband PK enzyme activity was 15% of normal and the proband queen's PK enzyme activity was 50% of normal.[26]

Affected Somali and Abyssinian cats usually have a normal lifespan, unlike dogs with this condition (see Beagles, Basenji, Westie, Dachshund). Dogs tend to develop liver failure and osteosclerosis while cats do not. Enzyme analysis and molecular genetic testing are available at the Deubler Laboratory—see below under Genetic Testing.

Anemia may be noted in cats as young as six months, and has been found in senior cats (12 yrs old) that were clinically normal.

A recent study showed not all cats between 1-11 years of age developed clinical signs, though a mortality rate of about 25% (presumed to be due to PK) occurred in the study group. In a little over half of the cats (median age 1.7 y), lethargy, diarrhea, poor appetite, and weight loss, pale mucous membranes and icterus were most commonly noted. Symptomatic cats had variable lab findings with increased bilirubin, globulins, liver enzymes and reticulocytes. The authors say "As PK-deficient cats can be asymptomatic testing for PK deficiency before breeding is strongly recommended."[27]

Disease Predispositions

Renal Failure: Renal failure rate for Abyssinian cats was identified to be more than double the baseline rate in a study of cats seen at veterinary colleges between 1980-1990 (189,371 cases in the Purdue University Veterinary Medical Database), at an odds ratio for risk of 2.42:1 (22 of 771 cats, prevalence 2.85%).[28]

Cervical Neck Lesions: Increased risk was reported. Abyssinians were one of two breeds (the other being Siamese) most commonly affected by feline odontoclastic resorptive lesions (FORLs).[29]

Gingivitis: Anecdotal evidence for increased prevalence.

Psychogenic Alopecia, Hyperesthesia: Anecdotal reports of increased prevalence.

Urinary Tract Infection (UTI): In a study of 22,908 cats with feline lower urinary tract disorders, Abyssinian cats were overrepresented for UTI.[30]

Feline Dilated Cardiomyopathy (FDC): Breed disposition was reported for FDC; the hypertrophic form is rarely reported in this breed.[31] Average age of onset is 7 years. Case rates have dropped since diet supplementation with taurine began but is still seen. Previously, mortality for FDC was about 85%, but with taurine supplementation mortality is currently in the 30%-50% range. Cats don't typically cough as in the dog; heart rate may range from bradycardic to tachycardia, and both ventricles are affected. Pleural effusion, cold extremities, weakness and azotemia are typical. Affected cats are prone to arterial thromboembolism. Systolic heart murmur or diastolic gallop can often be heard, and 61% have arrhythmias, usually ventricular. Echocardiography is the best modality for definitive diagnosis.[32]

Medial Patellar Luxation (MPL)/Hip Dysplasia (HD): In one study it was noted that of 69 Abyssinian cats, 26 (38%) had abnormal patella seating with easily induced luxation; a possible dominant (but polygenic) inheritance was suggested. Minimum age was 6 months; average age of the study group of cats was 4.3 years. This study group represented several US and European lines in the breed; diagnosis was by manual palpation to displace the patella.[33]

In a mixed breed study looking at medial patellar luxation and hip dysplasia at the University of Pennsylvania (1998) of 78 non-randomly selected cats over six months of age (average age 2.5 yr), Abyssinians were afflicted with MPL more frequently and severely than the average cat. Cats with MPL in the pooled group (including the Abyssinian) were three times as likely to have HD as those without MPL. Only 11 of the 78 cats had clinical signs of pelvic limb abnormalities so many cats are not being diagnosed in clinical practices. Norberg angle (NA) and distraction index (DI) in combination with OFA criterion were used to assess the cats. They found 80% of Abyssinian cats (8/10) had MPL and of these, 7/8 had bilateral MPL. And 33% (3/10) had HD, while 33% (3/10) had concurrent HD/MPL. A positive correlation between joint laxity and HD was identified.[34,35,36,37]

FIP Susceptibility: An American Study found that Abyssinian cats were significantly over-represented for a diagnosis of FIP when they analyzed data for a 16 year period at a veterinary teaching hospital.[38]

Rare and Isolated Reports

Congenital Hypothyroidism: Primary dyshormonogenesis has been diagnosed in a group of related Abyssinians that had early onset disproportionate dwarfism, goiter, constipation and retained kitten features. It was reported to be inherited as an autosomal recessive disorder. This trait results in thyroid peroxidase deficiency. By four weeks of age kittens were stunted, by six to nine months of age still immature, and by adulthood, variable expression was noted. Deciduous teeth were shed late and epiphyseal plate closure was delayed. Both TSH and TRH tests were abnormal, and the t-T4 and T3, and f-T4 low.[39] This was proposed to be an under-diagnosed cause of fading kittens. If detected early and treated with appropriate thyroid hormone supplementation, effects may be reduced or ameliorated.[40]

Myasthenia Gravis (MG) and Thymoma-associated Neuromuscular Disorder: Can be a congenital (Siamese) or acquired condition (Aby, Somali). One study reported that compared with mixed-breed cats, relative risk for acquired MG is highest in Abyssinian (and Somali) cats; relative risk also increased after three years of age. The MG is associated with dysphagia, megaesophagus, weakness, or weakness with a cranial mediastinal mass.[41] Acetylcholine receptor antibodies produced within/by the thymoma and in muscle cross reacted. Clinically, voice changes, tremor, ventroflexion of the neck and gait abnormalities were noted. Myasthenia gravis signs are typical of the acquired idiopathic form.[42] Acetylcholine receptor antibody titers of > 0.3 nmol/L are diagnostic for acquired MG. Some afflicted cats were noted to have been treated for hyperthyroidism with methimazole for 2-4 months prior to the diagnosis of MG in one report. The study did not attribute any causative effect though.[41]

Mycobacterium avium Susceptiblity: In North America and Australia, of a case series of 12 cats under 6 years old, 10/12 were Abyssinian, and 1/12 was Somali, a closely related breed. Clinical signs include weight loss, lower respiratory tract infection, and enlarged lymph nodes, with slow re-growing hair. A familial immune-compromise was suspected in certain lines. They were FeLV-FIV negative cats but developed disseminated infection.

Long term treatment with clarithromycin combined with another agent such as rifampicin and a fluoroquinolone, or doxycycline was somewhat effective. It was proposed that there are certain lines of Somali and Abyssinian cats that are predisposed due to a familial immunodeficiency.[43]

Glycogen Storage Disease: A 10-year old cat in Indiana was diagnosed with a storage disease that resulted in accumulation of what appeared to be unbranched glycogen in skeletal muscle, and minor deposits were in cardiac muscles, brain and spinal cord. Onset of signs occurred gradually, with paresis progressing to paralysis.[44]

Genetic Tests

Progressive Retinal Atrophy: Direct tests for **rdAc** and **Rdy** are available at the UC-Davis VGL.

Pyruvate Kinase Deficiency DNA Test: This is a direct test (not linkage) which identifies affected, carrier, and normal cats. Testing is recommended for anemic Abyssinian and Somali cats, relatives of affected or carrier animals and breeding stock unless all parents of the breeding pair have previously tested negative. Check with the local lab but generally, a minimum of 1-2 ml EDTA blood should be sent immediately (not frozen—cooling the sample is not essential). It should be processed within 48 hours. Test request form available online. A pair of buccal swabs can be used, but one must ensure cells are sampled, not just saliva. Concurrent blood typing can be carried out on the same blood sample. Available at PennGen and UC-Davis VGL.

Renal Function: Screen renal function (as a minimum, serum creatinine and urinalysis) in cats eight years and older since a breed propensity to renal failure has been identified.

Electroretinogram (ERG): Cats with inherited rod-cone degeneration can be screened using ERG in the pre-clinical phase to identify cats at risk for progression. A study comparing homozygous affected and heterozygous at risk cats confirmed that cats with the inherited condition will show the following changes:

Decreased a-wave amplitude
Increased b-wave implicit times
Abnormal ERG waveforms
b-wave:a-wave ratios high

A graphic representation of results can distinguish between genotypes, even before funduscopic changes are evident.[45]

Another study showed that short ERG protocol is more efficient than a long one in the identification of affected cats. A study using 12 parameters was adequate to discriminate rod-cone dystrophic cats from normal cats.[46]

Anti-acetylcholine receptor antibodies (serum) for MG: Send to Comparative Neuromuscular Laboratory, att: Diane Shelton, UCSC http://vetneuromuscular.ucsd.edu/

No genetic tests are yet available for rdAc or Rdy eye diseases.

Miscellaneous

- **Breed name synonyms:** Aby, Ticked Cat, Egyptian Cat, informal name "Bunny Cat"
- **Registries:** FIFé, TICA, CFA, ACFA, CFF, CCA, NZCF, WCF, ACF, GCCF
- **Breed resources: CFA Abyssinian Breed Council:** www.abyssinianbc.org
  The Abyssinian Cat Club of America: http://www.abyworld.com/
  Abyssinian Cat Association (UK): www.theabycat.com

References

1. Chew DJ, DiBartola SP, Boyce JT, et al. Renal amyloidosis in related Abyssinian cats. *J Am Vet Med Assoc* 1982;181(2):139-142.
2. DiBartola SP. Familial renal diseases of cats. *Proceedings.* The North American Veterinary Conference 1999:326-327.
3. van der Linde-Sipman JS, Niewold TA, Tooten PCJ, et al. Generalized AA-amyloidosis in Siamese and Oriental cats. *Vet Immunol Immunopathol* 1997;56:1-10.
4. Gruys E, Van de Stadt M, Blok JJ, et al. Feline Amyloidosis. First International Feline Genetic Disease Conference *Proceedings (abstr), in: Feline Practice Supplement,* 1999;15.
5. van Rossum M, van Asten FJAM, Rofina J, Lenstra JA, Benson MD, Gruys E. Analysis of cDNA sequences of feline SAAs. *Amyloid: J Protein Folding Disord* 2004;11:38-43.
6. Anderson RE, Maude MB, Nilsson SEG, et al. Plasma lipid abnormalities in 465 the Abyssinian cat with a hereditary rod-cone degeneration. Letter to the Editor, *Exp Eye Res* 1991;53:415-417.
7. Narfström K. Progressive Retinal Atrophy in Abyssinians. First International Feline Genetic Disease Conference Philadelphia June, 1998 *Proceedings (abstr) in: Feline Practice Supplement,* 1999;21.
8. Narfström K. Hereditary progressive retinal atrophy in the Abyssinian cat. *J Hered* 1983;74:273-276.
9. Wiggert B, van Veen T, Kutty G, et al. An early decrease in interphoto-receptor retinoid-binding protein gene expression in Abyssinian cats homozygous for hereditary rod-cone degeneration. *Cell Tissue Res* 1994;278:291-298.
10. Seeliger MW, Narfström K. Functional assessment of the regional distribution of disease in a cat model of hereditary retinal degeneration. *Invest Ophthalmol Vis Sci* 2000;41(7):1998-2005.
11. Nilsson SFE, Mäepea O, Alm A, Narfström K. Ocular blood flow and retinal metabolism in Abyssinian cats with hereditary retinal degeneration. *Invest Ophthalmol Vis Sci* 2001;42(5):1038-1044.

12. Narfström K, Ehinger B, Bruun A. Immunohistochemical studies of cone photoreceptors and cells of the inner retina in feline rod-cone degeneration. *Vet Ophthalmol* 2001;4(2):141-145.

13. May CA, Lutjen-Drecoll E, Narfstrom K Morphological changes in the anterior segment of the Abyssinian cat eye with hereditary rod-cone degeneration. Curr Eye Res. 2005;30(10):855-62.

14. Narfström K, David V, Jarret O, Beatty J, Barrs V, Wilkie D, O'Brien S, Menotti-Raymond M. Retinal degeneration in the Abyssinian and Somali cat (rdAc): correlation between genotype and phenotype and rdAc allele frequency in two continents. Vet Ophthalmol. 2009 Sep-Oct;12(5):285-91

15. Narfström K. Hereditary and congenital ocular disease. *J Fel Med Surg* 1999;1:135-141.

16. Menotti-Raymond M, Deckman KH, David V, Myrkalo J, O'Brien SJ, Narfström K. Mutation discovered in a feline model of human congenital retinal blinding disease. Invest Ophthalmol Vis Sci. 2010 Jun;51(6):2852-9.

17. Smith SA, Tobias AH, Jacob KA, et al. Arterial thromboembolism in cats: Acute crisis in 127 cases (1992-2001) and long-term management with low-dose aspirin in 24 cases. *J Vet Intern Med* 2003;17:73-83.

18. Bagdi N, Magdus M, Leidinger E, et al. Frequencies of feline blood types in Hungary. *Acta Vet Hung* 2001;49(4):369-375.

19. Giger U, Bucheler J, Patterson DF. Frequency and inheritance of A and B blood types in feline breeds of the United States. *J Hered* 1991;82:15-20.

20. Giger U, Griot-Wenk M, Bucheler J, et al. Geographical variation of the feline blood type frequencies in the United States. *Fel Pract* 1991;19(6):21-27.

21. Giger U. In: Bonagura J, ed. *Kirk's Current Veterinary Therapy XIII.* Philadelphia: WB Saunders Co, 2000;396-399.

22. Barrs VR, Giger U, Wilson B, Chan CTT, Lingard AE, Tran L, Seng A, Canfield PJ, Beattya JA. Erythrocyte pyruvate kinase deficiency and AB blood types in Australian Abysinnian and Somali cats. *Aust Vet J* 2009;87(1):39-44.

23. Giger U, Casal M, Niggemeier A. The fading kitten syndrome and neonatal isoerythrolysis. Proceedings. The 15th Annual ACVIM Medical Forum, Lake Buena Vista FL 1997;308-310.

24. Kohn B, Goldschmidt MH, Hohenhaus AE, et al. Anemia, splenomegaly, and increased osmotic fragility of erythrocytes in Abyssinian and Somali cats. *J Am Vet Med Assoc* 2000;217(10):1483-1491.

25. Giger U, Rajpurohit Y, Skelly B, et al. Erythrocyte pyruvate kinase deficiency in cats. In: First International Feline Genetic Disease Conference 1998. *Proceedings (abstr), Feline Practice Supplement,* 1999;8.

26. Ford S, Giger U, Duesberg C, Beutler E, Wang P. Inherited erythrocyte pyruvate kinase (PK) deficiency causing hemolytic anemia in an Abyssinian cat. 10th Annual Veterinary Medical Forum. San Diego CA. May 1992. Proceedings [abstr] in: *JACVIM* 1992;6:123.

27. Kohn B, Fumi C. Clinical course of pyruvate kinase deficiency in Abyssinian and Somali cats J Feline Med Surg. 2008 Apr;10(2):145-53.

28. Lulich JP, O'Brien TD, Osborne CA, et al. Feline Renal Failure: Questions, answers, questions. *Compend Contin Educ Pract Vet* 1992;14(2):127-152.

29. van Wessum R, Harvey, CE, Hennet P. Feline dental resorptive lesions-prevalence patterns. *Vet Clin North Am: Sm Anim Pract* 1992;22:1405-1416.

30. Lekcharoensuk C, Osborne CA, Lulich JP. Epidemiologic study of risk factors for lower urinary tract diseases in cats. *J Am Vet Med Assoc* 2001;May1;218(9):1429-1435.

31. Fox PR. Feline cardiomyopathy (Part I). Hypertrophic cardiomyopathy. *Proceedings.* 19th Annual ACVIM Forum Denver CO 2001;145.

32. Atkins CE. Feline dilated cardiomyopathy. Winter 2004 AAFP Meeting. Proceedings [abstr] in: *AAFP Newsletter* August 2004 22(2):29-30.

33. Engvall E, Bushnell N. Patellar luxation in Abyssinian cats. *Fel Pract* 1990;18(4):20-22.

34. Smith GK Lagenbach A, Giger U, et al. Patellar luxation and hip dysplasia in a group of cats. First International Feline Genetic Disease Conference Philadelphia June 1998 *Proceedings (abstr) in: Feline Practice Supplement,* 1999;23.

35. Little S. Feline hip dysplasia. Notes. Winn Feline Foundation Website.

Available at: www.winnfelinehealth.org/hip-dysplasia.html Accessed Sep 29, 2004.

36. Smith GK, Lagenbach A, Green PA, et al. Evaluation of the association between medial patellar luxation and hip dysplasia in cats. *J Am Vet Med Assoc* 1999;215(1):40-45.

37. Lagenbach A, Giger U, Green P, et al. Relationship between degenerative joint disease and hip joint laxity by use of distraction index and Norberg angle measurement in a group of cats. *J Am Vet Med Assoc* 1998;213(10):1439-1443.

38 Pesteanu-Somogyi LD, Radzai C, Pressler BM. Prevalence of feline infectious peritonitis in specific cat breeds. *J Feline Med Surg.* 2006 Feb;8(1):1-5

39. Jones BR, Gruffydd-Jones TJ, Sparkes AH, et al. Preliminary studies on congenital hypothyroidism in a family of Abyssinian cats. *Vet Rec* 1992;131:145-148.

40. Tobias S, Labato MA. Identifying and managing feline congenital hypothyroidism. *Vet Med* 2001;Sep:719-726.

41. Shelton GD, Ho M, Kass PH. Risk factors for acquired myasthenia gravis in cats: 105 cases (1986-1998). *J Am Vet Med Assoc* 2000;Jan1;216(1):55-57.

42. Bagley RS. Diseases of the peripheral nervous system, neuromuscular junction and muscle; Evaluation of weakness. *Proceedings.* AAFP Fall meeting. 1998:31-33.

43. Baral RM, Metcalfe SS, Krockenberger MB, Catt MJ, Barrs VR, McWhirter C, Hutson CA, Wigney DI, Martin P, Chen SC, Mitchell DH, Malik R. Disseminated Mycobacterium avium infection in young cats: overrepresentation of Abyssinian cats. *J Feline Med Surg.* 2006 Feb;8(1):23-44.

44. Langohr IM, Tanabe M Idiopathic complex polysaccharide storage disease in an Abyssinian cat. *Vet Pathol.* 2005 Jul;42(4):502-6.

45. Hyman JA, Vaegan, Lei B, Narfstrom KL Electrophysiologic differentiation of homozygous and heterozygous Abyssinian-crossbred cats with late-onset hereditary retinal degeneration *Am J Vet Res.* 2005 Nov;66(11):1914-21.

46. Vaegen, Narfstrom K Optimal discrimination of an Abyssinian cat recessive retinal degeneration: a short electroretinogram protocol is more efficient than a long one. *Clin Experiment Ophthalmol.* 2004 Dec; 32(6): 619-25.

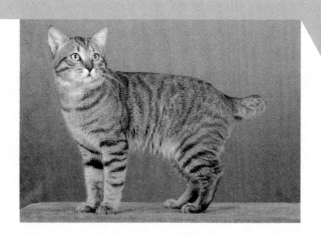

American Bobtail

The Breed History

This American breed is thought to have originated in Arizona in the 1960s, deriving from a cat named *Yodie*. A mutation in a cat led to the presence of a bobtail, and breeders used this cat as a foundation animal for the new breed.

Breed origins are poorly documented, and some consider Japanese Bobtail and Manx genes to have been in the source cat rather than this being a spontaneous mutation in a feral cat. The mutation is distinct in studies carried out so far comparing the American Bobtail with the Manx. Only American Bobtails with a standard tail length (just above the tarsus) are considered show stock. Almost tailless cats and those with short kinked tails are also born. CFA first accepted this breed in 2000 in the Miscellaneous Class, TICA registry accepted them in 1989. No outcrossing is allowed. These cats are larger than Japanese Bobtail cats.

Physical Characteristics

Weight: 7-15 lb (3-7 kg), females smaller than males in this weight range, and some males may exceed 15 pounds.

Coat: There are two coat varieties; Longhair **(autosomal recessive)** and Shorthair. The longhair type is a semi-long shaggy soft coat. The short haircoat stands out, and also has an unkempt appearance. It is a water resistant coat. The undercoat is soft and dense like rabbit fur. All colors are accepted.

Eyes: With a strong wild staring expression, eyes are oval-almond in shape, and all eye colors are accepted except odd eyes.

Points of Conformation: American Bobtail cats are well muscled medium-large cats with short heavy legs. There is a distinctive brow. Ears are medium in size, are high and wide set and have Lynx tufts and furnishings. The head is broad and is a modified wedge shape, and the nose has a moderate break which is slightly concave. There is a prominent whisker pinch. These cats have prominent scapulae, and large round paws. The bobtail is an **autosomal dominant** trait. The tail must be long enough to be seen above the back when the cat is active but be above the hock when resting. Average bobtail length ranges from 1-4" (2.5-10 cm) and straighter tails are preferred. The American Bobtail gait is smooth and rolling.

Grooming: Low to moderate grooming needs are typical for the Longhair, and there are low grooming needs for the shorthaired cats. Coats do not tend to mat easily.

Recognized Behavior Issues and Traits

Reported breed characteristics include: Curious, friendly, adaptable, high intelligence, "dog-like" personality; enjoy games such as fetch and hide and seek, get along well with most dogs, love children, are quiet voiced cats using chirps and trills mostly, many can learn to open doors, and are easy to leash train. Used for psycho-assistance therapy cats because of their excellent calm temperament, and do well in busy, noisy environments.

Normal Breed Variations

Slow to mature (three years of age before they fit the breed standard)

Drug Sensitivities

None reported in the literature

Inherited Diseases

Tails may range in length from full normal tail to a rumpy, though the latter is very rare.

Disease Predispositions

None reported in the literature

Genetic Tests

No commercial tests available.

Miscellaneous

- **Breed name synonyms:** AmBob, Bobtail
- **Registries:** TICA, CFA
- **Breed resources: American Bobtail Breeders Association:** http://www.angelfire.com/country/americanbobtails/ **American Bobtail CFA Breeders Club:** http://americanbobtailbreeders.com/

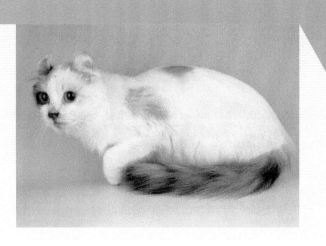

body is well muscled and the legs are moderate in length. Paws are moderately small and round.

Note that kittens are born with straight ears and they start curling at about 4-7 days of age. The curl does not set fully until about 16 weeks of age or even much later. There is still considerable regional variation in type due to continued outcrossing to domestic cats.

Grooming: The American Curl cat has low grooming needs, and is a low shedding cat.

The Breed History

This breed traces its origins to Lakeland California to a random autosomal dominant mutation in a black longhaired cat in 1981. The litter from this foundation cat Shulamith contained some curled ear kittens. One kitten was longhaired, the other shorthaired according to some sources, others report that they were both longhaired and that the shorthairs were introduced during subsequent outcrossing. The CFA first recognized this breed in 1986, provisional status was granted in 1991, and accepted for championship status in 1993. The TICA registry accepted the breed in 1985. The single litter origin of the American Curl breed has required that some outcrosses occur to maintain breed vigor. The outcrosses have been to domestic cats without pedigree and in CFA, books closed Jan 2010.

Physical Characteristics

Weight: females: 5-8 lb (2.5-3.5 kg), males 7-11 lb (3-5 kg)

Coat: A flat, silky coat with both long and shorthair types accepted. The tail is plumed in the longhair variety; all colors, patterns and color combinations are recognized. Minimal undercoat is present. In shorthairs, a striped pattern of legs, face and tail is described. Ears are well furnished inside.

Eyes: Moderately large, all colors are accepted; they are walnut shaped with a mascara line. In colorpoint cats the eyes are blue.

Points of Conformation: Moderate in all proportions, the ears which are the distinguishing breed feature have rounded tips curling smoothly back 90 to 180 degrees at the tip only and point towards the midline. They are graded as first degree if they are mildly turned (pet quality), second degree if they are moderately turned (breeding quality) and third degree if they are significantly curled (show quality-full crescent). Only the distal portion of the pinna should curl—the base cartilage should be firm—more like a human ear than a normal cat ear cartilage in texture. The repeated physical uncurling of the ear tip is not advised since the cartilage may be compromised .Use caution during physical examination so as not to tug on the ear.

The head is a modified wedge shape, nose is straight and moderate in length with a slight break, and the overall build is semi-foreign. Tail length equals body length and tapers from a wide base. The

Recognized Behavior Issues and Traits

Reported breed characteristics include: Even tempered, they like close human contact, friendly, curious, quiet though playful, get along with other pets, good with children, adaptable; somewhat of a "dog personality" since they like to follow the family around. The Curls keep a kitten-like playful attitude until late in life. Not particularly vocal.

Normal Breed Variations

Slow maturing (2-3 years)

Drug Sensitivities

None reported in the literature

Inherited Diseases

Curl: This is an autosomal dominant mutation (Cu).[1] It does not appear to affect cartilage in joints and so is not considered a deleterious mutation. Curls may be mated with curls. Degree of offspring curling does not seem to correlate closely with parents but curl X curl mating will usually produce offspring with some degree of curling in all kittens.

Disease Predispositions

None reported in the literature—reported to be hardy due to domestic shorthair vigor.

Genetic Tests

None commercially available

Miscellaneous

- **Breed name synonyms:** Curl
- **Registries:** CFA, ACFA (separate Longhair and Shorthair standards), TICA (separate Longhair and Shorthair standards), CFF, FIFé (Shorthair and Longhair separate), CCA
- **Breed resources: American Curl Cat Club (ACCC) [CFF]:** 100 Westmont Rd. Syracuse, NY 13219
  United Society of American Curls: 11691 Kagel Canyon, Lake View Terrace, CA 91342-7422
  Cat Club American Curl: http://www.american-curl.org/cariboost_files/statuts_20ccac_en.pdf

References

1. Robinson R. The American Curl cat. J Hered 1989;80(6):474-475.

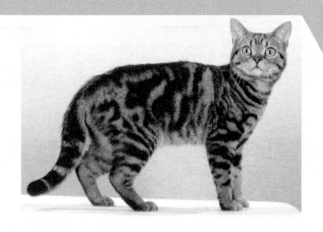

The Breed History

The American Shorthair derives from stock brought over from Europe with the pioneers. The British Shorthair is likely one of the main progenitors; the first registered cat (1904) was sired by a British Shorthair. Bred for rodent control, these hardy cats made do with a harsh outdoor lifestyle living in streets and barns. Common in North America, the registry allowed housecats without pedigree into the breed for many years but now the registry books are closed. The breed name changed from Domestic Shorthair to American Shorthair in 1966. The CFA accepted this breed first in 1906 and it has remained popular for many years (a top 10). The FIFé does not recognize the American Shorthair.

Physical Characteristics

Weight: females 8-12 lb (3.5-5.5 kg), males 11-15 lb (5-7 kg)

Coat: The dense coat is standoff and coat density increases during the cold weather. Accepted colors and patterns number about 80, with silver tabby being the most commonly seen. TICA and CFA standards differ in the types of tabby accepted. Hair texture is crisp.

Eyes: Most eye colors accepted. The eyes are a modified round shape.

Points of Conformation: Though not the largest of the cat breeds, the American Shorthair is particularly noted for sturdy bone and muscling. Overall, their conformation is moderate in every way (mesomorphic). The face is broad with prominent cheeks. The head is slightly longer when compared to the British Shorthair. Ears are medium sized and moderately wide set, with a rounded tip.

The tail is medium in length and thick, tapering to a blunt tip. Paws are round. The nose is medium in length and in profile, is slightly concave.

Grooming: Moderate grooming needs are met by a light brushing about two times a week. A bit more care is needed while shedding.

Recognized Behavior Issues and Traits

Reported breed characteristics include: Gentle, affectionate, quiet, playful and adaptable. An easy-going temperament is a breed characteristic. Good with children and dogs generally. They are robust and adaptable to both indoor and outdoor lifestyles. Not demanding of attention.

Normal Breed Variations

In one study, 100% of American Shorthair cats tested blood type A.[1]

Watch calorie intake to prevent obesity.

Good mothering ability.

Early sexual maturity.

Good longevity.

Drug Sensitivities

None reported in the literature

Inherited Diseases

Hypertrophic Cardiomyopathy (HCM): This is the most common cardiac condition in cats (10% prevalence), and is seen in some lines of American Shorthairs. It was reported that it was likely inherited in this breed but the mode of inheritance was unknown.[2]

An autosomal dominant mode of inheritance was considered most likely in a family of American Shorthair cats.[3] The condition was described as familial systolic anterior motion of the mitral valve and/or hypertrophic cardiomyopathy.

Onset of HCM is usually in middle age, and is more common in males, but this breed tends to have a milder form of the condition than some other breeds of cats such as the Ragdoll or Maine Coon. It is thought to be due to a mutation affecting the myosin protein in cardiac muscle.[4,5] No specific screening recommendations have been made to date for this breed.

Craniofacial Deformity: Some lines of the breed carry the gene for this condition *(best known in the Burmese cat: see that chapter for details)* though frequency is dropping due to careful breeding management. These cat families tend to have a more extreme facial feature set, as with the Contemporary Burmese. This is an autosomal recessive disorder.[6]

Nasal dermoids are sometimes present in some cats; these are also seen in Burmese cats carrying this gene. Eyelid colobomas and cleft lips have also been seen in the ASH. A shallow longitudinal furrow of tissue, or color change running along the nose has been found in almost 90% of American Shorthair carrier cats, and may be a phenotypic marker of a carrier, though sensitivity and specificity of this finding is not 100% so pedigree analysis should also be used.[7]

Disease Predispositions

None reported in the literature

Rare and Isolated Reports

Polycystic Kidney Disease (PKD): PKD is most common in Persian breeds, and those breeds having crossed out to Persians in their breeding programs. In screening programs carried out at the University of California, Davis in 2002, American Shorthair cat were found positive in two small test groups: In clinic I: 6 of 40 American Shorthair cats were positive, and in the second clinic, 2 of 8 American Shorthair cats tested positive by ultrasound screening of healthy cats from catteries. A genetic test is available.[8]

Ornithine Transcarbamylase Deficiency: One case report describes an 18 month old American Shorthair cat presented with stunted growth and postprandial depression. Elevated bile acids and ammonia were noted. Urea cycle enzyme deficiency is of sex linked dominant inheritance in humans, but of unknown mechanism in cats. Diagnosis is by urinary metabolite identification; a portosystemic shunt was ruled out.[9]

Hereditary Deafness: Is associated with the dominant gene for white cat (W); may be found in white cats of this breed.[10]

Genetic Tests

Though there are no published recommendations for screening this breed for HCM using echocardiography, one may consider screening breeding stock until further information is available.

Direct genetic test for PKD is available from the UC-Davis VGL.

Miscellaneous

- **Breed name synonyms:** Domestic Shorthair (historical name in use until 1960s), ASH, DASH
- **Registries:** ACFA, TICA, CFA, CFF, CCA, WCF
- **Breed resources:** National American Shorthair Club (CFA):
  781 Progress Street
  Macon, GA 31201
  http://www.ashclub.org/

References

1. Giger U. In: Bonagura J, ed. *Kirk's Current Veterinary Therapy XIII.* Philadelphia: WB Saunders Co, 2000;396-399.
2. Meurs KM. Inherited heart disease in the cat. *Proceedings.* Tuft's Canine and Feline Breeding and Genetics Conference Oct 2-4, 2003 Available at VIN: www.vin.com/tufts/2003. Accessed Nov 19, 2004.
3. Meurs K, Kittleson MD, Towbin J, Ware W. Familial systolic anterior motion of the mitral valve and or hypertrophic cardiomyopathy is apparently inherited as an autosomal dominant trait in a family of American Shorthair cats. *Proceedings.* 15th Annual ACVIM Veterinary Medical Forum, Lake Buena Vista FL [*abstr*] 1997;685.
4. Meurs KM, Kittleson MD, Towbin JA, Ware WA. Familial systolic anterior motion of the mitral valve and/or hypertrophic cardiomyopathy is apparently inherited as an autosomal dominant trait in a family of American shorthair cats. J Vet Intern Med 1997;11:138 (abstract)
5. Kittleson MD, Meurs KM, Kittleson JA, et al. Heritable characteristics, phenotypic expression, and natural history of hypertrophic cardiomyopathy in Maine Coon cats. In: First International Feline Genetic Disease Conference *Proceedings (abstr), Feline Practice Supplement,* 1999;7. Titled: Hypertrophic cardiomyopathy in Maine Coon cats. Notes of the lecture available at: www.winnfelinehealth.org/reports/cardiomyopathy.html Accessed Aug 6, 2004.
6. Erdman C, Lyons LA. Facial Development Study Update, (Aug 2003-Aug 2004). *Notes.* University of California (Davis) Feline Genetics Extravaganza II Aug 28-29, 2004.
7. Lyons LA. The Lyon's Den. Feline Genome Project: Cranio-facial Defect. Accessed at: http://faculty.vetmed.ucdavis.edu/faculty/lalyons/Sites/
burmese.htm. Accessed Nov 2004.
8. Lyons LA. The Lyons Den Website. Feline Genome Project: Polycystic Kidney Disease. Available at: http:faculty.vetmed.ucdavis.edu/faculty/lalyons/Sites/pkd.htm. Accessed Nov 6, 2004.
9. Washizu T, Washizu M, Zhang C, et al. A suspected case of ornithine transcarbamylase deficiency in a cat. *J Vet Med Sci* 2004;Jun;66(6):701-703.
10. Strain GM. Hereditary deafness in dogs and cats: Causes, prevalence, and current research. *Proceedings.* Tuft's Canine and Feline Breeding and Genetics Conference. Oct 2-4, 2003 Available at: http://www.vin.com/tuffs/2003. Accessed Nov 19, 2004.

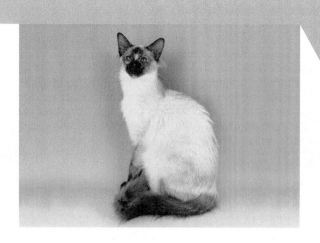

Balinese

The body coat color and points of the Balinese usually becomes darker as the cat ages. Intermediate (medium) length coats result from outcross mating. These shorter haired cats are termed *variants*. This type of coat is short and plush, somewhat in between the shorthair and semi-longhair. These variants are not shown.

Eyes: Medium in size, sapphire blue, almond shaped. Deeper blue is preferred.

Points of Conformation: These cats share most of the same conformation points as Siamese cats; the longer coat with well-plumed tail is the distinguishing feature. Because of the longer cover of hair though, these cats appear less angular to the eye than the Siamese. Ears are large, with some interior furnishings. The Balinese are built like the Siamese. The head is an elongated tapered wedge with a fine muzzle and straight long nose. Paws are delicate and oval. The tail is tapering, thin and ends in a point.

Grooming: For the Balinese cat, there are low-moderate grooming needs and a low matting tendency.

The Breed History
The gene for longer hair in Siamese cats is autosomal recessive in inheritance, and when these semi-longhaired cats were born into Siamese litters in the 1940s, they were selected for in a new breeding program. Prior to this time, they were considered an undesirable offspring type and called Longhaired Siamese. The early breed development occurred in California and New York during the 1950s. The TICA and CFA accepted this breed in 1970, and FIFé followed in 1972.

Javanese refers to semi-longhaired Siamese (e.g., Balinese) with lynx (tabby) and tortie point patterns instead of classic Siamese solid points (lilac, seal etc). The Javanese as a separate breed was accepted by CFA in 1979—in all other registries Javanese cats are part of the Balinese breed. Overseas the Javanese name is synonymous with **Oriental Longhair.**

Traditional (Applehead) Balinese cats are of a type derived from the Traditional (Applehead) Siamese. They are of heavier build with a much rounder face and head conformation, smaller ears, and longer haircoat over the body (>2") including ruff, pantaloons, and ear tufting. Most registries do not have a separate partition for this subtype. In the many registries, they are registered but are not generally show cats.

Falling somewhere in between the Traditional Balinese and Modern Balinese type is another intermediate type termed "Classic".

The name "Balinese" is thought to derive from these cats appearing as graceful as Balinese dancers.

Outcrossing to Siamese cats is still allowed in the CFA registry.

Physical Characteristics
Weight: 6-11 lb (2.5-5 kg).
Traditional subtype cats average 10-14 lb (4.5-6.5 kg)

Coat: The semi-longhair single coat is fine, silky and flat lying and not much longer than a short haircoat; the longest hairs are found on the tail. They have a dark face mask. All of the Siamese color point coats are represented in the Balinese. In CFA registry, recognition is extended only to blue, chocolate, lilac and seal point—other pointed cats are referred to as Javanese, a separate breed.

Recognized Behavior Issues and Traits
Reported breed characteristics include: Highly intelligent, friendly, though some individuals may be aloof. The Balinese are curious, playful and often less vocal, a bit softer voiced, and a bit less active than the Siamese cats. They are also highly social, and need plenty of human contact and mental stimulation; may follow favored people around the house. Balinese cats are content to be lap cats in between burst of activity. Climbing trees or perches are important for these athletic cats; they love being up high. Good with children and dogs; may even curl up and sleep with a favored dog and let themselves be groomed by that dog. If left alone all day, may benefit from another cat in the household. Not suited to an outdoor lifestyle.

Normal Breed Variations
Need to watch calorie intakes as can become obese more easily than some other breeds

Drug Sensitivities
None reported in the literature

Inherited Diseases
Because this breed originated primarily from Siamese cats, and outcrossing with Siamese continues, see **Siamese Pointed Cat** chapter for information on the pointing gene and its effects on coat and vision, and other Siamese breed conditions.

Disease Predispositions
None reported in the literature

Rare and Isolated Reports

Sphingomyelin Lipidosis (SYN: Sphingomyelinosis): This is a rare condition and reported only in Siamese and Balinese. This storage disease results in reduced activity of the enzyme sphingomyelinase that metabolizes lipids and when deficient, leads to lysosomal accumulation of sphingomyelin in many tissues. Cholesterol accumulates in the liver. Sphingomyelin lipidosis is similar to human Niemann-Pick disease Type A.

A case report of a Balinese kitten described onset of hind limb dysmetria at three months of age, with gradual progression of signs. Head tremor, mydriasis and nystagmus, and other signs developed. Visual deficits, weakness and progression to moribund state occurred; hepatosplenomegaly and plantigrade stance was also described in other reports. This type of storage disease is milder and more slowly progressive when compared with G_{M1} and G_{M2} gangliosidosis. Histologic lesions were present in kidney, spleen, lung, liver and brain.[1] It is inherited as an autosomal recessive trait in Siamese cats; likely the same in Balinese cats.[2]

Feline Mucopolysaccharidosis VI: A case report described two Balinese cats with paresis/paralysis, facial dysmorphia (flattened face, small ears, bulging forehead), skeletal abnormalities (fusion of cervical and lumbar region vertebrae, osteoporosis and widened IV spaces in T-L, flat-chested, long bone epiphyseal dysplasia, coxofemoral luxation).

Excessive urinary levels of dermatan sulphate (a glycosamino-glycan; mucopolysaccharide) were due to lysosomal arylsulphatase B enzyme deficiency. Onset of clinical signs was at 12-16 weeks old. Slow growth, smaller stature, abnormal gait progressing to posterior paresis within a few months, painful lumbosacral area, large paws, medial stifle deviation and over-flexed rear limbs were noted. In spite of supportive care, one cat died at 18 months of age. Diagnosis of disease requires dimethyl-methylene blue test of urine, and biopsy of skin with fibroblast assay of the enzyme confirmed reduction of arylsulphatase B. This trait has also been reported in three Siamese cat families. This is likely an inherited condition as it has only ever been reported in Siamese and Siamese-related cats.[3] In a colony of cats studied in Australia, two separate mutations were found.[4]

Genetic Tests

None commercially available

Miscellaneous

- **Breed name synonyms:** Javanese (the name applies to non-Siamese type points such as cream, tabby, tortie and red). In TICA and other non-CFA registries, the Balinese and Javanese are the same breed. In Europe, they may be classed as Oriental Longhairs.
- **Other breed synonyms include:** Bali, Longhaired Siamese, Lao-Tsun Cat.
- **Registries:** FIFé, TICA, CFA, ACFA, CFF, NZCF, CCA, WCF, GCCF, ACF
- **Breed resources: Traditional and Classic Cat International (including Applehead Siamese, Traditional Balinese):** http://www.tccat.org/
  Balinese Cat Society (UK): http://www.rantipole.demon.co.uk/bcs

Balinese and Siamese Cat Club (UK):
http://www.thebalineseandsiamesecatclub.co.uk/

References

1. Baker HJ, Wood PA, Wenger DA, et al. Sphingomyelin lipidosis in a cat. *Vet Pathol* 1978;24 (5):386-391.
2. Shell LG. A review of feline neuromuscular diseases. In: Symposium: Feline Neurologic Diseases. *Vet Med* Jun;1998;565-574.
3. Di Natale P, Annella T, Daniele A, et al. Animal models for lysosomal storage diseases : A new case of feline mucopolysaccharidosis VI. *J Inher Metab Dis* 1992;15:17-24.
4. Crawley AC, Yogalingam G, Muller V, et al. Inherited degenerative joint disease in cats due to mild Mucopolysaccharidosis Type VI. First International Feline Genetic Disease Conference Philadelphia June, 1998 *Proceedings (abstr)* in: *Feline Practice Supplement,* 1999:30.

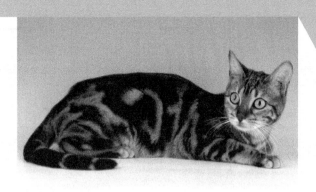

Bengal

an elongated modified wedge. Muzzle is broad, whisker pads are pronounced. Ears are short, wide set and rounded tips. The nose is broad and has a slight puff in profile. Limbs are long with good bone/ heavy muscling. The muscular body is long. Tail is thick and tapers. Paws are large and rounded.

Grooming: Low grooming needs; just provide weekly chamois rub down or light brushing.

Recognized Behavior Issues and Traits

Reported breed characteristics include: Affectionate, athletic, curious, happy, intelligent, and outgoing. Very active, they love to climb and jump; they need a climbing tree or post; a high energy pet; will fetch and will usually take to leash walks if introduced early. The Bengal likes lots of human contact. Though in shows, mild fear response is acceptable, those that show signs of challenge are disqualified. Bengal cats have variations in voice and other atypical vocalizations, and they are considered very vocal. They love water. They are good with older children. Some may learn to open doors.

Normal Breed Variations

Reduced fertility in early filial generations: F1 males are usually sterile, and F2 and F3 males have reduced fertility.

Bengal Kitten Information Project[1] An Internet-based breeder survey was carried out to establish normal baselines for reproduction.

 55 reporting breeders, 176 litters, 701 kittens,
 July 2003 to June 2004.
 Average litter size 4.0
 Stillbirth rate 6%
 C sections 3%
 Average birth weight: Male 94 g female 92 g
 Congenital defects included: flat-chested, cleft palate.

Blood Type: In a small study done in the UK, 4 of 8 cats tested as part of a survey were blood type AB, and the other four were type A.[2]

A group has been working to map over 500 genetic markers in Bengal cats. Study announced in 1998.[3]

Drug Sensitivities

None reported in the literature

Inherited Diseases

Flat-chested Kittens: Similar to the flat-chested condition in Burmese (see Burmese chapter), whereby reduced chest dorso-ventral dimension occurs. This trait is seen with some frequency in Bengal cats and is seen in F1 kittens, so it is not the result of inbreeding (Pers. Comm., Dr. Solveig Pflueger). Signs may include poor weight gain, exaggerated cranial thoracic vertebral kyphosis, vomiting, dyspnea, cyanosis, exercise intolerance and cough, and a ridge along the costo-chondral junction of the ribs.

The Breed History

This is a recently developed American breed. In 1963, hybridization of the Asian leopard cat (*Prionailurus bengalensis*) and domestic cat was carried out. The original cross arose out of a research initiative by geneticists to explore natural resistance to FeLV. The breed was derived from eight hybrids selected from this project. Outcrosses to Egyptian Mau, Indian Street cat and domestic cats occurred. Early hybrids were not easy to tame, but the breed has been progressively selected for amicability.

A five generation breeding history is necessary for registry as a Bengal, and within that pedigree a maximum of one Asian leopard cat may be present. Bengals with greater than four generations of inter-Bengal breeding are referred to as SBT (stud book tradition) Bengal cats. Earlier filial (F) generations are technically still referred to as Leopard cat crosses or hybrids, and are not typically sold for the pet market, though some placid fourth filial generation cats (F4s) may be sold to experienced cat owners. The F1 cats (F4 or later crossed back with wild cat) are referred to as foundation cats. Some states have restrictions in place against F1 and F2 cats. The TICA registry was the first to accept this breed but stipulated at that time that show cats be at least F4s.

Physical Characteristics

Weight: female 10-15 lb (4.5-6.75 kg), male 10-22 lb (4.5-9.5 kg)

Coat: The short, dense, soft coat is usually brown tabby, blue tabby and snow tabby, with marbled or spotted patterns with an autosomal dominant inheritance pattern. Marbling is a swirling of color produced by combination of the wild type rosette with domestic classic tabby. The spotted pattern is most common. Hair texture is silky. Spots should be very distinct and large, and a necklet or necklets should be present on the throat, with a "jawstrap" extending between the mandibles. Tail is spotted or ringed and the tip is black. In marbled cats, the marking color is enhanced by a darker outline color to the spots (rosettes). Belly must be spotted. Colors accepted may vary with the registry. *Glitter* refers to a high gloss gold or pearl sheen, and is not required, but is desirable. Kitten coats may not mature until 6 months of age.

Eyes: Variable colors; gold, hazel, green, and blue; large, wide set.

Points of Conformation: This large cat has a fairly small head with

As kittens mature, and the rib cage calcification completes, clinical signs abate in many of those kittens that were less severely affected and thus not euthanized in the neonatal period. Though recognized by breeders, the flat-chested kittens have not been reported in the literature. Signs are often first noted at 7-10 days of age.

Pyruvate Kinase (PK) Deficiency: Autosomal recessive disease causing hemolytic anemia. See under Abyssinian. A genetic test is available.

Disease Predispositions

FIP Susceptibility: An American study found that Bengal cats were significantly over-represented for a diagnosis of FIP when they analyzed data for a 16 year period at a veterinary teaching hospital.[4]

Rare and Isolated Reports

Ulcerative Nasal Dermatitis: Of 48 Bengal cats seen in a Sweden clinic between 1999 and 2003, six cats had fissured, crusted and ulcerated erosive changes to the nasal planum. Age of onset was between 4 months and 1 year. Cause of the condition was not elucidated. It was proposed to be an immune-mediated mechanism.[5]

Bengal Idiopathic Polyradiculoneuropathy: A case report detailed a motor function loss in a 16-month-old NM. The rapid progression of dysfunction began in pelvic limbs then spread to the thoracic limbs. The etiology was not determined. Studies confirmed a ventral motor root (primarily axonal) neuropathy. Cyclic tetraparesis occurred over a year interval. Prognosis for the disease is considered good.[6]

In a case retrospective study, Bengals represented 8.7% of the cases, with average age of presentation one and a half years of age. Abnormal EMGs, motor neuron velocities and action potential amplitudes were identified by the researchers. Axonal degeneration and demyelination were found, sometimes alone, sometimes together. To diagnose, they recommend both nerve and muscle biopsies. Weakness is the usual clinical complaint, with mostly lower motor neuron signs, though a small proportion had upper motor neuron function changes, megacolon, and less commonly, laryngeal paresis or normal neurologic examination. Over 50% of the cats had resolution but a small number recrudesced.[7]

Other miscellaneous conditions reported include predilection for Tritrichomonas foetus infections, PRA, hip dysplasia and patellar luxation.[8]

Genetic Tests

Since at least in one very small sample, some cats have the rare blood type AB, it may be prudent to screen breeding stock, and prior to transfusion to check for the B allele until further information is available about geographic and breed distribution of the blood types.

Direct genetic test for PK deficiency is available from PennGen and UC-Davis VGL.

Miscellaneous

- **Breed name synonyms:** Leopardettes (historical), Bengel, Spotted Cat
- **Registries:** FIFé, TICA, ACFA, CFF, GCCF, ACF, WCF, CCA, NZCF
- **Breed resources: International Bengal Cat Society Inc.:** http://www.tibcs.com/whatis.aspx
  The Bengal Cat Club (UK; GCCF): http://www.bengalcatclub.co.uk/
  The International Bengal Breeder's Association Inc.: http://www.webring.org/hub?ring=theinternation18

References

1. Little S. Bengal Kitten Information Project, Pers. Comm. March 2009.
2. Knottenbelt CM, Addie DD, Day MJ, Mackin AJ. Determination of the prevalence of feline blood types in the UK. *J of Small Anim Pract* 1999;40:115-118.
3. Lyons LA, Raymond MM, O'Brien SJ. The feline genome project: The role of the genetic map of the cat in fancy cat breeding. First International Feline Genetic Disease Conference *Proceedings (abstr), Feline Practice Supplement,* 1999;20.
4. Pesteanu-Somogyi LD, Radzai C, Pressler BM. Prevalence of feline infectious peritonitis in specific cat breeds. *J Feline Med Surg.* Vol 8(1):ppp1-5. 2006.
5. Bergvall K. A novel ulcerative nasal dermatitis of Bengal cats. Vet Dermatol 2004;15(Suppl. 1):20-40.
6. . Granger N, Stalin CE, Brown TB, Jeffery NDIdiopathic polyradiculoneuropathy in a Bengal cat: electrophysiological findings and 1 year follow-up. J Feline Med Surg. 2008 Dec;10(6):603-7.
7. Pettigrew R, Kent, M, Berry WL, Shelton AJ. Muscle and Nerve Biopsies in 138 Cats: Diagnosis and Outcome.
Online August 4th, 2010 at: http://www.vin.com/proceedings/Proceedings.plx?CID=WSAVA2002&Category=1319&PID=9729&O=Generic
8. Feline Advisory Board Website. Accessed May 2010 at: http://www.fabcats.org/breeders/inherited_disorders/bengal.php

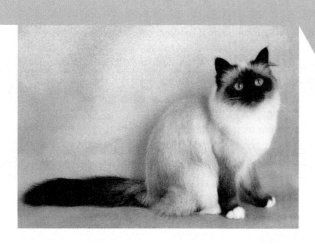

Birman

Roman-nosed, ears are small and wide set. Nose is medium in length, forehead. The tail is full and moderate in size and length, and the body of these cats is long. Limbs are heavily boned and medium in length giving these cats a somewhat stocky conformation. Paws are large and round.

Grooming: The Birman haircoat has low-moderate grooming requirements and looks best with daily brushing; hair has a very low matting tendency.

Recognized Behavior Issues and Traits

Reported breed characteristics include: Playful, friendly, calm, though not as docile as the Persian, less active and less vocal than the Siamese with a soft voice. A Birman may bond with one person, and they may be somewhat territorial. Very affectionate, they are somewhat of a lap cat. When upset, a Birman cat may make a huff sound. Getting along well with dogs, some will even offer to groom their favorite. If the people of the house are absent during the day, some sort of companion should be considered to help keep them content.

Normal Breed Variations

Good longevity

Good mothering ability

Slow maturing

See Azotemia below in Congenital and Inherited Diseases—some feel that this finding is a normal breed variation

Marked reduction in genetic diversity was identified in this breed when compared to random bred cats in a study of 20 domestic and 2 wild cat breeds.[1]

Birman Kitten Information Project:[2] An Internet-based breeder survey was carried out to establish normal baselines for reproduction. Report: 59 reporting breeders, with 204 litters, 735 kittens. Sept 2003-Aug 2004
  Average litter size 3.6
  Stillbirth rate 7%
  C-sections rate 9%
  Average birth weight: Male 98 g female 93 g
  Congenital defects:, seen in 8.3% of litters and included: epibulbar dermoids, syndactyly (an autosomal dominant trait with variable expressivity leading to a split paw), cleft palate, umbilical hernia and open abdomen.

Type B Blood: The prevalence was reported to be 60% in a very small study in Denmark.[3] In an American report, 38 of 216 tested were type B blood (17.5%).[4]

Elsewhere, 18%[5] and 16%[6] type B cats were reported.

There are some rare type AB cats in this breed. In a group of 24 cats

The Breed History

This Sacred Cat of Burma (Burma is now known as Myanmar) is a distinctively coated and colored cat. Birman cats were prized by priests and many legends surround their origin. A seal point queen named *Sita* exported to France about the year 1919 gave birth to a litter that became the foundation stock for the breed in the west. By the end of the Second World War, they became almost extinct in France and across Europe. Crosses with Persian and Siamese cats followed. First specimens arrived in England in the 1960s and the cats were first recognized in America by the CFA in 1967. No outcrossing is allowed and in most other registries, the cat must have five generations following an outcross in order to qualify. By 1999, with over 1000 cats registered, the breed entered the top 10 in CFA.

Traditionally, cats are named for the year of their birth by having a standard letter of the alphabet to start their name. In 2003, breeders started back at the letter "A" after cycling through the 26 years of the alphabet.

Physical Characteristics

Weight: 10-18 lb (4.5-8 kg)

Coat: Kittens are born white and the coat does not usually finish its development until maturity, though pigmentation begins to develop well before weaning. The medium-long single coat is full like the Persian coat, but shorter and silkier in texture. Championship CFA colors are the same as for Siamese breed cats. The gauntlet markings (or laces) consist of white extensions of the mittens running up the plantar surface of the metatarsals. This pattern is an autosomal recessive trait. Ideally, the laces are one-half to three-quarters of the height up to the tarsus.

Mittens do not extend above the point where the paw meets the vertical limb on the forelimb. A mask covers most of the face. The main coat is light in color and over the back and sides ideally looks as if misted with a gold, termed *golden mist*; this overlay is often absent in kittens.

Eyes: Large, wide set, sapphire blue. Deeper blue is better.

Points of Conformation: The face has a distinctive Siamese look, but the heavier boning and round full face distinguishes them. The face is more of a rounded-wedge. The profile is slightly

surveyed in the UK, 8% were AB in this group while 29% were B, 63% type A.[7]

Drug Sensitivities
None reported in the literature

Inherited Diseases

Azotemia: Birman cats were reported in a small British prospective survey (n=106) of healthy cats to have a higher than expected prevalence of azotemia, indicated by increased BUN and/or creatinine. They found 82% of cats less than 6 months old had creatinine levels above the feline laboratory reference range, and in adults of average age 4 years, 35% had elevated levels. The reason for the high frequency of azotemia in apparently healthy cats was not discovered. Though renal disease was not tested for by additional means, a serial blood test 18 months later for BUN/Cr did not confirm significant progression of azotemia except in two cats that succumbed to renal failure. It was suggested by the authors that "one should consider renal dysfunction when undertaking anesthesia, surgery or treatment" in this breed and test accordingly.[8]

Inherited Defect of Neutrophil Granulation: The condition was reported to be an autosomal recessive trait. A total of 46% of the cats in the study population (n=78) were affected. The dark eosinophilic cytoplasmic granules were functionally normal, but under the microscope they had noticeably increased dye affinity, so if this should be noted during diagnostic evaluation, it should be interpreted that the neutrophils are still functional (incidental finding).[9]

Neonatal Isoerythrolysis (NI): Prevalence of Type B blood type leads to a higher potential incidence of neonatal isoerythrolysis (NI) due to cold acting agglutinins. All B type cats have circulating anti-A antibodies and even primiparous queens can carry these. Type B queens bred to type A toms can result in fatal red cell lysis in AA or AB blood type offspring with undetected NI. Kittens with NI can be distinguished from other fading kittens because of pigmenturia; anemia and icterus will also be present; not all kittens at risk for NI will develop overt clinical symptoms. The proportion of matings at risk for NI was reported to be 0.145.[4] The proportion of matings at risk for NI was reported as 0.13.[5]

Breeders should be advised not to allow offspring resulting from mating where blood types are unknown to nurse on the queen for the first 18 hours. Breeders should be made aware of the importance of testing since in that same recent survey, it was reported that 52% of breeders had carried out at least one breeding without typing the tom and queen. Foster nurse young kittens with an A type queen or use milk replacer if blood types are unknown.

In one case report involving two litters, tail tip necrosis was identified.[10] High neonatal mortality or tail tip necrosis should trigger tests for possible presence of NI.

Disease Predispositions

Arterial Thromboembolism (ATE): Birman cats were overrepresented (odds ratio 10.52) in a population of 127 arterial thromboembolism (ATE) cats in a study done at the University of Minnesota Veterinary Medical Teaching Hospital from 1992-2001. Most cats had left atrial enlargement.[11]

Corneal Sequestration: Black body or cornea nigrum is often bilateral and Birman cats are over-represented. Usually in central cornea; it is a brown to black pigmented lesion; often surrounded by a loose collarette of poorly adherent corneal epithelium. Defect may extend into the middle or deep stroma—or even to Descemet's membrane. Sloughing and corneal healing may take 2-6 months; surgical debridement is another option. Epiphora, yellow-brown ocular discharge and blepharospasm may be seen.[12] This condition is corneal stromal necrosis and topical glucocorticoids are contraindicated; some cases may be linked to feline herpesvirus infection; if suspected, do PCR on the black body tissue. Recurrences or involvement of the second eye in previously unilateral cases may occur.[13]

FIP Susceptibility: Pedigree analysis indicated a heritability of 0.521 after correction for inbreeding in one cattery. It was proposed to be a polygenic inheritance for susceptibility to development of clinical FIP. Nine of 11 deaths occurred in cats related to one tom—so it was correlated with relatedness. Macrophage viral permissiveness may be the underlying functional defect.[14]

An American study found that Birman cats were significantly over-represented for a diagnosis of FIP when they analyzed data for a 16 year period at a veterinary teaching hospital.[15]

Respiratory Disease Propensity: There is anecdotal evidence of more than expected prevalence in some catteries.

Rare and Isolated Reports

Cataracts: Congenital (present at birth), juvenile (newborn to six years of age) forms have been reported with variable rate of progression.[16] Most cases have been noted in a Swedish family of cats, where onset of lens opacity was noted in 2-5 year old cats. Progressive worsening occurred and the problem was bilateral. These were considered to be primary cataracts and type of opacity varied. Two of the 6 observed cats had cataracts that normalized.[12]

Peripheral and Central Distal Axonopathy: In a report, three female littermates and a kitten from a previous litter with same parents were similarly affected. Onset as early as 10 days, to 8-10 weeks of age, and signs included tendency to fall due to posterior ataxia and weakness, and slowly progressive gait abnormalities such as hypermetria and plantigrade stance. Histologic changes included foamy axonal degeneration, myelinopathy, and both central and peripheral nervous system distribution was noted. Sciatic nerves were degraded, but spinal nerve roots were not. Two kittens were reported elsewhere with primarily cerebellar lesions. A sex-linked recessive gene with progressive penetrance was postulated.[17]

Epibulbar Dermoid: Lateral limbus is reported to be the usual location, and dermoids may be unilateral or bilateral. May or may not be hair covered. May encompass bulbar conjunctiva, eyelid margin and skin and may be associated with internal malformations so ophthalmoscopic evaluation should be thorough (include ophthalmoscope, biomicroscopy).[12] First reported in Birman cats in 1985; mode of inheritance uncertain.[16]

Eyelid Agenesis (frequently limited to upper and lateral eyelids): these cats may have concurrent iris, lens and optic nerve colobomas. This is the most common congenital eyelid defect in cats.[18]

Congenital Hypotrichosis and Thymic Aplasia: A condition where thymic aplasia of kittens and lack of haircoat occurred simultaneously; reflects both ectodermal and entodermal defect.

In reported cases, death occurred by 13 weeks and some kittens were born dead, some euthanized because of immune-compromised state. By pedigree analysis it was considered to be an autosomal recessive inheritance. The defect resulted in an overall reduced number of hair follicles; those that were present were hypoplastic with hairs generally in telogen, other lymph tissues such as Peyer's patches, spleen and nodes were hypoplastic. This group consisted of nine related kittens; all affected cats had a common great-great grandsire.[19,20]

Miscellaneous Reported Conditions:
Congenital portosystemic shunts: anecdotal, hepatic encephalopathy, signs starting at 10-12 weeks of age.

Factor IX deficiency.

Pelger–Huet Anomaly: Neutrophil dysmaturity, likely autosomal dominant. Heterozygotes clinically normal.[21]

Genetic Tests
Blood typing before transfusions or breeding is recommended. If kitten tail tip necrosis or neonatal mortality due to "fading kitten" like syndrome occurs, test after the fact.

Renal function test: screening of BUN and creatinine pre-op routinely for all cats is recommended.

Miscellaneous
- **Breed name synonyms:** Sacred Temple Cat of Burma, Temple Cat, Mitted Cat
- **Registries:** TICA, CFA, ACFA, CFF, FIFé (Sacred Birman; SBI), NZCF, CCA, WCF, GCCF, ACF
- **Breed resources: National Birman Fanciers:** http://www.nationalbirmanfanciers.com/
  Sacred Cat of Burma Fanciers: http://www.scbf.com/
  North American Birman Fanciers (ACFA): http://www.birman.org/newsletters/nabf.html

References

1. Lipinski MJ, Young AE, Lyons LA. Genetic diversity and population dynamics of domestic cat breeds. *Proceedings.* Tuft's Canine and Feline Breeding and Genetics Conference Oct 2-4, 2003 Available at VIN: www.vin.com/tufts/2003. Accessed Nov 19, 2004.
2. Little, S. Birman Kitten Information Project, Pers. Comm. March 2009.
3. Jensen AL, Olesen AB, Arnberg J. Distribution of feline blood types detected in the Copenhagen area of Denmark. *Acta Vet Scand* 1994;35:121-124.
4. Giger U, Bucheler J, Patterson DF. Frequency and inheritance of A and B blood types in feline breeds of the United States. *J Hered* 1991;82:15-20.
5. Giger U. In: Bonagura J, ed. *Kirk's Current Veterinary Therapy XIII.* Philadelphia: WB Saunders Co, 2000;396-399.
6. Giger U, Casal M, Niggemeier A. The fading kitten syndrome and neonatal isoerythrolysis. *Proceedings.* The 15th Annual ACVIM Medical Forum, Lake Buena Vista FL 1997;308-310.
7. Knottenbelt CM, Addie DD, Day MJ, et al. Determination of the prevalence of feline blood types in the UK. J of Small Anim Pract 40:115-118, 1999.
8. Gunn-Moore DA, Dodkin SJ, Sparkes AH. *J Fel Med Surg* Letter to the Editor. 2002;4:165-66.
9. Hirsch VM, Cunningham TA. Hereditary anomaly of neutrophil granulation in Birman cats. *Am J Vet Res* 1984;45(10):2170-2174.
10. Bridle KH, Littlewood JD. Tail tip necrosis in two litters of Birman kittens. *J Small Anim Pract* 1998;39:88-89.
11. Smith SA, Tobias AH, Jacob KA, et al. Arterial thromboembolism in cats: Acute crisis in 127 cases (1992-2001) and long-term management with low-dose aspirin in 24 cases. *J Vet Intern Med* 2003;17:73-83
12. Narfström K. Hereditary and congenital ocular disease in the cat. *J Fel Med Surg* 1999;1:135-141
13. Glaze MB. Feline corneal diseases: Part II. *Proceedings.* The 70th Annual AAHA Conference. 2003;1:367-368
14. Foley JE, Pedersen NC. The inheritance of susceptibility to feline infectious peritonitis in purebred catteries. *Fel Pract* 1996;24(1):14-22.
15. Pesteanu-Somogyi LD, Radzai C, Pressler BM. Prevalence of feline infectious peritonitis in specific cat breeds. *J Feline Med Surg.* Vol 8(1):ppp1-5. 2006.
16. Hoskins JD. Congenital defects in cats. *Compend Contin Educ Pract Vet* 1995;17(3):385-405.
17. Moreau PM, Vallat JM, Hugon J, et al. Peripheral and central distal axonopathy of suspected inherited origin in Birman cats. ACTA *Neuropathol* 1991;82:143-146.
18. Narfström K. Hereditary eye diseases. First International Feline Genetic Disease Conference Philadelphia June, 1998 *Proceedings (abstr)* in: *Feline Practice Supplement,* 1999;13.
19. Casal ML, Straumann U, Sigg C, et al. Congenital hypotrichosis with thymic aplasia in nine Birman kittens. *JAAHA* 1994;30:600-602.
20. Casal ML, Arnold S, Straumann U et al. Congenital hypotrichosis with thymic aplasia in Birman kittens. First International Feline Genetic Disease Conference Philadelphia June, 1998 *Proceedings (abstr)* in: *Feline Practice Supplement,* 1999;33-34.
21. Feline Advisory Beaureau Website Accessed May 2010 at: http://www.fabcats.org/breeders/inherited_disorders/birman.php

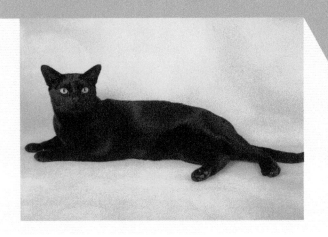

Bombay

The Breed History

This hybrid breed is thought to be named after the Indian city of Bombay, though its origins are in Kentucky, where in the 1950s, a breeder was attempting to breed true a black coated Burmese cat (a "parlor panther" to mimic the appearance of a black panther or Indian Black Leopard). The Bombay derived from a cross between an American Shorthair, (Black with copper eye color) and a Sable Burmese. The Bombay was accepted for championship status of CFA in 1976, and accepted by TICA in 1979. The European and American types are quite similar but in the British Isles, Black British Shorthairs were used instead to cross with sable Burmese, so the British Bombay reflects these origins. This is a rare cat. Some outcrossing to origin-type cats (Black American Shorthair, Sable Burmese) is still allowed, though it is usually the Burmese not the shorthair that is used so that the body type stays true. Sable Bombays are sometimes born, and they can be registered but not shown.

Physical Characteristics

Weight: 6-11 lb (2.5-5 kg)

Coat: The Bombay has a very high gloss jet black close-lying short single haircoat. Though generally breeding true, the odd mating will produce some sable kittens due to residual pointing gene from the Burmese origins. Kittens may not be fully black but will generally darken as they mature. Black is dominant and sable is the recessive gene. Some light tabby markings in kittens can sometimes be seen but will fade.

Eyes: Large round golden to copper eyes—darker is preferred (overseas, the accepted colors include yellow and green).

Points of Conformation: Conformation is quite similar to the Burmese cat, though the Bombay is a bit heavier built with longer limbs, and the rounded head is proportionally larger and both head and body longer due to American Shorthair influence. The angle of change in the nose profile is also less pronounced in Bombay cats than in Burmese. The tail is fine, moderate in length and tapers. The whisker pads are prominent. The muzzle is short-medium, ears are medium-small with rounded tips. The feet are small and round. Nose and pad leather is black.

Grooming: Minimal grooming is required for the Bombay cat. One can just use hands or chamois to maintain shine.

Recognized Behavior Issues and Traits

Reported breed characteristics include: Calm, friendly; gregarious, love climbing and jumping, playful as youngsters, placid as mature cats, the Bombay cats are lap cats, curious, thrive on human companionship and are very intelligent. Bombay cats are generally easy to leash train. Like to fetch ball and play other games and love the company of children. Get along with other pets well, particularly dogs. Not particularly vocal; and when they vocalize, this is a quiet voiced cat. Good for indoor lifestyle.

Normal Breed Variations

Large litters

Early sexual maturity

Reported to be a hardy cat

They possess a characteristic swaying walk and are very agile

Drug Sensitivities

None reported in the literature

Inherited Diseases

Craniofacial Deformity: Some lines of the breed carry the gene for this condition (best known in the Burmese- *see that chapter for details*). This is an **autosomal recessive** disorder.[1] This defect is less of a problem now due to careful breeding. As in the Burmese, this is often a lethal gene in utero, or necessitates euthanasia in newborns. There are some lines that are free of this disorder.

Disease Predispositions

See American Shorthair and Burmese chapters since Bombay cats may share some disorders with the progenitor breeds, though Bombay cats are generally very healthy cats; likely due to hybrid vigor.

Genetic Tests

No tests available commercially

Miscellaneous

- **Breed name synonyms:** Patent Leather Cat, Black Burmese, Black Leopard Cat, Asian Shorthair, Asian Selfs, nickname: "Patent leather kid with the copper penny eyes"
- **Registries:** TICA, ACFA, CFA, CFF, ACF, WCF, CCA
- **Breed resources:** The Bombay and Asian Self Breed Club (UK): http://www.bombayandasianselfbreedclub.org/
  International Bombay Society:
  Suzanne Zwecker, Secretary 5782 Dalton Drive
  Canandaigua, NY 14425

References

1. Erdman C, Lyons L. Facial Development Study Update (Aug 2003-Aug 2004) In: Notes, University of California (Davis) Feline Genetics Extravaganza II Aug 28-29, 2004.

2. Cat Fancy October 2008 Black Magic. E. Jordan. Pp 22-25.

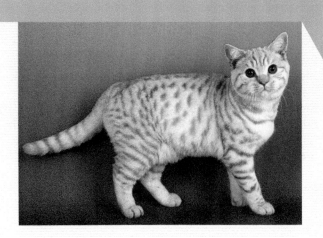

British Shorthair

every few days. When bathing, avoid blow drying. More frequent grooming needed while shedding.

Recognized Behavior Issues and Traits

Reported breed characteristics include: Likes human companionship but is not demanding and not considered a lap cat. Not known as jumpers and climbers. The British Shorthair is considered very appropriate with children and other pets. Quiet cats with a pleasant voice, they are suited for therapy cats, and travel well.

Normal Breed Variations

Slow to mature (three to five years), later sexual maturity compared with American Shorthair cats.

Easy birthing and litters average four to five kittens.

These cats may tend to become obese if not limit fed.

Blood Type B: Frequency of B blood type in a 1991 American study found 50 of 85 cats in that group to be type B (proportion was 0.588).[1] In another report, a frequency of 36% blood type B was reported.[2] In the UK, in a study group of 121 British Shorthair cats, 58.7% were type B, and 1.6% type AB.[3] These data show that there is considerable regional variation in the distribution of the B blood type allele.

Drug Sensitivities

None reported in the literature

Inherited Diseases

Feline Hypertrophic Cardiomyopathy (HCM): This is the most common cardiac condition in cats (10% prevalence), and a fairly common condition in some British Shorthairs; possibly inherited.[4] This condition affects mostly middle age to older cats, clinical signs seen more often in males.

Serum cardiac troponin 1 levels (cTnI), a marker of myocardial damage may be elevated in the face of normal echo findings according to early studies and may be useful in future screening for at-risk cats, though further studies are needed.[5]

Neonatal Isoerythrolysis (NI): Increased risk should be considered in this breed due to prevalence of type B blood; testing before mating especially in regions of higher prevalence may prevent adverse events. The proportion of matings at risk for NI was reported to be 0.24.[6]

Polycystic Kidney Disease (PKD): Can occur in the breed with the Persian mutation. (See under Persian). A genetic test is available.

Disease Predispositions

Transfusion Reactions: Increased risk should be considered in this population due to prevalence of type B blood. Before transfusion,

The Breed History

This is the National cat of the British Isles. These cats derived from British domestic shorthaired street cats ("moggies"), cats that may have first arrived in the region during Roman incursions. During WW II, most of these cats were lost. Rejuvenation of the breed occurred due to careful breeder outcrosses carried out for a period following the war. When compared with the American and European Shorthairs, this cat has a much rounder head. Lewis Carroll in "Alice in Wonderland" made the British Shorthair tabby the model for the Cheshire cat.

In Britain, this breed may be referred to as the "Shorthair". This breed is still rarely seen in North America. The CFA first recognized this breed in 1980. No outcrossing is allowed in CFA though some other registries still allow selected outcrossing to Persian, American and European Shorthair, and Chartreux; these may not be eligible for CFA registry.

Physical Characteristics

Weight: 9-18 lb (4-8 kg), females smaller than males

Coat: The short, dense, plush soft single coat is accepted in most colors and patterns. Lavender, chocolate, and Himalayan pointed coloring are not allowed in CFA, but TICA allows chocolate and lavender. Hair texture is hard, not wooly. By far, the most frequent color seen is the **British Blue:** tabby markings may fade after six months of age. This is a slate grey color.

Coat is water repellant.

Eyes: Large, round, and usually copper to gold. Silver, golden, and shaded silver cats have green to hazel eye color.

Points of Conformation: Cobby (heavily set), short thick boned limbs, with broad thorax, and a large round head. Ears are small with rounded tips. The muzzle is moderately short, nose is short and broad and with a slight dip, whisker pads are prominent (resulting in the so-called *"Cheshire grin"*). Paws are moderately sized and round, and they possess a thick medium length tail with a round tip.

Russian Blues have green eyes, they are less cobby, the coat is more open, and they are smaller cats than the British Blue.

Grooming: Low grooming needs; one can just hand groom quickly

blood typing will help identify cats at risk.

Calcium oxalate urolithiasis: A case control study of ~15,000 cats affected with urolithiasis and ~150,000 unaffected cats over 15 years reported British Shorthair cats at increased risk.[10]

Gingivitis: Anecdotal reports of increased prevalence.

FIP susceptibility: A study in Australia confirmed that the British Shorthair breed cats were over-represented.[11]

Rare and Isolated Reports

Congenital Cataracts: An older case report identified congenital cataracts in this breed and it was proposed by the original authors to have an autosomal recessive inheritance pattern.[7]

Factor IX Deficiency (Hemophilia B): A sex-linked recessive gene which produces mild to moderate bleeding tendencies in males and females, with normal carriers has been reported. In reference to one older case report, in one cat, clinical signs were reported first at surgery (had 27% of normal factor activity); in other cases, excessive spontaneous hemorrhage (n=2, with <5% factor activity) occurred. Cases reported were from one family of cats from Philadelphia in 1984.[8]

Another published report described onset of periodic shifting lameness at four months of age, with ongoing gingival bleeding at six months old in the index kitten. Relatives of this index cat were tested and pedigree analysis was carried out to confirm the inheritance pattern. Female carriers had intermediate Factor IX activity (One was 67%, one 88%, another 80%, though carriers typically have activity of the factor in the range of 40-60%); female carriers are usually clinically normal. Some of the male kittens in related litters died young. Subcutaneous hematomas may also been seen in affected individuals. Note that when getting blood samples to assay Factor IX, stress activation of the factor may artificially increase levels assayed. It was proposed to be the explanation for higher than expected factor activity levels in these assayed carrier females.[9]

Primary Hypoadrenocorticism: Single case reported in 1999; only 11 naturally occurring cases have been reported in the literature. The case involved a two year old female cat presented with lethargy, weakness, constipation, and hypothermia.[12]

Hereditary Deafness: Is associated with the dominant gene for white cat (W); may be found in white cats of this breed.[13]

Genetic Tests

Testing for B blood type would be prudent before mating and transfusions due to prevalence of B blood type in the breed. Also test young cats with episodes of bleeding, excessive gingival bleeding, periodic shifting lameness (hemarthrosis) and subcutaneous hematomas, for factor IX and coagulation profile for suspected Hemophilia B.[9]

HCM screening recommendations not set for this breed, but until further information is available, may consider echo screening for breeding animals.[4]

Direct genetic test for PKD is available from UC-Davis VGL.

Miscellaneous

- **Breed name synonyms:** for tipped cats—Chinchilla Shorthair, **Historical Synonym:** British Blue (since original cats were blues). Also: Brit, National Cat of Britain, Blue Cat
- **Registries:** FIFé (as the "British"), TICA (British Shorthair and British Longhair), CFA, ACFA, CFF, NZCF, WCF, ACF, GCCF (as the "British")
- **Breed resources:** Southern British Shorthair Cat Club: www.british-shorthairs.co.uk/
  CFA British Shorthair Breed Council:
  http://www.britishshorthairbc.org/bshbc001.htm
  Colourpointed British Shorthair Club:
  http://www.colourpointedbritish.co.uk/index.html

References

1. Giger U. Frequency and inheritance of A and B Blood types in feline breeds in the United States. *J Hered* 1991;82:15-20.
2. Giger U. In: Bonagura J, ed. *Kirk's Current Veterinary Therapy XIII.* Philadelphia: WB Saunders Co, 2000;396-399.
3. Knottenbelt CM, Addie DD, Day MJ, et al. Determination of the prevalence of feline blood types in the UK. *J Small Anim Pract* 1999;40:115-118.
4. Little S. Selected inherited diseases of the cat, in *Proceedings.* International Ragdoll Congress Oct, 2004. Available at: www.catvet. homestead.com/Inherited_Diseases_2004.pdf Accessed Nov 23, 2004.
5. Connolly DJ, Cannata J, Boswood A, et al. Cardiac troponin I in cats with hypertrophic cardiomyopathy. *J Fel Med Surg* 2003;5:209-216.
6. Giger U, Casal M, Niggemeier A. The fading kitten syndrome and neonatal isoerythrolysis. *Proceedings.* The 15th Annual ACVIM Medical Forum, Lake Buena Vista FL 1997;308-310.
7. Narfström K. Hereditary and congenital ocular disease. *J Fel Med Surg* 1999;1:135-141.
8. Brooks MB. Factor IX deficiency (Hemophilia B) in two male domestic shorthair cats. *JAAHA* 1989;25:153-55.
9. Maggio-Price L, Dodds WJ. Factor IX deficiency (Hemophilia B) in a family of British Shorthair cats. *J Am Vet Med Assoc* 1993;203(12):1702-1704.
10. Lekcharoensuk C, Lulich JP, Osborne CA, et al. Association between patient-related factors and risk of calcium oxalate and magnesium ammonium phosphate urolithiasis in cats. *J Am Vet Med Assoc* 2000;Aug15;217(4):520-525.
11. Norris JM, Bosward KL, White JD, et al Clinicopathological findings associated with feline infectious peritonitis in Sydney, Australia: 42 cases (1990-2002). *Aust Vet J.* 2005 Nov;83(11):666-73.
12. Tasker S, MacKay AD, Sparkes AH. A case of feline primary hypoadreno-corticism. *J Fel Med Surg* 1999,1:257-260.
13. Strain GM. Hereditary deafness in dogs and cats: Causes, prevalence, and current research. *Proceedings.* Tuft's Canine and Feline Breeding and Genetics Conference. Oct 2-4, 2003 Available at: http://www.vin.com/ tufts/2003. Accessed Nov 19, 2004.

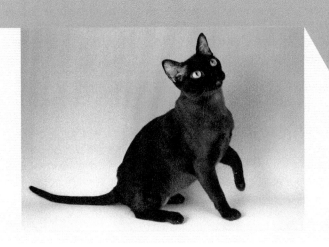

The Breed History

This breed is thought to have originated in Rangoon, Burma (now Myanmar) where brown cats referred to as "Rajahs" were documented. Thai 16th century writings portray similar cats. In North America, the foundation dark sable female named Wong Mau was brought over to California in the late 1920s. She is believed to have been a Tonkinese (Burmese-Siamese cross). Modern Burmese cats are thought to derive solely from Wong Mau. Her offspring were of three coat types; the type with sable coloring was selected for the next generation.

The American Burmese type is distinct from the European Burmese. The latter is found in Europe, Australasia and South Africa and is a much more angular cat—the head is more wedge shaped and these cats are longer, and lithe in build. Additional colors are accepted in non-CFA registries—those other colors were termed **Malayan** in the USA. The CFA considers the American and European as two breeds. In the American fancy, the Burmese is further subdivided into **Traditional** cats, with more elongated head and the **Contemporary** cats, with a rounder more brachycephalic head. The latter gained popularity in the 1970s. No outcrossing is allowed in CFA.

The CFA accepted the Burmese breed in 1936, disallowed them for a while, and again reinstated them in the early 1950s, with full championship status by 1957. Only sable coloring was accepted by CFA until the late 1980s, at which time the accepted color spectrum was expanded to four colors. Malayans were separately registered from 1979-1984.

Burmese cats have played a role in development of other breeds incuding the Burmilla (Chinchilla Persian X Platinum Burmese), Tiffany (Longhaired Burmese), Bombay (Black Shorthair X), and Tonkinese (Siamese X).

Physical Characteristics

Weight: 8-13 lb (3.5-6 kg); females smaller than males

Coat: A distinctive breed characteristic is their very high gloss and thick close-lying shorthaired coat; satin-like in texture. Colors include **sable** (also termed **usual**, or **brown**), frost or **platinum** (lilac), **champagne (honey-beige)**, and **blue** (a warm grey color). Minimal undercoat is present. All coat colors are lighter on the ventral aspect of the cat and darker fur is often found around the face (mask), tail, feet and ears. The mask and points should be minimal in mature cats. Burmese sable points are recessive (*cb cb*). Young sable cats will darken as they mature.

Eyes: They possess large yellow or gold eyes, round in shape. In CFA, green eyes penalize and blue eyes disqualify. The FIFé registry allows green eyes.

Points of Conformation: Conformation is similar to the Bombay cat, though Burmese are smaller, lighter in build and the rounded head is proportionately smaller. A medium-small sized cat; compact and heavy for their size, the Burmese's round head shape and nose break conformation is a breed characteristic. The body is short-coupled, the medium length tail is fine and tapers, whisker pads prominent, muzzle is short-medium, ears are medium-small, and round tipped. The feet are small, and round-oval. Most points of the cat's conformation are round.

Grooming: Low grooming needs are required for Burmese cats—just a hand or chamois wipe or soft brush weekly.

Recognized Behavior Issues and Traits

Reported breed characteristics include: Calm friendly temperament, intelligent, adaptable, love climbing, and playful as youngsters. May enjoy playing fetch, are very placid as mature cats; many are a lap or shoulder cat, thrive on human companionship, and they love warm places. Tend to follow their favored people around; some refer to them as "Velcro" kitties. Not particularly vocal; considered a quiet voiced cat. Good with children, seniors and pets. Not suited to outdoor lifestyle. Though uncommon, a few have a strong personality.

Normal Breed Variations

Epiphora: Secondary to face conformation rather than due to any unusual anatomic defects in the lower punctum.

Blood Type: Prevalence 100% A type was reported in American cats.[1]

There may be some differences in geographic distribution of blood types; in a very small survey in the UK, of 10 cats tested, one was type B blood.[2]

Good longevity

Good mothering ability

Males/stud cats easygoing

Burmese Kitten Information Project[3] An Internet based breeder survey was carried out to establish normal baselines for reproduction.

Reported: 67 reporting breeders, 206 litters. 927 kittens, June 2003-May 2004. [results below are averaged from the study where response were divided into the three subtypes of Burmese cat-Contemporary (20% of breeders), European (53% of breeders), Traditional (28%)]:

Average litter size: 4.5

Stillbirth rate: 8.7%
The stillbirth rate was higher in Contemporary subtype (12%), otherwise 7%

C section rate: The rate was higher in the European (11%) than in the others (<1%)

Average birth weight: Male 86 g, female 81 g

Congenital deformities: About 3% were Flat-chested (48% of flat-chested kittens did not survive to four weeks of age), also found craniofacial deformity, dermoids, cherry eye.

Drug Sensitivities

None reported in the literature

Inherited Diseases

Craniofacial (mid-facial) Deformity (breeder SYN: head defect): Over the last few decades, concerted efforts by breeders has resulted in the near elimination of this deformity, but it is of interest to the reader as an example of a genetic disorder linked to a perceived desired phenotype.

An inherited lethal deformity; homozygous status results in some kittens needing early pediatric euthanasia, as well as *in utero* mortality. Use of Burmese carrier cats in Bombay and American Shorthair breeding programs has resulted in a low frequency of the trait in those breeds also. Prevalence of this disorder has dropped considerably due to breeder efforts to eliminate the gene from the breed. Introduction of this defect coincided with the development of a very "round" emphasis in the American show ring; also termed the *contemporary, new look,* or *eastern* look. By the mid 1980s, almost 100 kittens from a number of catteries were afflicted, and efforts began to reduce the deformity prevalence.[4]

The autosomal recessive gene controlling the deformity is not in direct genetic linkage to the head phenotype, though the contemporary facial features are a strongly associated trait. Researchers continue to try to characterize the gene structure.[5] It should be noted that the more contemporary head phenotype seems to sort as an incomplete dominant, and that a contemporary phenotype head type cat of recent development may or may not carry the gene for the head defect.[4]

In an early report of one cattery, the condition was described as a complex of craniofacial abnormalities with hereditary meningoencephalocele and it was proposed that the autosomal recessive gene **(mc)** had incomplete penetrance because homozygotes sometimes did not express penetrated lethality—based on pedigree studies.[6] Malformations resulting from early embryonic defects in rostral neural tube closure include duplication of most of the maxillary processes derivatives including canine teeth and whiskers pad area, agenesis of medial fronto-nasal prominence derivatives, and meningoencephalocele (telencephalic). Secondary ocular degenerative processes may also occur.[7]

Nasal dermoids are also seen in some cats. These are also seen in American Shorthairs carrying this gene. A shallow longitudinal furrow of tissue or different color running along the nose has been found in almost 90% of American Shorthair carrier cats, and may be a phenotypic marker of a carrier, though sensitivity and specificity of this finding is not very high.[4]

Agenesis of Nares: Associated with dyspnea, mouth breathing, and snoring.[8]

Epibulbar Dermoids: Usually located in the lateral angle of the eye.[9] They are circular, hairy, and may involve the skin, bulbar conjunctiva and palpebral margin. May also have concurrent internal eye defects, so ophthalmoscopic and biomicroscopic examination should also be carried out in affected cats.[10]

Eyelid Agenesis: Frequently limited to upper and lateral eyelids.[9] Eyelid agenesis is the most common congenital eyelid defect in cats.[10]

Hypokalemic Polymyopathy: This is a chronic episodic condition of muscle weakness. It has been reported in cats from the U.S.A., Britain, New Zealand, and Australia. Though it was suspected to be inherited, the mode of inheritance was unknown as of 1995.[11] Recently, it was putatively suggested to be an autosomal recessive trait.[12] Attacks are often transient. In humans, a similar condition called familial hypokalemic periodic paralysis occurs, and at a cellular level and it is thought that these conditions are similar.

A series of 18 cases of episodic hypokalemia episodes in related kittens aged 2-6 months old was reported. About half of the cats had full resolution of the condition.[13] In another report, in addition to usual signs of weakness and neck ventroflexion, hind limb lameness, knuckled forelimbs and hind limbs, and abnormal hunched sitting posture were noted. These kittens were induced to have attacks of varying severity by exercising; resultant attacks lasted two to three weeks; youngest were 12 weeks old, oldest cat was 1 year of age; most were clustered around the age of 3-4 months. This condition may resolve without treatment; very high creatine kinase and low serum potassium were evident; changes mirrored the attack temporally.[14] Breeding cats with this condition is not recommended.[15]

Disease Predispositions

Renal Failure: Renal failure rate for the Burmese was more than double baseline in a study of cats from 23 veterinary colleges from 1980-1990 (189,371 cases in Purdue University Veterinary Medical Database) at an odds ratio for risk of 2.07:1 (2.45% prevalence).[16]

Diabetes Mellitus (Type 2): An early study of North American Burmese cats in a pooled study group of 333 cats with diabetes did not identify a breed predisposition in that population.[17] In another study in Australia, a breed predilection was established in a study group (n=4402) monitored over a 22 month period. Burmese cats accounted for 20% of diabetic cats of known breed, even though the population of Burmese was only 7% of the normoglycemic cat population.[18, 19]

In a 2004 review paper, in NZ, Australia, and the UK, the frequency of diabetes in Burmese was reported to be four times that of domestic cats, with 1:50 afflicted (compared to <1:200 domestic cats). In Burmese cats 8 years of age and older, the reported rate was 1:10. In some families over 10% of Burmese offspring developed diabetes.

If this is a genetic disorder, the mode of inheritance remains unknown; it is thought that mutation of genes that affect insulin sensitivity are responsible for the breed predilection. Most affected cats are over 6 years of age, with peak incidence at 12 years of age. Other factors that can enhance risk include low activity, obesity, dental disease and a high carbohydrate/low protein diet. It is interesting that Burmese cats put weight on in the internal abdomen first (this is a risk factor for people with that same propensity).[20]

In a recent study in Australia over 5 years, in 12,576 cats of all breeds, prevalence was 7.4:1000 cats and 22.4:1000 for Burmese cats.[21]

Flat-Chested Kittens: A series of young Burmese kittens in the U.K. was reported to have an increased risk of a flat-chested condition in the pediatric phase. Dorso-ventrally flat-chested kittens were usually born with normal phenotype, and then developed a form of chest deformity somewhat similar to pectus excavatum by about nine days of age. About 3%-4% of Burmese kittens were affected. The condition ranges in severity from mild and transient—to a severe form, sometimes overlapping with concurrent pectus.

Signs include poor weight gain, cranial thoracic vertebral kyphosis, vomiting, dyspnea, cyanosis, exercise intolerance and cough. Though recognized by breeders, flat-chested kittens have not been widely reported in the literature. Litter viability was 76% in one study of affected litters. In cats in this UK study group, both queens and kittens had higher levels of whole blood taurine than typical reference cat levels.

Kitten's levels in turn were significantly higher than the queens. Taurine has a negative effect on skeletal muscle contractility (hyperpolarization and anticholinergic effect) and this muscle weakness may contribute to the condition. Often as kittens mature and the rib cage calcification completes, the clinical signs abate in many that were less severe and thus not euthanized in the neonatal period. The paper did not elucidate further an established link between hypertaurinemia and the flat-chested condition.[22]

Presence of a dorsal spinal curvature, prominent horizontal rib ridge, and minimal dorsal deviation of sternum into the thoracic cavity in flat-chested kittens distinguish this condition from pectus excavatum.[23]

Calcium Oxalate Urolithiasis: This is one of the breeds identified as having a higher risk of developing this type of stone;[24, 25] Burmese cats were also reported to have lower risk of magnesium ammonium phosphate (struvite) uroliths.[24]

Wool Sucking: Onset is usually after weaning, this condition also affects other Oriental breeds. Target is commonly a blanket, sweater, socks; often the behavior terminates at sexual maturity, but some cases may have late onset or continue signs late into life. In one report 28% of fabric eating cats were Burmese breed in a group of 152 affected cats. Wool sucking is a stereotypic oral movement and though many cats begin by selecting wool as a substrate, many

go on to other types of fabric and even non-fabric substrates such as plastics. Early-weaned cats are over-represented but there is no clear causal relationship.[26]

Corneal Sequestration (Synonym: Black body or cornea nigrum): A condition with unknown cause, found more commonly than expected in this breed.[9] Lesion is usually in central or paracentral cornea. A brown to black pigmented lesion is frequently surrounded by a loose collarette of poorly adherent corneal epithelium. The lesion may extend into mid or deep stroma; even to Descemet's membrane. Sloughing and corneal healing may take 2-6 months; surgical debridement is an option for deeper lesions.[10]

Can be unilateral or bilateral but is most often unilateral; is a corneal stromal necrosis. Topical glucocorticoids are contraindicated; some cases may be linked to feline herpesvirus infection. If virus is suspected, a PCR on excised black body tissue may be helpful. Recurrences or involvement of the second eye in a previously unilateral lesion may occur. In early phases, an amber colored corneal stromal opacity may be noted. It gradually develops distinct raised borders; and the surrounding cornea is cloudy with neovascularization; chemosis, blepharospasm, mucopurulent ocular discharge and hyperemic conjunctivae may also be noted. The surface of sequestrum does not stain with flourescein dye but does retain Rose Bengal stain. Exophthalmic/brachycephalic head conformation is thought to play a role in susceptibility. May recur months or years later, or in a unilateral case the second eye may become affected.[27, 28]

Feline Dilated Cardiomyopathy (DCM): Increased breed predisposition to DCM and decreased risk of hypertrophic cardiomyopathy is reported in Burmese cats.[29] Case levels have dropped since dietary supplementation with taurine began. Previously, mortality for DCM was about 85% and with taurine supplementation the mortality is 30%-50%. Feline signs are not typically a cough as in the dog; heart rate may be bradycardic to tachycardia and both ventricles are affected. Affected cats are prone to arterial thromboembolism. Systolic heart murmur, or diastolic gallop can often be heard, and 61% have arrhythmias, usually ventricular.[30]

Propensity to FeLV Infection: Endogenous feline leukemia (enFeLVs) were studied in a single specimen of Burmese, Egyptian Mau and Persian breed cats to determine how many loci proviruses were typically inserted. This may indicate genetic propensity for leukemia genesis in these cats when exposed to the exogenous feline leukemia virus.

They found provirus on 12/18 autosomes, with an average 19 autosomal copies per cat. One specific locus contained both homologues in all 3 cats. They were also found on both X and Y chromosomes.[31]

Rare and Isolated Reports

Primary Glaucoma: Primary glaucoma is rare in cats when compared with dogs and humans. Findings in narrow angle glaucoma may include a moderately mydriatic pupil, reduced PLR, episcleral blood vessel congestion and buphthalmos. In a study of a small group of affected cats (1996-2001), closed or narrow irido-corneal angles, with reduced number and size of pectinate ligaments, and increased IOP were identified. Tapetal hyper-reflectivity, attenuated retinal vasculature and sometimes optic disc cupping occurred. This condition is still very rarely reported, but an early indication is that this breed may be somewhat predisposed to narrow angle glaucoma. With early diagnosis and appropriate therapeutic intervention, vision may be optimized. Routine screening of this breed may be deemed an appropriate wellness strategy.[32]

In a study of 1100 cases of feline glaucoma from 1992-2006, researchers found 8 cases of primary glaucoma, and of these eight, six were domestic cats and two were Burmese cats—no other purebreds were identified in that sample.[33]

Transient Opacity–Aqueous Humor: Suspected triglyceride rich material accumulated in Burmese cats less than one year old that had no other discernable health problems. Spontaneous recovery occurred within a day, a few recrudesced (2/6 cats).[34] Four additional cases were reported in that same year. Two were littermates.[35] It is not known whether this represented isolated cases of reaction to a foreign stimulant. Lipid aqueous humor changes are reported to be associated with hyperlipidemia according to a recent report.[36]

A 2009 report proved that Burmese cats of the Australian strain have reduced triglyceride clearance when compared to domestic or other pedigreed cats. Resting levels were normal. This study may shed light on altered fat metabolism in this genetic pool of Burmese.[37]

Severe Transient Hyperlipidemia and Anemia: In a study group of 12 litters of kittens of weaning age this condition was described; one of the litters was Burmese. A genetic defect in lipid metabolism was suspected.[38]

Endocardial Fibroelastosis: Reports in the older literature (1982) described a very rare condition where the endocardium was markedly thickened in a series of offspring from one Burmese queen and tom. This was thought to be an inherited disorder, characterized by diffuse fibrous and elastic thickening of the endocardium; the left side being dilated and hypertrophied concurrently; tachycardia, CHF, gallop or systolic murmur and terminal cyanosis and dyspnea were noted with onset at 3 weeks to 4 months of age.[39, 40]

Persistent Atrial Standstill: Bradycardia non responsive to medical management and a pacemaker may be needed.[8]

Synovial Osteochondromatosis: Burmese cats are overrepresented, and this condition can be confused with benign periarticular ossification, perhaps resulting in underreporting.[41]

FIP Susceptibility: Feline leukocyte antigen class II is important for control of immune response, and is represented by a set of genes, and polymorphism may play a role in susceptibility; further studies are needed. Burmese cats may be particularly susceptible to FIP. It was noted in this small study sample that related cats of this breed had fewer alleles compared to other breeds.[42]

Another study in Australia confirmed that the Burmese breed cats were over-represented and that they were more likely to develop dry FIP versus effusive FIP.[43]

An American study did not find that Burmese cats were over-represented for diagnosis of FIP when they analyzed data for a 16 year period at a veterinary teaching hospital.[44]

GM2 Gangliosidosis: See the Korat chapter for more detailed information about this condition. A GM2 gangliosidosis lysosomal storage disease with beta-subunit of hexosaminidase enzyme was reported in European Burmese cats. This condition is fatal. Accumulation was noted in brain tissue.[45]

A group of European breeders have formed the DEG or Data Exchange Group to share testing information. The mutation is a deletion (cytosine in HEXB).[46]

Medial Patellar Luxation: A very small study case reported that of eight clinically normal Burmese cats assessed as part of a larger study, two had abnormal patella seating with easily induced luxation. Compared with non pedigreed cats where the rate was two abnormal cats out of 31 cats, they were overrepresented.[47]

Genetic Tests

Burmese coat genes are the least extreme of the ts-tyrosinase partial albinism allele series. The mutation has been identified in the code for tyrosinase enzyme.[48]

New research shows that the c(b) allele of the albino locus gene are variants on the D1 chromosome specifying tyrosinase.and the chocolate (b) and cinnamon (b(9l)) a second allele at the B (brown) locus are nucleotide variants of TYRP1 (chromosome D4).[49]

The mutations are reported to most likely to be identical by descent rather than multiple mutation events occurring at the same site in another study.[50]

Glaucoma Screening: Ophthalmoscopic exam, gonioscopy, and tonometry are recommended for breeding stock.

Renal Function: Screen for renal function (minimum of Creatinine/ BUN and urinalysis) in cats eight years and older since a breed propensity to renal failure was identified.[16]

Scott-Ritchey Research Center web site at http://www.vetmed. auburn.edu/srrc and UC-Davis VGL for Gangliosidosis GM2 testing in European Burmese

Miscellaneous

- **Breed name synonyms:** Historically, dilutes were registered in CFA as Malayan cats—they are now accepted as Burmese in separate class
- **Other Synonyms:** Burm, Thai Copper Cats, Asian Shorthair
- **Registries:** FIFé, TICA, CFA, ACFA, GCCF, ACF, WCF, NZCF, CCA
- **Breed resources: United Burmese Cat Fanciers:** http://unitedburmese.com/
  The Burmese Cat Club: http://www.burmesecatclub.com/
  The Burmese Cat Society: http://www.burmesecatsociety.org.uk/
  National Alliance of Burmese Breeders (CFA): http://www.burmesecat.org/

References

1. Giger U. In: Bonagura J, ed. *Kirk's Current Veterinary Therapy XIII.* Philadelphia: WB Saunders Co, 2000;396-399.

2. Knottenbelt CM, Addie DD, Day MJ, et al. Determination of the prevalence of feline blood types in the UK. *J Small Anim Pract* 1999;40:115-118.

3. Little, S. Birman Kitten Information Project, Pers. Comm. March 2009.

4. Lyons LA. The Lyon's Den. Cranio-facial Deformity. Available at: http://faculty.vetmed.ucdavis.edu/faculty/lalyons/Sites/burmese.htm Accessed Nov 15, 2004.

5. Erdman C, Lyons LA. Facial Development Study Update (Aug 2003-Aug 2004) In: *Notes*, University of California (Davis) Feline Genetics Extravaganza II Aug 28-29, 2004.

6. Sponenberg DP, Graf-Webster E. Hereditary meningoencephalocele in Burmese cats. *J Hered* 1986;77(1):60.

7. Noden DM, Evans HE. Inherited homeotic midfacial malformations in Burmese cats. *J Craniofac Genet Dev Biol Suppl* 1986;2:249-266.

8. Hoskins JD. Congenital defects in cats. *Compend Contin Educ Pract Vet* 1995;17(3):385-405.

9. Narfström K. Hereditary eye diseases. First International Feline Genetic Disease Conference Philadelphia June, 1998 *Proceedings (abstr)* in: *Feline Practice Supplement,* 1999;13.

10. Narfström K. Hereditary and congenital ocular disease in the cat. *J Fel Med Surg* 1999;1:135-141.

11. Edwards CM, Belford CJ. Hypokalemic polymyopathy in Burmese cats. *Aust Vet Practit* 1995;25(2):58-60.

12. Gaschen F, Jaggy A, Jones B. Congenital diseases of feline muscle and neuromuscular junction. *J Fel Med Surg* 2004;6:355-366.

13. Gruffydd-Jones TJ, Sparkes AH, Caney SA, et al. Hypokalemic Episodic weakness in Burmese kittens. First International Feline Genetic Disease Conference Philadelphia June 1998 Proceedings (abstr) in: *Feline Practice Supplement,* 1999;29.

14. Blaxter A, Lievesley P, Gruffydd-Jones T, et al. Periodic muscle weakness in Burmese kittens. Vet Rec 1986;118(22):619-620.

15. Taboada J. Ventroflexion of the neck in cats. *Proceedings.* The 12th ACVIM Veterinary Medical Forum, San Francisco CA 1994:385-386.

16. Lulich JP, O'Brien TD, Osborne CA, et al. Feline Renal Failure: Questions, answers, questions. *Compend Contin Educ Pract Vet* 1992;14(2):127-152.

17. Panciera DL, Thomas CB, Eicker SW, et al. Epizootiologic patterns of diabetes mellitus in cats: 333 cases (1980-1986). *J Am Vet Med Assoc* 1990;197(11):1504-1508.

18. Rand J. Current understanding of feline diabetes: Part 1: Pathogenesis. *J Fel Med Surg* 1999;1(3):143-153.

19. Rand JS, Bobbermien LM, Hendrikz JK, et al. Over representation of Burmese cats with diabetes mellitus. *Aust Vet J* 1997;75(6):402-405.

20. Rand JS, Fleeman LM, Farrow HA, et al. Canine and feline diabetes mellitus: Nature or nurture? *J Nutr* 2004;134:2072S-2080S.

21. Lederer R, Rand JS, Jonsson NN, Hughes IP, Morton JM Frequency of feline diabetes mellitus and breed predisposition in domestic cats in Australia. *Vet J.* 2009 Feb;179(2):254-8.

22. Sturgess CP, Waters L, Gruffydd-Jones TJ, et al. Investigation of the association between whole blood and tissue taurine levels and the development of thoracic deformities in neonatal Burmese kittens. *Vet Rec* 1997;141:566-570.

23. Little S. Breed Specific Reproduction Projects. In: *Notes*, University of California (Davis) Feline Genetics Extravaganza I July, 2003.

24. Thumchai R, Lulich J, Osborne CA, et al. Epizootiologic evaluation of urolithiasis in cats: 3,498 cases (1982-1992). *J Am Vet Med Assoc* 1996;208(4):547-551.

25. Houston DM, Moore AEP, Favrin MG, Hoff B. Feline urethral plugs and bladder uroliths: A review of 5484 submissions 1998-2003. *Can Vet J* 2003;Dec;44(12):974-977.

26. Neilson J. Anxieties, phobias and compulsive disorders. *Proceedings.* AAFP Fall Conference. 2002;125-139.

27. Pentlarge VW. Corneal sequestration in cats. *Compend Contin Educ*

Pract Vet 1989;11(1):24-32.

28. Glaze MB. Feline corneal diseases: Part II. *Proceedings.* The 70th Annual AAHA Conference. 2003;1:367-368.

29. Fox PR. Feline cardiomyopathy (Part I). Hypertrophic cardiomyopathy. *Proceedings.* The 19th Annual ACVIM Veterinary Medical Forum, Denver CO 2001:1129.

30. Atkins CE. Feline dilated cardiomyopathy. Winter 2004 AAFP Meeting. Proceedings [abstr] in: *AAFP Newsletter* August 2004 22(2):29-30.

31. Roca AL, Nash WG, Menninger JC, Murphy WJ, O'Brien SJ. Insertional polymorphisms of endogenous feline leukemia viruses. *J Virol.* 2005 Apr;79(7):3979-86.

32. Hampson ECGM, Smith R, Bernays ME. Primary glaucoma in Burmese cats. *Aust Vet J* 2002;80(11):672-680.

33. Jacobi S, Dubielzig RR Feline primary open angle glaucoma. Vet Ophthalmol. 2008 May-Jun;11(3):162-5.

34. Gunn-Moore DA, Crispin SM. Unusual ocular condition in Burmese cats. *Vet Rec* 1998;142(12):376.

35. Eason P. Unusual ocular condition in Burmese cats. *Vet Rec* 1998;142(19):524.

36. Hardman C, et al. *Proceedings.* American College of Veterinary Ophthalmologists, 1999.

37. Kluger EK, Hardman C, Govendir M, Baral RM, Sullivan DR, Snow D, Malik R Triglyceride response following an oral fat tolerance test in Burmese cats, other pedigree cats and domestic crossbred cats. *J Feline Med Surg.* 2009 Feb;11(2):82-90

38. Gunn-Moore DA, Watson TDG, Dodkin SJ, et al. Transient hyperlipidaemia and anaemia in kittens. *Vet Rec* 1997;140:355-359.

39. Zook BC, Paasch LH. Endocardial fibroelastosis in Burmese cats. *Am J Pathol* 1982;106(3):435-438.

40. Rozengurt N. Endocardial fibroelastosis in common domestic cats in the UK. *J Comp Path* 1994;110:295-301.

41. Allan GS. Radiographic features of feline joint disease. *Vet Clin North Am: Sm Anim Pract* 2000;30(2):281-301.

42. Addie DD, Kennedy LJ, Ryvar R, et al. Feline leucocyte antigen class II polymorphism and susceptibility to feline infectious peritonitis. *J Fel Med Surg* 2004;6:59-62.

43. Norris JM, Bosward KL, White JD, et al Clinicopathological findings associated with feline infectious peritonitis in Sydney, Australia: 42 cases (1990-2002). *Aust Vet J.* 2005 Nov;83(11):666-73.

44. Pesteanu-Somogyi LD, Radzai C, Pressler BM. J Prevalence of feline infectious peritonitis in specific cat breeds. *Feline Med Surg.* 2006 Feb;8(1):1-5.

45. Bradbury AM, Morrison NE, Hwang M, Cox NR, Baker HJ, Martin DR Neurodegenerative lysosomal storage disease in European Burmese cats with hexosaminidase beta-subunit deficiency. Mol Genet Metab. 2009 Feb 20.

46. Feline Advisory Beaureau Website at: http://www.fabcats.org/breeders/inherited_disorders/burmese.php

47. Engvall E, Bushnell N. Patellar luxation in Abyssinian cats. *Fel Pract* 1990;18(4):20-22.

48. Lyons LA, Imes DL, Grahn RA. Investigation of albinism in domestic cats. *Proceedings.* The 2nd International Conference Advances in Canine and Feline Genomics. Utrecht Netherlands Oct 2004. Poster #18.

49. Schmidt-Kuntzel A, Eizirik E, O'Brien SJ, et al. Tyrosinase and tyrosinase related protein 1 alleles specify domestic cat coat color phenotypes of the albino and brown loci. *J Hered* 2005 Jul-Aug;96(4):289-301.

50. Lyons LA, Imes DL, Rah HC, et al Tyrosinase mutations associated with Siamese and Burmese patterns in the domestic cat (Felis catus). *Anim Genet.* 2005 Apr;36(2):119-26.

Recommended Reading

Glaze MB Congenital and hereditary ocular abnormalities in cats. *Clin Tech Small Anim Pract.* 2005 May;20(2):74-82.

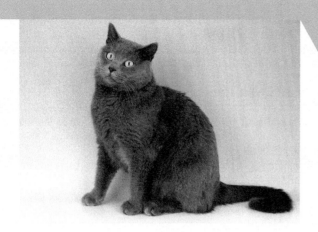

Chartreux

Grooming: Grooming needs are minimal; a quick rub with a chamois or work through with fingers generally suffices. Heavy seasonal shedding occurs so more frequent attention is needed while changing the coat.

Recognized Behavior Issues and Traits

Reported breed characteristics include: Gentle and placid but playful, they love climbing and are good mousers. Dog-like in behavior, intelligent, they like close human contact and may shadow their owners around the home, but are not demanding. Good with children and other pets.

They are known for a very gentle "smiling" expression. Not very vocal, they have a quiet high-pitched voice and a chirp—some do not meow. Adaptable, travel well. May play fetch, and love activities with family.

Normal Breed Variations

Slow maturing cats (about 24 months)

Gain weight easily so one must watch their caloric intake.

Strong hunting instinct so caution around pocket pets.

Drug Sensitivities

None reported in the literature

Inherited Diseases

None reported in the literature

Disease Predispositions

Overrepresented breed in a very small breed sample identifying risk of developing magnesium ammonium phosphate (MAP, struvite) uroliths.[1]

Genetic Tests

Hip and stifle screening to monitor prevalence of hip dysplasia and patellar luxation may be indicated as anecdotal evidence indicates that increased frequency occurs in this breed.

Miscellaneous

- **Breed name synonyms:** Historical: Cat of France, Chartruese, Blue Cat
- **Registries:** FIFé, TICA, CFA, ACFA, CFF, ACF, WCF, CCA
- **Breed resources:** Le Club du Chat des Chartreux (FIFé): www.club-du-chartreux.com/index2.html (in French)
  Les Amis des Chartreux (CFA): http://www.amisduchartreux.org/

References

1. Lekcharoensuk C, Lulich JP, Osborne CA, Koehler LA, Urlich LK, Carpenter KA, Swanson LL. Association between patient-related factors and risk of calcium oxalate and magnesium ammonium phosphate urolithiasis in cats. *J Am Vet Med Assoc* 2000;Aug15;217(4):520-525.

The Breed History

This is a rare breed. Sometimes confused with the Blue British Shorthair, the Chartreux originated in France, perhaps residing in the Monastery of La Grande Chartreuse near Grenoble, and some colonies from Belle Isle were recorded, but even earlier records may link them back to Syria (the Cat of Syria was similar in physical appearance). The name Chartreux may have arisen from the liquor or perhaps they were named after Spanish wool "pile de Chartreux" cloth that was similar in texture to the cat's fur. First records date back to 1558.

In those times they were valued for their pelts and also as ratters. First specimens arrived in America in the 1970s, and the CFA registry granted them championship status in 1987. In this breed, a naming convention results in all registered cats in any particular year having a name starting with the letter that has been assigned to that year. This breed almost became extinct following World War II, and outcrossing to Blue Persian and Blue British Shorthair was reportedly done overseas to regenerate the gene pool. No outcrossing is allowed currently. Some European registries may use the term *Chartreux* to apply to a Blue British Shorthair or European Shorthair with blue coloring, but they are distinct breeds. Pronounced *"Shart-rooh"*, or in some areas, *"shart-row"*.

Physical Characteristics

Weight: Female 7-10 (3.5-4.5), male 10-17 lb (4.5-7.5 kg)

Coat: Short-medium length double haircoat is dense and soft, with a plush, wooly standoff texture. Naturally water repellant, the coat can take up to five years to fully develop. It is light to dark blue-gray (ash to slate) in color, with silver tipping. Ghost barring may be seen in kittens, and tail rings may be seen in juvenile cats up to 24 months of age.

Eyes: Rounded large eyes are copper to gold in color. A vivid orange hue is favored.

Points of Conformation: Their rounded broad heads have full cheeks and well developed jaws. They possess a medium-short straight nose with a slight break. Ears are high set and medium sized, with minimal furnishings and rounded tips. This is a medium sized cat, less heavy in constitution than the Blue British Shorthair. They possess a short neck, deep chest, broad shoulders, short limbs with fairly fine leg bones; paws are small and round. Tail is fairly short, thick and tapers to a rounded tip.

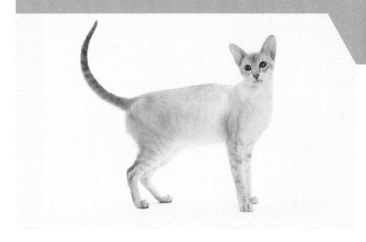

Colorpoint Shorthair

As geriatric cats, tend to lose weight.

The Breed History

Siamese cats were crossed with other breeds such as the American Shorthair and Abyssinian to develop new non-Siamese colors such as solid red point, solid cream point, red-lynx point and chocolate-tortie point. There are other additional point colors and patterns (16 in all). CFA registration occurred in 1974. Only Siamese outcrossing is allowed (book closes in 2019 for CFA).

Physical Characteristics

Weight: Female 6-8 lb (2.5-3.5 kg), male 8-12 (3.5-5.5 kg)

Coat: Glossy coat is very short with fine hair texture and lies close. Body of the coat is off-white in color with subtle shading which tends to darken as the cats age. The pointing and coat type are exactly the same as the Siamese; just the colors differ. Leather and paw pad pigmentation should be in sync with the coat coloring.

Eyes: Almond shaped medium sized eyes are close set, though greater than one eye width apart. Eyes are colored sapphire blue.

Points of Conformation: Siamese in conformation, though a slightly more muscular build is evident due to early outcrossing with American Shorthair. Head is long, a tapered wedge, with no stop and a straight profile. Ears are large and pointed, and their outer margin follows the wedge of the face in a straight continuation. Nose is long and straight. Body and limbs are lithe. Feet are oval and small. Neck is long and slim. Tail is long, fine, and tapers to a point.

Grooming: Coat is low maintenance except for periodic light brush or bath.

Recognized Behavior Issues and Traits

Reported breed characteristics include: High intelligence, high vocalizing tendency, like lots of attention, very affectionate, need playtime—this is an "other colored" Siamese cat. Need perches, cat trees and toys to keep entertained. Love to jump and do not like to be left alone for long periods of time.

Normal Breed Variations

Control calorie intake to counteract tendency to obesity

Drug Sensitivities

Increased tendency for post-vaccinal reactions (fever, lethargy) via anecdotal evidence only

Inherited Diseases

Corneal Sequestrum: Black body or cornea nigrum is often bilateral in Colorpoint cats. Usually in central cornea; brown to black pigmented lesion; often surrounded by a loose collarette of poorly adherent corneal epithelium. Lesion may extend into shallow or deep stroma, or even to Descemet's Membrane. Sloughing and corneal healing may take 2-6 months; surgical debridement is another option.[1]

Disease Predispositions

Many of Siamese conditions apply (*see Siamese Pointed Cat chapter*) though due to hybridization, the gene pool is broader and overall, the Colorpoint Shorthair cats are considered healthy and hardy.

Anecdotal reports of heart problems in some lines

Gingivitis and periodontal disease/periodontitis: anecdotal evidence of increased breed propensity

Genetic Tests

None commercially available

Miscellaneous

- **Breed name synonyms:** none
- **Registries:** CFA, CCA (in other registries such as GCCF, they are a color class of Siamese)
- **Breed resources: For clubs, contact the CFA at:** 1805 Atlantic Avenue, Manasquan NJ 08736-0805

References

1. Narfström K. Hereditary and congenital ocular disease in the cat. *J Fel Med Surg* 1999;1:135-141.

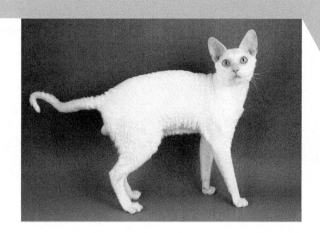

Cornish Rex

The Breed History

First described in 1950, these cats arose from a random mutation in the offspring of a shorthaired tortie and white barn cat in Cornwall, England. The first generation offspring rex male was mated back to the mother, and subsequent out-crossings to British Shorthair, Oriental Shorthair, and Siamese fixed the autosomal recessive haircoat gene and strengthened the breed. First brought to California in 1957, a female gave birth to the foundation kittens for the American lines.

The Cornish Rex was first registered with the CFA and GCCF in the 1960s. This is a different gene from the Devon Rex mutation (or the Selkirk Rex). No outcrosses currently allowed. The American Cornish Rex is longer in the head than the British type.

Physical Characteristics

Weight: 6-8 lb (2.5-3.5 kg)

Coat: The Cornish Rex comes in many colors and patterns Bi-colored is the most popular in the registry and show ring; smokes are also fairly common. The short coat is very soft and wavy, curly or rippled. There is a spectrum of hair length, thickness and curl. Longer coat is not as wavy (plush), shorter coat is "nappy" (termed suede). This mutation leaves only undercoat—there are no guard hairs. Uniform tight soft hairs lie close, organizing into "washboard" rows of wavy hairs much like the old-fashioned marcel hairstyle. Whiskers are curly.

Born curly coated, these cats go straight haired until about 16 weeks of age when they begin to curl, with coat quality finishing development at sexual maturity. Any bare areas apart from temples and ears are a serious show fault.

Eyes: Oval eyes, medium to large, many colors accepted.

Points of Conformation: English standard varies from the American standard. Small to medium cats, they possess a "racy" body, with a long wedge or "egg"-shaped small head, narrow muzzle, with hollow-cheeked look, very large high set ears lacking furnishings, with rounded tips. Brows are also crinkled. Chin is well developed, profile is lightly Roman nosed, whisker break is evident, and neck is long. Legs are long, with small oval feet. It is normal for them to stand with an arched back, creating a tucked-up abdomen appearance. The tail is long and slender, tapering to a point.

Grooming

Grooming: Does not mat. Minimal grooming is needed and this should be done with a chamois or fingers only. They do shed, but hairs are small.

Recognized Behavior Issues and Traits

Reported breed characteristics include: Very intelligent, get along well with dogs and children, high energy, enjoy close human contact, and will leash train. Love to play games, and keep kitten-like behaviors late into life. Like to jump very high—to tops of doors and fridges! May shadow a favored person around the house; sometimes referred to as "Velcro kitties". Cornish Rex are vocal cats. Good for indoor lifestyle and apartment living.

Normal Breed Variations

Low tolerance of temperature extremes

Easy birthing, good mothers, small-average litters averaging three, average birth weight is 100 g

Not predisposed to obesity; many owners free choice feed

Long lifespan

Blood Type B: Frequency of B blood type reported was 33%.[1]

Drug Sensitivities

None reported in the literature

Inherited Diseases

Neonatal Isoerythrolysis (NI): Published data support a high risk of complications if parent blood type is not tested prior to breeding. The proportion of matings reported at risk is 0.23.[2]

All B type cats have circulating anti-A antibodies and even primiparous queens can carry these. Breeding type B queens to type A toms can result in fatal red cell lysis in blood type A offspring with undetected NI. Kittens with NI can be distinguished from other fading kittens because pigmenturia; anemia and icterus will also be present; not all kittens at risk for NI will develop overt clinical symptoms.[3] Use a foster A type queen for the fist 18 hours or milk replacer if confirmed case of NI.

Disease Predispositions

Transfusion Reactions: Due to increased frequency of B blood type, an increased risk of transfusion reactions is expected.

Dystocia: A survey of 2,928 litters that included multiple cat breeds was carried out to ascertain prevalence of dystocia and over-representation of Cornish Rex cats was found, though only 16 Cornish rex litters were analyzed. Average dystocia rate in the study group was 5.8% of litters, with a low rate in a mixed breed colony of 0.4%, and for comparison, a rate of 12.5% in Cornish Rex.[4]

Hypertrophic Cardiomyopathy: The most common cardiac condition in all breeds of cats (10% prevalence), possibly inherited in the Rex breeds.[5]

Hereditary Deafness: Is associated with the dominant gene for white cat (W); may be found in white cats of this breed.[6]

FIP Susceptibility: A study in Australia confirmed that the Cornish Rex breed cats were over-represented.[7]

An American study found that Rex cats were significantly over-represented for a diagnosis of FIP when they analyzed data for a 16 year period at a veterinary teaching hospital.[8]

Patellar Luxation: A 1990 report noted a historical breed propensity for patellar luxation.[9]

Rare and Isolated Reports

Umbilical Hernia: In one early literature report, a family of Cornish rex cats had a high incidence of umbilical hernia and it was postulated to be a polygenic condition.[10]

Hypotrichosis: Thin hair progresses to baldness at two weeks of age. May re-grow by 6-9 weeks of age, but loss again occurs at sexual maturity leaving them permanently bald. An autosomal recessive inheritance was postulated.[11]

Genetic Tests

Though not specifically reported in the literature, blood typing prior to mating or transfusions would be prudent.

Miscellaneous

- **Breed name synonyms:** Curly-coat cat, Crex, Rexed cat.
- **Registries:** FIFé, TICA, CFA, ACFA, CFF, GCCF, ACF, WCF, NZCF, CCA
- **Breed resources: The Rex Cat Club (GCCF-U.K.):**
  http://www.sam.luxford-watts.zen.co.uk/home.html
  Cornish Rex Society: In the U.K.:
  http://www.cornish-rex.co.uk/
  In the U.S.:
  http://www.flickoff.com/wavelink.htm
  (Cornish) Rex Breeders United (CFA):
  446 Itasca Ct NW
  Rochester MN 55901
  CFA Cornish Rex Breed Council: http://www.cornishrexbc.org

References

1. Giger U. In: Bonagura J, ed. *Kirk's Current Veterinary Therapy XIII.* Philadelphia: WB Saunders Co, 2000;396-399.

2. Giger U, Casal M, Niggemeier A. The fading kitten syndrome and neonatal isoerythrolysis. *Proceedings.* The 15th Annual ACVIM Medical Forum, Lake Buena Vista FL 1997;308-310.

3. Giger U, Bucheler J, Patterson DF. Frequency and inheritance of A and B blood types in feline breeds of the United States. *J Hered* 1991;82:15-20.

4. Gunn-Moore DA, Thrusfield MV. Feline dystocia: prevalence, and association with cranial conformation and breed. *Vet Rec* 1995;136:350-353.

5. Little S. Selected inherited diseases of the cat, in *Proceedings.* International Ragdoll Congress Oct, 2004; Pers. Comm.

6. Strain GM. Hereditary deafness in dogs and cats: causes, prevalence, and current research. *Proceedings.* Tuft's Canine and Feline Breeding and Genetics Conference. Oct 2-4, 2003 Available at: http://www.vin.com/tufts/2003. Accessed Nov 19, 2004.

7. Norris JM, Bosward KL, White JD, Baral RM, Catt MJ, Malik R. Clinicopathological findings associated with feline infectious peritonitis in Sydney, Australia: 42 cases (1990-2002). *Aust Vet J.* 2005 Nov;83(11):666-73.

8. Pesteanu-Somogyi LD, Radzai C, Pressler BM. Prevalence of feline infectious peritonitis in specific cat breeds. *J Feline Med Surg.* 2006 Feb;8(1):1-5.

9. Engvall E, Bushnell N. Patellar luxation in Abyssinian cats. *Fel Pract* 1990;18(4):20-22

10. Robinson R. Genetic aspects of umbilical hernia incidence in cats and dogs. Vet Rec 1977;Jan1;100(1):9-10.

11. Hoskins JD. Congenital defects in cats. *Compend Contin Educ Pract Vet* 1995;17(3):385-405.

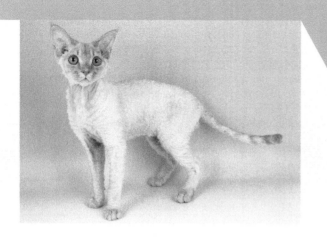

pads are evident. Other features include a moderately short nose, very large rounded ears which are set low, lending the cats an elfin look. The neck is fine. The tail is long and slender. Legs are long, straight and medium in bone. Paws are small and oval.

Grooming: Low shedding is standard for this breed. Devon cats have minimal grooming requirements. A light chamois or a hand is used to gently rub over the cat as needed. Not advised to blow dry. Oiliness in the coat can be controlled with chamois grooming but periodic bathing may be required. Ears tend to be greasy and require more regular cleaning than the average cat.

Recognized Behavior Issues and Traits
Reported breed characteristics include: Talkative but with quiet voice, playful, love to climb high and a cat tree and high perches help to keep the Devon exercised. They love warm places and are well suited to apartment life. Devon Rex cats like to play fetch and are active pets overall. Very people-oriented; can be lap cats and can demand attention.

Normal Breed Variations
They are not hardy in temperature extremes.

These cats will nurse their young longer than most cats.

They tend to gain weight easily.

They have naturally waxy ears, so may require more frequent cleaning than the average cat.

Blood Type B: In a study of blood type distribution in the US, Devon Rex cats (n=100) had 43% type B blood.[1] A prevalence of 41% type B was reported in another reference.[2]

Devon Rex Kitten Information Project:[3] An internet based survey was carried out to gather breed normal data. Data were for 30 breeders, 103 litters with 377 kittens. June 2001-May 2002.
   Average litter size 3.7
   Stillbirth rate 4%
   Dystocia 8% (1% of affected queens required C-section[4])
   Average birth weight: Male 88 g female 83 g
   Congenital deformities occurred in 12.4% of litters,[4] 2.3% born with umbilical hernias, others defects reported included flat chest, and cleft palate.

Drug Sensitivities
None reported in the literature

Inherited Diseases
Multiple Vitamin K-dependent Blood Coagulation Factor Deficiency: (Vitamin K-dependent factors II, VII, IX, X) (Breeder SYN: hemophilia). This condition has only been identified in the Devon Rex breed so far. The cluster of Devon cats in one report from

The Breed History
About the year 1960 in Devonshire England, a stray was found to carry this new "rex haircoat" gene. The first progenitor male was named *Kirlee*. This mutation is not related to Cornish Rex or Selkirk Rex and early crossings between them proved this; though some of these crossbreds were used in the early Devon Rex breeding program. The Devon Rex haircoat (*re*) is an autosomal recessive gene affecting normal hair follicle development.

The Devon Rex is more waved than curly haired; the latter being the type seen in the Cornish Rex. In 1967, the GCCF in Britain and FIFé in Europe accepted the breed. The CFA recognized Devon Rex as distinct from Cornish Rex in 1979, put the Devons into the provisional class in 1981, and championship status was granted in 1983. In 2013 outcrossing will no longer be allowed; until then, The Devon can be crossed with British Shorthair and American Shorthair cats only.

Physical Characteristics
Weight: 6-9 lb (2.5-4 kg)

Coat: Can be any color since hair mutation and color are not linked. The ventrum may be downy and of reduced hair density, but the texture of the coat is silky and fine like crushed velvet, and bare patches are penalized except the temples and ears. The coat overall is less dense than a Cornish Rex coat and is whirled or curled, crinkly rather than wavy, and about 1/2" long. The coat is very short, very soft and the hairs are fine; though normal guard hairs are lacking over the body, on the tail some full guard hairs may make the haircoat a little coarser there.

Hair cover on the limbs and head, abdomen, and neck is less curly and shorter. Brow and whiskers may be crinkled, and whiskers and coat hairs break easily. Whiskers are usually less than 1 in (2.5 cm) long. In kittens, waves are not fully developed and coat is not mature until about 16-24 weeks of age, with molting during development, though mature coats can sometimes be significantly delayed in re-growth, finishing well past sexual maturity. Rarely, longhairs are born.

Eyes: Large oval eyes can be any color and are wide set.

Points of Conformation: The head is a short modified wedge with a distinct break. Prominent cheekbones, and well defined whisker

Australia had a range of normal clotting profile/clinically normal findings, abnormal clotting profile/clinically normal, ranging to abnormal profile/abnormal clinical status.

Clinical cases presented with signs such as hematoma and conjunctival hemorrhage, post-operative bleeding, sudden death due to intra-thoracic hemorrhage, and it was reported that some had untested relatives (such as littermates) affected or that had died. The screening of cats revealed PT and APTT tests were substantially prolonged.[5]

Multiple Vitamin K-dependent blood coagulation factor deficiency was found in another report of two littermates with bleeding tendency. An underlying mutation in the vitamin K-dependent γ-glutamylcarboxylase enzyme was identified as the reason for the bleeding disorder; this enzyme plays an important role in reconstituting Vitamin K in the liver cycle.[6]

A report in a British Devon Rex cat indicated that the same coagulation factor deficiency combination was again present. Another cat with the same grandmother also died of post-operative hemorrhage. The cats responded to oral/subcutaneous vitamin K administration and transfusion.[7]

A likely autosomal recessive inheritance was reported. Age of onset is generally before one year of age.[8]

It is important to note that not all reported afflicted cats had clinically evident bleeding episodes. The prevalence of this defect is unknown in the breed, so testing Devon Rex cats by coagulation profile before surgery might be prudent until further data is available.

Devon Rex Hereditary Myopathy (Breeder Synonym: Spasticity):
A neuromuscular disease leading to muscle weakness, and is similar to limb girdle muscular dystrophy in humans. First reported in 1974, this condition presents as an unusual gait (high stepping), significant neck ventroflexion, head bobbing, limping, abnormal mastication due to pharyngeal muscle weakness, megaesophagus, difficulty drinking (nose may be inserted underwater), dorsal scapula protrusion, shaking, and collapse. Aspiration pneumonia or sudden death due to choke is a possible consequence of difficulty with prehension of food and water. Neck ventroflexion may worsen during micturition and defecation and while walking, and signs may wax and wane in intensity over days to weeks.[9] Blood count, serum biochemistry including CK and electrolytes are all within normal ranges. Histology is best performed on proximal limb and cervical muscles, and magnitude of changes is correlated with age and severity of clinical signs at time of biopsy.

Age at onset of signs varies but signs are often noted by breeders at 4-7 weeks, though some are delayed to about 13 weeks of age (range of onset 4-20 weeks).[8, 10] Though afflicted cats usually worsen, as an adult some may adapt to the disability. In a survey of cats from the UK, Australia, and New Zealand an autosomal recessive monogenic pattern of inheritance was proposed to explain the trait.[8] A recent report indicates that dystroglycan (DAG1) may be the gene causing this problem, and the researchers have attempted to sequence the mutation; apparently the same mutation is present in Sphynx Spasticity.[11]

Newest studies term this **Dystroglycanopathy (muscular dystrophy):** This disease results in a loss of glycosylated alpha-dystroglycan expression, but not reduced binding.[12]

Cervical Ventroflexion: In a study carried out in Great Britain, primary muscle weakness was diagnosed in young cats, with marked neck ventroflexion and normal Creatine Kinase and muscle biopsies. No therapy was found to be helpful.[13]

Hypotrichosis: Thin hair regresses to baldness at 2 weeks old. May re-grow by 6-10 weeks of age, but loss occurs again at sexual maturity leaving cats permanently bald.[14] It is thought to be an autosomal recessive mode of inheritance. Hair follicles are hypoplastic and hairs are in telogen.

Hereditary Deafness: Is associated with the dominant gene for white cat (W); may be found in white cats of this breed.[15]

Neonatal Isoerythrolysis (NI): High prevalence of B blood type makes this a concern in this breed; typed parents are now the standard for breeders. Published proportion of matings at risk for NI is 0.24 for this breed.[16] Also given as 0.246.[1] All B type cats have circulating anti-A antibodies and even primiparous queens can carry these. Type B queens bred to type A toms can result in fatal red cell lysis in A blood type offspring with undetected NI. Kittens with NI can be distinguished from other fading kittens because of pigmenturia; anemia and icterus will also be present; not all kittens at risk for NI will develop overt clinical symptoms.[1]

Disease Predispositions

Transfusion Reactions: Due to high prevalence of blood type B, natural allo-antibodies markedly increase the risk of transfusion reactions so donors and recipients should be blood typed.

Toe and Skin Fold Greasiness, Paronychia: Seborrheic dermatitis caused by M. Pachydermatis is more common in the breed (90% samples positive in a cross sectional survey comparing Cornish and Devon Rex cats with DSH cats).[17]

In a study the previous year, the same researchers isolated M. sloffiae from claw folds of seborrheic cats.[18]

Another study by the same authors that year explored the use of itraconazole to treat this seborrhea in a 21 day pulse treatment.[19]

Hypertrophic Cardiomyopathy (HCM): The most common cardiac condition in cats (10% prevalence). Suspected to be inherited in the breed, and cats with HCM should be removed from the breeding pool.[20]

Medial Patellar Luxation (MPL) and Hip Dysplasia (HD):
Historically, a proposed genetic predisposition to patellar luxation was reported, with hip dysplasia prevalence also increased in this breed.[21] In 1985, it was one author's early finding that prevalence of MPL was apparently much greater in the Devon Rex.[22]

A nonrandom group of 78 cats of different breeds including 25 Devon Rex cats were assessed. About 32% of this group of cats and 40% (10 of 25) of Devons had HD using OFA-like criteria and a positive correlation between joint laxity, DJD and HD was identified.

The majority of cats were not clinically lame, but diagnostic imaging tests showed pathologic changes.

The Devon Rex cats were affected more severely and with higher frequency than the average cat. In the pooled all-breed group with MPL in the study group, those with MPL were three times more likely to have concurrent hip dysplasia than those without MPL.[23, 24, 25, 26]

In the 1999 study done at University of Pennsylvania joint laxity measures included Norberg angle (NA), distraction index (DI)] as well as OFA criterion. Some degree of MPL was found in 58% of pooled cats and concurrent MPL and HP in 24%. Of the 25 Devon Rex cats, 16 had MPL (64%); eight Devon Rex cats had both HD and MPL (32%).[26]

Both HD and PL are more common than was previously presumed. Medial patellar luxation is thought to be congenital and can be unilateral or bilateral. Higher prevalence of MPL is suggestive of a hereditary basis.

Dystocia: A report summarizing a survey of 2,928 litters that included multiple cat breeds was analyzed to ascertain prevalence of dystocia, and over-representation of Devon Rex cats was found (22 Devon litters analyzed). Average dystocia rate in the study group was 5.8% of litters, with a low in mixed breed cat colony of 0.4%, to a high of 18.2% in the Devon Rex study group.[27]

Rare and Isolated Reports

Amyloidosis: Hepatic rupture in association with systemic amyloidosis was reported in a Devon Rex cat.[28] Hepatic amyloidosis has not previously been reported in this breed. Prior reports involved Orientals, Siamese, and primarily renal amyloidosis in Abyssinian cats.

Feline Urticaria Pigmentosa (papular eosinophilic/mastocytic dermatitis): Very similar to the condition described in Sphinx cats (as Urticaria pigmentosa-see *Sphynx chapter*) and in young Himalayan cats. Pruritis, wheals, and red-brown papules are termed cutaneous mastocytosis in humans; is also associated with eosinophilic infiltration.

Five unrelated Devon Rex cats aged 5 months to 4 years of age were afflicted with very specific dermatologic changes which waxed and waned over a period of 3 weeks, to many months (up to 10). Variably pruritic or non-pruritic wheals progressed to erythematous, normal or hyperpigmented crusted macular and papular lesions; some had seborrheic erosive dermatitis, others secondary pyoderma (pyoderma was associated with hyperpigmentation and pruritis). May be closely related to the other eosinophilic hypersensitivity disorders such as plaque and granuloma and may be an allergic hypersensitivity response or propensity.[29]

FIP Susceptibility: An American study found that Rex cats were significantly over-represented for a diagnosis of FIP when they analyzed data for a 16 year period at a veterinary teaching hospital.[30]

Recurrent Syncope: A case report described a cat that had 7-year history of recurring syncopal episodes that were associated with paroxysmal supraventricular tachycardia (SVT) and was diagnosed using an implantable loop recorder, and treated with sotalol.[31]

Swimmer Syndrome: After several weeks, a 3-week old showed response to bandaging and physiotherapy. Euthanasia is the usual veterinary recommendation for this condition.[32]

Genetic Tests

Coagulation profile and blood typing before surgery, transfusion, or in breeding animals is recommended.

Though no program is recommended in the literature, screening breeding animals for HD and MPL using radiography and orthopedic examination may be helpful to manage these conditions in the breed.

Miscellaneous

- **Breed name synonyms:** Curly-coated cat, Devon, Rexed cat, nickname: Poodle cat
- **Registries:** FIFé, TICA, CFA, ACFA, CFF, CCA, NZCF, WCF, ACF, GCCF
- **Breed resources: Devon Rex Breed Club:**
  http://www.devonrexbreedclub.com/
  The Rex Cat Club (GCCF–U.K.):
  http://www.sam.luxford-watts.zen.co.uk/home.html
  Rex Breeders United:
  446 Itasca Ct NW
  Rochester MN 55901

References

1. Giger U, Bucheler J, Patterson DF. Frequency and inheritance of A and B blood types in feline breeds of the United States. *J Hered* 1991;82:15-20.
2. Giger U. In: Bonagura J, ed. *Kirk's Current Veterinary Therapy XIII.* Philadelphia: WB Saunders Co, 2000;396-399.
3. Little S. Breed Specific Reproduction Projects. In: *Notes,* University of California (Davis) Feline Genetics Extravaganza I July, 2003.
4. Little S. Breed specific feline reproduction and kitten health data: A preliminary report. *Proceedings.* Tuft's Canine and Feline Breeding and Genetics Conference Oct 2-4, 2003 Available at VIN: www.vin.com/tufts/2003. Accessed Nov 19, 2004.
5. Maddison JE, Watson ADJ, Eade IG, et al. Vitamin K-dependent multifactor coagulopathy in Devon Rex cats. *J Am Vet Med Assoc* 1990;197(11):1495-1497.
6. Soute BAM, Ulrich MMW, Watson ADJ, et al. Congenital deficiency of all vitamin K-dependent blood coagulation factors due to a defective vitamin K-dependent carboxylase in Devon Rex cats. *Thrombosis and Hemostasis* 1992;68(5):521-525.
7. Littlewood JD, Shaw SC, Coombes LM. Vitamin K-dependent coagulopathy in a British Devon Rex cat. *J Small Anim Pract* 1995;36:115-118.
8. Malik R. Genetic Diseases of Cats (and Dogs). *Proceedings.* University of Sydney Post Graduate Foundation in Veterinary Science. Valentine Charlton Refresher Course for Veterinarians; Cats 2000. 2000;Jul;27-37.
9. Gaschen F, Jaggy A, Jones B. Congenital diseases of feline muscle and neuromuscular junction. *J Fel Med Surg* 2004;6:355-366.
10. Robinson R. "Spasticity" in the Devon Rex cat. *Vet Rec* 1992;130:302.
11. Suciu A, Lipinski M, Froenicke L, et al. Dystroglycan (DAG1) as a candidate gene for a feline hereditary myopathy "Spasticity". In: *Notes.* University of California (Davis) Feline Genetics Extravaganza II Aug 28-29, 2004.
12. Martin PT, Shelton GD, Dickinson PJ, Sturges BK, Xu R, LeCouteur RA, Guo LT, Grahn RA, Lo HP, North KN, Malik R, Engvall E, Lyons LA. Muscular dystrophy associated with alpha-dystroglycan deficiency in Sphynx and

Devon Rex cats. Neuromuscul Disord. 2008 Dec;18(12):942-52

13. Taboada J. Ventroflexion of the neck in cats. *Proceedings.* 12th Annual American College of Veterinary Internal Medicine Forum, San Francisco CA 1994;385-386.

14. Hoskins JD. Congenital defects in cats. Compend Contin Educ Pract Vet 1995;17(3):385-405.

15. Strain GM. Hereditary deafness in dogs and cats: causes, prevalence, and current research. *Proceedings.* Tuft's Canine and Feline Breeding and Genetics Conference. Oct 2-4, 2003. Available at: http://www.vin.com/tufts/2003. Accessed Nov 19, 2004.

16. Giger U, Casal M, Niggemeier A. The fading kitten syndrome and neonatal isoerythrolysis. *Proceedings.* The 15th Annual ACVIM Medical Forum, Lake Buena Vista FL 1997;308-310.

17. Bond R, Stevens K, Perrins N, Ahman S Carriage of Malassezia spp. yeasts in Cornish Rex, Devon Rex and Domestic short-haired cats: a cross-sectional survey. *Vet Dermatol.* 2008 Oct; 19(5):299-304.

18. Ahman S, Perrins N, Bond R Carriage of Malassezia spp. yeasts in healthy and seborrhoeic Devon Rex cats. *Med Mycol.* 2007 Aug;45(5):449-55.

19. Ahman S, Perrins N, Bond R. Treatment of Malassezia pachydermatis-associated seborrhoeic dermatitis in Devon Rex cats with itraconazole--a pilot study *Vet Dermatol.* 2007 Jun;18(3):171-4.

20. Meurs KM. Inherited heart disease in the cat. *Proceedings.* Tuft's Canine and Feline Breeding and Genetics Conference Oct 2-4, 2003 Available at VIN: www.vin.com/tufts/2003. Accessed Nov 19, 2004.

21. Little S. Selected inherited diseases of the cat, in *Proceedings.* International Ragdoll Congress Oct, 2004. Available at: www.catvet.homestead.com/Inherited_Diseases_2004.pdf, Accessed Nov 23, 2004.

22. Prior JE. Luxating patellae in Devon Rex cats. *Vet Rec* 1985; Au;17;117(7):154-155.

23. Lagenbach A, Giger U, Green P, et al. Relationship between degenerative joint disease and hip joint laxity by use of distraction index and Norberg angle measurement in a group of cats. *J Am Vet Med Assoc* 1998;213(10):1439-1443.

24. Smith GK Lagenbach A, Giger U, et al. Patellar luxation and hip dysplasia in a group of cats. First International Feline Genetic Disease Conference Philadelphia June 1998 *Proceedings (abstr)* in: *Feline Practice Supplement,* 1999;23.

25. Little S. Feline hip dysplasia. *Notes.* Winn Feline Foundation Website. Available at: www.winnfelinehealth.org/hip-dysplasia.html Accessed Sep 29, 2004.

26. Smith GK, Langenbach A, Green PA, et al. Evaluation of the association between medial patellar luxation and hip dysplasia in cats. *J Am Vet Med Assoc* 1999;215(1):40-45.

27. Gunn-Moore DA, Thrusfield MV. Feline dystocia: prevalence, and association with cranial conformation and breed. *Vet Rec* 1995;136:350-353.

28. Beatty JA, Barrs VR, Martin PA, et al. Spontaneous hepatic rupture in six cats with systemic amyloidosis. *J Small Anim Pract* 2002;43:355-363.

29. Noli C, Colombo S, Abramos F, et al. Papular eosinophilic/mastocytic dermatitis (Feline Urticaria Pigmentosa) in Devon Rex cats: A distinct disease entity or a histopathological reaction pattern? *Vet Dermatol* 2004;15:253-259.

30. Pesteanu-Somogyi LD, Radzai C, Pressler BM. Prevalence of feline infectious peritonitis in specific cat breeds. *J Feline Med Surg.* 2006 Feb;8(1):1-5.

31. Ferasin L. Recurrent syncope associated with paroxysmal supraventricular tachycardia in a Devon Rex cat diagnosed by implantable loop recorder. *J Feline Med Surg.* 2009 Feb;11(2):149-52.

32. Verhoeven G, de Rooster H, Risselada M, Wiemer P, Scheire L, van Bree H. Swimmer syndrome in a Devon rex kitten and an English bulldog puppy. *J Small Anim Pract.* 2006 Oct;47(10):615-9.

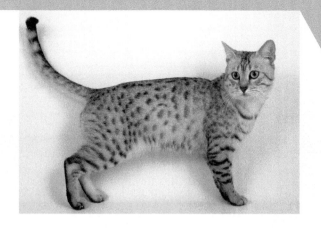

Egyptian Mau

are noted in the breed standards. Hair texture varies between coat colors but is silky and lustrous in general.

Eyes: Eyes are always a shade of light green (called gooseberry) in mature cats. Kittens may have amber overtones up to 18 months of age only. Almond shaped eyes are large.

Points of Conformation: Medium sized cats, they are well muscled, with rounded-wedge shaped head and medium length muzzle. There is no break, and ears are large, moderately pointed and positioned to continue the lines of the face, preferably tufted. Paws are small and round-oval in shape. Tail is medium-long, tapering from a thick base, and overall the cat is quite fine in appearance. They possess a loose skin flap, running from flank to stifle area.

Grooming: The Mau has low grooming needs; a periodic light brush or hand/chamois will suffice. Towel rather than blow dry if a bath is needed.

The Breed History

Mau is an Egyptian word for cat—perhaps originally this word was an approximation of the meow sound. This is the only naturally spotted domestic cat breed. The first scribed records of the Mau cat go back to 1400 BC which makes it one of the very oldest known breeds; they were represented in artwork dating much further back—about 3000 BC.

It is thought that they were domesticated from spotted African Wild Cats, Felis libyca *subsp. ocreata*. Egyptians used to hold cats in special regard, and frequently mummified them. At one cemetery site, 300,000 cat mummies were interred. Bastet, daughter of Ra was the Egyptian goddess of fertility and in statuary, was represented with a cat head.

Egyptian Mau spotted cats came from Cairo to America in 1956 via Italy. The breed was accepted by CFF in 1968 and accorded championship status by CFA in 1977. The FIFé approved them in 1992. In the UK, Shorthair Oriental Spotted Tabbies were called "Maus" for a while and this has caused some confusion regarding the two breeds. No outcrossing is currently allowed. The progenitor female for the North American lines was a silver cat named *Baba*.

Physical Characteristics

Weight: 5-12 lb (2-5.5 kg), males larger than females

Coat: The original coat was the spotted pattern in bronze (dark brown-black spots on bronze agouti), but now silver (charcoal spots on silver agouti) or smoke (black spots over silver-charcoal body hairs and white undercoat) are also accepted. Black and blue kittens occur and can be registered but are pet quality. Agouti hairs have at least two bands of color striping. Hair is short-medium in length.

Good sharp contrast between spots and background is highly valued. Spots of the silver and bronze coats can be any size or shape but should not form any tabby pattern. Bronze cats may have a pattern limited to the topline though. Some tabby markings are seen in the Smokes. Forehead pattern is in an M-shape, which had significance in ancient times, as it reminded the Egyptians of their sacred scarab. Dark lines extend between the ears back to the neck. These lines are termed frown marks. Mascara marking lines the eyes. A dorsal stripe goes down the topline extending to the tail base. Other specific coat markings such as tail and limb banding

Recognized Behavior Issues and Traits

Reported breed characteristics include: Variable personalities are present in the breed, from those demanding attention to aloof cats but overall, are considered well balanced. They are vigorously playful, and are lively and friendly with family in general. They chortle and talk softly. Tend to bond closely with one family member and be fiercely loyal. Can be taught tricks and many will leash train. Like to jump and sit in high places, so a perch or cat tree should be provided. Need time to explore new environments, so it is best to gradually introduce new people and places.

Normal Breed Variations

Are the fastest domestic cat runners checked so far—clocked at 30 mph (48 km/hr).

Deciduous teeth can be delayed in shedding.

May shake their tail when happy; appears as if spraying but no urine produced.

Slightly longer average gestation period—queens often go up to 70 days.

Best to limit feeding.

Some cats like water, but this does not necessarily translate into enjoying baths.

Kitten Internet Information Project:[1]
    52 litters
    192 kittens
    3.7 kittens/litter
    6% stillbirths
    10% C-sections
    Female average birth weight: 101 g, male 107 g

Drug Sensitivities
None reported in literature

Inherited Diseases
None reported in the literature

Disease Predispositions
Feline leukemia Virus: Endogenous feline leukemia (enFeLVs) were studied in a single specimen of Burmese, Egyptian Mau and Persian breed cats to determine how many loci and where proviruses were typically inserted. This may indicate genetic propensity for leukemia genesis in these cats when exposed to the exogenous feline leukemia virus. They found provirus on 12/18 autosomes, with an average 19 autosomal copies per cat. One specific locus contained both homologues in all 3 cats. They were also found on both X and Y chromosomes.[2]

Back in the time of early breed development, temperament problems, asthma and cardiomyopathy were mentioned in a fancy article as predispositions, but careful outcrossing and selective breeding has helped to control these traits in the breeding pool.

Anecdotal reports of food sensitivity in some lines

Rare and Isolated Reports
Hypomyelination/Dysmyelination: Case report described two inbred littermates at 7 weeks of age with clinical signs of progressive hypermetria/ataxia and bouts of reduced activity and periodic seizures. Brain and spinal cord had extensive vacuolation or spongy degeneration of grey and white matter. By 4 months of age, their overall status was poor, with some dsyphagia. One kitten was euthanized at 4 months of age, the other kitten gradually improved. In the litter, one other kitten was stillborn, another died very young, and yet another developed mild hind limb ataxia at 10 months of age. The parents had a common sire on both sides. The spongy degeneration was postulated to result from lowered ATPase activity in astrocyte mitochondria. A genetic basis was suspected.[3]

Genetic Tests
No commercially available tests

Miscellaneous
- **Breed name synonyms:** Mau, Egyptian Cat, Spotted Cat
- **Registries:** FIFé, TICA, CFA, ACFA, NZCF, CCA, WCF, GCCF
- **Breed resources: Egyptian Mau Breeders and Fanciers Club (CFA):** http://www.geocities.com/Petsburgh/2369/
  Global Egyptian Mau Society: http://www.egyptianmau.org/
  The Egyptian Mau Club (UK):
  http://www.egyptianmaus.co.uk/
  National Egyptian Mau Council (CFA):
  http://www.egyptianmaubc.org/records.html

References
1. Little, S. Pers. Comm. 2009
2. Roca AL, Nash WG, Menninger JC, Murphy WJ, O'Brien SJ. Insertional polymorphisms of endogenous feline leukemia viruses. J Virol. 2005 Apr;79(7):3979-86
3. Kelly DF, Gaskell CJ. Spongy degeneration of the central nervous system in kittens. Acta Neuropathol (Berl) 1976;35:151-158.

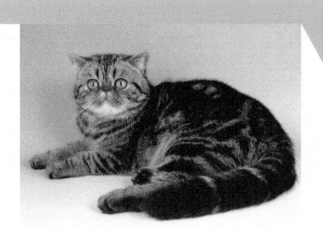

The Breed History

Exotic breed cats are essentially shorthaired Persians in type. The origins of the Exotics were from crosses of British Shorthairs with Persians. In America, breeders also crossed these cats with Burmese and American Shorthair cats in the 1960s. Though termed Exotic Shorthair in many places, in America they are usually referred to by the name Exotic. The CFA registry recognized the Exotic in 1967 and today, only Persian outcrosses are accepted.

Physical Characteristics

Weight: 8-14 lb (3.5-6.5 kg)

Coat: All Himalayan and Persian colors are allowed. The very soft dense plush double coat is a bit longer than the usual shorthair coat; almost a medium length.

Eyes: Large eyes are prominent and round. Color of eyes is in sync with color of the coat.

Points of Conformation: The conformation specifications for Exotics mirror those for the Persian. These are medium sized cobby cats, with a compact build, short heavy legs, and large round paws. The Exotic possesses a massive round head with full cheeks, and small rounded ears set far apart and low, with rounded tips. A distinct stop between the eyes is present. A short snub nose is also characteristic. Tail is short and thick with a rounded tip.

Grooming: Coat care consists of a brief daily grooming session. There is a much reduced matting tendency when compared with Persians. May need to cleanse away tears/debris at the medial canthus on an "as need" basis.

Recognized Behavior Issues and Traits

Reported breed characteristics include: Playful, friendly, curious, quiet and affectionate. Excellent compatibility with children and other pets. These cats are a bit livelier than the typical Persian cats, but share the small voice of the Persian. Many enjoy being lap cats. Not demanding of attention.

Normal Breed Variations

Tend to gain weight easily so there is an increased risk of obesity

Blood Type B: Prevalence of 27% type B was reported.[1]

Exotic/Exotic Shorthair

Drug Sensitivities

None reported in the literature

Inherited Diseases

See Persian chapter for more information about shared traits.

(An example of a condition shared by Exotic and Persian): Polycystic Kidney Disease (PKD): PKD is most common in Persian breed, and those breeds having out-crossed to Persians in their breeding programs. According to one study in France, prevalence of PKD was 39% in Exotic Shorthairs, in a healthy population screened for cysts in the kidney by ultrasonographic evaluation.[2]

Another study in Australia determined that in the population of healthy owned cats, 50% of the Exotics were positive for PKD.[3] In another study group of 17 Exotics there was a 41% positive rate.[4] In screening programs carried out at University of California at Davis in 2002, Exotics were assessed in three separate study groups (40%, 33% and 41% positive) by ultrasound screening of healthy cattery cats.[5]

Neonatal Isoerythrolysis (NI): All B type cats have circulating anti-A antibodies and even primiparous queens can carry these. Type B queens bred to type A toms can result in fatal red cell lysis in A blood type offspring with undetected NI. Kittens with NI can be distinguished from other fading kittens because of pigmenturia; anemia and icterus will also be present; not all kittens at risk for NI will develop overt clinical symptoms.[6]

Disease Predispositions

See Persian chapter for details regarding the many shared predispositions

(e.g., Brachycephalic—can be associated with sinus problems, breathing difficulties, corneal ulceration secondary to drying, epiphora.

Jaw and teeth anatomical abnormalities: (asymmetric jaw, crowded teeth)

Dystocia: Increased dystocia due to large domed skulls.

Transfusion Reactions: Due to high prevalence of blood type B, natural allo-antibodies markedly increase the risk of transfusion reactions so donors and recipients should be blood typed).

Calcium Oxalate Urolithiasis: In a case control study outlining risk of development of uroliths, Exotics were found to be at increased risk of forming calcium oxalate uroliths.[7]

Hereditary Deafness: Is associated with the dominant gene for white cat (W); may be found in white cats of this breed.[8]

Genetic Tests

Blood type cats before mating or transfusions recommended

Miscellaneous

- **Breed name synonyms:** Shorthaired Persian, Zot
- **Registries:** FIFé (Exotic), TICA (Exotic Shorthair), CCA, NZCF (Exotic) CFA, ACFA (Exotic Shorthair), CFF, WCF (Exotic Shorthair), ACF (Exotic Shorthair), GCCF (Exotic)
- **Breed resources: Exotic Cat Club (GCCF):**
  http://www.exotic-cat-club.org/
  Exotic Shorthair Cat Society (U.K):
  http://www.exoticcatsociety.co.uk/
  Exotic CFA Breed Council:
  http://www.exoticbc.org/
  United Silver and Golden Fanciers Online (Silver/golden Persians and exotics):
  http://www.unitedsilverandgoldenfanciers.com/

References

1. Giger U. In: Bonagura J, ed. *Kirk's Current Veterinary Therapy XIII.* Philadelphia: WB Saunders Co, 2000;396-399.

2. Barthez PY, Rivier P, Begon D. Prevalence of polycystic kidney disease in Persian and Persian-related cats in France. *J Fel Med Surg* 2003;5(6):345-347.

3. Beck C, Lavelle RB. Feline polycystic kidney disease in Persian and other cats: a prospective study using ultrasonography. *Aust Vet J* 2001;79(3):181-4.

4. Barrs VR, Gunew M, Foster SF, et al. Prevalence of autosomal dominant kidney disease in Persian cats and related breeds in Sydney and Brisbane. *Aust Vet J* 2001;79:257-259.

5. Lyons LA. The Lyon's Den. Feline Genome Project: Polycystic Kidney Disease. Available at: http://faculty.vetmed.ucdavis.edu/faculty/lalyons/Sites/pkd.htm Accessed Nov 6, 2004.

6. Giger U, Bucheler J, Patterson DF. Frequency and inheritance of A and B blood types in feline breeds of the United States. *J Hered* 1991;82:15-20.

7. Lekcharoensuk C, Lulich JP, Osborne CA, et al. Association between patient-related factors and risk of calcium oxalate and magnesium ammonium phosphate urolithiasis in cats. *J Am Vet Med Assoc* 2000;Aug15;217(4):520-525.

8. Strain GM. Hereditary deafness in dogs and cats: causes, prevalence, and current research. *Proceedings.* Tuft's Canine and Feline Breeding and Genetics Conference. Oct 2-4, 2003. Available at: http://www.vin.com/tufts/2003. Accessed Nov 19, 2004.

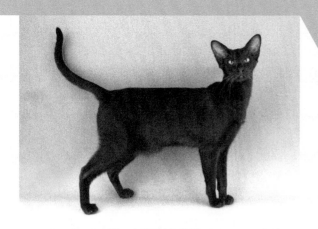

Havana Brown

Physical Characteristics

Weight: Females 6-8 lb (2.5-3.5 kg), males 8-10 lb (3.5-4.5 kg)

Coat: A rich shiny chocolate brown-mahogany color with no markings; brown pigmentation also include the whiskers, nose leather and pads. The coat is a medium short close lying coat. They may have ghost tabby markings as kittens; with reddish highlights. Note that TICA recognizes lilac colored cats also, but CFA does not.

Eyes: Oval eyes are medium in size, and are any shade of green with a darker richer color preferred.

Points of Conformation: The head is long and there is a distinct stop and distinct pinch behind the whisker pad, with a so-called "corn-cob" or "hour glass" muzzle—this is a breed distinguishing feature. Ears are large with rounded tips, tipping forward, and also lightly haired and furnished. They possess a lithe medium length body, medium size and length of neck, long legs, and a medium thickness, tapering long tail. A foreign type, the Havana Brown is not as tubular as Siamese or Oriental breed cats. Paws are small, compact and oval shaped.

Grooming: Little grooming needed. Quick weekly brush with rubber brush, chamois or soft cloth is fine.

Recognized Behavior Issues and Traits

Reported breed characteristics include: Very intelligent, affectionate, need close human contact, playful, these high activity cats love to jump up high, and are quiet voiced and very adaptable. Possessing a dog-like personality, Havana Browns may be trained to fetch and be leash trained. The Havana may bond closely with a favorite person. They prefer a tranquil home, and sometimes can be a bit standoffish towards people they do not know.

Normal Breed Variations

Caloric intake may need to be limited to prevent obesity.

Very low genetic diversity was found in a study carried out at the University of California, Davis. Cats from 13 different catteries and different breeds were assessed at multiple microsatellite DNA markers. Final assessment was that this breed had one third of the genetic diversity of random bred cats in this sample of 56 cats.[1, 2, 3] Havana and Korat were assigned moderate genetic diversity (0,53) in this study.

Kitten Internet Information Project:[4]
  21 litters
  83 kittens
  3.9 kittens/litter
  11% stillborn
  24% C-sections
  Average female birth weight 86 g, average male birth weight 95 g.

The Breed History

In Britain around the year 1951, a cross between a seal point Siamese and a black part-Siamese shorthair cat produced a solid brown offspring named *Elmtower Bronze Idol*, the first cat in the GCCF registry for the breed. Brown colored cats had already arrived from Europe much earlier (reported to be in the 1890s in a London cat show; perhaps the oldest being *Granny Grumps*). These chocolate solid foreign-type cats were called **Chestnut Brown Foreign** for a while. At some point, Russian Blues were reported to be introduced into the breed during outcrossing.

The name **Havana** may originate from the rabbit breed that has the same coloring, or perhaps they are so-named because they are brown like Havana cigars. The word *brown* was added to the **Havana** name when the breed was imported to the USA in 1956. American Havana Browns generally derive from one champion sire, *Quinn's Brown Satin of Sidlo*.

Roofspringer Mahogany Quinn was the foundation female in America, and Sildo's mother.

These cats were recognized first as the Chestnut Foreign Shorthair by GCCF in 1958 and the name was changed to Havana in 1970. In some registries, Havana is the preferred breed name since lilac color is now also accepted.

In the CFA the Havana Brown (as it is now called in America) was accepted for championship status in 1964. There is only very limited outcrossing (pre-approval required) allowed in CFA and none allowed in TICA. For a while (1974) CFA cut off outcrossing, but breeders petitioned the organization to help them diversify the gene pool in the late 1990s.

The British version, the Havana or Chestnut Brown Foreign cat is more like a Chestnut Oriental Shorthair cat of CFA in breed standard for conformation; the American cat is more moderate in build.

This is a very rare breed; in 1998, 1000 cats in total were registered, with 130 in the breeding pool at only 12 active CFA catteries, and in 1997 only 36 cats were registered in the CFA.

As a note aside, Havana and Serval (African Wildcat) hybridization has lead to a newer breed, Savannah.

Drug Sensitivities
Nothing reported in the literature

Inherited Diseases
Hemophilia: Has been reported in this breed with low prevalence; an X-linked recessive trait so males express the trait; only rarely seen in females when homozygous for this recessive gene.[4]

Disease Predispositions
Calcium Oxalate Urolithiasis: According to a case-control study[5] it was reported that Havana Brown cats are at increased risk of forming calcium oxalate uroliths.[6]

Rare and Isolated Reports
Floppy Pinnae: Two clinically normal cats were presented for sudden flop over of the ears in late maturity, bilateral; the distal one third of the pinna was bent over, ear tips cool and devoid of cartilage. There was a possibility that this condition may have been secondary to prolonged use of glucocorticoid therapy for pruritic ears resulting in iatrogenic hyperadrenocorticism.[7] The etiology was not conclusive. Compare with *floppy pinnae in Siamese* chapter.

Genetic Tests
If suspect hemophilia, run coagulation profile and specific factor assays (Hemophilia A: Factor VIII, Hemophilia B: Factor IX).

Miscellaneous
- **Breed name synonyms:** Havana, Chestnut Brown Foreign Cat, Swiss Mountain Cat (historical)
- **Registries:** TICA (as Havana--both lilac and brown colors accepted), CFA, ACFA, GCCF (in Oriental, as Havana)
- **Breed resources: Havana Brown Breed Council (CFA):** www.havanabrownbc.org
- **Havana Brown Fanciers (CFA NW USA):** http://www.havanabrownfanciers.net/
- **Havana and Oriental Lilac Cat Club (GCCF):** http://www.havanaandorientallilaccc.co.uk

References

1. Lipinski MJ, Young AE, Lyons LA. Genetic diversity and population dynamics of domestic cat breeds. *Proceedings.* Tuft's Canine and Feline Breeding and Genetics Conference Oct 2-4, 2003 Available at VIN: www.vin.com/tufts/2003. Accessed Nov 19, 2004.

2. Lyons LA. The Lyon's Den Website. Breed Diversity and Cat Domestication Project. Available at: http://faculty.vetmed.ucdavis.edu/faculty/lalyons/ Sites.... Accessed November 23, 2004.

3. Menotti-Raymond M, David VA, Pflueger SM, Lindblad-Toh K, Wade CM, O'Brien SJ, Johnson WE. Patterns of molecular genetic variation among cat breeds. Genomics. 2008 Jan;91(1):1-11.

4. Little, S. Pers. Comm. 2009.

5. Brooks MB. Feline hereditary coagulopathies. First International Feline Genetic Disease Conference Philadelphia June, 1998 *Proceedings (abstr)* in: *Feline Practice Supplement,* 1999;6,17,20.

6. Lekcharoensuk C, Lulich JP, Osborne CA, Koehler LA, Urlich LK, Carpenter KA, Swanson LL. Association between patient-related factors and risk of calcium oxalate and magnesium ammonium phosphate urolithiasis in cats. *J Am Vet Med Assoc* 2000;Aug15;217(4):520-525.

7. Scott DW. Feline dermatology 1986 to 1988: Looking through to the 1990s through the eyes of many counselors. *JAAHA* 1990;26:515-532.

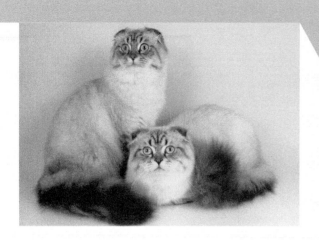

The Breed History

The Highland Fold, like the Scottish Fold traces back to a single white shorthaired ancestor from Scotland who in 1961 had a litter containing two folded kittens. *See Scottish Fold chapter for details.*

Longhaired Scottish Fold cats, apparently resulting from Persian outcrossing, are considered a separate breed called the Highland Fold in some registries, and in other registries are within a separate division in the Scottish Fold breed, the Scottish Fold Longhair. The GCCF first accepted the shorthaired breed, followed by most other major registries in the 1970s, and the longhaired variety followed in the 1980s. Outcrossing to American and British Shorthair cats is still allowed.

Because this breed is a division of the Scottish Fold breed in some registries, separate data are not always available in the literature. Many studies will consider a Highland Fold cat a Scottish Fold cat for study purposes because of the shared registry.

Physical Characteristics

Weight: female 6-9 lb (2.5-4 kg), male 9-13 lb (4-6 kg)

Coat: The Highland Fold is a medium-long haired cat, soft coated in texture, with ruff and britches, and "fluffy" on the tail. Note the Longhair is not accepted in all registries. All colors are accepted excluding pointed or Oriental colors (lilac, chocolate etc); except the CFF registry which allows pointed cats.

Eyes: Usually gold colored.

Points of Conformation: This is a medium sized cat with a rounded outline. The head is large, and the nose is broad and curved. The muzzle is short, with well-developed cheeks. A minimal stop is present only. The ears are small-medium with rounded tips; the fold results in ear tips sitting down and forward. Single fold ears loosely approximate the normal ear type, progressively more tightly folded ears are called double fold and triple fold; the latter being the show type.

The forward curved ear sitting cap-like over the temples results from an autosomal dominant mutation (Fd) with incomplete penetrance. Every litter will have some straight eared kittens. Folding of the ears occurs between 14 and 28 days and usually ears are set by 3-4 months of age. Not all ears stay folded; some pop back up to a straight position. The tail is medium long, tapering with a rounded tip. Legs are medium-short, and paws are round. A tail that is short, of reduced flexibility or kinked disqualifies.

Grooming: Weekly brushing is all that is required. During shedding season more frequent brushing may be needed. Pay attention to ear health because the canals are closely covered by the ears.

Recognized Behavior Issues and Traits

Reported breed characteristics include: These are moderately active cats. They possess gentle dispositions, and have low vocalizing tendency, with small chirping voice. They enjoy close human contact and may shadow their owners, and be a lap cat. A quirk in their posture is that they may sit up in a Buddha position. Adaptable, travel and do well in both quiet and noisy/busy households. Good with other pets.

Normal Breed Variations

Need to watch caloric input; tend to obesity.

Small litters are the norm.

B Blood Type: A prevalence of 19%, and in another report, four of 27 cats (~15%) tested had B blood type (reported for Scottish Fold cats).[1,2] Though Highlands have not been studied separately, Highland Fold cats will probably have similar rates because of their shared genetic pool.

Drug Sensitivities

None reported in the literature

Inherited Diseases

Osteochondrodysplasia Skeletal Deformities: This is a Fold breed-specific condition and should be understood before purchasing kittens or before professionally assessing this breed. *See Scottish Fold chapter for description and references.*

Neonatal Isoerythrolysis (NI): Apparent "fading" kittens from litters where the parents are not blood tested are seen in the Scottish Fold, and attributed to the presence of type B blood in one parent; by extrapolation one might expect this to be the case in the Highland Fold. All B type cats have circulating anti-A antibodies and even primiparous queens can carry these. Type B queens bred to type A toms can result in fatal red cell lysis in A blood type offspring with undetected NI. Kittens with NI can be distinguished from other fading kittens because of pigmenturia; anemia and icterus will also be present; not all kittens at risk for NI will develop overt clinical symptoms.[2]

Disease Predispositions

Transfusion Reactions: Increased probability of reactions due to prevalence of B blood type, extrapolated from Scottish Fold data.

Ear mite propensity: More difficult to treat effectively due to the folded ear structure. Anecdotal evidence.

Hereditary Deafness: Is associated with the dominant gene for white cat (W); may be found in white cats of this breed; extrapolated from Scottish Fold data.[3]

Calcium Oxalate Urolithiasis: A Scottish Fold breed propensity for this condition was reported.[4]

Rare and Isolated Reports

Polycystic Kidney Disease: *See Scottish Fold chapter for description and references.*

Genetic Tests

Blood typing before breeding or transfusions is advisable due to prevalence of B blood type in the breed.

Miscellaneous

- **Breed name synonyms:** Fold, Longhaired Scottish Fold, Lop-eared cat or Lop (historical), nickname: Foldie.
- **Registries:** TICA (Scottish Fold Longhair and Scottish fold separated), CFA, ACFA (Scottish Fold is a separate breed from Highland Fold), CFF, ACF (Scottish fold Longhair, Scottish Fold), CCA (Longhair and Shorthair are divisions within the Scottish Fold) —not accepted in GCCF
- **Breed resources: The Longhair Clan—Longhair Scottish Fold Breed Club (CFF):** Jean Viel III 49 Hancock St., Salem, MA 01970
- **Scottish Fold Fanciers:** http://www.ziplink.net/users/days/SFF.html

References

1. Giger U. In: Bonagura J, ed. *Kirk's Current Veterinary Therapy XIII.* Philadelphia: WB Saunders Co, 2000;396-399.
2. Giger, U, Bucheler J, Patterson DF. Frequency and inheritance of A and B blood types in feline breeds of the United States. *J Hered* 1991;82(1):15-20.
3. Strain GM. Hereditary deafness in dogs and cats: causes, prevalence, and current research. *Proceedings.* Tuft's Canine and Feline Breeding and Genetics Conference. Oct 2-4, 2003. Available at: http://www.vin.com/tufts/2003. Accessed Nov 19, 2004.
4. Lekcharoensuk C, Lulich JP, Osborne CA, et al. Association between patient-related factors and risk of calcium oxalate and magnesium ammonium phosphate urolithiasis in cats. *J Am Vet Med Assoc* 2000;Aug15;217(4):520-525.

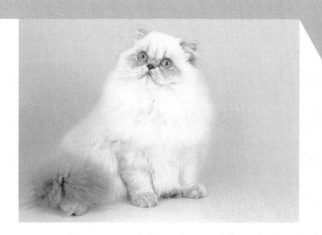

The Breed History

In the 1920s in Europe and in the 1930s in Britain, Siamese and Persian cats were crossed to obtain coloring of the points (called Himalayan pointing). As Colorpoint Longhair, first registry was in the GCCF in 1957. This cat was then further developed in the US and Canada and by the late 1950s they were accepted by the ACFA, and as part of the Persian standard by CFA in 1984. Note that the CFA and many other registries consider these cats part of the Persian breed, to be shown in different color classes called the Himalayan Division. The name Himalayan is derived from their similarity to rabbits by that name, with a similar pointed pattern.

These cats resulted from crosses of two Persian/Siamese crossbreds to give the desired Himalayan (colorpoint) type in the offspring. Overall, genetically this breed has more Persian than Siamese; outcross to Persians is allowed.

Physical Characteristics

Weight: 8-15 lb (3.5-7 kg)

Coat: This coat is the same as a Persian coat, just with Siamese *ts*-colored points. All colors of pointing are accepted. Note that the transition between point and body color is less distinct in the Himalayan because of the longer hairs, so the transition zone is softened. Also, the points take longer to evolve than in a shorthair and dilute points take a very long time to mature in appearance.

The ruff is very full and extends between legs; coat standard is as for Persian in length, texture, density. Possess a thick and silky haircoat, very plush without being wooly.

Eyes: Blue, though a softer blue than Siamese sapphire. More intense color is preferred. In CFA, any other color is a disqualification. Eyes large, round and wide set.

Points of Conformation: Structurally, they are very close in type to Persian. With a round large head, the nose is very short and upturned so as to view the leather straight on, stop up between the eyes, and solid body conformation. The small ears are round tipped. Tail is short and bushy, and legs short. Paws are round, large, with tufts of long fur between the toes.

Grooming: Has high grooming needs. The Himalayan needs a daily brush, or even twice daily especially during shedding season.

Tears need to be cleansed from the medial canthus regularly to prevent dermatitis and tear staining.

Recognized Behavior Issues and Traits

Reported breed characteristics include: Calm, outgoing and friendly cat, quiet voiced like Persian. Adaptable, and gets along well with children and other pets.

Normal Breed Variations

B Blood Type: Reported frequency of type B cats in one study was 20%.[1] A prevalence of 6% type B was reported elsewhere.[2]

Brachycephalic syndrome: Narrow nares, elongated soft palate, possible narrow trachea, tear duct overflow.

Drug Sensitivities

None reported in the literature

Inherited Diseases

Himalayan/Siamese Pointing Gene: *see the Siamese cat chapter for a summary of the effects of this gene on coat and vision (imperfect albinism trait; temperature sensitive tyrosinase enzyme mutation).*

Polycystic Renal Disease (PKD): PKD is most common in Persian breeds, and those breeds having out-crossed to Persians in their breeding programs.[3] *See the Persian cat chapter for details and references regarding this condition.*

Hereditary Cataracts: Bilateral lesions have been reported as early as 12 weeks of age in Himalayan kittens.[4] Two types occur: congenital or juvenile cataracts.[5]

Cataracts were of apparent autosomal recessive inheritance with variable expression in a line of Himalayan cats. By 12 weeks of age, complete lenticular opacity had developed. A littermate had bilateral posterior subcapsular triangular cataracts, and the tom had similar lesions.[6]

Disease Predispositions

Corneal Sequestration (Synonyms: black body, cornea nigrum): In early phases, an amber colored corneal stromal opacity is noted. Surrounding cornea is cloudy with neovascularization; chemosis, blepharospasm, mucopurulent ocular discharge, and hyperemic conjunctivae may be noted. The surface of the sequestrum does not stain with fluorescein dye but does retain rose bengal stain. The exophthalmic conformation is thought to play a role in susceptibility.[7] Often unilateral, Persian type cats are over-represented. Usually in central or para-central cornea; brown to black pigmented lesion; often surrounded by a loose collarette of poorly adherent corneal epithelium. The lesion may extend into the shallow or deep stroma, or even to Descemet's membrane. Sloughing and corneal healing may take 2-6 months; surgical debridement is another option.[1]

It is a corneal stromal necrosis and topical glucocorticoids are contraindicated; some cases may be linked to feline herpesvirus infection; if suspected, do PCR on excised black body tissue. Recurrences or involvement of the second eye in previously unilateral cases may occur.[8]

Feline Bronchial Asthma: (Synonyms: allergic bronchitis, chronic bronchitis, feline lower airway disease). Himalayan cats are overrepresented in studies of asthmatic cats. Cough does not always occur. Radiographs may be normal (normal in 23% of affected cats in multi-breed study). Earlier studies indicate Siamese and Himalayan cats are at higher risk, perhaps due to genetic susceptibility.[9]

Non-healing Corneal Ulcers: In a retrospective study this breed was found to be overrepresented in cases of refractory ulcers. These indolent ulcers involved only the superficial epithelium and unless complicated, did not extend into stroma. During extended treatment regimens averaging 5 weeks, these same cats were also predisposed to corneal sequestration.[10]

Urolithiasis: Retrospective case control study of 3,498 urolithiasis cases (1982-1992) indicated that Himalayan cats were at higher risk for calcium oxalate uroliths and at reduced risk for magnesium ammonium phosphate (MAP, struvite) crystals.[11] In another retrospective analysis of 22,908 lower urinary tract disease cases (1980-1997), Himalayan cats were reported to be at increased risk of urocystolithiasis.[12] In yet another study, Himalayan cats were found to be 5.8 times more likely to develop calcium oxalate stones, and 1.8 times as likely to develop MAP.[13]

Hip Dysplasia (HD): A University of Missouri-Columbia Veterinary Medical Teaching Hospital study (1991-1995) found that based on VD hip radiographs, (684 cats, 12 breeds); prevalence was 5.8% in unregistered versus 12.3% in purebred cats. Classic radiographic signs were found to be different than in dogs, with minimal remodeling of femoral neck and shallow acetabulum and remodeling of cranio-dorsal acetabular rim being the most common finding. Himalayan cats were reported to have a rate of 25% (4/16) HD.[14]

Rare and Isolated Reports

Primary Hereditary Seborrhea Oleosa: First signs at only 2-3 days old. It is severe, progressive, with no coat color predilection. Orthokeratotic hyperkeratosis is seen on biopsy. It is a primary keratinization defect without good treatment options.[15]

Congenital Portosystemic Vascular Shunts: In one report, Persian and Himalayan together accounted for 16% of cases out of 98 cats. Signs were noted by 6 months of age, and single extrahepatic portocaval anomaly was the most common type of defect.[16]

Hyperchylomicronemia: An autosomal recessive condition; in one report; it occurred in two siblings. Onset at 3 weeks of age, reported changes included poor growth, lipemia retinalis, hyperlipidemia (hypertriglyceridemia), anemia, peripheral neuropathy, xanthomata.[17]

Neonatal Isoerythrolysis (NI): Death usually at 12-24 hours of age; it was noted that queens were all primiparous, with retro-placental hemorrhage in late pregnancy being the proposed immune stimulator.[18] One report gives the proportion of matings at

risk for NI at 0.06 in this breed.[19]

Multiple Eyelid Cysts: In a very small study group of Persian and Himalayan cats, histology indicated a similar lesion to apocrine hidrocystomas; multilocular cysts. The PAS+, diastase resistant granules were seen in the cytoplasm of affected cells. Blepharospasm, epiphora and masses or color changes of eyelids were chief complaints.[20]

Von-Willebrand's Disease: A case of a 9 year old cat experiencing severe hemorrhage after dental extraction was reported; and had concurrent bladder hemorrhage and axilla hematoma. Iron deficiency anemia persisted during recovery; aPTT was abnormal, indicating decreased F VIII:C activity.[21]

Dermatosparaxis (Synonym: Cutaneous asthenia, dermal fragility syndrome): A case report of this genetic disease (mutated amino terminal of procollagen peptidase enzyme) described onset of signs beginning at 6 months old. Fragile and hyper-extensible thin skin with an abnormal feeling texture was palpated.[22] There was a marked tendency for abnormal skin to tear easily with minimal bleeding when wounded, healing quickly with major scar formation. Skin was only 1/3rd of the normal thickness, and attachment to underlying tissues minimal. By 9 months of age, this kitten would experience gaping holes in the skin due to routine self grooming behavior. In sheep, calves and man it is an autosomal recessive inheritance pattern. In man, termed Ehlers-Danlos Syndrome Type VII.[23]

In one report of this condition in a domestic shorthair cat, authors describe a way to ascribe numerical value to define the severity in an individual which could be used to document severity in this breed too:
- Extensibility index=height of skin fold over lumbar area (cm) divided by # of cm from occiput to tail base, then multiply by 100. Affected cats are expected to have index greater than 19%.[24]

Fibrodysplasia Ossificans: Case report of multifocal, non-symmetrical lesions started at the elbow joint as an apparent soft tissue swelling, not related to trauma, and progressing to ossification in 7 days. Heterotopic trilaminar or zonal pattern of ossification around the humerus, tibia and fibula was subsequently noted.[25]

Primary Hypoparathyroidism: A 6 month-old kitten with lethargy, tremors, loss of appetite, and seizures was reported. Stunted growth, thin body condition, and bilateral punctuate to linear cataracts were seen. Clinical signs began at 8 weeks of age.[26]

FIP Susceptibility: An American study found that Himalayan cats were significantly over-represented for a diagnosis of FIP when they analyzed data for a 16 year period at a veterinary teaching hospital.[27]

Genetic Tests

Polycystic kidney disease. Genetic test available from UC-Davis VGL.

Blood type prior to breeding or transfusion.

Radiographs hips to screen for hip dysplasia.

Miscellaneous

- **Breed name synonyms:** Colorpoint Longhair (Britain), Pointed Persian, Himmy, Persian Colorpoint, Persian-Himalayan, Khmer (historical)
- **Registries:** FIFé (within Persian), TICA (separate breed), AACE (separate breed) CFA (division within Persian), ACFA (separate breed), CFF, (division of Persian), GCCF (Colorpoint Longhair, subset of Persian), ACF (in Persian), WCF (provisional Persian/Himalayan), NZCF (within Persian), CCA (separate breed from Persian)
- **Breed resources: Atlantic Himalayan Club:** www.himalayan.org/links.htm
  Colorpoint Cat Club (GCCF): http://www.thecolourpointcatclub.co.uk/
  Colorpoint Society of Great Britain (GCCF): http://www.colourpointsocietygreatbritain.co.uk/
  Persian Cat CFA Breed Council: www.persianbc.org

References

1. Giger U, Bucheler J, Patterson DF. Frequency and inheritance of A and B blood types in feline breeds of the United States. *J Hered* 1991;82:15-20.
2. Giger U. In: Bonagura J, ed. *Kirk's Current Veterinary Therapy XIII.* Philadelphia: WB Saunders Co, 2000;396-399.
3. Lyons LA. The Lyon's Den. Feline Genome Project: Polycystic Kidney Disease. Available at: http://faculty.vetmed.ucdavis.edu/faculty/lalyons/Sites/pkd.htm Accessed Nov 6, 2004.
4. Narfström K. Hereditary and congenital ocular disease. *J Fel Med Surg* 1999;1:135-141.
5. Hoskins JD. Congenital defects in cats. *Compend Contin Educ Pract Vet* 1995;17(3):385-405.
6. Rubin LF. Hereditary cataract in Himalayan cats. *Fel Pract* 1986;16(1):14-15.
7. Pentlarge VW. Corneal sequestration in cats. *Compend Contin Educ Pract Vet* 1989;11(1):24-32.
8. Glaze MB. Feline corneal diseases: Part II. *Proceedings.* The 70th Annual AAHA Conference. 2003;1:367-368.
9. Adamama-Moraitou KK, Patsikas MN, Koutinas AF. Feline lower airway disease: a retrospective study of 22 naturally occurring cases from Greece. *J Fel Med Surg* 2004;6:227-233.
10. La Croix NC, van der Woerdt A, Olivero DK. Nonhealing corneal ulcers in cats: 29 cases (1991-1999). *J Am Vet Med Assoc* 2001;18(5):733-735.
11. Thumchai R, Lulich J, Osborne CA, et al. Epizootiologic evaluation of urolithiasis in cats: 3,498 cases (1982-1992). *J Am Vet Med Assoc* 1996;208(4):547-551.
12. Lekcharoensuk C, Osborne CA, Lulich JP. Epidemiologic study of risk factors for lower urinary tract diseases in cats. *J Am Vet Med Assoc* 2001;218(9):1429-1435.
13. Lekcharoensuk C, Lulich JP, Osborne CA, Koehler LA, Urlich LK, Carpenter KA, Swanson LL. Association between patient-related factors and risk of calcium oxalate and magnesium ammonium phosphate urolithiasis in cats. *J Am Vet Med Assoc* 2000;Aug15;217(4):520-525.
14. Keller GG, Reed AL, Lattimer JC, et al. Hip dysplasia: A feline population study. *Veterinary Radiology & Ultrasound* 1999;40(4):460-464.
15. DeManuelle T. Feline dermatopathies: Newly described disorders. Proceedings. 70th Annual AAHA Conference *Proceedings* 1:93-95, 2003.
16. Levy JK. Congenital Portosystemic vascular shunts in cats: 98 cases. First International Feline Genetic Disease Conference Philadelphia June, 1998 *Proceedings (poster abstr)* in: *Feline Practice Supplement,* 1999:30.
17. Jones BR. Inherited hyperchylomicronaemia in the cat. *J of Small Anim Pract* 1993;34:493-499.
18. Jonsson NN, Pullen C, Watson ADJ. Neonatal isoerythrolysis in Himalayan kittens. *Austr Vet J* 1990;67(11):416.
19. Giger U, Casal M, Niggemeier A. The fading kitten syndrome and neonatal isoerythrolysis. *Proceedings.* The 15th Annual ACVIM Medical Forum, Lake Buena Vista FL 1997;308-310.
20. Chaitman J, van der Woerdt A, Bartick TE. Multiple eyelid cysts resembling apocrine hidrocystomas in three Persian cats and one Himalayan cat. *Vet Pathol* 1999;36:474-476
21. French TW, Fox LE, Randolph JF, et al. A bleeding disorder (von Willebrand's disease) in a Himalayan cat. *J Am Vet Med Assoc* 1987;190(4):437-439.
22. Counts DF, Byers PH, Holbrook KA, et al. Dermatosparaxis in a Himalayan cat: I. Biochemical studies of dermal collagen. *J Invest Dermatol* 1980;74:96-99.
23. Collier LL, Leathers CW, Counts DF. A clinical description of Dermatosparaxis in a Himalayan cat. *Fel Pract* 1980;10(5):25-36.
24. Plotnick A, Brunt JE, Reitz B. Cutaneous asthenia in a cat. *Fel Pract* 1992;20(4):9-12.
25. Bradley WA. Fibrodysplasia ossificans in a Himalayan cat. *Aust Vet Practit* 1992;22(4):154-158.
26. Bassett JR. Hypocalcemia and hyperphosphatemia due to primary hypoparathoidism in a six-month-old kitten. *JAAHA* 1998;34:503-507.
27. Pesteanu-Somogyi LD, Radzai C, Pressler BM. Prevalence of feline infectious peritonitis in specific cat breed. *J Feline Med Surg.* Vol 8(1):pp1-5. 2006.

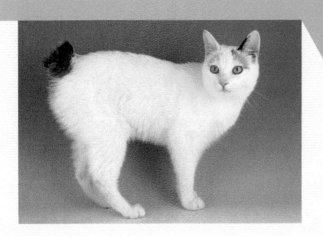

The Breed History

This is reported to be an ancient breed. The bobtail cat was widely distributed around Asia in ancient times. The Emperor of China may have sent the first cats to Japan. First records of this type of domesticated cat in Japan date to 1000 years ago. First representatives of the breed were imported to the USA in 1968. The CFA granted championship status in 1976 for the Shorthair, and in 1993 added the Longhair variety. The bobtail is present in all cats of this breed, instead of showing up as a range of tail lengths as in the Manx cat. The tail is distinctive for this breed, the terminus being less than three inches away from the body, and frequently is kinked or curved. Tail hairs form a "pom-pom" rabbit-like tail and each tail is unique. In Japan, the van "Mi-Ke" (pronounced Mee-Kay) is thought to bring good luck. Maneki-neko (beckoning cat) statues depict a Bobtail cat with one paw raised, and are often placed in the doorways of homes and businesses for good luck. No outcrosses are allowed in CFA.

Newest genetic studies surprisingly found that the breed is more closely aligned with the European and North American gene pool.[1]

Physical Characteristics

Weight: 6-9 lb (2.5-4 kg)

Coat: The traditional color is called Mi-ke (three-fur). That color is a tri-color red, black and white cat, but frequently the red areas have tabby markings and these are termed calico. A number of other colors and patterns are accepted but are much less common than Mi-ke; black and white coat is the second most prevalent. The single, short-medium length coat is silky in texture and flat-lying. The longhaired coat is really a semi-long hair, and this variety is also accepted by TICA and CFA, but by AFCA is judged as a separate breed. In the semi-longhair a ruff, britches and toe tufting is desirable. Both types of coat have minimal undercoat.

Eyes: The large eyes are oval and slanted, and their color is appropriate for the coat coloring. Blue and odd-eyes accepted.

Points of Conformation: These are small sized semi-foreign type cats, and there is no conformation difference between the Longhair and Shorthair varieties. They have a triangular head, a long straight nose and a small stop at eye level. Ears are large, tilting forward. Body is long and lithe with good muscling and long fairly fine boned legs. Feet are oval in shape and small sized.

Grooming: The Japanese Bobtail cat has low grooming requirements and low shedding tendency. This is a somewhat water resistant coat. Longhair cats require a bit more grooming, but have low matting tendency. Not recommended to blow dry this coat in Shorthairs.

Recognized Behavior Issues and Traits

Reported breed characteristics include: Quiet cats; meow is musical. Active, highly intelligent, friendly, enjoy close human contact and playing fetch. Very good with children and other pets/groups of cats, travel well, adaptable. Independent minded. Good mousers. Good to leash train. Likes shoulder rides. Some say that these cats are quite similar to Abyssinians in personality.

Normal Breed Variations

Bobtail is an **autosomal recessive** gene that all Bobtails carry *(compare with Manx dominant gene)*. Manx are not related to American Bobtail cats either in the mutation or by lineage. American Bobtail gene is also thought to be novel and not the same mutation as the Japanese Bobtail trait though further studies are needed.

The tail pom of fluffy hair should appear to arise next to body rather than a few inches along a straight tail base. A corkscrew tail is accepted. Tail may be rigid or flexible, but should be moveable at the base.

Litter size is reported to average four to five kittens, and birth weights are heavier than the average for other breeds of cats, with low kitten mortality, and precocious kitten development (walk early).

Considered very healthy and hardy

Blood Type B: A study of the prevalence of blood type B in a number of breeds found Japanese Bobtail cats had a prevalence of 5-25% B blood type.[2] A 16% prevalence of blood type B also reported elsewhere.[3]

Drug Sensitivities

None reported in the literature

Inherited Diseases

Neonatal Isoerythrolysis (NI): Moderate prevalence of B blood type is present in the breed so NI may be found in some litters. Blood typing before breeding is recommended.

Disease Predispositions

Transfusion Reactions: Prevalence of B blood type also leads to an increased risk of transfusion reactions. Blood typing for donor and recipient recommended.

Genetic Tests

Blood type determination: before breeding or transfusions

Miscellaneous

- **Breed name synonyms:** JBT, Bobtail, Mi-ke, Neko, Maneki Neko, Jibit
- **Registries:** FIFé (SH only), TICA (LH, SH variety separate in Japanese bobtail breed group), CFA (LH and SH variety in SH division), ACFA (LH and SH separate breeds), CCA, CFF, NZCF, WCF, ACF
- Breed resources: **Breeders of Bobtails Society (BOBS):**
  Lynne Berge,
  1069 Gridley Street, Bay Shore NY 28621
  Japanese Bobtail Breeders' Society: http://www.jbbs.org/
  Shorthair Japanese Bobtail Club (CFA):
  http://www.japanesebobtails.com/clubs.html

References

1. Lipinski MJ, Froenicke L, Baysac KC, Billings NC, Leutenegger CM, Levy AM, Longeri M, Niini T, Ozpinar H, Slater MR, Pedersen NC, Lyons LA
The ascent of cat breeds: genetic evaluations of breeds and worldwide random-bred populations.
Genomics. 2008 Jan;91(1):12-21
2. Giger U. Frequency and inheritance of A and B Blood types in feline breeds in the United States. *J Hered* 1991;82:15-20.
3. Giger U. In: Bonagura J, ed. *Kirk's Current Veterinary Therapy XIII.* Philadelphia: WB Saunders Co. 2000;396-399.

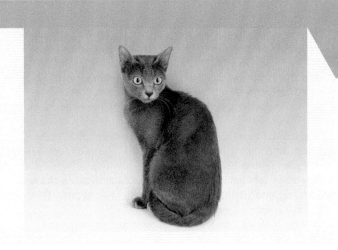

Korat

The Breed History
Considered a good luck symbol by the Thais, this breed to them symbolizes wealth and rain because of the soft silver color. First written records date to the Ayudhya Period of Siamese history which encompasses 1350-1767, where a cat of this description was identified as a good luck cat. First found in the Korat province in Northeastern Thailand (then Siam), Korat (Koh-**raht**) are more commonly referred to as Si-Sawat (see-sa-what) in Thailand, which means prosperity. First American imports occurred in 1959. The CFA accepted the Korat for championship status in 1966. TICA accepted them in 1969, FIFé in 1972. In Thailand, they were given in pairs as gifts, and especially valued as bride gifts; also cherished as gifts for visiting dignitaries. No outcrosses are allowed.

Physical Characteristics
Weight: 6-10 lb (2.5-4.5 kg)

Coat: The Korat possesses a single short coat; hairs are dark in the middle, and light blue-gray at the base, the ends are tipped with silver (coat color is termed silver-blue). The coat lies close, is silky and glossy, and the silver tipping produces a halo effect around the cat. Silver tipping is pronounced on feet and muzzle. In Thailand, the coat color is referred to a "rain cloud gray". Though the odd lilac or lilac point cat is born, they are not accepted as Korat for registration. In one study, Korat cats had a 21% carrier rate and 2% rate of pointed cats.[1]

Eyes: The Korat has very large eyes which gradually transition through yellow amber-amber-amber-green, then to peridot green by two to four years of age.

Points of Conformation: A small-medium sized cat, they are moderately compact (semi-cobby). The head is heart-shaped, and the profile has a slight stop and the nose curves down towards the terminus. Large ears have rounded tips, and have minimal furnishings. Oval feet are compact. The Korat has a medium length tapered tail with minor kink accepted (felt but not seen).

Grooming: Grooming needs are minimal, and a quick weekly brush will suffice.

Recognized Behavior Issues and Traits
Reported breed characteristics include: Gentle, affectionate. Considered sensitive to noise and handling, they should be exposed to various sounds and people/handling from a young age. Korats may resist being held up in the air or stretched/restrained. Playful, good with children, form a strong bond with their owners. High activity cats, territorial, may like to be a bit of a boss. May shadow people around the home, some like to play fetch and are quiet voiced around home, but vocal in strange environments such as a show ring.

Normal Breed Variations
Korat were assigned moderate genetic diversity (0.53) in one study.[2]

Drug Sensitivities
None reported in the literature

Inherited Diseases
G_{M2}-gangliosidosis: This condition is a lysosomal storage disease resulting from an autosomal recessive defect, a mutation (fHEXBKorat) in the gene for the β-hexosaminidase (HEXB) or α-hexosaminidase (HEXA) enzyme. In one study colony kittens showed disease by 4 weeks of age, and by 6 weeks, significant neuron and hepatocyte lysosomal storage vacuoles/inclusions were present.[3]

Progressive neurological deficits were noted at 4-7 weeks of age including fine head tremor, ataxia, and eventual loss of mobility. Reduced vision, myoclonus and dsyphagia were also described, with seizures and spastic quadriplegia late in the disease, leading to natural death by about 6-8 months of age. Livers grossly appeared pale and enlarged.[4]

G_{M1}-gangliosidosis: Periodic cases have been reported in the literature. In one report, a 7 month-old stunted kitten presented with slowly progressive neurologic signs (hind limb tremors, ataxia with hypermetria, spinal nerve hyper-reflexia, progressive paraparesis), mild dyspnea and regurgitation, and low β-galactosidase (GALB) enzyme activity. The activity of the enzyme, β-hexosaminidase was increased. Vacuoles in nervous tissue and liver were found to be filled with oligosaccharides and G_{M1}-gangliosides. The index cat was euthanized at 21 months old. Pedigree analysis was suggestive of an autosomal recessive trait.[5]

Studies show the same mutation is responsible for the G_{M1}-gangliosidosis condition in both Korat and Siamese cats; identification of the mutation has allowed carrier detection; international screening began in 1999.[6] Enzyme assays overlap between affected and normal cats so their diagnostic utility is limited compared with genetic testing.

The mutation for G_{M2}-gangliosidosis (fHEXBBaker), a distinct mutation, was recently elucidated and reported in the Domestic Shorthair cat.[7]

Therapy approaches for both of these conditions in the future could be similar but at this point, all are still experimental. Research includes modalities such as bone marrow cell transplantation and gene therapy.[8] Currently, there is NO effective therapy.

Because the clinical picture of the two distinct mutations in the Korat breed is similar, definitive diagnosis historically has been a challenge. Since the storage diseases have now been identified over a period of 4 decades, continued presence of clinical cases suggests this trait may have many carriers in this breed.[9]

Testing as of December 2004 of 500 Korat cats has provided a case frequency rate of carriers for both mutations of 20%, so it is important breeders do not cull carriers or the genetic diversity of the breed will be reduced significantly. It is recommended that breeders use programs where mating of known carriers exclusively occurs with cats that have tested negative. All offspring should be subsequently tested, and for the next generation, select only normal kittens for breeding stock, and neuter the carriers and direct them to pet quality adoptions. This will gradually eliminate the undesirable trait while maintaining the other excellent traits of quality cats. (Dr. H. J. Baker, pers. comm.)

Disease Predispositions
None reported in the literature

Genetic Tests

Korat Gangliosidosis Screening Program For G_{M1}– and G_{M2}–gangliosidosis:
Molecular screening program for both GM1 and GM2 disorders is available at the Scott-Ritchey Research Center at the College of Veterinary Medicine, Auburn University. Contact the laboratory for a kit containing sample tubes, instructions and the USDA letter. Results are confidential. Requires 1 ml of whole blood - EDTA, overnight delivery. The sample need not be refrigerated. There is no charge for the breeders to check their cats, and a certificate may be provided for those working within cat registries that require testing for registration (in Germany for example). If samples are sent from outside the USA, a USDA exemption letter must be filled out.

College of Veterinary Medicine, Auburn University AL 36849 Phone: (334) 844-5951 Fax: (334) 844-5850

Cheek swab testing is also available from the UC-Davis VGL.

Urine screening is done at University of Pennyslvania see: http://research.vet.upenn.edu/Default.aspx?alias=research.vet.upenn.edu/penngen

Miscellaneous
- **Breed name synonyms:** Blue Cat, Temple Cat, Thai Cat, Si-Sawat Cat.
- **Registries:** FIFé, TICA, CFA, ACFA, CCA, WCF, ACF, GCCF.
- **Breed resources: Korat Cat Fanciers Association:** http://www.koratworld.com/
  FiFe Korat breed council: http://www.fifekoratbc.com
  Si-Sawat (Korat) Society: http://www.si-sawat.org/

References

1. Grahn R, Grahn J. A practical application of the pointing test. *Notes*. University of California (Davis) Feline Genetics Extravaganza II Aug 28-29, 2004.
2. Menotti-Raymond M, David VA, Pflueger SM, Lindblad-Toh K, Wade CM, O'Brien SJ, Johnson WE
Patterns of molecular genetic variation among cat breeds. Genomics. 2008 Jan;91(1):1-11.
3. Muldoon LL, Neuwelt EA, Pagel MA, et al. Characterization of the molecular defect in a feline model for Type II G_{M2}-gangliosidosis (Sandhoff Disease). *Am J Pathol* 1994;144(5):1109-1118.
4. Neuwelt EA, Johnson WG, Blank NK, et al. Characterization of a new model of G_{M2}-gangliosidosis (Sandhoff Disease) in Korat cats. *J Clin Invest* 1985;76:482-490.
5. De Maria R, Divari S, Bo S, et al. β-galactosidase deficiency in a Korat cat: a new form of feline G_{M1}-gangliosidosis. *Acta Neuropathol* 1998;96(3):307-14.
6. Baker HJ. The molecular basis of feline G_{M1} and G_{M2} gangliosidoses. First International Feline Genetic Disease Conference Philadelphia June 1998 *Proceedings (abstr)* in: *Feline Practice Supplement*, 1999;11.
7. Martin DR, Krum BK, Varadarajan GS, et al. An inversion of 25 base pairs causes feline G_{M2} gangliosidosis variant 0. *Exp Neurol* 2004;187:30-37.
8. Haskins ME. Lysosomal storage diseases in cats: An overview. First International Feline Genetic Disease Conference Philadelphia June 1998 *Proceedings (abstr)* in: *Feline Practice Supplement*, 1999;22.
9. Baker HJ, Smith BF, Martin DR, et al. Molecular screening for the feline gangliosidoses in Korats. First International Feline Genetic Disease Conference Philadelphia June 1998 *Proceedings (abstr)* in: *Feline Practice Supplement*, 1999;22.

LaPerm

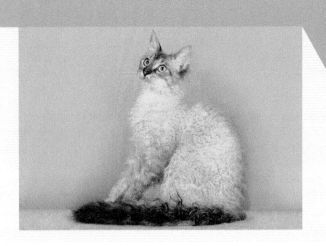

The Breed History

The La Perm coat is due to a curly haired mutation originating in Oregon in 1982. The name was reported given because the breeder thought the curly hair resembled a perm in human hair. The original female kitten was born bald and gradually developed a curly coat by 4 months of age. Subsequent kittens were born bald or with a slightly curly coat, though starting at two weeks of age and for another few months molting occurred in some kittens so that partial alopecia resulted. This rex mutation is an autosomal dominant mode of inheritance. TICA accepted the cat in 2003. The CFA registry accepted it in championship class in 2008. CFA allows outcrossing to Domestic Shorthair and Domestic Longhair cats—outcrossing ended January 2010.

Physical Characteristics

Weight: males 7-10 lb (3-4.5 kg), females 5-7 lb (2-3 kg); males tend to be larger

Coat: This coat mutation is unique since it provides good insulation. Both longhaired and shorthaired varieties exist. Even the furnishings at the ear base are somewhat curled. Curls are strongest under the neck and on the ventral body wall. Curlier coats are preferred, and in longer coats, ringlets or waves can be present. Short coats are usually wavy; generally not as curled as much as in the longer-coated cats. The tail is covered by a tapered plume in the longhairs and is more a bottle-brush, though still wavy in shorthairs. The longhair coat is actually more of a medium length. Both sexes may have a ruff. Unique coat texture is described as light and airy, and soft.

Kittens are born with variable coat cover and at about 14 days old, may start to go variably alopecic. All coats are shorter over the shoulders, and some cats never re-grow a full density coat, though most recover the full coat by four to five months of age. As the cat matures, the curls get tighter in longhairs. All colors are accepted, including colorpoint.

Coat is double, with the undercoat being dense, and the outer hairs curly and soft in texture. When stroked, it feels springy; hair texture is variable between cats. Eyebrow and whisker pad hairs are curly. Seasons may affect coat density and length.

Eyes: Eyes are large, and not necessarily coat related in color.

Points of Conformation: The La Perm is a semi-foreign cat in type, though they are still presumed to be of Domestic Shorthair cat in origin. Neck is fine, body is medium; they possess a medium-sized rounded modified wedge head that is carried quite erect. The ears are medium sized with well-developed furnishings, ideally including lynx tipping in longhairs. The tail is tapering, and is long. They have compact rounded feet.

Grooming: The La Perm has minimal grooming needs and low shedding tendency, though regular bathing and brushing is suggested. Towel drying should be carried out rather than blow drying.

Recognized Behavior Issues and Traits

Reported breed characteristics include: Very active, playful, and curious. Need close human contact, bond strongly, generally quiet voiced. Excellent hunters, and many will train to leash. Some may be lap cats and seem to adjust well to any family's activity level.

Normal Breed Variations

None reported in the literature

Drug Sensitivities

None reported in the literature

Inherited Diseases

None reported in the literature

Disease Predispositions

None reported in the literature

Genetic Tests

None commercially available

Miscellaneous

- **Breed name synonyms:** Dalles La Perm, Curly-coated cat, Poodle Cat. Common nickname: Alpaca cat
- **Registries:** CFA (Miscellaneous Category), TICA (1995 as Dalles La Perm, now two divisions-LaPerm, and LaPerm Shorthair), GCCF, NZCF
- **Breed resources:** The Rex Cat Club (GCCF-U.K.): http://www.rexcatclub.com/
  The La Perm Society of America: http://www.lapermcats.com/

References

1. Jordan, E. Breed Profile: LaPerm Pp 22-25. Cat Fancy September 2008

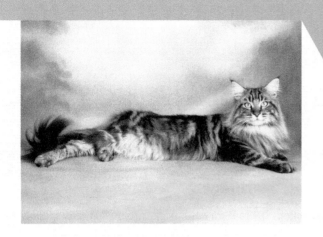

Maine Coon

The Breed History

A hardy hunter, this is the only North American longhair cat. Originating in Maine, this breed is now designated as the State Cat of Maine. Perhaps resulting from crosses between domestic cats and Angora and other longhaired imported cats, their large size and a luxurious haircoat are breed hallmarks. It is possible that Pilgrims brought longhaired cats with them that were the progenitor cats, and natural selection resulting from harsh winters favored a long dense coat. Some also credit the origins of the coat type to outcrossing with imported longhaired Siberian Forest Cats or Norwegian Forest Cats. A valued working farm cat, the Maine Coon was used extensively for rodent control. They are one of the first American breeds (first records date to the 1860s), and also one of the largest domestic cats anywhere. Very popular, they usually rank near the top in CFA. Championship status in CFA was awarded in1976. No outcrossing is allowed.

Physical Characteristics

Weight: Range 10-22 lb (4.5-10 kg) Females smaller and more refined than the males.

Coat: Glossy haircoat is longer over the body than on the head and shoulders and longer on stomach and the legs. Ruff is present, especially in males. The Maine Coon is double-coated and fur is thick, shaggy, but soft in texture and waterproof. Most colors and patterns are accepted though brown tabby is the best known. Chocolate, lavender, cinnamon, pointed and agouti are not accepted.

Eyes: Eyes are large, and all colors are accepted. Blue and odd eyes are found in the white cats.

Points of Conformation: Powerful musculature characterizes these large cats that are also endowed with a large wedge shaped head. The tapering tail is very long and this thick hairy tail, with rings in tabbies may have given rise to the Coon part of the breed name. The Maine Coon possesses a profile with the medium-length nose that is slightly concave. Well haired ears are large, with pointed tips and lynx tufts. Paws are round and well haired. Tail is long and tapering from a broad base.

Grooming: Though the Maine Coon coat does not tend to mat, regular grooming is needed. Preferably a quick daily session, but many find once weekly brushing will suffice.

Recognized Behavior Issues and Traits

Reported breed characteristics include: Sometimes called the "Gentle Giant" Maine Coon cats are adaptable, and require regular exercise and branches or ledges for climbing and jumping. Playful, and keeping kitten attitude until late in life, these cats like to play fetch. Most will leash train. Agile, powerful, calm, intelligent, good with children and dogs, these cats vocalize with a chirping trill, and the meow is very soft. Some enjoy swimming, and Maine Coon cats enjoy human companionship, and make very good companions. Not considered a lap cat.

Normal Breed Variations

They are slow to mature (~3-4 years), and puberty finishes late.

They have excellent tolerance to harsh cold climates.

They normally have have small litters with just two to three kittens but are noted for good mothering.

They tend to gain weight easily.

Blood type B: Prevalence of 3% type B cats was reported.[1]

The long hair phenotype in cats is a recessive characteristic so how it is distributed in the different longhaired breeds, and coded for is of interest. Mutation (AM412646:c.194C>A) is responsible for long hair in Persian and Maine Coon. Mutation 3 AM412646:c.474delT) is only present in Maine Coon cats.[2]

Drug Sensitivities

None reported in the literature

Inherited Diseases

Hypertrophic Cardiomyopathy (HCM): The most common cardiac condition in cats (10% prevalence); in Maine Coon the inheritance is consistent with an autosomal dominant gene with high penetrance. In cats, this heart condition is often associated with arterial systemic thromboembolism and congestive heart failure; specific changes occurring in this breed include papillary muscle hypertrophy, left atrial dilatation, left ventricular wall thickening and mitral valve systolic anterior motion. In cats, pulmonary edema is not necessarily perihilar as in dogs.

Offspring from crossing affected to unaffected cats developed clinical signs between 1-2 years of age, with severe disease by 2-4 years old. If both parents were affected, offspring became symptomatic at about 3 months of age, and severe disease was established by 6-18 months of age. Sudden death and heart failure are terminal sequelae. A sarcomere gene mutation leading to coronary arteriosclerosis and interstitial fibrosis with sarcomere myofibrillar disarray was postulated to be the pathophysiologic mechanism of failure. This condition closely mimics light chain mutations in man.[3]

In man, a number of myosin mutations have been identified, so some HCM cats may be testing negative because their mutation is yet unidentified.

In one earlier report, myomesin (M band sarcomeric protein) was found to be reduced or absent within the myocardium of cats with familial HCM and increased anomalous β-myosin heavy chain protein was also found.[4] Affected cats were used to propagate a colony for characterization, and echocardiogram serial studies confirmed 55% of the offspring were affected.[5]

The newest research has now elucidated the genetic defect to be myosin-binding protein C (MYBPC3-A31P). A survey of cats from many geographic areas confirmed the dominant mutation is widespread in the breed, with a worldwide rate of 34%, with 90% being heterozygous.[6]

A prospective ultrasound screening of a group including homozygotes and heterozygotes for the mutation demonstrated regional diastolic dysfunction but left ventricular hypertrophy was also found in wild type cats.[7]

Once severe HCM is established, progression to terminal endpoints occurs within a few months to several years at the most.[8] Typical clinical signs of feline heart disease can be seen but significant disease can be present in the absence of any clinical signs.[9]

Serum cardiac troponin 1 levels (cTnI), a sensitive and specific marker of myocardial damage may be elevated according to early studies and may be useful in future, though further studies are needed. Levels increased to a peak 12-48 hours after an episode of damage, and stayed elevated for 8 days.[10]

Overall, left ventricular outflow obstruction, left ventricular diastolic dysfunction, left ventricular wall (less commonly asymmetric septal) hypertrophy and interstitial fibrosis and ischemia lead to typical heart failure.[11]

Papillary muscle hypertrophy is another finding.[6] Average age of onset is 6-1/2 years, and more cases are seen in males. It has been postulated that growth hormone excess may have a role in some cases. Prognosis for asymptomatic cats is good (5-10 year survival), poor for those with arterial thromboembolism (6 months) and moderate survival time of 18 months is typical (with appropriate management) for heart failure.[12]

Report recommendations include: investigate all murmurs in kittens over four months old, screen breeding stock annually during their breeding career using auscultation and echocardiography starting at age 2 for males, and 3 for females; ECG, thoracic radiographs and blood pressure determination may also be recommended if signs suggestive of clinical heart disease such as heart murmur are present. It is very important to note disease may be present without a murmur.

If it is suspected that the cat has died of heart disease, it is recommended to conduct a necropsy. Average heart weight at post mortem is 20 g for moderately affected cats, and 30 g for severely affected patients; myofibrillar disarray is a hallmark histologic lesion.[13]

Spinal Muscle Atrophy (SMA): Autosomal recessive genetic disease causing tremor, proximal muscle weakness, and muscle atrophy beginning at ~4 mo of age. Apparent loss of function is rapid initially, but progresses slowly after 7-8 mo of age, and variably disabled cats lived for at least 8 y. Electromyography and microscopic examination of muscle and nerve biopsies are consistent with denervation atrophy as a result of a central lesion. A genetic test is available.[14]

Disease Predispositions

Hip Dysplasia (HD) +/-Patellar Luxation (PL): Hip dysplasia is more common in cats than was previously thought and almost all cats are clinically normal—clinical signs do not correlate with radiographic changes. A few reports suggest a predilection in females in cats, unlike dogs where no sex predilection exists and a polygenic mode of inheritance is proposed.[15]

In one report in a non random group of 78 cats, 45% of Maine Coon cats had PL and 18% had concurrent HD/PL; overall, the pooled group of cats were three times more likely to have these conditions concurrently than either alone.[16]

In a University of Missouri Veterinary Medical Teaching Hospital study, in 684 cats representing 12 breeds and non-registered domestic cats, domestic cats had hip dysplasia prevalence of 5.8%, pooled purebred cats had 12.3% prevalence, and an overall frequency of HD of 6.6% was found in the entire study group. Unlike dogs, minimal remodeling of the femoral neck was noted. Shallow remodeled acetabulum, with the cranio-dorsal acetabular margin most significantly affected was reported as the primary lesion instead in cats. Reported OFA database survey results (1974-1995) for 284 Maine Coon cats between 12 and 23 months of age showed 21% were positive for HD according to OFA protocol standards.[17,18]

In another non random group of 121 Maine Coon cats, using the Norberg Angle (NA) and Distraction Index (DI) it was determined 50.4% of Maine Coon cats had HD using OFA guidelines, 85% of these cats had bilateral changes; 57% had concurrent degenerative joint disease. Mean DI for affected cats was 0.64, while the mean NA was 80 degrees. The DI in normal cats averaged 0.55, and NA 92 degrees. If these were dogs, the affected cat scores would be typical of dog breeds with high prevalence of HD such as Newfoundland and Saint Bernard.[19] It was notable that most cats are clinically normal. Owner complaints may include reduced height of jumping, walking tucked under, and not running as much.[20]

Thought to be a polygenic trait, it is assumed to be moderately to highly heritable. It is not yet known if limited feeding/weight control has a role as in dogs, but larger framed cats more commonly have hip dysplasia. Until further studies are done, it might be prudent to avoid overfeeding young growing cats.[20,21,22]

Renal Failure: The renal failure rate for Maine Coon cats was more than double the baseline rate in a study of cats from 23 veterinary colleges from 1980-1990 (189,371 cases from Purdue University Veterinary Medical Database) at an odds ratio for risk of 2.44:1.[23]

Rare and Isolated Reports

Glycogenosis Type IV (GSD IV) Mimicking Disorder: Though GSD IV is a condition of Norwegian Forest cats, a very similar condition has been noted in a report of 7 Maine Coon cats. It was thought to be an autosomal recessive disorder leading to the neuromuscular disease in that small group of cats. Muscle atrophy, gait deficits, rear weakness and reluctance to jump were signs noted by about 4 months of age. Progression to dsyphagia, and rear limb paraplegia occurred over a year. Elevated creatine phosphokinase enzymes and nervous tissue conduction abnormalities were not evident; iodine stain did not reveal abnormal glycogen accumulation but histology of nervous tissue was abnormal.[29]

Flat-chested Kittens: Flat-chested Kittens: Similar to the flat-chested condition in Burmese (see Burmese Chapter), whereby reduced dorso-ventral chest dimension occurs. This trait is only seen in some lines. (Dr. Solveig Pflueger, Pers. Comm.) Signs may include poor weight gain, exaggerated cranial thoracic vertebral kyphosis, vomiting, dyspnea, cyanosis, exercise intolerance and cough, and a ridge along the costo-chondral junction of the ribs. As kittens mature and the rib cage calcification completes, clinical signs abate in many of those kittens that were less severely affected and thus not euthanized in the neonatal period. Though recognized by breeders, the flat-chested kittens have not been reported in the literature. Generally, it is first noted at 7-10 days of age.

Muscular Dystrophy (laminin α 2): A case affecting a 12 month-old cat in Belgium was reported in 2003. The kitten had never walked normally subsequent to adoption at 10 weeks old. No relatives were affected so a genetic basis was not identified, though a de novo mutation could have occurred. Generalized muscle atrophy, limited extension and flexion of limb joints, marked CK elevation and weakness were noted. Euthanasia was necessary due to a progressive condition.[24]

Superficial Necrolytic Dermatitis with Hepatopathy: A 5 year-old cat presented with hepatocutaneous syndrome. Pruritis, alopecia, and liver enzyme increases were noted. Mean survival after diagnosis is about 6 weeks in dogs and was similar here; etiology is unknown.[25]

Hereditary Deafness: Is associated with the dominant gene for white cat (W); may be found in white cats of this breed. Brainstem Auditory-evoked Responses (BAER) can be used to evaluate hearing, as in dogs. Hearing loss may be bilateral or unilateral.[26]

Motor Neuron Disease: In a review paper, a juvenile onset MND case was relayed, affecting Maine Coon cats. An autosomal recessive inheritance was postulated. At 4 months of age, onset of severe weakness and muscle atrophy occurred and by late juvenile phase, kittens would walk with a "pelvic limb sway".[27]

Genetic Tests

Hip Radiographs: With OFA testing, 24 months of age is the minimum age for certifying hips but evaluations can be carried out earlier. Note that the Penn Hip system picks up joint laxity (can determine DI). Joint laxity is correlated with DJD. Consider checking patellar luxation propensity by manual palpation, and if positive, take stifle radiographs at the same time. Recommendations given were to recheck breeding cats annually for HD since some may develop radiographic signs only later in life.[12]

Renal Function: Screening for renal function using serum creatinine and urinalysis in cats 8 years or older is recommended since a breed propensity to renal failure was found.[23] Microalbuminuria and Urine P:C ratio may also be used for early screening.

HCM Monitoring: Yearly auscultation by a veterinarian to check for murmurs/arrhythmias is a minimum in normal cats. Breeding cats should be checked annually by echocardiogram since some may develop HCM later in life. Monitor starting at age 2 for males, and 3 for females; ECG, thoracic radiographs and blood pressure determination may also be recommended if signs suggestive of clinical heart disease such as heart murmur/arrhythmia are present.[12, 13]

Normal M-mode echo parameters reported for Maine Coon cats differ somewhat from the typical domestic cat, so these means should be used for reference when screening healthy cats and are provided in this report.[28]

HCM Genetic testing is available at NC State-Meurs Lab.

Direct genetic test for SMA is available from MSU-Fyfe Lab.

Miscellaneous

- **Breed name synonyms:** Coon Cat, Maine Cat, American Longhair, Forest Cat. (Historical) Maine Shag was used for the cats with colors other than brown tabby.
- **Registries:** FIFé, TICA, CFA, ACFA, CFF, CCA, NZCF, WCF, ACF, GCCF.
- **Breed resources: CFA Maine Coon Cat Breed Council:** www.mainecoonbc.org
  Maine Coon Cat Club: http://www.maine-coon-cat-club.com/
  The Maine Coon Breeders and Fanciers Association: http://www.mcbfa.org/
  United Maine Coon Cat Association (CFF): http://www.cffinc.org/umcca/main.htm
  Orthopedic Foundation for Animals (OFA): www.offa.org

References

1. Kittleson MD, Meurs KM, Kittleson JA, et al. Heritable characteristics, phenotypic expression, and natural history of hypertrophic cardiomyopathy in Maine Coon Cats. First International Feline Genetic Disease Conference Philadelphia PA June 1998. In: Feline Practice Supplement. (abstr) 1999:7. and Abstract: *JVIM* 12:198, 1998.
2. Drögemüller C, Rüfenacht S, Wichert B, Leeb T. Mutation within the FGF5 gene are associated with hair length in cats. Animal Genet 2007 JUN;38(3):218-221.
3. Meurs KM, Kittleson MD, Reiser PJ, et al. Myomysin, a sarcomeric protein is reduced in Maine Coon cats with familial hypertrophic cardiomyopathy. 19th Annual ACVIM Medical Forum. Denver CO May 2001 (abstr) in: *JVIM* 2001;15(3):281. Also abstract is in AAFP August 2001 Newsletter p 19.
4. Kittleson MD, Meurs KM, Munro MJ, et al. Familial hypertrophic cardiomyopathy in Maine Coon Cats: An animal model of human disease. *Circulation* 1999;99:3172-3180.
5. Kittleson MD, Kittleson JA, Mekhamer Y. Development and progression of inherited hypertrophic cardiomyopathy in Maine Coon cats. 14th Annual ACVIM Medical Forum, San Antonio TX May 1996 [abstr] in: *JVIM* 1996;12(3):165.

6. Fries, R., Heaney, A.M., Meurs, K.M. Prevalence of the Myosin-Binding Protein C Mutation in Maine Coon Cats. Vet Intern Med 2008;22:893-896.

7. Carlos Sampedrano,C., Chetboul, V. Et al. Prospective echocardiographic and tissue Doppler imaging screening of population of Maine Coon cats tested for the A31P mutation in the myosin-binding protein C gene: a specific analysis of the heterozytous status. J Vet Intern Med 23(1):91-99. 2009.

8. Rodriguez DB, Harpster N. Feline hypertrophic cardiomyopathy: Etiology, pathophysiology and clinical features. *Compend Contin Educ Pract Vet* 2002;24(5):364-372.

9. Connolly DJ, Cannata J, Boswood A, et al. Cardiac troponin I in cats with hypertrophic cardiomyopathy. *J Fel Med Surg* 2003;5:209-216.

10. Medinger TL, Bruyette DS. Feline hypertrophic cardiomyopathy. *Compend Contin Educ Pract Vet* 1992;14(4):479-490.

11. Atkins CE. Feline hypertrophic cardiomyopathy. Winter 2004 AAFP Meeting. Proceedings [*abstr*] in: *AAFP Newsletter* August 2004 22(2):30-31.

12. Little S. Selected inherited diseases of the cat, in *Proceedings*. International Ragdoll Congress Russelheim Germany Oct, 2004. Available at: www.catvet.homestead.com/Inherited_Diseases_2004.pdf, Accessed Nov 23, 2004.

13. Kittleson MD, Gompf R, Little S. Winn Feline Foundation Website. Special Report to the Winn Feline Foundation: Feline Hypertrophic Cardiomyopathy Advice for Breeders. Notes. Available at: www.winnfeline-health.org/health/hypertrophic-cariomyopathy.html Accessed Sept 29, 2004.

14. He Q, Lowrie C, Shelton GD, et. al.: Inherited motor neuron disease in domestic cats: a model of spinal muscular atrophy. Pediatr Res. 2005 Mar;57(3):324-30.

15. Giger U. In: Bonagura J, ed. *Kirk's Current Veterinary Therapy XIII.* Philadelphia: WB Saunders Co, 2000;396-399.

16. Allan GS. Radiographic features of feline joint disease. *Vet Clin North Am: Sm Anim Pract* 2000;30(2):281-302.

17. Smith GK, Langenbach A, Green PA, et al. Evaluation of the association between medial patellar luxation and hip dysplasia in cats. *J Am Vet Med Assoc* 1999;215(1):40-45.

18. Keller GG, Reed AL, Lattimer JC, et al. Hip dysplasia: A feline population study. *Veterinary Radiology & Ultrasound* 1999;40(4):460-464.

19. Keller GG, Corley EA. Hip Dysplasia: Orthopedic Foundation for Animals Data on the Maine Coon Cat. Maine Coon Breeders and Fanciers Association Scratch Sheet 1996:18.

20. Murphy TP, Biery DN, Fordyce HH, et al. Radiographic prevalence of hip dysplasia in 121 Maine coon cats. *Abstracts.* 27th Annual Conference of the Veterinary Orthopedic Society. Val d'Isère France, March 3-12, 2000. In: *Vet Comp Orthop Traumatol* 2000;13(3):A12.

21. Murphy T. Feline hip dysplasia - where are we? *Maine Coon International Information Network Magazine* 1999;19:3.

22. Little S. Winn Feline Foundation Website. A Winn Foundation Health Article Online: Feline hip dysplasia. *Notes.* Available at: www.winnfeline-health.org/hip-dysplasia.html Accessed Sept 29, 2004.

23. Lulich JP, O'Brien TD, Osborne CA, et al. Feline Renal Failure: Questions, answers, questions. *Compend Contin Educ Pract Vet* 1992;14(2):127-152.

24. Poncelet L, Résibois A, Engvall E, et al. Laminin alpha 2 deficiency associated muscular dystrophy in a Maine Coon Cat. *J Small Anim Pract* 2003 Dec 44(12):550-52.

25. Kimmel SE, Christiansen W, Byrne KP. Clinicopathological, ultrasonographic and histopathological findings of superficial necrolytic dermatitis with hepatopathy in a cat. *J Am Anim Hosp Assoc* 2003;39:23-27.

26. Fischer A, Kraus G. Brainstem auditory-evoked responses (BAER) for diagnosis of congenital deafness in white cats. Poster. In: First International Feline Genetic Disease Conference Philadelphia PA June 1998. *Feline Practice Supplement* (abstr) 1999:28.

27. Gaschen F, Jaggy A, Jones B. Congenital diseases of feline muscle and neuromuscular junction. *J Fel Med Surg* 2004;6:355-366.

28. Drourr L, Lefbom BK, Rosenthal SL, Tyrrell WD Jr. Measurement of M-mode echocardiographic parameters in healthy adult Maine Coon cats. *J Am Vet Med Assoc* 2005;226(5):734-737.

29. Fyfe JC. Glycogenosis Type IV of Norwegian Forest Cats. *Proceedings.* 17th Annual Medical Forum of the American College of Veterinary Internal Medicine. 1999:281-283.

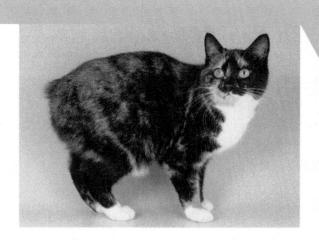

The Breed History

It is reported by some that Manx cats were originally brought from Japan to North America by traders. The tailless trait is autosomal dominant in this breed and recessive in the Japanese Bobtail thus refuting the theory that these tail mutants share a common origin. Another theory places breed origins on the Isle of Man. The original cats were both long and shorthaired. Records on the Isle of Man document their origin from domestic cats by a process of spontaneous mutation. CFA recognized the bred in the 1920s; longhairs in 1990. In some registries, longhaired Manx are termed **Cymric**. The CCA recognized the Cymric (*"kim-rick"*) in 1976. In 1994, longhairs became a division within Manx in the CFA. In some registries they are still separate breeds. No outcrosses allowed.

Physical Characteristics

Weight: 8-12 lb (3.4-5.5 kg); males a bit larger than the females

Coat: Short dense double haircoat is less full in warm weather. The outer coat hairs are hard in texture except in the white and dilutes. Longhair coat hairs are medium in length, silky but not cottony in texture, with breeches and ruff. Many coat colors and patterns accepted.

Eyes: Eyes are large and round; color conforms to coat.

Points of Conformation: The Manx is of medium size and cobby (stocky) conformation; features tend to roundness. A large, rounded head, with full cheeks is the standard. Ears are small-medium, round tipped, and angled outward (so-called "cradle" set). The nose is broad, medium length, and straight in profile. Neck is short. They possess round feet. Spine forms a gradual upward arch.

Recognized Behavior Issues and Traits

Reported breed characteristics include: Gentle sweet cats, playful, love close contact with people, adapt well to other pets. Gait tends to be rolling behind; a hop somewhat like a rabbit in rumpies. Easygoing, some learn to open door knobs, many like water, and willingly leash train. Some say that Manx have dog-like traits, such as toy burying. Some cats are like one-man dogs and follow a favored person around the house and may act like "watchdog" cats in the home. Good hunters. Quiet voiced and often use a trilling vocalization. Good with children if raised with them; they like a quiet home.

Grooming: Daily grooming is needed to prevent build-up of undercoat, may need to blow dry after bath in longhairs due to thick double coat.

Normal Breed Variations

Different degrees of "taillessness" exist:
Rumpy (SYN: rumpies): no protuberance, so is level or hollow (dimple) where tail usually originates (show quality); no caudal vertebrae
Rumpy riser (SYN: risers): when one runs a hand down over tail base, a small fused protuberance is felt—not penalized in show if it does not act as a stop to a hand caress; one to seven caudal vertebrae
Stumpy (SYN: stubbies): short bobtail, a stumped tail less than 1/2 the usual length and eligible for AOV classes, can move it laterally; two to 14 caudal vertebrae, may have a kink.
Longy (SYN: tailies, longies [pl]): half tail (blunt ended) and full tail (regular tapered end); sometimes kinked; are not shown though they are used in breeding programs.

They are long-lived.

They are slow to mature.

They gain weight easily.

Drug Sensitivities

None reported in the literature

Inherited Diseases

Sacrocaudal Dysgenesis: The variable phenotype resulting from the autosomal dominant (M) gene for taillessness/sacrocaudal dysgenesis is likely due to incomplete penetrance, variable expressivity, or there is a modifying gene at work due to the spectrum of the phenotypic expression.

Reduced tail length, and especially reduced lower spine length are correlated with abnormalities of the sacrocaudal area leading to deleterious effects in addition to the breed specific trait of taillessness being selected for. Heritability for the gene was reported to be 0.4.[1] There is a progression of severity of abnormalities as the gene expression becomes fuller. Since homozygosity of alleles at the Manx tailless gene locus appears to be lethal *in utero*, an informed breeding program will produce kittens with tails of all lengths. The heterozygote may be semi-lethal; there is an excess of females in viable Manx gene carriers; the sex ratio change is not well characterized.[2] Abnormalities of fetuses as young as 5 weeks gestation include gross malformation of the CNS.[3]

Associated M gene abnormalities include:
Myelodysplasia/Anury/Spinal Dysraphism: The lower spinal column does not form normally. The spectrum includes:
- vertebral defects (missing or irregular vertebrae) in lumbar and sacral area;
- taillessness, an absence of caudal vertebrae **(SYN: anury)** –*this is the characteristic being selected for;*
- neuronal defect **(myelodysplasia)**, leading to cavitation of

dorsal white matter and tract degeneration which may begin as high as the mid-lumbar cord;[3]

- neural tube and notochord defect leading to incomplete early embryologic closure, with sacral and caudal dysgenesis or partial agenesis **(spinal dysraphism)**. Resulting in: **Spina Bifida, Hydromyelia, Myelocele, Tethered Cord,** and **Syringomyelia;** these occur with low frequency in live born kittens.

Vesicourethral Dysfunction: Those with incontinence problems tend to be euthanized early. A published case report outlined detailed status of a cat afflicted with detrusor muscle atonia, pelvic floor EMG deficits, proximal urethra malfunction and total lack of adrenergic enervation of the bladder and proximal urethra.[4] According to that report, 50% of rumpy cats have urinary incontinence and sacral cord abnormalities. Bladder may be grossly distended with neurogenic dysfunction.[3]

In a case control study of 285,000 records of cats with and without urinary tract disease, the Manx was reported to be at increased risk for congenital urinary tract defects and urinary incontinence.[5]

Gait Abnormalities: Ataxia progressing to paraplegia; sometimes kittens bunny hop. Bunny hopping is strongly associated with syringomyelia, and plantigrade posture while walking or standing can occur.[3] Gait deficits may be of neurogenic origin, or alternatively, be a mild lameness associated with pelvic bony malformation. Club foot is sometimes also present. Gait changes are not present in all cats.

Colon Dysfunction: Constipation/obstipation; neurogenic. Not present in all cats. Hyaline degeneration of the smooth muscle layers is evident and reduced ganglion cell numbers in Meissner's plexus noted; grossly a megacolon, with associated abdominal distention and fecal perineal staining in afflicted cats. Some cats may also have mild rectal prolapse.[3]

Structural or functional deficits may remain stable or may deteriorate. Associated pathologic changes may show up *in utero*, at birth, before weaning, or in the first 4 months of life in less severely affected kittens. Severely affected kittens will show fecal or urinary incontinence, reduced perineal cutaneous sensation, and significant pelvic limb weakness before weaning, and vertebral abnormalities are commonly noted on imaging studies.[6]

Breeders often hold kittens until 16 weeks of age because usually if a kitten is going to have difficulties, problems generally manifest by 4 months of age. In tailed Manx crosses, birth defect rates are low-normal, with rates in the same range as humans and other cat breeds.[7]

Litter size is also low normal in this breed. An internet-based survey[8] found that in:
    39 litters, 121 kittens
    Average number of kittens per litter: 3.1
    Stillbirths: 8%
    C-sections: 15%
    Average birth weight: males 95, females 91 g

Disease Predispositions

Hereditary Deafness: Is associated with the dominant gene for white cat (W); may be found in white cats of this breed.[12]

Tail Arthritis: Some cats with stumpy or longy tails left undocked may develop arthritis later in life if the caudal vertebrae malformed - anecdotal.

Rare and Isolated Reports

Corneal Dystrophy: An inherited condition resulting from local metabolic defects. This is an autosomal recessive trait. Signs are often noted at about 16 weeks of age and progress from anterior stromal edema to diffuse bullous keratopathy.[9] Stromal dystrophy may lead to epithelial rupture at a young age; Descemet's membrane is also abnormal.[10] This is usually a bilateral condition.[11]

Genetic Tests
None commercially available

Miscellaneous

- **Breed name synonyms:** Tailless Cat, Cymric (for longhaired in some registries), Man's Cat, Isle of Man Cat
- **Registries:** FIFé, TICA, CFA, ACFA, GCCF (short haired), ACF, WCF (provisional), NZCF, CCA, CFF. In some registries, longhairs or semi-longhairs are called Cymric (TICA), in others they are termed longhaired Manx (CFA).
- **Breed resources: The American Manx Club:**
  http://www.americanmanxclub.com
  The International Manx & Cymric Society (ACFA):
  254 S. Douglas
  Bradley IL 60915
  Cymric Cat Club (CFA):
  PO Box 917
  Snohomish WA 98291
  The Breed Club Europe Manx and Cymric:
  http://www.raskatt.com/emc/emc.html

References

1. Robinson R. Expressivity of the Manx gene in cats. J Hered 1993; May-Jun;84(3):170-172.
2. Basrur PK. Genetics in Veterinary Medicine. Vaspar s.1. 1999:205.
3. DeForest ME, Basrur PK. Malformations and the Manx Syndrome in cats. Can Vet J 1979;20:304-314.
4. Woodside JR, Dail WG, McGuire EJ, et al. The Manx cat as an animal model for neurogenic vesical dysfunction associated with myelodysplasia: A preliminary report. J Urol 1982;127(1):180-183.
5. Lekcharoensuk C, Osborne CA, Lulich JP. Epidemiologic study of risk factors for lower urinary tract diseases in cats. J Am Vet Med Assoc 2001;218(9):429-435.
6. Shell LG. Spinal cord diseases in cats. In: Symposium: Feline neurologic diseases. Vet Med Jun 1998;553-563.
7. Pflueger SMV. Feline genetic disorders-Frequent questions and answers. Proceedings. Tuft's Canine and Feline Breeding and Genetics Conference. Oct 2-4, 2003 Available at: http://www.vin.com/tufts/2003. Accessed Nov 19, 2004.
8. Little, S. Pers. Comm. March, 2009)
9. Peiffer RL. Inherited ocular diseases of the dog and cat. Compend Cont Educ Pract Vet 1982;4(2):152-164.
10. Cooley PL, Dice PF II. Corneal dystrophy in the dog and cat. Vet Clin North Am: Small Anim Pract 1990;20(3):681-692.
11. Hoskins JD. Congenital defects in cats. Compend Contin Educ Pract Vet 1995;17(3):385-405.
12. Strain GM. Hereditary deafness in dogs and cats: causes, prevalence, and current research. Proceedings. Tuft's Canine and Feline Breeding and Genetics Conference. Oct 2-4, 2003 Available at: http://www.vin.com/tufts/2003. Accessed Nov 19, 2004.

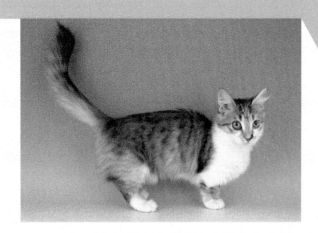

The Breed History

The Munchkin is a newer breed, with acceptance in TICA since 1995. The autosomal dominant gene mutation producing shortened limbs arose in 1983 in a black cat born in Louisiana. Outcrossing is limited to non-pedigreed cats only. Periodically, this mutation has arisen in cats unrelated to the *foundation cat*—approximately 30 cats have been reported since 1990. Sometimes the mutation has occurred in other purebred cats as well as in domestic cats. The name derives from the "Munchkins" in The Wizard of Oz movie of 1939. The actual breed name was cemented following a comment to a reporter about the cats being "cute little munchkins", used in the generic sense.

Physical Characteristics

Weight: females 4-8 lb (1.8-3.6 kg) males 6-10 lb (2.75-4.5 kg)

Coat: Medium and semi-longhaired varieties exist. Texture of the shorter coat is plush with a minimal undercoat. The texture of the longer coat is medium and in the undercoat it is silky, and a ruff, britches and plume are present. All colors and patterns accepted.

Eyes: All colors accepted, and coat and eye colors do not have to be correlated. Eyes are large and walnut shaped.

Points of Conformation: Long bones are significantly shorter than a typical cat and may be slightly bowed and somewhat thickened. Though carpal deviation is not written into the breed standard, some may appear somewhat deviated because of the radius bone conformation. The Munchkin has a medium sized, rounded wedge-shaped head. Ears are medium sized and slightly rounded at tips, the nose is moderate in length, and a slight convexity in profile is accepted. Tail is long, medium, and tapered. The body is medium length with stocky build. Munchkins are about 40% longer than they are high. Feet are compact and round. Normal mobility is present, though sometimes the gait can appear to have a waddling appearance.

Grooming: The Munchkin is a low maintenance cat. Weekly brushing usually suffices. Longhaired cats may need periodic bathing.

Munchkin

Recognized Behavior Issues and Traits

Reported breed characteristics: These cats are not recommended for outdoor living. Curious, playful, very affectionate, they keep their kitten personalities late into life. Get along well with other pets and take to leash training. Movement is described as "ferret like". They like to stash their special toys.

Normal Breed Variations

Munchkin Kitten Information Project:[1]
An Internet based breeder survey to establish normal baselines for reproduction was carried out.

    54 litters. 221 kittens. Oct 2003-Sept 2004.
    Average litter size 4.1
    Stillbirth rate 6 %, 5% C-sections
    Average birth weight: Male 87 g female 78 g

These cats tend not to jump as high as some athletic normal leg phenotype cats but can easily jump as high as a typical Persian cat—about 3-4 feet (Pflueger, S. Pers. Comm.). Dr. Pflueger also reports the incidence of congenital anomalies is in the same range as for other cat breeds.

Drug Sensitivities

None reported in the literature

Inherited Diseases

Chondrodysplasia: The short-legged trait of Munchkin cats is similar in phenotype to the short-legged Dachshund mutation and in humans, achondroplasia. Short-legged cats do not seem to be more susceptible to intervertebral disc disease and as they age, do not develop a higher than expected incidence of degenerative joint disease or other back or leg pathology. The trait is lethal in the homozygote; probably an early embryonic death.

Flat-chested Kittens: Similar to the flat-chested condition in Burmese *(see Burmese Chapter)*, whereby reduced dorsoventral chest dimension occurs. This trait is only seen in some lines of Munchkin cats. Signs may include poor weight gain, exaggerated cranial thoracic vertebral kyphosis, vomiting, dyspnea, cyanosis, exercise intolerance and cough, and a ridge along the costo-chondral junction of the ribs. As kittens mature and the rib cage calcification completes, clinical signs abate in many of those kittens that were less severely affected and thus not euthanized in the neonatal period. Though recognized by breeders, the flat-chested kittens have not been widely reported in the literature. Generally, it is first noted at 7-10 days of age.

In Burmese cats it has been reported that the condition could possibly be a muscle defect associated with changes in taurine rather than an inherited deformity.[2]

This condition is not apparently linked to the short limb characteristic since the flat-chested kittens can be found in long-legged Munchkin offspring.

Compared with pectus excavatum, this condition results in less pronounced dorsal deviation of the sternum up into the chest.

Disease Predispositions
None reported in the literature

Rare and Isolated Reports
"Twisty Cat": Historically, there was some concern that this trait was linked to the short-legged trait but this is now disproved. Twisty cat refers to cats born polydactyl with radius hypoplasia, resulting in localized absent or attenuated bone development. (Dr. Solveig Pflueger, Pers. Comm.)

Genetic Tests
None commercially available

Miscellaneous
- **Breed name synonyms:** Munchie, Munchk, nicknames "Dachshund Cat", "Basset Cat"
- **Registries:** TICA (Munchkin and Munchkin Longhair), AACE
- **Breed resources: Munchkin Breed Club:** http://www.munchkin.net/

References
1. Little S. Dr. Little's Website. Munchkin Kitten Information Project. Pers. Comm. March, 2009
2. Sturgess CP, Waters L, Gruffydd-Jones TJ, et al. Investigation of the association between whole blood and tissue taurine levels and the development of thoracic deformities in neonatal Burmese kittens. Vet Rec 1997;141:566-570.

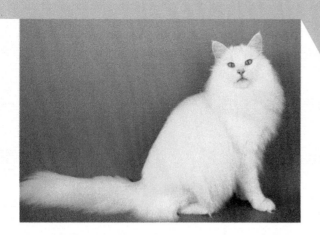

Norwegian Forest Cat

The Breed History

These large cats evolved in Norway but their ancient roots may trace back to importation by sailors from other regions of the world, with progenitor domestic cats from countries such as Turkey (perhaps Turkish Angora). They were reported to be distinctive in Norway by about 1000 AD. Natural selection in the harsh climate lead to heavily coated, large rugged cats that thrived as farmer's working cats. In the 1930s the breed was first recognized, and by the late 1970s as first exports to the UK and America began, formal breeding programs were instituted. FIFé accepted the breed in 1977, and the CFA for championship status in 1993. Outcrossing is not allowed. These are still rare in North America; CFA in 2000 registered only 561 cats.

Physical Characteristics

Weight: 12-24 lb (5-10 kg); females are considerably smaller than males in this range

Coat: The very heavy double coat in semi-longhair is more or less dense depending on the season of the year. Water resistant, it is hard in texture. Texture of the hair is a bit softer in non-solid colored cats. Ruff, collar, chops and mane are the furnishings around the neck, full britches are present at the rear limbs. Ears are tufted and heavily furnished. All colors and patterns except those containing fawn, cinnamon sable, (FIFé) and lilac, chocolate and colorpoint (FIFé and CFA) are accepted. Brown tabby and white is the most common color/pattern. The coat is naturally a bit oily.

A recent study reported that a separate genetic mutation is responsible for the long hair in this breed.[1]

Eyes: Medium sized, almond shaped, the color is not necessarily synchronized to coat color; those with white in the coat may have blue and odd-eyed colors.

Points of Conformation: The NFC is not stocky, but is very strongly built. The triangular head is large but long and angular, with a long straight nose on profile. The broad ears are medium sized, round tipped. Lynx tipping is preferred. Paws are large and round, with some tufting of hair. Tail is long, tapering and well plumed, especially in winter. Compared to the Maine Coon, this breed has a shorter body.

Grooming: Grooming generally consists of a quick brush every few days and they do not tend to mat like some of the longhair breeds. They may need daily grooming while shedding.

Recognized Behavior Issues and Traits

Reported breed characteristics include: Easy-going, affectionate, calm but some are aloof with strangers, reserved, territorial, love to climb and jump, and are good hunters. Outdoor cats may fish. Not demanding of their owner's affections. Not considered lap cats. Soft voiced. If indoors, a climbing tree will help to keep the cat off the fridge and door tops.

Normal Breed Variations

Considered slow to mature (4-5 yrs).

Blood type B: In one study of American Norwegian Forest Cats, prevalence of blood type B was zero.[2] Prevalence of 7% Type B was reported in later references.[3, 4]

Norwegian Forest Cat Kitten Information Project:[5]
An Internet based breeder survey to establish normal baselines for reproduction was reported.

49 reporting breeders, 124 litters, 562 kittens.
Nov 2003 - Oct 2004.

October 2004 Report:
Average litter size 4.5
Stillbirth rate 5 %
C-sections: 6 %
Average birth weight: Male 106 g female 103 g

Drug Sensitivities

None reported in the literature

Inherited Diseases

Glycogenosis Type IV: (SYN: Type IV Glycogen Storage Disease). This storage disease is reported exclusively in this breed of cat and is an abnormality of glucose metabolism. An **autosomal recessive** pattern of inheritance of the trait occurs; affected cats are homozygous. This condition carries a very poor prognosis; affected cats will die—either in utero, around birth or by 10-14 months of age. There is no known treatment.[6]

Primary signs usually reflect the atrophy/degeneration in muscle and nervous tissues, though cytoplasmic inclusions containing abnormal glycogen deposits are evident in multiple body systems and organs. Type IV storage disease is due to a deficiency of the glycogen branching enzyme (GBE) that, as the name implies, produces normal glycogen branching. The efficient addition or removal of glucose from glycogen stores is dependent on the normal branched structure.

Variable expression of the condition occurs, with two main age ranges of onset: at birth, or at late juvenile phase, with presentation ranging from normal appearing stillborn kittens, collapse in neonates (hypoglycemia, cardiopulmonary collapse), and in the late phase form, with progressive neuromuscular and cardiac degeneration in between 5 and 7 months of age, or a sudden cardiac decompensation in cats about 9 months to 1 year of age. In the neonate, this condition might be confused with fading kitten syndrome.[7]

Sequencing of the exon deletion producing the disorder was carried out and by 1999 testing for carriers had begun, with subsequent efforts by breeders to eliminate the mutant allele in breeding stock.

Clinical signs may initially include muscle tremors and a creatine kinase spike typically occurs with onset at 5 months of age. By 8 months of age, severe tremors, hyperthermia, poor stamina and muscle wasting noted. Mild ataxia (some describe it as "bunny hopping", and difficulties with prehension and deglutition noted. Abnormal EEG, EMG and ECG, and progressively, abnormal echocardiograms noted. Progressive neurological signs (tetraplegia), and tonic-clonic seizures and hypoglycemia preceded euthanasia.[8]

As the disease progresses, histologic studies have shown that muscle fibers are replaced by fibrosis; this contracture can lead to permanent flexion of digits and carpi, and extension of the tibiotarsal and femorotibial joints.[9] According to this same author, pedigree analysis indicates that this gene originated in 2 cats imported to the US from Norway and Germany, but that these two cats were not found by pedigree analysis to be related, though the mutation is the same.

Branching enzyme activity was confirmed to be very low in an inbred family of NFC, and a breeding colony to further study this condition was established. Activity was less than 1/10th normal in liver and muscle, and less severely reduced in parents of that cat.[10]

Three related cats were closely studied and clinical signs had progressed to tetraplegia, generalized muscle atrophy and contracted tendons by 8 months old. One cat died suddenly before any clinical signs were noted, and another cat succumbed to left sided heart failure at 13 months old. Nervous, cardiac and skeletal tissues were primarily affected by storage products, with degenerative changes noted on histology.[11]

GBE activity is 25-75% of normal in unaffected carriers, and is 5% of normal activity (in liver, muscle) in affected cats. In the late juvenile onset version of the condition, progression takes 10-15 weeks, and the concurrent hyperthermia is still poorly understood. Perhaps endogenous pyrogens are released during tissue degeneration, or ongoing general tremors may generate heat. Echocardiographs confirm that fibrosis of the subendocardium occurs (focal hyperechoic areas noted), and there is left ventricular hypertrophy. Mild elevation of alanine aminotransferase activity may reflect hepatopathy but only small amounts of abnormal storage products are found in hepatocytes in histopathology preparations. Cranial nerve function is normal with the exception of a reduced swallowing reflex. For diagnosis of the perinatal onset form, note that abnormal glycogen can be found in ventricular myocytes and in many CNS neurons at that age. In both normal and affected kittens at birth, muscle glycogen stores are depleted—no other abnormalities are found here. Detailed report of histologic changes can be found in this reference.[12]

Neonatal Isoerythrolysis (NI): Proportion of matings at risk for NI was reported to be 0.06.[3]

Disease Predispositions

Hypertrophic Cardiomyopathy (HCM) is of increased prevalence, but not proven to be inherited.

Genetic Tests

Glycogenosis Type IV DNA Test

Josephine Deubler Genetic Testing Laboratory (PennGen) University of Pennsylvania Veterinary Hospital. Minimum of 1-2 ml EDTA blood should be sent immediately (not frozen); cooling the sample is not essential. Should be processed within 48 hours. Test request form, service fees and other information available online at: http://w3.vet.upenn.edu/research/centers/penngen/services/deublerlab/gsd4.html. This is a direct test not a linkage test and can identify carriers.

The lab will do concurrent blood typing on that sample. One can also submit two buccal swabs.

Miscellaneous

- **Breed name synonyms:** "Wegie"; an American Nickname, Forest Cat, National Cat of Norway, Norwegian Cat, NFC, Norst Skogkatt (Nordic for Norwegian forest cat), Skaukatt, Skoggkatt, Wegrie, Norwegische Waldkatze (German), Chat des Bois Novegien (French).
- **Registries:** FIFé, TICA, CFA, ACFA, CFF, GCCF, ACF, WCF, NZCF (Norwegian), CCA .
- **Breed resources: CFA Norwegian Forest Cat Breed Council:** http://www.nfcbc.org/
  Norwegian Forest Cat Club (UK): http://www.nfcc.co.uk/
  Norwegian Forest Cat Fanciers' Association: http://www.forestcats.net/
  National Norwegian Forest Cat Club:
  17 Ashwood Rd.
  Trenton NJ 08610
  The Viking Cat Club: http://www.vikingcatclub.co.uk/

References

1. Drögemüller C, Rüfenacht S, Wichert B, Leeb T Mutations within the FGF5 gene are associated with hair length in cats. Anim Genet. 2007 Jun;38(3):218-21. (A)
2. Giger U, Bucheler J, Patterson DF. Frequency and inheritance of A and B blood types in feline breeds of the United States. J Hered 1991;82:15-20.
3. Giger U. In: Bonagura J, ed. Kirk's Current Veterinary Therapy XIII. Philadelphia: WB Saunders Co, 2000;396-399.
4. Giger U, Casal M, Niggemeier A. The fading kitten syndrome and neonatal isoerythrolysis. Proceedings. The 15th Annual ACVIM Medical Forum, Lake Buena Vista FL 1997;308-310.
5. Little S. Dr. Susan Little's Website. Norwegian Forest Cat Kitten Information Project, Pers. Comm. March, 2009.
6. Gaschen F, Jaggy A, Jones B. Congenital diseases of feline muscle and neuromuscular junction. J Fel Med Surg 2004;6:355-366.
7. Fyfe JC. Glycogen storage disease Type IV in Norwegian Forest Cats:

Molecular detection of carriers. In: First International Feline Genetic Disease Conference 1998. *Proceedings (abstr), Feline Practice Supplement,* 1999;10.

8. Coates JR, Paxton R, Cox NR, et al. A case presentation and discussion of Type IV glycogen storage disease in a Norwegian Forest Cat. *Progress in Veterinary Neurology* 1996;7(1):5-11.

9. Fyfe JC. Glycogenosis Type IV of Norwegian Forest Cats. *Proceedings.* 17th Annual Meeting of the American College of Veterinary Internal Medicine. 1999:281.

10. Fyfe JC, Giger U, Van Winkle TJ, et al. Glycogen storage disease type IV: Inherited deficiency of branching enzyme activity in cats. *Pediatr Res* 1992;Dec;32(6):719-725.

11. Fyfe JC, Giger U, Van Winkle T, et al. Familial glycogen storage disease (Type IV GSD IV). *Proceedings.* 8th Annual Meeting of the American College of Veterinary Internal Medicine Veterinary Medical Forum. Washington, DC 1990:1129.

12. Fyfe JC, Van Winkle TJ, Haskins ME, et al. Animal model of human disease: Glycogen Storage Disease Type IV. *Comp Path Bullet* XXVI 1994;(3):3-6.

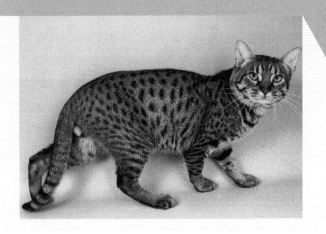

Ocicat

The Breed History

A Ruddy Abyssinian and Seal Point Siamese breeding was carried out to try to produce a new type of pointed Siamese. The outcome in the F1 resulted in the desired pattern, but after backcross to another Siamese cat, they produced a second, unusually coated offspring in that second generation—a light spotted cat. This was an unexpected outcome. This cat looked a lot like an extinct Egyptian type cat. Other breeding programs were begun to replicate this combination of coat genes, so the breed now has a broad genetic base with the *Dalai* line being prominent.

Early breed development also involved American Shorthair cats. The breed name is derived from the **Ocelot**, a wild spotted feline in combination with the word **cat**. The CFA first recognized these cats in 1966. The registries CFA and TICA accepted the breed for championship status in 1987-88. In 1986, the CFA closed the registry to American Shorthair and Siamese outcross breeding. This continues to be a rare breed. Outcrosses to Abyssinian were no longer allowed as of 2005.

Physical Characteristics

Weight: 6-14 lb (2.5-6.5 kg), females are smaller than males

Coat: The coat is very short, dense, flat lying and smooth with a pronounced gloss. The bull's eye agouti dark spot markings on a lighter background coat may not be distinct in young kittens, but will sharpen as they mature. Distinct spots are very important. Classic tabby markings are pet quality. Tip of tail hairs color reflects base coat color; other hairs are all agouti. Twelve colors are shown in five divisions. A distinct "M" mark is on the forehead and mascara markings are present.

Eyes: Colors are accepted in gold, green and copper spectrum but not blue.

Points of Conformation: The Ocicat head is a modified wedge shape with broad nose and muzzle. The Ocicat is a long bodied cat. Ears are large and angle outward. The tail is slightly tapering and long. Feet are compact and oval.

Grooming: Minimal grooming is needed for the Ocicat; a soft brush, chamois or hands will keep the coat well maintained.

Recognized Behavior Issues and Traits

Reported breed characteristics include: Affectionate, curious, active, playful; some can be lap cats. Need human companionship, devoted but not clinging, easy to train; can leash train, fetch, and are adaptable in new environments. They are good with children and other pets, and also with strangers. Sociable; they behave a bit like a dog. Ocicats like to talk but are less vocal than Siamese.

Normal Breed Variations

Known for easy birth and good mothering

Ocicat Kitten Information Project:[1] An Internet based breeder survey was carried out to establish normal baselines for reproduction.

40 reporting breeders, 136 litters, 581 kittens,
Nov 2003-Oct 2004;
   Average litter size 4.3
   Stillbirth rate 4 %
   C-sections 4%
   Average birth weight: Male 101 g female 95 g

Drug Sensitivities

None reported in the literature

Inherited Diseases

Progressive Retinal Atrophy (rdAc): Auto recessive disease causing blindness. See under Abyssinian breed. A genetic test is available.

Disease Predispositions

None reported in the literature

Genetic Tests

Direct genetic test for rdAc-PRA is available from UC-Davis VGL.

Miscellaneous

- **Breed name synonyms:** Oci, Spotted Cat, Ocelot
- **Registries:** FIFé, TICA, CFA, ACFA, ACF, GCCF, WCF, CCA, NZCF
- **Breed resources: CFA Ocicat Breed Council:**
  http://www.ocicatinfo.org
  Ocicats of North America (CFA):
  http://www.catoninetail.com/ona/
  Ocicats International: http://www.ocicatsinternational.com/

References

1. Little S. Ocicat Kitten Information Project, Pers. Comm. March 2009.

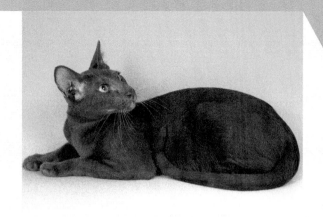

The Breed History

Orientals, or Oriental Shorthairs/Longhairs are strikingly similar to the Siamese apart from the lack of points. Thailand is the original source of the progenitors of this breed. These self-colored Orientals were previously termed **Foreign Shorthairs** in the UK and Europe. In the UK, the Oriental White still retains the designation Foreign White. The Oriental breed is relatively recently developed; in the 1950s in Britain and in the early 1960s in America, Siamese were crossed with domestic shorthairs to produce the original Oriental Shorthair specimens. Foreign Shorthairs were also imported to the USA. The CFA accepted this breed for championship status in 1977. The Longhair division was established in CFA in 1995 after 10 years of breed development in America. In other associations they are sometimes not placed in separate divisions. If offspring of Orientals are born with points, they cannot be shown as Siamese in CFA. Outcrossing to Siamese and Colorpoint is allowed in the Shorthair division. Oriental Longhair cats may be outcrossed to Siamese, Colorpoint, Balinese or Javanese.

Physical Characteristics

Weight: males 9-12 lb (4-5.5 kg), females are a bit smaller

Coat: All colors and patterns (300) are recognized except pointed cats, sepia, and mink. Pointed cats can be registered as Orientals, but not shown. Smoke, tabbies, solid, and shaded are the four major show divisions of patterns in UK, while in CFA, bi-color and parti-color classes also exist. The color black in this breed is termed **Ebony**. The Oriental Shorthair coat is very short, flat lying and soft textured, and in Oriental Longhairs, it is a short-medium length single coat, close lying and hairs are fine in texture. Hairs are longer on the tail.

Eyes: Eyes are medium sized, and almond in shape. Cross-eyed cats are penalized.Eyes may be green, though in white and bi-color cats in America, they may also be odd-eyed, green or blue, and in the UK, white cats are accepted with blue eyes only.

Points of Conformation: Medium sized cats, the limbs are long. The conformation is a classic foreign Oriental tubular cat. The head is a tapering-wedge shape with a long nose; on profile head and nose are completely flat with no break. No whisker pad pinch. The flared ears are large with pointed tips, and the neck is long and slender. Tail is long and thin; almost whip like, and tapers to a point;

in longhairs, is well plumed. The paws are small, compact and oval.

Grooming: Minimal grooming needed. Some do not recommend bathing. Rubber curry and chamois are adequate.

Recognized Behavior Issues and Traits

Reported breed characteristics include: Siamese-like in temperament; need human companionship and do not thrive if left alone for long periods. Playful, almost dog-like, agile, like to climb and jump, very vocal, curious, active, and with very high intelligence. Can sometimes demand attention, some youngsters extroverted. Not a lap cat—more like a "Velcro" kitty. Remain kitten-like late into life.

Normal Breed Variations

Large litters

Blood Type: 100% blood type A was reported[1]

Drug Sensitivities

None reported in the literature

Inherited Diseases

See the Siamese cat chapter -- Because this breed is a color variant, Orientals and Siamese share many conditions.

Disease Predispositions

See the Siamese cat chapter -- Because this breed is a color variant, it shares most of the same conditions.

MAP Urolithiasis: The risk of developing magnesium ammonium phosphate uroliths was reported to be increased in this breed.[2]

Lymphosarcoma (LSA): A mediastinal form of LSA in young, FeLV negative cats—significantly overrepresented in Orientals and Siamese. Three months to 2 years of age is peak incidence. Dysphagia and dyspnea are hallmark signs. Very aggressive tumors, and regress rapidly with early chemotherapy. Most cases descend from a single male who died of LSA in the 1980s. By pedigree analysis it was determined that this form of LSA has many of the characteristics of an **autosomal recessive** inheritance trait.[3]

In a retrospective case study of 7,159 sick and healthy cats at a Veterinary Medical Teaching Hospital in Australia over a decade, 60 cats had LSA. As a percent of all types of LSA, Siamese and Orientals when pooled accounted for 33.3% of the cases, though they made up only 2% of the hospital population. Mediastinal form was most common (86% were Siamese) and all were FeLV negative.[4]

This condition has been reported from Australia, Europe and the USA. A recent study report describes pedigree analysis of two families that also seems to confirm that this is indeed an AR trait.[5]

A study is underway with candidate genes BCL2 and MYC being subjected to mapping of genetic markers surrounding them.[5,6]

Hereditary Deafness: Is associated with the dominant gene for white cat (W); may be found in white cats of this breed.[7]

Rare and Isolated Reports

Transient Hyperlipidemia and Anemia: One litter of Oriental kittens reported.[8]

Genetic Tests

None commercially available

Miscellaneous

- **Breed name synonyms:** OSH, POSH, Oriental Shorthair, Oriental Longhair, Solid Siamese, Foreign. Historical: Chestnut Foreign Shorthair; Lavender Foreign Shorthair; White Foreign Shorthair.
- **Registries:** FIFé (Oriental LH, Oriental SH), TICA (Oriental SH, Oriental LH), CFA, ACFA (Oriental LH, Oriental SH), CFF, CCA, NZCF, WCF (in with Siamese), ACF (Oriental SH, Oriental LH), GCCF (just oriental LH)
- **Breed resources: CFA Oriental Breed Council:**
  www.orientalbc.org
  Oriental Shorthairs of America:
  http://home.comcast.net/~OSA_club/index.htm

References

1. Giger U. In: Bonagura J, ed. *Kirk's Current Veterinary Therapy XIII.* Philadelphia: WB Saunders Co, 2000;396-399.
2. Lekcharoensuk C, Lulich JP, Osborne CA, et al. Association between patient-related factors and risk of calcium oxalate and magnesium ammonium phosphate urolithiasis in cats. *J Am Vet Med Assoc* 2000;Aug15;217(4):520-525.
3. Lorimer HE. Hereditary lymphosarcoma in Oriental shorthair cats. First International Feline Genetic Disease Conference Philadelphia June, 1998 Proceedings (abstr) in: *Feline Practice Supplement,* 1999:29.
4. Court EA, Watson ADJ, Peaston AE. Retrospective study of 60 cases of feline lymphosarcoma. *Aust Vet J* 1997;75(6):424-427.
5. Geary LA, Lyons LA. Lymphosarcoma in Siamese/Oriental Shorthair breeds. *Notes.* University of California (Davis) Feline Genetics Extravaganza II Aug 28-29, 2004.
6. Lyons LA, Geary LA. Lymphosarcoma in Siamese/OSH populations. Proceedings of the 2nd International Conference Advances in Canine and Feline Genomics. Oct 2004 Utrecht Netherlands. Poster #30.
7. Strain GM. Hereditary deafness in dogs and cats: causes, prevalence, and current research. *Proceedings.* Tuft's Canine and Feline Breeding and Genetics Conference. Oct 2-4, 2003 Available at: http://www.vin.com/tufts/2003. Accessed Nov 19, 2004.
8. Gunn-Moore DA, Watson TDG, Dodkin SJ, et al. Transient hyperlipidaemia and anaemia in kittens. *Vet Rec* 1997;140:355-359.

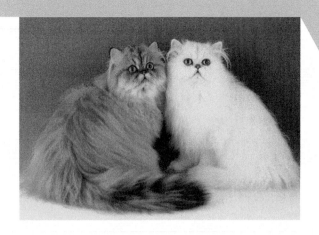

Persian

The Breed History

The early Persian type cats likely reached us via European trade originating in Iran (formerly Persia) during the 1600s. The **Himalayan** was the result of crossing Persian with Siamese later in breed development (1920s-1930s) to add the colorpoint pattern, and is a division of Persian in some registries—a separate breed in others *(see Himalayan chapter)*.

The Persian cat is always amongst the most popular of cat breeds. Historically, Persian cats had a less foreshortened face. The current British Longhair (Persian) standard has more moderate facial features. Persians were first registered in CFA in 1909. No out-crossing is allowed.

Physical Characteristics

Weight: 8-15 lb (3.5-7 kg)

Coat: The thick soft undercoat is overlain by a profuse standoff outer coat of long soft hairs. Well-developed ruff and frill, and tail is heavily haired. Coat texture should not be wooly.

Eyes: The large wide-set eyes are copper or orange. In shaded silver, golden and chinchilla, they are blue-green or emerald green. In Europe, a copper-eyed shaded silver is termed Pewter. Variable colored eyes are present in Persian white cats.

Points of Conformation: Persians have a heavy cobby build, small ears with rounded tips. A very short upturned nose and muzzle, with a well defined stop or break between the eyes is present. Persian cats have a large rounded broad head. Paws are rounded, tufted, and large. Tail is short, and carried low. The neck is short. Peke-faced is a subtype that is extremely foreshortened, similar to a Pekingese dog, while doll-faced cats are more moderate in their brachycephalic head conformation. The Peke subtype is specifically described in only certain registries. In ACFA for example, the Peke-faced is recognized as a head indented between eyes, creases following cheekbone; forehead, nose and chin form a perpendicular line.

Grooming: High grooming requirements are typical for Persian cats. Once to twice daily grooming to prevent matting is helpful; allow 15 minutes minimum daily. Regular baths are also used to help maintain the coat in excellent condition. Daily removal of tears to prevent staining and dermatitis in medical canthus area and facial folds may be required.

Recognized Behavior Issues and Traits

Reported breed characteristics include: Gentle, easygoing, placid, affectionate, quiet voiced, adaptable, playful, not big jumpers and climbers, get along well with children and other cats, and best as indoor cats. Himalayan cats are considered on average a bit more active than Persian cats due to infusion of Siamese blood.

Normal Breed Variations

Need to watch food intake and exercise to prevent obesity.

Heavy shedding especially when coat changes.

B Blood Type: There is geographic variation in prevalence of B blood type cats, but overall, the trait is present at sufficient rates that blood typing should be done prior to mating or transfusions. In a study of blood type distribution in the USA, Persian cats (n=230) had 9.6% type B blood.[1] In another American study, 41/170 or 24% were B type.[2] Prevalence of 14% type B was also reported.[3] In a small UK survey, 12% were type B cats.[4]

Epiphora: Secondary to face conformation rather than due to any unusual anatomic defects in the lower punctum.[5]

B Blood Type: There is geographic variation in prevalence of B blood type cats, but overall, the trait is present at sufficient rates that blood typing should be done prior to mating or transfusions. In a study of blood type distribution in the USA, Persian cats (n=230) had 9.6% type B blood.[1] In another American study, 41/170 or 24% were B type.[2] Prevalence of 14% type B was also reported.[3] In a small UK survey, 12% were type B cats.[4]

Epiphora: Secondary to face conformation rather than due to any unusual anatomic defects in the lower punctum.[44]

Hair coat genetics: The long hair phenotype in cats is a recessive Mutation (AM412646:c.194C>A) Somali, Persian, Maine Coon, Ragdoll.[6]

Drug Sensitivities

None reported in the literature

Inherited Diseases

Autosomal Dominant Polycystic Kidney Disease (ADPKD): This condition leads to formation of cysts within the kidney parenchyma, and is often associated with eventual renal failure. Cyst size and number gradually increase over time in most cats. PKD is the most commonly seen inherited disorder in cats, affecting approximately 38% of Persian cats worldwide, and since there is a large population of Persian cats (Persian and Persian-related cats are about 80% of the cat fancy), about 6% of all cats have this disorder.

Recently the gene for autosomal dominant PKD (ADPKD) has been identified. No homozygotes have been seen which suggests two copies of this gene lead to *in utero* lethality.[5] A genetic test is available.

Signs of the condition are variable in age of onset and degree of expression/rate of progression. Even within closely related families, expression can be significantly different. Multiple cysts may be found in both medulla and cortex. Smooth and round, and of variable size, these hypoechoic structures can be easily visualized with ultrasound using a 7.5 MHz transducer (10 MHz in kittens). By ultrasound evaluation, it was determined that in some kittens as young as 7 weeks old, cysts were already present. Many cats have good longevity, while about one quarter of seriously affected cats die before 5 years of age. Those living a full lifespan may harbor a few small cysts, so normal health does not preclude presence of cystic condition.[7]

Age of onset of clinically significant renal disease ranges from 3-10 years, with a mean of 7 years of age. Concurrent tubulo-interstitial nephritis of variable severity and distribution occurs. Neither the brachycephalic head conformation nor longhair genes segregate with the PKD gene. No increased probability of hypertension was reported associated with ADPKD.[8]

Another study reported increased mean arterial pressure (MAP) and aldosterone:renin ratio in Persians over 4 years of age with PKD.[9]

Note that absence of cysts at 6 months of age is strongly correlated with a low risk of development of cysts in the future.[10] Note that cysts may also be found in the liver and pancreas in some cats.[5] In a study in the Netherlands, of 27 affected cats, 68% had cystic changes in the liver or congenital hepatic fibrosis, and pancreatic cysts or pancreatic fibrosis.[11] One report mentions associated peritoneoperi-cardial hernias.[12] That same report suggests that for screening purposes, the cutoff for positive PKD status be set at three or more cysts found in two kidneys by US evaluation. Cysts range in size from 1 mm to over 1 cm, and as they grow, pressure on the surrounding tissues leads to dysfunction—renomegaly and renodynia may occur. Late stage, the surface of the kidney may become irregular.[13] Cysts derive from both distal and proximal nephron.[14] Persian cat ADPKD strongly resembles ADPKD in humans.[15]

Feline Hypertrophic Cardiomyopathy (HCM): The pattern of inheritance is unclear in this breed. Left ventricular outflow obstruction, left ventricular (LV) diastolic dysfunction, LV wall/septum hypertrophy, myocardial hypertrophy, interstitial fibrosis and ischemia lead to typical signs of heart failure; also may see aortic thromboembolism. Dyspnea and crackles, arrhythmias, and murmurs are typical findings.[16] Persian cats are overrepresented so perhaps there is a genetic influence. Average age of onset is 6.5 years. Over 75% of cases are in males, usually sudden death or acute left sided heart failure is the terminal event. Concurrent pulmonary edema is distributed in a patchy pattern diffusely through the lung field (not necessarily perihilar, as is typical in dogs), and they are not usually hypothermic. Histologic examination shows one quarter of cats have myofiber disarray. Growth hormone excess may play a role in this condition.[17]

In a study of a partially inbred colony of cats with Persian ancestry, plasma atrial natriuretic factor was elevated; an autosomal dominant inheritance was suspected.[18]

PDA: Increased breed incidence was reported; may be associated with septal and valvular defects.[19]

Congenital Portosystemic Vascular Shunts: Persian and Himalayan together accounted for 16% of cases out of 98 cats in one report. Signs were noted by 6 months of age; a single extrahepatic portocaval anomaly was the most common type of defect seen.[20]

Neonatal Isoerythrolysis (NI): Prevalence of B blood type makes NI a concern in this breed. All B type cats have circulating anti-A antibodies and even primiparous queens carry these. Type B queens bred to type A toms can result in fatal red cell lysis in A blood type offspring with undetected NI. Kittens with NI can be distinguished from other fading kittens because of pigmenturia; anemia and icterus will also be present; not all kittens at risk for NI will develop overt clinical symptoms.[2] The proportion of matings at risk for NI was reported to be 0.12.[21]

FIP Susceptibility: Pedigree analysis indicated a high heritability (> 0.54) in a selection of catteries, with perhaps a polygenic trait controlling susceptibility to development of clinical FIP. There was no correlation between FIP death and inbreeding.[22]

FeLV Susceptibility: Feline leukocyte antigen (FLA), important for control of immune response, is represented by a set of genes and polymorphism here may play a role in susceptibility.[23]

Disease Predispositions

Corneal Sequestration (SYN: Black body or cornea nigrum): In early phases, an amber colored corneal stromal opacity may be noted. It gradually develops distinct raised borders; the surrounding cornea is cloudy and neovascularized; chemosis, blepharospasm, mucopurulent ocular discharge, and hyperemic conjunctivae may also be noted. Surface of sequestrum does not stain with fluorescein dye but does retain rose bengal stain. Exophthalmic conformation is thought to play a role in susceptibility.[24] It is central or paracentral in distribution, and Persian cats are over-represented. When matured, this is a brown to black pigmented lesion; often surrounded by a loose collarette of poorly adherent corneal epithelium. Lesions may extend into shallow or deep stroma, or even to Descemet's membrane. Sloughing and corneal healing may take 2-6 months; surgical debridement is an option.[44] Most often they are unilateral, but can be bilateral; it is a corneal stromal necrosis.

Topical glucocorticoids are contraindicated; some cases may be associated with feline herpesvirus infection; if suspected, do a PCR test for the virus on excised black body tissue. Recurrence, or involvement of the second eye in previously unilateral cases may occur.[25] Mean age of affected Persians is 5 1/2 years.[26]

Non-healing Corneal Ulcers: In a retrospective study of cats with refractory ulcers, the Persian was found to be overrepresented. These indolent ulcers involve only the superficial epithelium and unless complicated, do not extend into the stroma. During extended treatment regimens averaging 5 weeks, the same cats were also predisposed to corneal sequestration.[27]

Cervical Neck Lesions: Increased risk for Persian cats was reported. Of cats with in one study, 47% afflicted were Persians.[28]

Lower Urinary Tract Disease: Increased risk of calcium oxalate urolithiasis was reported.[29] A retrospective study (3,498 urolithiasis cases) found increased risk for calcium oxalate (CaOx) uroliths but reduced risk for forming Magnesium Ammonium Phosphate (MAP or struvite) crystals.[30] Persian cats were found to be 3.2 times more likely to develop CaOx stones, and 1.4 times as likely to develop MAP as cats of other breeds in another report.[31]

In a retrospective analysis of 22,908 LUTD cases (1980-1997), Persian cats were reported to be at increased risk of congenital defects as well.[32] A new type of uroliths was reported, consisting of Mg, K, and inorganic pyrophosphate; a possible dysfunction of the pyrophosphate-hydrolyzing alkaline phosphatase enzyme was proposed (perhaps a genetic defect) as a reason for the novel stone structure.[33]

Dystocia: A survey of 2,928 litters of multiple cat breeds was carried out to ascertain prevalence of dystocia, and over-representation of Persian breed cats was found. There were 939 Persian litters analyzed. Average dystocia rate in a mixed breed colony was 0.4%, and 7.5% in the Persian group.[34]

Cryptorchidism: There is some variation between practitioners on the cutoff age to be considered failure to descend. A common definition of cryptorchidism is when testes fail to descend into the scrotum by 7-8 months of age. Persian cats were the breed with the highest reported incidence of cryptorchidism, accounting for 20% of cases in one study.[35] In a study (1980-89) of 1,345 cats admitted for orchiectomy, 29% of Persians were cryptorchid versus 1.4% in non-Persians.[36]

Brachycephalic Syndrome: A flat-face conformation and rounded skull can result in stenotic nares, jaw changes, elongated soft palate, and distorted nasopharynx.[37] Because of the sedentary lifestyle of cats, many cats can live with this conformational defect, but in severe cases surgical therapy is required.

Transfusion Reactions: Due to prevalence of B blood type, natural allo-antibodies markedly increase the risk of transfusion reactions so donors and recipients should be blood typed.

Idiopathic Facial Dermatitis (Dirty Faced Persians): In the UK, and sporadically in the US, black exudates that mat in hair and on skin, with frequent self excoriation secondary to pruritis, and associated skin erythema have been noted. Often ceruminous otitis externa is present simultaneously. A genetic basis is suspected; histology shows dyskeratotic basal epithelial cells, acanthosis and crusting with mixed inflammatory infiltrate and sebaceous hyperplasia.[38] Mean age of onset is 1 year of age, with a symmetric pattern around eyes, mouth, chin and ears, and may be associated with submandibular lymphadenopathy. Mucoid ocular discharge may be noted. Though inflammatory cells are often noted, and bacteria and yeast may be isolated, the condition is not antibiotic or glucocorticoids responsive.[39]

Separation Anxiety Syndrome: Of a study group of 136 cats, Persians accounted for 12% of the cats. Associated clinical signs in Persians were that females urinated, and males urinated and defecated out of place.[40]

Hereditary Deafness: Is associated with the dominant gene for white cat (W); may be found in white cats of this breed.[41]

Hip Dysplasia (HD): This condition is much more prevalent than was previously thought. In a 1998 report, in a nonrandom group of 78 cats of different breeds, 32% of this pooled group of cats, and 60% of Persians had HD using OFA-like criteria. A positive correlation with joint laxity and HD was identified.[42] A study (1991-1995) found that based on VD hip radiographs, (684 Cats, 12 breeds) HD prevalence was 5.8% in unregistered versus 12.3% in purebred cats. Persian cats had a 15.8% rate (3/19). Classic radiographic signs were found to be different than in dogs, with minimal remodeling of the femoral neck. Instead, shallow acetabulum and remodeling of the cranio-dorsal acetabular rim were noted.[43]

Rare and Isolated Reports

Chédiak–Higashi Syndrome: Chediak-Higashi has an autosomal recessive inheritance pattern. This condition affects dilute blue smoke Persian cats. Iris is pale and yellow-green, thin, and the fundus hypopigmented due to loss of retinal pigmented epithelial cells. CHS also leads to tapetal cell dysmaturity and gradual loss of tapetal cells leading to lack of visible tapetum. Cataracts may also form. A membrane defect is thought to be the underlying defect in CHS, leading to increased unsaturated fatty acid levels.[44]

Essentially a lysosomal defect is associated with this dilute partial oculocutaneous albinism. CHS is associated with bleeding tendency, and granules staining pink to magenta with Romanowsky stain in leukocytes. Also granules are present in melanocytes. Bleeding tendency is due to a platelet storage pool deficiency.[45] Cats may be photophobic, and mild neutrophilia may also occur. Cats with this condition should not enter breeding programs. Normal lifespan is expected.

Alpha Mannosidosis: Lysosomal enzyme α-mannosidase deficiency, an autosomal recessive disorder, leads to progressive storage disease. Leukocyte morphology changes include vacuolation of lymphocytes and monocytes. Cells such as neurons accumulate partially processed N-linked oligosaccharides.[46] Signs begin in the first month of life and are progressive, with death frequently occurring a few months later. Tremors, facial dysmorphia, ataxia, seizures, reduced vision (cataracts), organomegaly, behavior changes and skeletal deformities may occur. Three families of Persians have been reported with this rare storage disease (in the USA, Switzerland, and Belgium). The mutation was characterized, and resulted in zero enzyme activity.

In DSH cats, milder phenotype and 2% enzyme activity has been reported.[47]

Corneal opacification may result in frosted appearance of the eyes by 11 weeks of age; marked pathology occurs in the RPE, but is not visualized clinically. Lens shows characteristic Y-suture pattern of cataract—appearance is granular to feathery.[48]

Entropion: Suspected to be hereditary, present at an early age; high prevalence in Persian; all or part of lower palpebral margin is affected, and is often bilateral.[44,49]

Eyelid agenesis: Most commonly seen in the temporal upper palpebral.[44]

Cataracts: Congenital or juvenile cataracts have been reported.[44]

Heterochromia Iridis: Variations in iris and retinal pigment epithelium and choroid may occur.[44]

Retinal Degeneration: Begins as foci of hyperreflective tapetum, then coalesce to become generalized; leading to blindness.[44] In one report, two litters from the same parents developed visual deficits, and fundus abnormalities on ophthalmoscope exams were noted by a few months of age. Diffuse outer segment degeneration occured.[49]

A recent report strongly suggests this is an autosomal recessive rod cone dysplasia. By 3 weeks of age in offspring of homozygous cross with heterozygous parents, pupillary light reflexes were abnormal, by 6 weeks the tapetum hyperreflective, and by 15 weeks of age, the retinal degeneration was advanced; all were blind by 16 weeks old.[50]

Hyperlipoproteinemia/Hyperlipidemia: Pattern is familial. High circulating triglycerides and hyperchylomicronemia occur. Signs may include: iridocyclitis, lipemia retinalis (pink or creamy retinal vasculature), xanthomata (lipid granulomas of skin), and lipid aqueous humour. Nerves may become impinged due to xanthomata, leading to paresis or paralysis.[51]

Anterior chamber contents may have a creamy or white appearance when hyperchylomicronemia is present, and opalescence when hypertriglyceridemia alone is present. Arcus lipoids cornea and lipid keratopathy can also be seen with hyperlipoproteinemia.[52] Uveitis has also been described.

Concurrent atherosclerosis of abdominal vessels, aorta and coronary vessels also occurred. Deficiency of lipoprotein lipase enzyme is thought to be the underlying defect responsible for the hyperlipoproteinemias.[53]

In another report of kittens with severe hypertriglyceridemia, anemia was also evident.[54]

Dystrophic Epidermolysis Bullosa: This is a collagen VII defect leading to reduced anchoring fibrils, so trauma leads to formation of blisters that progress to ulcers; an easily torn off skin is the result. Sloughing of foot pads and oral mucosa occurs in addition to loss of hairy skin.[55]

Primary Hereditary Seborrhea Oleosa: First signs are noted at only 2-3 days of age and are severe and quickly progressive, with no coat color predilection. Greasy, scaly skin and a rancid odor are present. Orthokeratotic hyperkeratosis is found on biopsy. A primary keratinization defect is thought to be the underlying condition. To date, no effective treatment options have been reported.[56]

Multiple eyelid cysts: Histology is similar to apocrine hidrocystomas of humans. In one report, these were described as multilocular cysts; PAS+, diastase resistant granules were seen in the cytoplasm of affected cells. Blepharospasm, epiphora and masses/color changes of eyelids were the chief complaints.[57] In another case, unilocular cysts in a senior Persian were reported and were characterized as cystadenomas.[58]

Progressive Retinal Atrophy PRA: Kittens are 2-3 weeks of age at onset, autosomal recessive. By about 4 months of age, they have severe photoreceptor loss.[59]

Miscellaneous: Dermatophytosis, Otitis Externa, Umbilical Hernia, Peritoneopericardial hernia, Portosystemic Shunt, Cryptorchidism, Lymphocytic Cholangitis, Hemophilia A.[60]

Genetic Tests

Mannosidosis Genetic (Direct) Test

Josephine Deubler Genetic Testing Laboratory, (PennGen) at the University of Pennsylvania Veterinary Hospital offers testing.

Minimum of 1-2 ml EDTA blood processed within 48 hours. Is not necessary to cool; and do avoid freezing. Test request form is available online. Can do concurrent blood typing on the same sample. Can also submit a pair of buccal swabs for testing. http://research.vet.upenn.edu/SubmitaSample/tabid/554/Default.aspx

PKD: Direct genetic test is available at UC-Davis VGL and the Animal Health Trust.

Ultrasound screening of kidneys should be done with transducer of 7.5 MHz for adults, 10 MHz for kittens. In older cats, cysts are larger and thus easier to detect. Typical findings are spherical cysts with smooth sharp outline, anechoic internally, with through transmission of larger cysts.[9] Recommend scan breeding stock at 10 months of age in 2 planes; both kidneys, and again at 2 years old if early US is equivocal (single cyst or a few in one kidney only), or if negative since may not pick up PKD at 10 months of age if very small cysts or no changes. In some patients, renomegaly may be visible on routine radiographs. Because of prevalence, breeding PKD positive cats to negative cats may be necessary for a while to prevent gene pool diversity loss.[61]

Blood type before transfusions or mating are recommended.

Miscellaneous

- **Breed name synonyms:** Himalayan, Himalayan-Persian, Longhair, Longhaired Exotic, Khmer (historical, Europe), British Longhair
- **Registries:** FIFé, TICA (separate from Himalayan here), CFA, *ACFA (separate from Himalayan), *CFF (separate from Himalayan here; chocolate and lavender are known as Kashmir). GCCF (division includes colourpoint, exotic SH), ACF (includes colourpoints), WCF (provisional Persian/Himalayan category), NZCF (colourpoints in here), CCA (Himalayan separate)
  CFF and ACFA distinguish between Peke-faced and standard Persian.
- **Breed resources:** The Atlantic Himalayan Club: http://www.himalayan.org/links.htm
  CFA Persian Breed Council: www.persianbc.org
  The Feline PKD Homepage: www.felinepkd.com/
  United Silver and Golden Fanciers Online: http://www.unitedsilverandgoldenfanciers.com/

References

1. Giger U, Griot-Wenk M, Bucheler J, et al. Geographical variation of the feline blood type frequencies in the United States. *Fel Pract* 1991;19(6):21-27.

2. Giger U, Bucheler J, Patterson DF. Frequency and inheritance of A and B blood types in feline breeds of the United States. *J Hered* 1991;82:15-20.

3. Giger U. In: Bonagura J, ed. *Kirk's Current Veterinary Therapy XIII.* Philadelphia: WB Saunders Co, 2000;396-399.

4. Knottenbelt CM Addie DD Day MJ Mackin AJ. Determination of the prevalence of feline blood types in the UK. *J Small Anim Pract* 1999;40:115-118.

5. Lyons LA, Biller DS, Erdman CA, et al.. Feline polycystic kidney disease mutation identified in PKD1. *J Am Soc Nephrol* 2004;15:2548-2555.

6. Drögemüller C, Rüfenacht S, Wichert B, Leeb T. Mutation within the FGF5 gene are associated with hair length in cats. *Animal Genet* 2007 JUN;38(3):218-221.

7. Cooper KC, Piveral P. Autosomal dominant polycystic disease in Persian cats. *Fel Pract* 2000;28(2):20-21.

8. DiBartola SP. Autosomal dominant polycystic kidney disease. *Proceedings.* 18th Annual ACVIM Forum. Seattle WA 2000:438-440.

9. Pedersen KM, Pedersen HD, Häggström, J, et al. Increased mean arterial pressure and aldosterone-to-renin ratio in Persian cats with polycystic disease. *JVIM* 2003;17(1):21-27.

10. DiBartola SP. Familial renal diseases of cats. *Proceedings.* The North American Veterinary Conference 1999:326-327.

11. Bosje JT, van den Ingh TSGAM, van der Linde-Simpson JS. Polycystic kidney and liver disease in cats. *Vet Q* 1998;20(4):136-140.

12. Malik R. Genetic Diseases of Cats (and Dogs). *Proceedings.* University of Sydney Post Graduate Foundation in Veterinary Science. Valentine Charlton Refresher Course for Veterinarians; Cats 2000. 2000;Jul;27-37.

13. Lyons LA, Biller DS. Autosomal dominant polycystic disease in Persian and Persian-related cats. *Proceedings.* Tuft's Canine and Feline Breeding and Genetics Conference Oct 2-4, 2003 Available at VIN: www.vin.com/tufts/2003. Accessed Nov 23, 2004.

14. Eaton KA, Biller DS, DiBartola SP, et al. Autosomal dominant polycystic kidney disease in Persian and Persian-cross cats. *Vet Pathol* 1997;34:117-126.

15. Biller DS, DiBartola SP, Eaton KA, et al. Inheritance of polycystic kidney disease in Persian cats. *J Hered* 1996;87:1-5.

16. Medinger TL, Bruyette DS. Feline hypertrophic cardiomyopathy. *Compend Contin Educ Pract Vet* 1992;14(4):479-490.

17. Atkins CE. Feline hypertrophic cardiomyopathy. Winter 2004 AAFP Meeting. Proceedings [*abstr*] in: *AAFP Newsletter* August 2004 22(2):30-31.

18. Martin L, VandeWoude S, Boon D, et al. Left ventricular hypertrophy in a closed colony of Persian cats. 12th Annual ACVIM Veterinary Medical Forum, San Francisco CA. [*abstr*] in: *JVIM* 1994;8(2):143.

19. Hoskins JD. Congenital defects in cats. *Compend Contin Educ Pract Vet* 1995;17(3):385-405.

20. Levy JK. Congenital Portosystemic vascular shunts in cats: 98 cases. First International Feline Genetic Disease Conference Philadelphia June, 1998 *Proceedings (abstr)* in: *Fel Pract Suppl,* 1999:30.

21. Giger U, Casal M, Niggemeier A. The fading kitten syndrome and neonatal isoerythrolysis. *Proceedings.* The 15th Annual ACVIM Medical Forum, Lake Buena Vista FL 1997;308-310.

22. Foley JE, Pedersen NC. The inheritance of susceptibility to feline infectious peritonitis in purebred catteries. *Fel Pract* 1996;24(1):14-22.

23. Addie DD, Kennedy LJ, Ryvar R, et al. Feline leucocyte antigen class II polymorphism and susceptibility to feline infectious peritonitis. *J Fel Med Surg* 2004;6:59-62.

24. Pentlarge VW. Corneal sequestration in cats. *Compend Contin Educ Pract Vet* 1989;11(1):24-32.

25. Glaze MB. Feline corneal diseases: Part II. *Proceedings.* The 70th Annual AAHA Conference. 2003;1:367-368.

26. Featherstone HJ, Sansom J. Feline corneal sequestra: a review of 64 cases (80 eyes) from 1993 to 2000. *Vet Ophthalmol* 2004;Jul-Aug;7(4):213-227.

27. La Croix NC, van der Woerdt A, Olivero DK. Nonhealing corneal ulcers in cats: 29 cases (1991-1999). *J Am Vet Med Assoc* 2001;18(5) :733-735.

28. van Wessum R, Harvey, CE, Hennet P. Feline dental resorptive lesions-prevalence patterns. *Vet Clin North Am: Sm Anim Pract* 1992;22:1405-1416.

29. Houston DM, Moore AEP, Favrin MG, Hoff B. Feline urethral plugs and bladder uroliths: A review of 5484 submissions 1998-2003. *Can Vet J* 2003;Dec;44(12):974-977.

30. Thumchai R, Lulich J, Osborne CA, et al. Epizootiologic evaluation of urolithiasis in cats: 3,498 cases (1982-1992). *J Am Vet Med Assoc* 1996;208(4):547-551.

31. Lekcharoensuk C, Lulich JP, Osborne CA, Koehler LA, Urlich LK, Carpenter KA, Swanson LL. Association between patient-related factors and risk of calcium oxalate and magnesium ammonium phosphate urolithiasis in cats. *J Am Vet Med Assoc* 2000;Aug15;217(4):520-525.

32. Lekcharoensuk C, Osborne CA, Lulich JP. Epidemiologic study of risk factors for lower urinary tract diseases in cats. *J Am Vet Med Assoc* 2001;218(9):1429-1435.

33. Frank A, Norrestam R, Sjodin A. A new urolith in four cats and one dog: composition and crystal structure. *J Biol Inorg Chem* 2002;Apr;7(4-5):437-44.

34. Gunn-Moore DA, Thrusfield MV. Feline dystocia: prevalence, and association with cranial conformation and breed. *Vet Rec* 1995;136:350-353.

35. Richardson EF, Mullen H. Cryptorchidism in cats. *Compend Contin Educ Pract Vet* 1993;15(10):1342-1369.

36. Millis DL, Hauptman JG, Johnson CA. Cryptorchidism and monorchism in cats: 25 cases (1980-1989). *J Am Vet Med Assoc* 1992;200(8):1128-1130.

37. Griffon DJ. Upper airway obstruction in cats: Pathogenesis and clinical signs. *Compend Contin Educ Pract Vet* 2000;22(9):822-827.

38. Bond R, Curtis CF, Ferguson EA, et al. An idiopathic facial dermatitis of Persian cats. *Vet Dermatol* 2000;11(1):35-41.

39. Takle GL, Hnilica KA. Eight emerging feline dermatoses. *Vet Med May* 2004:456-467.

40. Schwartz S. Separation anxiety syndrome in cats. 136 cases (1991-2000). *J Am Vet Med Assoc* 2002;220(7):1028-1033.

41. Strain GM. Hereditary deafness in dogs and cats: causes, prevalence, and current research. *Proceedings.* Tuft's Canine and Feline Breeding and Genetics Conference. Oct 2-4, 2003. Available at: http://www.vin.com/tufts/2003. Accessed Nov 19, 2004.

42. Lagenbach A, Giger U, Green P, et al. Relationship between degenerative joint disease and hip joint laxity by use of distraction index and Norberg angle measurement in a group of cats. *J Am Vet Med Assoc* 1998;213(10):1439-1443.

43. Keller GG, Reed AL, Lattimer JC, Corley EA. Hip dysplasia: A feline population study. *Veterinary Radiology & Ultrasound* 1999;40(4):460-464.

44. Narfström K. Hereditary and congenital ocular disease in the cat. *J Fel Med Surg* 1999;1:135-141.

45. Callan MB, Griot-Wenk M, Hackner S, et al. Hereditary thrombopathies ca using bleeding in two domestic shorthair cats. First International Feline Genetic Disease Conference Philadelphia June, 1998 *Proceedings (abstr)* in: *Fel Pract Suppl,* 1999:32.

46. Alroy J, Freden GO, Goyal V, Raghavan SS, Schunk KL. Morphology of leukocytes from cats affected with alpha-mannosidosis and Mucopolysac¬charidosis VI (MPS VI). *Vet Pathol* 1989;26:294-302.

47. Berg T, Tollersrud OK, Walkley SU, et al. Purification of feline lysosomal alpha-mannosidase, determination of its cDNA sequence and identification of a mutation causing alpha-mannosidosis in Persian cats. *Biochem J* 1997;328:863-870.

48. Aguirre G, Ray J, Haskins M. Ocular manifestations of inherited metabolic diseases in cats. *Proceedings.* The 25th Annual Meeting of the ACVO, Oct 26-30, 1994:28-29.

49. Peiffer RL. Inherited ocular diseases of the dog and cat. *Compend Cont Educ Pract Vet* 1982;4(2):152-164.

50. Rah HC, Maggs DJ, Blankenship T, et al. Characterization of early onset of retinal degeneration in Persian cats. *Proceedings.* Tuft's Canine and Feline Breeding and Genetics Conference. Oct 2-4, 2003. Available at: http://www.vin.com/tufts/2003. Accessed Nov 19, 2004.

51. Jones BR. Inherited hyperchylomicronaemia in the cat. *J Small Anim Pract* 1993;34:493-499.

52. Crispin SM. Ocular manifestations of hyperlipoproteinaemia. *J Small Anim Pract* 1993;34:500-506.

53. Wisselink MA, Koeman JP, Wensing TH, et al. Hyperlipoproteinaemia associated with atherosclerosis and Cutaneous Xanthomatosis in a cat. *Vet Q* 1994;16(4):199-202.

54. Gunn-Moore DA, Watson TDG, Dodkin SJ, Blaxter AC, Crispin SM, Gruffydd-Jones TJ. Transient hyperlipidaemia and anaemia in kittens. *Vet Rec* 1997;140:355-359.

55. Olivry T, Dunston SM, Markinkovich MP. Reduced anchoring fibril formation and collagen VII immunoreactivity in feline dystrophic epidermolysis bullosa. *Vet Pathol* 1999;36:616-618.

56. DeManuelle T. Feline dermatopathies: Newly described disorders. *Proceedings.* 70th Annual AAHA Conference Proceedings 2003;1:93-95.

57. Chaitman J, van der Woerdt A, Bartick TE. Multiple eyelid cysts resembling apocrine hidrocystomas in three Persian cats and one Himalayan cat. *Vet Pathol* 1999;36:474-476

58. Cantaloube B, Raymond-Letron I, Regnier A. Multiple eyelid apocrine hidrocystomas in two Persian cats. *Vet Ophthalmol* 2004;Mar-Apr;7(2):121-125.

59. Rah H, Maggs DJ, Blankenship TN, Narfstrom K, Lyons LA. Early-onset autosomal recessive progressive retinal atrophy in Persian cats. *Invest Ophthalmol Vis Sci.* 2005;46(5):1742-7.

60. Feline Advisory Beaureau accessed online August 2010 at: http://www.fabcats.org/breeders/inherited_disorders/persian.php

61. Little S. Selected inherited diseases of the cat, in *Proceedings.* International Ragdoll Congress Oct, 2004. Pers. Comm., 2005.

Recommended Reading

Glaze MB Congenital and hereditary ocular abnormalities in cats. *Clin Tech Small Anim Pract.* 2005 May;20(2):74-82.

Pixiebob

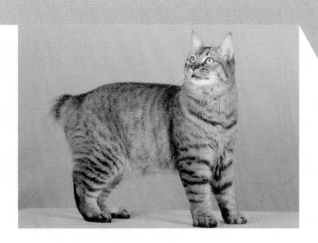

The Breed History

This breed was developed in America to be a bobcat look-alike. The breed was developed from domestic cats. Though some report wild Bobcat blood in the breed, DNA evidence does not support inclusion of wildcat blood. In 1984 *Pixie*, a founding female was bred in Washington State. Outcrossing to wild cats and pedigreed cats is not allowed, though outcrossing to approved **legend** cats (native brown tabby unregistered domestic cats with appropriate traits) is allowed. TICA first accepted them as a provisional breed in 1994, with full championship status in 1998.

Physical Characteristics

Weight: 10-18 lb (4.5-8 kg), some males larger.

Coat: The Pixie-Bob coat has extensive ticking and in the shorthair, is quite short and dense. The coat is soft, and has elastic resilience. There is a longhaired (actually a medium length coat) Pixie-Bob, and the texture of that coat is soft and close lying. The longhair should not have any ruff but mutton chops may be present. Random light to medium brown tabby spotting is ideal; base color is mouse grey; color may change quite a bit with the changing of the seasons. Spots should be small, plus or minus a rosette. Classic and marble tabbies also occur and are considered pet quality. Coat is water resistant.

Eyes: A softly triangular shape, the eyes are deep-set with an intense gaze, are medium sized, and hooded brows above are prominent. A gold or brown eye is preferred though the green color referred to as Gooseberry is accepted.

Points of Conformation: The large Pixie-Bob head is pear shaped, with strong mascara markings and spectacles around the eyes. Chin is white. Ears are set wide, with round tips; lynx tipping is preferred; moderate in size. Nose is wide and slightly convex in profile, and the muzzle is moderate in length; break is evident. Body is a heavy build, prominent scapulae, flank is deep, chest is wide, and they are large in overall size. Limbs are long and well boned and muscled. Polydactyl cats are accepted (seven digit maximum). The tail is usually about two inches long, but may extend to a maximum of six inches; a kink or curl does not disqualify. When rear limbs are extended, the tail should not reach past the tarsus. Paws are large, round and compact. Pixie-bobs possess a typical rolling gait. A belly pouch is evident.

Grooming: Low grooming needs for this breed, low tendency to mat.

Recognized Behavior Issues and Traits

Reported breed characteristics include: Affectionate, quiet, "one man dog" cat, not particularly adaptable to changing homes; seem to wag their short tail during play. They like to rule the home, so sometimes best not to be with other pets. Curious, easily trained; play fetch and leash walks. Good with children. Tend to make chatter and chirp noises rather than typical cat meows. May be somewhat cautious with strangers, and requires more attention than some other breeds of cats.

Normal Breed Variations

None reported in the literature

Drug Sensitivities

None reported in the literature

Inherited Diseases

None reported in the literature

Disease Predispositions

Pancreatitis-anecdotal

Genetic Tests

None available commercially

Miscellaneous

- **Breed name synonyms:** Bobcat
- **Registries:** TICA (LH and SH separated), CCA
- **Breed resources: The Official Pixie-Bob Site:** http://www.pixie-bob.org/

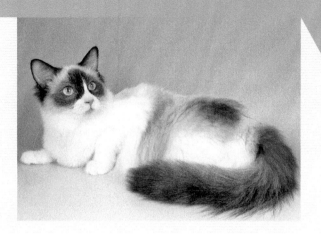

The Breed History

For this recently developed breed there is a considerable lack of consensus as to the exact origins of early progenitors. What is proposed is that in the 1960s this breed arose in California as a result of a breeder starting with two foundation males, *Raggedy Ann Daddy Warbucks* and another she called *Blackie*. Both of these were offspring of *Josephine*, a white (Persian or Turkish Angora type) cat; *Warbucks* and *Blackie* were fathered by two different sires. Those sires continue to be an unknown, with one theory reporting that it was a Persian that had Birman type markings and others saying the white Persian was crossed with a seal point Birman in one of the progenitor crosses, and that this offspring was bred with a sable Burmese. The coat texture does not match Persian cats, so at some point it is likely either Birman or Burmese, or perhaps both were crossed with the white Persian-type, or perhaps this occurred at another point in breed development.

The Ragdoll name derives from the tendency to be calm, resulting in relaxed muscle tone when handled. They have become a popular breed. In TICA, 2002 registration numbers topped 23000 and this breed was fourth in popularity in that registry behind Maine Coon, Persian, and the Bengal. In CFA, recent registration placed this breed twelfth in popularity with much smaller numbers registered (761). No outcrosses are allowed in CFA. The FiFé recognized the breed in 1992 and the GCCF in 1991. The Ragamuffin is a more recently developed breed of cats that utilized some Ragdoll influence in development. Though the Ragdoll breed has a resemblance to the Birman, the latter is a smaller cat, is produced in only the mitted pattern and possesses a less angulated face.

Physical Characteristics

Weight: Female 10-14 lb (4.5-6 kg), male 12-20 lb (5.5-9 kg)

Coat patterns include:

Pointed: Colorpoint is accepted in CFF in Siamese colors of chocolate, seal, lilac and blue. The CFA adds red and cream. The TICA registry adds others such as cinnamon, and fawn. Hairs may be solid, shaded, or smoke; points solid, lynx, tortie.
Van: Ears, tail and upper mask pigmented, ideally the rest of the cat is white though up to 20% body colored is accepted in CFA. This pattern can be shown in CFA.
Mitted: (white on forefeet to carpus-gloving gene), on rear limbs up and over the hock (gauntlet) and white at ruff and chin (not shown in CFA, but are registered)

Ragdoll

Bi-color: (inverted moderately symmetrical V mask on forehead, in white, that includes whisker pads and extends contiguously under chin, chest, along underside). White feet are mitted due to the gloving gene. The color of the point of the ears determines the assigned coat color. This pattern may be shown in CFA.

Haircoat: The semi-long haircoat is fine and glossy. Hair is shorter on head and forelimbs. Some describe the coat as having a minimal wooly undercoat (CFA profile), but other sources describe the coat as single. This coat is described as "rabbit fur" in texture because it is so fine. The coat can take up to two years to mature. Body color can be deeper than in the traditional colorpoint breeds. Coat color tends to darken with age.

Eyes: Blue-vivid, moderately large sized, oval.

Points of Conformation: These are large cats, heavy-set build both in fore and rear. A modified wedge shaped medium sized skull, full muzzle and a medium to short straight nose, and wide set ears are medium - large sized with rounded tips. Paws are large, round, and body musculature is well developed. Tail is long and bushy and tapers slightly. Legs are long, with hind limbs being longer than the forelegs.

Grooming: These cats have low tendency to mat. They have low-moderate grooming needs. They have a moderate shedding tendency only. A steel comb or other tool can be used gently twice a week.

Recognized Behavior Traits

Reported breed characteristics include: Very quiet cats, affectionate, extremely docile, playful, and enjoy human contact. Reduced hunting and fighting instincts are apparently selected for in a typical Ragdoll cat. Name derives from their tendency to be very placid and relax when handled (though they do not "flop", or lose all muscle tone). Some may follow people around and are sociable with children and other pets. Adaptable, and will leash train easily. Excellent pets in households with seniors, other pets and children. Not much for climbing and jumping around the home, more accurately a lap cat. They are also soft voiced cats. Good for apartment life.

Normal Breed Variations

Tend to obesity so need to watch caloric intake

Slow to mature (takes three to four years)

B Blood Type: Ragdoll cats tested as part of a survey in the UK were found to be 28.6% blood type B, though the number of cats of this breed tested was very small (n=7).[1]

Ragdoll Kitten Information Project:[2] An internet based survey was carried out to determine breed normal reproductive parameters.

232 litters, 121 litters, total kittens, 1,030
   Average litter size 4.4
   Stillbirth rate 5%
   C-sections 3.5%
   Average birth weight: Male 101 g female 96 g
   Congenital deformities, in 8.5% of litters: included cleft palate, split eyelid

The long hair phenotype in cats is a recessive so how it is distributed in the different longhaired breeds, and coded for is of interest.[3] Mutation (AM412646:c.194C>A) Somali, Persian, Maine Coon, Ragdoll.

Drug Sensitivities
None reported in the literature

Inherited Diseases

Feline Hypertrophic Cardiomyopathy (HCM): HCM is the most common cardiac condition in cats (10% prevalence). The only sign may be sudden death; also associated with arterial thromboembolisms.

A severe early onset form of HCM was identified in a retrospective study group of 10 Ragdoll cats (1997-1999). Cats were young (5 months to 2 years; mean age 15 months), and had severe concentric left ventricular hypertrophy. Six were in heart failure, the other 4 were asymptomatic. Seven of 10 cats were male. Most had interventricular septal hypertrophy, a bit less than half of the group had systolic anterior motion of the mitral valve, and in 7 cats, average left atrial systolic dimension was 1.97 cm; aortic root dimension was less than 0.85 cm in the same cats. Eight of ten cats had a systolic murmur upon auscultation.[4,5]

A novel MYBPC3 mutation has been found in Ragdoll cats. This mutation is in a different domain than that of the Maine Coon cat (see that chapter for more details). Two distinct and separate mutations in this gene have been identified in unrelated breeds so this is not likely a founder effect, but rather a novel mutation.[6]

Disease Predispositions

Arterial Thromboembolism: Ragdoll cats were overrepresented (odds ratio 14.4) in a population of 127 affected cats in a retrospective study of records done at the University of Minnesota Veterinary Medical Teaching Hospital (1992-2001). Most cats in the study had left atrial enlargement.[7]

Calcium Oxalate Urolithiasis: In one case control study from the University of Minnesota Urolith Center (1981-1997), it was reported that Ragdoll cats had an increased risk of developing this type of uroliths.[8]

FIP Susceptibility: An American Study found that Ragdoll cats were significantly over-represented for a diagnosis of FIP when they analyzed data for a 16 year period at a veterinary teaching hospital.[9]

Rare and Isolated Reports

Polycystic Kidney Disease (PKD): Is most common in Persian breeds and those breeds having out-crossed to Persians in their breeding programs. In screening programs carried out at University of California at Davis in 2002, a small group of Ragdoll cats was checked in a study (Clinic 3); two of 11 cats were positive for PKD; assessed by ultrasound screening of healthy cats from catteries.[10]

Genetic Tests

Though data are limited on prevalence breed-wide, ultrasound screening (annual) of breeding cats for hypertrophic cardiomyopathy starting before one year of age is recommended.

A genetic test for HCM is available from UC-Davis VGL and NC State Meurs Lab.

Blood type cats before transfusion or mating would be prudent—but this is also based on limited breed-wide data.

Miscellaneous

- **Breed name synonyms:** Rag, Mitted Cat, Josephine's Daughter, Daughters of Josephine, Cherubim, Doll.
- **Registries:** FIFé, TICA, ACFA, CFF, ACF, GCCF, WCF, CCA, NZCF, CFA
- **Breed resources: Ragdoll Fanciers Club International:** http://www.rfci.org/
  Ragdoll International (TICA): http://www.ragdollinternational.org/
  Ragdoll Fanciers Worldwide Club: http://rfwclub.org/
  The British Ragdoll Cat Club: http://www.tbrcc.co.uk/
  Ragdoll Connection Network: http://www.ragdoll-cats.com/
  Ragdolls of America Group: http://ragdollscfa.org/about_rag.shtml
  Ragdoll Breed Club (CFA): www.ragdollbreedclub.org

References
1. Knottenbelt CM, Addie DD, Jay MJ, et al. Determination of the prevalence of feline blood types in the UK. *J Small Anim Pract* 1999;40:115-118.
2. Little S. Breed Specific Reproduction Projects. In: *Notes*, University of California (Davis) Feline Genetics Extravaganza I July, 2003.
3. Drögemüller C, Rüfenacht S, Wichert B, Leeb T. Mutation within the FGF5 gene are associated with hair length in cats. Animal Genet 2007 JUN;38(3):218-221.
4. Ferguson GJ, Lefbom BK, Rosenthal SL, et al. Severe hypertrophic cardiomyopathy in 10 young Ragdoll cats, 19th Annu Meet ACVIM Vet Med Forum 2001 (abstr) In: *J Vet Intern Med* 2001;15(3):308.
5. Little S. Selected inherited diseases of the cat, in *Proceedings*. International Ragdoll Congress Oct, 2004. Available at: www.catvet. homestead.com/Inherited_Diseases_2004.pdf Accessed Nov 19, 2004.
6. Meurs KM, Norgard MM, Ederer MM, et al. A substitutionmutation in the myosin binding protein C gene in Ragdollhypertrophic cardiomyopathy. Genomics 2007;90:261–264
7. Smith SA, Tobias AH, Jacob KA, et al. Arterial thromboembolism in cats: Acute crisis in 127 cases (1992-2001) and long-term management with low-dose aspirin in 24 cases. *J Vet Intern Med* 2003;17:73-83.
8. Lekcharoensuk C, Lulich JP, Osborne CA, et al. Association between patient-related factors and risk of calcium oxalate and magnesium ammonium phosphate urolithiasis in cats. *J Am Vet Med Assoc* 2000;Aug15;217(4):520-525.
9. Pesteanu-Somogyi LD, Radzai C, Pressler BM. Prevalence of feline infectious peritonitis in specific cat breeds. *J Feline Med Surg.* 2006 Feb;8(1):1-5
10. Lyons LA. The Lyon's Den Feline Genome Project. http://www.vetmed. ucdavis.edu/Catgenetics/Feline_Genome_Project.html content present in 2004 now offline.

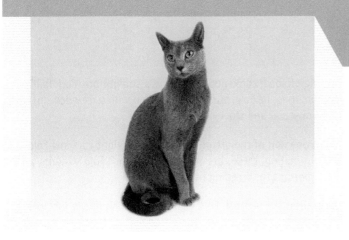

Russian Blue

families; need close human contact. Docile in nature, they get along well with other pets and children, and may shadow their owners. Easily startled, and some individuals are shy; many have a cautious nature; may be aloof with strangers. Not demanding of attention. A "smiling" demeanor is reported.

The Breed History

Originally thought to be from the Russian sea port of Archangel (Archangelsk Isle), first recorded specimens were brought to Western Europe in the late 1800s. The ancient Russian stock was feral. First show records in England date to 1875 where Russian Blues were shown in a generic blue cat class. After WW II there were very few cats in England and up to 1966, some outcrossing with Siamese produced a much more foreign type of cat. Most breeders began working to restore the old type, and since then Siamese-type has been considered less desirable. Scandinavian lines were integrated to help fix excellent eye color and head conformation traits in the breed. No outcrosses are allowed in CFA. The European type is larger and stockier than the American type. First registrations in CFA occurred in 1949. This is an uncommon breed.

Physical Characteristics

Weight: 8-12 lb (3.5-5.5 kg)

Coat: The very dense, short haircoat is plush and double with a glossy finish and silky texture. The only accepted color is a distinctive blue coat (a type of grey) with silver tipping of the guard hairs—a lighter shade of base color is preferred. The silvery sheen is highly desirable. No white is allowed in the coat. Kittens sometimes have a faint tabby marking pattern but this usually fades with time. Nose leather is grey, and pads lavender to mauve.

Eyes: Oval wide-set eyes are vivid green, though in kittens they start out a yellow color.

Points of Conformation: A medium sized cat, the body is lithe and long. The head is a medium wedge, and has a blunt muzzle without a break producing a flat profile, nose is straight and long. The large ears are wide set with little hair cover and slightly rounded tips. Neck is long and tail is fine and tapers, round feet are compact and small. Coat color, texture and eye color do not usually reach their zenith until at least 2 years of age.

Grooming: Low shedding and low grooming needs; gentle occasional attention is sufficient.

Recognized Behavior Issues and Traits

Reported breed characteristics include: These athletic cats love to jump and climb, and are very playful. The Russian Blue cats are not big talkers, and have a soft voice. They are intelligent; may learn to open doors. They form a strong bond with their human

Normal Breed Variations

Need to watch caloric intake because they gain weight easily.

Very low genetic diversity was found in a study at the University of California, Davis. Cats from 20 different cat breeds (per breed n=30 or greater) were assessed using 30 microsatellite markers. Final assessment was that this breed had marked decrease in genetic diversity compared with random bred cats in this sample.[1]

Drug Sensitivities

None reported in the literature.

Inherited Diseases

None reported in the literature.

Disease Predispositions

Urolithiasis: Increased risk for development of urolithiasis was reported.[2]

Renal Failure: Renal failure rate for Russian Blue cats was more than double the baseline in a study of cats from 23 veterinary college records between 1980-90 (189,371 cases, Purdue University Veterinary Medical Database), at an odds ratio of 2.17:1.[3]

Genetic Tests

None commercially available

Miscellaneous

- **Breed name synonyms:** Archangel Cat, Foreign Blue, Maltese Cat, Spanish blue, Russian, Blue Cat
- **Registries:** FIFé, TICA, CFA, ACFA, CFF, CCA, WCF, GCCF (as Russian) The Australia (ACF) and New Zealand (NZCF) registries call this breed "the Russian" and also accept blue, black and white coated cats.
- **Breed resources: Russian Blue Breeders' Association (GCCF):** http://www.russianblue.org.uk/
  Russian Blue Fanciers (CFA): http://www.russianblue.info/RBF/rbf.htm

References

1. Lipinski MJ, Young AE, Lyons LA. Genetic diversity and population dynamics of domestic cat breeds. *Proceedings.* Tuft's Canine and Feline Breeding and Genetics Conference Oct 2-4, 2003 Available at VIN: www.vin.com/tufts/2003. Accessed Nov 19, 2004.
2. Lekcharoensuk C, Osborne CA, Lulich JP. Epidemiologic study of risk factors for lower urinary tract diseases in cats. *J Am Vet Med Assoc* 2001;May1;218(9):429-435.
3. Lulich JP, O'Brien TD, Osborne CA, Polzin DJ. Feline Renal Failure: Questions, answers, questions. *Compend Contin Educ Pract Vet* 1992;14(2):127-152.

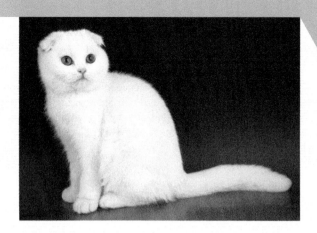

ears stay folded; some pop back up to a straight position. Tail is medium long, flexible, bushy and tapering with a rounded tip. Folds have muscular and stocky conformation.

About one half of the offspring will have straight ears in a Fold X straight mating; these cats are termed Scottish Fold Variants, and are important for breeding not showing.

Grooming: The Scottish Fold has low grooming needs, just weekly brushing is required, though more frequent care may be needed during shedding. One should monitor ear health.

Recognized Behavior Issues and Traits
Reported breed characteristics include: These are moderately active cats. They possess placid dispositions, and have low vocalizing tendency, with small chirping voice. They enjoy close human contact, may shadow their owners, and be a lap cat. A quirk is that they may sit up in "Prairie dog stance" and when getting a better view, "sitting Buddha". The Scottish Fold cats are adaptable, and do well in both quiet and noisy/busy households. Good with other pets, excellent hunters.

Normal Breed Variations
Small litters are the norm.

Need to watch caloric input; tend to obesity.

B Blood Type: Prevalence of 19% blood type B was reported.[1] Four of 27 cats (~15%) tested had B blood type in another report.[2]

Drug Sensitivities
None reported in the literature

Inherited Diseases
Osteochondrodysplasia: On average, 1:3 of folded ear kitten offspring from a fold (Fd) X fold (Fd) breeding will have serious degenerative joint disease, resulting in prognathia, vertebral and appendicular joint and bone abnormalities. Caudal vertebrae are particularly affected, resulting in a tail with reduced or absent flexibility. Metacarpals, metatarsals and phalanges may also be shortened and phalanges abnormally splayed. Age of onset of clinical signs in homozygotes is usually between 4 and 6 months of age. No cure is available, symptomatic management is done. Hubler et al reported that radiotherapy is useful as a palliation.[3] Affected individuals tend to have shorter, thicker tails and gentle palpation of the tail can often identify affected cats early (clinical signs: reduced mobility, pain).

In a retrospective Australian study of a small population of cats between 5 months and 6 years of age, signs of afflicted cats included lameness, reduced ability to jump and swelling of the plantar metatarsal region, thick short tails, and stilted gait.[4] In this study, pedigree analyses (where available) showed that almost

The Breed History
Originating from Pertshire in Tayside Scotland, the first Folds were reported in 1961. The progenitor white cat had two folded kittens that were then crossed to British Shorthair and British Isles domestic shorthair cats to establish the breed. Later, crosses to American Shorthair cats were carried out.

First cats were exported to America in 1971. The GCCF in Britain discontinued registry of the breed in 1973 due to the effects of the gene on cartilage elsewhere in the body. The CFA granted provisional status in 1977 and accepted the Scottish Fold for championship status later. Breeders are still allowed to outcross to American and British Shorthairs, and in some registries, Exotic Shorthairs.

The longhaired Scottish Fold, resulting from Persian-type outcrossing is a separate breed called the **Highland Fold** in some registries, and in other registries is a division termed **Scottish Fold Longhair**.

Physical Characteristics
Weight: Female 6-9 lb (2.5-4 kg), male 9-13 lb (4-6 kg)

Coat: Both a longhair and a shorthair type occur in this breed where registries have not split the Highland Fold out into a separate breed. In the shorthaired cat, the coat is dense, short-medium, standoff, and very soft and plush. Texture may vary somewhat. Note the Longhair is not accepted in all registries. All colors are accepted excluding pointed or Oriental colors; except the CFF registry which allows pointed cats.

Eyes: Large, round and all colors accepted, and eye pigmentation corresponds to coat color.

Points of Conformation: This is a medium-sized cat. The head is large, round, and the nose is short, and broad. Muzzle is short, with well-developed cheeks. The ears are small-medium with rounded tips, the fold results in ears sitting down and forward with tips towards the nose. Single fold ears approximate the original wild type, progressively more tightly folded ears are called double fold and triple fold; the latter being the show type. The forwardly curved ear sitting cap-like over the temples resulted from an **autosomal dominant** mutation (*Fd*) with incomplete penetrance. Every litter will have some straight ears. Folding of the ears occurs between 14-28 days and usually is set by 3-4 months in the kittens. Not all

all affected cats purportedly resulted from a mating of a normal eared cat with a folded ear cat which implied to the authors that heterozygotes were afflicted by a less severe form of this defect which expressed later in life. Defective systemic cartilage maturation, including defective endochondral osteogenesis/ossification may be the underlying mechanism for this abnormality according to these and other authors.[4,5]

This is an autosomal dominant mutation with variable penetrance, appearing to be the very same one inducing abnormal cartilage in the ears. Progressive lameness is due to changes in the distal appendicular skeleton, including ankylosing polyarthropathy, exostoses, soft tissue calcification, sometimes osteopenia leading to reduced overall bone density, and thickened dysmature articular cartilage with focal necrosis. Onset does not always occur early in life; clinical signs may not be noted until 6 years of age; may be crippling at the most penetrant expression, and clinically insignificant at the other end of the spectrum in some heterozygotes. Caudal vertebrae of cats with abnormal tails are shortened and thickened.[5,6]

Informed breeding programs focus on Fold (*Fd*) crossed with straight eared Folds (*fd*), or another alternative, Fd cats bred (approved outcrossing) to American or British Shorthairs.[7] Selection of breeding stock carrying fold (*Fd*) with long flexible tails and acceptable survey radiographs is an adjunctive breeding strategy.

At the veterinary post purchase examination, the veterinarian includes gentle check of tail and toes for normal mobility. Clients are advised to discuss the health guarantee with their breeder prior to purchase regarding their options if the kitten should develop system-wide evidence of cartilage defects.

Neonatal Isoerythrolysis (NI): "Fading" kittens due to NI are a concern in this breed because of prevalence of Type B blood. All B type cats have circulating anti-A antibodies and even primiparous queens can carry these. Type B queens bred to type A toms can result in fatal red cell lysis in A blood type offspring with undetected NI. Kittens with NI can be distinguished from other fading kittens because of pigmenturia; anemia and sometimes icterus will also be present; not all kittens at risk for NI will develop overt clinical symptoms.[2] The proportion of matings at risk for NI is reported to be 0.15.[8]

Disease Predispositions

Transfusion Reactions: Increased probability of reactions due to prevalence of B blood type.[2]

Ear mite propensity: More difficult to treat effectively due to the folded ear structure. Anecdotal.

Hereditary Deafness: Is associated with the dominant gene for white cat (W); may be found in white cats of this breed.[11]

Calcium Oxalate Urolithiasis: A breed propensity for this condition was reported.[12]

Rare and Isolated Reports

Early Onset Osteodystrophy: A 10 week-old Scottish Fold kitten was examined because of early onset of signs of osteodystrophy/osteochondrodysplasia. The kitten's litter was the result of an inadvertent mating of two folded individuals. This report identifies an early onset form of skeletal deformity in this breed.[9] (see above section on Osteochondrodysplasia for comparison)

Polycystic Kidney Disease (PKD): This condition is most common in Persian breeds, and those breeds having crossed out to Persians in their breeding programs. In screening programs carried out at University of California, Davis in 2002, Scottish Fold cats were positive in one study group: in a second study group, 3 of 14 cats tested positive by ultrasound screening of healthy cats from catteries. A genetic test is available.[10]

Genetic Tests

Blood typing before breeding or transfusions is advisable due to prevalence of B blood type in the breed.

Direct genetic test for PKD is available from UC-Davis VGL.

Though no breed recommendations have been published, based on the results of the Australian study of heterozygotes, additional selection measures for suitable healthy breeding stock by radiographic means (for the Fold-eared parent) may be prudent in addition to breeder phenotypic screening (normal long tails, normal gait, normal feet and legs).

Miscellaneous

- **Breed name synonyms:** Fold, Highland Fold for the Longhaired cats, Historical SYN: Lops, Lop-ears. Nickname: Foldie
- **Registries:** TICA (Scottish Fold Longhair and Scottish Fold separated), CFA, ACFA (separate breed from Highland Fold), CFF, ACF (Scottish Fold Longhair, Scottish Fold are separate), WCF (provisional), CCA (Longhair and Shorthair together), NZCF
- **Breed resources: Scottish Fold Rescue Inc:**
  http://scottishfoldrescue.homestead.com/
  The Longhair Clan—Longhair Scottish Fold Breed Club (CFF):
  49 Hancock St
  Salem MA 01970
  Scottish Fold Fanciers (CFF):
  http://www.ziplink.net/users/days/SFF.html

References

1. Malik R, Allan GS, Howlett CR, et al. Osteochondrodysplasia in Scottish Fold cats. *Aust Vet J* 1999;77(2):85-92.
2. Allan GS. Radiographic features of feline joint disease. *Vet Clin North Am: Sm Anim Pract* 2000;30(2):281-301.
3. Hubler M, Volkert M, Kaser-Hotz B, Arnold S. Palliative irradiation of Scottish Fold osteochondrodysplasia. Vet Radiol Ultrasound. 2004;45(6):582-5.
4. Malik R. Genetic Diseases of Cats (and Dogs). *Proceedings*. University of Sydney Post Graduate Foundation in Veterinary Science. Valentine Charlton Refresher Course for Veterinarians; Cats 2000. 2000;Jul;27-37.
5. Miller J. Strategies to avoid detrimental breed characteristics. First International Feline Genetic Disease Conference *Proceedings (abstr)*, in: *Feline Practice Supplement*, 1999;20-21.
6. Giger U. In: Bonagura J, ed. *Kirk's Current Veterinary Therapy XIII*. Philadelphia: WB Saunders Co, 2000;396-399.
7. Giger, U, Bucheler J, Patterson DF. Frequency and inheritance of A and B blood types in feline breeds of the United States. *J Hered* 1991;82:15-20.
8. Giger U, Casal M, Niggemeier A. The fading kitten syndrome and neonatal

isoerythrolysis. *Proceedings.* The 15th Annual ACVIM Medical Forum, Lake Buena Vista FL 1997;308-310.

9. Paugh Parthington B, Williams JF, et al. What is your diagnosis? *J Am Vet Med Assoc* 1996;209(7):1235-1236.

10. Lyons LA. The Lyon's Den. Feline Genome Project: Polycystic Kidney Disease. Available at: http://faculty.vetmed.ucdavis.edu/faculty/lalyons/Sites/pkd.htm Accessed Nov 6, 2004.

11. Strain GM. Hereditary deafness in dogs and cats: causes, prevalence, and current research. *Proceedings.* Tuft's Canine and Feline Breeding and Genetics Conference. Oct 2-4, 2003. Available at: http://www.vin.com/tufts/2003 Accessed Nov 19, 2004.

12. Lekcharoensuk C, Lulich JP, Osborne CA, et al. Association between patient-related factors and risk of calcium oxalate and magnesium ammonium phosphate urolithiasis in cats. *J Am Vet Med Assoc* 2000;Aug15;217(4):520-525.

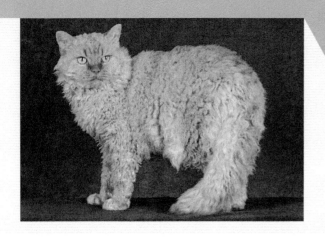

The Breed History

In 1987 a straight-coated female in a Wyoming shelter gave birth to a curly coated shorthaired cat. This cat was crossed with a black Persian and of the first filial generation, three had curly coats. One of the curly offspring, a male black and white cat was bred back with another; 50% curlies, one a long hair resulted. The next (repeat) breeding produced a red point. This is an autosomal dominant mutation, unlike that for the Devon and Cornish Rex genes. No crosses with these other types of rexes are allowed. Outcrossing to British Shorthair, Exotic, and Persian breeds is still allowed, though a phase out is planned so that by 2015, there will be no outcrosses. First accepted by TICA, then ACFA, and finally in CFA.

Physical Characteristics

Weight: 7-11 lb (3-5 kg); males a bit larger

Coat: The shorthair coat is soft, wavy and plush, curled with a wavy tail; the longhair coat is thick but with loose curl ringlets, like a lamb's; the main difference in the two coats is that the longhair is less plush, has a longer ruff, and the tail hairs are longer and plumed.

Homozygotes are more sparsely coated and have tighter curls (the breed standard is closest to the heterozygote cat). Whiskers are curly and short and may break off. Coat colors include pointed, smoke, shaded, solids. Coats are curled at birth, but then they go straighter and remain that way until sexual maturity. The final adult coat matures at 18-24 months of age. The Selkirk Rex coat is a bit fuller than the Devon or Cornish Rex cat, with some guard hairs. They do not tend to molt like the young Devon and Cornish cats. Climate and seasons may affect the coat.

Eyes: Round, wide set, accepted in all colors.

Points of Conformation: These are medium built cats. The head is rounded, cheeks and whisker pads prominent, ears medium sized with pointed tips. The nose is convex and short with a moderate break. The tail is thick with a rounded tip. Good muscling and bone is evident with a broad chest, and tending to cobby. Overall, in type the Selkirk Rex is closer to the British Shorthair than an American Shorthair.

Grooming: Need regular GENTLE combing and brushing. There is a moderate shedding tendency. Rough grooming may break hairs or straighten curls.

Recognized Behavior Issues and Traits

Reported breed characteristics include: Gregarious cats, with good tolerance of other pets and children, and a laid back attitude. They are playful, curious, and possess very affectionate personalities. The Selkirk Rex makes a good apartment cat.

Normal Breed Variations

None reported in the literature

Drug Sensitivities

None reported in the literature

Inherited Diseases

None reported in the literature

Disease Predispositions

None reported in the literature

Genetic Tests

None commercially available

Miscellaneous

- **Breed name synonyms:** Rexed cat, Rex Cat, Curly-coated cat. Informal name: *"cat in sheep's clothing"*
- **Registries:** TICA (Longhair, Shorthair), CFA, ACFA (Longhair, Shorthair), CFF, ACF, GCCF, NZCF
- **Breed resources: The Rex Cat Club (GCCF-U.K.):** http://www.sam.luxford-watts.zen.co.uk/home.html

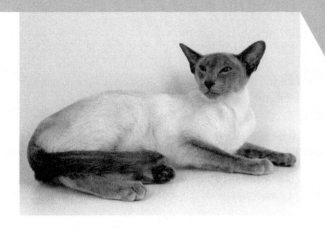

Siamese Pointed Cat or Siamese

The Breed History

This ancient breed, a perennial favorite, is often referred to simply as the Siamese. Evidence of their development was first recorded in Siam (now Thailand) in the fifteenth century, though only in seal point variety. These cats were keenly treasured by royalty, and for a while, ownership was limited to royalty. Early cats were of the Traditional Applehead conformation, and had a heavier body build than the modern version of the Siamese cat. They were first exported to America around 1878. The first breed standard was drawn up in 1892. CFA accepted the breed in 1927. Blue point did not become a recognized breed color until 1934.

Physical Characteristics

Weight: Female 6-8 lb (2.5-3.5 kg), Male 8-12 lb (3.5-5.5 kg)

Coat: Sleek, short, fine, single, close lying. Accepted colors in North America registries include:
- **Seal point** [fawn body with brown-black points]
- **Blue point** [deep silver-slate blue points with gray body]
- **Lilac point** [white body and gray-pink points; is frost]
- **Chocolate point** [ivory body with rich chocolate points]

Points include a masked face, tail, paws, and ears. In some registries, particularly in Europe, the Siamese can be registered in additional colors. These other colors are recognized in America as the **Colorpoint Shorthair** breed. The Himalayan factor is the basis for the pointing pattern (cs cs), and is an autosomal recessive. Coloring darkens somewhat with age. High ambient temperatures lead to lighter pointing.

Eyes: Always an intense sapphire blue. Eyes are close-set, almond shaped and moderate in size.

Points of Conformation: The distinctly wedge-shaped long head is triangular, and large ears are placed to continue that facial plane along their outer margins. Ear tips are pointed. No break; the face is flat on profile, the nose is long and straight. The body is long, lithe, fine-boned, and the neck is fine. The limbs are long and paws are small and oval. The tail is fine, long and tapering with no kinks, reaching the tip of the hind paw when drawn downwards.

The Traditional or Applehead Siamese is a distinct subtype within the breed. The Traditional has a rounder body and head, and is not a show type but is registered as a Siamese cat in almost all registries.

The Tonkinese is quite close in body type to the Applehead.

Grooming: The Siamese cat has low grooming needs. Just a quick wipe with hand or chamois is needed.

Recognized Behavior Issues and Traits

Reported breed characteristics include: Playful; even exuberant, affectionate, talkative with a loud voice, at some times when yowling is said to be like a baby crying. High intelligence, and have high attention needs, forming a very strong bond with their favorite person. Excellent jumpers, they need play time. Some can be demanding at times. They are really gregarious; good with pets and children. Will more readily leash train than most other breeds; often referred to as dog-like in their personality traits.

Normal Breed Variations

They reach sexual maturity early.

100% type A blood type was reported.[1]

Drug Sensitivities

None reported in the literature.

Inherited Diseases

Imperfect (temperature sensitive, t-s) Albinism/Himalayan Pointing Gene: This genetic change produces a so-called imperfect albino condition because of the partial loss of tyrosinase function—where the skin is cooler, the pigment production is normal and in warm areas, melanin production does not occur as the enzyme does not function at the higher temperatures. Siamese pointed cats are homozygous (cs cs) at the pointing gene locus. This genotype is part of an allele series [true albinism (ca ca)], Siamese (cs cs), Mink Tonkinese (cb cs), Burmese (cb cb)] listed in sequence here from more to less heavily expressed phenotype.[2] Albinism has other expression apart from pointing effects.

Gene effects on Coat: Kittens are born white. They gradually develop points starting before weaning and it is not until about one year of age for many cats that the points are fully developed. Note that if the veterinary health care team members shave for intravenous access anywhere but in the darkest fur, the fur will grow back in as a dark patch initially, and only very gradually will it begin to match the surrounding coat color. This is a consideration for show cats. Older cats become gradually darker.

Gene effects on Vision: Congenitally abnormal visual pathways are associated with ts-albinism in the Siamese:
A. **Reduced binocular vision and reduced visual acuity** due to excess decussation of fibers at the optic chiasma. Melanin pigment in retinal pigmented epithelium normally plays a supporting role in axonal growth from the eye to the brain and so central pathways (retino-geniculo-cortical) are altered when this regulator is absent as in Siamese ts-albinism. Retinal X cells

have a role in spatial resolution and altered numbers lead to reduced spatial resolution/contrast sensitivity in vision.[3] A few functional binocular cells are left in the brain, and more in the supra-sylvian areas allow for coarse stereopsis.[4, 5]

These aforementioned congenitally abnormal pathways are associated with:

Convergent Strabismus (Esotropia): So-called "cross-eyed" cats used to be more common. This condition does not appear to adversely affect functional vision because cats are compensating for impaired stereopsis, even though the visual pathways remain abnormal.[6] Affected Siamese newborns have divergent strabismus; a normal finding in neonates, but as they mature, by a few months of age eyes are parallel but then migrate inward to compensate for deviated central vision pathways. The abnormal eye position helps the cat compensate for visual pathway defect.[7]

Nystagmus: Also a compensating strategy that allows the cats to work around the hard wired defect. Nystagmus may improve with age and disappear briefly when a cat focuses on a subject of interest.[6]

Both of these secondary signs result from the compensation for abnormal processing of unconscious light responses and are not primary structural defects, just responses . Abnormalities in the visual pathways occur in all Siamese pointed cats but the phenotype varies. The resulting changes in vision are complex, but it is notable that a portion of the cat's visual field is inverted/opposite to the normal display. All Siamese cats lack normal binocular vision.[7]

New research shows that the c(b) allele of the albino locus gene are variants on the D1 chromosome specifying tyrosinase and the chocolate (b) and cinnamon (b(9l)) a second allele at the B (brown) locus are nucleotide variants of TYRP1 (chromosome D4).[8]

The mutations are reported to most likely to be identical by descent rather than multiple mutation events occurring at the same site in another study.[9]

Familial AA Amyloidosis: Systemic amyloidosis is an inherited disorder leading to amyloid deposition in various organs and tissues, including liver and kidney. The liver is commonly the significant organ involved in Siamese cats (compare with amyloidosis in Abyssinians where significant signs are mostly renal). Cats 1-5 years of age are typically affected. Considered to be familial, Siamese cats account for ~95% of reported cases of AA amyloidosis. Spontaneous hepatic rupture associated with hepatic amyloid deposition can occur.[10]

In a case report, two cats from one cattery with amyloidosis were described. This condition led to spontaneous liver hemorrhage in one cat, and chronic renal failure in another, so signs vary depending on which organ is most affected.[11]

In one report (1987-1994), 6.2% of Siamese/Oriental cats presented for post mortem were affected by generalized AA amyloidosis. The amyloid fibril protein (AA) amino acid sequence is different than that found in the Abyssinian form of this condition. Clinical signs of amyloidosis include anorexia, vomiting, stomatitis, anemia, emaciation, painful distended abdomen and diarrhea. Post mortem changes may include pale friable engorged liver and spleen, and

dilation of intestines. A few cases in the retrospective study were found to have had concurrent FIP, and a few had recently gone through parturition.[12]

In a study of cats (1983-1987) in the Netherlands, 1.5% of 710 Siamese referrals were diagnosed with AA-amyloidosis. In 36% of the Siamese cats with amyloidosis, inflammatory conditions were present (rhinitis, FIP).[13]

The apolipoprotein, apo-serum amyloid A (AA) amyloidosis propensity is still not certainly a solely genetically problem. Recent sequencing of the proteins shows mutations in amino acids related to a particular breed present in other breeds, and this may mean that in addition to the presence of amyloid-associated genes, other factors such as chronic inflammation or certain infections are involved in the genesis of phenotypic clinical amyloidosis. At least three genes or gene clusters may be responsible for the trait.[14]

Mucopolysaccharidosis Type VI (MPS VI): This is an autosomal recessive lysosomal storage disease resulting from deficiency of the enzyme N-acetyl-galactosamine-4-sulfatase (aryl sulfatase B) leading to the accumulation of the glucosaminoglycan (GAG), dermatan sulfate. The central nervous system appears to be spared in this condition even when expressed in its most severe form. The skeletal system is the primary target. A test has identified a mutation (label: L476P) leading to the condition.[15] Note that in the past, the Berry urinary spot test (toluidine blue) was used as a screening test to identify excess GAGs in the urine, and remains useful.[16]

Three distinct phenotypes from two separate distinct mutations (L476P, D520N) were reported in a study. The L476P homozygote cats have coarse facial features (broad face, short nose, small ears), dwarfism, degenerative joint disease (DJD), widespread leukocyte and other cellular lysosomal inclusions, and dermatan sulfaturia. The two other genotypes (D520N homozygous, and L476P/D520N) have normal growth and appearance but internal changes. The L476P/D520N is the mildest in expression.[17] Skeletal disorders such as DJD are primary endpoints of the MPS VI trait.

In a screening study of three continents, the mutation D520N was found in 11.4% of the open Siamese cat population from 5 of 6 countries. It was concluded that the genotypes D520N/D520N and D520N/L476P are likely widely distributed in the general population. These cats will be normal except for an increase in DJD, particularly at the caudal aspect of the proximal humeral epiphysis, and mild changes in the femorotibial joints may also occur. Radiographic hallmarks of the condition include: generalized osteopenia, severe vertebral epiphyseal dysplasia, coarse trabeculae and irregular subchondral bone development. Facial dysmorphia and stunted growth are evident starting at about 8 weeks of age in severe genotype kittens. Hind limb paresis or paralysis may develop due to compression of the spinal cord. A stiff gait and reduced activity may be noted. Mild basophilic granulation in neutrophils routinely prepared for blood films can be useful as a screening test. Definitive diagnosis requires specialized testing available at the University of Pennsylvania, or one can run the urine dermatan sulfate test.[18]

In North America, at least seven families have produced clinical cases of MPS VI. Presence of atypical DJD or other skeletal disease in Siamese should place MPS VI on the differential list.

This trait can affect the eyes also. Corneal opacification occurs; frosted appearance of the eyes may be noted by 11 weeks of age, progressing until one year of age; marked pathology occurs in the RPE, but is not visualized clinically.[19]

In man this disease is termed Maroteaux-Lamy Syndrome.

Progressive Retinal Atrophy (rdAc): Autosomal recessive genetic disease causing blindness. Found at a gene frequency of 33% in the breed. See under Abyssinian. A genetic test is available.

Disease Predispositions

Wool Sucking: Onset is usually after weaning, also affects Siamese crosses. Target is commonly a blanket, or knitted clothing. Compulsive behavior often ends at sexual maturity, but some cases may have late onset or continue signs late into life. A study found 55% of fabric eating cats were Siamese in a group of 152 affected cats. Behavior is characterized by compulsive stereotypic oral movement. Though many cats begin with substrate of wool, many add other types of fabric, and even non-fabric substrates (plastics). Early weaned cats are over-represented but there is no clear causal relationship.[32]

Separation Anxiety Syndrome: Of a study group of 136 cats with SAS symptoms, Siamese accounted for 6 % of the cats. In this breed, most commonly the females defecated, and males expressed excessive vocalization.[33]

Floppy Pinnae: With a middle adulthood age of onset, normal ears become floppy ears (just the upper portion of the pinna). This condition can resolve without treatment.[22] One theory is that flopping is due to relapsing polychondritis, which requires a biopsy for diagnosis.[34,35]

Corneal Sequestration (Synonym: Black body or cornea nigrum): Siamese cats are over-represented. Usually in central or paracentral cornea; brown to black pigmented lesion; often surrounded by a loose collarette of poorly adherent corneal epithelium. Stromal necrosis may extend into shallow or deep stroma, or even to Descemet's membrane. Sloughing and corneal healing may take 2-6 months; surgical debridement is another option. Material may be tear concretion mixed with stroma and inflammatory cells.[36]

Progressive Retinal Atrophy (PRA): A breed predilection for diffuse bilateral PRA was reported. First changes include attenuation of retinal blood vessels, retinal thinning in the area centralis (tapetal glow), then generalized tapetal hyperreflectivity, and progressing to ghosted or absent dorsal vessels with attenuated optic disc. Vision loss occurs late in the process and night vision is retained. Client complaints include the cat bumping into things, reluctance to jump, and mydriasis.[37,38]

Open Angle Glaucoma: A chronic primary glaucoma that may have Siamese breed predilection. Affected cats gradually progress in severity of clinical signs, and may develop luxation of lens.[6]

Hyperthyroidism: Reduced risk for this breed was reported.[39] Siamese cats were almost 10x less likely to develop hyperthyroidism (Odds Ratio 9.6) than non-Siamese.[40]

Pancreatitis: In a retrospective case study (40 cases) Siamese cats were overrepresented (15% of the cases). Necrosis and suppurative inflammation were two distinct forms. Hypokalemia occurred in about half of the cats, and normal lipase and amylase were found. In a previous report, 39% of pancreatitis cases were Siamese breed.[41]

Dsytocia: A survey of 2,928 litters (multiple cat breeds) was carried out to ascertain prevalence of dystocia, and an over-representation of Siamese cats was found. A total of 571 Siamese litters were analyzed. The average rate in a mixed breed colony for dystocia was 0.4% of litters. A rate of 10% was found in Siamese cats.[42]

Cervical Neck Lesions: Increased risk was reported in a survey where Siamese were one of two breeds (the other being Abyssinian) most commonly affected by Feline Odontoclastic Resorptive Lesions.[43]

Gingivitis and Periodontal Disease: Anecdotal evidence of increased prevalence.

Slipped Capital Femoral Epiphysis: Siamese breed cats were 23% of affected cats (3/13) in a survey, though they made up only 5% of the population (of 13,250). Average body weight in the pooled study group was 5.6 kg, significantly over the normal average for cats. A physeal dysplasia was characterized by diffusely widened physis with disorganized cartilage. Though this condition is typically associated with trauma in dogs, in this set of cases there was no history of any trauma. It is likely the growth plate cannot handle normal shear stresses due to the dysplasia. This condition affected cats 4.5-24 months of age. A genetic etiology is suspected. Insulin levels or insulin receptor resistance in obesity was proposed to play a role in physeal dysplasia.[44]

Medial Patellar Luxation (MPL): A study reported that of 12 Siamese cats assessed as part of a larger study, five had abnormal patella seating with easily induced luxation. Compared with the rate of affected cats in non-pedigreed (2/31), Siamese had an increased MPL prevalence in this particular study.[45]

Hip Dysplasia (HD) may be associated with luxating patellas.[46]

In another report, Siamese cats had a frequency of 7.1% hip dysplasia.[47]

Adenocarcinoma (small intestine): Breed associated risk was reported to be eight times that for other cat breeds.[48] In a population where 7.8% of cats in the group were of Siamese breed, 71% of the cases were diagnosed in Siamese cats.[36] In 100 previously published cases 42% were Siamese breed. In retrospective case study at MSU (1975-1985) for GI adenocarcinoma in cats, 6/11 cases were Siamese. In this report tubular adenocarcinoma case survival time was an average of 11 months, while mucinous and undifferentiated type had average survival times of 4 months. Overall, a survival time of 5 months with metastasis, and 10 months for patients without metastases was the reported average.[49]

Lymphosarcoma (LSA): In a retrospective case study of 7,159 admissions over a decade, 60 cats had LSA; Siamese cats were predisposed. Young Siamese and Orientals when pooled accounted for 33.3% of LSA cases, though they made up only 2% of the hospital population. Mediastinal LSA (thymus, mediastinal lymph nodes) was most common in Siamese cats, and 86% of mediastinal cases were diagnosed in Siamese, with mean age 2 years. All were FeLV negative. Breed lines diagnosed with early onset LSA had origins in Europe and Australia.[50] A recent report describes analysis of two families that supports the hypothesis that this is an autosomal recessive trait, and homozygous in affected patients.[51]

Feline Dilated Cardiomyopathy (DCM): Siamese cats may be predisposed. Incidence has dropped since dietary supplementation with taurine began, but cases still occur. Average age of onset is 7 years. Previously, mortality for DCM was ~85%, but with taurine supplementation the mortality is in ~30%-50% range. Feline clinical signs are not typically a cough as in the dog; heart rate may range from bradycardia to tachycardia. Systolic heart murmur or diastolic gallop can often be heard, and 61% have arrhythmias, usually ventricular. Echocardiography is the best modality for definitive diagnosis.[52]

Renal Failure: Rate for Siamese was identified to be more than double baseline in a study (1980-1990, 189,371 cases. Purdue Veterinary Medical Database) at an odds ratio for risk of 2.6:1, with prevalence of 2.8%.[53]

Lower Urinary Tract Disease: Higher than expected rates of cystine urolithiasis reported in a small study group (3/18 were Siamese).[54] Oxalate uroliths have been reported to be the most common type of stones in Siamese cats (especially males), and urate and cystine stones also more common than expected.[55]

Myasthenia Gravis: The congenital form seen in the breed is not associated with antibodies against the acetylcholine receptor (as in Abyssinian and Somali cats). Same symptoms as the acquired form are seen.[56]

Feline Bronchial Asthma: (Synonyms: allergic bronchitis, chronic bronchitis, feline lower airway disease). Siamese breed cats are overrepresented—in a retrospective study, of 22 cats with lower airway disease, Siamese made up 55% of afflicted cats. Cough was seen in most but not all cats. Radiographs were normal in 23% of affected cats. These authors summarize earlier findings that indicate Siamese and Himalayan cats are at higher risk, perhaps due to genetic susceptibility. Siamese may have a more prolonged clinical course, and a relapsing tendency.[57]

Rare and Isolated Reports

Sphingomyelinosis: (Feline Neimann-Pick Disease): An autosomal recessive polyneuropathy resulting from the reduction of the enzyme sphingomyelinase. This results in a storage disease characterized by accumulation of cholesterol, gangliosides and sphingomyelin. Head and fine generalized tremors, stunted growth, progressive lower motor neuron tetraparesis, hypermetria and ataxia begin at about 8-20 weeks of age. Signs are slowly progressive over months. Anisocoria and blindness are usually present by 5 months of age. Head tremors lead to dysphagia. Late stage signs include plantigrade/palmigrade stance, weakness, and hepatosplenomegaly. Onset of polyneuropathy is usually before 1 year of age.[20] Diagnosis is by nerve biopsy, lysosomal enzyme and lipid testing in skin, liver and or brain tissue, and EMG (slow conduction velocity).[21]

Congenital Hydrocephalus: A genetic basis for Siamese cats with this trait was proposed. The hydrocephalus leads to dilated ventricles, with resulting pressure necrosis of the nervous tissue surrounding them. Clinically, domed skulls, lateral strabismus (setting sun sign), vision defects, and spastic gait problems result. Aggression, dullness, circling, and seizures may also be seen.[20]

Neuroaxonal Dystrophy: A degenerative neurologic condition in two littermates has been described. The condition resulted in swollen distal ends/pre-terminal segments of the axons in the central nervous system. This is an autosomal recessive condition. Ataxia starts at about 2 weeks of age; head tremor occurs first, then hypermetria and rear limb paralysis. In these 2 kittens, coat pigmentation was normal.[22]

Hypomyelination of the Central Nervous System (Congenital Tremors): Two littermates were reported to be affected by early onset tremors, seizures and ataxia. A third kitten died at three days of age. By four weeks of age, the surviving littermates had tremors with frenzied biting episodes when active; normal at rest. Peripheral myelin was normal, while CNS myelin was abnormal/reduced. The unusual frenzied biting behavior has not been reported in other species with this condition and is thought to be associated with paresthesia secondary to inappropriate responses of hypo-myelinated nerves.[23]

Inherited Hyperchylomicronemia: Presenting signs include weakness, loss of appetite and severe anemia by 4 weeks of age. This defect in lipoprotein lipase enzyme activation was seen in two related litters. The clinically normal parents and related kittens had reduced enzyme activity also. This is suspected to be an autosomal recessive inheritance.[24]

Fasting hyperchylomicronemia, hypertriglyceridemia, lipemia retinalis, splenomegaly, and xanthomata of skin, and liver and kidney, and sometimes anemia are also described. Xanthomata (fat granulomas) in the vicinity of the nerves lead to nerve compression and subsequent dysfunction such as rear limb paresis (with plantigrade stance) and cranial nerve dysfunction. If the levels of lipid and lipoproteins are high, the blood may take on the gross appearance of cream of tomato soup.[25]

A transient hyperlipidemia and anemia was described in three litters of Siamese kittens. Severe hypertriglyceridemia and anemia were noted around the time of weaning, and 3 of 4 siblings and 1 of 5 half siblings from the litters were affected. Marked elevation of chylomicrons and VLDL were identified. Anorexia, ataxia, and lethargy were predominant clinical signs.[26]

Hemophilia B (Christmas Disease, Factor IX Deficiency): A sex-linked recessive hemorrhagic disorder with resulting hemarthrosis, excessive post-surgical hemorrhage, gingival hemorrhage and spontaneous hematoma formation. Females are asymptomatic carriers, males are affected.[16]

GM1-Gangliosidosis: A beta-galactosidase deficiency.[16] Recent studies show the same mutation is responsible for this condition in both Korat and Siamese cats.[27]

Ceroid Lipofuscinosis: This is a lysosomal storage disease, with lipofuscin accumulation. Signs may include seizures and weakness.

An autosomal recessive inheritance has been postulated.[14,28]

Copper Storage Disease: Peri-acinar (centrilobular) copper accumulation in liver of cats has been reported (as in Bedlington terriers). In one affected cat, at post mortem at 2 years of age, granules were found to have accumulated in proximal convoluted tubules/collecting ducts of kidney and in the macrophages/alveolar epithelium of the lung as well.[29]

Merosin (laminin α-2) Deficient Myopathy/Muscular Dystrophy: Mode of inheritance of laminin α-2 deficiency is unknown. Rear limb weakness begins at 6 months of age, progressively worsening atrophy and contracture occurs by one year old; those in the report were euthanized before reaching 24 months of age.[30]

Porphyria: Porphyrin (porphobilinogen) accumulates in bones, teeth, urine making them stain brown, and fluoresce. In regular light, urine appears brown.[16] Affected cats may be sensitive to sunlight; porphyria is not usually life threatening. Refractile bodies occur in erythrocytes; may also develop hemolytic anemia. Concurrent nephropathy (tubular ischemia, mesangial proliferation) occurred.[31] Due to deficiency of uroporphyrinogen III synthetase, porphobilinogen deaminase. An autosomal dominant pattern of inheritance is reported.[28]

Endocardial Fibroelastosis: An elastic thickening extending diffusely through the endocardium. Left atrium and left ventricle affected, reported age of onset in early postnatal period, or alternatively, middle age in Siamese cats. This is a very rare condition. Genetic basis was suggested.[58]

Persistent Atrial Standstill: Siamese may have a breed predisposition to this rare problem.[59] Bradycardia is poorly responsive to medical management; a pacemaker may be needed.[16]

Cutaneous Mastocytoma: Locally recurring, usually in younger Siamese cats; this presentation is a rare subtype of cutaneous mastocytoma. Usually multiple nodules (> 5) in deep dermis and subcutis; histiocytic-like cells, noted to cluster in household in siblings, mostly on head; a genetic predisposition possible. These have low metastatic potential.[60,61]

Vitiligo: Symmetrical pigment loss on the footpads, nose and eyelids. May be immune mediated (melanocyte surface marker antibodies found).[61]

Feline Hyperesthesia Syndrome: (Synonyms: rolling skin disease; psychomotor epilepsy.

Junctional Epidermolysis bullosa: A recessive condition with skin blisters where the weak collagen breaks down. It is first seen pre-weaning and may result in claw loss.[61]

Other conditions reported in the breed include:
Psychogenic Alopecia, Malignant Mammary Tumors (early onset tendency), Food Hypersensitivity, Familial Cleft Palate, Congenital Portosystemic Shunts (usually extrahepatic), Insulinoma, PTH tumors, hydrocephalus, congenital deafness, pyloric stenosis, intestinal polyps, hemophilia B, mycobacterium avium-intracellulare complex (MAC), hereditary porphyria, kinked tails, mast cell tumors, congenital

peripheral vestibular disease, juvenile ataxia, aortic stenosis.[62]

Genetic Tests
Mucopolysaccharidosis Type VI

Josephine Deubler Genetic Testing Laboratory (PennGen). At the University of Pennsylvania veterinary hospital.

Minimum of 1-2 ml EDTA blood processed within 48 hours—express mail service in padded mailer adequate. Is not necessary to cool; avoid freezing. Test request form available online. Can do concurrent blood typing. Can submit a pair of buccal swabs for testing. http://research.vet.upenn.edu/SubmitaSample/tabid/554/Default.aspx UC Davis Feline Genome Project (Dr. Lesley Lyons) Submit buccal swabs for research on possible autosomal recessive inheritance for lymphoma. http://www.vetmed.ucdavis.edu/Catgenetics/Feline_Research_Projects.html

Older cats should be screened for renal function using serum creatinine and urinalysis (as a minimum) in cats 8 years and older since there is a breed propensity for renal failure.[41]

Direct genetic test for rdAc-PRA is available from UC-Davis VGL.

Miscellaneous
- **Breed name synonyms:** Temple cat of Siam, Royal cat of Siam, Thai cat, Meeser, Meesy
- **Registries:** FIFé (Siamese), TICA (Siamese), CFA, ACFA (Siamese), CFF (Siamese), GCCF (includes Balinese as Longhaired Siamese), ACF, WCF (with Oriental Shorthair), NZCF (Siamese), CCA (Siamese)
- **Breed resources: National Siamese Cat Club:** http://nationalsiamese.com
  Seal Point Siamese Cat Club (GCCF): http://sealpointsiamesecatclub.org/

References
1. Giger U. In: Bonagura J, ed. *Kirk's Current Veterinary Therapy XIII.* Philadelphia: WB Saunders Co, 2000;396-399.
2. Lyons LA, Imes DL, Grahn RA. Investigation of albinism in domestic cats. *Proceedings.* (Poster #18) 2nd International Conference Advances in Canine and Feline Genomics. Oct 2004, Utrecht Netherlands.
3. Girelli M, Campara D, Tassinari G, et al. Abnormal spatial but normal temporal resolution in the Siamese cat: a behavioral correlate of a genetic disorder of the parallel visual pathways. *Can J Physiol Pharmacol* 1995;73:1348-1351.
4. Bacon BA, Lepore F, Guillemot J. Binocular interactions and spatial disparity sensitivity in the superior colliculus of the Siamese cat. *Exp Brain Res* 1999;124:181-192.
5. Bacon BA, Mimeault D, Lepore F, et al. Spatial disparity sensitivity in area PMLS of the Siamese cat. *Brain Res* 2001;906:149-156.
6. Peiffer RL.. Inherited ocular diseases of the dog and cat. *Compend Cont Educ Pract Vet* 1982;4(2):152-164.
7. Johnson BW. Congenitally abnormal visual pathways of Siamese cats. *Compend Contin Educ Pract Vet* 1991;13(3):374-378.
8. Schmidt-Kuntzel A, Eizirik E, O'Brien SJ, et al. Tyrosinase and tyrosinase related protein 1 alleles specify domestic cat coat color phenotypes of the albino and brown loci. *J Hered* 2005 Jul-Aug;96(4):289-301.
9. Lyons LA, Imes DL, Rah HC, et al. Tyrosinase mutations associated with Siamese and Burmese patterns in the domestic cat (Felis catus). *Anim Genet.* 2005 Apr;36(2):119-26.
10. Beatty JA, Barrs VR, Martin PA, et al. Spontaneous hepatic rupture in six cats with systemic amyloidosis. *J Small Anim Pract* 2002;43:355-363.
11. Godfrey DR, Day MJ. Generalised amyloidosis in two Siamese cats:

spontaneous liver haemorrhage and chronic renal failure. J Small Anim Pract 39:442-447, 1998.

12. van der Linde-Sipman JS, Niewold TA, Tooten PCJ, et al. Generalized AA-amyloidosis in Siamese and Oriental cats. Vet Immunol Immunopathol 1997;56(1-2):1-10.

13. Gruys E, Van de Stadt M, Blok JJ, et al. Feline Amyloidosis. First International Feline Genetic Disease Conference Proceedings (abstr), in: Feline Practice Supplement, 1999:15.

14. van Rossum M, van Asten FJAM, Rofina J, et al. Analysis of cDNA sequences of feline SAAs. Amyloid: J Protein Folding Disord 2004;11:38-43.

15. Yogalingam G, Litjens T, Bielicki J, et al. Feline Mucopolysaccharidosis Type VI. J Biol Chem 1996;271(44):27259-27265.

16. Hoskins JD. Congenital defects in cats. Compend Contin Educ Pract Vet 1995;17(3):385-405.

17. Crawley AC, Yogalingam G, Muller VJ, et al. Two mutations within a feline Mucopolysaccharidosis type VI colony cause three different clinical phenotypes. J Clin Invest 1998;101:109-119.

18. Crawley AC, Muntz FH, Haskins ME, et al. Prevalence of Mucopolysaccharidosis Type VI mutations in Siamese cats. J Vet Int Med 2003;17:495-498.

19. Aguirre G, Ray J, Haskins M. Ocular manifestations of inherited metabolic diseases in cats. Proceedings. The 25th Annual Meeting of the ACVO, Oct 26-30, 1994:28-29.

20. Shell LG. A review of feline neuromuscular diseases, Seizures in the cat In: Symposium: Feline neurologic diseases. Vet Med Jun 1998:542-574.

21. Cuddon PA. Feline neuromuscular disease. Fel Pract 1994;22(2):7-13.

22. Rodréguez F, Espinosa de los Monteros A, Morales M, et al. Neuroaxonal dystrophy in two Siamese kittens. Vet Rec 1996;138:548-549.

23. Stoffregen DA, Huxtable CR, Cummings JF, et al. Hypomyelination of the central nervous system of two Siamese kitten littermates. Vet Pathol 1993;30:388-391.

24. Watson TDG, Gaffney D, Mooney CT, et al. Inherited hyperchylomicronaemia in the cat: Lipoprotein lipase function and gene structure. J Small Anim Pract 1992;33:207-212.

25. Jones BR. Inherited hyperchylomicronaemia in the cat. J of Small Anim Pract 1993;34:493-499.

26. Gunn-Moore DA, Watson TDG, Dodkin SJ, et al. Transient hyperlipidaemia and anaemia in kittens. Vet Rec 1997;140:355-359.

27. Baker HJ. The molecular basis of feline GM1 and GM2 gangliosidoses. First International Feline Genetic Disease Conference Philadelphia June, 1998 Proceedings (abstr) in: Fel Pract Suppl 1999:11.

28. Giger U, Haskin ME. Inherited disorders. In: August, JR ed. 2nd ed. Consultations in Feline Medicine Philadelphia: WB Saunders. 1994:183-191.

29. Haynes JS, Wade PR. Hepatopathy associated with excessive hepatic copper in Siamese cats. Vet Pathol 1995;32:427-429.

30. Gaschen FP. Feline myopathies. Proceedings. NAVC 2002 16:437-438.

31. Watson ADJ. Feline precursor porphyria, characterized by persistent delta aminolevulinic aciduria. J Small Anim Pract 1990;31:393-397.

32. Neilson J. Anxieties, phobias and compulsive disorders. Proceedings. AAFP Fall Conference. 2002:125-139.

33. Schwartz S. Separation anxiety syndrome in cats. 136 cases (1991-2000). J Am Vet Med Assoc 2002;220(7):1028-1033.

34. Pearson T. Floppy pinnae in Siamese cats. Letter to the Editor. Vet Rec 1998;143(16):456.

35. Rest JR. Floppy pinnae in Siamese cats. Letter to the Editor. Vet Rec 1998;143(20):568.

36. Narfström K. Hereditary and congenital ocular disease. J Fel Med Surg 1999;1:135-141.

37. Giuliano EA, van der Woerdt, A. Feline retinal degeneration: Clinical experience and new findings (1994-1997). J Am Anim Hosp Assoc 1999;35:511-514.

38. Carlile JL. Feline Retinal atrophy. Vet Rec 1981;108:311.

39. Kass PH, Peterson ME, Levy J, et al. Evaluation of environmental, nutritional, and host factors in cats with hyperthyroidism. JVIM 1999;13:323-329.

40. Scarlett JM, Moise NS, Rayl J. Feline hyperthyroidism—a descriptive and case-control study. Prev Vet Med 1988;6:295-309.

41. Hill RC, van Winkle TJ. Acute necrotizing pancreatitis and acute suppurative pancreatitis in the cat: A retrospective study of 40 cases (1976-1989). JVIM 1993;7:25-33.

42. Gunn-Moore DA, Thrusfield MV. Feline dystocia: prevalence, and association with cranial conformation and breed. Vet Rec 1995;136:350-353.

43. van Wessum R, Harvey, CE, Hennet P. Feline dental resorptive lesions-prevalence patterns. Vet Clin North Am: Sm Anim Pract 1992;22:1405-1416.

44. Craig LE. Physeal dysplasia with slipped capital femoral epiphysis in 13 cats. Vet Pathol 2001;38:92-92.

45. Engvall E, Bushnell N. Patellar luxation in Abyssinian cats. Fel Pract 1990;18(4):20-22.

46. Keller GG, Reed AL, Lattimer JC, Corley EA. Hip dysplasia: A feline population study. Veterinary Radiology & Ultrasound 1999;40(4):460-464.

47. Gardner CH, Hicks SL, Puette JR, et al. What is your diagnosis? J Am Vet Med Assoc 2003;223(6):783-784.

48. Birchard SJ. Nonlymphoid intestinal neoplasia in 32 dogs and 14 cats. JAAHA 1986;22:533-537.

49. Cribb AE. Feline gastrointestinal adenocarcinoma: A review and retrospective study. Can Vet J 1988;29:709-712.

50. Court EA, Watson ADJ, Peaston AE. Retrospective study of 60 cases of feline lymphosarcoma. Aust Vet J 1997;75(6):424-427.

51. Lyons LA, Geary LA. Lymphosarcoma in Siamese/OSH populations. 2nd International Conference Advances in Canine and Feline Genomics. Proceedings. Poster #30.

52. Atkins CE. Feline dilated cardiomyopathy. Winter 2004 AAFP Meeting. Proceedings [abstr] in: AAFP Newsletter August 2004 22(2):29-30.

53. Lulich JP, O'Brien TD, Osborne CA, et al. Feline Renal Failure: Questions, answers, questions. Compend Contin Educ Pract Vet 1992;14(2):127-152.

54. Osborne C, Lulich J, Sanderson S, et al. Feline cystine urolithiasis-18 cases. First International Feline Genetic Disease Conference Philadelphia June, 1998 Proceedings (abstr) in: Fel Pract Suppl, 1999:31-32.

55. Houston DM, Moore AEP, Favrin MG, et al. Feline urethral plugs and bladder uroliths: A review of 5484 submissions 1998-2003. Can Vet J 2003;Dec;44(12):974-977.

56. Bagley RS. Diseases of the peripheral nervous system, neuromuscular junction and muscle; Evaluation of weakness. Proceedings. AAFP Fall meeting. 1998:31-33.

57. Adamama-Moraitou KK, Patsikas MN, Koutinas AF. Feline lower airway disease: a retrospective study of 22 naturally occurring cases from Greece. J Fel Med Surg 2004;6:227-233.

58. Rozengurt N. Endocardial fibroelastosis in common domestic cats in the UK. J Comp Path 1994;110:295-301.

59. Itoh N, Itoh S, Kawara S, et al. Persistent atrial standstill in a Siamese cat. Fel Pract 1994;22(4):14-17.

60. Chastian CB, Turk MAM, O'Brian D. Benign Cutaneous mastocytomas in two litters of Siamese kittens. J Am Vet Med Assoc 1988;193(8):959-960.

61. Scott DW. Feline dermatology 1986-1988: Looking to the 1990s through the eyes of many counselors. J Am Anim Hosp Assoc 1990;26:515-523.

62. Feline Advisory Beaureau Website accessed at: http://www.fabcats.org/breeders/inherited_disorders/siamese.php

Recommended Reading

Glaze MB Congenital and hereditary ocular abnormalities in cats. Clin Tech Small Anim Pract. 2005 May;20(2):74-82

Miller MS, Tilley LP, et al. In: Kirk RW, Bonagura JD, eds. Current Veterinary Therapy XI. Philadelphia: WB Saunders Co. 1992:786-791.

Tilley LP, Liu SK. Persistent Atrial Standstill in the dog and cat. Proceedings. The Annual ACVIM Veterinary Medical Forum NY (abstr) 1983:43.

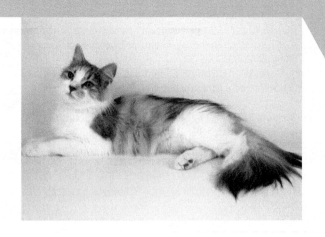

Siberian Forest Cat

cats and children. Soft voiced. They are good climbers, excellent jumpers, and are suited for indoor-outdoor and outdoor lifestyles. These cats can also live in apartment if proper climbing and entertainment equipment is provided.

The Breed History

This is an ancient indigenous street cat from Russia. Controlled breeding towards a uniform breed standard began only in the 1900s. This is the National Cat of Russia. Early records of a cat meeting this description trace back to 1000 AD. No outcrosses are allowed. First specimens arrived in the United States in 1990, but the Siberian Forest Cat breed is still very rare in the USA. TICA accepted them in 1998. The CFA had accepted this breed in the Miscellaneous Class in 2000 and they achieved championship status in 2006.

Physical Characteristics

Weight: 10-20 lb (4.5-9 kg), females smaller than males

Coat: Many coat colors and patterns are accepted. Brown tabby is the most common. It is a very thick medium to semi-longhair plush double-triple coat. Ruff, britches and tail are much longer haired. Ears have full furnishings. The coat is a bit oily, a feature that helps the coat repel water. Hair texture can vary somewhat with color but is described as crispy.

In one study, Siberian forest cats had a 49% carrier rate for carriage of the gene for pointing. This is a trait that is being gradually eliminated from this breed.[1] This variant is known as Neva Mascarade.

Eyes: Medium sized, and round.

Points of Conformation: This is a medium-large "rounded" cat with a distinctively wild appearance. Skull is rounded and broad in a modified wedge shape. Wide and low set medium-sized ears have rounded tips. Ear furnishing is well developed, and ear tipping is accepted. Paws are compact, round and large with toe tufting. The tail is short to medium in length and is wide at the base, tapering to a blunt tip.

Grooming: Moderate grooming needs, they have increased shedding propensity in spring and fall; tending to blow their coat. Need to watch for mats forming under limbs in axilla and groin.

Recognized Behavior Issues and Traits

Reported breed characteristics include: Not suited to lap cat lifestyles. Siberian Forest cats are active and playful, though they have a fairly passive personality. Siberians are friendly with other

Normal Breed Variations

They are slow maturing (~4-5 years)

1/3rd of the American cats tested are low allergen protein (FeL d1) which makes these cats suitable for some allergy sufferers.[2]

Drug Sensitivities

None reported in the literature

Inherited Diseases

None reported in the literature

Disease Predispositions

None reported in the literature

Rare and Isolated Reports

Hypertrophic Cardiomyopathy (HCM): A single Siberian cat tested positive for the Maine Coon cat (myosin binding protein C) mutation.[3]

Genetic Tests

None commercially available

Miscellaneous

- **Breed name synonyms:** Siberian, Sibirian, Sibirskaya Koshka (historical SYN), Sibi
- **Registries:** FIFé (Siberian Cat), TICA (Siberian), CFA (Miscellaneous class), ACFA (Siberian Cat), CFF, WCF (Siberian), GCCF (Siberian), ACF (Siberian)
- **Breed resources: Comrade Cat Club:**
  RR 1 Box 2460
  Bowdoinham, ME 04008
  TAIGA Siberian Cat Breed Club (CFA, TICA, ACFA, AACE):
  www.homestead.com/taigasiberians

References

1. Grahn R, Grahn J. A Practical Application of the Pointing Test. In: *Notes.* University of California (Davis) Feline Genetics Extravaganza II Aug 28-29, 2004.
2. Marek R. D. Russian Beauty. Cat Fancy March 2008 pp47-49.
3. Feline Advisory Bureau at: http://www.fabcats.org/breeders/inherited_disorders/siberian.php

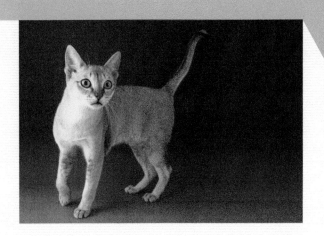

Singapura

The Breed History

This diminutive and rare breed derives its name from Singapore where this breed originated. An informal synonym used for them is "drain" or "river" cat because of their previous feral life in the city streets by the waters of Singapore River where they were renowned for controlling vermin. This is their national cat.

In Singapore the cat is now affectionately known as "Kucinta", deriving from their words for cat and love. Three specimens were first imported into the USA in the early 1970s. Another from a Singapore SPCA came to the US in 1980. The Singapura breed was accepted for championship status by CFA in 1988 and by TICA in 1984. The modern registered Singapura cat breed in North America is thought to have arisen from only the four progenitor cats mentioned above, and another pair imported in 1987. No outcrosses are allowed in CFA.

Physical Characteristics

Weight: Females 4-7 lb (2-3 kg), males 5-8 (2.5-3.5 kg); average less than 3 kg.

Coat: Haircoat is dense and very short and lies close to the body. Hair has a fine texture. Sepia brown agouti is the sole acceptable color and it is ivory body color with warm dark brown ticking (genetically a sable ticked tabby). Each hair has banding with a minimum of two dark bands; light next to body and a dark tipped extremity. Tail tip and upper topline aspect are darker. Barring pattern may be present inside the legs and lightly on the face. Mascara eyeliner, and dark lines from inner canthus to nose (cheetah lines) and nose liner marks are present. Lighter non-agouti color coat is evident on the chest and underside.

Eyes: Coloring of the eyes includes green, yellow or hazel. Eyes are very large in size and almond-rounded in shape.

Points of Conformation: This is the smallest domestic cat; a moderately built cat. Head is rounded with blunt nose and broad muzzle, with well-defined whisker pads and prominent chin. Ears are large and wide set, lightly pointed, with little hair covering. Neck is short and thick. Small oval feet are present. Tail is short to medium in length, and blunt tipped but slender.

Grooming: Low grooming needs for the Singapura cat—just a chamois cloth or hand petting is sufficient.

Recognized Behavior Issues and Traits

Reported breed characteristics include: A playful, friendly, curious and intelligent cat with a strong need for close human contact. They possess a soft quiet voice with low tendency to vocalization and are gentle lap cats. Some can open doorknobs; are quite trainable, and most remain playful until late in their lifespan. They get along well with other cats—an unusual observation is that some stud cats get along well and sleep together peacefully.

Normal Breed Variations

Reportedly slow to fully mature; up to two years of age; females may not reach sexual maturity until past one year of age and males may not breed until 15 months of age.

Queens are good at mothering, and kittens may not leave nesting boxes until about four weeks of age.

Drug Sensitivities

More than expected adverse vaccine reactions reported in one source.

Inherited Diseases

None reported in the literature

Disease Predispositions

None reported in the literature

Genetic Tests

None commercially available

Miscellaneous

- **Breed name synonyms:** Pura, National Cat of Singapore, Singapore, Sing, drain cat, river cat
- **Registries:** TICA, CFA, ACFA, ACF, GCCF, WCF (provisional), CCA
- **Breed resources: Singapura Fancier's Society:** CFA, 1805 Atlantic Avenue, Manasquan NJ 08736
  The International Singapura Alliance (CFA):
  http://singapura-alliance.org/pageID_5906292.html
  United Singapura Society and Founders' International Singapuras (CFA): 82 W Catalina Dr. Oak View CA 93022
  Independent Singapura Fanciers:
  http://sh1.webring.com/people/fs/singapuracats/
  Progressive Singapura Cat Club (UK):
  http://www.singapuracatclub.co.uk/

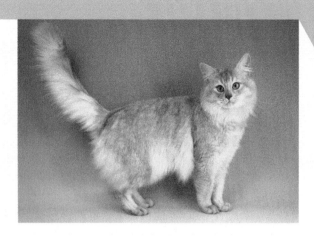

Somali

The Breed History

Somali are a semi-longhaired Abyssinian cat. First records date back to Britain in the 1930s when a spontaneous mutation in Abyssinians occurred, or perhaps the different haircoat was introduced by crossing with longhaired breeds. Outcrossing did occur at some point since the Abyssinian gene pool was seriously depleted in wartime. Historical studies of some lines indicated an autosomal recessive gene for the longhaired coat was present, and periodically, longhaired kittens were born into litters. An American breeder in the 1960s selected **Somali** for a name because Somalia bordered Abyssinia (now Ethiopia). The CFA granted championship status to the Somali breed in the late '70s, and FIFé followed in 1982. Outcrossing to Abyssinian is still allowed.

Physical Characteristics

Weight: Female 8-10 lb (3.5-4.5 kg), male 10-12 lb (4.5-5.5 kg)

Coat: Ruddy cats are the most common color but blue, fawn and sorrel colors are also accepted. Some registries also allow newer colors.

Ruddy is also termed usual. The base color is a rich golden brown sometimes referred to as burnt sienna. Ticking pigment is black. Ticking on the Somali hair consists of 6-12 bands (in comparison to the lesser number in Abyssinians). The root of the hair is the lighter color. Kittens are darker, and their hair base color may be light or gray. Markings include spectacles, mascara eyeliner and a pencil line extending in line towards the ears. Tabby markings on forehead are usually present to some extent. Underside and legs and tail should be unmarked.

Coat is medium in length, a very soft and dense double coat. It is longer on ruff, britches and on the tail. It is a very bushy tail (part of the reason Somali cats have a nickname of "fox cat"). Coat is darker along topline and white is only found around mouth and chin.

The coat doesn't finish maturing until about 18 months of age so ticking evaluation is compromised until then.

Eyes: Eyes are hazel, green or amber colored. Almond shaped eyes are large and slanting.

Points of Conformation: Medium-large sized cat, lithe and semi-foreign build, and the back is long. "Fox-like" is a frequent descriptor. Tail is thicker at the base and tapers slightly. Toe tufts are present and feet are compact and oval.

The head is a rounded wedge shape, large ears are placed wide set and set well back, with interior furnishings and slightly rounded tips.

Grooming: Low grooming requirements; a gentle brushing every other day should suffice. Shedding occurs spring and fall and daily grooming is best at those times.

Recognized Behavior Issues and Traits

Reported breed characteristics include: Friendly, affectionate, active and playful, these cats like to be close to people. They are soft voiced and don't vocalize often. Curious, with a strong personality, and very alert, some are a bit shy, though most get along well with children, strangers and other pets. Some like to groom their owner's hair. They do fine indoors if given climbers, perches and toys. May shadow their favorite person, and be a lap cat. Compared with the Abyssinian, they are calmer and less active, though a few times a day they may get strong bursts of energy. Some like water and learn to turn on faucets. Others open drawers and cupboards. An indoor-outdoor lifestyle is fine, but Somali cats may not tolerate the cold as well as some other breeds of cats.

Normal Breed Variations

Slow maturing kittens

Litters of about 3-4 kittens on average

B Blood Type: In Somali cats, was reported to be a 22% prevalence.[1] A prevalence of 18% type B has also been reported.[2] In the UK as part of a survey, nine cats were tested and two were Type AB while the rest were type A. Type AB cats are very rare.[3]

Long Hair Genetics: The long hair phenotype in cats is a recessive so how it is distributed in the different longhaired breeds, and coded for is of interest. A recent study determined a mutation (AM412646:c.194C>A) in Somali, Persian, Maine Coon, and Ragdoll Cats was responsible for the long hair genotype.[4]

Drug Sensitivities

None reported in the literature

Inherited Diseases

They share many conditions with the Abyssinian-see that chapter.

Pyruvate Kinase (PK) Deficiency and Increased Osmotic Fragility of Red Blood Cells (RBCs): Autosomal recessive. The PK enzyme is involved in anaerobic glycolysis pathway of erythrocytes. Reduced activity of the enzyme results in energy depletion and premature red cell destruction. Cats with this condition may experience recurrent severe hemolytic anemia and splenomegaly.

In one report of 18 Somali and Abyssinian cats, osmotic fragility occurred in the absence of PK deficiency. Onset of anemia in one report ranged from 6 months to 5 years of age (mean 23 months) and PCV ranged from 15%-25% (some as low as 5%). Hepatic enzymes were elevated in some cats. Macrocytosis that persisted when anemia resolved was noted. It was suggested that this condition may have a heredity basis since affected cats were closely related (affecting both Somali and Abyssinian).[5]

In another study of both Abyssinian and Somali cats aged 1-10 years old, chronic intermittent macrocytic regenerative hemolytic anemia and mild splenomegaly was reported. Pyruvate kinase activity ranged from 6%-20% of the normal activity. Osmotic fragility of RBCs was normal to slightly increased.[6]

Affected Somali and Abyssinian cats usually have a normal lifespan unlike dogs with this condition (seen in Beagles, Basenji, West Highland White Terrier, Dachshund). Dogs tend to develop liver failure and osteosclerosis while cats do not. Enzyme analysis and molecular genetic tests are available.[7]

Anemia may be noted in cats as young as 6 months old, and has been found in senior cats (12 yr) that were clinically normal.

A case was described in which the index cat developed a 100% bilirubin cholelith which was thought to be due to chronic hemolysis. (link to reference A on the reference page.[8]

A recent study showed high variability in age of onset and severity of clinical signs so testing before breeding was strongly recommended.[9]

In Australia, 24 cats were tested for the gene and the mutant allele frequency was 0.29.[10]

Amyloidosis: See Abyssinian chapter for details

Neonatal Isoerythrolysis (NI): The prevalence of B blood type can lead to increased incidence, and the proportion of matings reported to be at risk for NI is 0.14.[11]

All B type cats have circulating anti-A antibodies and even primiparous queens can carry these. Type B queens bred to type A toms can result in fatal red cell lysis in A blood type offspring with undetected NI. Kittens with NI can be distinguished from other fading kittens because of pigmenturia; anemia and icterus will also be present; not all kittens at risk for NI will develop overt clinical symptoms.[1]

Progressive Retinal Atrophy (rdAc): Autosomal recessive genetic disease causing blindness. See under Abyssinian. A genetic test is available.

Proressive Retinal Atrophy (Rdy): Autosomal dominant genetic disease causing blindness. See under Abyssinian. A genetic test is available.

Disease Predispositions

Gingivitis: anecdotal over-representation in this breed.

Transfusion Reactions: B blood type similarly results in increased risk of transfusion reactions so donors and recipients should be typed ahead of a transfusion.

Rare and Isolated Cases

Retinal Dysplasia (RD): Abnormal retinal development can affect focal, multifocal or diffuse areas of the retina. Retina degeneration and subsequent scarring interferes with vision. In Sweden, a suspected hereditary form of RD (multifocal) was seen in related Somali cats.[12]

Malignant Histiocytosis: A case report described a multisystem histiocytosis, including neurologic signs, inappetence, and vomiting. Other cases have occurred, but this is a variant of the condition.[13]

Thymoma-associated Neuromuscular Disorder: Can occur as a primary condition (no antibodies—see Siamese) or an acquired form for which Abyssinian and possibly Somali cats are predisposed; Acetylcholine receptor antibodies produced within/by the tumor and in muscle cross react resulting in voice changes, myasthenia gravis, tremor, ventroflexion of the neck and gait abnormalities –myasthenia gravis signs are as for the idiopathic form.[14]

Myasthenia Gravis (MG, acquired): Highest relative risk for acquired MG compared with a baseline of mixed breed cats was reported for Abyssinians and related Somali cats, with relative risk increasing after 3 years of age. The MG was commonly associated with cranial mediastinal mass (not always).[15] See Abyssinian chapter for more information. See above also: Thymoma-associated Neuromuscular Disorder.

Genetic Tests

Pyruvate kinase deficiency

Direct test is available from PennGen.

Minimum of 1-2 ml purple top EDTA blood and should be sent immediately (don't freeze). Test within 48 hrs of sampling.

The lab can do concurrent blood typing on that sample. They can also use 2 buccal swabs.

Direct genetic tests for rdAc PRA and Rdy are available from UC-Davis VGL.

Blood typing done before mating and transfusions

Miscellaneous

- **Breed name synonyms:** Longhaired Abyssinian, Longhaired ticked cat, Fox cat.
- **Registries:** FIFé, TICA, CFA, ACFA, CFF, CCA, NZCF, WCF, GCCF
- **Breed resources:** The Association for Somali Cats: http://tasc.freeservers.com/
  Somali breeders and Fanciers Association Inc: http://www.somalibreeders.com/
  Somali Cat Club of America: www.ladybear.com/Somalis
  Somali Cat Club of Great Britain (GCCF): http://www.somalicatclub.com/

Grand Somali Society:
238 Church St
Poughkeepsie NY 12601
CFA Somali Breed Council: http://www.somalibc.org

References

1. Giger, U, Bucheler J, Patterson DF. Frequency and inheritance of A and B Blood types in feline breeds in the United States. *J Hered* 1991;82:15-20.

2. Giger U. In: Bonagura J, ed. *Kirk's Current Veterinary Therapy XIII.* Philadelphia: WB Saunders Co, 2000;396-399.

3. Knottenbelt CM, Addie DD, Day MJ, et al. Determination of the prevalence of feline blood types in the UK. *J of Small Anim Pract* 1999;40:115-118.

4. Drögemüller C, Rüfenacht S, Wichert B, Leeb T. Mutation within the FGF5 gene are associated with hair length in cats. *Animal Genet* 2007 JUN;38(3):218-221.

5. Kohn B, Goldschmidt MH, Hohenhaus AE, et al. Anemia, splenomegaly, and increased osmotic fragility of erythrocytes in Abyssinian and Somali cats. *J Am Vet Med Assoc* 2000;217(10):1483-1491.

6. Giger U, Rajpurohit Y, Skelly B, et al. Erythrocyte pyruvate kinase deficiency in cats. In: First International Feline Genetic Disease Conference *Proceedings (abstr), Feline Practice Supplement,* 1999:8.

7. Deubler Lab Website. Available at: http://research.vet.upenn.edu/ SubmitaSample/tabid/554/Default.aspx

8. van Geffen C, Savary-Bataille K, Chiers K, Giger U, Daminet S. Bilirubin cholelithiasis and haemosiderosis in an anaemic pyruvate kinase-deficient Somali cat. *J Small Anim Pract.* 2008 Sep;49(9):479-82. Need full text article still

9. Kohn B, Fumi C. Clinical course of pyruvate kinase deficiency in Abyssinian and Somali cats *J Feline Med Surg.* 2008 Apr;10(2):145-53.

10. Barrs, V.R., Giger, U., Wilson, B., Chan, C.T.T., Lingard, A.E., Tran, L., Seng, A., Canfield, P.J., Beattya, J.A. Erythrocytic pyruvate kinase deficiency and AB blood types in Australian Abyssinian and Somali cats. *Aust Vet J.* 2009;87(1):39-44

11. Giger U, Casal M, Niggemeier A. The fading kitten syndrome and neonatal isoerythrolysis. *Proceedings.* The 15th Annual ACVIM Medical Forum, Lake Buena Vista FL 1997:308-310.

12. Narfström K. Hereditary and congenital ocular disease. *J Fel Med Surg* 1999;1:135-141.

13. Reed N, Begara-McGorum IM, Else RW, Gunn-Moore DA. Unusual histiocytic disease in a Somali cat. *J Feline Med Surg.* 2006 Apr;8(2):129-34.

14. Bagley RS. Diseases of the peripheral nervous system, neuromuscular junction and muscle; Evaluation of weakness. *Proceedings.* AAFP Fall meeting. 1998:31-33.

15. Shelton GD, Ho M, Kass PH. Risk factors for acquired myasthenia gravis in cats: 105 cases (1986-1998). *J Am Vet Med Assoc* 2000;Jan1;216(1):55-57.

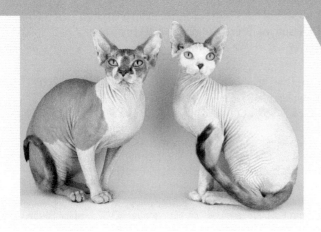

Sphynx/Sphinx

Eyes: Lemon-gold eyes, slanted and large. Other colors are uncommon but accepted.

Points of Conformation: This medium sized lithe cat is characterized by the lack of haircoat guard hairs. Skin around the face, neck and shoulders is somewhat loose and wrinkled. The head is a modified wedge and long, high cheekbones are prominent. A moderate break is present, and nose is moderately long, and whisker pads are distinct. Ears are very large with no furnishings. The neck is long. The paws are oval-round and toes are long with thick pads. Tail is thin, long and tapered. Belly is full and potty, not a tubular profile like Oriental type breeds.

Grooming: These are oily cats and they require frequent sponge baths (weekly or bi-weekly). Some cats may require a seborrhea shampoo. Daily rubbing with a chamois is helpful to prevent oil buildup.

Recognized Behavior Issues and Traits

Reported breed traits include: Intelligent, playful, people-oriented, affectionate, curious, easy-going, and they love to purr. Gentle cats, they are not prone to being excessively vocal. They do well with other pets in the household. Some may be a bit demanding of attention and may follow people around the home. Very athletic, love to jump and climb. Enjoy the company of children.

Normal Breed Variations

High calorie intake is needed to counteract energy lost for warming.

Sphynx cats exhibit poor temperature tolerance and need to wear sweaters in cool ambient temperatures; suitable for an indoor lifestyle only.

They are vulnerable to sunburn.

Has active sebaceous glands on body—oily secretions can have a brown color, skin may give off a rancid odor if oiliness is not controlled by wipes and baths.

The body of the cat usually feels quite warm to touch

Females may cycle less frequently than other queens; kittens may be born with some hair along the spine, which disappears

Blood Type B: Frequency of B blood type was reported to be 17%.[1]

Sphynx Kitten Information Project:[2] An Internet based survey was carried out to determine breed reproduction normal parameters April 2002-March 2003.

Survey involved 18 breeders, 50 litters (mostly from Canada, US), 201 kittens:
    Average litter size 4
    Stillbirth rate 5%
    Dystocia < 1%, of those 7% required C-section

The Breed History

Hairless cats were reported long ago in Central America, and in Russia (Peterbald), but modern Canadian Sphynx (also spelled Sphinx) breed history began in Ontario Canada in 1966 with a mutation leading to alopecia universalis. This autosomal recessive mutation (hr) occurred again in Canada in 1978 where in Toronto, a Siamese breeder found two stray bald cats, and from this stock the modern breed was derived. These were first bred to a white Devon Rex male. Another mutation reportedly arose in Minnesota in 1975 and this cat was used for breeding. The breed made a cameo appearance in the Austin Powers movie as Dr. Evil's cat.

Though early registration occurred when the initial mutation occurred, the breed was withdrawn from the fancy and reintroduced to the registry in the 1980s. TICA accepted them for championship status in the year 1986. The CCA accepted the breed in 1991 for championship status also. The CFA accepted the breed in the Miscellaneous Class in 1998 and it is now in Championship. This is the only widely recognized breed of hairless cat.

Though early registration occurred when the initial mutation occurred, the breed was withdrawn from the fancy and reintroduced to the registry in the 1980s. TICA accepted them for championship status in the year 1986. The CCA accepted the breed in 1991 for championship status also. Currently, outcrossing to American Shorthair cats is allowed (books in CFA close for this breed in 2010). The CFA accepted the breed in the Miscellaneous Class in 1998 and it is now in Championship. This is the only widely recognized breed of hairless cat.

Physical Characteristics

Weight: females 6-8 lb (2.7-3.6 kg), males 8-12 lb (3.6-5.4 kg)

Coat: This cat breed is not truly hairless as many believe. There is a fine down cover described as "peach fuzz" or suede. Hairs must be less than 1/8th" long, and sometimes small short tufts of hair are found on tail tip, scrotum, brow, bridge of nose, back of ears, or outside of paws. All colors and patterns are accepted.

Heterozygotes have more down than do homozygotes. May or may not have whiskers or brows. If present, whiskers may be short or break off easily.

Average birth weight: Male 96 g female 95 g
Congenital deformities (2.5% of litters) included: cleft palate, umbilical hernias.

Drug Sensitivities
None reported in the literature

Inherited Diseases
Alopecia Universalis: This is the condition that these cats have been selected for. Note that it is not accompanied by adnexal abnormalities as in hypotrichosis.[3]

Neonatal Isoerythrolysis (NI): The presence of B blood type in the breed would be expected to increased risk of NI reactions in kittens. The reported proportion of matings at risk for NI is 0.16.[4]

Disease Predispositions
Transfusion Reactions: The presence of B blood type in the breed leads to increased risk of adverse reactions.

Malassezia dermatitis: Especially paronychia HCM (anecdotal)[9]

Rare and Isolated Cases
Spasticity/Hereditary Myopathy: An autosomal recessive mutation in the Devon Rex, a similar phenotypic presentation has been seen in Sphynx leading to abnormal deglutition; frequently leads to aspiration pneumonia—very similar to the Devon Rex Hereditary Myopathy, also termed Spasticity. A recent report indicates that a change in dystroglycan (DAG1) may be causing this problem in both Devon Rex and Sphynx, and the authors attempted to sequence the mutation.[5]

Urticaria Pigmentosa: This condition has been found in related Sphynx cats. Dermal infiltration with mast cells is noted. In one report, three young cats developed multifocal lesions which in one cat led to significant pruritis that could be controlled with combined antihistamine (hydroxyzine) and glucocorticoids (prednisone) therapy.[6] These cats had a common grandsire (clinically normal). The condition was of juvenile onset, was bilaterally symmetrical, erythematous, and trunk, limbs, neck and head were most affected. Some macules were dark brown and skin lesions tended to be linear. Peripheral eosinophilia and/or basophilia was often present. This was a cutaneous mastocytosis, not associated with systemic disease. Afflicted cats were negative for dermatographism.[7]

Genetic Tests
Blood typing before breeding and transfusions

Miscellaneous
- **Breed name synonyms:** Hairless Cat (historical), Bald Cat, Sphinx, Canadian Hairless
- **Registries:** TICA, CCA, CFA, ACFA, CFF, NZCF, CCA, FIFé, ACF
- **Breed resources:** International Sphynx Society (CFA):
  www.classytouch.net
  International Sphynx Breeders and Fanciers Association:
  HC66, Box 70035
  Pinetop AZ 85935

Sphynx Cat Association:
http://www.hoosierkitties.com/breed/sphinx.htm
CFA Sphynx Breed Council: www.sphynxbc.org/

References
1. Giger U. In: Bonagura J, ed. *Kirk's Current Veterinary Therapy XIII.* Philadelphia: WB Saunders Co, 2000;396-399.
2. Little S. Breed Specific Reproduction Projects and Kitten Health Data. In: *Poster.* Tuft's Canine and Feline Breeding and Genetics Conference. Oct 2-4, 2003 Available at: http://www.vin.com/tufts/2003. Accessed Nov 19, 2004. University of California (Davis) Feline Genetics Extravaganza I July, 2003.
3. Hoskins JD. Congenital defects in cats. *Compend Contin Educ Pract Vet* 1995;17(3):385-405.
4. Giger U, Casal M, Niggemeier A. The fading kitten syndrome and neonatal isoerythrolysis. *Proceedings.* The 15th Annual ACVIM Medical Forum, Lake Buena Vista FL 1997;308-310.
5. Suciu A, Lipinski M, Froenicke L, et al. Dystroglycan (DAG1) as a candidate gene for a feline hereditary Myopathy "Spasticity". In: *Notes.* University of California (Davis) Feline Genetics Extravaganza II Aug 28-29, 2004.
6. DeManuelle T. Feline dermatopathies: Newly described disorders. *Proceedings.* 70th Annual AAHA Conference Proceedings 2003;1:93-95.
7. Vitale CB, Ihrke PJ, Olivry T, et al. Case Report: Feline urticaria pigmentosa in three related Sphinx cats. *Vet Dermatol* 1996;7:227-233.
8. Jordan, E. Less is More. Pp. 26-27. Cat Fancy September 2008.
9. Feline Advisory Beaureau: http://www.fabcats.org/breeders/inherited_disorders/sphynx.php

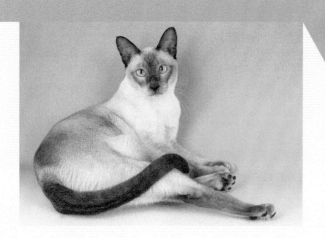

Tonkinese

The Breed History
The breed foundation female is Wong Mau, a Siamese cross originally from Burma (now Myanmar). She is also the progenitor female of the Burmese breed of cats. The foundation offspring from the 1930s litter was split into Burmese for brown coated kittens, and those with Wong Mau's pointed pattern were assigned to the Tonkinese breed. Crosses between Siamese and Burmese cats continued, which led to the formation of the Tonkinese breed. Then the books were closed to prevent too much Siamese type influence. The Tonkinese name may have derived from the word Tonkin, possibly an ancient name for Viet Nam, and the name is used for Gulf of Tonkin in that region. First recognized by CCA in the year 1971, and CFA in 1978, with championship status granted in 1984. The European standard is somewhat different than the North American one. No outcrossing is allowed in the CFA.

Physical Characteristics
Weight: Female 6-8 lb (2.5-3.5 kg), male 8-12 lb (3.5-5.5 kg)

Coat: They possess a short thick coat of fine silky glossy hairs that lay close to the body. A small cowlick is usually present on the chest. A small number of colors are accepted: Platinum (termed Lilac in Siamese), Blue, Natural (termed Brown outside North America), and Champagne (Chocolate in Siamese). The Natural or Brown color is the same as the Sable Burmese or Seal Point Siamese. Other colors are accepted in some registries.

Three Patterns can be Registered:
1. **Mink:** Ideal show type. Delineation between points and body color should be visible but not be sharp. *(cb cs)*. Note that cb and cs are co-dominant which results in this intermediate phenotype.[1]
2. **Pointed:** Sharp transition of points; as in Siamese cats *(cs cs)*.
3. **Solid:** Very weak transition to points; only slight lightening on the body, as in Burmese cats *(cb cb)*.

Latter two types are pet quality (AOV registered), and occasional honeys or fawns are also AOV.

Tonkinese points are **autosomal recessive** inheritance. These patterns reflect three types of partial temperature sensitive (ts) oculocutaneous albinism, there is a spectrum of mutation effects at one locus.[2]

In the Natural mink the body is a light brown. This is intermediate between the light body of Siamese, and the dark body of the Burmese. Coat tends to darken further with age. Allow up to 16 months for dilute coats to fully develop.

Eyes: Aqua in the Minks (this is an intense aquamarine green-blue), blue in other pointed cats but not the Siamese blue. Should not be Burmese chartreuse green. Eyes are almond shaped, moderate in size.

Points of Conformation: Medium build and size, with moderate to heavy stature. Modified softened wedge shaped head, like Siamese traditional "apple head" conformation. High cheeks, slight break. The medium-large ears have rounded tips. Leather of the ear may show due to minimal hair covering. Paws are oval and small. Tail is moderate in length and tapers at the tip.

Grooming: Minimal grooming—just a weekly or twice weekly pass through with a rubber brush will suffice.

Recognized Behavior Issues and Traits
Reported breed characteristics include: Active, playful, moderately vocal, very social, get along well with other pets and children, intelligent, curious, like to jump, adaptable, need close human contact, strong willed and strong personality; have some of the Siamese and Burmese traits. Can be leash trained and love to play fetch. Suited for indoor lifestyle and will happily ride shoulders and head butt for attention. Have been featured in the past as therapy cats in a National Geographic special—Tonkinese are well suited to AAA because of their gentle, gregarious nature.

Normal Breed Variations
Watch calorie intake due to tendency to obesity

A prevalence of 100% blood type A was reported.[3]

Drug Sensitivities
None reported in the literature

Inherited Diseases
See Siamese and Burmese chapters—share many of their conditions but generally quite hardy and healthy; likely due to hybrid vigor.

Disease Predispositions
Medial Patellar Luxation: A study in 1990 noted that of 22 Tonkinese cats assessed as part of a larger study, 4 had increased patella mobility/less secure seating. Minimum age in the overall mixed breed study group was 6 months; average age of the cats was 3.6 years. Compared with non pedigreed cats in this study group with a rate of 2:31 cats affected, this breed had a greater laxity rate.[4]

Genetic Tests

No tests available commercially but now that the mutations of the tyrosinase gene leading to the ts-albinism (pointing) have been identified, checking for carriers of pointing alleles will follow, reducing the number of test crosses needed by breeders.[1]

Miscellaneous

- **Breed name synonyms:** Tonk, Tonkanese, Golden Siamese (historical), Old-fashioned Siamese, Pointed Burmese
- **Registries:** CCA, TICA, CFA, ACFA, CFF, GCCF, ACF, NZCF, CCA
- **Breed resources: Tonkinese Breed Association:**
  Website: http://www.tonkinesebreedassociation.org/
  Tonkinese Cat Club (GCCF): http://www.tonkinesecatclub.co.uk/

References

1. Imes DL, Young AE, Grahn RA, Lyons LA. Get to the point: Identifying albinism mutations in cats. *Proceedings*. Tuft's Canine and Feline Breeding and Genetics Conference Oct 2-4, 2003 Available at VIN: www.vin.com/tufts/2003. Accessed Nov 19, 2004.

2. Lyons LA, Imes DL, Grahn RA. Investigation of albinism in domestic cats. *Proceedings*. 2nd International Conference Advances in Canine and Feline Genomics. Oct 2004. Utrecht Netherlands. Poster #18.

3. Giger U. In: Bonagura J, ed. *Kirk's Current Veterinary Therapy XIII.* Philadelphia: WB Saunders Co, 2000;396-399.

4. Engvall E, Bushnell N. Patellar luxation in Abyssinian cats. *Fel Pract* 1990;18(4):20-22.

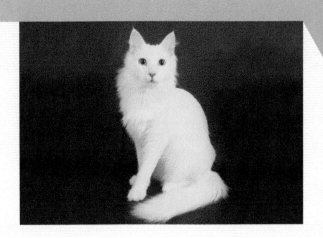

Turkish Angora

intelligent, curious, possess good hunting instincts, love to jump, and are able to jump very high. They like close human contact and some will shadow their owners. They like a regular routine and are noted to have a strong personality.

The Breed History

This ancient longhair breed originated in Turkey. First written records date to the 1800s. These graceful, tall, slender cats almost became extinct in the early 1900s due to extensive crossing with Persians.

In Turkey a special breeding program was maintained to preserve the original cat type. Only the Turkish cats originating from that breeding program in the Ankara zoo have been accepted into the modern registry. In 1963, the first pair was brought to America. First CFA registrations occurred in the year 1970. Note that in Britain, Angora cats are registered (GCCF) but are not the same breed as the Turkish Angora, but are in fact closer in breeding and type to the Oriental longhair in the US. No outcrossing is allowed in CFA.

Physical Characteristics

Weight: Females 5-9 lb (2.3-4 kg), males 6-11 lb (2.5-5 kg)

Coat: Many colors are accepted, but not Oriental shades such as lavender, chocolate or the Himalayan pointed pattern. Single layer coat is medium long, glossy and silky, lying close to the body, and hairs have a slight wave. White is the most common color. The full features of the coat are not developed until 18 to 24 months of age. Longer hair is present on ruff and britches and the tail is a full bottle brush-plume tail.

Variation occurs between registries in accepted coloring. This applies to shading and silver (genetics: inhibitor gene plus agouti gene) which is not allowed in CFA but is allowed in TICA and FIFé.

Eyes: The large eyes are almond shaped and colors include green, copper, gold, green-gold, blue and odd-eyed.

Points of Conformation: These are small-medium sized cats, lithe, with long bodies, are fine boned, and possess a fine wedge shaped head. Nose is medium in length and straight with no break, ears are large, tufted, and close set. Tail is long and tapering, and paws are compact, small and round. Toe tufting is preferred.

Grooming: Low matting tendency compared with Persians, daily light brush or combing is sufficient. Shedding is usually seasonal.

Recognized Behavior Issues and Traits

Reported breed characteristics include: Affectionate, active,

Normal Breed Variations

Blood Type: In a survey in Turkey of 28 cats, 46.4% were B type.[1]

Drug Sensitivities

None reported in the literature

Inherited Diseases

Neonatal Isoerythrolysis (NI): Increased risk of NI is present due to considerable prevalence of blood type B. Authors recommend typing cats before breeding; even the first breeding since primiparous females' offspring can be affected.[1]

Congenital Deafness: Sometimes seen in white coat with blue-eyed and odd-eyed pigmentation.[2]

Disease Predispositions

Transfusion Reactions: High risk of reactions due to presence of type B blood type in this breed, and blood typing should be done before transfusions according to the authors.[1]

Genetic Tests

Blood typing before breeding and transfusions

Miscellaneous

- **Breed name synonyms:** Turk, Angora, Turkish Longhair, Ankara cats (historical syn)
- **Registries:** FIFé, TICA, CFA, ACFA, CFF, WCF, CCA
- **Breed resources:** Turkish Angora Fanciers International: http://turkishangora.org/
  The Turkish Cat Society (UK): www.turkishcatsociety.co.uk

References

1. Arikan S, Duru SY, Gurkan M, Agaoglu ZT, Giger U. Blood type A and B frequencies in Turkish Van and Angora cats in Turkey. *J Vet Med A Physiol Pathol Clin Med.* 2003;Aug;50(6):303-306.
2. Strain GM. Hereditary deafness in dogs and cats: causes, prevalence, and current research. *Proceedings.* Tuft's Canine and Feline Breeding and Genetics Conference. Oct 2-4, 2003, Available at: http://www.vin.com/tufts/2003. Accessed Nov 19, 2004.

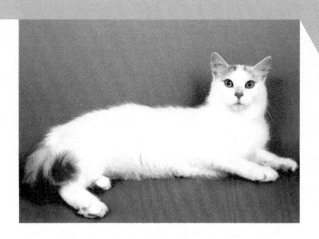

Turkish Van

Coat texture is very soft (like cashmere) and plush; it is a semi-longhaired single silky coat. Coat lies flat, with britches and feathers on belly, feet and legs. Length and fullness of coat depends on the season. This is a water resistant coat.

Eyes: Colors include blue, odd-eyed or yellow-amber (the original auburn van eye color). Eyes are moderately large, wide set, oval-almond shaped. Color may become less intense with age.

Points of Conformation: These are medium-large cats with sturdy conformation. Head is a broad wedge shape, with prominent cheekbones, and moderately long straight nose. Face has a slight break. Ears are high set, medium-large in size, well furnished, and tips are somewhat rounded. Tail has "bottle brush" hair cover and the tail is the same length as the body, with a blunt tip. Body and chest are both broad, and the feet are large, round and compact with tufting of hair between the toes.

Grooming: Moderate grooming needs—just a quick daily brush or combing required. Much reduced matting tendency compared with Persians. Though they are known as swimming cats, this does not necessarily translate into a love of baths.

Recognized Behavior Issues and Traits
Reported breed characteristics include: Highly intelligent—the hallmark of the breed is their love of swimming, though not all individuals are water-loving. Gait of the male cats can appear to swing due to the wide pelvis. They are active cats, friendly and independently minded, vocal and love climbing but not jumping; they like to keep their feet on the ground. Good for leash training and love to play fetch. Some can open cupboard doors. Can be startled with certain sounds; some don't travel well and may resist carrying. Not considered lap cats. Vans are often described as "dog like".

Normal Breed Variations
Litter average size 4 kittens
These are slow maturing cats (~3-5 years)

Blood Type: In a survey of 85 cats in Turkey, 60% were B blood type.[1] In a recent survey of 78 Van cats in Turkey, naturally occurring alloantibody titers were measured; in this study 57.7% of the cats were type B (n=45 cats). In this subset, all the B type cats had grossly evident agglutinating anti-A antibodies in plasma. Type A cats (n=33) were also checked and 78% had anti-B antibody in their plasma; of these 18% had microscopic agglutination only.[2]

Drug Sensitivities
None reported in the literature

Inherited Diseases
Neonatal Isoerythrolysis (NI): Increased risk due to high prevalence of B blood type; Neonatal isoerythrolysis occurs when A or AB type kittens of a B type queen are allowed to nurse in the

The Breed History
Eastern Turkey surrounding Lake Van is the place of origin of the breed. Vans are not closely related to Turkish Angora cats and are larger and more heavily built than the Angora. Many of the Turkish Van cats love to swim! Vans were first exported in 1955 to England, then to America where interest took off in 1982. The distinguishing white and red markings in this breed are known as *van*, and this term is now used to describe other cats in other breeds with the same color pattern. These other similarly marked cats are referred to as van cats also, but this should not be confused with them being related. No outcrosses are allowed.

In Turkey, indigenous people often refer to "van" cats as all white cats with odd-eyes; perhaps a description more in line with what the fancy organizations have labeled the Turkish Angora. The CFA accepted this breed in Miscellaneous Class in 1988, provisional in 1993, and for Championship status in 1994. The GCCF and FIFé both recognized the breed in 1969.

Physical Characteristics
Weight: Breed standard specifies both weight and length.
Males- > 28" height, > 10 lb to 19 lb (4.5-8.5 kg)
Females > 25" height, > 8 lb (3.5 kg)

Coat: The most common color is van, a chalk white body with dark orange-red (auburn) tail and lighter red-orange colored blazed marking over the skull. Sometimes head markings extend up onto the ears (considered ideal). Ideally, a white blaze should extend up the middle of the forehead. The tail is faintly ringed in orange or cream cats, but not in blue or tortie cats. The other color markings are combined with a white body in a van pattern. Some registries (CFA) allow for up to 20% of the body to be the colored hairs (in "thumbprints"). Cream is a dilute of the orange color.

Point restricted or Oriental colors (lilac, chocolate) are not accepted in any registries. Van is piebald spotting genetically *(SS)*, a **dominant gene with incomplete penetrance**. Different grading systems have been published to describe the differing degrees of white, with grades 2-9 having some variation of the piebald; with ideal Van markings being around 8-9 on the scales. If there is more than 20% color on body, or lacking van color on head or tail it will be a pet quality cat.

immediate postnatal period. Authors recommended typing male and female cats before breeding, even the first breeding, since a primiparous females' offspring can be affected.[1,2]

Disease Predispositions

Transfusion Reactions: High risk of reactions due to presence of type B blood type in this breed, so blood typing should be done before transfusions according to the authors.[1] Where there was an A type donor and B type recipient, if not typed, the recipient had a 8.9% probability of an acute severe reaction, while another 77.8% could be expected to have acute mild reactions, with the balance having premature red cell destruction post-transfusion.

Genetic Tests

Blood typing should be performed before transfusion or breeding due to high prevalence of blood type B.

Miscellaneous

- **Breed name synonyms:** Van cat, Swimming Cat, Water Cat, Turk, National Cat of Turkey, Turkey, White Ringtail (historical SYN), Russian Longhair, White Russian
- **Registries:** FIFé, TICA, CFA, ACFA, GCCF, ACF, WCF, NZCF
- **Breed resources: Vantastix Turkish Van Breed Club:** www.vantastixcatclub.com
  Classic Turkish Van Cat Association: http://www.vantasia.org/
  Turkish Van Cat Club (UK):
  http://www.turkishvancatclub.co.uk/index1.htm

References

1. Arikan S, Duru SY, Gurkan M, Agaoglu ZT, Giger U. Blood type A and B frequencies in Turkish Van and Angora cats in Turkey. *J Vet Med A Physiol Pathol Clin Med.* 2003; Aug; 50(6):303-306.
2. Arikan S, Akkan HA. Titres of naturally occurring alloantibodies against feline blood group antigens in Turkish Van cats. *J Small Anim Pract* 2004; Jun;45(6):289-292.

Available Genetic Tests for Breed Specific Canine and Feline Genetic Disorders

Disorder	Breeds	Type of Test	Test Facility
AB Blood Groups	Cats	Direct	UC-Davis VGL
Benign Familial Juvenile Epilepsy	Lagotto Romagnolo	Direct	Canigen
Black Hair Follicular Dysplasia	Large Munsterlander	Direct	HealthGene
Bobtail (Canine Brachyury)	Australian Shepherd Australian Stumpy Tail Cattle Dog Austrian Pinscher Bourbonnais Pointer Brazilian Terrier Brittany Spaniel Croatian Sheepdog Danish/Swedish Farmdog Jack Russel Terrier Karelian Bear Dog Mudi Polish Lowland Sheeplog Pyrenean Shepherd Savoy Sheepdog Schipperke Spanish Waterdog Swedish Vallhund	Direct	ANTAGENE Genoscoper Animal Health Trust (some breeds)
Canine Leukocyte Adhesion Deficiency (CLAD)	Irish Red and White Setter Irish Setter	Direct	Optigen Animal Health Trust
Cardiomyopathy, Arrhythmogenic Right Ventricular (ARVC)	Boxer	Direct	North Carolina State University - Meurs Lab
Cardiomyopathy, Dilated (DCM)	Doberman Pinscher	Direct	North Carolina State University - Meurs Lab
Cardiomyopathy, Juvenile	Portuguese Water Dog	Direct	PennGen
Cataract, Juvenile (Early Onset Hereditary Cataract – EHD)	Boston Terrier French Bulldog Staffordshire Bull Terrier	Direct	Animal Health Trust VetGen
Cataract	Australian Shepherd	Direct – Susceptibility Gene	Animal Health Trust
Cerebellar Ataxia	Spinone Italiano	Linkage	Animal Health Trust
Cerebellar Ataxia	Finnish Hound	Direct	Genoscoper
Cerebellar Ataxia (NCL-A)	American Staffordshire Terrier	Direct	ANTAGENE Optigen
Ceroid lipofuscinosis	Border Collie	Direct	Animal Health Trust Optigen
Ceroid lipofuscinosis	American Bulldog Dachshund English Setter Tibetan Terrier	Direct	OFA (Am. Bulldogs and Tibetan Terrier) U Missouri (Dachshund and English Setter)
Chondrodysplasia	Norwegian Elkhound	Direct	Genoscoper

Disorder	Breeds	Type of Test	Test Facility
Coat Color and Nose Color Variation	Afghan Hound Australian Shepherd Belgian Shepherd Border Collie Briard Brittany Cardigan Welsh Corgi Chinese Shar Pei Collie (Rough, Smooth) Cocker Spaniel Curly-Coated Retriever Dachshund Dalmatian Doberman Pinscher English Cocker Spaniel English Setter English Springer Spaniel Field Spaniel Flat-coated Retriever French Bulldog German Shepherd German Longhaired Pointer German Shorthaired Pointer German Wirehaired Pointer Great Dane Greyhound Groenendael Japanese Chin Labrador Retriever Laekenois Large Munsterlander Lowchen Malinois Miniature Schnauzer Newfoundland Pointer Pomeranian Poodle Portuguese Water Dog Pudelpointer Pug Shetland Sheepdog Staffordshire Bull Terrier Tervuren Whippet Wirehaired Pointing Griffon	Direct	HealthGene
Coat Color Gene Variations	Most Dog Breeds – see VetGen website	Direct	VetGen
Coat Color Genes - Cats	Most Cats	Direct	UC-Davis VGL
Coat Length (FGF5)	Alaskan Malamute Border Collie Cats (all breeds) German Shepherd Pembroke Welsh Corgi Weimeraner	Direct	Animal Health Trust UC-Davis VGL
Cobalamin Malabsorption (Methylmalonic Aciduria)	Australian Shepherd Giant Schnauzer	Direct	PennGen

Disorder	Breeds	Type of Test	Test Facility
Cobalamin Malabsorption (Methylmalonic Aciduria)	Basset Hound Beagle Border Collie DSH Komodor Shar Pei	Phenotypic	PennGen
Collie Eye Anomaly (Choroidal Hypoplasia)	Australian Shepherd Border Collie Boykin Spaniel Lancashire Heeler Nova Scotia Duck Tolling Retriever Rough Coated Collie Shetland Sheepdog Smooth Coated Collie Whippet, Longhair	Direct	Optigen
Cone (Retinal) Degeneration	Alaskan Malamute Australian Shepherd German Shorthaired Pointer	Direct	Optigen
Congenital Hypothyroidism with Goiter (CHG)	Rat Terrier Toy Fox Terrier	Direct	Michigan State University – Fyfe Lab. PennGen
Congenital Keratoconjuntivitis Sicca and Ichthyosiform Dermatitis	Cavalier King Charles Spaniel	Direct	Animal Health Trust
Congenital Macrothrombocytopenia	Cavalier King Charles Spaniel	Direct	Auburn Univ. – Boudreaux Lab
Congenital Stationary Night Blindness (RPE65-CSNB)	Briard	Direct	Optigen Animal Health Trust
Copper Toxicosis	Bedlington Terrier	Direct	VetGen Animal Health Trust
Cyclic Neutropenia (Grey Collie Syndrome)	Smooth Coated Collie Rough Coated Collie	Direct	HealthGene
Cystinuria	Newfoundland Labrador Retriever	Direct	Optigen (Newf only) PennGen VetGen (Newf only)
Degenerative Myelopathy (DM)	American Eskimo Dog American Water Spaniel Bernese Mountain Dog Borzoi Boxer Canaan Dog Cardigan Welsh Corgi Chesapeake Bay Retriever Collie French Bulldog German Shepherd Dog Irish Setter Kerry Blue Terrier Kuvasz Mixed-breed/Other breeds Pembroke Welsh Corgis Poodle, Standard Pug Rhodesian Ridgeback	Direct - Susceptibility Gene	OFA

Disorder	Breeds	Type of Test	Test Facility
Encephalitis, Pug Dog (PDE)	Pug	Direct – Susceptibility Gene	UC-Davis
Episodic Falling	Cavalier King Charles Spaniel	Direct	Animal Health Trust
Exercise Induced Collapse (EIC, Dynamin 1 Mutation)	Boykin Spaniel Chesapeake Bay Retriever Curly Coated Retriever German Wirehaired Pointer Labrador Retriever Pembroke Welsh Corgi	Direct	UMinn VDL
Factor VII Deficiency	Alaskan Klee Kai Beagle Scottish Deerhound	Direct	PennGen Animal Health Trust (Beagle and Scottish Deerhound)
Facor IX Deficiency (Hemophilia B)	Airdale Terrier Bull Terrier German Wirehaired Pointer Labrador Retreiver Lhasa Apso	Direct	Cornell Univ. Comparative Coag. Lab (GWP) HealthGene (Others)
Factor XI Deficiency	Kerry Blue Terrier	Direct	PennGen
Fanconi Syndrome	Basenji	Linkage	OFA
Fanconi Syndrome	Basenji Norwegian Elkhound	Phenotypic	PennGen
Fucosidosis	English Springer Spaniel	Direct	PennGen Animal Health Trust
Glanzmann's Thrombasthenia (Type I)	Great Pyrenees Otterhound	Direct	Auburn Univ. – Boudreaux Lab.
Globoid cell leukodystrophy	Cairn terrier West Highland White Terrier	Direct	Jefferson Medical Coll.
Glycogenosis (GSD) Type IIIa	Curly Coated Retriever	Direct	Michigan State University – Fyfe Lab.
Glycogenosis (GSD) Type IV	Norwegian Forest Cat	Direct	PennGen
GM1-Gangliosidosis	Portuguese Water Dog	Direct	New York University Neurogenetics Lab
GM1 (GLB1) and GM2 (HEXB) Gangliosidosis	Korat	Direct	UC-Davis VGL
GM2-Gangliosidosis	Burmese Japanese Chin	Direct	UC-Davis VGL (Burmese) OFA (Japanese Chin)
Hypersarcosinemia	Portuguese Water Dog	Phenotypic	PennGen
Hyperuricosuria (SLC2A9)	American Staffordshire Terrier Australian Shepherd Bulldog Black Russian Terrier Dalmatian German Shepherd Dog Giant Schnauzer Jack/Parson Russel Terrier Large Munsterlander Labrador Retriever Pomeranian Weimaraner	Direct	UC-Davis VGL Animal Health Trust
Hypertrophic Cardiomyopathy	Maine Coon Cat Ragdoll	Direct	North Carolina State University - Meurs Lab UC-Davis VGL (Ragdoll)

Disorder	Breeds	Type of Test	Test Facility
Ichthyosis	Golden Retriever Norfolk Terrier	Direct	Antagene (Goldens) Optigen (Goldens) Venta Lab-MSU 517-355-6463 x1552 (Norfolks)
Improper Coat (IC13)	Portuguese Water Dog	Direct	Optigen
Ivermectin Sensitivity (MDR1)	Australian Shepherd Collie German Shepherd Dog Old English Sheepdog Shetland Sheepdog Other breeds	Direct	Washington State U – Pharm Lab
L-2-HGA (L-2-hydroxyglutaric aciduria)	Staffordshire Bull Terrier	Direct	Animal Health Trust
Mannosidosis	DSH Persian	Direct	PennGen
Merle Gene (SILV)	Australian Shepherds Beauceron Sheepdog Border Collie Cardigan Welsh Corgi Catahoula Leopard Dog Chihuahua Cocker Spaniel Collie Dachshund Great Danes Norwegian Hound Pitt Bull Pomeranian Pyrenean Shepherd Shetland Sheepdogs	Direct	(GenMark has been bought by Idexx, who will be offering again in the future)
Mitochondrial Myopathy	Cocker Spaniel Old English Sheepdog	Phenotypic	PennGen
Mucolipidosis II (I-Cell Disease)	DSH	Direct	PennGen
Mucopolysaccharidosis (MPS)	DSH German Shepherd Dog Miniature Pinscher Miniature and Toy Poodle Miniature Schnauzer Plotthound Schipperke Siamese Wirehaired Dachshund	Direct	PennGen
Mucopolysaccharidosis (MPS)	Cardigan Welsh Corgi Pembroke Welsh Corgi Rottweiler	Phenotypic	PennGen
Musladin-Lueke Syndrome	Beagle	Direct	UC-Davis VGL
Muscular Myopathy (Centronuclear myopathy)	Labrador Retriever	Direct	Alfort School of Veterinary Medicine, France Animal Health Trust
Myostatin Mutation (Gross Muscle Hypertrophy, Bully Whippets)	Whippet	Direct	DDC Veterinary

Disorder	Breeds	Type of Test	Test Facility
Myotonia Congenita	Miniature Schnauzer	Direct	Optigen PennGen
Myotonia Hereditaria	Australian Cattle Dog	Direct	U-Guelph AHL
Narcolepsy	Dachshund Doberman Pinscher Labrador Retriever	Direct	Optigen
Neonatal Ataxia	Coton de Tulear	Direct	Antagene Univ. Missouri
Neonatal Encephalopathy	Standard Poodle	Direct	OFA
Nephropathy (Hereditary N., Familial N.)	English Cocker Spaniel	Direct	Optigen
Oculoskeletal Dysplasia (OSD)/ Retinal Dysplasia (RD)	Labrador Retriever Samoyed	Direct	Optigen
Perianal Fistula/Anal Furunculosis	German Shepherd	Direct Susceptibility Gene	Genoscoper
Persistent Muellerian Duct Syndrome	Miniature Schnauzer	Direct	Cornell:Meyers-Wallen Lab
Phosphofructokinase Deficiency (PFK)	American Cocker Spaniel English Springer Spaniel Whippet (VetGen only)	Direct	Optigen PennGen VetGen Animal Health Trust (ESS)
Polycystic Kidney Disease (PKD)	American Shorthair British Shorthair Himalayan Persian Scottish Fold	Direct	UC-Davis – VGL Animal Health Trust
Polyneuropathy (Leonberger Polyneuropathy)	Leonberger	Direct	UMinn VDL U Bern
Polyneuropathy (NDRG1)	Greyhound	Direct	Optigen
Primary Hyperoxaluria	Tibetan Spaniel	Phenotypic	PenGen
Primary Hyperparathyroidism	Keeshond	Linkage	Cornell – Goldstein Lab
Primary Lens Luxation (PLL)	Australian Cattle Dog Chinese Crested Jack Russell Terrier Lakeland Terrier Lancashire Heeler Miniature Bull Terrier Parson Russell Terrier Patterdale Terrier Rat Terrier Sealyham Terrier Tenterfield Terrier Tibetan Terrier Toy Fox Terrier Volpino Italiano Welsh Terrier Wire Fox Terrier	Direct	Animal Health Trust OFA
Progressive Retinal Atrophy	Papillon	Direct	Genoscoper
Progressive Retinal Atrophy (cord1)	Dachshund, Miniature Longhaired and Smooth haired English Springer Spaniel	Direct Susceptibility Gene	Animal Health Trust U-Missouri
Progressive Retinal Atropy (crd2)	American Pit Bull Terrier	Direct	Optigen

Disorder	Breeds	Type of Test	Test Facility
Progressive Retinal Atrophy (crd3)	Glen of Imaal Terrier	Direct	Optigen
Progressive Retinal Atrophy - Dominant	Bullmastiff (English) Mastiff	Direct	Optigen
Progressive Retinal Atrophy (GR-PRA1)	Golden Retriever	Direct	Animal Health Trust Optigen
Progressive Retinal Atrophy (prcd)	American Cocker Spaniel American Eskimo Dog Australian Cattle Dog Australian Shepherd Chesapeake Bay Retriever Chinese Crested Cockapoo English Cocker Spaniel Entelbucher Mountain Dog Finnish Lapphund Golden Retriever Goldendoodle Kuvasz Labradoodle Labrador Retriever Lapponian Herder Norwegian Elkhound Nova Scotia Duck Trolling Retriever Poodle; Miniature & Toy Portuguese Water Dog Silky Terrier Spanish Water Dog Stumpy Tail Cattle Dog Swedish Lapphund Yorkshire Terrier	Direct	Optigen
Progressive Retinal Atrophy (rcd1)	Irish Red and White Setter Irish Setter	Direct	Optigen Animal Health Trust VetGen (Irish Setter)
Progressive Retinal Atrophy (rcd1a)	Sloughi	Direct	Optigen Animal Health Trust
Progressive Retinal Atrophy (rcd2)	Collie – Smooth and Rough	Direct	Optigen
Progressive Retinal Atrophy (rcd3)	Cardigan Welsh Corgi	Direct	Michigan State Univ. - Peterson-Jones Lab. Optigen VetGen
Progressive Retinal Atrophy (rcd4)	Gordon Setter Irish Setter	Direct	Animal Health Trust
Progressive Retinal Atrophy (rdAc)	Abyssinian Ocicat Siamese Somali	Direct	UC-Davis VGL
Progressive Retinal Atrophy (Rdy)	Abyssinian Somali	Direct	UC-Davis VGL
Progressive Retinal Atrophy – Type A	Miniature Schnauzer	Direct	Optigen
Progressive Retinal Atrophy – X-Linked	Samoyed Siberian Husky	Direct	Optigen

Disorder	Breeds	Type of Test	Test Facility
Pyruvate Dehydrogenase Phosphatase Deficiency (PDH or PDP1)	Clumber Spaniel Sussex Spaniel	Direct	U-Missouri Animal Health Trust
Pyruvate Kinase Deficiency (PK)	Abyssinian American Eskimo Dog Basenji Beagle Bengal Cairn Terrier Chihuahua Dachshund DSH Somali West Highland White Terrier	Direct	Optigen (Basenji) PennGen (All) VetGen (Basenji) Animal Health Truist (Westies) UC-Davis VGL (Cats)
Renal Dysplasia	Lhasa Apso Shih Tzu Soft Coated Wheaton Terrier	Direct Susceptibility Gene	DOGenes
Retinal Dysplasia – Canine Multi-focal Retinopathy (CMR)	Australian Shepherd Bullmastiff Cane Corso Coton de Tulear Dogue de Bordeaux Great Pyrenees Lapponian Herder Mastiff (English and French) Perro de Presa Canario	Direct	Optigen
Severe Combined Immunodeficiency (SCID)	Bassett Hound Cardigan Welsh Corgi Pembroke Welsh Corgi	Direct	PennGen
Spinal Muscular Atrophy	Maine Coon Cat	Direct	Michigan State University – Fyfe Lab.
Thrombopathia	Bassett Hound Landseer Spitz	Direct	Auburn Univ. – Boudreaux Lab.
Trapped Neutrophil Syndrome (TNS)	Border Collie	Linkage	Optigen Univ. New South Wales
Von Willebrand's Disease – Type I	Bernese Mountain Dog Coton de Tulear Doberman Pinscher Drentsche Patrijshound German Pinscher Kerry Blue Terrier Manchester Terrier Papillion Pembroke Welsh Corgi Poodle	Direct	VetGen
Von Willebrand's Disease – Type I	Irish Red and White Setters	Direct	Animal Health Trust
Von Willebrand's Disease – Type II	Collie Deutsch Drahthaar German Shorthaired Pointer German Wirehaired Pointer Pointer	Direct	VetGen
Von Willebrand's Disease – Type III	Kooikerhondje Scottish Terrier Shetland Sheepdog	Direct	VetGen

Genetic Testing Centers

Alfort School of Veterinary Medicine – CNM
7 avenue du General de Gaulle
F-94704 Maisons-Alfort
CEDEX – FRANCE
http://www.labradorcnm.com/

Animal Health Trust Genetics Dept
Lanwades Park Kentford Newmarket,
Suffolk, CB8 7UU, U.K.
Telephone: 08700 50 24 24 Fax: 08700 50 24 25
http://www.aht.org.uk/genetics_tests.html

ANTAGENE
Immeuble Le Meltem
2 allée des Séquoias
69578 Limonest cedex – France
Tél: +33 (0)4 37 49 90 03
Fax: +33 (0)4 37 49 04 89
www.antagene.com

Auburn University – Boudreaux Lab
Mary Boudreaux, DVM
Dept of Pathobiology
166 Greene Hall
College of Veterinary Medicine
Auburn University, AL 36849
(334) 844-2692
http://www.vetmed.auburn.edu/faculty/pathobiology-faculty/
boudreaux

Cornell University Goldstein Molecular and Genetics Laboratory
Richard E. Goldstein, DVM
NYSCVM – Cornell University
Ithaca, New York 14853-6401
Phone: 607-253-4480
Fax: 607-253-3534
http://www.vet.cornell.edu/labs/goldstein/

Cornell University – Meyers-Wallen Lab
Vicki Meyers-Wallen, VMD, PhD
Baker Institute – Cornell University
Ithaca, New York 14853
Phone 607-256-5683
Fax: 607-256-5608
http://bakerinstitute.vet.cornell.edu/faculty/page.php?id=206

Cornell Univ. Comparative Coagulation Lab
Animal Health Diagnostic Center
NYSCVM – Cornell University
Ithaca, New York 14853-6401
607-275-0622
http://www.diaglab.vet.cornell.edu/coag/test/hemopwh.asp

DDC Veterinary
225 Corporate Court
Fairfield, OH 45014
800-625-0874
www.vetdnacenter.com/canine-bully-test-whippets.html

DOGenes
161 Sherin Ave
Peterborough, ON, K9J 7V5 CANADA
705-748-0089
www.dogenes.com

Genoscoper
Karvaamokuja 3
FI-00380 Helsinki Finland
+358 9 737 823, +358 44 5747 434
http://www.genoscoper.com/in_english2/

HealthGene
2175 Keele St.
Toronto, ON M6M 3Z4 Canada
877-371-1551
http://www.healthgene.com/

Jefferson Medical College
Dr. David Wenger
Dept of Neurology
Jefferson Medical College
1020 Locust St, 394
Philadelphia, PA 19107
215-955-1666
David.wenger@mail.tju.edu

Michigan State University – Peterson-Jones Lab
Dr Petersen-Jones - Corgi Test.
Michigan State University,
D-208 Veterinary Medical Center,
East Lansing, MI 48824-1314
517-353-3278
http://www.cardigancorgis.com/documents/Acrobat/membersPRA-
SubmissionForm.pdf

Michigan State University – Fyfe Lab
Dr. John C. Fyfe
Laboratory of Comparative Medical Genetics
2209 Biomedical Physical Sciences Bldg
Michigan State University
East Lansing, MI 48824-4320
517-355-6463x1559
http://mmg.msu.edu/92.html

New York University Neurogenetics Laboratory
Dr. Bai Jin Zeng
NYU Medical Center
New York, NY 10016
212-263-2943
http://www.pwdca.org/health/tests/information/GM1TestInstruc-
tions.html

North Carolina State University – Meurs Lab
ATTN: Veterinary Cardiac Genetics Laboratory
Research Building 460
4700 Hillsborough Street
Raleigh, NC 27606
Tel: 919-513-8279
http://www.cvm.ncsu.edu/vhc/csds/vcgl/

OptiGen
Cornell Business & Technology Park
767 Warren Road, Suite 300
Ithaca, NY 14850
Phone: 607-257-0301
Fax: 607-257-0353
http://www.optigen.com/

Orthopedic Foundation for Animals
2300 E Nifong Boulevard
Columbia, Missouri, 65201-3806
Phone: (573) 442-0418
Fax: (573) 875-5073
www.offa.org

PennGen Laboratories
3850 Spruce Street
Philadelphia, PA 19104-6010
215-898-8894
www.vet.upenn.edu/penngen

Texas A&M Comparative Dermatology Lab
Texas A&M College of Vet Med
442 University Drive
College Station, TX 77845
979-845-2651
compderm-NFT@cvm.tamu.edu

University of Bern
Institute of Genetics
PO-Box 8466
CH-3001 Bern, Switzerland
Tel +41 (0) 31 631 2322 Fax +41 (0) 31 631 2640
www.vetsuisse.unibe.ch/genetic/content/service/dog/index_eng.html

University of California – Davis Veterinary Genetics Laboratory
One Shields Ave.
Davis, CA 95616-8744
530-752-2211
http://www.vgl.ucdavis.edu/services/index.php

U-Guelph Animal Health Laboratory
University of Guelph
P.O. Box 3650, 95 Stone Road West
Guelph, Ontario
N1H 8J7 CANADA
519-824-4120 ext 54502
www.labservices.uoguelph.ca/units/ahl/

Univ. Minnesota Veterinary Diagnostic Laboratory
College of Veterinary Medicine, University of Minnesota
1333 Gortner Ave
St. Paul, MN 55108
612-625-8787
http://www.vdl.umn.edu/ourservices/canineneuromuscular

University of Missouri – Animal Molecular Genetics Lab
Univ of MO College of Vet Medicine
320 Connaway Hall
Columbia, MO 65211
http://www.caninegeneticdiseases.net/

University of New South Wales – Wilton Lab
Dr. Alan Wilton
School of Biotechnology and Biomolecular Sciences
University of New South Wales
New South Wales 2052, Australia
E-mail: a.wilton@unsw.edu.au

VetGen
3728 Plaza Drive, Suite One
Ann Arbor, MI 48108
800-483-8436
www.vetgen.com

Washington State University – Pharm Lab
Veterinary Clinical Pharmacology Lab (WSU-VCPL)
PO Box 2280
Pullman, WA 99165-2280
Phone/FAX: 509-335-3745
www.vetmed.wsu.edu/depts-VCPL/

Quick Reference to Conditions by Breed: Breed Specific Conditions in Dogs

This list is not exhaustive or complete, but recognizes the published conditions as presented in the breed chapters.

Subject	Condition	Breed-Dog
Behavioral	Aggression	Bedlington Terrier Cairn Terrier Chinese Shar Pei Chow Chow Cocker Spaniel Dalmatian English Cocker Spaniel English Springer Spaniel German Shepherd Dog Portuguese Water Dog Rottweiler Scottish Terrier Silky Terrier West Highland White Terrier
	Aggression, Dog To Dog	German Shorthaired Pointer
	Anxiety	Dalmatian Vizsla
	Flank Sucking	Doberman Pinscher
	Fly Catching Behavior	Cavalier King Charles Spaniel
	Nervousness	Pointer
	Noise Phobia	German Shorthaired Pointer
	Separation Anxiety	Border Collie
	Spinning/Tail Chasing	Bull Terrier Miniature Bull Terrier
Cardiovascular	2nd and 3rd Degree Heart Block	Cocker Spaniel
	Acepromazine Collapse	Boxer
	Aortic Stenosis	Dogue De Bordeaux German Shepherd Dog Glen of Imaal Terrier Golden Retriever
	Aortic Thromboembolism	Cavalier King Charles Spaniel
	Arrhythmias	German Shepherd Dog Greyhound
	Atherosclerosis	Doberman Pinscher Miniature Schnauzer
	Atrial Septal Defect	Boxer Poodle
	Atrial Stenosis	Bull Terrier
	Atrioventricular (AV) Block	Afghan Hound Chow Chow English Springer Spaniel German Wirehaired Pointer Labrador Retriever
	Atrioventricular Valve Dysplasia	Mastiff
	Cardiomyopathy, Arrhythmogenic	Boxer

Subject	Condition	Breed–Dog
	Cardiomyopathy, Dilated	Airedale Terrier Borzoi Cocker Spaniel Doberman Pinscher English Cocker Spaniel Great Dane Irish Wolfhound Leonberger Newfoundland Poodle Saint Bernard Scottish Deerhound Standard Schnauzer
	Cardiomyopathy, Juvenile Dilated	Manchester Terrier Portuguese Water Dog
	Chronic Myxomatous Valvular Endocarditis	Yorkshire Terrier
	Conotruncal Defect	Beagle Border Terrier Keeshond
	Heart Murmur	Airedale Terrier Bedlington Terrier Border Terrier Brussel's Griffon Cairn Terrier Greyhound Vizsla
	Hypotension, Physiologic Mild	Irish Wolfhound
	Left Ventricular Outflow Obstruction	Bull Terrier Miniature Bull Terrier
	Mitral Valve Stenosis	Bull Terrier
	Mitral Valvular Disease	American Water Spaniel Cavalier King Charles Spaniel Dachshund Great Dane Greyhound Japanese Chin Miniature Schnauzer Norfolk Terrier Pekingese Pomeranian Poodle Saluki West Highland White Terrier Yorkshire Terrier
	Patent Ductus Arteriosis (PDA)	American Water Spaniel Bichon Frisé German Shepherd Dog Maltese Pembroke Welsh Corgi Pomeranian Poodle Pyrenean Shepherd Shetland Sheepdog

Subject	Condition	Breed-Dog
	Pericardial Effusion, Idiopathic	Golden Retriever
	Portosystemic (Liver) Shunt	Australian Cattle Dog Bernese Mountain Dog Bichon Frisé Border Collie Cairn Terrier Chihuahua Dandie Dinmont Terrier Havanese Irish Wolfhound Lhasa Apso Maltese Miniature Pinscher Miniature Schnauzer Norfolk Terrier Norwich Terrier Old English Sheepdog Papillon Parson Russell Terrier Pekingese Pug Scottish Deerhound Shih Tzu Silky Terrier Standard Schnauzer Tibetan Spaniel West Highland White Terrier Yorkshire Terrier
	Pulmonic Stenosis	American Water Spaniel Beagle Boxer Bulldog Chihuahua Chow Chow French Bulldog Mastiff Miniature Schnauzer Nova Scotia Duck Tolling Retriever Parson Russell Terrier Samoyed Smooth Fox Terrier Wire Fox Terrier
	Sick Sinus Syndrome	Cocker Spaniel English Springer Spaniel Miniature Schnauzer West Highland White Terrier
	Subaortic Stenosis	Black Russian Terrier Bouvier Des Flandres Boxer Curly Coated Retriever Newfoundland Rottweiler
	Tricuspid Valve Dysplasia	Borzoi Curly Coated Retriever Labrador Retriever

Subject	Condition	Breed–Dog
	Vascular Ring Anomaly/ Persistant Right Aortic Arch (PRAA)	Boston Terrier German Pinscher German Shepherd Dog
	Vasculitis, Necrotizing	Boxer
	Ventricular Septal Defect	Bloodhound Shiba Inu
Dermatological	Acrodermatitis, Lethal	Bull Terrier
	Actinic Keratosis	American Staffordshire Terrier Bull Terrier Dalmatian
	Alopecia X	Chow Chow Finnish Spitz Keeshond Pomeranian Poodle Samoyed Siberian Husky
	Alopecia, Endocrine	American Eskimo Dog Chesapeake Bay Retriever
	Alopecia, Focal	Silky Terrier
	Alopecia, Seasonal Flank	Affenpinscher Airedale Terrier Bearded Collie Boxer Manchester Terrier Wirehaired Pointing Griffon
	Anal Gland Disease	Manchester Terrier Pekingese Scottish Deerhound
	Atopic/Allergic Dermatitis	Akita Airedale Terrier Australian Terrier Bedlington Terrier Bernese Mountain Dog Bichon Frisé Boston Terrier Bouvier Des Flandres Boxer Briard Brussel's Griffon Bull Terrier Cairn Terrier Cavalier King Charles Spaniel Chesapeake Bay Retriever Chinese Shar Pei Chinook Clumber Spaniel Cocker Spaniel Collie Dalmatian English Cocker Spaniel English Setter Field Spaniel French Bulldog

Subject	Condition	Breed–Dog
		Glen of Imaal Terrier
		German Shepherd Dog
		German Shorthaired Pointer
		Golden Retriever
		Great Dane
		Great Pyrenees
		Greyhound
		Ibizan Hound
		Irish Setter
		Keeshond
		Kerry Blue Terrier
		Labrador Retriever
		Lhasa Apso
		Mastiff
		Newfoundland
		Norwegian Elkhound
		Norwich Terrier
		Old English Sheepdog
		Otterhound
		Petit Bassett Griffon Vendéen
		Portuguese Water Dog
		Pug
		Rhodesian Ridgeback
		Rottweiler
		Scottish Deerhound
		Scottish Terrier
		Sealyham Terrier
		Shiba Inu
		Silky Terrier
		Soft Coated Wheaten Terrier
		Spinone Italiano
		Sussex Spaniel
		Tibetan Spaniel
		Tibetan Terrier
		Toy Fox Terrier
		Vizsla
		Welsh Terrier
		West Highland White Terrier
		Wirehaired Pointing Griffon
		Whippet
		Yorkshire Terrier
	Black Hair Follicular Dysplasia	Saluki
		Schipperke
	Bullous Pemphigus	Great Dane
	Calcinosis Circumscripta	German Shepherd Dog
		Labrador Retriever
		Rottweiler
	Color Dilution Alopecia	Dachshund
		Doberman Pinscher
		German Pinscher
		Italian Greyhound
		Miniature Pinscher
		Whippet
	Comedomes	Chinese Crested
		Miniature Schnauzer
		Xoloitzcuinti

Subject	Condition	Breed–Dog
	Cutaneous And Renal Glomerular Vasculopathy (CRGV)	Greyhound
	Cutaneous Lupus Erythematosus (Nasal Solar Dermatitis)	Brittany Collie German Shorthaired Pointer Shetland Sheepdog
	Cutaneous Mucinosis	Chinese Shar Pei
	Cutaneous Vasculopathy	German Shepherd Dog
	Demodicosis	Afghan Hound Basenji Boxer Bull Terrier Bulldog Cane Corso Chinese Shar Pei Collie Dalmatian Doberman Pinscher French Bulldog German Shorthaired Pointer Great Dane Italian Greyhound Manchester Terrier Miniature Pinscher Old English Sheepdog Pointer Rottweiler Schipperke Scottish Terrier Staffordshire Bull Terrier Tibetan Spaniel Vizsla Whippet Wire Fox Terrier
	Dermatomyositis	Beauceron Collie Shetland Sheepdog Yorkshire Terrier
	Dermoid Sinus	Rhodesian Ridgeback
	Digital Keratoma (Corns)	Greyhound
	Discoid Lupus Erythematosus (DLE)	German Shepherd Dog
	Epidermolysis Bullosa	Beauceron
	Follicular Dysplasia	Boxer Doberman Pinscher Irish Water Spaniel Portuguese Water Dog Weimaraner
	Hepatocutaneous Syndrome (Superficial Necrolytic Dermatitis)	Scottish Terrier Shetland Sheepdog West Highland White Terrier
	Hyperkeratosis, Digital	Irish Terrier

Subject	Condition	Breed–Dog
	Ichthyosis	Cavalier King Charles Spaniel Golden Retriever Norfolk Terrier Parson Russell Terrier
	Lawn Chemical Hypersensitivity	Xoloitzcuinti
	Lichenoid-Psoriasiform Dermatosis	English Springer Spaniel Shetland Sheepdog
	Malassezia Pachydermatis	Parson Russell Terrier West Highland White Terrier
	Mucocutaneous Pyoderma	German Shepherd Dog
	Nasal Parakeratosis	Labrador Retriever
	Otitis Externa	Boykin Spaniel Brittany Cane Corso Chinese Shar Pei Clumber Spaniel Cocker Spaniel English Springer Spaniel Golden Retriever Great Pyrenees Greyhound Poodle Portuguese Water Dog Spinone Italiano Wirehaired Pointing Griffon
	Otitis Media	Cavalier King Charles Spaniel
	Palmar Hyperkeratosis	Dogue De Bordeaux
	Pattern Baldness	Chihuahua Curly Coated Retriever Greyhound Whippet
	Pemphigus Foliaceus	Akita Bearded Collie Chinese Shar Pei Chow Chow Collie English Springer Spaniel Finnish Spitz Newfoundland Schipperke
	Perianal Fistula/Furunculosis	German Shepherd Dog Leonberger
	Pigmented Plaques	Pug
	Pilomatricoma	Soft-Coated Wheaten Terrier
	Pododermatitis/Interdigital Cysts	Bulldog
	Sebaceous Adenitis	Akita Chow Chow English Springer Spaniel Lhasa Apso Old English Sheepdog Poodle Samoyed Vizsla

Subject	Condition	Breed–Dog
	Sebaceous Cysts	Bouvier Des Flandres Cavalier King Charles Spaniel Golden Retriever Gordon Setter Kerry Blue Terrier Norwegian Elkhound Otterhound Portuguese Water Dog Rottweiler
	Sebaceous Gland Hyperplasia	Border Terrier
	Seborrheic Dermatitis	Airedale Terrier Basset Hound Cairn Terrier Chinese Shar Pei Cocker Spaniel English Springer Spaniel Golden Retriever Irish Setter
	Spiculosis	Kerry Blue Terrier
	Sunburn	Xoloitzcuinti
	Superficial Suppurative Necrolytic Dermatitis	Miniature Schnauzer
	Symmetrical Lupoid Onchodystrophy (SLO)	Bearded Collie English Setter Giant Schnauzer Gordon Setter Greyhound
	Systemic Lupus Erythematosus (SLE)	German Shepherd Dog Nova Scotia Duck Tolling Retriever
	Uveodermatologic (VKH-Like) Syndrome	Akita Old English Sheepdog Samoyed Shetland Sheepdog Siberian Husky
	Vit A-Responsive Dermatosis	Cocker Spaniel
	Zinc Responsive Dermatosis	Alaskan Malamute Siberian Husky
Endocrine/Metabolic	Ceroid Lipofuscinosis	American Staffordshire Terrier Australian Cattle Dog Border Collie Cocker Spaniel Dachshund Dalmatian English Setter Miniature Schnauzer Polish Lowland Sheepdog Saluki Tibetan Terrier
	Cobolamin Deficiency	Chinese Shar Pei
	Cobalamin Malabsorption	Border Collie Giant Schnauzer

Subject	Condition	Breed–Dog
	Copper Storage Disease	Bedlington Terrier Skye Terrier West Highland White Terrier
	Copper Toxicosis	Dalmatian Doberman Pinscher
	Diabetes Mellitus	Australian Terrier Beagle Bichon Frisé Border Collie Border Terrier Cairn Terrier Cavalier King Charles Spaniel Collie Finnish Spitz Keeshond Labrador Retriever Manchester Terrier Miniature Pinscher Miniature Schnauzer Norwegian Elkhound Poodle Pug Puli Samoyed Schipperke Silky Terrier Standard Schnauzer Tibetan Terrier West Highland White Terrier Yorkshire Terrier
	Eosinophilic Diseases	Cavalier King Charles Spaniel Siberian Husky
	Fucosidosis	English Springer Spaniel
	Globoid Cell Leukodsytrophy	Cairn Terrier West Highland White Terrier
	Glucocerebrosidosis	Silky Terrier
	Glycogenosis Type IIIa	Curly Coated Retriever
	GM1-Gangliosidosis	English Springer Spaniel Portuguese Water Dog Shiba Inu
	GM2-Gangliosidosis	Japanese Chin
	Hyperadrenocorticism (Cushing's Disease)	Australian Terrier Bedlington Terrier Boston Terrier Cairn Terrier Dachshund Dandie Dinmont Terrier Miniature Schnauzer Poodle West Highland White Terrier Yorkshire Terrier Silky Terrier Standard Schnauzer
	Hyperlipoproteinemia/Hyperlipidemia	Miniature Schnauzer Shetland Sheepdog

Subject	Condition	Breed–Dog
	Hyperparathyroidism, Primary	Keeshond
	Hyperuricosuria	American Staffordshire Terrier Australian Shepherd Black Russian Terrier Bulldog Dalmatian German Shepherd Dog Giant Schnauzer Jack Russell Terrier Labrador Retriever Parson Russell Terrier Pomeranian Weimaraner
	Hypoadrenocorticism (Addison's Disease)	American Eskimo Dog Bearded Collie Great Dane Great Pyrenees Leonberger Nova Scotia Duck Tolling Retriever Poodle Portuguese Water Dog Rottweiler Soft Coated Wheaten Terrier West Highland White Terrier
	Hypoglycemia	Yorkshire Terrier
	Hypothyroidism, Autoimmune	All Breeds
	Hypothyroidism, Congenital	Giant Schnauzer
	Hypothyroidism, Congenital With Goiter	Toy Fox Terrier
	IgA Deficiency	German Shepherd Dog Irish Setter
	Immunodeficiency, Inherited	Cavalier King Charles Spaniel Weimaraner
	L-2 Hydroxyglutaric Aciduria	Staffordshire Bull Terrier
	Malignant Hyperthermia	Greyhound
	MDR1 Mutation (Drug & Ivermectin Sensitivity)	Australian Shepherd Border Collie Collie German Shepherd Dog Old English Sheepdog Shetland Sheepdog
	Metabolic Vitamin E Deficiency	English Cocker Spaniel
	Mitochondrial Myopathy (Pyruvate Dehydrogenase)	Clumber Spaniel Sussex Spaniel
	Mucopolysaccharidosis I	Plott Hound
	Mucopolysaccharidosis IIIa	Dachshund
	Mucopolysaccharidosis IIIB	Schipperke
	Mucopolysaccharidosis VI	Cardigan Welsh Corgi Miniature Pinscher Miniature Poodle Miniature Schnauzer
	Mucopolysaccharidosis VII	German Shepherd Dog

Subject	Condition	Breed-Dog
	Phosphofructokinase (PFK) Deficiency	English Springer Spaniel
	Pituitary Dwarfism	German Shepherd Dog
	Primary Immunodeficiency	Chinese Shar Pei
	Pyruvate Kinase Deficiency	American Eskimo Dog Basenji Beagle Cairn Terrier Dachshund West Highland White Terrier
	Severe Combined Immunodeficiency (SCID)	Parson Russell Terrier
	Severe Combined Immunodeficiency (SCID) -X Linked	Basset Hound
	Spectrin Deficiency	Golden Retriever
	Sulfonamide Hypersensitivity	Doberman Pinscher Miniature Schnauzer Samoyed
	Xanthomatosis (Dalmatian Bronzing)	Dalmatian
Gastrointestinal	Atrophic Gastritis	Norwegian Lundehund
	Colitis	Chinook Kerry Blue Terrier
	Colorectal Polyp	Collie
	Cricopharyngeal Dysfunction/Achalasia	Golden Retriever
	Esophageal Achalasia	Miniature Schnauzer
	Exocrine Pancreatic Insufficiency	Bedlington Terrier Cavalier King Charles Spaniel Chow Chow Collie German Shepherd Dog Weimaraner
	Gallbladder Disease	Shetland Sheepdog
	Gastic Dilitation/Volvulus (GDV)	Akita Airedale Terrier Bernese Mountain Dog Beauceron Bloodhound Borzoi Bouvier Des Flandres Briard Bullmastiff Cane Corso Chesapeake Bay Retriever Chinese Shar Pei Chow Chow Collie Curly Coated Retriever Doberman Pinscher Dogue De Bordeaux Flat-Coated Retriever German Shepherd Dog German Shorthaired Pointer Giant Schnauzer Golden Retriever

Subject	Condition	Breed–Dog
		Gordon Setter
		Great Dane
		Great Pyrenees
		Irish Red and White Setter
		Irish Setter
		Irish Wolfhound
		Komondor
		Leonberger
		Mastiff
		Neopolitan Mastiff
		Newfoundland
		Old English Sheepdog
		Poodle
		Rottweiler
		Saint Bernard
		Samoyed
		Scottish Deerhound
		Spinone Italiano
		Sussex Spaniel
		Weimaraner
	Gluten Enteropathy (Sensitivity)	Irish Setter
	Hepatitis	Cairn Terrier
		English Cocker Spaniel
		English Springer Spaniel
		Labrador Retriever
	Histiocytic Ulcerative Colitis	Boxer
		French Bulldog
	Immunoproliferative Enteropathy	Basenji
	Inflammatory Bowel Disease (IBD)	Clumber Spaniel
		German Shepherd Dog
		Greyhound
		Norwegian Lundehund
		Portuguese Water Dog
		Rottweiler
		West Highland White Terrier
	Irritable Bowel Syndrome	Norwegian Elkhound
	Megaesophagus	Chinese Shar Pei
		German Shepherd Dog
		Golden Retriever
		Great Dane
		Irish Setter
		Miniature Schnauzer
		Wire Fox Terrier
	Pancreatitis	Airedale Terrier
		Australian Terrier
		Boxer
		Cavalier King Charles Spaniel
		Collie
		Miniature Schnauzer
		Standard Schnauzer
	Protein Losing Enteropathy (PLE)	Maltese
		Norwegian Lundehund
		Rottweiler
		Soft Coated Wheaten Terrier
		Yorkshire Terrier

Subject	Condition	Breed-Dog
	Xanthogranulomatous Inflammation of the Small Bowel	American Staffordshire Terrier
	Vacuolar Hepatopathy	Scottish Terrier
	Villous Atrophy	Bouvier Des Flandres
Hematological	Auto-Immune Hemolytic Anemia (AIHA/IMHA)	Airedale Terrier Bichon Frisé Cairn Terrier Cocker Spaniel Collie English Springer Spaniel Finnish Spitz Labrador Retriever Maltese Miniature Pinscher Miniature Schnauzer Old English Sheepdog Parson Russell Terrier Saluki Shetland Sheepdog Vizsla
	C3 Compliment Deficiency	Brittany
	Cyclic Neutropenia	Collie
	Dalmatian RBC Type	Dalmatian
	Factor I Deficiency	Vizsla
	Factor VII Deficiency	Beagle Scottish Deerhound
	Factor XI Deficiency	Kerry Blue Terrier
	Glanzmann's Thrombasthenia	Great Pyrenees Otterhound
	Hemophagocytic Syndrome	Tibetan Terrier
	Hemophilia A (Factor VIII)	German Shepherd Dog Golden Retriever
	Hemophilia B (Factor IX)	Airedale Terrier Black & Tan Coonhound French Bulldog German Wirehaired Pointer Lhasa Apso Rhodesian Ridgeback
	Hypereosinophilia	Rottweiler
	Hyperkalemia, Benign	Shiba Inu
	Hyperphosphatasemia, Benign	Scottish Terrier Siberian Husky
	Immune-Mediated Thrombocytopenia (ITP)	Airedale Terrier Old English Sheepdog
	Leukemia	Golden Retriever
	Leukocyte Adhesion Deficiency (CLAD)	Irish Red And White Setter Irish Setter
	Leukopenia, Physiologic	Belgian Tervuren
	Microcytosis, Benign	Shiba Inu
	Platelet ADP Deficiency	Cocker Spaniel

Subject	Condition	Breed–Dog
	Platelet Procoagulant Deficiency	German Shepherd Dog
	Stomatocytosis	Miniature Schnauzer Standard Schnauzer
	Thrombocytopenia, Physiologic	Cavalier King Charles Spaniel
	Thrombopathy, Hereditary	Basset Hound
	Trapped Neutrophil Syndrome (TNS)	Border Collie
	von Willebrand's Disease	Airedale Terrier Basset Hound Bernese Mountain Dog Chesapeake Bay Retriever Collie Doberman Pinscher German Pinscher German Shepherd Dog German Shorthaired Pointer German Wirehaired Pointer Golden Retriever Irish Red And White Setter Kerry Blue Terrier Manchester Terrier Papillon Pembroke Welsh Corgi Pointer Poodle Scottish Terrier Shetland Sheepdog Toy Fox Terrier
Musculoskeletal	Atlantoaxial Subluxation	Japanese Chin
	Atlanto-Occipital Subluxation	Pekingese Pomeranian
	Calvarial Hyperostotic Syndrome	Bullmastiff
	Central Tarsal Bone Fracture	Greyhound
	Centro-Nuclear Myopathy	Labrador Retriever
	Cervical Vertebral Arthrosis	Scottish Deerhound
	Chondrodysplasia	Norwegian Elkhound
	Chondrodystrophy (Dwarfism)	Beagle
	Cranial Cruciate Ligament (ACL) Rupture	Akita Australian Terrier Bernese Mountain Dog Boxer Chesapeake Bay Retriever Chow Chow Dogue De Bordeaux German Shepherd Dog Giant Schnauzer Golden Retriever Greyhound Labrador Retriever Leonberger Mastiff Neopolitan Mastiff Newfoundland Rottweiler Saint Bernard

Subject	Condition	Breed–Dog
	Craniomandibular Osteopathy (CMO)	Cairn Terrier Scottish Terrier West Highland White Terrier
	Disikospondylitis	Airedale Terrier Great Dane
	Distal Tibial Valgus Deformity	Shetland Sheepdog
	Dwarfism, Hypochondroplastic	Irish Setter
	Elbow Dysplasia	All Breeds
	Eosinophilic Myositis	Belgian Sheepdog
	Episodic Myokymia	Jack Russell Terrier
	Exercise Induced Collapse (EIC)	Boykin Spaniel Chesapeake Bay Retriever Curly Coated Retriever Labrador Retriever
	Gross Muscle Hypertrophy (Bully Whippets)	Whippet
	Hemivertebra	Boston Terrier French Bulldog German Shorthaired Pointer Pug
	Hemivertebra, Kinked Tail	Cairn Terrier Scottish Terrier
	Hip Dysplasia	All Breeds
	Humeral Condyle Dysplasia	Cocker Spaniel
	Hypertrophic Osteodystrophy (HOD)	German Shepherd Dog Golden Retriever Great Dane Irish Setter Kuvasz Labrador Retriever Weimaraner
	Incomplete Ossification Of The Humeral Condyle	Brittany
	Inflammatory Myopathy	Boxer Newfoundland
	Lateral Luxation Of The Superficial Digital Flexor Tendon	Shetland Sheepdog
	Leg Fractures	Italian Greyhound
	Legg-Calve-Perthes Disease	Affenpinscher American Eskimo Dog Australian Shepherd Australian Terrier Border Terrier Cairn Terrier Cavalier King Charles Spaniel Chihuahua Chinese Crested Dachshund Lakeland Terrier Lhasa Apso Löwchen Maltese

Subject	Condition	Breed–Dog
		Manchester Terrier
		Miniature Pinscher
		Miniature Schnauzer
		Parson Russell Terrier
		Pekingese
		Poodle
		Pug
		Schipperke
		Shih Tzu
		Silky Terrier
		Smooth Fox Terrier
		Toy Fox Terrier
		West Highland White Terrier
		Wire Fox Terrier
		Xoloitzcuinti
		Yorkshire Terrier
	Lumbosacral Transitional Vertebrae	Great Pyrenees
	Metacarpal Sesamoid Disease	Rottweiler
	Muscular Dystrophy	Bouvier Des Flandres
		Cavalier King Charles Spaniel
		Irish Terrier
	Myasthenia Gravis, Acquired	Akita
		Chihuahua
		German Shepherd Dog
		German Shorthaired Pointer
		Golden Retriever
		Newfoundland
		Scottish Terrier
	Myasthenia Gravis, Congenital	Dachshund
		English Springer Spaniel
		Parson Russell Terrier
		Smooth Fox Terrier
	Myopathy, Inherited	Great Dane
	Myotonia Congenita	Chow Chow
		Miniature Schnauzer
	Occipital Bone Hypoplasia (Chiari-Like Malformation)	Brussels Griffon
		Cavalier King Charles Spaniel
	Osteoarthritis	Bernese Mountain Dog
		Bouvier Des Flandres
		Great Pyrenees
		Greyhound
		Rottweiler
		Vizsla
	Osteochondritis Dessicans (OCD)	Bernese Mountain Dog
		Border Collie
		Bouvier Des Flandres
		Boxer
		Bulldog
		Chesapeake Bay Retriever
		English Setter
		German Shepherd Dog
		German Shorthaired Pointer
		German Wirehaired Pointer
		Golden Retriever
		Great Dane

Subject	Condition	Breed–Dog
		Great Pyrenees Irish Wolfhound Kuvasz Labrador Retriever Leonberger Mastiff Newfoundland Old English Sheepdog Rottweiler Saint Bernard Tibetan Mastiff
	Osteochondrodysplasia/Chondrodysplasia	Alaskan Malamute Great Pyrenees Havanese
	Osteogenesis Imperfecta	Dachshund
	Panosteitis	Bernese Mountain Dog German Shepherd Dog Golden Retriever Great Dane Great Pyrenees Leonberger Mastiff Rottweiler Tibetan Mastiff
	Patella Luxation	All Breeds
	Polyarthritis, Juvenile-Onset	Akita
	Polymyositis	Vizsla
	Sesamoid Disease	Greyhound
	Shoulder Instability	Poodle
	Skeletal Dysplasia	Nova Scotia Duck Tolling Retriever
	Spinal Muscle Atrophy	Brittany
	Spondylosis Deformans	Boxer
	Temporomandibular Joint (TMJ) Dysplasia	Basset Hound Cavalier King Charles Spaniel
	Tibial Tuberosity Avulsion	Staffordshire Bull Terrier
Neurological	Axonal Dystrophy	Ibizan Hound
	Axonopathy	Boxer
	Canine Epileptoid Cramping Syndrome (Spike's Disease)	Border Terrier
	Canine Multiple System Degeneration (CMSD)	Chinese Crested Kerry Blue Terrier
	Cerebellar Abiotrophy	Airedale Terrier American Staffordshire Terrier Border Collie Gordon Setter Harrier Old English Sheepdog Scottish Terrier Spinone Italiano
	Cerebellar Ataxia, X-Linked	Pointer

Subject	Condition	Breed–Dog
	Cervical Spondylomyelopathy/Vertebral Instability (Wobbler Syndrome)	Bernese Mountain Dog Borzoi Dalmatian Doberman Pinscher Great Dane Mastiff Rottweiler Weimaraner
	Congenital Hydrocephalus w/Cerebellar Ataxia	Bullmastiff
	Coonhound Paralysis (Polyradicuoneuritis)	Black and Tan Coonhound Bluetick Coonhound Redbone Coonhound
	Deafness, Congenital	American Eskimo Dog American Foxhound Australian Cattle Dog Australian Shepherd Australian Terrier Beagle Bedlington Terrier Border Collie Boston Terrier Bull Terrier Cavalier King Charles Spaniel Chinese Crested Cocker Spaniel Dachshund Dalmatian Doberman Pinscher English Cocker Spaniel English Foxhound English Setter Great Pyrenees Havanese Ibizan Hound Icelandic Sheepdog Italian Greyhound Kuvasz Löwchen Maltese Manchester Terrier Miniature Bull Terrier Norwich Terrier Nova Scotia Duck Tolling Retriever Old English Sheepdog Papillon Parson Russell Terrier Pointer Puli Sealyham Terrier Smooth Fox Terrier Tibetan Terrier Toy Fox Terrier Whippet
	Deafness, Juvenile	Rhodesian Ridgeback

Subject	Condition	Breed-Dog
	Degenerative Myelopathy (DM)	American Eskimo Dog American Water Spaniel Bernese Mountain Dog Bloodhound Borzoi Boxer Canaan Dog Cardigan Welsh Corgi Chesapeake Bay Retriever Collie French Bulldog German Shepherd Dog Irish Setter Kerry Blue Terrier Kuvasz Old English Sheepdog Pembroke Welsh Corgi Poodle Pug Rhodesian Ridgeback
	Distal Juvenile Myelopathy	Rottweiler
	Dysmyelinogenesis	Welsh Springer Spaniel
	Encephalopathy, Neonatal	Gordon Setter Poodle
	Episodic Collapse	Cavalier King Charles Spaniel
	Hepatocerebellar Degeneration	Bernese Mountain Dog
	Hereditary Ataxia	Parson Russell Terrier Smooth Fox Terrier
	Hereditary Quadriplegia And Ambylopia	Irish Setter
	Hereditary Sensory Neuropathy	Pointer
	Horner's Syndrome, Idiopathic	Collie Golden Retriever
	Hydrocephalus	Chihuahua Maltese Pomeranian
	Hypertrophic Neuropathy	Tibetan Mastiff
	Hypomyelination/Dysmyelination	Bernese Mountain Dog Chow Chow English Springer Spaniel
	Idiopathic Epilepsy/Inherited Seizures	Airedale Terrier American Eskimo Dog American Water Spaniel Australian Shepherd Australian Terrier Beagle Bedlington Terrier Belgian Sheepdog Belgian Tervuren Bernese Mountain Dog Border Collie Boxer Brittany Brussel's Griffon

Subject	Condition	Breed–Dog
		Canaan Dog
		Cane Corso
		Cavalier King Charles Spaniel
		Chesapeake Bay Retriever
		Chinook
		Collie
		Dalmatian
		Dogue De Bordeaux
		English Cocker Spaniel
		English Springer Spaniel
		Field Spaniel
		Flat-Coated Retriever
		Finnish Spitz
		German Shepherd Dog
		German Shorthaired Pointer
		Giant Schnauzer
		Golden Retriever
		Great Pyrenees
		Greyhound
		Ibizan Hound
		Irish Setter
		Irish Water Spaniel
		Irish Wolfhound
		Italian Greyhound
		Keeshond
		Labrador Retriever
		Mastiff
		Miniature Pinscher
		Norwegian Elkhound
		Norwich Terrier
		Nova Scotia Duck Tolling Retriever
		Otterhound
		Papillon
		Petit Bassett Griffon Vendéen
		Poodle
		Portuguese Water Dog
		Pyrenean Shepherd
		Rottweiler
		Saint Bernard
		Schipperke
		Scottish Terrier
		Shetland Sheepdog
		Siberian Husky
		Silky Terrier
		Spinone Italiano
		Standard Schnauzer
		Tibetan Mastiff
		Tibetan Terrier
		Vizsla
		Welsh Terrier
		Wirehaired Pointing Griffon
	Intervertebral Disc Disease (IVDD)	Basset Hound
		Beagle
		Cardigan Welsh Corgi
		Cavalier King Charles Spaniel
		Clumber Spaniel
		Dachshund
		French Bulldog

Subject	Condition	Breed-Dog
		Greyhound Lhasa Apso Pekingese Pembroke Welsh Corgi Rottweiler Shih Tzu Tibetan Spaniel
	Juvenile Polyarteritis (Pain Syndrome)	Beagle Petit Bassett Griffon Vendéen
	Laryngeal Paralysis, Aquired	Afghan Hound Irish Setter Labrador Retriever Newfoundland
	Laryngeal Paralysis, Congenital	Bouvier Des Flandres Staffordshire Bull Terrier
	Leukodystrophy, Spinal Cord	Bullmastiff
	Leukoencephalomyelopathy	Rottweiler
	Lissencephaly	Lhasa Apso
	Lumbosacral Stenosis/Cauda Equina Syndrome	Belgian Malinois German Shepherd Dog Greyhound
	Meningoencephalitis	Greyhound
	Myoclonic Epilepsy	Basset Hound Beagle Dachshund
	Narcolepsy	Dachshund Doberman Pinscher Labrador Retriever
	Necrotizing Meningitis	Bernese Mountain Dog
	Necrotizing Meningoencephalitis	Chihuahua French Bulldog Maltese Pekingese Pomeranian Pug Yorkshire Terrier
	Necrotizing Myelopathy (Afghan Myelopathy)	Afghan Hound
	Neuroaxonal Dystrophy	Papillon Parson Russell Terrier Rottweiler
	Peripheral Neuropathy	Doberman Pinscher
	Polioencephalomyopathy (Spongiform Leukoencephalomyelopathy)	Australian Cattle Dog Shetland Sheepdog
	Polymicrogyria	Poodle
	Polyneuropathy	Alaskan Malamute Bouvier Des Flandres Dalmatian Great Pyrenees Greyhound Leonberger
	Progressive Neuronopathy	Cairn Terrier

Subject	Condition	Breed–Dog
	Rosenthal Fiber Encephalopathy	Bernese Mountain Dog
	Scottie Cramp	Scottish Terrier
	Seizures, Fly Biting Partial	Great Pyrenees
	Sensorimotor Axonopathy	Golden Retriever
	Spina Bifida	Bulldog
	Spinal Dysraphism/ Myelodysplasia	Weimaraner
	Spinal Muscle Atrophy	Pointer
	Spinal Subarachnoid Cysts	Rottweiler
	Spinocerebellar Degeneration	Brittany
	Steroid Responsive Meningitis/Arteritis	Nova Scotia Duck Tolling Retriever Pembroke Welsh Corgi
	Syringomyelia	Brussel's Griffon Cavalier King Charles Spaniel English Toy Spaniel
	Vestibular Disease	Tibetan Terrier
	White Shaker Syndrome	Maltese West Highland White Terrier
Oncology/Cancer	Adenocarcinoma, Nasal	Collie
	Bladder and Urethral Tumors	Beagle
	Choroid Plexus Brain Tumor	Golden Retriever
	Cutaneous Plasmocytoma	Yorkshire Terrier
	Gastric Carcinoma	Belgian Sheepdog Belgian Tervuren Chow Chow Collie Norwegian Lundehund Staffordshire Bull Terrier
	Glial Tumors	Boston Terrier
	Hemangioma, Synovial	Belgian Sheepdog
	Hemangiosarcoma	Airedale Terrier German Shepherd Dog Golden Retriever Greyhound Italian Greyhound Portuguese Water Dog Saluki Vizsla Whippet
	Histiocytic Sarcoma	Rottweiler
	Histiocytoma, Cutaneous	Dachshund
	Histiocytosis, Malignant	Bernese Mountain Dog Flat-Coated Retriever Golden Retriever Labrador Retriever
	Intracutaneous Cornifying Epithelioma	Norwegian Elkhound
	Iridociliary Epithelial Tumors	Labrador Retriever
	Lingual Fibrosarcoma	Golden Retriever
	Liver Cancer	Standard Schnauzer

Subject	Condition	Breed-Dog
	Lymphosarcoma	Airedale Terrier Bernese Mountain Dog Briard Dogue De Bordeaux Golden Retriever Gordon Setter Greyhound Labrador Retriever Old English Sheepdog Portuguese Water Dog Rottweiler Vizsla West Highland White Terrier
	Mammary Cancer	Borzoi Brittany English Setter English Springer Spaniel German Shorthaired Pointer
	Mammary Gland Osteoma	Poodle
	Mast Cell Tumor	Airedale Terrier Australian Terrier Bernese Mountain Dog Boxer Chinese Shar Pei German Shorthaired Pointer Golden Retriever Maltese Norwegian Elkhound Pug Rhodesian Ridgeback Staffordshire Bull Terrier Vizsla Weimaraner
	Melanoma	Cocker Spaniel Gordon Setter
	Melanoma, Limbal	Golden Retriever Labrador Retriever
	Melanoma, Lingual	Chinese Shar Pei Chow Chow
	Meningioma	Boxer Golden Retriever
	Multifocal Renal Cystadenocarcinoma And Nodular Dermatofibrosis	German Shepherd Dog
	Oral Cancer	Boxer German Shorthaired Pointer Golden Retriever
	Osteosarcoma	Airedale Terrier Boxer Golden Retriever Great Dane Great Pyrenees Greyhound Irish Setter Irish Wolfhound

Subject	Condition	Breed-Dog
		Leonberger Mastiff Newfoundland Old English Sheepdog Rottweiler Saint Bernard Scottish Deerhound
	Plasma Cell Tumor	Cocker Spaniel
	Prostate Carcinoma	Bouvier Des Flandres
	Sertoli Cell Tumor	Cairn Terrier Pekingese
	Soft Tissue Sarcoma	Rhodesian Ridgeback
	Squamous Cell Carcinoma, Digit	Bouvier Des Flandres Briard Giant Schnauzer Labrador Retriever Poodle
	Squamous Cell Carcinoma, Lingual	Labrador Retriever Poodle Samoyed
	Synovial Myxoma	Doberman Pinscher
	T Cell Lymphoma (Mycosis Fungoides)	Boxer
	Testicular Tumors	Maltese
	Thyroid Cancer	Golden Retriever Siberian Husky
	Transitional Cell Carcinoma	Airedale Terrier Scottish Terrier West Highland White Terrier
	Uveal Spindle Cell Tumor	Siberian Husky
Ophthalmological	Blindness, Congenital	Doberman Pinscher
	Cataracts	All Breeds
	Chorioretinopathy	Borzoi
	Choroidal Hypoplasia	Bearded Collie
	Chronic Superficial Keratitis (Pannus)	Australian Shepherd Belgian Malinois Belgian Sheepdog Belgian Tervuren Bloodhound Bulldog Chinese Shar Pei Chow Chow Dachshund German Shepherd Dog Greyhound Irish Red And White Setter Pekingese Pug Shih Tzu Siberian Husky
	Collie Eye Anomaly/Choroidal Hypoplasia/ Coloboma (CEA/CH)	Australian Shepherd Border Collie Collie

Subject	Condition	Breed-Dog
		Nova Scotia Duck Tolling Retriever
		Pyrenean Shepherd
		Shetland Sheepdog
	Cone Degeneration	Alaskan Malamute
		Australian Shepherd
		German Shorthaired Pointer
	Corneal Dystrophy	Affenpinscher
		Afghan Hound
		Airedale Terrier
		Alaskan Malamute
		Basenji
		Beagle
		Bearded Collie
		Bedlington Terrier
		Bichon Frisé
		Boston Terrier
		Boykin Spaniel
		Briard
		Brussel's Griffon
		Cavalier King Charles Spaniel
		Chow Chow
		Collie
		Dachshund
		Dalmatian
		Dandie Dinmont Terrier
		Dogue De Bordeaux
		English Toy Spaniel
		German Pinscher
		German Shepherd Dog
		Great Pyrenees
		Irish Wolfhound
		Kuvasz
		Labrador Retriever
		Lhasa Apso
		Mastiff
		Miniature Bull Terrier
		Miniature Pinscher
		Norwich Terrier
		Nova Scotia Duck Tolling Retriever
		Pointer
		Polish Lowland Sheepdog
		Puli
		Rottweiler
		Saint Bernard
		Samoyed
		Scottish Terrier
		Shetland Sheepdog
		Shih Tzu
		Siberian Husky
		Standard Schnauzer
		Tibetan Terrier
		Weimaraner
		Vizsla
		Weimaraner
		We lsh Springer Spaniel
		Welsh Terrier
		Wirehaired Pointing Griffon
		Yorkshire Terrier

Subject	Condition	Breed–Dog
	Corneal Epithelial Defects, Spontaneous	Keeshond
	Corneal Ulcer	Boxer Golden Retriever
	Distichiasis	Airedale Terrier Alaskan Malamute American Staffordshire Terrier American Water Spaniel Australian Shepherd Australian Terrier Basset Hound Beagle Bedlington Terrier Bichon Frisé Black and Tan Coonhound Boston Terrier Boxer Boykin Spaniel Brittany Brussel's Griffon Bulldog Bullmastiff Canaan Dog Cavalier King Charles Spaniel Chesapeake Bay Retriever Clumber Spaniel Cocker Spaniel Collie Curly Coated Retriever Dachshund Dalmatian Dandie Dinmont Terrier Doberman Pinscher Dogue De Bordeaux English Cocker Spaniel English Setter English Toy Spaniel Field Spaniel Flat-Coated Retriever French Bulldog German Shorthaired Pointer Glen Of Imaal Terrier Golden Retriever Great Dane Great Pyrenees Havanese Icelandic Sheepdog Irish Red And White Setter Irish Setter Irish Water Spaniel Irish Wolfhound Japanese Chin Keeshond Kerry Blue Terrier Kuvasz Labrador Retriever Leonberger Lhasa Apso

Subject	Condition	Breed–Dog
		Löwchen
		Maltese
		Miniature Schnauzer
		Neopolitan Mastiff
		Norwegian Elkhound
		Nova Scotia Duck Tolling Retriever
		Old English Sheepdog
		Papillon
		Parson Russell Terrier
		Pekingese
		Pembroke Welsh Corgi
		Pharaoh Hound
		Poodle
		Portuguese Water Dog
		Pug
		Saint Bernard
		Samoyed
		Schipperke
		Scottish Terrier
		Sealyham Terrier
		Shetland Sheepdog
		Shiba Inu
		Shih Tzu
		Soft Coated Wheaten Terrier
		Swedish Vallhund
		Staffordshire Bull Terrier
		Standard Schnauzer
		Sussex Spaniel
		Tibetan Spaniel
		Tibetan Terrier
		Vizsla
		Weimaraner
		Welsh Springer Spaniel
		Welsh Terrier
		Yorkshire Terrier
	Early Retinal Degeneration (Erd)	Norwegian Elkhound
	Ectopic Cilia	Shih Tzu
	Ectropion	Basset Hound
		Black and Tan Coonhound
		Bloodhound
		Boxer
		Bulldog
		Cane Corso
		Chesapeake Bay Retriever
		Chinese Shar Pei
		Chow Chow
		Clumber Spaniel
		Cocker Spaniel
		Dogue De Bordeaux
		Gordon Setter
		Great Dane
		Leonberger
		Mastiff
		Neopolitan Mastiff
		Newfoundland
		Saint Bernard
		Spinone Italiano
		Sussex Spaniel

Subject	Condition	Breed–Dog
	Entropion	Akita Bedlington Terrier Bernese Mountain Dog Black and Tan Coonhound Bloodhound Bulldog Bullmastiff Cane Corso Chesapeake Bay Retriever Chinese Shar Pei Chow Chow Clumber Spaniel English Toy Spaniel French Bulldog German Shorthaired Pointer Great Dane Great Pyrenees Icelandic Sheepdog Irish Setter Irish Water Spaniel Japanese Chin Komondor Labrador Retriever Leonberger Lhasa Apso Mastiff Neopolitan Mastiff Newfoundland Pekingese Pug Rottweiler Saint Bernard Shih Tzu Spinone Italiano Tibetan Spaniel Welsh Springer Spaniel Wirehaired Pointing Griffon
	Epiphora	Poodle
	Episcleritis	Cocker Spaniel
	Everted Cartilage of Third Eyelid	Giant Schnauzer Great Dane Irish Wolfhound Leonberger Newfoundland Weimaraner
	Exposure Keratopathy	Chow Chow Lhasa Apso Shih Tzu
	Eyelid Cysts	Newfoundland
	Glaucoma, Primary	Akita Alaskan Malamute Australian Cattle Dog Basset Hound Beagle Bichon Frisé Boston Terrier

Subject	Condition	Breed–Dog
		Bouvier Des Flandres
		Cairn Terrier
		Chinese Shar Pei
		Chow Chow
		Cocker Spaniel
		Dalmatian
		Dandie Dinmont Terrier
		English Cocker Spaniel
		Entlebucher Mountain Dog
		Flat-Coated Retriever
		Golden Retriever
		Great Dane
		Lakeland Terrier
		Lhasa Apso
		Newfoundland
		Norwegian Elkhound
		Norwich Terrier
		Parson Russell Terrier
		Pekingese
		Poodle
		Samoyed
		Shiba Inu
		Shih Tzu
		Siberian Husky
		Vizsla
		Welsh Springer Spaniel
		Welsh Terrier
		Wire Fox Terrier
	Glaucoma, Secondary	Australian Cattle Dog
		Border Collie
		Bull Terrier
		Chinese Crested
		English Springer Spaniel
		Golden Retriever
		Great Dane
		Labrador Retriever
		Newfoundland
		Norfolk Terrier
		Parson Russell Terrier
		Poodle
		Rhodesian Ridgeback
		Smooth Fox Terrier
	Goniodysplasia	Bouvier Des Flandres
		Vizsla
	Iris Coloboma	Dachshund
		Dalmatian
		Sussex Spaniel
	Iris Cysts	Golden Retriever
		Great Dane
		Irish Red And White Setter
		Irish Wolfhound
		Newfoundland
	Iris Sphincter Dysplasia	Dalmatian
	Keratoconjunctivitis Sicca (KCS)	Australian Terrier
		Bedlington Terrier
		Bulldog

Subject	Condition	Breed–Dog
		Cavalier King Charles Spaniel Cocker Spaniel English Cocker Spaniel Kerry Blue Terrier Lhasa Apso Pekingese Portuguese Water Dog Shih Tzu West Highland White Terrier Yorkshire Terrier
	Lacrimal Gland Hypersecretion	Bichon Frisé
	Lens Luxation	Australian Cattle Dog Bearded Collie Brittany Chinese Crested Chinese Shar Pei Greyhound Italian Greyhound Japanese Chin Lakeland Terrier Miniature Bull Terrier Parson Russell Terrier Petit Bassett Griffon Vendéen Pyrenean Shepherd Sealyham Terrier Tibetan Terrier Toy Fox Terrier Welsh Terrier Whippet Wire Fox Terrier
	Macroblepharon	Great Dane Mastiff Pug Shih Tzu
	Microphthalmia	Australian Shepherd Beagle Cavalier King Charles Spaniel Collie Dachshund Doberman Pinscher Old English Sheepdog
	Nystagmus	Belgian Sheepdog
	Optic Nerve Coloboma	Basenji Brussel's Griffon Norfolk Terrier
	Optic Nerve Hypoplasia	Bullmastiff Dachshund German Pinscher Irish Wolfhound Miniature Pinscher Norfolk Terrier Poodle Shih Tzu

Subject	Condition	Breed-Dog
	Pectinate Ligament Dysplasia	English Springer Spaniel Flat-Coated Retriever
	Persistent Hyaloid Artery	Australian Shepherd Basset Hound Boykin Spaniel Brussel's Griffon Cairn Terrier Dachshund English Toy Spaniel Irish Setter Japanese Chin Soft Coated Wheaten Terrier Sussex Spaniel
	Persistent Hyperplastic Primary Vitreous	Bouvier Des Flandres Staffordshire Bull Terrier
	Persistent Hyperplastic Tunica Vasculosa Lentis	Doberman Pinscher German Pinscher German Shorthaired Pointer Japanese Chin
	Persistent Pupillary Membranes (PPM)	All Breeds
	Photoreceptor Dysplasia, Type-A PRA (Partially Dominant)	Miniature Schnauzer
	Pigmentary Keratitis	Japanese Chin
	Progressive Retinal Atrophy (PRA), Central	Polish Lowland Sheepdog
	Progressive Retinal Atrophy (PRA), Dominant	Bullmastiff Mastiff
	Progressive Retinal Atrophy (PRA), Recessive	Airedale Terrier American Eskimo Dog Australian Cattle Dog Australian Shepherd Basenji Belgian Sheepdog Belgian Tervuren Bernese Mountain Dog Border Collie Borzoi Boykin Spaniel Briard Brussel's Griffon Cardigan Welsh Corgi Chesapeake Bay Retriever Chinese Crested Cocker Spaniel Collie Dachshund English Cocker Spaniel English Springer Spaniel Entlebucher Mountain Dog Glen Of Imaal Terrier Golden Retriever Gordon Setter Harrier Irish Red And White Setter Irish Setter

Subject	Condition	Breed-Dog
		Irish Terrier
		Irish Wolfhound
		Italian Greyhound
		Kuvasz
		Labrador Retriever
		Lhasa Apso
		Löwchen
		Miniature Pinscher
		Norfolk Terrier
		Papillon
		Pekingese
		Pomeranian
		Poodle
		Portuguese Water Dog
		Pyrenean Shepherd
		Rottweiler
		Schipperke
		Shih Tzu
		Standard Schnauzer
		Tibetan Mastiff
		Tibetan Spaniel
		Tibetan Terrier
		West Highland White Terrier
		Yorkshire Terrier
	Progressive Retinal Atrophy (PRA), Unknown	Canaan Dog
		Greyhound
		Silky Terrier
	Progressive Retinal Atrophy (PRA), X-Linked	Samoyed
		Siberian Husky
	Prolapsed Gland Of The Nictitans (Cherry Eye)	Beagle
		Bloodhound
		Bulldog
		Cane Corso
		Cocker Spaniel
		Lhasa Apso
		Neopolitan Mastiff
		Shih Tzu
		Tibetan Spaniel
	Proliferative Keratoconjunctivitis	Collie
	Punctate Keratitis	Dachshund
	Retinal Degeneration, Unknown Inheritance	Belgian Malinois
		Black Russian Terrier
		Black and Tan Coonhound
		Briard
	Retinal Dysplasia	Akita
		Affenpinscher
		Airedale Terrier
		Alaskan Malamute
		American Staffordshire Terrier
		American Water Spaniel
		Australian Shepherd
		Basset Hound
		Beagle
		Bearded Collie
		Bedlington Terrier
		Belgian Sheepdog
		Belgian Tervuren

Subject	Condition	Breed–Dog
		Black & Tan Coonhound
		Bloodhound
		Border Collie
		Boykin Spaniel
		Briard
		Bull Terrier
		Bulldog
		Bullmastiff
		Cane Corso
		Cardigan Welsh Corgi
		Cavalier King Charles Spaniel
		Chinese Shar Pei
		Chinook
		Clumber Spaniel
		Cocker Spaniel
		Collie
		Doberman Pinscher
		Dogue De Bordeaux
		English Cocker Spaniel
		English Springer Spaniel
		English Toy Spaniel
		Field Spaniel
		French Bulldog
		German Shepherd Dog
		German Shorthaired Pointer
		Giant Schnauzer
		Golden Retriever
		Gordon Setter
		Great Pyrenees
		Ibizan Hound
		Icelandic Sheepdog
		Irish Red And White Setter
		Irish Wolfhound
		Labrador Retriever
		Lhasa Apso
		Maltese
		Mastiff
		Miniature Schnauzer
		Miniature Schnauzer
		Newfoundland
		Norfolk Terrier
		Old English Sheepdog
		Pembroke Welsh Corgi
		Petit Bassett Griffon Vendéen
		Pharaoh Hound
		Pointer
		Puli
		Rottweiler
		Samoyed
		Schipperke
		Scottish Terrier
		Sealyham Terrier
		Silky Terrier
		Swedish Vallhund
		Standard Schnauzer
		Sussex Spaniel
		Welsh Springer Spaniel
		West Highland White Terrier
		Yorkshire Terrier

Subject	Condition	Breed–Dog
	Rod Dysplasia	Norwegian Elkhound
	Sudden Acute Retinal Degeneration (SARDS)	Dachshund Miniature Schnauzer
	Tapetal Degeneration	Beagle
	Uveal Cysts	Labrador Retriever
	Uveitis	Golden Retriever
	Uveitis, Cataract Resorption Induced	Boston Terrier
	Vitreous Degeneration	Brussel's Griffon Bull Terrier Chihuahua Chinese Crested Curly Coated Retriever Greyhound Havanese Italian Greyhound Kerry Blue Terrier Löwchen Miniature Bull Terrier Miniature Pinscher Papillon Pomeranian Poodle Saluki Schipperke Scottish Terrier Sealyham Terrier Shih Tzu Silky Terrier Smooth Fox Terrier Swedish Vallhund Whippet
Oronasal	Ankyloglossia, Ventral	Anatolian Shepherd
	Brachygnathism	Chihuahua Norwich Terrier
	Cleft Palate	Bernese Mountain Dog Boston Terrier Boxer Brussel's Griffon Chihuahua Portuguese Water Dog
	Dental Problems	Italian Greyhound
	Gingival Hypertrophy	Boxer
	Hypodontia	Chinese Crested Kerry Blue Terrier
	Inverted Canines	Bull Terrier Staffordshire Bull Terrier
	Malocclusion	German Shorthaired Pointer
	Missing Teeth	Airedale Terrier Bedlington Terrier Cairn Terrier Chinese Crested Kerry Blue Terrier Manchester Terrier

Subject	Condition	Breed–Dog
		Norwich Terrier Soft Coated Wheaten Terrier Swedish Vallhund Tibetan Terrier Xoloitzcuinti
	Periodontal Disease	Beagle Poodle
	Prognathism	Chihuahúa Norwich Terrier
	Retained Deciduous Teeth	Tibetan Spaniel
	Rostrally Displaced Mxillary Canine Teeth	Shetland Sheepdog
	Supernumerary Teeth	Greyhound
	Undershot	Bedlington Terrier Cairn Terrier Portuguese Water Dog Soft Coated Wheaten Terrier
Respiratory	Brachycephalic Complex	Boston Terrier Bulldog Cavalier King Charles Spaniel French Bulldog Lhasa Apso Norwich Terrier Pekingese Pug Shih Tzu Staffordshire Bull Terrier Tibetan Spaniel
	Bronchiectasis	Cocker Spaniel English Springer Spaniel Poodle Rottweiler Siberian Husky
	Chronic Interstitial Lung Disease	Staffordshire Bull Terrier West Highland White Terrier
	Chylothorax	Afghan Hound
	Ciliary Dyskinesia	Bichon Frisé English Springer Spaniel Old English Sheepdog
	Collapsing Trachea	Chihuahua Norwich Terrier Pomeranian Poodle Schipperke Silky Terrier Yorkshire Terrier
	Lung Lobe Torsion	Afghan Hound Pug
	Pneumothorax, Spontaneous	Siberian Husky
	Pyothorax	English Springer Spaniel
	Rhinitis/Bronchopneumonia	Irish Wolfhound
Systemic and Deformities	Anasarca	Bulldog Clumber Spaniel

Subject	Condition	Breed–Dog
	Atresia Ani	Boston Terrier Chow Chow Finnish Spitz German Shorthaired Pointer Maltese Poodle
	Hiatal Hernia	Bulldog Chinese Shar Pei French Bulldog
	Hydrops Fetalis	Pug
	Imperforate Nasal Puncta	Bedlington Terrier
	Inguinal Hernia	Cairn Terrier Tibetan Spaniel
	Leishmaniasis	American Foxhound
	Molera (Open Fontanel)	Chihuahua
	Musladin-Leuke Syndrome	Beagle
	Nasopharyngeal Dysgenesis	Dachshund
	Perineal Hernia	Boston Terrier Bouvier Des Flandres Cardigan Welsh Corgi Collie German Shepherd Dog Old English Sheepdog Pekingese Pembroke Welsh Corgi Poodle
	Recurrent Limb Edema	Great Dane
	Recurrent Fever of Unknown Origin (Shar Pei Fever)	Chinese Shar Pei
	Splenic Torsion	Great Dane
	Umbilical Hernia	Airedale Terrier Bernese Mountain Dog Bichon Frisé Cairn Terrier Cavalier King Charles Spaniel Chesapeake Bay Retriever Chihuahua Cocker Spaniel German Shorthaired Pointer Great Pyrenees Irish Setter Leonberger Manchester Terrier Nova Scotia Duck Tolling Retriever Portuguese Water Dog Rottweiler Shih Tzu Tibetan Spaniel Tibetan Terrier Vizsla Wirehaired Pointing Griffon
Urogenital	Bladder Stones, Calcium Oxalate	Cairn Terrier Dandie Dinmont Terrier Poodle Standard Schnauzer

Subject	Condition	Breed-Dog
	Bladder Stones, Not Categorized	Australian Terrier Bichon Frisé Brussel's Griffon Keeshond Pekingese Portuguese Water Dog Pug Shih Tzu West Highland White Terrier Yorkshire Terrier
	Bladder Stones, Silica	Old English Sheepdog
	Bladder Stones, Urate	Black Russian Terrier Bulldog Dalmatian
	Bladder Stones, Xanthine	Cavalier King Charles Spaniel Dachshund
	Cryptorchidism/Retained Testicles	Airedale Terrier Australian Shepherd Australian Terrier Beagle Bedlington Terrier Belgian Tervuren Bichon Frisé Boxer Brussel's Griffon Cairn Terrier Canaan Dog Chihuahua Chinook Clumber Spaniel French Bulldog German Shorthaired Pointer Icelandic Sheepdog Italian Greyhound Manchester Terrier Nova Scotia Duck Tolling Retriever Old English Sheepdog Papillon Poodle Portuguese Water Dog Rottweiler Siberian Husky Silky Terrier Swedish Vallhund Tibetan Spaniel Toy Fox Terrier Vizsla Wirehaired Pointing Griffon Whippet Xoloitzcuinti Yorkshire Terrier
	Cystinuria and Cystine Bladder Stones	Australian Cattle Dog Australian Shepherd Basenji Basset Hound Cardigan Welsh Corgi

Subject	Condition	Breed–Dog
		Dachshund Irish Terrier Labrador Retriever Mastiff Miniature Pinscher Newfoundland Pembroke Welsh Corgi Scottish Deerhound Silky Terrier Smooth Fox Terrier Staffordshire Bull Terrier Tibetan Spaniel Wire Fox Terrier
	Dystocia	Boston Terrier Boxer Chihuahua Scottish Terrier
	Ectopic Ureters	Entlebucher Mountain Dog Siberian Husky Skye Terrier Soft-Coated Wheaten Terrier
	Fanconi Syndrome	Basenji
	Glomerulonephritis	Greyhound
	Gomerulonephropathy	Bullmastiff
	Hereditary Nephritis	Bull Terrier English Cocker Spaniel Samoyed
	Hermaphrodism	German Shorthaired Pointer
	Hypospadias	Boston Terrier
	Juvenile Nephropathy	Boxer
	Juvenile Renal Disease	Chow Chow Doberman Pinscher Miniature Schnauzer Norwegian Elkhound Poodle Rottweiler
	Kidney Disease, Not Catergorized	American Eskimo Dog Shetland Sheepdog
	Polycystic Kidney Disease	Bull Terrier
	Prostate Disease	Doberman Pinscher
	Protein Losing Nephropathy	Soft Coated Wheaten Terrier
	Renal Amyloidosis	Beagle Chinese Shar Pei English Foxhound
	Renal Arteriosclerosis	Greyhound
	Renal Dysplasia	Lhasa Apso Shih Tzu Skye Terrier Soft Coated Wheaten Terrier Tibetan Terrier West Highland White Terrier

Subject	Condition	Breed–Dog
	Renal Dysplasia, Juvenile	Bernese Mountain Dog Golden Retriever Gordon Setter
	Urinary Incontinence, Hormonal	Doberman Pinscher Giant Schnauzer Great Pyrenees Irish Setter Weimaraner
	XX Sex Reversal	Cocker Spaniel German Shorthaired Pointer Norwegian Elkhound Soft-Coated Wheaten Terrier Weimaraner

Quick Reference to Conditions by Breed Breed Specific Conditions in Cats

Subject	Condition	Breed–Cat
Behavior	Wool Sucking	Burmese Siamese
	Separation Anxiety Syndrome	Persian Siamese
B Blood type/NI/Transfusion reactions		Abyssinian Bengal Birman British SH Cornish Rex Devon Rex Exotic/Exotic SH Highland Fold Himalayan Japanese Bobtail Norwegian Forest Cat Persian Ragdoll Scottish Fold Somali Sphynx Turkish Angora Turkish Van
Cardiac/Vascular	Dilated Cardiomyopathy	Abyssinian Burmese Siamese
	Congenital Portosystemic Vascular Shunts	Himalayan Persian
	Hypertrophic Cardiomyopathy	American SH British SH Cornish Rex Devon Rex Maine Coon Persian Ragdoll
	PDA	Persian
	Endocardial Fibroelastosis	Burmese Siamese
	Persistent Atrial Standstill	Burmese Siamese
	Arterial Thromboembolism	Abyssinian Birman Ragdoll
Dental/Oral/Nasal Cavity	Cervical neck lesions	Abyssinian Persian Siamese
	Brachycephalic Syndrome (stenotic nares, long palate, exophthalmos, asymmetric jaw, tooth crowding, breathing problems etc)	Exotic/Exotic SH Persian

Subject	Condition	Breed–Cat
Ears and Hearing	Curl ear Floppy Pinna	American Curl Havana Brown Siamese
	Hereditary deafness (associated with White haircoat gene)	American Shorthair British Shorthair Cornish Rex Devon Rex Exotic/Exotic SH Highland Fold Maine Coon Manx Oriental Persian Scottish Fold Turkish Angora
Endocrine/Metabolic Includes Storage diseases	Systemic AA amyloidosis (renal form)	Abyssinian Somali
	Systemic AA Amyloidosis (hepatic form)	Devon Rex Siamese
	Mucopolysaccharidosis VI	Balinese Siamese
	Alpha Mannosidosis	Persian
	GM1-Gangliosidosis	Korat Siamese
	GM2-Gangliosidosis	Burmese Korat
	Hypokalemic Polymyopathy	Burmese
	Diabetes Mellitus (Type II)	Burmese (Australian lines)
	Congenital Hypothyroidism	Abyssinian
	Glycogenosis Type IV	Norwegian Forest Cat
	Glycogenosis Type IV Mimicking Disorder	Maine Coon
	Primary Hypoadrenocorticism	British Shorthair
	Primary Hypoparathyroidism	Himalayan
	Pyruvate kinase deficiency/erythrocyte Fragility	Abyssinian Bengal Somali
	Transient hyperlipidemia and anemia	Burmese Oriental
	Hyperchylomicronemia	Himalayan
	Sphingomyelin lipidosis (Sphingomyelinosis)-Neimann-Pick	Balinese Siamese
	Ornithine Transcarbamylase deficiency	American Shorthair
	Chediak-Higashi Syndrome	Persian
	Hyperlipoproteinemia/Hyperlipidemia	Persian
	Ceroid Lipofuscinosis	Siamese
	Copper Storage Disease	Siamese
Gastrointestinal Hematology and Immune	Inherited defect of Neutrophil Granulation	Birman
	Hemophilia B (Factor IX) Christmas Disease	British Shorthair Siamese

Subject	Condition	Breed–Cat
	FIP Susceptibility	Birman Burmese Persian
	Multiple Vitamin-K dependent blood coagulation factor deficiency	Devon Rex
	Congenital hypotrichosis and thymic aplasia	Birman
	Hemophilia	Havana Brown
	Von Willebrand's Disease (FVIII)	Himalayan
	Transient hyperlipidemia and anemia	Burmese Oriental
	Hyperlipoproteinemia/Hyperlipidemia	Persian
	Inherited Hyperchylomicronemia	Siamese
Integument and Haircoat	Ulcerative nasal dermatitis	Bengal
	Congenital hypotrichosis and thymic aplasia	Birman
	Hypotrichosis	Cornish Rex Devon Rex
	Papular Eosinophilic/Mastocytic dermatitis=Urticaria Pigmentosa	Devon Rex Sphynx
	Primary Hereditary Seborrhea Oleosa	Himalayan Persian
	Dermatosparaxis (cutaneous asthenia, dermal fragility)	Himalayan
	Hepatocutaneous syndrome (superficial necrolytic dermatitis)	Maine Coon
	Dystrophic epidermolysis Bullosa	Persian
	Idiopathic Facial dermatitis	Persian
	Himalayan/Siamese Pointing Gene [Imperfect (temperature sensitive) oculocutaneous albinism]	Siamese
	Cutaneous Mastocytoma	Siamese
	Vitiligo	Siamese
	Alopecia Universalis	Sphynx
Liver and Pancreas	Pancreatitis	Siamese
	Hepatocutaneous syndrome	Maine Coon
Musculoskeletal	Hip Dysplasia	Himalayan Persian
	Hereditary Myopathy (Spasticity)	Devon Rex Sphynx
	Hypokalemic Polymyopathy	Burmese
	Osteochondrodysplasia	Highland Fold Scottish Fold
	Luxating Patella	Abyssinian (medial) Burmese (medial) Cornish Rex Siamese (medial) Tonkinese (medial)
	Synovial Osteochondromatosis	Burmese
	Hip Dysplasia +/- Luxating Patella	Devon Rex Maine Coon

Subject	Condition	Breed–Cat
	Fibrodysplasia Ossificans	Himalayan
	Muscular Dystrophy (laminin alpha 2)	Maine Coon Siamese
	Chondrodysplasia	Munchkin
	Early Onset Osteodystrophy	Scottish Fold
	Slipped Capital Femoral Epiphysis	Siamese
Nervous	Peripheral and central distal axonopathy	Birman
	Hypomyelination/Dysmyelination	Egyptian Mau Siamese
	Congenital hydrocephalus	Siamese
	Neuroaxonal Dystrophy	Siamese
	Congenital Myasthenia Gravis	Siamese
	Motor Neuron Disease/Spinal Muscle Atrophy	Maine Coon
	Acquired Myasthenia Gravis	Somali
Oncology	Thymoma associated neuromuscular disorder (incl. MG)	Abyssinian Somali
	Mediastinal LSA	Oriental Siamese
	Intestinal Adenocarcinoma	Siamese
Ophthalmic	Recessive PRA	Abyssinian Ocicat Persian Siamese Somali
	Cataracts (Congenital or Juvenile)	Birman British SH Himalayan Persian
	Epibulbar dermoids	Birman Burmese
	Dominant PRA	Abyssinian Somali
	Eyelid agenesis	Birman Burmese Persian
	Corneal Sequestration	Birman Burmese Colorpoint SH Himalayan Persian Siamese
	Primary Glaucoma (narrow angle)	Burmese
	Non-healing corneal ulceration	Himalayan Persian
	Transient Aqueous Humor opacity	Burmese
	Eyelid Cysts (hidrocystomas)	Himalayan Persian
	Corneal Dystrophy	Manx
	Entropion	Persian

Subject	Condition	Breed–Cat
	Nystagmus	Siamese
	Convergent Strabismus	Siamese
	Himalayan/Siamese Pointing Gene [Imperfect (temperature sensitive) oculocutaneous albinism]	Siamese
	Glaucoma (open angle)	Siamese
	Retinal Degeneration	Somali
Respiratory	Bronchial Asthma (feline lower airway disease=FLAD)	Himalayan Siamese
Systemic and Deformities (include tail mutants)	Tail mutations	American Bobtail Japanese Bobtail
	Flat-chested kittens	Bengal Burmese Maine Coon Munchkin
	Sacrocaudal Dysgenesis/Taillessness	Manx
	Mid-facial (Craniofacial) deformity +/-nasal dermoids +/-Nares agenesis	American Shorthair Bombay Burmese
	Twisty cat	Munchkin
Urogenital	Polycystic Kidney Disease	American Shorthair British Shorthair Exotic/Exotic SH Highland Fold Himalayan Persian Scottish Fold
	Predisposition to renal failure	Abyssinian Burmese Maine Coon Russian Blue Siamese
	Kitten and Juvenile Azotemia	Birman
	CaOx urolithiasis	British Shorthair Burmese Exotic/Exotic SH Havana Brown Highland Fold Himalayan Persian Ragdoll Scottish Fold Siamese
	Predisposition to UTI	Abyssinian
	MAP urolithiasis predisposition	Chartreux Oriental
	Cystine Urolithiasis	Siamese
	Cryptorchidism	Persian
	Dystocia predisposition	Cornish Rex Devon Rex Exotic/Exotic SH Persian Siamese

Cat Fancy Registries and Kennel Clubs

Kennel Clubs

A kennel club is the repository for breeding records, generates registration certificates, organizes dog shows, and awards. The clubs set judging standards, and whether it's a job or a hobby, their mission is to help the owners, breeders and handlers protect and promote the breeds.

American Kennel Club (AKC)
260 Madison Ave
New York, NY 10016
212.696.8200
http://www.akc.org/

United Kennel Club (UKC)
100 E Kilgore Rd
Kalamazoo, MI 49002-5584
269.343.9020 Fax: 269.343.7037
http://www.ukcdogs.com

National Kennel Club (NKC)
255 Indian Ridge Rd, PO Box 331
Blaine, TN 37709
865.932.9680 Fax: 865.932.2572
http://www.nationalkennelclub.com/

Kennel Club of Great Britain (KCGB)
1 Clarges Street
London UK W1J 8AB
Tel: 0870.606.6750 Fax: 020.7518.1058
http://www.the-kennel-club.org.uk/

Canadian Kennel Club (CKC)
89 Skyway Avenue, Suite 100
Etobicoke, Ontario Canada M9W 6R4
416.675.5511 Fax: 416.675.6506
http://www.ckc.ca/

Australian National Kennel Council (ANKC)
http://www.ankc.org.au/
Contact the relevant State or Territory Controlling Body listed on the website.

New Zealand Kennel Club (NZKC)
Prosser Street, Private Bag 50903, Porirua 6220
Tel: (04) 237.4489 Fax: (04) 237.0721
http://www.nzkc.org.nz/

Cat Fancy Associations

The term cat fancy refers to the promotion, breeding and showing of cats whether as hobby or job. Cat breed associations were formed to protect and promote purebred cats. They maintain breeding records and provide pedigrees and registration certificates, cat show coordination and standards, and awards for championships. A cat's registration can be moved to an association in another country, but championships do not transfer with the cat into the new registry.

Cat Fanciers' Association (CFA)
1805 Atlantic Ave, PO Box 1005
Manasquan, NJ 08736-0805
732.528.9797
http://www.cfainc.org

The International Cat Association (TICA)
PO Box 2684
Harlingen, TX 78551
956.428.8046 Fax: 956.428.8047
http://www.tica.org

Cat Fanciers' Federation (CFF)
PO Box 661
Gratis, OH 45330
937.787.9009 Fax : 937.787.4290
http://www.cffinc.org

American Cat Fanciers' Association (ACFA)
Box 1949
Nixa, MO 65714
417.725.1530 Fax: 417.725.1533
www.acfacat.com

American Association of Cat Enthusiasts (AACE)
Box 213
Pine Brook, NJ 07058
973.335.6717 Fax: 973.334.5834
www.aaceinc.org

American Cat Association (ACA)
8101 Katherine Ave
Panorama City, CA 91402
National Cat Fanciers' Association (NCFA)
10215 Mt. Morris
Flushing MI 48433

Fédération International Féline (FIFé)
c/o The General Secretary
Little Dene, Lenham Heath
Maidstone, Kent ME17 2BS UK
Tel: +44 (0)1622 850913
Fax: +44 (0)1622 850908
http://www.fifeweb.org

Canadian Cat Association/Association Féline Canadienne
(CCA, AFC)
289 Rutherford Road S Suite 18
Brampton, ON Canada L6W 3R9
905.459.1481 Fax: 905.459.4023
www.cca-afc.com
*(in the US)
CANADIAN CAT ASSOCIATION (CCA)
83 Kennedy Rd Unit 1806
Lookout, MO 65726

Governing Council of the Cat Fancy (GCCF)
4-6 Penel Orlieu,
Bridgewater Somerset, TA6 3PG UK
Tel:+44(0) 1278.427575
http://www.gccfcats.org/

Australian Cat Federation (ACF)
PO Box 331
Port Adelaide, BC SA 5015
Tel: 08.8449.5880
http://www.acf.asn.au/

New Zealand Cat Fancy (NZCF)
Fancy Private Bag 6103
Napier, NZ
Tel: +64 (0) 6.839.7881
www.nzcatfancy.gen.nz

World Cat Federation (WCF)
Geisbergstr.2
D-45139 Essen, Germany
Tel: +49.201 / 555724 Fax: +49.201/509040
http://www.wcf-online.de/en/index.html

World Felinological Federation (WFF)
(CFA, CFF, FIFe, TICA, WCF)
PO Box 68
123458 Moscow, Russia
Tel: +7 095.502.2430
http://www.wff-portal.org/

Feline Federation Europe (FFE)
(Germany)
Tel: +49.911.244.81.07 Fax: +49.911.244.81.08
www.bavarian-cfa.de/data/ffe/ffe1.htm

Other Resources

Cornell Feline Health Center
New York State College of Veterinary Medicine
Cornell University
Ithaca, NY 14853
Dr. Louis J Camuti Memorial Feline Consultation
and Diagnostic Service
800.548.8937
http://www.vet.cornell.edu/fhc/

The Robert H. Winn Feline Foundation
1805 Atlantic Ave Box 1005
Manasquan NJ 08736
732.528.9797
http://www.winnfelinehealth.org

American Veterinary Medical Association (AVMA)
1931 N Meacham Rd. Suite 100
Schaumburg, IL 60173
800.248.2862
http://www.avma.org

American Association of Feline Practitioners (AAFP)
390 Amwell Road
Suite 403
Hillsborough, NJ 08844
phone: 800-874-0498
phone: 908-359-9351
fax: 908-292-1188
http://www.catvets.com

American Animal Hospital Association (AAHA)
12575 W Bayaud Ave
Lakewood, CO 80228
303.986.2800
http://aahanet.org

Morris Animal Foundation
45 Inverness Dr
E Englewood CO 80112
Tel: 800.243.2345 or 303.790.2345
Fax: 303.790.4066
http://www.morrisanimalfoundation.org

Orthopedic Foundation for Animals
2300 E Nifong BoulevardColumbia, Missouri, 65201-3806
Phone: (573) 442-0418
Fax: (573) 875-5073 www.offa.org

AKC Canine Health Foundation
P.O. Box 900061Raleigh, NC 27675-9061
888-682-9696
www.akcchf.org

American Society for the Prevention of Cruelty to Animals
(ASPCA)
424 92nd St
New York, NY 10128
212.876.7700
http://www.aspca.org

ASPCA Animal Poison Control Center
888.426.4435
http://www.aspca.org/pet-care/poison-control/

Humane Society of the United States
2100 L St NW
Washington, DC 20037
202.452.1100
http://www.hsus.org

The Delta Society
580 Naches Ave SW Suite 101
Renton, WA 98055
425.226.7357
http://www.deltasociety.org/

Canadian Veterinary Medical Association
339 Booth Street
Ottawa ON K1R 7K1
Email: admin@cvma-acmv.org
http://canadianveterinarians.net/

Feline Advisory Bureau
Taeselbury
High Street
Tibbury, Wiltshire SP3 6LD
United Kingdom
+44 (0) 1747 871 872
http://www.fabcats.org

Appendix F

General References for the Dog

1. AKC at http://www.akc.org/index.cfm
2. UKC http://www.ukcdogs.com/WebSite.nsf/WebPages/Home
3. OFA www.offa.org
4. Canine Health Information Center www.caninehealthinfo.org
5. Journal of the American Animal Hospital Association www.jaaha.org
6. Journal of Veterinary Internal Medicine www.acvim.org/websites/acvim/index.php?p=76
7. The Genetic Connection: A guide to health Problems in Purebred Dogs. Ackerman, L. AAHA Press 1999.
8. Canadian Kennel Club http://www. ckc.ca
9. Pub Med http://ncbi.nlm.nih.gov/PubMed accessed for research papers.
10. VIN www.vin.com
11. University of Montreal Veterinary Medical Database www.medvet.umontreal.ca/bibio/vetjr.html
12. IVIS www.ivis.org
13. Canadian Guide to Dogs http://www.canadasguidetodogs.com/breederinfo6.htm
14. National Kennel Club http://www.nationalkennelclub.com/
15. The Kennel Club U.K. http://www.the-kennel-club.org.uk/services/
16. Ketring, K.L., Glaze, M.B. Atlas of Breed-Related Canine Ocular Disorders. VLS Books, 1998.
17. The Complete Dog Book 20th Ed. The American Kennel Club. Howell Book House, NY, 2000.

General References for the Cat

1. Bell J. The Genetic test for Persian-related PKD: Will it be constructive or destructive? *Notes.* University of California (Davis) Feline Genetics Extravaganza II Aug 28 2004.
2. *The Encyclopedia of the Cat.* Bruce Fogle, Firefly Books Ltd. Willowdale Canada,1997.
3. Baker HJ, Smith BF, Martin DR et al. *Molecular diagnosis of gangliosidosis: A model for elimination of inherited disease in Pure Breeds. In: August, JR. Consultations In Feline Internal Medicine. 4th ed.* Philadelphia, WB Saunders 2001:615-620
4. Giger U. *Clinical Genetics. In: Ettinger SJ, Feldman EC Eds, 5th Ed. Textbook of Veterinary Internal Medicine.* W.B. Saunders, Philadelphia 2000:2-5.
5. *Complete Cat Breeds.* Alan Edwards, Southwater (Anness Publishing Limited, NY USA), 2001.
6. Clark RD. *Medical, Genetic and Behavioral Aspects of Purebred Cats.* Forum Publications, Inc., St. Simons Island GA, 1992.
7. *Breed Predispositions to Disease in Dogs & Cats.* Gough, Alex and Thomas, Alison. Blackwell Publishing Ltd. Oxford, U.K., 2010.
8. Giger, U. In: Bonagura J, ed. *Kirk's Current Veterinary Therapy XIII.* Philadelphia: WB Saunders Co, 2000;396-399, 1999.
9. *The Royal Canin Cat Encyclopedia,* Aniva Publishing, Paris France, 2000.
10. Pub Med http://ncbi.nlm.nih.gov/PubMed accessed for research papers.
11. VIN www.vin.com accessed for general medical research.
12. OMIA (Online Mendelian Inheritance in Animals), Australian Genetics Database http://omia.angis.org.au/
13. CFA website www.cfainc.org
14. TICA website www.tica.org
15. FIFé website www.fifeweb.org
16. NZCF website www.nzcatfancy.gen.nz/
17. CFF website www.cffinc.org
18. CCF website www.cca-afc.com
19. GCCF website www.gccfcats.org
20. ACFA website http://www.acfacat.com
21. Fanciers Breeder Referral List www.breedlist.com
22. Cat Fancy Magazine breed articles in print and at: www.catfancy.com
23. Vet Clin North Am: Sm Anim Pract http://www.vetsmall.theclinics.com/
24. J Am Anim Hosp Assoc www.jaaha.org
25. Compend Contin Educ Pract Vet http://www.vetlearn.com/Veterinarians.aspx
26. J Fel Med Surg www.elsevier.com/locate/jfms
27. FAB Feline Advisory Bureau UK http://www.fabcats.org/

Glossary of Terms

This list of terms primarily encompasses genetic definitions and brief descriptions of breed standard terminology.

Readers are referred to Stedman's Medical Dictionary, veterinary edition or another veterinary medical dictionary for general medical terms.

Agouti

A wild type hair banded with different colors. Symbol is A.

Albinism

Autosomal recessive gene set leading to lack of visible pigmentation in skin, iris, and haircoat. Different alleles sort to produce four phenotypes:

1. **Full albinism (ca or cc):** An all white cat; the pure albino gene results in complete lack of melanin pigmentation in many organs, including the skin and haircoat. A true albino animal has pink skin and mucous membranes and eyes without pigmented iris giving a pink tinge (c), or china bluish color (ca).
2. **Siamese albinism (cs cs):** Oculocutaneous partial albinism is a temperature sensitive tyrosinase enzyme mutation seen in cats such as Siamese and Siamese-related cats carrying the "pointing" gene.
3. **Burmese albinism (cb cb):** less complete albinism, same enzyme but minimal difference in coat color from points to base coat color.
4. Tonkinese cats have three genotypes of albinism depending on their type of pointing:

   Mink Tonkinese albinism (cb cs)

   Note aside: Solid Tonkinese—like the Burmese cats (cb cb)
   Point Tonkinese—like the Siamese cats (cs cs)

True White animals (W) result from an autosomal dominant gene, and are not albinos.

Deafness does not always occur on the same side with the blue eye in albino cats if heterochromia iridis; odd-eyed iris pigmentation is present.

Albino

An animal expressing the genes for albinism (see *albinism*).

Allele

One of many different versions of the same trait at the same locus. For example, a gene may have a dominant and a recessive version coding for coat color. (e.g., B=black coat is dominant and b=brown coat is recessive). Each individual animal can carry a maximum of two of these versions of the same gene, as long as their genome has a standard number of chromosomes. If both alleles are the same (BB) they are said to be homozygous, and if the alleles are different, containing one dominant and one recessive (Bb), they are said to be heterozygous.

Applehead

Also termed *traditional* in the Siamese breed; an old-fashioned head conformation that is less extreme than the typical modern American show specimen.

Atopy

Allergic dermatitis and pruritis secondary to inhalant allergy or other antigenic stimulant.

Auto-Immune Hemolytic Anemia (AIHA)

An auto-immune destruction of red blood cells leading to severe anemia.

Autosome

All chromosomes except for the pair of sex chromosomes; the homologous pairs of chromosomes in somatic cells; somatic cells encompass all body cells except gametes.

Bi-Color

A coat of a white background with solid patches pattern interspersed.

Brachycephalic Head

Short muzzle and domed skull conformation. The Persian cat breed is an example of this type of head conformation.
Brachycephalic Complex: The brachycephalic complex includes stenotic nares, elongated soft palate, everted laryngeal saccules, laryngeal collapse, and occasionally hypoplastic trachea. Can cause respiratory distress, laryngeal collapse and cyanosis, especially with heat stress or activity.

Break

In the head in profile, describes a change in the angle of the nose/head junction around the level of the eyes.

Breed

Denotes a consistent type of animal that when bred within that population produces a reproducible phenotype, and shares genetically determined characteristics, one or more of which set that animal apart from other breeds. Is only a breed if recognized by a breed or fancy registry.

Brindle

Hairs of a different color interspersed between another solid coat hair color; admixing in tortoiseshell cats is an example.

Britches

Long hair on the back of limbs, longer than the average hair coat length; sometimes termed pantaloons.

Calico
A coat color consisting of a mix of tortoiseshell and white (calico is an American term); also tri-color, parti-color. SYN: Chintz, Tortoiseshell.

Canthus
Medial and lateral canthus refers to the inner and outer corner junctions respectively, of the upper and lower eyelids; the palpebral fissure angles.

Carrier
In the context of inherited disease, is a dog which carries a recessive, mutant allele that is matched by the presence of a normal allele. On average, it will pass on this mutant allele to half of its offspring.

Chinchilla
In the cat, describes a coat of white, with very minimal tipping; compare with **smoke** where tipping covers a much greater portion of the hair shaft, and **shaded** where pigment is in between in its distribution.

Chocolate
Brown pigment is a precursor of the normal eumelanin (black) hair pigment due to a mutation of the tyrosinase-related protein 1 (TYRRP1).

Chromatin
In between cell divisions (interphase), the mammalian DNA resides in a loose filamentous pattern within the cell nucleus.

Chromosome
Chromosomes are DNA strands that are coiled up into a discrete cylindrical unit that appears in the nucleus as an X-shaped body (two chromatids joined at a centromere) early in cell division (starting in prophase). Dogs have 78 (38 pairs of autosomes and 2 sex chromosomes; written as 78XX or 78XY), cats have 38 chromosomes (38XX or 38XY).

Chronic Superficial Keratitis
Pannus refers to this process when accompanied by pigment deposition on the normally clear cornea.

Co-Dominant
In genetics, co-dominance is when both alleles play a role in the expression of a trait, a phenotype/protein product, so the alleles are said to be co-dominant. (e.g.,* Blood types AB and B, and spotting gene (S) are co-dominant in cats).

Cobby
Stout, compact body with short heavy limbs and tail, broad shoulders and hips such as in the Manx. In Persian and British Shorthair cat breeds some refer to them as cobby, while others class them as semi-cobby since they are not quite so short coupled.

Codon
A set of three nucleotide pairs located together on a DNA or RNA strand that code for an amino acid or a stop sequence. SYN: triplet.

Colorpoint Longhair
Is synonymous with **Himalayan** in America; a long haired Persian cat having the restricted Himalayan pointing gene.

Congenital
A condition present at birth. Note that this term does not specify the etiology of the problem, just that the animal was born with it.

Crisp
Describes a haircoat texture in cats that is firm, not soft or silky. It is typical of the Shorthair breeds.

Crossbreeding
The mating together of two individuals from different breeds.

Cryptorchidism
Retained testes, may be intra-abdominal or pre-scrotal.

Demodicosis (generalized)
Overgrowth of normal populations of demodex mites in hair follicles causing areas of hair loss and inflammation. This disorder has an underlying immunodeficiency in its pathogenesis.

Deoxyribonucleic Acid (DNA)
The double helix structure that contains the genetic code for an organism. Base pairs (adenine/thymine and cytosine/guanine) are joined by hydrogen bonds on rungs running between a backbone of two ladders of support (a phosphorylated deoxyribose strand). DNA is also present in the mitochondria within the cytoplasm where it is of circular structure, and termed extra-chromosomal DNA.

Dilute
A coat color that is a pale version of another full intensity pigmented coat color. The dilute gene is recessive to the full intensity color. Examples include: blue is dilute of black, and cream is the dilute of red.

Diploid
The normal number of chromosomes in body cells (except germ cells, sperm and ova); each species has a normal characteristic diploid chromosome count.

Distichiasis
Abnormally placed eyelashes that irritate the cornea and conjunctiva.

DNA Testing SYN: DNA Typing, DNA Fingerprinting, DNA Profiling
A procedure whereby DNA strands are split into small segments by restriction enzymes, then duplicated many times using PCR, subjected to electrophoresis to produce bands that are melded with radioactive probes specific to an area of interest. Sources of DNA

|* ref: Griot-Wenk et al, Blood type AB in the feline AB blood group system. Am J vet Res 57:1438,1996

can include cheek swabs, blood, hair follicles, and can be done on any age of animal. Parentage testing may be developed based on 10-15 microsatellites.

Domestic Cat
Any non-registered cat--Felis domesticus; usually referred to as domestic longhair and domestic shorthair.

Dominant
A gene is considered dominant when it is always expressed. This expression results in expression of that characteristic in those offspring receiving either one or two copies of this type of gene. The homozygous dominant mutant animal may be more severely affected than one with only one copy; penetrance can also be variable. Alleles may be co-dominant (see co-dominant).

Double Coat
Top coat of longer hair overlies a downy undercoat layer.

Ectropion
Rolling out of eyelids, often with a medial canthal pocket. Can also cause conjunctivitis.

Entropion
Rolling in of eyelids, often causing corneal irritation or ulceration.

Eumelanin
Black pigment; wild type.

Extreme
Any conformation points that deviate from the traditional; often used to describe a more foreign appearance of cat.

Familial
A pattern of a characteristic whereby clusters of affected individuals appear within a pedigree, and the condition is found to be more common in this group than in the general population. Not always a genetic trait.

Fibrocartilaginous Embolic Myelopathy (FCEM)
Disorder of acute spinal cord infarction caused by embolization of fibrocartilage.

Filial
The offspring of a mating; subsequent generations. The F1 or fist filial generation of a mating is like the "children" of that mating and F2, the second filial generation is like the "grandchildren" etc.

Foreign Type
A cat of longer, leaner, finer body type with wedge or modified wedge head conformation, long limbs, and long tail such as in Abyssinian and Russian Blue breeds (cf cobby type), and a bit heavier in the body and flank, less finely built cf oriental type such as in Siamese. Some breeds are a bit heavier than a foreign cat, but not cobby and these are sometimes classed as semi-foreign

(examples include Havana Brown, Egyptian Mau).

Forest Type
A cat with long, large rangy body type, long limbs, heavily boned but not cobby. Seen in Siberian Forest, Norwegian Forest, and Maine Coon cats.

Furnishings
The presence of hair in and around the ears.

Gametes
Sex cells (in the male, spermatozoa and in the female, ova or eggs); haploid cells.

Gastric Dilatation/Volvulus/Bloat (GDV)
Volvulus is a life-threatening twisting of the stomach within the abdomen and requires immediate veterinary attention.

Gene
The "code" for a particular characteristic; the unit of inheritance with a physical location (locus) on a particular chromosome. A gene directs formation of amino acids that make up proteins such as enzymes through an intermediate step involving ribosomes and RNA in the cytoplasm of the cell.

Genetic Linkage
The case when two or perhaps more loci are inherited together because they are located close together on a gene. Linkage is assessed by identifying genetic markers and assaying for the known marker, with the presumption that the marker and the gene of interest will normally segregate together.

Gene Pool
All of the genes that exist within an interbreeding population.

Genome
The complete set of DNA an animal inherits.

Genotype
The genetic makeup of an individual; the sum inheritance of all genes on all chromosomes.

Glaucoma
Ocular condition causing increased pressure within the eyeball, and secondary blindness due to damage to the retina. Can also predispose to lens luxation.

Glitter
An effervescent light glow resulting from bubbles in the hair shaft, reflecting light more than the hairs in a typical cat haircoat, as seen in the Bengal cat.

Glove
Cat coat marking where white covers forepaws but does not extend further up on the limb.

Guard Hairs
Refers to the long outer coat hairs.

Harlequin
In cats, the marking is color on head and tail and a maximum of three small patches of color on the body on a white background.

Hemivertebra and Butterfly Vertebra
Misshapen or malformed vertebrae. May cause scoliosis, pain or spinal cord compression if severe.

Hereditary Defect
A genetic defect or inherited disorder that may also be present at birth (congenital) or may develop later in life, in which case the onset of the condition often develops at a fairly consistent time, with a fairly consistent presentation.

Heritability
The measurement of the proportion of a trait expression (phenotype) due to inheritance (genotype). Heritability is represented by the symbol h^2.

Heterochromia Iridis
Different color irises.

Heterozygous (Heterozygote)
A heterozygote has a genetic constitution for a specific trait where one allele is recessive and the other is dominant.

Heterozygous
Individuals that have two different alleles in a gene pair for a particular characteristic.

Himalayan
An American term for a Colorpoint Persian cat. Also describes the dark pointed trait in the Persian-related breeds.

Homozygous (Homozygote)
A homozygote is an organism that has both alleles of a trait of interest present as either recessive or dominant versions (so the organism is homozygous for a trait).

Homozygous
Individuals that have identical alleles in a gene pair for a particular characteristic.

Hybrid
The crossing of two species (e.g., Bengal is breeding a domestic cat to an Asian leopard cat). This term is also sometimes used to describe crosses between two different breeds.

Hyperadrenocorticism
SYN: Cushing's disease. Hyper-function of the adrenal gland caused by a pituitary or adrenal tumor. Clinical signs may include increased thirst and urination, symmetrical truncal alopecia, and abdominal distention.

Hypoadrenocorticism
SYN: Addison's Disease. Disease causing autoimmune destruction of the adrenal gland.

Immune-Mediated Thrombocytopenia (ITP)
Autoimmune destruction of platelets causing subcutaneous hemorrhage and bleeding.

Inbreeding
The mating of first degree relatives such as mother to son, or full-brother to full-sister.

Inbreeding Coefficient, Wright's Coefficient
A numerical indication of the relatedness between the sire and dam of an individual. The proportion of all variable gene pairs that are likely to be homozygous due to inheritance from ancestors common to the sire and dam. Also, the probability of an individual being homozygous at a given gene pair for a gene received from an ancestor common to the sire and dam.

Incidence
The number of new measured conditions within a set time frame (e.g., per annum) identified in a defined population.

Incomplete Penetrance
When a dominant gene does not always express fully, incomplete penetration of the effects of the gene occur.

Inflammatory Bowel Disease (IBD)
Inflammatory disorder causing chronic diarrhea and weight loss. Affected dogs or cats can usually be controlled with diet and/or medications.

Intervertebral Disc Disease (IVDD)
A disorder causing back pain, weakness, or paralysis due to prolapse of intervertebral disk material into the spinal cord.

Keratoconjunctivitis Sicca (KCS)
SYN: Dry Eye. An ocular condition causing lack of tear production and secondary conjunctivitis, corneal ulcerations, and vision problems.

Leather
In cats, this is the surface of the outer nose and the term is usually combined with a color of the nose in the breed standard; this and paw pad color are often required to be correlated with the appropriate coat color.

Line Breeding
A breeding strategy whereby mating occurs between a male and female that are more closely related to each other than the average (inbreeding coefficient) of the population. This is a breeding strategy that results in concentration of desirable genes due to crosses of vertically related individuals in a pedigree. This can result in concentration of undesirable recessive traits so judgment is important when using this technique.

Linkage

When genes are in close proximity on the chromosome (on loci close together), these loci are likely to be passed on to an offspring together during meiosis, and this allows a linked marker to identify the passage of a yet unidentified gene that is of importance, with reasonable probability.

Locus (pl. loci)

A locus is the physical location of a gene on the chromosome. This actually encompasses a pair of locations for each set of alleles on the homologous chromosomes, but on the sex chromosomes, in the male, loci are unpaired.

Longie/Longy

Manx tail in longest conformation; most normal appearance and used in breeding program but not shown.

Lynx Tufts

At the tip of the ear, the hairs follow the margins and extend straight up over the tip of the ear.

Marbled

A coat pattern whereby spots have a dark margin; for example, in Bengal coats.

Marker

A component of a genetic map which uniquely identifies a locus.

Mask

A pattern on the haircoat over the front of the head; darker color on the face, extends over muzzle and whisker pads, and may continue at the top with tracings to the ears.

Megaesophagus

Dilation and loss of contractility of the muscles of the esophagus. Causes food regurgitation and secondary aspiration pneumonia.

Meiosis

The two-stage cell division process that results in one half of the normal cell chromosome number; this type of cell division occurs in testes or ovaries to produce the gametes for reproduction. Homologous chromosome pairs separate along the cell midline so that each offspring cell at the end of the meiosis II process has 1/2N chromosomes; this way when egg and sperm fuse to make the offspring, the N (normal chromosome number) is maintained through subsequent generations.

Microsatellite

A special region of DNA which possesses an unusual base sequence where two, three or four bases are repeated over and over again, for example CACACACA etc or GCGCGCGC etc. these microsatellites have proved to be very useful markers in developing the canine genetic map.

Mitosis

This is the cell division process that occurs in body cells, (excepting the gametes, egg and sperm). Prophase, metaphase, anaphase and telophase are the main event sequences in mitosis. Cell division results in a full complement (2N or diploid chromosome number) in the two daughter cells. *See meiosis.*

Monogenic

A characteristic controlled by a single gene.

Mutation

A permanent change in the base sequence of DNA. This may be the result of changing a single base to another one, the removal of part of the base sequence or the addition of extra bases in the sequence. When a mutation occurs within a gene, it may alter the genetic plan that is embedded within that gene.

Necklace

Tabby markings on the neck that may be broken or unbroken.

Nucleotide

The building blocks of DNA consisting of nucleic acids bound to phosphorylated deoxyribose or in RNA, to phosphorylated ribose.

Nucleus

A structure present within most cells which contains the DNA in the form of chromosomes.

Odd-Eyes

Where two different colors of iris are present; usually blue or less commonly green; the other usually gold, or sometimes copper or orange.

Orange

Red/ginger X-linked coat color in cats (O). Pigment is phaeomelanin rather than wild type eumelanin.

Oriental Type

Describes the body type typical of breeds such as the Siamese. These cats are long, tubular, lean, angular, and the head is long and wedge-shaped with large ears, limbs long and fine, tail fine and tapering; sometimes called whip-like, minimal flank depth. Finer than Foreign Type and much finer than Cobby Type.

Outbreeding

The mating of two individuals who are less related than the average (inbreeding coefficient) of the population.

Outcrossing

Breeding using two individuals that are less closely related than the average population; no common ancestors in previous three generations.

Pannus, Chronic Superficial Keratitis

Chronic corneal inflammatory process that can cause vision problems due to corneal pigmentation.

Parti-Color
A coat color pattern whereby more than one color is superimposed on a white background (e.g., calico)

Patellar Luxation
Slipping kneecaps that can move out of their normal position either medial or lateral.

Patent Ductus Arteriosus (PDA)
Polygenically inherited congenital heart disorder, where a fetal vessel remains open after birth, causing a mixing of oxygenated and un-oxygenated blood.

Pedigree
A record of an animal's ancestry that provides details about several generations of a family. Presented as a chart, and is used for genetic analysis.

Peke-Faced
Describes a type of Persian cat with extreme short face conformation; ears are higher set, nose is pushed in between the eyes, and muzzle is wrinkled. Round skull and head, strong chin.

Penetrance (Incomplete)
This term refers to the proportion of afflicted individuals where a gene does not express 100% of the genotypic potential. If there is complete penetrance, this means all offspring carrying the allele are afflicted to the same degree.

Phenotype
The physical appearance or biochemical attributes of an individual that result from the expression of the genotype or the sum effect of their paired genes, as well as environmental influences interacting with that genotype.

Pleiotropic
One gene with multiple effects (blue eyes, deafness in white coated cat).

Plumed
The cat's tail has longer hair than the body, and appears as a thick layer of fluffy hair.

Pointing/Pointed
Refers to the pigmentation of distal limbs, mask, ears and tail; in cats with the Siamese/Himalayan pointing gene they will develop much darker pigmentation than the base coat color in these locations. Pointing gene leads to a fairly sudden sharp demarcation between point color and base color.

Polygenic
More than one gene at multiple loci code for a characteristic.

Polymerase Chain reaction (PCR)
The procedure used to reproduce small segments of DNA quickly. Using a polymerase enzyme, one can reproduce many copies in the laboratory; used in DNA testing.

Prevalence
The measured number of ongoing cases (not new cases as with incidence) for a characteristic or disease/disorder in a population; not counted over a time frame- just how many are present at a particular point in time.

Progressive Retinal Atrophy (PRA)
Inherited degeneration of the retina, progressing to blindness.

Prolapsed Gland of the Nictitans (Third Eyelid)
SYN: Cherry eye

Pulmonic Stenosis
Inherited congenital heart anomaly (narrow pulmonary root) that can cause heart failure.

Pyo-Traumatic Dermatitis
SYN: Hot spots

Recessive
A gene is said to be recessive when it only expresses when in the presence of a paired recessive gene. When paired with a dominant gene, the dominant will override the recessive one. An autosomal recessive trait may skip generations.

Rex
A type of haircoat that consists of wavy/curly/crinkled/kinked hairs, and coded for by the genes found in Cornish Rex (*r r*) and Devon Rex cats (*re re*) for example.

Rims
Palpebral (eyelid) margins; part of the breed standard where the usual requirement is dark pigmentation at the margins.

Roman Nose
On profile, the nose sticks out to the front of a straight line; convex profile.

Rosettes
Irregular spots; a tabby pattern variant.

Ruff
A collar of longer hairs; seen in the longhaired cats. Similar in appearance, but less distinct than a lion's ruff.

Rumpy
The shortest of the Manx tail conformations whereby the caudal vertebrae are absent outside of the body and no protuberance can be palpated; a dimple is found instead of a tail.

Rumpy Riser
An extremely short tail stump, a protuberance can be palpated; not usually mobile.

Seborrheic Dermatitis
Skin disorder presenting with greasy skin and haircoat.

Self
Another term meaning a solid colored coat; a coat without patterns.

Semi-Foreign
A cat with a build that is somewhat slender but not as elongated and fine as the oriental type cat such as Siamese. Japanese Bobtail is an example of semi-foreign type.

Sex Chromosomes
There are two chromosomes (X and Y) that are non-homologous; determine sex in the offspring (female XX, Male XY)

Sex-Influenced
Traits that are expressed based on genetic interaction with a substances such as sex hormones. Examples are masculinization from androgens, and breast development from estrogens.

Sex-Limited
Shows up in one sex only. Retained testicles is an example of a sex-limited trait.

Sex-Linked
When recessive genes are carried on the X chromosome, females are carriers (though when both parents carry the gene, rarely a female may be clinically affected). The latter occurs only in highly inbred lines as a rule. Males will be affected because they only get one X chromosome so the recessive gene will not have a dominant gene partner on another sex chromosome to override it as long as affected sex chromosome numbers are standard. If there is a dominant allele on an X chromosome, both male and female offspring can show the trait. Males always receive their X chromosome from their dam, so these X-linked traits are dam-male offspring lineage.

There is a small portion of the Y chromosome that does not match up with the X chromosome and the inheritance of genes in this section is termed **holandric**-all male progeny get these genes, and females get none, not even as a carrier since they do not possess Y chromosomes in normal configurations. These are **very rare** traits compared with X linked traits.

Shaded
A tipping pattern with color on the hair shaft with pigment distribution somewhere between the chinchilla (minimal) and smoke (greater).

Smoke
A haircoat produced by the silver inhibitor gene acting on the non-agouti base coat color which results in the hair being grey-silver at the base of each hair, extending up onto the hair a variable extent, but often about 30-50% of the hair is light. Tipping color determines the type of smoke (blue, black, red smoke); *see shaded and chinchilla.*

Somatic
All cells in a body apart from the reproductive cells (gametes).

Spectacles
Outside of the rims (see rims), the lighter coat color provides a round appearance of glasses around the eyes.

Standoff
A haircoat that sits up away from the skin, rather than laying flat and following along the curves of the body.

Stop
In the profile of a face, the profile deviates from flat when a stop is present; there is a dip below the eyes where the muzzle starts; in cats the concavity is at or below eye level.

Stumpy
The Manx tail conformation that is the second longest of the mutation tail phenotypic expression, with a small stump evident outside the body that is short (3-4 cm or 1.2-1.6 inches) and usually moveable, though may be malformed.

Tabby
A coat pattern with different expressions. Symmetrical curved markings or mackerel, an elongated striped "fishbone" pattern, spotted patched, blotched (tb) and others all have in common a variable striping and spotting pattern over a base color. Silver, red and brown are common base colors.

Ticked/Ticking
Presence of the agouti wild type gene produces bands on the hairs and the ticking in the coat results in overlay color at the hair tips; seen in Abyssinian cats.

Tipped
Describes colored hair tips—different color is at the base of the hair; variations in the amount of pigment along the hair shaft determines nomenclature--*see shade, smoke or chinchilla.*

Topline
The ridge along the top of the cat; following the spine column in the midline.

Torbie
A patched tabbie.

Tortie
An abbreviation for the word tortoiseshell; see tortoiseshell.

Tortoiseshell
A cat with black and orange and brown hairs admixed in a variable pattern. Seen in female cats, and rarely in males if sex chromosome numbers are abnormal.

Tri-Color
Term for the haircoat with three colors (e.g., calico cat (tortie and white).

Umbilical Hernia
Congenital opening in the body wall from where the umbilical cord was attached.

Undercoat
The short wooly or down hairs.

Urolithiasis
Mineral concretions (stones), also called calculi present in the urinary tract, including nephroliths (kidney stones), and bladder stones.

Usual
In some cat breeds it refers to the most common coat color and pattern. (e.g., in the Abyssinian, the ruddy agouti coat is termed "usual").

Van
A coat pattern whereby the main coat color is white, the tail is colored, and the head has colored markings also. Van pattern is piebald spotting genetically (SS), a dominant gene with incomplete penetrance.

The term originated with the Turkish Van cat coloration, but now is used in a generic sense for other breeds with similar color patterning.

Van is also the shortened synonym for the Turkish van breed.

Ventricular Septal Defect
VSD is a congenital heart anomaly presenting with a hole which communicates between the two ventricular chambers.

Walnut Shaped Eyes
Cats possessing oval top palpebral margin, and rounded bottom palpebral margin.

Wedge
The term used to describe a head conformation when it is a quite elongated triangle; the Siamese, Colorpoint Shorthair or Balinese heads are good examples. Ear bases to outside of muzzle form a straight line, no obvious whisker break, flat skull, and straight profile characterize this head. Modified or rounded wedge head conformation is a softer triangle, and examples include Birman, Egyptian Mau, Ocicat and Abyssinian; a short wedge—the Devon Rex. British Shorthair, Himalayan, Bombay and Burmese are breed examples, would be described as rounded heads for comparison. Semi-foreign type cats such as Japanese Bobtail and Norwegian Forest cats are described as having triangular heads.

Whisker Break
The junction between whisker pad and face at the muzzle to cheekbone area.

Wool Hairs
Form the soft undercoat in double coated breeds; also called down hairs.